Sports
Injury
Assessment and
Rehabilitation

Sports Injury Assessment and Rehabilitation

David C. Reid, B.P.T., M.D., M.Ch.(orth), M.C.S.P., M.C.P.A., F.R.C.S.(C)

Professor, Division of Orthopedic Surgery
Faculty of Medicine
Adjunct Professor
Faculty of Rehabilitation Medicine
Honorary Professor
Faculty of Physical Education and Sports Study
University of Alberta

Director
Glen Sather University of Alberta Sports Medicine Clinic
Orthopedic Consultant
University of Alberta Intervarsity Athletic Programs
Edmonton Oilers Hockey Club, N.H.L.
Edmonton Eskimoes Football Team, C.F.L.
Alberta Ballet Company
Edmonton, Alberta, Canada

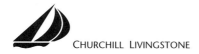

CHURCHILL LIVINGSTONE

New York, Edinburgh, London, Madrid, Melbourne, San Francisco, Tokyo

Library of Congress Cataloging-in-Publication Data
Reid, David C.
   Sports injury assessment and rehabilitation / David C. Reid.
     p. cm.
  Includes bibliographical references and index.
  ISBN 0-443-08662-1
  1. Sports medicine. I. Title.
  [DNLM: 1. Athletic Injuries—diagnosis. 2. Athletic Injuries-
-therapy. QT 260 R354s]
RC1210.R43 1992
617.1'027—dc20
DNLM/DLC
for Library of Congress

91-34085
CIP

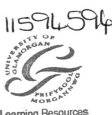

Learning Resources
Centre

Distributed in the United Kingdom by Churchill Livingstone, Robert Stevenson House, 1–3 Baxter's Place, Leith Walk, Edinburgh EH1 3AF, and by associated companies, branches, and representatives throughout the world.

Accurate indications, adverse reactions, and dosage schedules for drugs are provided in this book, but it is possible that they may change. The reader is urged to review the package information data of the manufacturers of the medications mentioned.

The Publishers have made every effort to trace the copyright holders for borrowed material. If they have inadvertently overlooked any, they will be pleased to make the necessary arrangements at the first opportunity.

Acquisitions Editor: *Leslie Burgess*
Copy Editor: *David Terry*
Production Designer: *Jill Little*
Production Supervisor: *Sharon Tuder*
Production services provided by Bermedica Production, Ltd.
Cover design by Paul Moran

Printed in the United States of America

First published in 1992   7

To my father, Robert,
whose example allowed me to set worthy goals,
and to my wife, Kaye,
who helped me achieve them.

Foreword

Over the last four decades a plethora of textbooks on the subject of sports medicine has appeared in the medical literature. Some of the books have been good, some bad, but many have been indifferent; these mainly suffer from lack of details on the rehabilitation of sports injuries, which practitioners throughout the world appreciate as being of critical importance. Too many highly specialized and often highly respected authors have written extremely erudite articles and textbooks that have been somewhat incomprehensible to the average sports medicine practitioner. Veritable tomes on complex procedures abound in the sports medicine literature, but very little detail exists on how to return an athlete to the field of his endeavors by accurately planning his treatment and functional testing before permitting full activity. Having known David Reid as therapist, medical student, and finally orthopaedic surgeon with a major interest in sports medicine, I realized that this book would be different, and indeed I was not disappointed.

Dr. Reid's well-structured text begins with the philosophy of sports medicine and follows with clearly defined sections on common problems. Each area is covered, beginning with its anatomic and physiologic considerations, which are most surely the basis for the scientific approach to athletic injuries that practitioners in this field strive to attain. Dr. Reid stresses the importance of early consultation and accurate diagnosis, without which logical treatment cannot be instituted, and he describes the functional, rather than academic, evaluation of the patient that is made before a return to the chosen sport is permitted.

Particularly enjoyable and helpful in this eminently readable and commendably logical book is the detail of the clinical examination, as well as the clearly delineated summary boxes in each area, which point out "quick facts," "practice points," and "clinical points." The contents of the summary boxes will be most helpful to those who read the text and those who might wish, for instance, to provide information packages to other practitioners involved with the treatment of sports medicine. Doubtless, we shall see their contents on many slides at future sports medicine lectures.

In conclusion, I feel that sports medicine practitioners from the fields of family practice, orthopaedics, rehabilitation medicine, and physiotherapy, as well as coaches and trainers will all derive benefit from the clear, concise style of David Reid.

A.L. Bass, M.B., F.R.C.P.(Ed), F.R.C.P.(C)
Chief
Department of Rehabilitation Medicine
Greater Victoria Hospital Society
Victoria, British Columbia
Late Clinical Professor
Department of Medicine (Rehabilitation)
McMaster University Faculty of Health Sciences
Hamilton, Ontario, Canada

Preface

It is impossible for a text to serve all needs and all interest groups; the danger in trying to please too wide an audience is that eventually no one is truly satisfied. This book is intended to serve as a working guide for the therapist, the orthopaedic surgeon, the primary care physician, and, to a lesser extent, other specialists who have an interest in sports medicine, therapy, and science. It is a practical book founded on science and experience, and it emphasizes diagnosis, treatment decisions, surgical indications, and the guidelines for progression of therapy—areas so often neglected in sports medicine texts.

The first section supplies the basic science and philosophies upon which to develop and adapt treatment from principles. The second section uses a regional approach in outlining the management of different clinical entities. The text is arranged to facilitate finding specific concepts for review by the reader. Thus, it should serve as a good course text. Boxes that highlight clinical points and data are used liberally throughout the text, and numerous tables and figures ensure clarity of diagnostic and therapeutic approaches. The handling of emergency situations, the knowledge of contraindications, and the indications for operative versus nonoperative treatment are areas that are stressed. Original papers are cited to allow the appreciation of the development of current concepts and the contribution of many of the significant figures in sports medicine.

Practitioners of sports medicine and sports therapy are pressured to allow the athlete to compete, whatever the cost. Our specialty is replete with aphorisms such as, "If the doctor says rest, he either doesn't know or doesn't care," and "If you miss one practice, you know it; miss two practices and your colleagues know it; miss three practices and the audience will see the difference." Covered stadiums, extended playing seasons, preseason camps, increasingly complex sports organization, and other factors have led to an "everlasting season." Thus, the ability to evolve programs of modified rest and the knowledge of when and how to gradually and safely allow return to practice and competition are emphasized. Furthermore, when using this knowledge, the long-term health of the limb and the whole athlete is paramount. Conviction, courage, experience, and professionalism are the attributes that will allow the appropriately timed advice to the athlete to change or quit a sport or recreation before permanent disability ensues.

This is a single-authored text based on over twenty-five years of involvement in sports, first as a national-level athlete, then as a physical educator, therapist, physician, and surgeon. Thus, it has the advantage of presenting a cohesive philosophy. For the beginner, this book represents a series of safe, well-tried management strategies. Experts may take what they feel useful and appropriate and meld it into their own treatment philosophies. Ideas evolve and change; this text should therefore serve as a springboard for the development of concepts and new approaches, not simply as a comfortable shell to live within.

David C. Reid, B.P.T., M.D., M.Ch.(orth)

Acknowledgments

I would like to thank the many colleagues who knowingly or unknowingly have shared ideas, given me the benefit of their experience, or served as inspirations over the years: Professor Duthie, Doctors Alan Bass, Olav Rostrop, John Goodfellow, Robert Jackson, Peter Fowler, Rich Hawkins, Robert Larson, and Doug Clement, therapists Norman Pilgrim, Ray Kelly, Clyde Smith, and Davis Magee, as well as, more recently, Doctors Gordon Matheson, Andrew Pipe, Pat McConkey, and Gordon Cameron.

In the actual production of this book, I must mention the unselfish time and energy given by my wife, Kaye; our sports medicine fellows, Doctors Gordon Russell, Ahmed Shaker, and Don Newhouse; therapists Shirley Kushner, Bob Dunlop, Mary Young, Judy Chepeha, and Nancy Jette Chisholm; as well as the other staff at the Glen Sather Sports Medicine Clinic at the University of Alberta in reviewing the manuscripts and sharing their experience. Artist Samuel (Sam) Motyka and photographer Patricia Marston of the University of Alberta Hospitals Media Services gave a special brand of professionalism, and my models Sharon Way Nee and Bob Dunlop, being therapists, knew what was required to emphasize the clinical points in the photographs.

Mary Kerber, my secretary, has worked endlessly in typing and making sure that the manuscripts, tables, and graphs were accurate and appropriately organized.

Contents

Basic Principles

Regional Considerations

Appendices

Sports Medicine and Therapy

1

We see so far because we stand on the shoulders of giants.
— *Sir Isaac Newton*

Sports science and sports medicine are terms used by individuals from numerous disciplines, including exercise physiologists, physicians, psychologists, physical therapists, athletic therapists, coaches, and physical educators.[1] Each of these groups has a specialized field of study and naturally places major emphasis in accordance to their specific interests. Furthermore, although musculoskeletal injuries form a large component of sports medicine, it must be appreciated that there are many other areas that are vitally important. Sports medicine encompasses (1) all aspects of the pathophysiology of activity acquired trauma; (2) injury treatment and prevention; (3) the implication of disease on activity; and (4) the impact of normal processes such as growth, pregnancy, and aging on performance (Fig. 1-1).

This book focuses mainly on musculoskeletal problems and particularly rehabilitation. Many physicians mistakenly believe that rehabilitation is not important. Nothing could be farther from the truth in any branch of musculoskeletal care, but it is a particularly inappropriate statement in relation to sports medicine. Hughston has stated that rehabilitation frequently accounts for 50 percent of a successful outcome after injury or surgery.[2] In sport, the construction of functional progressions allows safe reintegration into activities.[3] It involves designing progressively more difficult sequences of exercises based on an analysis of the stresses involved in the athlete's particular sport. Therefore knowledge of many aspects of performance is as important as knowledge of rehabilitation techniques for effective, efficient therapy. This book stresses the relations between exercise physiology, training techniques, sport-specific requirements, and therapy.

PRINCIPLES OF MUSCULOSKELETAL REHABILITATION

Ruskin and Rebecca analyzed the prevalence of orthopaedic abnormalities in a normal population.[4] They noted that 70.8 percent of the normal population had a previous history of injury, and 37.0 percent demonstrated residual problems due to previous sports trauma. It is tempting to suggest that a more prompt diagnosis and the institution of intensive therapy would reduce this unacceptable statistic of troublesome and sometimes permanent pathology acquired through activity.

As world records continue to be broken and competition assumes ever increasing intensity under the burden of social, financial, and political pressures, athletes push themselves to the limits of their endurance and performance parameters. This situation may lead to many injuries in the elite athlete. More frequently, injuries stem from simple training errors, which is an important concept, as the training regimen is theoretically more readily adjustable than game or competition situations (Fig. 1-2).

Sports medicine encompasses the care of participants of all ages, from the young, skeletally immature child to the elderly, as well as at the multiple levels of both organized and recreational sports. Each subset has its specific vulnerabilities.

The increasing awareness of the value of regular exercise has produced millions of individuals participating in numerous athletic pastimes. Because many of these recreational athletes eventually sustain injuries, it is to be expected that the practice of sports medicine will assume an increasingly important role.

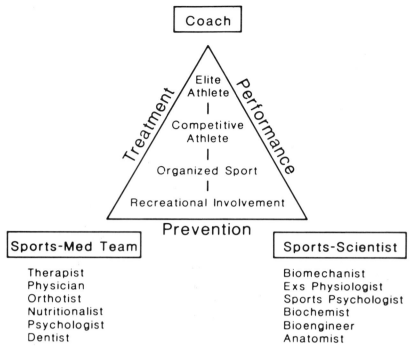

Fig. 1-1. Sports medicine and sports science are multispecialty disciplines that support the various echelons of recreation and sport. The basic principles evolve from the need for enhancement of performance, prevention of injuries, and efficient, effective treatment when injury does occur.

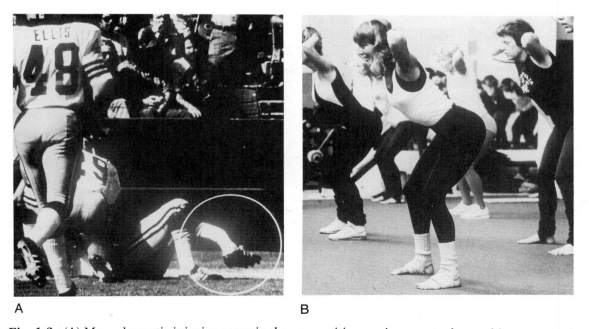

A   B

Fig. 1-2. (**A**) Many dramatic injuries occur in the competition environment where athletes are pushing themselves to their limits; (**B**) however, most problems are overuse injuries, often due to training errors such as training in inadequate footwear or on poorly sprung surfaces.

Mellion surveyed a large number of family physicians; 65 percent performed preparticipation examinations for schools or community leagues, and 45 percent served as team physicians for one or more sports.[5] This survey emphasizes the impact of sports medicine on medical practice and there has been a concurrent exponential rise in the involvement of therapists in the care of the injured athlete at all levels of participation.

For physician and therapist alike, the main parameters of sports medicine include the following.[6,7]

1. Knowledge of the mechanisms of injury, which assists in diagnosis and the development of preventive strategies
2. Early consultation to minimize the development of chronic intractable pathologic changes in tissues
3. Accurate assessment and diagnosis of the condition, which allows correct therapeutic decisions and realistic prognosis
4. Appropriate, imaginative, goal-oriented intensive treatment
5. Objective and functional assessment techniques that take into account the parameters of the specific sport
6. Safe plan for return to activity in order to avoid early reinjury
7. Development of injury prevention programs to minimize the risk of participation.

These principles form a recurring theme throughout the text.

MECHANISMS OF INJURY

Detailed analysis and knowledge of the mechanisms of injury allow an understanding of the injury patterns and factors that lead to the risk of trauma.[8] This information enables coaching and medical staff to modify training and competition situations in order to reduce these risk factors. Unfortunately, the more disabling injuries caused by collisions or falls are often the most difficult to control by changes in rules or the introduction of protective equipment. Nevertheless, there have been considerable efforts to do so over the last few years, with some success. The classification offered below may form a useful starting point for the analysis of data collected at sports medicine clinics. There is no attempt to prioritize these categories as each activity has its own inherent pattern of risk factors.

Collision with Another Athlete

Collisions may occur accidentally or as part of the design of a sport such as boxing or football. It leads to the designations "contact" and "noncontact" activities, a classification that assists in the decision making regarding judgments about athletes being fit during preseason medical examinations. In reality, many contact sports are collision activities (Fig. 1-3).

This point raises the issue of violence in sport and allows three further subdivisions of collision.

1. Brutal body contact. This contact occurs within the rules and therefore is considered a legal collision. It is an important component in such sports as hockey and may occur accidentally in others.
2. Organized brutality. This category involves impacts within the rules of the sport. However, these legal collisions frequently take on a life of their own when the athlete applies them with an intent to hurt. Although boxing may be offered as an example, such violence occurs in many contact sports and manifests the personality of the player or the coach. In these situations, although straining against the rules of the sport, it does not trespass on them. These impacts possibly transgress the criminal law, but they rarely come to court because they are dealt with by the sport officials.
3. Criminal violence. These incidents are so obvious the law should immediately be evoked. Such situations, e.g., slashing maliciously with a hockey stick across the head, may lead to permanent injury or even death. Unfortunately, there is a certain amount of folk theory associated with this type of action in some sports, and such violence may even be passed off as part of the game. It usually means that financially this violence pays more than it

> **Quick Facts**
>
> **PARAMETERS OF MUSCULOSKELETAL SPORTS MEDICINE**
>
> - Mechanisms of injury
> - Early consultation
> - Accurate diagnosis
> - Intensive goal oriented treatment
> - Objective and functional assessment
> - Safe plan for return to activity
> - Injury prevention strategies

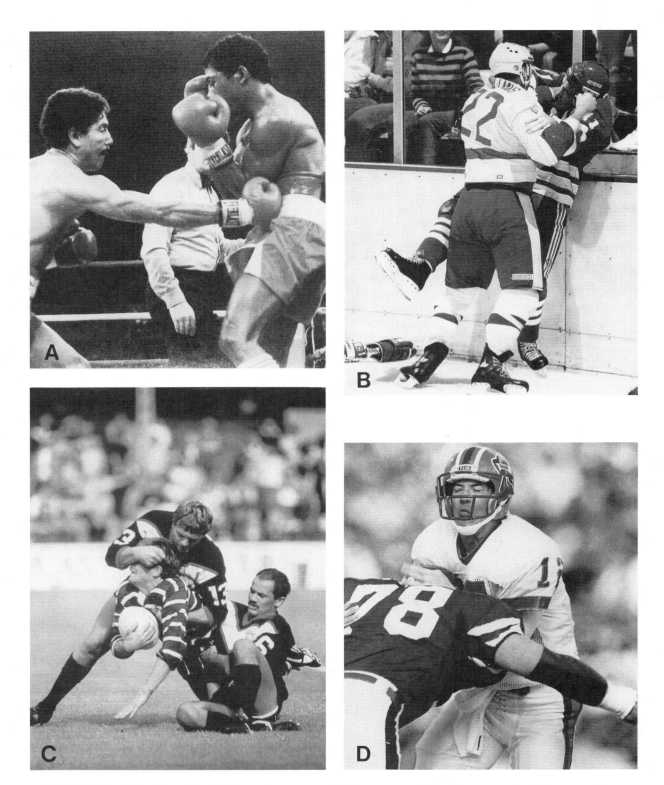

Fig. 1-3. Brutal body contact is integral to many collision-type activities; however, the injury rate rises as it merges imperceptibly into organized brutality and criminal violence according to the intent of the athlete. (**A**) In boxing, organized brutality is made worse by a low blow. (**B**) Fighting in hockey is perhaps organized brutality. (**C**) In rugby, brutal body contact magnified by gouging. (**D**) Football tackle complicated by spearing.

costs. It is an unfortunate element seen as frequently in amateur as in professional sport.

Collision with an Object

Hard impacts against the boards in hockey, contact with the goal posts in soccer, or falls on hard playing surfaces are examples of collision with an object. One of the parameters of sports medicine is to ensure that playing areas are as safe as possible prior to the commencement of competition. An experienced practitioner always appraises the venue on arrival in order to spot unnecessary hazards, such as inadequately padded football goal posts, and attempt to eliminate them.

Infringement of the Rules

Unfortunately, deliberate or accidental breaking of rules forms a major source of injury in some sports. In many instances, these infringements are extensions of the situations alluded to under the heading of collision with another athlete. In ice hockey, for instance, more than 80 percent of head and neck injuries and approximately 90 percent of hand injuries are due to fighting and highsticking. This source of injury is unacceptable and could be radically altered. Medical input into rule changes and pressure to enforce existing regulations have done much to make sports safer. Some of the best examples include the introduction of "no spearing" in football and depowering of the scrum in rugby, with the resultant decreased incidence of cervical spine trauma.

Dangerous Techniques

Some maneuvers used in sport may leave a specific body part vulnerable, such as the low tackle in football. An unusual example is the recent modification of the technique of long jumping designed to maximize the momentum gained during the run up. The takeoff is incorporated into a forward somersault. Although the evolution of this technique was perhaps based on sound biomechanical principles, in practice it led to a sudden increase in injuries, the most serious of which was trauma to the cervical spine. This technique was rapidly banned owing to the efforts of individuals involved with sports medicine.

Force Overload

Force overload may occur in situations where the athlete carries out a movement that produces an overwhelming mechanical force concentrated on one body part and leading to anatomic failure. For instance, with skiing the anterior cruciate ligament can be torn by the anterior shearing force generated by the quadriceps contraction, levering the body upright over the skis, while recovering from a backward fall.[9] Injuries may also occur in situations such as accelerating out of the starting blocks or decelerating at the end of a sprint, where muscle tightness may be a contributing factor in producing a torn hamstring muscle.

The force overload mechanism of injury, however, frequently occurs in situations where the anatomy is abnormal. As an example, ruptures of the Achilles tendon are most prevalent in athletes who have degenerative or involutional changes in their tendons due to aging, prolonged inactivity, a long history of tendinitis, or steroid injections.

Missile Injuries

Missiles abound in sport and recreation. The combination of small, hard materials and high velocity is particularly dangerous. Certain examples rapidly spring to mind, such as eye injuries or facial lacerations from the pucks in ice hockey. However, larger objects, such as rackets, javelins, and the discus, can be just as deadly. The ball in many sports travels at velocities greater than 62.5 mph (100 kph) and so constitutes a formidable object if the athlete is unable to take avoiding action or is inadequately protected. Indeed, at close range neural reflex arcs and the associated mechanical lag in moving body segments are much too slow for avoidance action, emphasizing the importance of protective equipment (Fig. 1-4).

Environmental Factors

Environmental factors include heat-induced illness during distance running events or training for other sports in hot climates. Other environmental influences include artificial turf increasing knee injuries, the problems of decompression in scuba diving, and difficulties encountered with altitude, cold conditions, and travel to other countries for competition with accompanying jet lag and traveler's gastroenteritis. Often a thorough knowledge of physiology is necessary to reduce the environmental risks. In other instances, modification of the rules or equipment forms part of the answer.

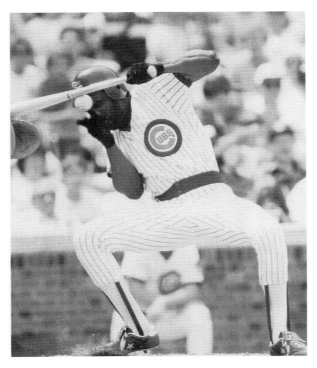

Fig. 1-4. With many sports, delivery of the missile is so fast that the normal reflex protective actions are too slow to take sufficient avoiding maneuvers. Hence protective equipment is essential.

Equipment Factors

Traditionally, protective equipment is assumed to reduce the risk of injury. However, there are several instances where it may contribute to the injury statistics.

1. Equipment failure is exemplified by a running shoe spike piercing the sole of a shoe and sticking into the foot of the runner. This injury is now rare owing to improved shoe design, although a fellow competitor may still be impaled in crowded races.
2. Occasionally equipment incorrectly worn, ill-fitting, or with ill-conceived modification may lead to problems, such as with acromioclavicular injuries and poorly fitting shoulder pads in hockey. Another example is the individual who enlarges the eye holes of a solid hockey face mask to improve the field of vision but increases the apertures sufficiently that a puck can reach the eye orbit.
3. Equipment may also change the nature of the game by protecting an individual sufficiently to allow heavier impacts at higher velocities. Unfor-

tunately, without an entire suit of armor some body part is always left vulnerable on either the attacker or the athlete receiving the blow. The most devastating joint injuries are produced by this contributing factor.
4. Failure to wear the available range of equipment may allow unnecessary injury, such as eye or tooth injuries during court games, hockey, and football.

Vehicular Accidents

Examples of vehicular accidents are numerous, but a fall from a horse serves as a case in point. Equestrian accidents, for instance, form the fourth leading cause of serious lumbar spine fractures in sport and recreation in North America. Cycling is also a rising concern.

Unsafe Manipulation of Physiology

In an effort to gain an advantage over opponents, there has evolved a battle of physiology and pharmacology. Theoretic advantages brought about by dietary manipulations, fluid restriction, weight loss, and prolonged exercise bouts are examples of activities that may have a negative as well as a positive aspect. Occasionally, these practices culminate in serious physical disorders. It is in this area that the coach has the greatest influence; and it is here that the most communication between coach, sports scientist, physician, and therapist is required.

Quick Facts
MECHANISMS OF INJURY

- Overuse or poor training parameters
- Collision with another athlete
- Collision with an object
- Infringement of rules
- Dangerous techniques
- Force overload
- Missile injuries
- Environmental factors
- Equipment factors
- Vehicular accidents
- Unsafe manipulation of physiology
- Drug abuse
- Failure to treat existing pathology
- Complications of treatment

Drug Abuse

Drug abuse is unfortunately becoming an important aspect of sport and sports injuries. It may produce some drastic examples of pathology, ranging from hypertension and genital changes due to steroid abuse to sudden death caused by stimulants such as cocaine. Drug use in sport presents one of the greatest challenges to sports medicine personnel—from the research and documentation perspective as well as with the evolution of effective educational campaigns.

Failure to Treat Existing Pathology

Long-standing inflammation may produce secondary degenerative changes and accompanying structural weakness. The medical advice may have to shift from minor modification of activity to prolonged absence from sport or even permanent restriction of a specific activity. Similarly, unattended ligament instability may result in gross articular surface damage. Prompt, effective care is the key to minimizing the above sequences; unfortunately, in reality this situation does not always occur. Delayed treatment is prevalent in sports medicine and is touched upon frequently in this book (Table 1-1).

Complications of Treatment

An undesirable outcome of any therapy is a superimposed complication that may be directly attributed to the treatment received. Such examples include frostbite from the use of cryotherapy, tendon rupture from steroid injection, or gastric ulceration from the use of nonsteroidal anti-inflammatory medication. Similarly, an error in the rate of progression of

TABLE 1-1. Delay in Seeking Treatment

Delay	No.	%
Same day	135	32
Second day	49	12
Third day	18	4
Fourth day	20	5
5–7 Days	23	6
1–2 Weeks	36	9
2–4 Weeks	29	7
1–2 Months	35	9
2–4 Months	22	6
5–12 Months	27	7
>1 Year	13	3

(Data from Kent,[12] with permission.)

therapy can lead to further tearing of a ligament, reinjury, or flaring up of a resolving tendinitis. In most instances, accumulated experience and careful ongoing assessment minimize these episodes.

An area that needs special mention concerns the therapist and physician involved with professional sport or elite athletes. All medical decisions must be made with the athlete's short- and long-term welfare in mind. The medical staff's approach to the athlete's problem should be in no way compromised by any contract with the team. It is sometimes impossible to serve two masters, and in these circumstances the obligation is only to the athlete.

Overuse Syndromes

From the point of view of mechanisms of injury, the most dramatic situations are usually those that occur during participation in competition. However, on reviewing the injury patterns of many athletic endeavors, the overuse or overstress syndrome predominates in its multitude of presentations. It frequently occurs as a result of training methods rather than participation in competition events (Fig. 1-2). Part of the problem stems from the fact that large numbers of recreational athletes are their own coaches, and training errors are easily introduced into their programs. Nevertheless, it should be easier to modify practice or training factors than to alter game and competition events. In theory, then, these overuse injuries should be potentially easier to treat. However, for a variety of reasons, including lack of patient compliance, they often are not.

Overuse syndromes include stress reaction and stress fractures of bone, tendinitis, bursitis, and chronic stretching of ligaments. An interesting sport-specific example would be stretching of the medial collateral ligament and chronic inflammation of the associated bursa at the knee suffered by swimmers practicing the whip kick.[10,11] This stroke produces a repetitive significant valgus stress on the medial aspect of the knee joint.

Overuse injuries are also a product of the disappearing "off season."[12] Covered stadiums, field houses, and increasingly complex sport organization has extended the length of seasons and eroded the "lay off" time between season. For this reason many young athletes never have a chance to take a complete break from their sport. As a result, injuries that would have traditionally healed during the off season now go on to chronicity.

It is important to plan a specific period of layoff or rest period during each athlete's year, so the stresses are reduced on the particular body part that has been subjected to the most repetitive forces during the long season of training and competition. This point is particularly important for the juvenile and adolescent athlete.

EARLY CONSULTATION

Early treatment is frequently something that is more talked about than practiced in the world of sports.[12,13] It may be due to the athlete underestimating the severity of the problem, the unavailability of experienced help, or because of resistance to seeking help subsequent to previous poor experiences with the medical profession. Sometimes pressure to continue training by the coach may contribute to the problem of delayed diagnosis. Data from my clinic indicates that only one-third of individuals are diagnosed and treated within 2 weeks of sustaining an injury (Fig. 1-5). Surprisingly, 20 percent of injuries were not seen until 6 months had elapsed.[12] Similarly, nearly half of the patients seen at the Toronto Western Hospital's Sports Medicine Clinic trained 5 days or longer before seeing a physician (Table 1-1). The worst procrastinators were often those who had set the highest personal performance standards. Because 62 percent of these individuals were being coached at the time of their injury, it may once more reflect, in part, the attitude of the coach.[13] About 30 percent of those who delayed seeking appropriate treatment eventually required immobilization or surgery. When speculating about the cause for delay, several factors were identified, including misinterpretation of the pain they encountered and assuming it was a normal part of increased training. Many reported ignoring swelling and discomfort. Striving for unrealistic goals produced injury and was a factor in failure to seek advice.[13]

In any event, the statistics point to the need for education of athletes and coaches at all levels, as well as the importance of generating an atmosphere of confidence in the treatment team. The latter factor is engendered only by constant good treatment and liaison with both coaches and athletes. Unfortunately, the net result of the current situation is that, for many therapists, treatment of the injured athlete is treatment of chronic pathology. This fact is contrary to the popular notion that sports medicine is primarily treatment of the acute injury.

Chronic problems are often more difficult to handle than acute pathology, which puts the physician and therapist at a disadvantage and is a key factor usually overlooked by the coach and athlete. The consequent frequent need for significant modification of training and prolonged treatment of these chronic injuries is often used as an unjust criticism of the treating staff. Nevertheless, once these injuries are identified, accurate diagnosis and intensive treatment should be the goals. Whenever the problem lies outside the expertise of the primary care person, referral to a more specialized individual or environment will obviate further delays in the appropriate management of the problem. Whatever the expectation of the athlete, however, there is a finite speed to resolution of inflammation and progress of healing for each tissue. Tissues heal in the shortest time when all conditions are made optimal, which is the task of the physician and therapist. Regardless, the most frequent question posed by the athlete, often before the initial examination is complete, is "When will I be fit to resume full activity?" It is a natural concern, as loss of time due to injury may delay well planned goals and dreams of success. Furthermore, loss of time due to injury may become more permanent in the young athlete because of persisting physical or psychological problems. A delay in presenting for treatment, however, can only compound these situations.

ACCURATE DIAGNOSIS

The establishment of an accurate diagnosis is a prerequisite in all branches of medicine, but there are some special implications in association with musculoskeletal athletic injuries. Only by separating liga-

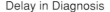

Delay in Diagnosis

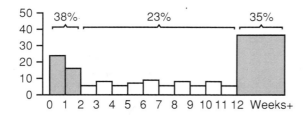

Fig. 1-5. Injured athletes presenting for diagnosis and treatment within 2 weeks of being injured. Note that only 61 percent present by 3 months.

ment injuries, tendon pathology, and muscle trauma into stages and degrees is it possible to draw up logical treatment programs and assess the timing for safe resumption of training and competition.[6,7,14,15]

Underestimating or misdiagnosing an injury may lead to reinjury. When a body part is reinjured, the subsequent healing and recovery time is usually double that for the initial injury. Not only does this factor influence the amount of training time lost, but the eventual tissue reaction and scarring that ensue may leave an increased susceptibility to reinjury. Nowhere is this point more classically illustrated than with repetitive hamstring tears or chronic Achilles tendinitis.

For some injuries, the immediate assessment is not always accurate. If recovery does not take place within the expected time, the diagnosis must be reassessed. For instance, with an 11-year-old boy who has been treated for a knee strain that does not recover in the expected time, the associated diagnosis of slipped capital femoral epiphysis at the hip should be ruled out by examination and roentgenography. If on close scrutiny the diagnosis still stands and the athlete is not responding to an apparently well planned and appropriate treatment regimen, other possibilities should be entertained. Perhaps the athlete is not following instructions. This area should be investigated, as communication may have been poor or instructions misunderstood, or the coach or parent are putting undue pressure on the individual to perform despite the injury. Alternatively, the athlete may have misinformed the coach as to the therapist's instructions in order to continue training and ostensibly not lose time.

Clinical Points

REASONS FOR FAILURE TO RESPOND TO TREATMENT

- Incorrect diagnosis
- Incorrect treatment
- Inadequate treatment
- Failure of athlete to follow plan
- Undue pressure from coach
- Undue pressure from parent
- Poor communication

Therefore
- Set goals
- Reassess early

The clinical points in the box stress the importance of communication as well as the establishment of confidence in the treatment team with all individuals involved in the athlete's progress.

INTENSIVE TREATMENT

There are circumstances where an athlete ideally should be treated several times a day. For most individuals, formal visits to a clinic may not be possible, cost-effective, or required. The physician or therapist should be in a position to outline specific home programs using simple exercises and easily available modalities such as ice or heat in the form of warm baths or hot water bottles. These home treatments can supplement the treatment sessions carried out at a clinic. The role of the therapist as teacher and motivator can perhaps never be overstressed.

A basic tenet of sports medicine is that athletes should be working harder to recover from the injury than they would be during their normal training program. The treatment room must never be allowed to become an escape from the rigors of training. The aim of the sports physician and therapist is to return the athlete to the coach in better all-round condition than when first seen after the injury.[7] It requires imagination, inspiration, a thorough knowledge of the sport, and an awareness of the limits of the athlete with any given injury.

FUNCTIONAL ASSESSMENT

Role of Pain

In some areas of medicine pain is an excellent indication of the severity of injury and the rate at which treatment should progress. Unfortunately, because of the enormous and often repetitive stresses involved in athletic activity, pain may be an unreliable guide. Reaction to pain is individualistic, and some athletes are stoic whereas others seem to feel the slightest change in their physiology. The former may hide their injury and their pain, and the latter may complain at the smallest setback. Indeed, some athletes use the injury situation to manipulate their parents, coach, or teammates.

Apart from the athlete, the individual clinical staff may be affected differently by a specific athlete's pain. Despite the fact that one definition of pain is "a personal, subjective feeling of hurt," it should be realized that the athlete presents different faces to different individuals. The level of pain reported to one practitioner may not be the same as that conveyed to the therapist, coach, or parent. For these reasons the concept of functional assessment is important.[16]

Unreliability of Nonfunctional Measurements

Functional assessment principles aim to use objective and functional tests as the guide to safe reintegration of the athlete into training and competition.[6,7,17,18] Many of the parameters are sport-specific. Just as pain levels may be inadequate as a sole guide to progress, so it should be realized that the tape measure and goniometry may not give a true picture. This point has been emphasized in studies showing that, despite adequate girth, isokinetic testing after completing a rehabilitation program may still show a deficiency in endurance parameters.[16,17] Moreover, muscle biopsies, ultrasonography, and computed tomographic studies have confirmed the inaccuracies of simple tape measurements of limb girth.[19-21]

Functional Principles

To minimize the risk of reinjury, an athlete should not be considered ready for full training or return to game situations under most circumstances until the following conditions are met.

1. Full, painless, active range of motion at the joint involved
2. Full passive range of motion at the appropriate joint
3. Adequate return of strength
4. Sufficiently rehabilitated muscle and cardiovascular endurance
5. Return of normal movement patterns
6. Psychologically ready.

When planning the progression of rehabilitation steps along the way it is essential to know, for any given athlete and sport, the cardiovascular and strength requirements in detail.[3,17] The therapist must also be cognizant of the biomechanical stresses involved in practice and competition situations, the skills and movement patterns, the vulnerability and frequency of injury of any specific joint, and the potential for modifying protective equipment.

With the above information the goals of rehabilitation become clear, and a step by step plan of progression may be initiated. Objective tests indicate when sufficient progress has been made for safe reintegration into light, moderate, and full training.

This chapter has emphasized the parameters of musculoskeletal sports medicine and therapy. The successful application of these principles requires considerable knowledge of each sport and recreational activity and an imaginative approach to the individual athlete's specific problem.

REFERENCES

1. Reid DC: Canadian Encyclopaedia. Mel Hurtig Publishing, Edmonton, 1987
2. Hughston JC: Knee surgery—a philosophy. Am Phys Ther 60:1611, 1980
3. Fleck SJ, Falkel JE: Value of resistance training for the reduction of sports injuries. Sports Med 3:61, 1986
4. Vinger PF, Hoerner EF (eds.): Sports Injuries: The Unthwarted Epidemic. 2nd Ed. PSG Publication Co. Massachusetts, 1986
5. Mellion MB (ed): Office Management of Sports Injuries and Athletic Problems. CV Mobsy, St. Louis, 1988
6. Bass AL: Football injuries. World Med 2:17, 1967
7. Bass AL: Athletic and soft tissue injuries. Physiotherapy 51:112, 1965
8. Williams JGP: A Color Atlas of Injury in Sport. Wolfe Medical Publishing, Smeats-Weert, Holland, 1980
9. McConkey JP: Anterior cruciate ligament rupture in skiing: a new mechanism of injury. Am J Sports Med 14:160, 1986
10. Kennedy JC, Hawkins R, Krissoff WB: Orthopaedic manifestations of swimming. Am J Sports Med 6:309, 1978
11. Reid DC: The everlasting season. I. The overuse syndrome. J Can Acad Sports Med 7:29, 1987
12. Kent F: Athletes wait too long to report injuries. Physician Sports Med 10:127, 1982
13. Noyes FR, De Lucas JL, Torvicle PJ: Biomechanics of anterior cruciate ligament failure: an analysis of strain-rate sensitivity and mechanisms of failure in primates. J Bone Joint Surg [Am] 56:236, 1974
14. Paulos L, Noyes FR, Grood E et al: Knee rehabilitation after anterior cruciate ligament reconstruction and repair. Am J Sports Med 9:140, 1981
15. Garrick JG: When can I? A practical approach to rehabilitation illustrated by treatment of an ankle injury. Am J Sports Med 9:67, 1981

16. Kegerreis S: The construction and implementation of functional progression as a component of athletic rehabilitation. J Orthop Sports Phys Ther 5:14, 1983

17. Hage P: Prescribing exercise: more than just a running program. Physiother Sports Med 11:123, 1983

18. Roy S, Irvine R: Sports Medicine: Prevention, Evaluation, Management and Rehabilitation. Prentice-Hall, Englewood Cliffs, NJ, 1983

19. Young A, Hughes I: Ultrasonography of muscle in physiotherapy practice and research. Physiotherapy 68:187, 1982

20. Matoba H, Sollnick PD: Muscle physiology: response of skeletal muscle to training. Sports Med 1:241, 1984

Principles of Treatment 2

To be uncertain is uncomfortable.
To be certain is ridiculous.
— Author Unknown

The spectrum of sporting and recreational activities is vast and the accompanying injuries diverse. Nevertheless, some common denominators form the essential principles of successful therapy: (1) accurate diagnosis and understanding of the accompanying underlying pathophysiologic processes; (2) comprehensive knowledge of the functional requirements of the athletes in their specific sport; (3) establishment of treatment goals and the probable rate of progression; and (4) a realistic evaluation of the possible prognosis of a specific injury. From these principles emanate the plan of treatment. For effective therapy of the injured athlete there must also be provision for maintaining cardiovascular fitness, maintenance or recovery of strength, the development of functional progressions, and the implementation of objective testing. This chapter focuses on the treatment of the initial inflammatory reaction and the subsequent implication of the above principles of treatment.

INFLAMMATION AND THE INJURY CYCLE

The central feature of trauma is inflammation. Without the inflammatory response normal healing would be slow or even nonexistent. The function of inflammation is to signal tissue damage and trigger the local and systemic factors to initiate the appropriate defense and repair processes. Inflammation, then, is a necessary condition. However, it is a primitive response usually excessive in magnitude for its function in soft tissue injury. Excessive inflammation produces pain, spasm, and edema, and it may delay healing and lead to chronic adverse tissue changes.[1,2] Poor or inadequate treatment may predispose to all the negative outcomes of inflammation in the injury cycle, whereas effective treatment is designed to enhance the positive features (Fig. 2-1).

Clinical Points

PRINCIPLES OF TREATMENT

- Accurate assessment of pathology
- Specific treatment of pathology
- Analysis of functional requirements
- Maintenance of cardiovascular fitness
- Maintenance or recovery of strength
- Development of functional progressions
- Implementation of objective testing

MODALITIES AND ANTI-INFLAMMATORY MEDICATIONS

The basis of physical therapy is exercise, but for the treatment of soft tissue trauma several physical modalities may assist in creating optimal conditions for healing. Much has been written on speeding up the healing process, but in reality there is no therapy that accelerates this phenomenon. All treatment is aimed at maximizing the ideal conditions for the tissues' own regenerative capability.[3,4] Ice, compression, and the nonsteroidal anti-inflammatory medications form the basis for early treatment, and their modes of action are discussed here. The therapeutic modalities are dealt with in Chapter 3.

Compression and Elevation

To understand the importance and effectiveness of the simple measures of elevation and compression during the early management of soft tissue injury, it is necessary to examine the pathophysiology of edema development.

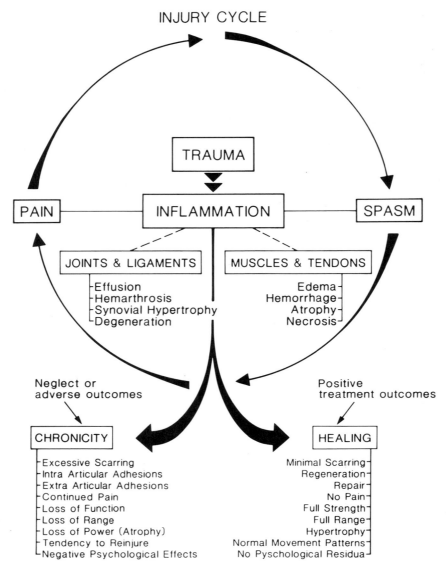

INJURY CYCLE

Fig. 2-1. Injury cycle illustrates the range of outcomes of trauma in response to treatment. Inflammation should be minimized to assist in allowing the events of healing to assume positive pathways as rapidly as possible.

Normal Tissue Fluid Flow

Fluid movement in the capillary bed depends on the state of the capillary wall, the degree of vessel dilation, the cardiac output, and the efficiency of venous and lymphatic return to the central circulation (Fig. 2-2). The endothelial cells and the basement membrane with its pores serve as a selective membrane. Water, oxygen, and carbon dioxide may diffuse directly through the cell membrane. Some plasma proteins and other substances filtrate through the pores, which are on average 20 times wider than the diameter of a water molecule and slightly less than that of most plasma proteins.[5]

Hydrostatic pressure which is supplied by cardiac output and peripheral resistance, is approximately 15 to 20 mmHg higher at the arteriole than the venule end of the capillary bed. Osmotic (oncotic) pressure is the pulling force of a solution for water and is higher at the venule end of the capillary bed, as all of the electrolytes and proteins are concentrated (averaging 28 mmHg). Albumin, the smallest of the plasma pro-

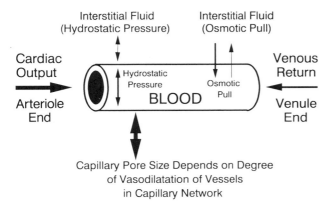

Fig. 2-2. At the arteriole end the hydrostatic capillary pressure is high and osmotic tissue pull relatively low, allowing movement of serum minus most of its proteins into the tissue spaces. The venous end allows return because of the enhanced osmotic pull in the vessels. Inflammation allows excessive motion of fluid and proteins into the interstitium.

teins, accounts for about 75 percent of the osmolality of the blood. The average interstitial osmotic pressure is 5 mmHg.[2]

The balance of these forces generates slightly more filtration into the tissue spaces than resorption, and this small discrepancy is dealt with by the lymphatic system (Fig. 2-3). Approximately one-tenth of the fluid filtering out of the capillaries enters the lymphatic system.

Tissue Reaction to Trauma

With tissue damage the mediators of inflammation are generated and released.[6,7] The result is capillary vasodilation and enhanced permeability, particularly via large intercellular gaps. The net effect is the passage of more plasma proteins into the interstitium and a decreased osmotic gradient. Small pockets of free fluid may then develop, and edema may become apparent clinically (Fig. 2-3). Depending on the degree of tissue damage, amount of motion, dependency of the limb, and ingrowth of capillaries, the degree of edema may interfere with tissue nutrition and oxygenation. It is obvious that limiting this collection of extracapillary fluid and enhancing its return to the circulation is a vital part of the early treatment of traumatic or ongoing inflammatory conditions. Apart from the pain that is generated by the excessive tissue pressure and chemical stimulation of the sensory nerve endings, the net result of prolonged edema is deposition of fibrinogen into the tissue spaces and thickening, adhesions, and decreased normal tissue fluid flow. Untreated this may take many months to reorganize and resorb.

Limiting Edema

Minimizing the initial trauma and inflammation are obvious ways of decreasing the ultimate morbidity generated by the edema. Any factor that tends to increase the rate of lymph flow assists resolution, as

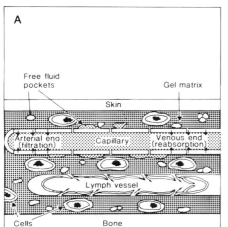
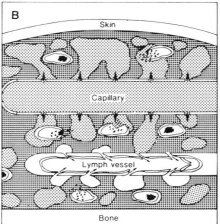
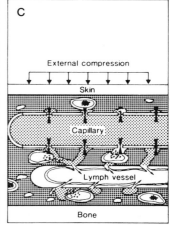

Fig. 2-3. (A) Interstitial fluid balance under normal conditions. Lymphatic vessels cope with the excess fluid. **(B)** With capillary dilation large amounts of fluid pass into the interstitium, creating a stagnant, edematous situation. **(C)** External compression helps force fluid into the vessels by increasing interstitial hydrostatic pressure. (Adapted from Barnes.[7])

the osmolality gradient between capillaries and tissue has been reduced. Elevation and compression are reasonable mechanisms for increasing the hydrostatic gradients from tissue to circulation. The lymphatic vessels have valves, and gentle range of motion during elevation produces an efficient milking action that may increase lymph flow up to 5 to 15 times the resting level.[7] Hence there is a sound rationale for the early application of pressure and elevation.

Cryotherapy

Cryotherapy, the local application of cold for therapeutic reasons, is believed to diminish the inflammatory reaction to trauma, reduce edema, minimize hemorrhage, and produce some analgesia. The therapeutic effects may be achieved via a range of physiologic changes including vasoconstriction, decreased blood flow, altered nerve conduction, and reduced muscle spasm.

Cold Versus Pressure

The effectiveness of ice therapy for reducing pain, swelling, and the duration of disability is well established.[4,5] The edema that follows injury complicates recovery by splinting or stiffening of the involved joint, increasing pain on movement, and reducing the ability of the circulation to support healing by slowing tissue perfusion. However, although cooling alone may temporarily reduce pain, bleeding, and swelling during the immediate postinjury period, its effects on the longer-term tissue changes are not clear.[6] Sloan et al., using a 40-minute cooling period to treat artificially induced acute inflammatory reactions in human tissue, showed that cooling alone produced a transient decrease in response at 15 minutes but not at 1 hour.[5] The addition of mild pressure (10 mmHg) to mild cooling (15° to 25°C) produced a highly significant reduction in swelling from 15 minutes onward. Pressure alone did not have a significant effect (Fig. 2-4). This experiment lends support to the time-honored belief that some form of cooling with compression is important after injury. Furthermore, cooling alone is not as likely to be as effective as it is in combination with pressure.

Mechanism of Inducing Analgesia

The mechanism by which ice produces analgesia is probably that it decreases the size of the nerve action potentials and, if sufficient cooling takes place, by

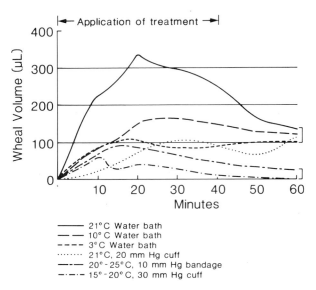

Fig. 2-4. Influence of cold and pressure, together and independently on an artificially induced acute inflammatory reaction. Pressure and cooling combined produced the most lasting effect on edema.[5]

blocking conduction (Table 2-1).[6-8] This analgesia is maximal immediately after ice therapy and declines rapidly over a 30-minute period.[9,10] Cryokinetics is the system of inducing analgesia with cooling followed by range of motion exercises.[3] The effectiveness of the analgesic action should introduce a certain amount of caution into the mobilization component, which should always be carried out with due regard to the magnitude of the initial injury and the probable effect of early motion on the eventual function of the body part involved.

TABLE 2-1. Analgesia Induced by Cold Therapy

Stage	Response	Time from Initiation of Therapy (minutes)
1	Cold sensation	0–3
2	Burning, aching	2–7
3	Local numbness, anesthesia	5–12
	Reflexes decreased	
	Pain spasm cycle interrupted	
4	Deep tissue vasodilation not accompanied by increased metabolism	12–15

(Adapted from Waylonis,[11] with permission.)

TABLE 2-2. Temperature Reduction with Various Cryotherapy Agents

Modality	Intramuscular Temperature Decrease (°C), by Time After Application			
	15 Min	30 Min	45 Min	60 Min
Ice[a]	3.4	6.9	9.2	11.3
Gel	1.8	4.4	6.5	3.4
Chemical	1.6	2.9	3.0	3.5
Freon	0.2	0.9	1.2	1.7

[a] Supporting studies show decrease of temperature in tissues of 3.0° to 12.5°C at 2 cm after 10 minutes of ice massage.

(Adapted from McMaster et al.,[10] with permission.)

Methods of Application

There are a variety of methods for applying cryotherapy, which is one of its attractions. It is usually an inexpensive, readily available modality that can be applied in the form of sophisticated gels, chemicals, or Freon sprays as well as by less sophisticated methods, including ice chips or ice blocks (popsicle therapy) or frozen bags of peas. The latter are malleable, available at home, and reusable (Table 2-2). The superiority of ice is manifest in most studies, but the other cryotherapeutic agents may be convenient during travel or in specific clinical situations (Table 2-2). Freon sprays and chemical cold packs may lower the tissue temperature sufficiently to run the risk of creating frostbite.

Temperature Distribution

The temperature distribution is not uniform throughout the tissues, and it is necessary to vary the duration of the therapy with the depth of the lesion being treated.[8] This treatment principle is important (Table 2-3). Intramuscular temperature depends on

TABLE 2-3. Temperature Decrease After 10 Minutes of Ice Massage

Depth (CM)	Temperature Decrease (°C)
Skin	6.4
Subcutaneous	5.8
0.5	6.0
1.0	5.8
2.0	3.6
4.0	1.7
8.0	1.2

(Adapted from Matsen et al.,[6] and Benson and Copp.[8])

the length of the cold therapy, the depth in the muscle, and the application modality.[11]

Other Physiologic Effects

The ability to alter viscoelastic properties of collagen, induce vasodilation, and minimize spasm are physiologic effects that have potential clinical application at various stages of soft tissue healing.[12] The exact initial changes in the tissues in response to cryotherapy may vary from subject to subject, and the subsequent reflex vasodilation responses are unpredictable. For this reason the treatment principles are more important than strict adherence to prearranged dosages. Clinical judgment must be exercised in each case with careful observation of the existing pathologic and anatomic parameters. With acute injuries, early application is probably more effective than delayed therapy.

Cold Therapy Applications

1. During the immediate postinjury period, 20-minute application of ice during each hour combined with compression, rest, and elevation seems to be the most clinically efficacious regimen for minimizing hemorrhage and edema. There are advocates of longer and shorter periods of ice application.
2. After the first 24 to 28 hours, various cold therapy regimens may be used to reduce discomfort and muscle spasm prior to range of motion and strengthening work.
3. In cases of acute and chronic tendinitis, ice massage is frequently used prior to exercise and after training bouts. It certainly reduces pain and discomfort, but the ability to control inflammation and edema in these situations is difficult to quantify.
4. During attempts to stretch out contractions or muscle tightness, cooling down on the stretch helps to stabilize collagen bonds in the lengthened position gained by prior warming or exercise.

Cold Therapy Techniques

1. Ice massage: The injured area is massaged with an ice cube. The simplest method is to freeze water in small Dixie Cups. The injured part and surrounding area are usually massaged for 5 to 10 minutes.
2. Ice bath: The injured part is immersed in a solution of water and crushed ice. The temperature

should be around 40°–50° F. This method is suitable for cryokinetics because it is easy to carry out range of motion exercises in the tanks. The effects of dependency are negated by the water pressure, so it is still possible to treat edematous areas by this technique.

Combining cold immersion alternately with hot water baths is effective therapy for mobilizing stiff joints. The resultant alternate vasoconstriction, dilatation, and mild analgesia are particularly effective. For small joints 15 seconds of cold followed by 45 seconds of warmth with exercise, repeated for 10 minutes may be used. For larger joints 1 minute of cold followed by 1 minute of heat is a more practical regimen.

3. Ice packs: The injured area is covered with a blanket or pack for 15 to 20 minutes. This method has the advantage of covering a large area, and it may allow simultaneous range of motion. Commercial ice packs are convenient; however, shaved or crushed ice between layers of terry towel cloths are equally effective and are frequently more moldable around the joint. Commercial chemical packs should be reserved for first aid and used with considerable caution, as the temperature with these packs may be lower than that achieved by ice packs.

4. Freon sprays, ethyl chloride, or other vapocoolants: Usually reserved for rapid cooling after direct contusions, this method of application is also potentially dangerous. It is recommended that these sprays should be used only for "spray and stretch" techniques as adopted for pain relief, trigger areas, and range of motion work.

Contraindications

Contraindications to the use of cryotherapy include Raynaud's phenomenon, peripheral vascular disease, cold allergy, severe cold-induced urticaria, cryoglobulinemia, and paroxysmal cold hemoglobinuria.[5] Awareness of the potential for frostbite and observing precautions such as limiting the time of direct application of cold should minimize this risk. Prolonged periods of cryotherapy directly over superficial nerve trunks has been occasionally associated with transient paralysis. Limiting the exposure time over the peroneal nerve at the fibula neck and the ulna nerve of the elbow, for instance, helps avoid this complication. Usually the nerve lesion is transient, and full recovery is the norm.

Precaution should be observed in individuals with very low hemoglobin levels if large areas are covered repeatedly, as there may be some accelerated red blood cell breakdown. Massage over the carotid sheath may stimulate the vagus nerve and thus produce significant bradycardia. Some individuals have a severe sensitivity to cold and may respond to ice pack therapy with an elevation of blood pressure, systolic and diastolic, in the range of 15 to 20 mmHg. These elevations should be treated with some caution. Preferably, alternative modalities are selected if the pressure changes are of a large magnitude. The use of ice over skin lesions must be considered carefully. Maceration of small lesions is prevented by the application of petroleum jelly. There is also discussion as to the advisability of ice over an area that has received a cortisone injection within the previous 24 hours, although there is little reason why it should be a problem. Knowledge of pathologic processes, common sense, adequate patient instruction, and careful observation for adverse reactions minimize the danger from ice application. Freon sprays have the most potential for abuse. Used sensibly, cryotherapy is one of the safer modalities, although carelessness may produce some severe circulatory problems.

Clinical Point

CONTRAINDICATIONS AND PRECAUTIONS

- Raynaud's phenomenon
- Cold hypersensitivity
- Diabetes with vascular involvement
- Peripheral vascular disease
- Malignancies
- Impaired sensation
- Ice massage over the carotid sheath
- Elderly patients with fragile skin
- Children or other individuals unable to comprehend warnings

---

Other Modalities

The other physical modalities include (1) those generating heat or mechanical effects in the tissues, e.g., hot packs, laser, ultrasound, and shortwave diathermy; (2) those using the special properties of electrical currents or the electromagnetic spectrum in an athermic mode, e.g., interferential currents, pulsed athermic shortwaves, transcutaneous electrical nerve stimulation, or direct currents; and (3) those recording and stimulating motor nerves and muscle, e.g., modifications of the muscle-stimulating currents, sinusoidal waves, and electromyographic biofeedback units. Each of these modalities may be selected for use in the subacute phase of inflammation or for dealing with the complications of trauma. Essentially, their rational use requires a sound understanding of the pathophysiologic processes underlying the specific diseases and injury situations. Attention to small details and the subtleties of the changing physical signs and symptoms allows maximum benefit. Applied without thought or consideration to the changing physiologic state wastes the athlete's and the therapist's time and is potentially harmful. In this regard, thorough knowledge of the specific contraindications is mandatory, and it is these points that are stressed in

Chapter 3, along with a more in-depth look at specific modalities.

Nonsteroidal Anti-Inflammatory Medication

Mechanism of Action

The nonsteroidal anti-inflammatory drugs (NSAIDs) are the most commonly used drugs for the management of acute soft tissue injury.[13,14] Prostaglandins, particularly E_1 and E_2, are central to the acute inflammatory response to trauma, helping initiate vasodilation and chemotaxis and increasing vascular permeability (Fig. 2-5).[14] However, if it is accepted that the magnitude of this initial inflammatory reaction is usually far in excess of what is needed to set the scene for healing, it is logical to use some therapy that minimizes this phase.[1] The NSAIDs are a reasonable choice because of their antiprostaglandin effect (Fig. 2-5).

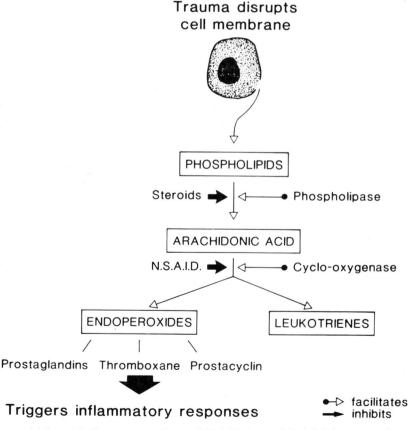

Fig. 2-5. Nonsteroidal anti-inflammatory drugs (NSAIDs) possibly inhibit prostaglandin synthesis by blocking cyclo-oxygenase, limiting arachidonic acid breakdown and therefore the formation of by-products known to enhance the inflammatory response and pain.

Choice of Medication

NSAIDs are most effective if given soon after the injury; they have maximal effect over a period of 3 to 10 days. Nevertheless, there are some situations where they may be continued longer, but specific attention must be paid to the appearance of side effects. The risk versus benefit ratio of prolonged therapy must be taken into consideration. Long-term administration must be monitored by blood tests including a complete blood count and metabolic screen of liver and renal function (Table 2-4).

There should be some basis for the choice of a particular NSAID, and onset of action, analgesic property, plasma half-life, renal status, and patient compliance may be such factors.[14,15] The convenience, in some instances, of a "one per day" medication may produce better patient compliance than medication that needs to be taken four times per day. Of the "one per day" medications, the slow-release type may produce less gastric irritation, but the continued release throughout the intestines occasionally precipitates diarrhea. Therefore in some situations preparations with a long plasma half-life, e.g., piroxicam and naproxen, may be more appropriate. All of these medications are idiosyncratic in terms of their therapeutic efficacy and undesirable side effects. Frequently it is necessary to try several medications, particularly for the more chronic inflammations, in order to establish the one that is most beneficial for

any given patient or to circumvent the side effects. It is logical to try NSAIDs from different generic categories in this search for efficacy (Fig. 2-6). There is no evidence to suggest that a combination of two or more NSAIDs is any more effective than the full recommended dose of any individual agent.[12]

In situations where NSAIDs would be highly desirable but there is poor gastric tolerance by the patient, it may be possible to give a cytoprotective agent, an H_2 blocker, or a pH buffer along with the anti-inflammatory medication. In any event, the importance of taking the NSAID with food or milk must be constantly stressed. The therapist may be the first person to be aware of the adverse effects of any medication taken by the patient and should be alert to these symptoms, making sure that they are brought to the attention of the prescribing physician. Prompt attention to early complaints frequently obviates catastrophic events, such as a significant gastric breed.

PROGRESSION OF ACTIVITIES

Components

At an early juncture in the treatment, an analysis of functional requirements must be carried out to focus more clearly the rehabilitation goals and allow planning of the steps in the progression of activity. Chapter 1 introduced the concept of functional assessment, which stressed an "in depth" analysis of the

TABLE 2-4. Dosage and Adverse Effects of Nonsteroidal Anti-inflammatory Medications[a]

Generic Name	Trade Name	Usual Dose (mg)	Freq.	Plasma Half-Life (hours)	Adverse Reactions (%)					
					Dyspepsia	GI Bleed	Rash	Blood Dyscrasia	Renal Failure	Other
Piroxicam	Feldene	20	QD	40	5	<1	2	<1	0	Dizziness
Ibuprofen	Motrin	600	TID	2	5	<1	5	<1	<1	Dizziness
Naproxen	Naprosyn	250	TID	15	5	<1	5	<1	<1	Dizziness
Naproxen Na	Anaprox	275	TID							
Flurbiprofen	Ansaid	100	TID	4	5	<1	5	<1	<1	Dizziness
Ketoprofen	Orudis	100	TID	2	5	<1	5	<1	<1	Dizziness
Phenybutazone	Butazolidine	100	TID	75	5	<1	2	>1	<1	Aplastic anemia
Indomethecin	Indocid	25	QID	3	10	<1	<1	<1	<1	Headaches
Sulindac	Clinoril	200	BID	10	5	<1	5	<1	0	Dizziness
Diclofenac	Voltarin	50	TID	2						Dizziness
	Voltarin SR	100	QD	2						Diarrhea
Diflusinal	Dolobid	500	BID	15	5	<1	5	0	0	Nausea
Acetylsalicylic acid	Aspirin	1000	TID	3						Tinnitus

Figures averaged from sample of literature.

[a] Many of the significant side effects are idiosyncratic.

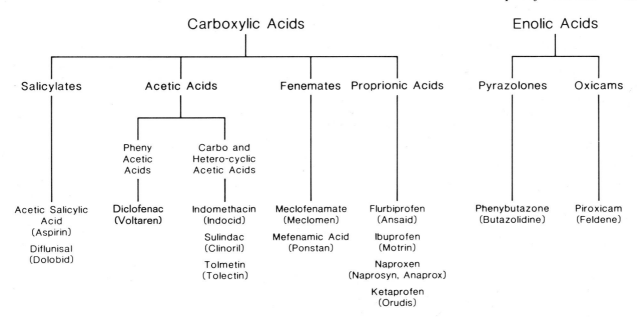

Fig. 2-6. Arrangement of NSAIDs by classes allows rational selection of alternate medication should adverse side effects occur.

sport. The physician or therapist must think of the activity in terms of its elements, including cardiovascular requirements, skills, biomechanics, anatomic ranges, flexibility, strength, balance of power and the psychologic requirements.[16-22]

Clinical Point

FUNCTIONAL PROGRESSION

- Evaluate cardiovascular requirements of activity
- List skills inherent in the sport
- Arrange skills according to stress
- Assess flexibility requirements
- Set strength goals for activity

Incorporation of this knowledge into the treatment plan decreases the risk of reinjury and ensures maintenance of maximum fitness and skill while the patient undergoes intensive local therapy to the injured body part.

Cardiovascular Requirements

The aerobic requirements of a specific sport, or even position on a team, sets fitness goals to be strived for and maintained throughout the treatment program.[9,21] These goals must be transferred to alternative activities that preserve the level of fitness while not overstressing the injured body segment. Table 2-5 outlines a rough guide to energy expenditures in some common fitness activities. Tables such as this one allow selection of appropriate alternate activities during rehabilitation programs.

Skills

The patient's skills must be analyzed to elucidate the proportion of stress imposed on each anatomic region and, in some cases, on specific anatomic structures. The list of skills may then be organized into a series of progressions based on these stresses. Depending on the site of the injury, specific skills that produce undesirable stresses can be either omitted or modified. As recovery takes place, these skills may be added sequentially in a reasonably safe manner. Such a program requires excellent communication with the athlete or coach.

Biomechanical Forces and Anatomic Ranges

Knowledge of the elements of an activity must be amalgamated with the known biomechanical and functional anatomy of the injured area. For instance, when rehabilitating knee injuries, it must be appre-

TABLE 2-5. Approximate Energy Expenditures and Fitness Values of Basic Rehabilitation Activities

Activity	Expenditure (kcal/hr)[a]	Comment	Cardioresp. Endurance	Strength	Flexibility
Cycling					
5 mph	240–250	Non-weight-bearing	−	−	−
10 mph	400–420	Even stresses on joints	+	−	+
11 mph	450–500	Good for early lower limb rehab	+	−	+
12 mph	600–620	Easy to control & progress	++	+	+
Skipping					
Leisurely	300–400	Weight bearing	+	−	+
Vigorous	750–800	Difficult to control Restores "spring" in gait	++	−	++
Rowing machine					
Leisurely	400–420	Non-weight-bearing	+	+	+
Vigorously	800–850	May stress lumbar spine Difficult to control	+	++	+
Jogging/running					
5 mph	600–620	Weight bearing	+	−	+
6 mph	750–780	Difficult to control	++	−	+
7 mph	850–880	Progression better on treadmill	++	−	+
8 mph	1000–1020	Basic activity for most sports	++	−	+
9 mph	1100–1200		++	−	+
10 mph	1250–1300	With starts & stops, large	++	−	+
Stair running	1000–1100	Stresses on lower limb joints	++	+	+
Skating					
Leisurely	400–450	Minimize joint stress	+	−	+
Vigorously	700–750	Difficult to control	++	+	++
Swimming					
Leisurely	350–500	Major non-weight-bearing activity	+	−	+
Crawl[b]	360–750	Can be combined with water	++	+	+
Back stroke[b]	360–750	Running program	++	+	+
Breast stroke[b]	360–750	Difficulty controlling effort	++	+	++
Butterfly[b]	400–850		++	+	++
Walking					
Level 1–2 mph (stroll)	120–150	Adaptable	−	−	−
Level 3 mph	300–350	Progression simple	−	−	−
Level 3.5 mph (brisk)	360–400	Stresses controlled	+	−	−
Level 4.0 mph (fast)	420–450	May add extremity weights	+	−	+
Level 5.0 mph	480–500	Weight bearing	++	−	+
Downstairs	400–425		−	−	+
Upstairs	600–1000		++	−	−
Uphill 3.5 mph	480–900		++	+	+
Downhill 2.5 mph	200–250		−	−	−

Symbols: −, no significant benefit; +, moderate benefit; ++, significant benefit.
This table gives only approximate values and can be used as a guide for planning substitute rehabilitation activity levels.

[a] Caloric consumption based on a 70 kg (150 lb) individual. Add or substitute 10% for each 7 kg (15 lb) above or below this body weight.
[b] About 25–50 yard-minimum^{-1}.
(Data from Shelton.[21])

ciated that forces up to five times body weight are generated by the quadriceps muscles,[16,18] which produces, in turn, retropatellar forces of two to three times body weight during running. Furthermore, these retropatellar forces increase to five to six times body weight with squatting and jumping.[18,19] The

therapist must bear these facts in mind when progressing the individual to these activities.[20,21]

In addition to recognizing the forces acting on a joint, attention should also be paid to the required functional range that allows the performance of a task in a smooth, uninhibited fashion.[17,19] To walk without a limp it is usually necessary to have 75 degrees of flexion in the swing leg, and stair climbing requires 90 degrees of flexion. Jogging and running need 105 to 125 degrees and sprinting 140 degrees of motion.[23] To allow the athlete to resume activities with insufficient range of motion precipitates effusions and joint pain.[23] Basically the individual requires some 5 to 10 degrees more range of static measurement than is needed for the comparable dynamic movement if smooth, functional motion is to be achieved. This rehabilitation concept is important.

Flexibility

In many ways flexibility is linked to the previous concept, although there is a subtle distinction to be drawn between functional range of motion, flexibility, and joint and ligamentous laxity. This area is controversial at the present time.[23-25] Although most physicians accept and agree that lack of flexibility following an injury predisposes to reinjury, the role of ligamentous laxity, loose and tight jointedness in the normal individual, and their injury-prone potential have not been clearly defined.[22,25] The pathologic extremes obviously fit into a different category.[7] Nevertheless, all training and competition necessitate establishment of a full active and passive range of motion if reinjury is to be avoided. Functional tests are superior to goniometric measurements, e.g., testing the ability to flex the knee and stretch the quadriceps after a rectus femoris tear.[21] The ability to sit with both buttocks firmly on the heels is a guideline for full training in most situations. Stretching the muscle across the hip and the knee by tilting the body backward, thereby extending the hip, is an indication that the quadriceps are sufficiently stretched to allow resumption of game or competition participation providing other parameters are rehabilitated.[21]

Strength and Balance of Power

The ratio of strength between muscle groups may ultimately prove to be more important than attainment of a specific power level.[26,27] Athletes with previous joint injuries and those whose injuries have necessitated surgery are particularly predisposed to muscle weakness, muscle imbalance, and a high rate of reinjury. In this regard, preseason testing and a planned preseason training program is essential for previously injured individuals.

Inadequate rehabilitation and poorly designed training programs can also contribute to muscle imbalance, poor flexibility, and susceptibility to injury

as exemplified by a study of hockey players sustaining groin injuries.[21,28,29] Adductor strains comprise 10 to 20 percent of muscular injuries in hockey.[30] In those individuals identified as having previously sustained these tears, nearly all had a force-power imbalance of at least 25 percent between the contralateral adductor muscles. There was also a significant ipsilateral adductor, quadriceps, and hamstring imbalance recorded in 80 percent of the players.[30,31] Lastly, 75 percent of injured players had decreased range of motion on the injured side prior to sustaining their injury. These examples illustrate the need for full rehabilitation and preseason preparation. The literature supports the concept that rehabilitation and conditioning programs may decrease injury rates.[16,30,31]

Activity Guidelines

Strength and flexibility requirements, estimated tissue healing times for the injured anatomic structure, injury patterns, and vulnerability to injury are the factors to be considered during progression from light training to moderate training and then to full training and fitness for competition.[32] In general, for lower limb injuries, permission for light training assumes that the player or athlete can perform specific strength training, has recovered functional range of motion, can perform non-weight-bearing endurance work, and has commenced jogging (Table 2-6).

Moderate training means that the athlete has reached the point at which the injury has sufficiently

TABLE 2-6. Progression of Lower Limb Joint Injuries

Training Level	Criteria and Mode of Progression
Light training	Specific-strength work established Functional range of motion present Non-weight-bearing endurance regimen begun Jogging commenced
Moderate training	Range of motion at least 75% normal Strength values at least 75% normal Skipping and jumping on rebounder begun Figure-of-eights commenced
Full training & game fit	Range of motion 95% normal Strength 90% normal Adequate endurance Sprinting and starts and stops practiced Repetitive jumping with no adverse effects

recovered that it is safe to start "figure-of-eight" runs and skipping. Double leg jumping skills may be added. The injured joint should have almost full range of motion, and the athlete's strength should have been rehabilitated to at least 75 percent of normal.

When full training or game fitness is declared, it is assumed the athlete's range of motion, passive and active, is within 5 percent of normal. Strength should be within 10 percent, and the individual can do wind sprints, fast starts and stops, and repetitive single- and double-legged jumps with no ill effect. Just as significant as strength recovery is the reestablishment of adequate endurance from the cardiovascular aspect and the metabolic activity of the muscle, specifically the type I (aerobic, slow twitch) fibers (Table 2-6).[32] Specific attention should be paid to training and testing this last aspect of muscle recovery.

The previous discussion is meant simply as an example for progression of lower limb joint injuries in a sport such as football, soccer, racquetball, and field hockey or court sports such as squash and racket ball. Adaptations are necessary for every athlete, as each injury has its unique characteristics. Indeed, one of the hallmarks of the experienced and successful sports physicians and therapists is that they recognize these distinctive or even subtle differences among their patients. Table 2-7 serves as a supplementary guide to the progression of activities in running sports, with special reference to the introduction of

cycling, walking, jogging, running, wind sports, and sports drills.[32]

Throughout the progression, the classic signs and symptoms of pain, swelling, and range of motion are observed. An increase in pain or swelling and reversal of a previous trend from increasing to decreasing range of motion are indications that the progress is too rapid.

Clinical Point

SIGNS OF TOO RAPID PROGRESSION

- Increasing pain
- Increasing swelling
- Decreasing range of motion

Even when not fit for training, athletes are encouraged to attend team practices so they benefit from tactical and coaching advice and remain an integral part of the team. However, to safely reintegrate the individual with a graduated training load requires full cooperation and communication with the coach.

Isokinetic Testing

The concept of isokinetic exercise was published initially by Hislop and Thistle in 1967.[26,33,34] It was

TABLE 2-7. Progression in Running-Based Sports After Joint Injuries

Step	Progression	Caution
Cycle	Build up to 30–45 minutes	Need adequate range of motion
Walk	Aim at 2 miles in <30 minutes	Need to be full weight-bearing
Jog	Alternate 50 yards jogging and walking. Increase ¼ mile each session Decrease walking, increasing jogging At 2 miles plateau for a period	Minimal effusion or pain Hold or decrease distance if increased pain, increased swelling, decreased range of motion
Run	When jogging 2 miles commence to increase pace to preinjury Build up distance by adding ¼ mile increments	Need adequate power Full flexibility
Windsprints	Add figure-of-eights, circuits, and appropriate start and stop drills, crossovers, cutting, power jumping activities	Strength bilaterally symmetric No residual effusion No pain—increase intensity carefully Only add one activity each session
Sports drills	Arrange skills in order of increasing stress on injured body part Add individual's skill at appropriate time	When able to do all appropriate drills without adverse effects, then ready for return to sport

(Adapted from Shelton.[21])

followed by the appreciation that torque values could be graphed, accurately measured, reproduced, and computerized, giving a more objective assessment method than the time-honored manual muscle tests and free weight systems.[24,30,31,34,35] The standard isokinetic parameters are strength, power, and power-endurance.

Strength, or slow torque, is defined as the maximum torque in foot-pounds or newton-meters, developed at velocities of less than 90 degrees per second, usually at 60 degrees per second. *Power* is represented by the maximum torque developed at faster velocities than 90 degrees per second. Traditionally, the speed of 240 degrees per second is used as a standard. *Power-endurance* is considered to be represented by the number of repetitions of an arc of motion at fast velocities, usually 240 degrees per second, from maximum torque to a point where the torque has decreased to 50 percent of the initial maximum torque value.[25] However, of all the measurements, this parameter is the most confusing in that it is influenced by the initial peak torque and the overall fitness level. A satisfactory standard of endurance has yet to be developed (Fig. 2-7). In addition to these measure-

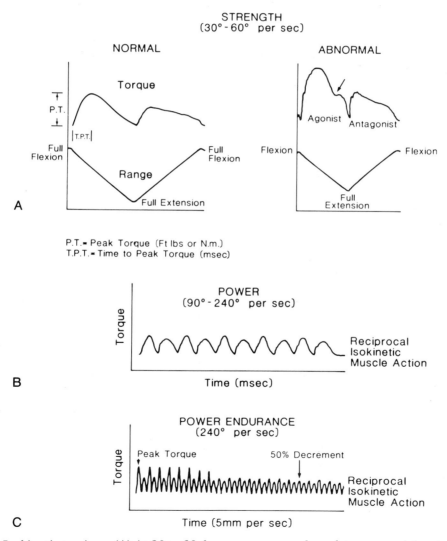

STRENGTH
(30°-60° per sec)

NORMAL

ABNORMAL

Torque

P.T.

T.P.T.

Full Flexion

Range

Full Flexion

Full Extension

A

Agonist Antagonist

Flexion

Flexion

Full Extension

P.T. = Peak Torque (Ft lbs or N.m.)
T.P.T. = Time to Peak Torque (msec)

POWER
(90°-240° per sec)

Torque

Reciprocal Isokinetic Muscle Action

B

Time (msec)

POWER ENDURANCE
(240° per sec)

Torque

Peak Torque

50% Decrement

Reciprocal Isokinetic Muscle Action

C

Time (5mm per sec)

Fig. 2-7. Isokinetic tracings. **(A)** At 30 to 60 degrees per second, peak torque and time to peak torque are indications of strength. **(B)** Reciprocal contraction at higher speeds measure power. **(C)** Measurements of the decrement by 50 percent gives an indication of endurance.

ments, both the torque developed over a specific increment of time and the time interval to the development of maximum torque in a single effort may reflect neuromuscular efficiency.

The implications of these measurements are not universally accepted, and to confuse the issue further new parameters have been added. These parameters are generated by several omnikinetic instruments that allow reciprocal varying speed muscle action and devices that allow both omnikinetic eccentric and concentric muscle action. Each company has developed an accompanying computer package. It would be fair to say that our ability to generate numbers has far surpassed our grasp of what they mean in terms of function, performance, and safe return to activity.[25,35]

Normal values are being established for specific populations, specific muscle actions, and specific speeds of limb segment movement. Such normals must be developed for each exercise and testing system, as values are not directly transferable. This problem is circumvented, to a small degree, by considering ratios of strength between muscle groups, both within a limb and between the two sides.[25,28,35]

Only in asymmetric sports such as archery, tennis, and baseball and in situations of previous injury or trauma do the data from the contralateral limb tend to be misleading.

Specificity of Training and Testing

Exercise physiologists have stressed the specific nature of exercise. It appears that after injury or immobilization there is a preferential wasting and loss of Type I muscle fiber.[32] These fibers have also been referred to as slow twitch, red, or oxidative fibers.[27] They are characterized by resistance to fatigue and are important in endurance activities (Fig. 2-8).

In the past, many rehabilitation efforts have been directed at developing strength, but today endurance work is gradually assuming greater significance. There is an adage in sports therapy that states "the athlete will go as far as the good leg will take him." Therefore after an injury, if there is inadequate restoration of the endurance fibers, the muscles of the injured limb tend to become fatigued and the joints are left susceptible to reinjury toward the end of game or practice situations.

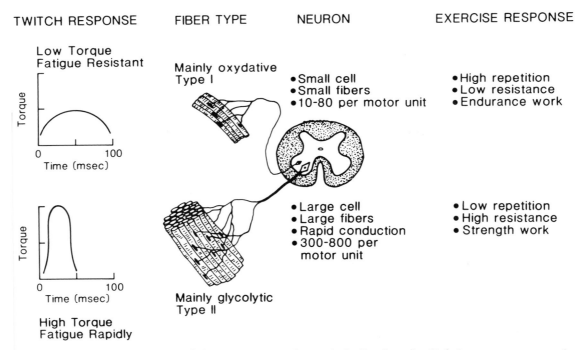

Fig. 2-8. Simplified division of the neuromuscular unit indicating the link between neuron size, conduction velocity, motor unit characteristics, and response to exercise. These concepts are important to the specificity of training.

Because the training is specific, all rehabilitation programs should include high repetition work in a controlled situation and eventually incorporate movements that mimic the specific limb motions of the sport.[21] Testing is likewise specific and is a factor to consider when measuring progress and setting goals.[28-30]

Substitute Activities

Even with a severely injured limb, training does not necessarily have to cease. For instance, a volleyball player with a leg in a cast can still practice serving the ball on a daily basis. Over the period of immobilization this activity would accumulate to several hundred serves and considerably improve the skill level of that particular element of the game. Similarly, a basketball player could practice shooting, or a wrestler could concentrate on an upper limb and neck strengthening program. With stress fractures in joggers or runners, cycling or, alternatively, a running program in the water, with most of the patient's weight supported by buoyancy, can be effective.

Whatever the injury, some modification is frequently necessary to allow healing and resolution. In some cases the modification may be minor, as with a swimmer with early shoulder tendinitis. In this situation, reduction in the number of strokes plus elimination of dry land training exercises in the fully abducted position may be sufficient. In this way, the strength training does not compound the stresses induced by the repetitive abduction maneuver of the swimming stroke on the rotator cuff. If increased leg work with a float board is not appropriate, cycling may be added to make up the energy equivalent and maintained cardiovascular fitness (Table 2-5).

Table 2-5 gives some appropriate energy expenditures of a few of the basic rehabilitation and training activities, e.g., cycling, skipping, rowing, swimming, skating, walking, jogging, and running. It can assist therapists in their quest to substitute activities and yet maintain appropriate fitness levels for the athlete.

Specific Instructions

It is possible that the most dangerous instruction given to an athlete after injury is that "you may now slowly resume training." The athlete, the coach, and the parent rarely have an accurate conception of what is meant by "slowly." Specific instructions must be given.

As an example, the instructions for a recreational runner, who may be used to doing 3 miles a day prior to developing a significant lower limb tendinitis, might be as follows. Training sessions should be no more than three times per week for the first 6 weeks. At any sign of return of symptoms, revert to the previous level and stay there for 1 week before recommencing the progression. Review the program with a physician or therapist should any significant symptoms return. Running should commence with an alternate ¼ mile jogging followed by a ¼ mile fast walk to cover a total of 1 mile. Maintain this distance, increasing the speed of jogging for 1 week; then add a ¼ mile of jogging every second training session until 2 miles are reached. Hold at 2 miles for at least one full week and do not progress until the speed is built up to preinjury level. At this point continue to add a ¼ mile each second training session until preinjury distance is achieved. In this example it would be 3 miles.

Clinical Point
RESUMING RUNNING AFTER TENDINITIS

(Runner accustomed to training 2 to 5 miles per session prior to injury)

1. Start at three or four sessions per week for 6 weeks.
2. Commence alternate ¼ mile run and walk.
3. Do no more than 1 mile total for 1 week.
4. Slowly increase speed over that week.
5. Then add ¼ mile every second session.
6. Hold at 2 miles at least 1 week.
7. Then increase ¼ mile every second session.
8. Hold at preinjury distance for 3 months.
9. Back off to next lower level if any discomfort ensues.

Unless the athlete is a serious competitor, he or she should probably be urged to avoid resuming daily running for a protracted period, as a good level of fitness can be maintained on an alternate-day training basis. This regimen provides an adequate recovery period should the athlete have a weak anatomic structure or a stress riser, or should the technique be such that the stresses are always concentrated on one anatomic structure. Should the individual believe it necessary to do some activity every day, one could suggest an alternate activity, e.g., cycling or swimming, or a program of flexibility exercises.

Whenever compatible with training goals, preinjury distances and times should be maintained, when reached, for at least 3 months, as there is frequently a propensity for injury recurrence. These decisions depend on the level of competition and degree of involvement of the individual.

If recreational athletes keep reinjuring themselves, it should be pointed out to them that an excellent level of fitness may be achieved by mixing running, walking, and calisthenics, and that their current choice of activity and intensity level may be inappropriate. Alternating jogging and walking, or stopping every ¼ to ½ mile for a series of vigorous exercises may maintain the training heart rate while relieving the tendons of the lower limb from the repetitive stresses of heel strike. This type of running program, based on "exercise stops," is a safer form of activity as far as the general musculoskeletal system is concerned and becomes progressively more important in the older athlete. The basic principles outlined above may be adapted to many injury situations and are presented merely as examples of giving specific instructions.

A modification of these principles adapted for lower limb joint injuries is outlined in Table 2-7. Progressions for the upper limb are given in the appropriate chapters.

SUMMARY

The basic treatment principles that have been outlined should be supplemented by analysis of the individual's anatomy and biomechanics, the stresses involved in the sport, and the magnitude and potential permanence of some of the injuries. The role of orthoses and protective devices is decided by these factors. The need for an in depth knowledge of each activity has been repeatedly stressed, so an appropriate analysis can be made in order to separate the sport into its respective cardiovascular elements, skills, strength, and ranges of motion. Rehabilitation is then directed at minimizing the inflammatory response, protecting the particular body part from stresses during early recovery, and slowly reintegrating the athletes into their respective activity. Based on anticipated healing times of the involved tissues, attention is paid, in turn, to flexibility, strength, balance of power, endurance, substitute activities, and finally objective and functional tests in order to return the athlete to training and competition with minimal chance of reinjury.

REFERENCES

1. Fisher BD, Baracos VE, Shnitka TK et al: Ultrastructural events following acute muscle trauma. Med Sci Sports Exerc 22:185, 1990
2. Walters JB, Isreal MS: General Pathology. 4th Ed. Churchill Livingstone, Edinburgh, 1974
3. Hocutt JE, Jaffe R, Rylander CR et al: Cryotherapy and ankle sprains. Am J Sports Med 10:316, 1982
4. Kellett J: Acute soft tissue injuries—a review of the literature. Med Sci Sports Exerc 18:489, 1986
5. Sloan JP, Giddings P, Hain R: Effects of cold and compression on edema. Physician Sportsmed 16:116, 1988
6. Matsen FA, Questad K, Matsen AL: The effect of local cooling on post fracture swelling: a controlled study. Clin Orthop 109:201, 1975
7. Barnes L: Cryotherapy—putting injury on ice. Phys Sports Med 3:130, 1979
8. Benson TB, Copp WP: The effects of therapeutic forms of heat and ice on the pain threshold of the normal shoulder. Pharmacol Rehabil 13:101, 1974
9. Cahill BR, Griffith EH: Effect of preseason conditioning on the incidence and severity of high school football knee injuries. Am J Sports Med 6:180, 1978
10. McMaster WC, Liddle S, Waugh TR: Laboratory evaluation of various cold therapy modalities. Am J Sports Med 6:291, 1978
11. Waylonis GW: The physiological effects of ice massage. Arch Phys Med Rehabil 48:42, 1967
12. Calabrese LH, Rooney TW: The use of non-steroidal anti-inflammatory drugs in sports. Physician Sportsmed 14:89, 1986
13. Clyman B: Role of non-steroidal anti-inflammatory drugs in sports medicine. Sports Med 3:242, 1986
14. Wagenhauser FJ: Benefit and risks of anti-inflammatory drugs: an introduction from the clinicians viewpoint. EMLAR Bull 3:84, 1986
15. Duncan JJ, Farr JE: Comparison of diclofenac sodium and aspirin in the treatment of acute sports injuries. Am J Sports Med 16:656, 1988
16. Campbell DE, Glenn W: Foot-pounds of torque of the normal knee and the rehabilitated post meniscectomy patient. Phys Ther 59:418, 1979
17. Burdett RG: Forces predicted at the ankle during running. Med Sci Sports Exerc 14:308, 1982
18. Smith SJ: Estimates of muscle and joint forces at the knee and ankle during jumping activity. J Hum Movement Stud 1:78, 1975

19. Ficat RP, Hungerford DS: Disorders of the Patello-femoral Joint. Williams & Wilkins, Baltimore, 1979
20. Perry J: Anatomic and biomechanics of the shoulder in throwing, swimming, gymnastics and tennis. Clin Sports Med 2:247, 1983
21. Shelton GL: Principles of musculoskeletal rehabilitation. In Mellion MB (ed): Sports Injuries and Athletic Problems. Hanley & Belfus, Philadelphia, 1988
22. Mann RA: Biomechanics of running. In Mack RP (ed): American Academy of Orthopedic Surgeons, Symposium on the Foot and Leg in Running Sports. CV Mosby, St. Louis, 1982
23. Godshall RW: The prediction of athletic injury: an eight year study. J Sports Med 3:50, 1975
24. Grace TG: Muscle imbalance and extremity injury: a perplexing relationship. Sports Med 2:77, 1985
25. Heiser TM, Weber J, Sullivan G et al: Prophylaxis and management of hamstring muscle injuries in intercollegiate football players. Am J Sports Med 12:368, 1984
26. Marino M, Gleim GW: Muscle strength and fibre typing. Clin Sports Med 3:85, 1984
27. Nicholas JA: Injuries to the knee ligaments. JAMA 212:2236, 1970
28. Gilliam TB, Sady SP, Freedson PA et al: Isokinetic torque levels for high school football players. Arch Phys Med Rehabil 60:110, 1979
29. Molner GE, Alexander J: Objective quantitative muscle testing in children. Arch Phys Med Rehabil 55:490, 1974
30. Mira AJ, Carlisle HM, Greer RB: A critical analysis of quadriceps function after femoral shaft fractures in adults. J Bone Joint Surg [Am] 62:61, 1980
31. Reid DC, Kelly R: Selected problems of the thigh and knee to illustrate some basic techniques of rehabilitation. In Taylor AW (ed): The Scientific Aspects of Sports Training. Charles C Thomas, Springfield, IL, 1975
32. Häggmark T, Jansson E, Eriksson E: Fibre type area and metabolic potential of the thigh muscle in man after knee surgery and immobilization. Int J Sports Med 2:12, 1981
33. Hislop H, Perrine JJ: The isokinetic concept of exercise. Phys Ther 47:114, 1967
34. Thistle HG, Hislop HJ, Moffroid M et al: Isokinetic contraction: a new concept of exercise. Arch Phys Med 48:279, 1967
35. Wikholm JB, Bohannon RW: Hand held dynamometer measurements: Tester strength makes a difference. J Orthop Sports Physiother 13:191, 1991

Physical Modalities 3

When the only tool you have is a hammer,
It's amazing how quickly everything becomes a nail.
—Unknown

The physical therapy modalities are presented under the headings of ultrasound, the muscle-stimulating currents including interferential therapy and transcutaneous electrical nerve stimulation, and the electromagnetic spectrum including laser light. Emphasis is placed on the biologic effects with special attention paid to the precautions and contraindications. The main purpose of the chapter is to present enough material to enable physicians to understand the potential of these modalities and assist in intelligent prescription. For the therapist the chapter reviews the basic parameters and evaluates some of the claims for efficacy. It is in no way meant to be an exhaustive dissertation on the techniques of application. The effects of heat, as well as the problems of spasm and scar, are discussed at length in the ultrasound section, as most of the principles apply equally to other heating modalities. Indications for selection of a modality are expanded on in the chapters devoted the various body parts and specific conditions.

Properly harnessed these modalities are powerful tools. Unfortunately, they are frequently used badly and ineffectively in sports medicine. It must be stressed that even used skillfully in experienced hands, they are only adjunctive measures to the cornerstones of sports therapy, which are (1) exercise modification, (2) biomechanical evaluation of the activity, and (3) carefully planned progression of athletes' specific training regimens. Under no circumstances must the application of a passive modality be considered total treatment. Electrical modalities should always be viewed in the perspective of what they may do to enhance the healing process and supplement the other aspects of therapy.

THERAPEUTIC ULTRASOUND

Although therapeutic ultrasound has been in use for half a century, it is still a modality for which knowledge of the fundamentals lags considerably behind its application. The upper limits of man's audibility is in the range of 15 to 20 kilocycles per second (kc/s), and these limits decrease gradually with age. Frequencies above the audible upper limits are referred to as ultrasound, although many animals can hear in these ranges. Therapeutic ultrasound is in the frequency range of 750 kc/s to 3 megahertz (MHz).

Therapeutic ultrasound is a physical agent providing both heating and mechanical phenomena within the tissues. The energy is produced via the piezoelectric effect of voltage applied to a ceramic disk or crystal contained within a probe of treatment head that is applied to the patient's skin. Some form of liquid or gel coupling medium is used to exclude air and ensure good contact of the treatment head with the tissues (Fig. 3-1).

Quick Facts

THERAPEUTIC ULTRASOUND

- Frequency range 750 kc/s to 3 MHz
- Pressures in tissues up to 4 atmospheres
- Accelerating and decelerating forces $10^5 \times g$
- Propagates by longitudinal waveform

The speed at which sound propagates is characteristic of the medium through which it is passing, which in human tissue is about 1,500 feet per second. With therapeutic sound in the region of 1 MHz, a wavelength of about 1.5 mm results.

High frequency sound propagates by longitudinal waveform (Fig. 3-2).[1] With pressure amplitudes of 1 to 4 atmospheres and small cells and elementary particles subjected to rapidly accelerating and decelerat-

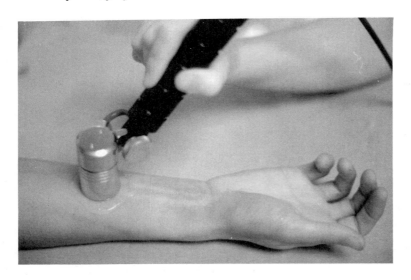

Fig. 3-1. Piezoelectric crystal is contained within the treatment head. A coupling agent is used to reduce impedance mismatch.

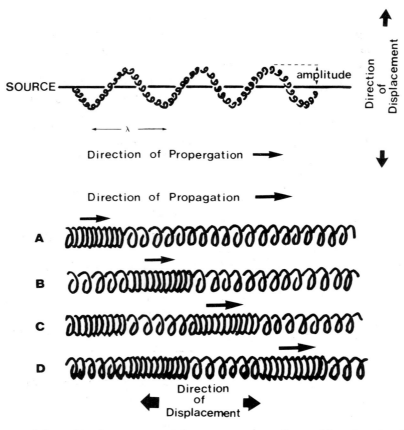

Fig. 3-2. Spring model used to demonstrated the propagation of sound by a longitudinal waveform. The band of compression moves through the medium and has an effect of oscillating the molecules around a mean position. Displacements are in the plane of transmission. A, B, C, and D show successive movement of a particular band of compression in the direction of propagation. (After Ward.[1])

ing forces of up to 10^5 times that of gravity ($10^5 \times$ g), it is not surprising that specific physiologic effects may be generated within the tissues.[2] These properties influence the type and magnitude of the response of the various tissues to ultrasound.

Modulation of Ultrasound

Ultrasound therapy, given as a continuous beam (continuous mode), tends to produce a rise in tissue temperature (Fig. 3-3). Indeed, of the diathermic modalities commonly used for therapy, ultrasound is the most efficient for heating localized areas of deeply placed tissue.[3] However, there are clinical situations where tissue heating may not be desirable and in which it is conceived that the therapeutic effects are due to the vibrational energy, independent of heating.[4,5] In these cases a pulsed mode of application may be selected (Fig. 3-3).[6] In most apparatus, the pulse frequency is 100 Hz; thus the time that elapses from the start of one pulse to the start of the next is one-hundredth of a second, or 10 milliseconds (ms) (Fig. 3-4).

Pattern of the Ultrasonic Field

Sound waves above 500 kc/s are propagated differently from audible frequencies. Sound tends to travel as a succession of concentric spheres spreading out from the source, rather like the ripples generated by dropping a pebble into a pond.[7] As the frequency of sound increases, the pattern of sound emission tends to become more unidirectional. With therapeutic ultrasound the pattern is restricted to a cone spreading out in front of the transducer head (Fig. 3-5). About 70 percent of the total beam energy is confined to an area with a diameter about one-half the transducer diameter (Fig. 3-6). Close to the sound head there are distinctive maxima and minima intensity patterns, but the pattern tends to become more

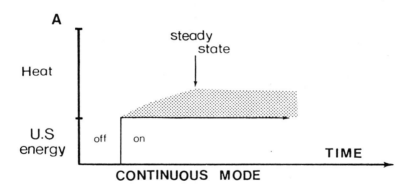

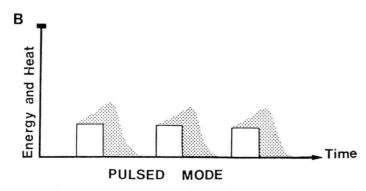

Fig. 3-3. (A) With a continuous mode, the heat gradually rises after commencement of treatment until a steady state is reached. Thus ultrasound used in this mode is often classed as diathermic. **(B)** With a pulsed mode, the heat generated by one pulse train may be wholly or partly dissipated before the next pulse train. In this way the heating potential is minimized.

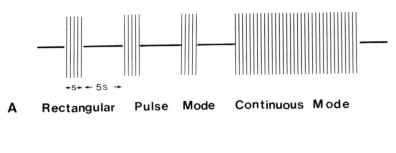

A Rectangular Pulse Mode Continuous Mode

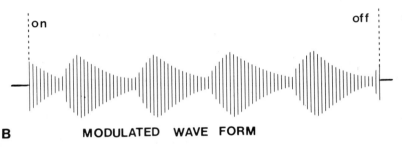

B MODULATED WAVE FORM

Fig. 3-4. (A) Rectangular pulse is the ideal waveform, as the various parameters can be accurately calculated. In these diagrams, the mark/space ratio is 1 : 5, the duty cycle is 1 : 6, and the power ratio is 1 : 6 (0.1667). When switched to continuous mode the power ratio is 1 : 1. **(B)** Modulated waveform from one ultrasound machine. Duty cycle on this machine was nominally 1 : 1. Power ratio was theoretically 0.5, but the calculated power ratio was actually only 0.35 ± 0.04. It illustrates that the experimentally calculated power ratio may be different from the theoretical one obtained using the duty cycle information stamped on the machine.

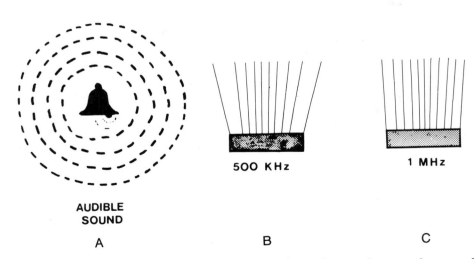

AUDIBLE
SOUND

A   B   C

Fig. 3-5. (A) Audible sound, as from a bell, gives sound waves that tend to travel outward from the source like ripples made by dropping a pebble in a pond. **(B)** Ultrasound source emitting 500,000 cycles per second (500 KHz). Considerable dispersion is seen. As the frequency increases, the dispersion decreases. **(C)** Slight dispersion is produced by 1 MHz. Deviation from the true parallel is less than 10 degrees of an arc.

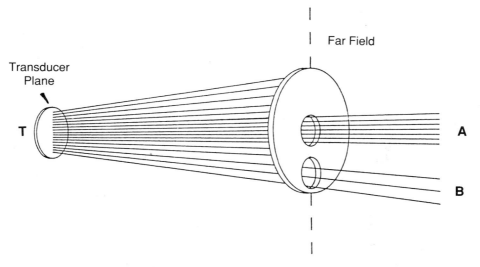

Fig. 3-6. Energy decreases in intensity toward the edge of the beam. Energy from the transducer (T) passing through the center of disk A is much greater than that passing through the perimeter of disk B. Thus intensity in disk A is much greater than that in disk B. It is measured in watts per square centimeter. These values are point intensities. The intensity across the whole plane would be the spatial average intensity at that particular depth in the far field.

uniform the farther it is away from the energy source (Fig. 3-7). The narrow beam and the complex interference pattern make it essential to move the treatment head continuously. In this way the energy bution becomes more uniform, and the potential for focusing and hot spots in the tissues is diminished.

Attenuation

Intensity is a parameter of ultrasound that reflects the strength of the vibrations occurring at a given location in the medium or tissues being treated. It describes the flow of energy through a small cross-sectional area of the beam (Fig. 3-7). It is measured in watts per square centimeters and the total energy in watts per given time. The common therapeutic intensities, at least at the radiating source, are 0.1 to 3.0 W/cm². The total power output depends on the surface area of the radiating crystal.

As the sound beam passes through tissue, some of the energy is reflected at each tissue interface. As the beam is transmitted on, tissue molecules are made to vibrate; this energy represents the absorptive component. Such total loss of energy due to reflective and absorptive components is called *attenuation*. Attenuation increases directly with frequenty (Table 3-1). Thus there is decreasing depth of penetration with increasing frequencies. Stated another way, as the

wavelength decreases, so does the depth of penetration because wavelength and frequency are inversely proportional to each other.

Attenuation generally increases with depth according to an exponential law. This situation obviously has an influence on the selection of dosage to treat tissues of different depths within the body.[8] Clinically, this exponential relation is referred to as the "half-value thickness." The half-value thickness (depth) is the thickness of material required to absorb 50 percent of the incident wave energy (Fig. 3-8).

Frequency

Different tissues absorb differing amounts of ultrasound at any given frequency (Table 3-1). Fat is relatively poor at absorbing sound, whereas muscle and connective tissue are better; their absorption rate increases proportionally with increasing frequencies.

Reflection and Refraction

When the sound wave strikes the boundary between tissues (tissue interfaces), reflection and refraction occur unless the acoustic impedance of the media is identical. Reflected waves can focus and produce a potentially dangerous standing wave pattern. Moving the sound head minimizes this problem. If

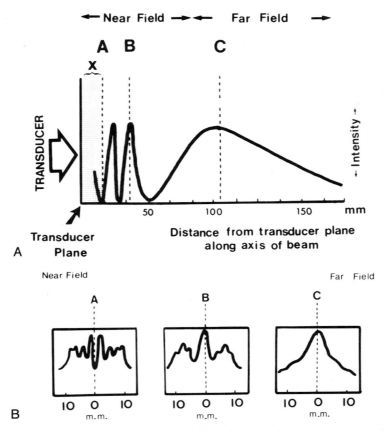

Fig. 3-7. (A) Intensity distribution in the sound field, which depicts the theoretic distribution for an ideal circular transducer of radiating area 5 cm² operating at 1 MHz in water. The area (X) close to the transducer has intensity changes too rapid to illustrate. The near field is approximately 100 mm in depth. A, B, and C are planes cut transversely across the sound beam. **(B)** Transverse sections across the beam.

the sound beam strikes the tissue interface at angles of more than 15 degrees, reflection rather than refraction takes place, and the energy is not transmitted to the deeper tissues. It is for this reason that the sound head must be kept as perpendicular to the skin surface as possible during treatment.

Coupling Agents

There is a large impedance mismatch between the sound head and tissues (Table 3-2). The use of a coupling agent reduces this mismatch, minimizes sound reflection, and maximizes penetration and potential absorption within the tissues.

There has been considerable controversy as to the efficacy of the various couplants, but in most studies the commercially available thixotropic agents and distilled water are most efficient.[9] When active ingre-

dients such as steroid creams are added to the couplant, there does not seem to be an effect on transmission. However, when mixed manually by therapists, large quantities of air bubbles are inevitably introduced that significantly interfere with transmission. Indeed, with all these agents it is important to reduce the air bubbles to a minimum, as they increase the acoustic impedance mismatch. The im-

TABLE 3-1.   Half-Value Thickness

Ultrasound Radiation	$\delta_{1/2}$ (cm)[a]		
	Fat	Muscle	Bone
1 MHz	15.28	2.78	0.040
2 MHz	5.14	1.25	0.010
3 MHz	2.64	0.76	0.004

[a] Half-value depth ($\delta_{1/2}$) for ultrasound. At 1 MHz the half-value thickness for average tissue is clinically assumed to be 5 cm.

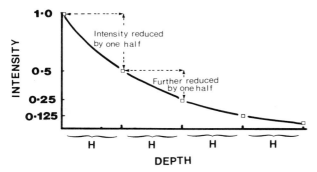

Fig. 3-8. Exponential attenuation. The intensity falls as the depth in the medium increases. The intensity is halved each time a depth of "one-half value thickness (H)" is traversed. In clinical situations, the average value of H is 5 cm.

portance of good technique, keeping the sound head firmly in contact with the skin, is therefore paramount.

The problem of accumulating bubbles on the sound head when using water baths must be borne in mind. They frequently can be removed by intermittently touching the head against the patient's tissues.

Because of the absorption in the coupling agent, the reading on the power indicator may not represent the exact amount of energy entering the patient's tissues, but it does bear a linear relation to it. Pressure, angle of application, and duration of treatment to any specific area are probably greater variables. So long as the coupling agents used are kept constant, attention to good technique is the best way for generating a reproducible dosage between treatment sessions.

Mechanisms of Action

Traditionally, the tissue effects of ultrasound have been categorized as thermal and mechanical effects. The mechanical phenomena may be further regarded

TABLE 3-2. Acoustic Impedance

Material	Velocity (ms^{-1})	Density (kg^{-3})	Impedance (kg^{-1}s^{-1})
Air	340	0.625	213
Fat	1,450	940.0	1.4×10^6
Muscle	1,550	1,100.0	1.7×10^6
Bone	2,800	1,800.0	5.1×10^6
Water	1,500	1,000.0	1.5×10^6
Steel	5,850	8,000.0	47.0×10^6
Aluminum	6,300	2,700.0	17.0×10^6

Clinical Point

IDEAL PROPERTIES OF COUPLING AGENTS

- Sufficient fluid to fill undulations between sound head and skin and exclude air bubbles
- Sufficiently viscous to remain in the treatment area
- Acoustic impedance that approximates that of the tissues
- Should absorb relatively little sound
- Should be easily removed from skin and odorless
- Should not stain clothes
- Nonirritating and hypoallergenic
- Nontoxic and noncorrosive
- Inexpensive and easily available

as cyclic and cyclic averaging effects. Cyclic effects are serially repeated tissue movements. Cyclic averaging phenomena are dependent on streaming, i.e., movement of the particles that are free to move within the sound beam.[10]

Ultrasound may produce physiologic and therapeutic effects at both a cellular and a tissue level; however, the absorption of sound is probably primarily a molecular phenomenon. Furthermore, long molecules, particularly in an organized form as is found in the protein chains of collagen in ligaments, tendons, and muscles, increase the absorption.

Thermal Effects

Production of Heat

Sound waves tend to produce oscillations of the tissue molecules, and the resultant internal stresses, motions, and collisions convert the sound energy to heat. At tissue interfaces the reflected energy increases the heating effects.[11] The ultimate temperature rise in the tissues depends a great deal on the associated physiologic changes for dealing with heat buildup in the body. However, initial heat production is related to the number and type of tissue interfaces and the half-value thickness laws of absorption (Fig. 3-9). Heating occurs efficiently in muscle and tendon. Furthermore, because of the reflection and absorp-

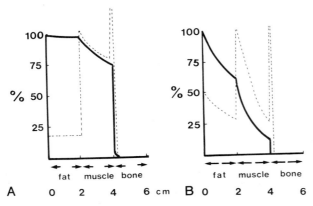

Fig. 3-9. Dotted line is the relative rate of heating; solid line is the wave intensity. **(A)** Most rapid decrease in wave intensity occurs in bone, so heating occurs mainly at the periosteum and bone surface. **(B)** At the higher frequency, heat production is greater in the more superficial structures. (After Ward.[1])

tion from bone, there may be a substantial rise in periosteal temperature. It can be calculated that the heating rate at the bone surface is about 30 times greater than anywhere in the muscle tissue. The heating is confined to a depth of a few millimeters; and, in practice, it is this muscle–periosteum–bone interface that may limit the intensity or duration of the ultrasound that can be used for therapeutic application. The patient may experience severe discomfort, probably periosteal in origin, if the bone is near the skin surface, such as at the back of the hand. By the same token, this concentration of energy adjacent to bone may be useful for heating ligaments and tendons.

Heat Dissipation and Transfer

As soon as there is an appreciable tissue temperature rise, mechanisms for heat dispersion are brought into play, including selective vasodilation and shunting of blood via reflexes in the microcirculation. In addition, heat is conducted through the tissues and dispersed. The low specific heat capacity and poor thermal conductivity of fat results in a greater tissue temperature rise than is anticipated. The efficient heat transfer through muscle tissue and the heat loss via its ample circulation results in a uniform heating pattern. Fortunately, bone is also a good conductor of heat, which counteracts some of the heat rise. As a result of these mechanisms, a new steady state is often

achieved after the initial rise in tissue temperature (Fig. 3-10).

Physiologic Effects of Tissue Temperature Rise

The physiologic effects of the tissue temperature rise are discussed in some detail because they apply to all thermal modalities, not just ultrasound. At the cellular level, an increase in tissue temperature increases the rate of metabolism. Hence there is a potential increase in cellular activity. This fact also implies an increase in metabolite production. The Arnt-Schultz principle states that a subthreshold quantity of energy does not cause demonstrable physiologic change, whereas application of threshold (and above) energy stimulates the absorbing tissue to normal function. Finally, application of a supramaximal quantity of energy destroys the absorbing tissue or prevents it from functioning normally.[12] Although this principle seems to state the obvious, it is an important reminder that most physiologic and biochemical reactions have kinetics that may be plotted on a bell curve. To push the reaction over the top of the curve is, in effect, to reverse the speed of the reactions. It has implications in terms of dosages, which are difficult to assess with many modalities.

At the tissue level the blood supply is increased, which is partly a response to the increase in tempera-

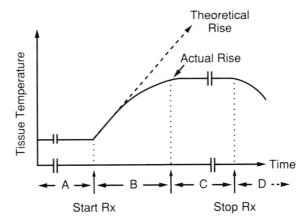

Fig. 3-10. Achievement of a steady state. As heat is introduced into the tissues at the start of the treatment, the temperature rises. However, heat conduction and physiologic adaptations allow for heat loss, so eventually a steady state is reached where heat gained equals heat lost. The duration of an elevated temperature and circulation flow after cessation of treatment is not fully known.

ture and partly due to the chemical effects of the increased production of metabolites. The effect is mainly at the microcirculatory level. Potentially this reaction delivers increased amounts of oxygen and chemical nutrients to the area as well as overcoming any venous stagnation. The flow of tissue fluid is probably made more efficient. Without this accompanying vasodilatation, increased tissue temperature would not only be ineffective but potentially harmful, as demands for nutrients and production of waste products would exceed their delivery and disposal.

However, although these vasodilatory phenomena undoubtedly take place, the magnitude of the response and its effectiveness are open to discussion. The change in blood flow following application of ultrasound to a limb is usually in the region of a three- to fourfold increase, proportional to the intensity. An average temperature elevation of 2.8°C may be produced at a depth of 3 cm in the muscle, and the effects of the hyperemia may persist some 20 to 30 minutes into the post-treatment period. Increased oxygen uptake accompanies this phenomenon.[13,14]

It should be emphasized that as far as muscle is concerned the potential increase in blood flow over basal levels produced by physical modalities can never approach the 30- to 40-fold increase that results from maximal exercise. This point serves to illustrate that even if the effects of ultrasound are related to temperature rise and blood flow the relation is not likely to be a simple one.

The effect of heat at a therapeutic level may induce muscle relaxation. The factor that contributes to this relaxation is possibly the sedative effect on sensory nerves decreasing neural excitability and hence gamma input. In addition, vasodilatation has a direct effect on removal of metabolites, which further decreases muscle excitability and allows relaxation.

Clinically, a pathologic focus secondary to trauma may give rise to muscle spasm. Intense prolonged protective spasm then impedes local circulation through the muscle. It is well recognized that intermuscular forces generated during muscle contraction can exceed the systolic pressure in local blood vessels. Hence the hydrostatic pressure maintaining normal blood flow is overcome. A situation then exists of muscle spasm decreasing local blood flow while at the same time increasing metabolic requirements owing to sustained contraction. The metabolites produced are not readily dissipated and may stimulate free nerve endings, giving rise to further pain. This sequence is, in effect, an ischemic-type stimulation superimposed on the previous traumatic pain. It may in turn produce further muscle spasm, and a pain cycle is established (Fig. 3-11). In summary, this cycle is one of pain producing spasm leading to further pain. It is suggested that relaxation of the muscle may be induced by heating, thereby interrupting the pain cycle. Naturally, ultrasound may not be the method of choice for this effect in all clinical situations because of the limited amount of muscle that may be heated at a given time. If small pathologic foci exist, however, it may be indicated. For larger areas short-wave diathermy may be a more practical method for inducing this effect. Heat may have a direct effect on decreasing the excitability of sensory nerves and hence have a primary pain relieving effect.

It has been demonstrated that the extensibility of connective tissue can be influenced by heat. Connective tissue, a combination of collagen and ground

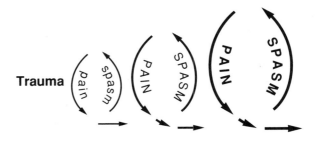

Relative Ischemia

Fig. 3-11. Trauma or some other tissue insult triggers pain. Pain, in turn, causes muscle spasm, which results in relative ischemia and a buildup of metabolites. This event, in turn, triggers more pain, and the cycle of pain–spasm–pain is set up. Sonating muscle may induce hyperemia and relaxation, breaking this cycle and thus bringing pain relief.

Clinical Point

HEATING EFFECTS OF ULTRASOUND

- The relation between temperature rise and therapeutic effect is not a simple one.
- Oxygen delivery may be facilitated.
- Microcirculation is enhanced.
- Pain and spasm are reduced.
- Plasticity of collagen is increased.

substance, appears in slightly different arrangements in tendons, ligaments, muscle sheaths, intermuscular septa, joint capsules, fascia, and even scar tissue. Therefore the fact that ultrasound may influence its extensibility is an important property. Normally, connective tissue exhibits the phenomenon of plasticity; that is, it deforms if stretched slowly over a period of time. The amount of extensibility may be increased considerably by physiologic temperature rise, which has obvious implications for using heat as a prerequisite for other stretching techniques. Particularly where the pathology is localized, pretreatment with ultrasound may be an effective means of achieving mobilization of a contracted or scarred connective tissue structure.

Mechanical Effects of Sound

Forces Generated by Ultrasound

The basic physical properties of ultrasound are similar to those for sonic energy. However, effects that are quantitatively minimal at sonic frequencies may become marked at ultrasonic levels and produce different effects. In the audible range, the threshold level of intensity for hearing is in the region of 10^{-16} W/cm². By contrast, it has been seen that dosages in the order of 0.5 to 3.5 W/cm² are used. This figure represents an intensity that is some ten thousand trillion times greater than what we are accustomed to in normal speech.

The sound waves propagate through the tissues as bands of rapidly alternating compression and rarefaction. For a wave intensity in the clinical range of 0.5 to 3.5 W/cm², the pressure amplitude may be in the range of 10 to 40 newtons/cm². For ultrasound of 1 to 3 MHz frequency, the regions of high pressure are separated by 1.5 to 2.0 mm, the distance of one wavelength,[15] which means that the pressure extremes, i.e., the peak of highs and lows, are separated by only the distance of one-half a wavelength (0.75 to 1.0 mm).[15] The implication is that any tissue component with dimensions of about one wavelength or more is subjected to considerable mechanical stresses, alternating rapidly at a frequency of 1 to 3 MHz.

Smaller structures experience less, but still substantial, stress and are vibrated back and forth by the pressure changes. Therefore the small cells and elementary particles of the medium are subjected to rapidly alternating accelerating and decelerating forces of about $10^5 \times g$. The maximal displacement of the individual molecules and particles from their equilibrium positions is proportional to the voltage applied to the crystal. At the clinical intensity, this displacement is small in the region of 10^{-7} to 10^{-6} cm. However, subjected to the accelerating and decelerating forces of the magnitude mentioned above, the velocity is fast. It is in fact in the order of 10 cm/s.[16] Thus one can visualize the molecules of the tissues and some subcellular particles oscillating backward and forward in the direction of propagation of the sound energy with minimal displacement but extremely high acceleration.

Effects on Cell Membranes

The rate of diffusion of ions across cell membranes is found to increase on exposure to ultrasound. This effect is observed over and above that which can be explained by heating alone.[16] It is possible that the agitation of molecules and ions increases the concentration gradients of ions and other materials and hence increases their rates of diffusion. In any diffusion process there is a narrow region either side of the membrane where the ion concentrations are not the same as in the bulk of the interstitial or intercellular fluid. It is the result of the buildup of materials or ions as they are diffused. If this area adjacent to the membrane is agitated, mixing and diffusion occur more rapidly, and therefore the concentration gradients are more efficiently maintained. It follows therefore that potentially the rate of diffusion is increased.[16]

Quick Facts

MECHANICAL EFFECTS

Pressure amplitudes of 10 to 40 newtons/cm² result in small displacements at high velocities.
- Cell membrane diffusion is affected.
- There is streaming of some small particles.
- Gaseous cavitation occurs.

It is also possible that the fluidity of the cell membranes is influenced. If one considers the cell membrane as having certain thixotropic properties, it could be predicted that the fluidity, and hence the permeability, of the cell membrane would increase in response to the mechanical agitation of ultrasound waves.

Radiation Pressure and Streaming

Whenever there is a tissue interface, the possibility of an impedance mismatch exists. In this case, a portion of the sound energy is reflected. One effect of reflection of energy at an interface is the exertion of an undirectional force at this point. This force is referred to as radiation pressure, and it depends on the amount of reflection that takes place and the intensity of the ultrasound. The role that radiation pressure may play in physiologic and clinical phenomena is not known; but when it is applied to particles free to move, it may result in their migration. This phenomenon is referred to as the *streaming effect*.[17] It is not a simple vibration of molecules around their equilibrium points, nor is it the convection effect of heated fluid.[17] It is a process that involves movement of molecules over great distances along the path of sound transmission.

The movement of molecules and particles in tissues by streaming could have a therapeutic effect. Certainly it would influence exchange of fluid in the ground substance of connective tissue, and it could conceivably affect nutrition of cells. Its role is largely uninvestigated.

Cavitation

One of the more controversial effects associated with ultrasound is a process called cavitation. Whether this phenomenon is truly active in therapeutic ultrasound is a matter of speculation.

In regions of rarefaction in the sound field, when the ultrasound intensities are great enough and the negative pressures sufficiently high, cavities may form. Acoustic cavitation involves the pulsation of gas- or vapor-filled voids in the sound field.[16] If gas is present in the liquid, bubbles form containing this gas. This process is known as *degassing*, or *gaseous, cavitation*. It is possible that this type of cavitation may exist in clinical situations. Sheer and microstreaming forces are significant close to boundaries of gas-filled cavities. With some cells, the effects of these and related phenomena may be lethal. However other sublethal changes, e.g., diffusion rates and altered membrane permeability, may affect metabolic activity in a positive way.

A second type of cavitation may take place if dissolved gas is not present within a medium, provided the intensities are sufficiently high. These cavities contain the vapor of the liquid through which the ultrasonic energy is passing. This type of cavitation requires intensities at least as high as 20 W/cm² and sometimes as high as 500 W/cm². This intensity is obviously well above any of those achieved in therapeutic situations. It is referred to as *true*, or *hissing, cavitation*.

It is not known to what extent some of the effects of gaseous cavitation may occur in specific tissues with therapeutic ranges. Traditionally, all cavitational effects have been considered in a negative light, and most investigators have denied their existence in the therapeutic range. However, in view of the literature cited above, it can be appreciated that at least gaseous cavitation not only may occur frequently but indeed may be a functional mechanism of action of therapeutic ultrasound.

Clinical Point

MECHANISMS OF ACTION OF ULTRASOUND

Thermal effects

- Heating of tissues
- Compensating circulatory adjustments
- Alteration in metabolic rates
- Change in tissue excitability
- Altered extensibility of connective tissue

Mechanical effects

- Cyclic effects
  - Vibration of cells and subcellular particles
  - Altered permeability
  - Alteration in ionic gradients
  - Internal stressing of large molecules and cells
  - Cavitation
- Cyclic averaging effects
  - Streaming

Therapeutic Potential

The main therapeutic goals of ultrasound application in sports therapy are to reduce inflammation, accelerate hematoma absorption, reduce pain and spasm, promote healing, increase extensibility of scar, and perform phonophoresis (movement of a whole molecule, rather than a charged particle, through the skin by means of ultrasonic radiation pressure). Heating and nonthermal effects play a role; unfortunately, all of the effects of ultrasound on living tissue are not fully delineated, and frequently it is necessary to hypothesize why this modality appears to have clinical efficacy.

Clinical Point

THERAPEUTIC POTENTIAL OF ULTRASOUND

- Reduce inflammation
- Accelerate hematoma resorption
- Reduce pain and spasm
- Promote healing
- Increase extensibility of scar
- Perform phonophoresis

Inflammation

Ultrasound is frequently used for the treatment of acute and subacute tenosynovitis, tendinitis, and synovitis. It has been suggested that it is a potent anti-inflammatory agent. Nevertheless, scrutiny of the literature reveals mainly clinical reports, uncontrolled studies, poorly formulated patient populations and designs, and little substantial backing for this claim.[7,8,18-20] Clinical experience still dictates that under certain circumstances and for specific pathologic conditions ultrasound may be a reasonable anti-inflammatory agent. However, identifying the clinical indications is difficult. The lower dosage range of 0.5 to 1.0 W/cm² seems to feature in most of the positive studies.

In 1980 I departed from the traditional explanations of the possible mechanisms of action of ultrasound and suggested that it may be possible to influence prostaglandin (PG) production. Some initial experiments proved this possibility to be the case. Subsequently we quantified this effect in muscle healing. Treatment of injured rat muscle in vivo reduced the normal rise in tissue PGE_2 by 71 percent and subsequently enhanced protein production. This enhanced protein production was thought to occur via reduction of the negative impact of an intense inflammatory response to the experimental tissue injury.[21] The ultrasound was delivered with a moving head technique, using continuous wave ultrasound at 1.5 W/cm² for 3 minutes per day from day 3 after

injury to day 9. It is difficult to extrapolate animal experimental data to the human situation, but ultrasound at low clinical dosages probably enhances the other anti-inflammatory therapies, e.g., modified rest and nonsteroidal anti-inflammatory medication. Ultrasound is indicated for acute localized lesions immediately following the initial ice routines of the first 24 to 48 hours. Its effectiveness in chronic inflammation is less spectacular.

Hematoma Resorption

Trauma, by either direct violence or stretching and twisting strains, is invariably accompanied by some degree of hemorrhage and edema. Such hemorrhage may contribute to the functional impairment of the affected body part. Ultrasound is frequently recommended as the physical agent of choice for accelerating the resolution of hematomas and tissue edema. Studies on experimental hematomas have shown more rapid dispersal with dosages above 0.8 W/cm² for ultrasound over control animals[22] (Fig. 3-12). Twice-daily treatment was more effective than one treatment per day. If the hematoma is in a small enough area, this treatment is practical. The mechanism of action is probably related in part to the vasodilation effect of heating the tissues. In addition, one

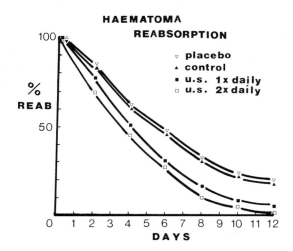

Fig. 3-12. Initial hematoma size was given the value 100 percent. The percent resorption was plotted over a 12-day period. The control and placebo groups had just over 20 percent of the original hematoma present at day 12. The treated groups had nearly complete resolution. The animals treated twice daily did marginally better than the once-daily group.

should consider the effects of acoustic or fluid streaming and decreasing the viscosity of the ground substance.[23,24] The recommended dosage range is 0.5 to 1.5 W/cm². The pulsed mode could be used during the period 24 to 36 hours after injury when the existing intense inflammatory effect would make additional heating undesirable.[4] A continuous mode could be utilized after this time, when any additional vasodilatation may in fact prove useful for enhancing hematoma resolution.

Reducing Pain and Spasm

Treatment with ultrasound has been reported to reduce pain and muscle spasm secondary to trauma and joint disease (Fig. 3-11). It may be via direct effects on nerve conduction or by the response of the tissues to heating. Nerve absorbs sound well, and it may be that it affects transmembranal electrolyte exchange. Lehman et al. demonstrated reduced pain threshold using dosages in the range of 0.88 to 1.50 W/cm².[25]

Work on small mammals has shown that ultrasound can affect isolated, directly stimulated muscle in several ways. It can reduce tension output, shorten contraction time, and prolong relaxation time.[26] The magnitude of these effects depends directly on the intensity of sound.

Ultrasound is usually an impractical modality of choice for humans with large muscle masses in spasm. Similar effects may be achieved more readily with hot packs, shortwave diathermy, and infrared radiation. Ultrasound should be reserved for the treatment of isolated lesions or small "trigger" areas. Dosages in the range of 0.5 to 1.0 W/cm² in the continuous mode may relieve local congestion, improve circulation, and decrease muscle and nerve irritability, which in turn may reduce muscle spasm.

Stimulation of Tissue Healing

There have been several reports in the literature that ultrasound may increase enzyme activity and thus generally increase anabolic function (Fig. 3-13). In 1971 Dyson and Pond observed the effects of ultrasound on defects made in the pinna of rabbit's ears.[6,24] They demonstrated that plane wave ultrasound, at certain dosages, may significantly increase the rate at which tissue regeneration takes place. The stimulation was not due to the thermal effect but to mechanical phenomena.[24] They also noted that H-thymidine uptake was increased in cultures of fibro-

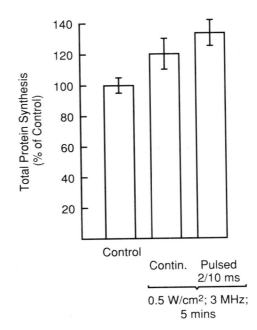

Fig. 3-13. Effects of pulsed versus continuous standing waves on synthesis of protein. The beneficial effects of pulsed over continuous waves may in fact not be present if a moving head treatment is used. (Adapted from Pond et al.[24])

blasts subject to low intensity sonation. They took this finding to indicate that DNA synthesis was probably being stimulated.

Further studies were made on the ability of fibroblasts in single-cell suspensions to synthesize and secrete protein. Ultrasound-treated cells were compared with mock-sonated controls. Because tissue integrity had to be destroyed to obtain these cells, any factor in the production of collagen needing tissue integrity was eliminated. Therefore any changes observed in the fibroblasts would result from the direct action of the ultrasound on either the fibroblasts themselves or the culture medium in which they were suspended. No other cell types could be involved, as none were present.[24] These studies presented fairly good experimental evidence of accelerated healing due to ultrasound. However, in most of these studies, standing wave conditions were used. This feature is not necessarily a negative one, as almost certainly most of the destructive features noted in the cell and ribosomal membranes were due to standing wave intensity. A moving sound head would avoid most of these negative features while preserving the positive ones.

Several facts emerge concerning the method of administering ultrasound in order to have the best chance of producing the effects demonstrated in vitro (Fig. 3-14).

1. A pulsed mode is probably better for the initial stages of healing.
2. The most effective frequency appeared to be 1 MHz. The higher frequencies are usually less effective. This point is fortunate, as ultrasound at 1 MHz has good penetration into the tissues, allowing adequate treatment of deep structures.
3. The lower dosage range (0.2 to 1.0 W/cm²) is most efficatious. In fact, at dosages above 1.5 W/cm² there may be reversal of the positive effects with retardation of collagen production and healing.

Ultrasound used carefully in the manner set out above may be a useful stimulus to optimal healing of freshly traumatized tissue as seen with ligament and muscle injuries.

Increasing Plasticity of Scars

The use of ultrasound to treat or "soften" scar tissue is standard physical therapeutic practice.[7] It is frequently justified by reference to the work of Bierman.[27] In fact, Bierman drew few definite conclusions from his careful but uncontrolled study of only four patients. He suggested only the possibility of softening of scar tissue by ultrasound. Although subsequent investigators have often been less critical than Bierman, there may be a firm basis for believing ultra-

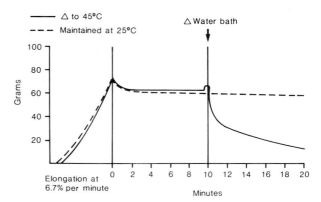

Fig. 3-15. Tendons elongated by a load of 73 g in 25°C baths. The length of the tendons was then maintained, and it is seen that at 25°C both the experimental specimen and the control showed slight decay in tension. After 10 minutes the temperature was increased in one bath to 45°C. A rapid drop in tension occurred. The control tendon, maintained at 25°C, did not show such a change in tension. (After Kottke et al.,[28] with permission.)

sound may assist in mobilizing contracted scar. There is, however, little evidence for the concept that ultrasound reduces the amount of scarring other than by possibly indirect methods, such as minimizing posttraumatic edema and accelerating hematoma resorption.

The concept of the plasticity of collagen is central to the discussion in this section. Collagenous tissue is considered to be the major element of contractures, and therefore the load-deformation or stress-strain characteristics of this tissue should be looked at in detail. It is apparent that collagenous tissue is viscoelastic and thus is susceptible to prolonged moderate stretching.[28] It shows the property of plasticity; i.e., the collagen fibers "creep" with respect to each other, thereby achieving elongation. It has also been shown that heating the tissues prior to stretching allows greater increases in length with less trauma.[28] Naturally, the less trauma the less tissue reaction, so there is a decreased tendency to produce further scar. This increased viscoelasticity is proportional, to an extent, to the tissue temperature (Fig. 3–15). Tissues with high protein content absorb sound selectively over tissues with a high water content. Because scar has a high protein content, it should follow that ultrasound is potentially a good modality for heating scar.

Reflection may also play an important role in the heating effects of ultrasound because the soft tissues

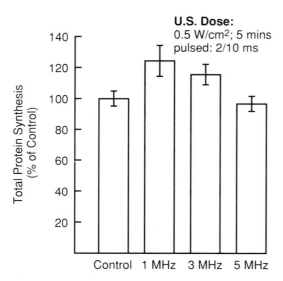

Fig. 3-14. Effects of frequency on protein synthesis. It can be seen that the lower frequency was the most efficient. (Adapted from Pond et al.[24])

adjacent to bone receive higher doses than those tissues near the transducer. In short, the acoustic impedance mismatch at the soft tissue – bone interface is such that periosteum, tendons, capsules, and ligaments receive a disproportionately large dosage, provided they are not too deeply situated and the appropriate ultrasound frequency is chosen (Fig. 3 – 16).[16]

In summary of this section, it might be said that ultrasound is probably beneficial as a preliminary treatment for stretching contracted soft tissue and scar in small anatomic areas. Although the nonthermal effects are undoubtedly contributory, it is in this area that the thermal effects of ultrasound are most beneficial. For this reason the higher intensities of 1.5 to 3.0 W/cm² are probably most suitable. The acoustic property of reflection is particularly important clinically when considering sonation of periarticular and deep soft tissues adjacent to bone. This feature enables efficient deep heating provided the treatment area is sufficiently localized. Most of all, it should be re-emphasized that ultrasound is used only as a preliminary treatment to the important mobilizing techniques of prolonged stretching and exercise.

Phonophoresis

In 1951 Hollander and his coworkers demonstrated the usefulness of intra-articular injections of hydrocortisone into selected arthritic joints. A search

for a method of topical application was then sought. Because there were reports of the possible effectiveness of ultrasound in the management of osteoarthritis at about the same time that steroid injections were becoming popular, it was natural that the possibility of combining the two agents was considered.

In addition, at about this time several papers were published regarding the effects of ultrasound on the transport of ions through biologic membranes as well as its ability to drive topically applied anesthetics through the skin. In fact, in 1966 Cameroy reported using ultrasound-driven carbocaine into the wrist prior to reducing Colles' fractures as an aid to anesthesia. The process of driving ions through the skin is called *iontophoresis*. It is not surprising that phonophoresis of steroid was soon used to supplement oral or infiltrated cortisone. It has been shown that measurable quantities of hydrocortisone can be driven to a subcutaneous depth of at least 2 inches.[29]

A series of papers by Griffin confirmed that phonophoresis of cortisone was possible. He carried out a double-blind study on a series of 102 patients with various musculoskeletal disorders.[29] Of the 66 patients who received topical hydrocortisone plus ultrasound, 68.1 percent were considered much improved, and another 18.1 percent were partially improved. By contrast, only 27.7 percent of the placebo group were considered improved and another

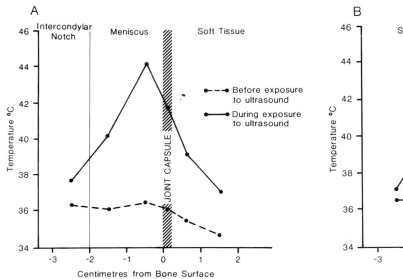
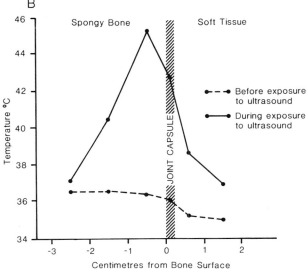

Fig. 3-16. Pigs' limbs were sonated using the moving head technique at 1.5 W/cm² for 5 minutes. Temperature distribution at the level of the joint space (**A**) and at 2 cm proximal to the joint space (**B**). (Redrawn from Lehmann and Krusen.[11])

16.8 percent partially improved. These results were impressive in view of the prior failure of response to injected steroid in some of the patients. Griffin hypothesized that the established ability of ultrasonic energy to increase the permeability of cells would allow more of the active hydrocortisone molecule into the cell interior, which then allowed the hydrocortisone to be more effective as an anti-inflammatory agent. Phonophoresis of steroid creams for allergic and irritative skin rashes has also been shown to be effective.

More recently topically applied non-steroidal anti-inflammatory agents have become available and there may be a role for phonophoresis with these medications.

In summary, it can be seen that phonophoresis of hydrocortisone and its derivatives is possible. The active molecules may be driven into the tissues by the radiation force in measurable quantities up to a depth of 2 inches. There is a possibility of a synergic anti-inflammatory effect of the ultrasound itself. Dosages of 0.5 to 1.0 W/cm^2, used in the continuous mode, are adequate to achieve phonophoresis of accessible joints. The tendency of noncommercially prepared cortisone preparations to contain air bubbles, which may totally negate sound transmission and hence phonophoresis secondary to acoustic mismatch, was discussed earlier in the chapter.

Contraindications

For the most part, therapeutic ultrasound has been considered a relatively safe modality. A series of standard precautions and contraindications have been developed. The vulnerable tissues are neural, reproductive, and fluid-filled cavities—the latter because of the danger of cavitation. There are conflicting reports of the effects of ultrasound on open epiphyses, and prolonged exposure is probably inadvisable. Although metal in the tissue is not a direct contraindication because of its excellent ability to dissipate heat, good protective sensation is required. The potential for ultrasound to loosen implants is an unanswered issue. Most of the harmful effects of ultrasound are reduced by the low output of the therapeutic range. The risks are further minimized by continuously moving the treatment head during therapy. This action eliminates most standing waves, smooths out extremes of energy intensity in the near and far fields, and prevents the formation of "hot spots."

Summary

An attempt has been made to outline the major therapeutic effects of ultrasound as they may apply to the treatment of musculoskeletal disorders. The lack of adequate studies has been a constant theme and is disappointing. Nevertheless, it can be seen that ultrasound has some definite potential in the area of tissue regeneration and hematoma resorption (Table 3-3).

The area of scar softening and contracture mobilization illustrates a major role for the heating effect of ultrasound. The potential for modifying an inflammatory response is the area with most contradictions and least experimental support. Paradoxically, it is the area in which ultrasound is most frequently used. A potentially exciting area of research is the possibility of modifying prostaglandin release and hence directly influencing inflammation.

Throughout this section, specific dosage ranges have been suggested, but in reality these guidelines are largely empiric. Because of its ease of access and its use by physical therapists, athletic therapists, chiropractors, and podiatrists, ultrasound will continue to be one of the main therapeutic modalities. Its limitations and contraindications, however, must be kept clearly in mind in order to give safe, effective treat-

---

Clinical Point

CONTRAINDICATIONS AND PRECAUTIONS

- Pregnant uterus and gonads
- Malignancies and precancerous lesions
- Tissues previously damaged by radiation therapy
- Vascular diseases including deep vein thrombosis and severe atherosclerosis
- Acute infections
- Eye or other fluid-filled cavities
- Overexposed spinal cord, major nerve trunks, stellate ganglion
- Hemophiliacs not covered by factor replacement
- Prolonged treatment over epiphyseal plates
- Anesthetic areas
- Around metal and plastic implants (with care)

TABLE 3-3. Selection of Ultrasound Dosages

Effect	Dosage (W/cm²)	Comment
Stimulation of tissue healing	0.1–1.0	Pulsed mode Frequency 1 MHz
Relief of pain and spasm	0.5–1.0	Continuous mode Treat only if small trigger area or small area of pathology
Anti-inflammatory action	0.5–1.5	Continuous mode For trauma after first 24–48 hours
Hematoma resorption	0.5–1.5	Pulsed mode for acute inflammation Continuous mode for subacute or chronic inflammation
Increased plasticity of connective tissue, contractures, and scars	1.5–3.0	Continuous mode Frequency according to depth: 3 MHz superficial, 1 MHz deep

ment. There have been numerous reports of poorly calibrated equipment. Indeed in some surveys, many instruments have been totally nonfunctioning. Regular checks for safety and calibration are necessary if the potential of this modality is to be realized.

ELECTRICAL STIMULATION

Electricity is a form of energy that can be made to exhibit magnetic, chemical, mechanical, thermal, and electrostatic effects. The net movement of electrons through any material, when a potential difference exists between the ends of the conducting pathway, is referred to as an electric current. Its unit of measurement is an ampere (A), which is the flow of 6.24×10^{18} electrons per second. A volt (V) is the electrical pressure required to send a current of 1 ampere through a conductor with a resistance of 1 ohm (Ω). Watts (W) are the unit of electrical power. One watt is the power used when a current of 1 A at an electromotive force of 1 V flows for 1 second. These are the basic terms on which the understanding of electrical modalities and their dosage calculations and designation depend.

There are many types of waveform available. Furthermore, pulse frequency (adjustable on many units) may be 4 to 50 pulses per second in the low frequency range and 90 to 160 pulses per second in the high frequency units (Fig. 3-17). The most significant therapeutic range is probably between 50 and 100 pulses per second.

The pulse width ranges from 9 to 350 microseconds (μs), which may have a significant effect on the amount of stimulation received at the nerve fiber. It is not uncommon to combine high amplitudes with low pulse widths, particularly if the latter is to stimulate muscle contraction.

The waveform seems to cause a significant amount of controversy but is likely to be the least important characteristic. First, the waveform as recorded by oscilloscopy is usually grossly distorted by the tissues; second, the "all or none" stimulation effect of nerve seems to depend mainly on the amount of charge per unit of time.

Tetanic currents or interrupted direct currents are used to produce a sustained tetanic type contraction by direct stimulation of muscle. They are reserved for situations where the nerve supply to muscle is dam-

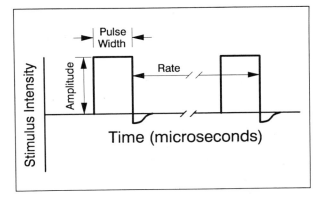

Fig. 3-17. Electrical modalities produce different waveforms with differing physiologic effects. They are characterized by their shape, pulse amplitude, pulse width, and pulse rate. A rectangular waveform is depicted.

aged. The method is usually too uncomfortable to use on intact neuromuscular units, and there are better options for this situation.

The original muscle stimulator produced a faradic current that is an uneven alternating current with a pulse duration of 1 ms and a frequency of 50 Hz. From this beginning was derived the more versatile and comfortable muscle stimulating currents with a variety of pulse shapes and widths that generate muscle contraction via the motor nerve.

Other currents have been adapted for their effect on sensory nerve and their ability to alter the intensity of pain impulses. They include the transcutaneous nerve stimulators, interferential currents, and high voltage pulsed galvanic stimulators.

Electrical Muscle Stimulation

Electrical muscle stimulation, or electromyostimulation (EMS), is used clinically to: (1) enhance contraction where there is reflex inhibition; (2) supplement contraction in postinjury or postsurgical states when the limb is immobilized; (3) re-enforce contraction, particularly toward the end of a training session when voluntary effort may decline; (4) as an adjunct to strengthening programs; and (5) as a means of promoting normal physiology in paralyzed muscle. In addition, EMS may be used to maintain or gain range of motion and to break down or stretch adhesions. Indirectly, it may also influence pain, particularly when the pain is secondary to muscle spasm.

Clinical Point
ELECTRICAL MUSCLE STIMULATION

- Overcome reflex inhibition
- Minimize atrophy with immobilization
- Use as an adjunct to strengthening programs
- Re-enforce voluntary contraction
- Maintain health of paralyzed muscle
- Increase range of motion
- Break down adhesions within muscle
- Assist in relieving pain and spasm

Low frequency stimulation usually ranges from 10 to 500 Hz and high frequency from 500 to 10,000 Hz. The literature confusingly designates 1,000 to 10,000 Hz "medium frequency," which gives overlapping terminology.

Muscle Stimulation

There are numerous protocols in the literature but two recurring themes. The typical muscle strength training routine is the 10/50/10 design of Kots and Chuilm.[30] It is the so-called Russian faradism, which consists in 10 seconds of peak amplitude electrical stimulation followed by 50 seconds of rest for 10 repetitions. Usually high frequencies are used, at least in the range of 2,500 Hz.

A regimen more biased toward endurance training includes relatively short intervals between contractions, with the contraction and rest intervals being approximately equal. These protocols are frequently 4 to 15 seconds on and off for a total of 6 to 15 minutes of electrical stimulation each session at the lower frequencies of 50 to 200 Hz.[31]

Most of the literature reports on the use of the sine wave pattern of electrical stimulation at 50 bursts per second (10 ms on, 10 ms off) or 25 bursts per second.[31,32] Furthermore, nearly all of the experimental and clinical data are derived from stimulation of the quadricep muscle groups.

Muscle contraction induced by EMS is different from voluntary contraction in that the area stimulated is usually localized to the area of current flow, and this area may be relatively small and superficial. Furthermore, there tends to be synchronous nerve recruitment and hence an unphysiologic mode of firing of motor units. This situation, with the constant nerve discharge frequency, may lead to fairly rapid fatigue, a fact that should be remembered when planning treatment protocols.

The use of EMS implies that there should be a distinct advantage over voluntary activation of the muscle. In healthy normal individuals it would require that a stronger force could be generated by EMS, increasing muscle contraction overload and hence resulting in more effective strengthening of muscle.[32] However, there have been few reports indicating that EMS can consistently cause a contraction that exceeds maximal voluntary contraction.[30,33] More recent studies suggest that the isolated EMS contraction force is less than the maximal voluntary isometric contraction,[34–36] which implies that the use of EMS must be combined with voluntary contraction protocols to be effective in strengthening muscle in the normal healthy individual and in most circum-

---

Clinical Point

BASIC MUSCLE STIMULATION REGIMENS

Strength Training
- Frequency 2,500 + Hz
- Peak amplitude for 10 seconds
- Rest for 50 seconds

- Duration: 10 repetitions
- Repeat sets

Endurance Bias
- Frequency 50 to 200 Hz
- Rest and work intervals approximately even
- On for 4 to 15 seconds
- Off for 4 to 15 seconds
- Duration: 6 to 15 minutes

---

stances in the pathologic state. Its role in enhancing less than optimal contraction, in overcoming inhibition, and as a training tool, however, is firmly established.

Reflex Inhibition and Muscle Wasting

During a period of reflex inhibition, muscle is either unable, or has a greatly diminished ability, to contract as a result of decreased stimuli from the nervous system.[32] This reflex inhibition may be provoked by joint capsule pain, distention, or immobility.[37,38] Inhibition is most frequently seen during the early stages of recovery from trauma or surgery to the joints. Some muscles seem to be more affected than others, and the proximity to the joint seems to have an influence. The quadriceps femoris group, particularly the vastus medialis, are the most significantly involved because of either susceptibility or the frequency of injury or surgery to the knee joint. EMS in conjunction with attempted voluntary contraction usually rapidly restores control and strength.

With patellar pathology or peripatellar pain, reflex inhibition or wasting of the vastus medialis may contribute to patellar tracking problems. The use of functional electrical stimulation, frequently in conjunction with biofeedback techniques, may assist in preferentially influencing the vastus medialis. This approach may supplement the McConnell taping techniques and provide a prelude to selective voluntary control of the vastus medialis oblique muscles.

Joint effusion is a particularly potent stimulus to reflex inhibition and muscle atrophy. Tense effusion should probably be aspirated and other significant swelling treated by NSAIDs, interferential currents, and adjustment of activity. EMS is particularly useful during the period of modified activity and minimizes the muscle wasting effect of the swelling.

Joint Stimulation and Disuse Atrophy

It is difficult to adequately exercise an immobilized limb, and the combined effect of disuse atrophy and reflex inhibition may result in a torque deficit as high as 80 percent for maximum isometric quadriceps contraction. There is good evidence that EMS superimposed on voluntary contraction may minimize wasting and reduce loss of strength.[39] The exact amount of EMS required to produce optimal effects is not fully documented, with some regimens requiring stimulation for many hours a day. The practicality and cost may outweigh the usefulness, and much more basic research is necessary before the potential of this important application of EMS can be maximized.

There is some discussion as to the major muscle fiber type involved in wasting. The slow twitch type I endurance fiber is certainly affected after surgery. However, there is also evidence that selected atrophy of type II fibers, important in fast velocity movement, can occur. The use of medium frequency stimulation may selectively activate these fast fibers.[40,41]

Important Consideration in EMS

Different positions seem to affect the ability of the quadriceps to generate torque when trained with associated EMS. However, patient comfort, pathology, and functional goals are more important than strict adherence to a set protocol. Although there may be some differences in response between men and women to EMS, the evidence is equivocal at the present time. There is also little known about the fatigue induced by EMS, and the limits of training potential may indeed be related to neuromuscular and muscle fiber fatigue factors. Furthermore, the dramatic changes in isometric strength in atrophied or untrained muscle following intensive EMS training may be related to motor learning effects as much as to an increase in muscle fiber size.

Electrical Muscle Stimulation Under Pressure

With significant tissue edema there may be a role for combining elevation, electrical muscle stimulation, and pressure as a treatment protocol. Reciprocal contraction of the major muscle groups of the affected limb enhances the pumping action and assists resolution of edema. In most situations voluntary contraction alone is sufficient, but when it is not possible EMS supplementation may be used. Elevation of the limb should not be such that the major veins are compressed in the groin. Usually 30 degrees of hip flexion is sufficient. The compression bandages applied over the electrodes should be wrapped in such a way as to produce slight enhancement of the pressure gradient from distal to proximal positions in the limb.

Electrical Muscle Stimulation Under Tension

After muscle trauma, healing may occur with a certain amount of deep scarring. Such healing patterns may have the effect of giving a slight pulling or tight sensation within the muscle on contraction, particularly when ballistic-type activity is performed. Such deep intramuscular adhesions predispose to retearing the muscle on resumption of training or competition. It must be realized that such localized adhesions or scars are not always associated with a gross, measurable loss of range of motion of the associated joint. There may or may not be deep tenderness to firm local palpation. It is difficult to mobilize these areas, and the old technique of faradism under tension may be adapted for the more modern muscle stimulators.

The area to be treated is thoroughly warmed using either exercise or a heating modality. The muscle with the adhesion is then placed on full stretch by appropriately positioning the limb. The limb is then secured so muscle contraction is isometric and joint motion impossible. The electrodes are placed on either side of the painful, offending section of muscle, and a slow tetanic-type contraction is induced. The intensity is gradually increased within the tolerance of the athlete. The rationale of this therapy is to attempt to localize the stretch within the muscle to the main area of adhesion formation. The treatment is followed by full range, high repetition exercises and then a cooldown, with ice packs on the stretched part, which is placed fully on stretch. This technique has proved successful in cases of repetitive tearing of the quadriceps or hamstrings but is certainly not needed as a routine treatment for all muscle tears.

Precautions and Contraindications

1. There is some danger of interference with cardiac pacemakers, particularly those with demand, rather than fixed, rates. Treatment of the lower extremities in the patients is probably acceptable, but the situation should be checked carefully.
2. Stimulation over the pregnant abdomen is not warranted and is potentially dangerous.
3. There is possibly some danger of aggravating ischemia in limbs affected by atherosclerosis; and although not documented, there may be some risk of generating emboli.
4. Localized infection may be spread by activity, and EMS produced motion is no exception.
5. Care should be taken when there is subcutaneous metal, fragile skin, or open cuts. Although none of these factors is a definite contraindication, each may led to painful and sometimes ineffective therapy.

In summary, there appears to be little advantage of functional electrical stimulation over resisted voluntary exercise unless there are some mitigating factors such as reflex inhibition, disuse atrophy with immobilization, edema, intramuscular adhesions, or some degree of denervation. Whenever possible, the electrical stimulation should be combined with voluntary muscle contraction. In the correct clinical circumstances, however, the effect of EMS may be dramatic.

Transcutaneous Electrical Neural Stimulation

Transcutaneous electrical neural stimulation (TENS) is also known as transcutaneous neural stimulation (TNS). The observation that certain fish, especially the torpedo fish and electric eel, could bring about stimulus-induced analgesia with jolts of 100 to 150 V, was well known to the Romans. Numerous machines were made to duplicate this effect during the late 1800s and early 1900s.

Many treatments in medicine receive wide acclaim, only to disappear as disenchantment with their efficacy sets in. Subsequently many of these old treatment concepts are rediscovered and campaigned to a new generation of health professionals. Success is frequently achieved because of improved equipment design, better knowledge of pathophysiology, and less-exaggerated claims. Even so, with each introduction of a new therapy there seem to be "messiahs" who believe the modality will solve all problems. Fortunately, calmer heads eventually prevail, good basic and clinical research is performed, and the modality is evaluated in the correct light and slotted into its appropriate place in our armamentarium. Such a modality is the transcutaneous nerve stimulator. During the 1960s, TENS was used as a screening test to identify patients who might benefit from implanted dorsal column stimulators for the treatment of chronic pain. Many patients, however, experienced considerable relief after TENS application itself, thus raising interest in the modality.

Gate Control Theory of Pain Reduction

The gate control theory proposes peripheral modulation of central pain stimulus transfer and interpretation. Melzack and Wall suggested that the perception of pain depended on the balance of large- and small-diameter fiber activity.[42] These fibers synapsed with T cells in the dorsal horn, which projected nerve activity toward the brain.[43] However, cells within the substantia gelatinosa section of the dorsal horns are believed to be capable of modulating the afferent volleys before they reach the transmission cells (Fig. 3-18). Small-fiber nociceptive input stimulates the T cells and opens the gate by inhibiting the modulating influence of the cells of the substantia gelatinosa (Table 3-4). An increase in large-fiber activity can preferentially close the gate via stimulation of the substantia gelatinosa cells, which in turn inhibit the transmission cells. Large-fiber activity can minimize nociceptive sensation even in the presence of increasing small-fiber input because of their faster conduc-

tion velocity (Table 3-4). High frequency TENS, according to the gate theory, provides increased large-fiber input and thus suppresses small-fiber activity.[44] The gate control theory, however, does not explain how TENS may reduce or alleviate pain after stimulation is stopped, and so there must be other mechanisms for blocking pain perception.

Endogenous Chemical Analgesia

Electrical stimulation may produce pain relief via endorphin production.[44] Endorphin is a term that describes biologic activity rather than chemical structure or class. Endorphins are formed in the brain and anterior pituitary gland and are produced along with adrenocorticotropic hormone (ACTH) and enkephalins when the more complex molecule ACTH–β-lipotropin is broken down.[43,45] Endorphins are probably also involved at the sites of tissue injury and inflammation. The conversion of arachidonic acids to the pain- and inflammation-mediating prostaglandin E (PGE) group may be modified by endorphins and enkephalins. They may indeed be involved in the breakdown of peripheral irritators. Thus if endorphin and enkephalin production can be stimulated by TENS, its chemical affect could outlast the period of stimulation.

Stimulation Variables

A controversy exists concerning the correlation between the efficacy of the various combinations of pulse frequencies, waveforms, and output intensities

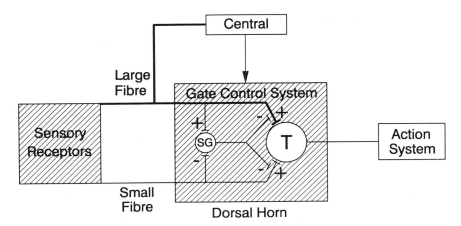

Fig. 3-18. Cells of the substantia gelatinosa (SG) serve as a modifying or gating system for sensory input. Large-fiber activity closes the gate, and an increase in small fiber activity opens the gate to the transmission of nociceptive information by the transmission cells (T) and brain. (After Melzack and Wall.[42])

TABLE 3-4. Classification and Function of Nerve Fibers

Type	Group	Function	Diameter (μm)	Conduction Velocity (meters/s)
A fibers				
A-α	I	Largest motor nerves Innervate skeletal muscle fibers	12–20	72–120
A-β	II	Largest sensory fibers Largely fast touch and proprioception Transmit sensory information rapidly	6–12	36–72
A-γ	III	Fibers innovating the muscle spindle and Golgi tendon Primarily proprioception	1–6	6–36
A-δ	III	Transmit quick pain, temperature, and light touch sensation	1–6	6–36
B fibers		Preganglionic autonomic fibers	—	—
C fibers		Mechanoreceptors Transmit slow pain and temperature Transmit postganglionic autonomic impulses	1	0.5–2.0

(Fig. 3-16). There is a belief that high frequency TENS may work through the gate control mechanism, whereas low frequency stimulation may be more effective in promoting endorphin.[46] However, the one common denominator of all TENS units is that of pulse intensity, and it is probably the most important variable.[47] Maximum amplitudes range from a low of 30 milliamps (mA) to a high of 120 mA.

Clinical Application

From the parameters above have evolved two basic forms of TENS: low and high intensity and low and high frequency. Low intensity TENS is applied at a high pulse rate (up to 100 pulses/s), does not cause muscle contraction, and is usually comfortable and barely perceivable. High intensity TENS is applied at a tolerable level of approximately 10 pulses/s. This stimulus is likely to be less comfortable and usually is modulated to achieve the desired pain-relieving effect (Table 3-5).

Pain Relief

High frequency TENS, mainly between 100 and 500 Hz, is set at a frequency that produces a distinct tingling sensation at the lowest pulse width possible, usually less than 200 μs and preferably around 60 μs. The pulse rate should be high ($\sim$60 to 80 pulses/s) and is referred to as conventional high frequency TENS or high TENS. Its object is to close the gate by large-fiber stimulation. This frequency gives the fastest pain relief of all techniques of TENS application, although it may be of short duration. In this regard it is often used as a pretreatment for other exercise

modalities. It should never be used in the acute situation to replace the traditional ice, rest, elevation, and compression, although it may supplement these treatments. It is an excellent means of interrupting the pain–spasm cycle. For chronic pain it may be applied for 30 minutes up to 24 hours (Tables 3-3, 3-4, and 3-5).

If the desired objective is to activate pituitary β-endorphin release and descending pain inhibition by the periaqueductal gray and raphe nucleus, low frequency, high intensity stimulation should be given (sometimes referred to as acupuncture-like low frequency TENS.)[48] Frequently an intensity strong enough to bring about muscle contraction may be necessary to induce this type of analgesia via the deep afferents. Ideal stimulation parameters for this effect are intensities that are nonpainful, with the frequency kept between 1 and 50 Hz and pulse widths of 200 to 500 μs. These low frequency treatments are usually of shorter duration, not exceeding 20 to 30 minutes. The duration of this pain relief may last several hours because of the 4-hour half-life of β-endorphin (Tables 3-3, 3-4, and 3-5).

It should be realized that any given patient may achieve pain relief from specific frequencies and intensities, and the therapist should search for these idiosyncratic patterns during clinical application. There are many studies available attesting to the efficacy of TENS for pain relief following surgery, and it has been used extensively following knee ligament repairs, shoulder stabilization procedures, and arthroscopy.[43,48]

When using TENS during the perioperative period for pain relief, the electrodes are usually placed

TABLE 3-5. Clinical Application of Transcutaneous Neural Stimulation

Mode	Frequency (Hz)	Pulse Width (μs)	Pulses/s	Intensity	Comments
High TENS (conventional TENS)	100–500	60–120	75–150	Submotor	Should produce distinct tingling sensation Close gate by large fiber stimulation Short duration Duration: 30 minutes to 24 hours
Low TENS (acupuncture-like TENS)	1–50	200–500	2–4	Produces contraction	Descending pain inhibition Endorphin and enkephalin mediated Longer duration of pain relief Duration: 15–30 minutes
Electroacupuncture (brief intense TENS)	1–50	150–500	2–4	Submotor through to tetanic contraction	Stimulation of acupuncture points along meridians Applied as strong as tolerated Duration: 30–60 seconds per point
Burst mode	50–100	75–100	2–4	Muscle contraction	Pain relief via endorphins Occasionally chosen to get associated strong but relatively comfortable muscle contraction Duration: 20–60 minutes

around the wound. For nonsurgical problems or less isolated traumatic pathology, the most effective placement of electrodes may be judged by using a neuroprobe to locate the trigger points.

With subacute injuries, treatment may be commenced using high frequency TENS to obtain rapid pain relief. After 10 to 20 minutes of this mode, low frequency TENS is administered to achieve a more lasting effect. There is less nerve accommodation with this transition protocol; and in the acute situation it may be painful owing to muscle stimulation, so it not indicated for this purpose.

Electroacupuncture

Depending on the desired effect, electrodes may be placed directly around the painful area, over perplexed nerve trunks, and most commonly over motor, trigger, and acupuncture points. The latter technique is referred to as electroacupuncture. The frequency, pulse width, and pulse amplitude are similar to, or of lower frequency than, those used in conventional units; however, the output is perceived as being greater by the patient because the electrode is smaller. This technique is sometimes referred to as acupuncture-like low frequency TENS, and pain relief is obtained via descending tract inhibition mediated by the neural hormones previously mentioned (serotonin and enkephalin). This mode is called hyperstimulation analgesia or brief intense analgesia. Interrupted direct current at 1 to 5 pulses/s or TENS at 150 pulses/s are used. The intensity is adjusted to allow muscle fasciculation or tetanic contraction. The duration of application can be up to 15 minutes, and the treatment may be repeated after a 2- to 3-minute rest period. If point stimulators are being used, trigger points are stimulated for 30 to 60 seconds per point at maximum tolerance. Alternatively, treatment may follow the meridians for acupuncture points.

Burst Mode TENS

The final general method of applying TENS is the burst mode. A carrier frequency of 50 to 100 Hz is packaged into bursts of current with a frequency of two to four bursts per second. The individual bursts are imperceptible, so a single pulse is felt by the athlete. This mode then uses a carrier frequency such as the conventional high TENS, which is modulated to produce a low TENS effect. The intention is to allow a strong muscle contraction at a low intensity of current, thus providing a more comfortable sensation. The pulse rate is usually 50 to 100 pulses per second and the pulse width around 75 to 100 μs. The intensity is adjusted for a strong, comfortable contraction and a duration of 20 to 60 minutes. Pain relief is achieved via endorphin pathways.

Contraindications

There are few contraindications for use with athletes. Occasionally the patient develops mild skin irritation from the electrodes, tape, or gel, which may be alleviated by changing the electrode system and by conscientious skin care. Sometimes individuals have true allergies to the electrode system, which requires careful analysis and changes if the treatment is important enough to continue. Caution must be taken with demand pacemakers and treatment over the chest is contraindicated. There should be no stimulation over the carotid sinus, the pregnant abdomen, the chest with cardiac problems, the eyes, or mucosal membranes. Caution should be applied to TENS use when there is undocumented pathology and particularly if analgesia might lead to unguarded use and potentially further harm. Some individuals experience unusual adverse sympathetic reaction, and although rare it is wise not to persist with the treatment.

In summary, TENS treatment is a safe, versatile method of inducing some analgesia and hence is a useful adjunct for other therapies. When used during the acute phase of injury, it is not a substitute for the standard therapy of ice, elevation, and compression. There are endless combinations of frequencies, pulse shapes, and methods of modulation; and to some extent the patient response is idiosyncratic. Unsuccessful treatment should lead to early adjustment of the treatment regimen; and if it is not productive after careful trials by an experienced therapist, early abandonment in favor or other modalities should be considered.

High Voltage Pulsed (Galvanic) Stimulation

High voltage pulsed (galvanic) stimulation (HVPGS) must be able to transmit a voltage in excess of 100 to 150 V, and usually it is up to 500 V. Because most electrical stimulators can exceed this value, the twin peaked monophasic waveform becomes the main distinguishing feature. The major claim for these units is that there is little cutaneous stimulation, and hence the treatment is more comfortable. This method has been used clinically for pain relief, tissue healing, reduction of muscle spasm, and muscle re-education. The frequency range offered by most HVPGS is 2 to 100 Hz, which allows incorporation of low or high TENS principles. Although the voltage is high, the average current generated is minimal, and it is thus a relatively safe modality. Although the word galvanic is incorporated in the title because a monophasic current is used, the short pulse duration of 20 to 200 μs does not qualify it for this term.

Usually applied with a large dispersive electrode and a small negative active electrode, this unit is easily adapted to submersion treatments for the limbs. The athlete can then combine HVPGS with an exercise program. Some therapists select it as the initial method of stimulation during the postinjury period.

Interferential Therapy

Inferential therapy is another form of transcutaneous nerve stimulation used particularly for pain relief. Two simultaneously applied medium frequency currents (generally in the range of 4,000 to 5,000 Hz) with sinusoidal waveforms are utilized. The waveforms become superimposed on each other, which causes interference with points of augmentation and attenuation. The interference results in the production of a "beat" mode with a frequency that ranges from 1 to 100 beats/s. The frequency of the beats can be altered by varying one of the two carrier frequencies (Fig. 3-19).

There are mechanisms for causing rhythmic changes in the frequency or rotating the electrical field for reducing nerve accommodation. Nevertheless, this machine is just another form of stimulator that may be used like a high TENS unit for pain control at 100 beats/s as well as for muscle contraction at less than 60 beats/s. Other than the possibility of deeper penetration and comfort, it is difficult to document distinct advantages for this system.

Intelligent TENS

There is a class of electrical stimulators referred to by the manufacturers as intelligent TENS (Electro-Acuscope and Myopulse). These instruments purportedly monitor the levels of electrical stimulation the injured tissue requires and return these tissues to a normal homeostatic state. They rely on a tissue resonance theory which implies that when injury occurs the normal electrical potentials generated by healthy metabolic function are disrupted. This altered activity affects the resonant frequency. The Acuscope is referred to as an electrical neural stimulator, and the Myopulse is a muscle stimulator; little,

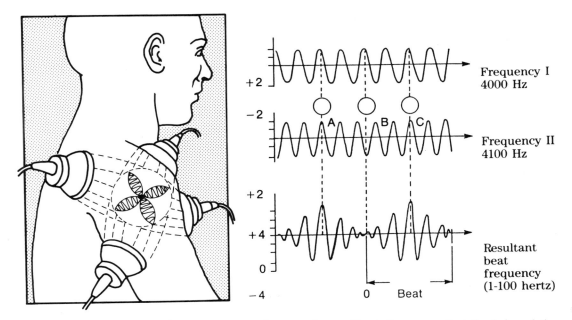

Frequency I
4000 Hz

Frequency II
4100 Hz

Resultant
beat
frequency
(1-100 hertz)

Fig. 3-19. Interferential devices are arranged to produce a "beat frequency" at the injured tissue. (Redrawn from Gieck and Saliba,[54] with permission.)

however, is known about the programming of the microchips of these instruments. Theoretically, whereas conventional TENS disrupts pain impulse propagation, the Acuscope measures electrical activity present in an area and compares it to a preprogrammed reference level. It then adjusts the waveform to deliver a specific amount of current or electromagnetic energy. The Auscope incorporates both a regular and the sophisticated TENS modes.

Galvanic (Direct) Current

Galvanic current allows stimulation of denervated muscle as well as the possibility of driving ions into the tissues, i.e., iontophoresis, and is classed in the low voltage category of apparatus. A galvanic current is a unidirectional (monophasic) current flowing for an indefinite duration; i.e., for convention, the duration is more than 300 ms. When used for muscle stimulation, the slow rise and fall of the pulse pattern stimulates muscle directly if the nerve supply is not intact. The iontophoretic effect is not frequently used, but it is favored by some therapists. On the principle that like charges repel and opposites attract, ions of various substances are placed under their similar polarity electrode and driven through tissues by currents usually less than 5 mA. In the past, histamine and renotin were used to provide a counterirritant effect, copper sulfate for cleaning and stimulation of

indolent wounds, sodium chloride for softening scars, and salicylate for analgesia. Currently, a combination lidocaine (Xylocaine) and a corticosteroid, usually dexamethasone sodium phosphate, are the only ions used with any frequency in sports medicine. Corticosteroid (1 ml) and anesthetic agent (2 ml) are ionized under the anode for approximately 20 minutes for treatment of edema and pain during acute spasms. This technique has also been recommended with epicondylitis, bursitis, and myofascial trigger points with myalgia or fasciitis. The efficacy of these treatments is questionable in the face of potent oral NSAIDs and injectable cortisone, but there are circumstances where local galvanic iontophoresis may enhance, supplement, or replace these other regimens. Gastric intolerance to medications, allergy, and the problem of skin atrophy serve as examples.

ELECTROMAGNETIC SPECTRUM

The electromagnetic spectrum consists in an array of energies that, delivered in suitable ways, may influence the molecules of the tissues biologically, mechanically, and frequently thermally. At one end of this spectrum are the radio waves adapted for shortwave diathermy application and the visible spectrum including laser light. As the wavelength gets shorter, ultraviolet emissions are encountered (Fig. 3-20).

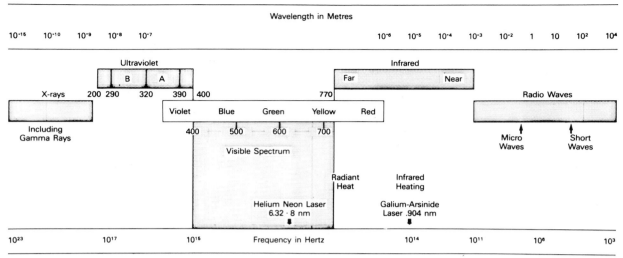

Fig. 3-20. Electromagnetic spectrum. It is not drawn to scale, and some of the placements of frequencies and wavelengths are approximate.

These waves are emitted in discrete packages called photons. Photons of a particular energy have a characteristic wavelength and frequency.[2]

Physical modalities are adapted to utilize the effects of the electromagnetic spectrum, particularly heat. Some of the features of these rays are discussed as they relate to sports medicine.

Infrared Modalities

Only the heating modalities, which include moist hot packs, heating pads, whirlpools, infrared lamps, and wax baths, are dealt with in this section. Thermal energy may be considered as vibration of the molecules and their electrons that make up the substance, in this case the tissues.

The choice of modality depends largely on the size and shape of the body part, the depth of the injured tissue from the surface, convenience factors, and the absence of specific contraindications. Usually, heat is applied after bleeding has stopped, the immediate postinjury edema and inflammatory stage stabilized, and mobilization begun. These conditions are usually met 24 to 48 hours after injury. Heat may also be used to assist pre-exercise warm-up and prior to stretching routines where the effects on increasing collagen plasticity are well documented.[28]

The electromagnetic spectrum has a relatively large area designated as infrared. Penetration depends on the wavelength and hence the source. Far infrared

---

> **Clinical Point**
>
> **POSSIBLE PHYSIOLOGIC EFFECTS OF HEAT**
>
> - Increased local temperature
> - Increased metabolic rate
> - Greater flux in tissue fluid, oxygen, and nutrients
> - Vasodilatation
> - Reduction of spasm
> - Mild analgesia
> - Increased tissue plasticity

---

wavelengths are between 111,000 and 28,860,000 Å and penetrate up to 2 mm of skin. The near infrared spectrum is between 7,500 and 14,430 Å and may penetrate up to 5 to 10 mm of skin.

Analgesia may be produced via the direct effect on sensory nerves, by dispersal of metabolites, or by decreasing tissue fluid flux and hence improving nutrition and decreasing edema. The hyperemia induced in the capillary bed, combined with the infrared radiation, raises the tissue temperature, which in turn increases the metabolic rate about 10 to 13 percent for each 1°C rise in temperature.

Warm Whirlpool Bath

The temperature range for the arm and hand should be 98° to 110°F (37° to 45°C), for the leg 98° to 104°F (37° to 40°C), and for full body treatment 98° to 102°F (37° to 39°C). Application is usually for 15 to 20 minutes. This treatment is versatile because of the large body areas that may be immersed. It also has the advantage that it is conducive for simultaneous exercise. The problem of dependent edema during the subacute stage is partly counteracted by the hydrostatic effect of the water and repetitive motion. Although one of the most useful modalities in sports medicine, the practice of leaving an individual in a whirlpool bath, particularly without adequate assessment, is not an accepted method of therapy. Regular checks of the equipment, tank, jets, and drains for bacterial and fungal growth are necessary. Folliculitis is an unusual but serious complication of whirlpool use. Specifically, *Pseudomonas* folliculitis presenting with either an erythematous papulovesicular or maculopapular rash is problematic. Occasionally the athlete is systemically sick, with general malaise, headache, and fever 6 hours to 5 days after whirlpool use. Other symptoms include sore throat, ear pain, rhinitis, sore eyes, and axillary lymphadenopathy.[49] *Pseudomonas* is not readily killed by chlorine, so particular attention should be paid to the presence of this organism.

Hydrocollator Packs

Hydrocollator packs are frequently pouches of petroleum distillate that may be heated in a tank and that maintain a temperature of around 170°F. There are a variety of shapes and sizes, which allows adaptation to different body parts and shapes. Before application they are surrounded with toweling of approximately 1 inch thickness, which is usually six layers of regular towel. The treatment time is 20 minutes. This treatment, classed as moist heat therapy, enables tolerance of a slightly higher temperature. It is usually used as a convenient, comfortable method of applying heat prior to some other therapy.

Infrared Lamps

Infrared lamps are infrequently used because of the limited depth of penetration and the danger of superficial burns. A warm, slightly moist towel spread over the part to be treated may decrease this risk. Nonluminous infrared lamps are no longer manufactured, as radiation at around 12,000 Å gives the best penetration, which is achieved with the luminous tungsten or carbon filaments. Application is at a minimum of 20 inches from the patient to decrease the risk of burning and is usually of 15 to 20 minutes' duration. The skin must be carefully and regularly checked.

Paraffin Wax Baths

Paraffin wax baths are sometimes inconvenient and messy, but they are effective for treating hand and wrist injuries. Paraffin wax treatments supply approximately six times the amount of heat that would be available from water baths because the mineral oil in the paraffin lowers its melting point. The bath is set at 126°F, and provisions must be made for periodically sterilizing and cleaning the wax.

A technique for repeated dipping of the hands allows application of 10 layers of wax. The heat is then held in using a plastic bag and several layers of toweling. A treatment lasts approximately 20 to 30 minutes. Although extra care is required with this treatment modality, it is superb for treating finger sprains, hand contusions, recovering digit fractures, and wrist injuries.

Contraindications and Precautions to Heat Therapy

There are some general contraindications to all modalities that produce heat: (1) impaired skin sensation; (2) the use of strong narcotic analgesics, which may alter both sensation and judgment; (3) circulatory dysorders, which prohibit the necessary vasodilation; (4) poor quality, fragile skin; (5) deep x-ray therapy during the preceding 3 months with atrophic skin and altered sensation; and (6) inability of the patient to comprehend adequately the dangers of the specific therapy.

In addition, special consideration is necessary before treating open or contaminated wounds, particularly with wax baths. The presence of certain dermatologic conditions may also present difficulties. Some linaments and creams may increase the risk of damage to the skin, and the area must be appropriately prepared. Essentially, most of these modalities are safe if the therapist takes sufficient care and the patient is adequately instructed.

Lasers

Lasers (light amplification by stimulated emissions of radiation) are light amplifiers that emit energy in the visible and infrared regions of the electromag-

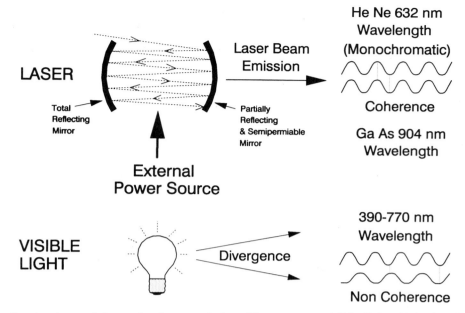

Fig. 3-21. Comparison of the main characteristics of laser versus visible light. (Adapted from Gieck and Saliba.[54])

netic spectrum (Fig. 3-21). Since Maiman successfully induced this form of emission in a ruby crystal, laser light has been produced from several gases and diodes.[50] Gallium-arsenide (GaAs) and helium-neon (HeNe) have proved most useful therapeutically. Initial experience with high doses produced only negative effects. Currently, cold or soft lasers with a maximal output of less than 1 mW are used therapeutically in sports medicine and have essentially an athermic effect. These lower doses may have a positive effect on wound healing and may be beneficial in pain reduction.[50-52]

Laser light is generated by the stimulated emission

of photons or light energy. Energy in the form of photons is released as ionized gas, is raised to a higher valence, and attempts to reach a more stable configuration. HeNe and GaAs are the atoms most commonly used to elicit the stimulated emission and resultant production of a coherent, monochromatic, collimated beam.[53]

Characteristics of Lasers

The three main characteristics of laser light are monochromaticity, coherence, and divergence.[48] Monochromaticity means that the light is of a single well defined wavelength. The infrared GaAs laser has a specific wavelength of 904 nm, which is beyond the visible spectrum of 400 to 770 nm (nm $= 10^{-9}$ meters). The emitted beam is therefore invisible. Frequently a filter is introduced to make a visible beam. The HeNe laser has a wavelength of 632.8 nm, taking it into the visible spectrum; and it is characterized by a colored beam often associated with laser (Fig. 3-21).

Normal light is made up of numerous wavelengths superimposing their phases on one another. By contrast, lasers with a single specific wavelength travel with the phases in synchrony. The beam progresses unidirectionally and symmetrically, which produces the second characteristic of coherence or phase relation. The third characteristic is the minimal diver-

---

Quick Facts

GASES USED FOR LASER

• Helium-neon	HeNe
• Carbon dioxide	CO_2
• Argon	Ar
• Neodymium yttrium aluminum garnet	NdYAG
• Krypton	Kr
• Gallium-aluminum-arsenide	GaAlAs
• Gallium-arsenide	GaAs

gence of the emitted light, so it maintains a concentrated beam.

Laser devices emit their energy in pulses that correspond to some degree to the natural resonating frequencies of tissues. Both GaAs and HeNe lasers have pulse frequencies of 73,142 and 292 Hz. The average power is inversely proportional to the frequency.

Physiologic Effects

The specific effect of laser light at a subcellular level is still a subject of some speculation. The resonance of human tissue is such that it absorbs laser emission well, although there is some reflection and dispersion. Generally, the higher the water content of the tissue, the greater is the absorption.[54]

The HeNe laser may have a direct penetration of 0.8 mm and indirect penetration and absorption up to 10 to 15 mm. The GaAs laser with the longer wavelength has a direct penetration of 15 mm and an indirect penetration of up to 5 cm. Hence penetration is directly proportional to wavelength.

The following tissue effects have been reported in the literature.[54,55]

1. Possible alteration in the levels of the various prostaglandins and hence modifying the inflammatory phase of trauma
2. Reduction of edema possibly secondary to effects on membrane potentials and active transport across the cell walls
3. Increased mitochondrial activity and associated elevated production of energy-rich phosphate, adenosine triphosphate (ATP), possibly related to enhancing electron transfer in the inner membrane of the mitochondria
4. Increased levels of RNA in the endoplasmic reticulum of animals
5. Stimulation of fibroblast proliferation and early increase in collagen production in wounds, the mechanism for which is unknown
6. Increased vascularization of wounds

Application of Lasers

When attempting to reduce edema, stimulate tissue function, and promote healing, a technique called gridding is used. Essentially the area to be treated is divided into approximately 1 cm squares, or grids. The unit of therapy is then applied to each square, usually 10 to 15 seconds per unit area for the GaAs laser and 20 to 30 seconds with the HeNe device. Other techniques or patterning of application have their advocates. Multiple head lasers are available that reduce treatment time. Because of the minimal divergence the applicator need not touch the skin, which is useful for open wounds. A distance of 1 to 2 cm is acceptable, but usually the closer it is the more efficient it becomes. Absorption is poor directly through scar, and it is common to laser around an incision or scar rather than through it. There are few definitive data concerning the best time for applying the laser, the correct dose for a desired effect, or the optimal exposure. Although the traditional short periods are well accepted, there are proponents of treatments that last much longer. Realistically, the limited depth of penetration of the laser beam makes it an unsuitable modality for many soft tissue lesions. Although the indirect effects of the laser have been reported to depths of 2 cm, 99 percent of the beam is absorbed directly by about 0.8 mm of the epidermis.[55]

If reduction of pain is the main aim, the painful site, appropriate nerve root, trigger points, or acupuncture points may be lasered. The power, duration, frequency, and spacing of treatments are individual, and a certain amount of adjustment is made for each clinical situation and depends on the therapist's experience.

Contraindications and Precautions

The U.S. Food and Drug Administration (FDA) still classifies lasers as investigational devices in the low risk category. Lasers probably should either not be used or precautions taken in the following situations.

1. Overstimulation: Exposing tissue to laser energy densities of more than 8 or 9 joules/cm² during one treatment session may have adverse effects.
2. The effects of laser application during the first trimester of pregnancy have not been established.
3. Photosensitizing medications may enhance or produce an unpredictable effect.
4. Lasers should never be applied over the unclosed fontanels of infants.
5. The results of lasers applied over tumorous tissue are unknown and hence contraindicated.
6. Treatment should be suspended in situations where prolonged or repeated nausea or dizziness is experienced either during or immediately after treatment.
7. It is undesirable to stare into the laser beam for any significant period of time, as it may affect the retina.
8. It is unwise to apply the laser to tissue if the underlying pathology has not been established.

In summary, the laser is like many physical therapy modalities in that there is a potentially powerful energy source being harnessed in the hope of producing a desirable therapeutic effect. The ability to calculate optimal dosages and deliver this quantum of energy to the appropriate tissue, however, is a formidable task and still in its infancy. It means that empiric application of these modalities requires experience, keen observation, and careful record keeping if successful results are to be duplicated.

Ultraviolet Light

Ultraviolet radiation has been used extensively in the past for the treatment of skin disorders but now is rarely used. With the increasing use of tanning booths, there is an obligation for the therapist and physician to be able to deliver sound scientific advice to counteract the inaccurate, misleading, often dangerous statements made by manufacturers and owners of these facilities.

Athletes use tanning beds or booths to acclimatize themselves to the sun and hence prevent sunburn (or just to acquire a tan). Body building competitors particularly believe that a darker color enhances muscle definition. The increase in popularity in tanning beds parallels claims that modern lamps emit ultraviolet A (UVA) radiation of wavelength 320 to 400 nm instead of the ultraviolet B (UVB) radiation of 290 to 320 nm (Fig. 3-20). However, UVA radiation is by no means innocuous, even though it is less likely to cause sunburn. UVA tends to suppress the immune system and is linked to eye damage, skin aging, and skin cancer (Table 3-6).[56]

The most immediate problem is severe corneal damage and conjunctivitis — hence the need for protective filtered glass goggles. Closing the eyes is not sufficient because UVA radiation can easily penetrate the width of the thin skin of the eyelids. The eyes, unlike the skin, do not develop a tolerance to the ultraviolet light.

Ultraviolet A exposure does not totally protect the athlete from the burning effect of natural sunlight. The tan produced by UVA gives much less protection from burning than the UVB-induced tan: UVB radiation increases the production of keratinocytes and melanocytes, increases the transfer of pigment, and thickens the stratum corneum of the epidermis. The use of sunscreens and a cautious, gradual increase in exposure is still the most effective way to minimize the chance of a sunburn. It is also important to keep in

TABLE 3-6.   Ultraviolet Radiation Emission

Gas or Element	Spectrum (nm)	Comments
Carbon arc	350–400	Mainly UVA, formerly considered biotic Difficult to maintain Impractical
Compressed xenon	220–400	Gas at 20 times atmospheric pressure Dangers of rupture if damaged
Mercury (low pressure)	184–253	Mainly UVB, abiotic Emission at 184 nm blocked mainly by the quartz envelope Main emission at 253 nm: germicidal, used to counteract bacteria
Fluorescent blacklight	300–400	Low pressure mercury coated with phosphors High UVB and entire UVA

mind the effects of photosensitizing agents whether considering tanning booths or natural exposure.

The technique of application is not described here but being familiar with skin testing techniques, having knowledge of contraindications, and carefully protecting the eyes are essential. Although ultraviolet radiation is important to health, only limited doses are required and are easily obtained by natural means.

Despite the attraction of a tan, most of the effects of ultraviolet radiation are abiotic (Table 3-6). Each athlete should be fully aware of the possible cumulative harmful effects of commercially available means of tanning.

Radio Waves

The therapeutic application of high frequency currents, the frequencies of which are high enough that electrolytic dissociation of the tissue does not occur, is possible with shortwave diathermy, microwaves, and pulsed electromagnetic energy.[57] The first two of these modalities are diathermic, meaning they are heat producing; others ostensibly produce therapeutic effects via biophysical phenomena induced by the alternating magnetic field.

Shortwave Diathermy

Shortwave diathermy provides the most efficient way of applying deep heat to a relatively large area of tissue (Fig. 3-22). Its use would be more accepted if it were safer and easier to adjust the dose. Full knowledge of its potential effects and meticulous attention to detail are required to produce the desired heating and the correct depth of penetration in a safe manner.

Shortwave diathermy has a frequency of 27.12 mHz and a wavelength of 11 meters. Two basic techniques are employed: electrostatic (condenser) and electromagnetic (induction) fields. With the condenser plate technique the patient's tissues form the dielectric in an electromagnetic field. The two condenser plates are selected by size and adjusted by spacing in order to produce maximum effect at the required depth in the tissues. If the induction technique is used, a diathermic coil is wrapped around the limb or a special monode electrode is required. The tissues within the field are magnetically stressed rapidly, with dipoles oscillating and distortion of electron orbits. The net result of this magnetic flux is enough molecular disturbance to generate heat. Treatments should last a minimum of 20 minutes and up to 40 minutes for large body areas. It is not possible to assess the dosage accurately. For sports injury a mild thermal application is usually required.

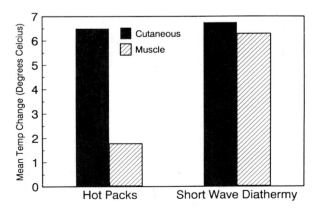

Fig. 3-22. Mean cutaneous and soleus temperature changes after 20 minutes of hot pack and shortwave diathermy. (After Verrier et al.,[58] with permission.)

In addition to the extreme care required during application, precautions must be observed when it is used in the following situations.

1. Over any part of the body in the presence of a cardiac pacemaker
2. Over malignant tumors (because of the danger of increasing metastasis)
3. In areas where circulation is not sufficient to disperse heat or accommodate increased metabolism
4. Over wet dressings or adhesive tape or through casts
5. If there is metal in the tissues
6. If there is impaired thermal sensation
7. Over the pregnant uterus or over the abdomen during menstruation
8. In cases of severe cardiac conditions where increased output may be a problem secondary to vasodilation
9. Over the chest with pulmonary tuberculosis
10. In unreliable patients or those who are unable to concentrate

Microwave Diathermy

Microwave has two assigned frequencies, 2456 and 915 MHz, giving it a higher frequency and shorter wavelength than shortwave diathermy (Fig. 3-19). The microwave antenna, or director, beams energy that is both absorbed and reflected. The limiting factor with heating may be the temperature rise of the superficial fat, which then produces discomfort. The tissue heating is generated by much the same mechanisms as with shortwave diathermy, and the same contraindications should be observed. Microwave diathermy is best used to treat areas of the body that are relatively flat (so reflection is minimized) and that have low subcutaneous fat content (so penetration is adequate).

Pulsed Electromagnetic Energy

It has never been conclusively demonstrated that the many mechanical and nonthermal effects that undoubtedly occur with shortwave diathermy and microwave therapy have any specific isolated therapeutic functions. However, the rationale behind the nonthermal pulsed electromagnetic equipment, e.g., Diapulse, suggests that there may be useful clinical effects other than heating. Therefore the shortwaves are pulsed in packages, with a sufficient rest interval that the small amounts of heat are rapidly dissipated and there is no cumulative rise in tissue temperature. All apparatus in this category use a base frequency of 27.12 MHz. There are a large number of instruments available, each with a number of output options in terms of pulse widths, pulse repetition rates, intensity settings, and shape of the electromagnetic field generated. Each requires a period of familiarization for effective use. These apparatus are used to promote healing, decrease inflammation, reduce muscle spasm, and produce some analgesia. Although there is a large body of basic research on subcellular and cellular effects, the efficacy, cost-effectiveness, and superiority of these apparatus have yet to be conclusively demonstrated.[59] Each has its special advocates and champions, and it remains for more carefully generated research to elicit their true place in the physiotherapeutic armamentarium.

SUMMARY

This chapter has looked briefly at some of the more commonly used physiotherapy modalities. There is no doubt that many of the instruments described utilize potent forces. We are still, however, a long way from effectively harnessing these powers to maximize any therapeutic potential they have. For the present it is worth re-emphasizing that the basis of sports medicine is still modification of exercise, therapeutic exercise, and functional rehabilitation. The modalities described herein are best used in preparation for the activity component of therapy.

REFERENCES

1. Ward AR: Electricity, Fields and Waves in Therapy. Lincoln Institute of Science Press, Melbourne, 1979
2. Licht SH: Therapeutic Electricity and Ultraviolet Radiation. 2nd Ed. Litcht Publishing, New Haven, 1967
3. Herrick JF: Temperature produced in tissues by ultrasound: experimental study using various techniques. J Acoust Soc Am 25:943, 1953
4. Reid DC: Therapeutic ultrasound. MCh thesis, University of Liverpool, 1980
5. Allen KGR, Battye CK: Performance of ultrasonic therapy instruments. Physiotherapy 64:174, 1978
6. Dyson M, Pond JB: The effect of pulsed ultrasound on tissue regeneration. Physiotherapy 56:136, 1970
7. Summer W, Patrick MK: Ultrasonic Therapy. Elsevier Press, London, 1964
8. Reid DC, Cummings G: Factors in selecting the dosage of ultrasound. Phys Ther Can 25:5, 1973

9. Reid DC, Cummings G: Efficacy of ultrasound complying agents. Physiotherapy 63:255, 1975
10. Dyson M, Pond JB, Joseph J et al: The stimulation of tissue regeneration by means of ultrasound. Clin Sci 35:273, 1968
11. Lehmann JF, Krusen FH: Therapeutic application of ultrasonic energy in physical medicine. Am J Phys Med 37:173, 1958
12. Griffin JG: Physiological effects of ultrasonic energy as it is used clinically. J Am Phys Ther Assoc 46:18, 1966
13. Paaske WP, Hovind H, Sejrsen P: Influence of therapeutic ultrasonic irradiation on blood flow in human cutaneous, subcutaneous and muscular tissue. Scand J Clin Invest 31:388, 1973
14. Wyper DJ, McNiven DR, Donnelly TJ: Therapeutic ultrasound and muscular blood flow. Physiotherapy 64:321, 1978
15. Ludwig GD: The velocity of sound through tissue and the acoustic impedances of tissue. J Acoust Soc Am 22:862, 1950
16. Webster DF, Pond JB, Dyson M et al: The role of cavitation in the "in vitro" stimulation of protein synthesis in human fibroblasts by ultrasound. Ultrasound Med Biol 4:343, 1978
17. Nyborg WL: Acoustic streaming. p. 265. In Mason WP (ed): Physical Acoustics. Academic Press, London, 1965
18. Middlemast S, Catterjee DS: Comparison of ultrasound and thermography for soft tissue. Physiotherapy 64:331, 1978
19. Makulolume RT, Mouzas GL: Ultrasound in the treatment of sprained ankles. Practitioner 218:586, 1977
20. Downing DS, Weinstein A: Ultrasound therapy of subacromial bursitis: a double blind trial. Phys Ther 66:194, 1986
21. Fisher B, Reid DC, Chan N et al: Effects of therapeutic ultrasound in skeletal muscle following acute blunt trauma. 1989 (in press)
22. Reid DC, Redford JB, King P: The influence of ultrasound and high frequency radiowaves on the rate of resorption of experimental hematomas. In Taylor KW (ed): Training: Scientific Basis and Application. Charles C Thomas, Springfield, IL, 1972
23. Reid DC: Selecting the dosage of ultrasound. Med Electronics Data 6:52, 1975
24. Pond JB, Woodward B, Dyson M: A microscopic viewing ultrasonic irradiation chamber. Phys Med Biol 18:521, 1971
25. Lehman JF, Brunmer GD, Stow RW: Pain threshold measurements after therapeutic application of ultrasound, microwaves and infrared. Arch Phys Med Rehabil 39:560, 1958
26. Gersten JW: Thermal and non-thermal charges in isometric tension, contractile protein and injury potential produced in frog muscle by ultrasonic energy. Arch Phys Med Rehabil 34:675, 1953
27. Bierman W: Ultrasound in treatment of scars. Arch Phys Med Rehabil 35:209, 1954
28. Kottke FJ, Pamby DL, Ptak RA: The rationale for prolonged stretching for correction of shortening of connective tissue. Arch Phys Med Rehabil 47:347, 1966
29. Griffin JG: Physiological effects of ultrasonic energy as it is used clinically. J Am Phys Ther Assoc 46:18, 1966
30. Kots VM, Chuilm VA: The Training of Muscular Power by Method of Electrical Stimulation. State Central Institute of Physical Culture, Moscow, 1975
31. Selkowitz DM: High frequency electrical stimulation in muscle strengthening. Am J Sports Med 17:103, 1989
32. Morrissey MC: Electromyostimulation from a clinical perspective: a review. Sports Med 6:29, 1988
33. Ikai M, Yabe K, Iischii K: Musekraft muskulare ermundung bei wilkorificher anspannungelektrischer reizung des muskels. Sportarzt Sportsmed 5:197, 1967
34. De Domenico G, Strauss GR: Maximum torque production in the quadriceps femoris muscle group using a variety of electrical stimulators. Aust J Physiother 32:51, 1986
35. Kramer J, Lindsay D, Magee D: Comparison of voluntary and electrical stimulation contraction torques. J Orthop Sports Phys Ther 5:324, 1984
36. Walmsley RP, Letts G, Vooys J: A comparison of torque generated by knee extension with a maximal voluntary muscle contraction vis-à-vis electrical stimulation. J Orthop Sports Phys Ther 6:10, 1984
37. Häggmark R, Eriksson E: Cylinder or mobile cast brace after knee ligament surgery. Am J Sports Med 7:48, 1979
38. Stokes M, Yong A: The contribution of reflex inhibition to arthrogenous muscle weakness. Clin Sci 67:7, 1984
39. Gould N, Donnermeyer D, Gammon GG et al: Transcutaneous muscle stimulation to retard disuse after open meniscectomy. Clin Orthop 178:190, 1983
40. Grimby G, Nordwill A, Atulten B: Changes in histochemical profile of muscle after long term electrical stimulation in patients with idiopathic scoliosis. Scand J Rehabil Med 17:191, 1985
41. Eriksson E: Sports injury of the knee ligaments: their diagnosis, treatment, rehabilitation and prevention. Med Sci Sports 8:133, 1976
42. Melzack R, Wall PD: Pain mechanisms: a new therapy. Science 50:971, 1965
43. Jensen JE, Ertheridge GL, Hazelrigg G: Effectiveness of transcutaneous electrical nerve stimulation in the treatment of pain: recommendations for use

in the treatment of sports injuries. Sports Med 3:79, 1986

44. Kleinkort JA, Foley RA: Laser acupuncture: its use in physical therapy. Am J Acupuncture 12:15, 1984

45. Cheng R, Pomeranz B: Electroacupuncture analgesic could be mediated by at least two pain relieving mechanisms: endorphin and non-endorphin systems. Life Sci 25:1957, 1979

46. Spiegel EA: Relief of pain and spasticity by posterior column stimulation: a proposed mechanism. Arch Neurol 39:184, 1982

47. Mannheimer C, Carlsson CA: The analgesic effects of transcutaneous electrical nerve stimulation (TNS) in patients with rheumatoid arthritis: a comparative study of different pulse patterns. Pain 6:329, 1979

48. Smith MJ: Electrical stimulation for relief of musculoskeletal pain. Physician Sportsmed 11:47, 1983

49. Rondt GA: Hot tub folliculitis. Physician Sportsmed 11:74, 1983

50. Krikorian DJ, Hartshorne MF, Stratton SA: Use of He-Ne laser for treatment of soft tissue trauma: evaluation by gallium-67 citrate scanning. J Orthop Sports Phys Ther 8:93, 1986

51. Ewemeka CJ: Laser biostimulation of healing wounds: specific effects and mechanisms of action. J Orthop Sports Phys Ther 9:333, 1988

52. Mester AF, Mester A: Clinical data of laser biostimulation in wound healing. Lasers Surg Med 7:78, 1987

53. Mester E, Mester AF, Mester A: The biomedical effects of laser application. Lasers Surg Med 5:31, 1984

54. Gieck JH, Saliba EN: The Athletic Trainer and Rehabilitation in the Injured Athlete. 2nd Ed. JB Lippincott, Philadelphia, 1988

55. Askoryan GA: Enhancement of transmission of laser and other radiation by soft turbid physical and biological media. Sov J Quantum Electron 12:877, 1982

56. DeBenedette V: Health club tanning booths: risky business. Physician Sportsmed 15:59, 1987

57. Lehmann JF, Warren CG, Scham SM: Therapeutic heat and cold 99:207, 1974

58. Verrier M, Ashby P, Crawford JS: Effects of thermotherapy or the electrical and mechanical properties of human skeletal muscle. Physiother Can 30:117, 1978

59. Reid DC: Treatment by pulsating athermic short waves. Physiother Can 22:183, 1970

Connective Tissue Healing and Classification of Ligament and Tendon Pathology

4

Reading is sometimes an ingenious device for avoiding thought.
—Sir Arthur Helps, 1850

Tendons and ligaments are examples of organized connective tissue that share many common features, including their attachment to bone, their response to immobilization, their reaction to slowly increased stress over time, and their response to trauma and the subsequent healing events. A logical approach to rehabilitation of tendon and ligament injuries demands a knowledge of the behavior of connective tissue at the microscopic and biochemical levels. A useful clinical classification of these injuries is presented, as is a discussion of the connective tissue responses to trauma and their implications for treatment planning and progression.

CONNECTIVE TISSUE

Connective tissue functions as (1) a fibrous container for soft tissues, (2) a vehicle for transmitting mechanical forces, and (3) a highway for blood vessels and nerves. Connective tissue is composed of a variety of cells in a complex matrix of collagen and ground substance, each appearing in various proportions and combinations, making classification difficult.[1] Distinct connective tissue types are linked by transitional forms; and even in the adult one type of connective

tissue may be directly transformed into another, to some degree, with the appropriate stimulus. There is a continual turnover by breakdown and replacement of the various components of connective tissue as well as subsequent reorganization of their connections and relations to each other enhanced by the stresses of activity.

The descriptive terms are usually derived from the arrangement of the fibrous components of connective tissue. If the fibers are loosely woven or densely packed, we speak of "loose" or "dense" connective tissue, respectively. The fibers in tendons and ligaments are arranged regularly and are referred to as "dense, organized connective tissue."

Quick Facts

CONNECTIVE TISSUE COMPONENTS

- Collagen
- Ground substance
  -Protoglycans
  -Water
- Cells

In addition, there are a number of connective tissue types with special properties that are modifications of the basic loose connective tissue, e.g., mucous connective tissue, elastic tissue, and adipose tissue. To understand the pathology that occurs in joints and tendons, it is helpful to examine more closely the three main elements that make up connective tissue: fibers, ground substance, and cells.

Connective Tissue

Fibers

The key to the strength of connective tissue is the unique configuration of the collagen molecule. Collagen is a connective tissue protein that has a triple helical structure and a repetitive amino acid sequence (glycine-x-y) in which x is often proline and y frequently hydroxyproline.[2,3] The individual collagen polypeptide chains assemble into the basic building block of the collagen fiber (Fig. 4-1). This soluble

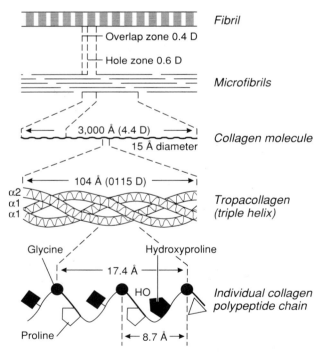

Fig. 4-1. Relation between a single α-polypeptide chain, a triple helix, the collagen molecule, and the fully developed fibril. The characteristic feature of a collagen molecule is its rigid, long, narrow, rod-like structure that is created by tight winding of three α-chains into a triple helix, termed ''tropocollagen.'' (Adapted from Prockop et al.,[2] with permission.)

triple-helix molecule was traditionally referred to as tropocollagen.[3] Strands of collagen molecules (tropocollagen) are assembled to form microfibrils, which in turn amalgamate into the orderly aggregate known as the collagen fibril.[3] The one-fourth overlap or staggering of the collagen molecules in the fibril gives a distinctive appearance. The zones between the overlap form important sites for crystal production in calcified connective tissues, e.g., bone. The attachment between fibers, giving strength to the tissue, is influenced by mechanical tension, motion, or the lack of these stimuli.

Ground Substance

The ground substance, although appearing amorphous, has important chemical and physical properties. It binds all the other elements together. It is through the ground substance that nutrition must diffuse to keep the connective tissue viable and adaptable to stress. Furthermore, the charged particles on the side chains of the molecules produce much of the shock-absorbing quality of the specialized connective tissue framework seen in articular cartilage. The main ground substance elements are the proteoglycans, formerly called protein polysaccharides.

Glycosaminoglycans, which form the major carbohydrate component of all proteoglycans, are composed of repeating disaccharide molecules.[3] Chondroitin sulfate A, dermatan sulfate (formerly called chondroitin sulfate B), keratan sulfate, and hyaluronic acid (hyaluronate) are the predominant glycosaminoglycans in the extracellular matrix of organized connective tissue.[3]

> ## Quick Fact
> ### GLYCOSAMINOGLYCANS OF GROUND SUBSTANCE
>
> Hyaluronic acid forms a core for binding proteoglycan subunits of keratan sulfate and chondroitin sulfate.

Whereas all of the glycosaminoglycans show varying degrees of polymerization, hyaluronic acid has the longest chain length, with 40 to 4,000 disaccharide units.[4] This hyaluronic acid frequently forms a core to which proteoglycan subunits of keratan or chondroitin sulfate may bind through link proteins to form large aggregates (Fig. 4-2).

In general, tissues such as ligaments and tendons, which are composed mainly of type I collagen and subjected to tensile forces, do not contain appreciable amounts of the huge proteoglycan aggregates that are characteristic of articular cartilage. By contrast, articular cartilage has mainly type II collagen and an abundance of proteoglycan aggregates. The charged molecules on the side chains, in affiliation with water, combine to give much of the resilience, low friction, and wear characteristics of joint surfaces.

The protein core is synthesized in the rough endoplasmic reticulum of the fibroblast in ligaments and tendons and the chondrocyte of articular cartilage. Extension and sulfation of the glycosaminoglycan chains commence in the smooth endoplasmic reticulum and are completed and transported in the Golgi apparatus. These chains are then excreted into the extracellular matrix.

The ground substance is clinically significant to the clinician in at least three ways: First, the proportions

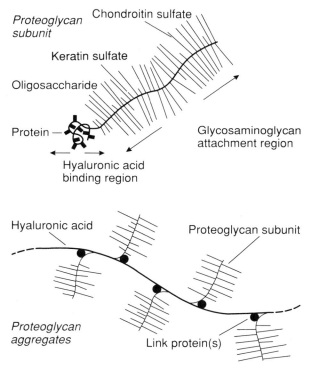

Fig. 4-2. (A) Typical proteoglycan subunit, whose protein core consists of a hyaluronic acid-binding region and a glycosaminoglycan attachment region. Chondroitin sulfate and keratan sulfate are the dominant proteoglycans and are found only in the latter region; short oligosaccharides are present in both regions. **(B)** Proteoglycan aggregate consists of a central hyaluronic acid filament to which numerous proteoglycan subunits attach via their binding regions. This interaction is strengthened by the presence of link proteins.

Quick Facts

CONNECTIVE TISSUE

Fibers	• Triple helix collagen molecule
	• Assemble into microfibrils
	• Amalgamate into collagen fibers
	• Mainly type I in ligaments and tendons
	• High tensile strength
Ground Substance	• Main elements: proteoglycans and water
	• Glycosaminoglycans comprise major carbohydrate component
	• Acts as barrier to some substances
	• Allows passage of others
	• Facilitates nutrition
	• Gives mechanical properties in compression
Cells	• Fibroblast is main cell in dense connective tissue
	• Produce collagen and ground substance
	• Essential for healing
	• Specific cell populations give the unique characteristics of specialized connective tissue

of the elements making up the ground substance change with age. With advancing years, a gradually larger proportion of chondroitin sulfate is laid down, and water content is reduced. Nutrition is impaired, the mobility of the part is reduced, and the facility for repair is affected. Second, infections, particularly if acute, spread through the ground substance, and movement may enhance this spread. The need for immobilization and rest for acute infections thus becomes obvious and the careful handling of acutely inflamed, noninfected areas a natural sequel. Finally, many of the physiotherapy modalities influence the viscosity of the ground substance by their heating effect. Even without raising the tissue temperature, ultrasound has been shown to decrease the viscosity of colloidal substances, particularly hyaluronic acid, although the exact mechanism is unknown.

Cells

There are numerous varieties of cells that may be found in the ground substance of connective tissue. Some are a fixed, permanent population, whereas others come and go at random or in response to some tissue need. This subject is dealt with only briefly here. For a full account, one must turn to the many excellent texts on histology that are available.[5]

Fibroblasts are regarded as the fixed cells of connective tissue. They are numerous and are responsible for the formation of the fibrous components of connective tissue. They are also implicated in the elaboration of the amorphous ground substance. Fibroblasts assume many morphologic forms but for the most part are spindle shaped. They retain the ability to grow and regenerate throughout life and may show a certain mobility in response to trauma and inflammation. They are intimately involved in the healing process.

Macrophages, variously termed histiocytes, are particularly numerous in loose connective tissue. They are freely mobile and play an important role in the reticuloendothelial system. They are active scavengers, engulfing dead cells, bacteria, and foreign particles. They may amalgamate to form the various giant cells seen in pathologic conditions. They also release many of the mediators that generate the inflammatory response.

Mast cells, usually found near blood vessels, are the center of much speculation. They produce the anticoagulant heparin, or at least a substance similar to it. They have also been shown to contain histamine and serotonin. These vasoactive substances are known as kinins and are important in the control of blood flow through an area, particularly in the inflammatory process.

In addition to the cells outlined above, most circulating blood cells may be found in the connective tissue under various circumstances. Most noteworthy are the lymphocytes and polymorphonuclear neutrophils, which are so vital in the cellular and humoral defense systems.

Quick Facts

CONNECTIVE TISSUE CLASSSIFICATION

Tissue Class	Example
Loose	Subcutaneous tissue
Dense	Fascia, muscle sheaths
Organized	Ligaments, tendons
Specialized	Cartilage, bone

Organization

Loose Connective Tissue

Loose or areolar connective tissue forms between organs and other structures where motion is necessary, such as small joint capsules, fascia, thin intermuscular layers, and subcutaneous tissue (Fig. 4-3). It allows movement through limited distances. It is important to realize that loose connective tissue adapts by shortening if there is no motion and, conversely, elongates slowly under prolonged tension. It varies considerably in its strength depending on the proportion of fibers present, which is largely dictated by the functional needs of the anatomic site.

Loose connective tissue develops from the mesenchyme, which remains after all the other types of connective tissue have been formed. Like a collapsed sponge, in some sites it contains innumerable potential cavities that can easily be filled artificially with liquid or air.[5] These structures are the "cells" of the early anatomists, who coined the term "areolar tissue." The network of collagen and reticular fibers runs in all directions and forms a loose mesh that allows great flexibility for movement. When these fibers are laid down or replaced, their length and mobility between attachments depend on the motion of the part during the period of formation (Fig. 4-3).

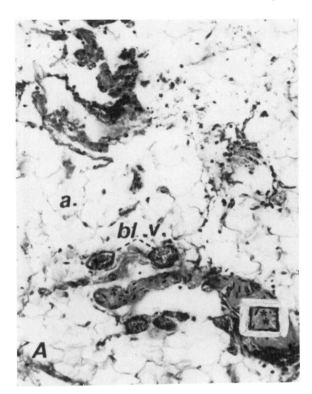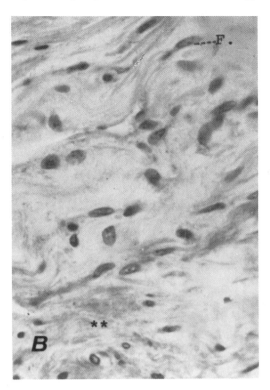

Fig. 4-3. Human loose connective tissue from two regions of the thigh. **(A)** Large proportion of adipose tissue is present. ×125. **(B)** More densely packed collagen. ×300. Adipose, bl.v-blood vessel; F-fibroblast; ** = collagen.

In certain anatomic locations the loose connective tissue contains networks of highly branched reticular or reticulin fibers. This situation occurs where connective tissue is adjacent to other tissues. For instance, reticular fibers are attached over the entire external surface of the sarcolemma of each muscle fiber so that some resistance to motion is provided through the reticular fibers to the surrounding connective tissue. How much of the force of muscular contraction is dissipated through these reticular fibers is unknown, but in conditions of fibrosis it is increased significantly. It is worth restating that when a part is immobilized the collagenous reticular fibers become contracted, with shortening of the distance between attachments within the network. As a result, the tissue becomes dense and hard, with loss of the suppleness of normal areolar tissue.

Dense, Irregular Connective Tissue

Dense, irregular connective tissue is found in areas where relatively little motion of a tissue is desired. It is prominent in the dermis of the skin and in the large

fascial planes and thick muscle sheaths (Fig. 4-4). The collagenous bundles form a dense meshwork, are thick, and are accompanied by more elastic fibers than the loose connective tissue (Fig. 4-5). This type of connective tissue is also laid down in scars. If motion is maintained during healing of a wound, connective tissue of the areolar type develops. If the wound is immobilized, dense, contracted scar forms. In edematous, immobilized areas there is a likelihood of dense connective tissue developing. It follows therefore that edema must be minimized and movement started early and continued during the period of healing if normal motion is to be restored efficiently after injury or surgery.

Dense, Organized Connective Tissue

Structurally, dense connective tissue is 78 percent water, 20 percent collagen, and 2 percent glycosaminoglycans (GAGs). Essentially, collagen forms 70 percent of the dry weight, turning over slowly with a half-life of 300 to 500 days.[4]

It is this tissue that makes up tendons and ligaments

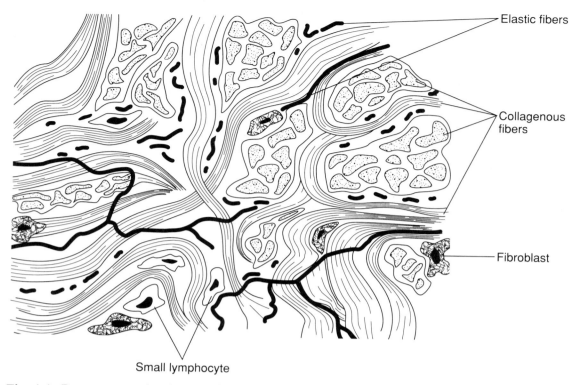

Fig. 4-4. Dense connective tissue as found in the dermis of the skin, large fascial planes, and muscle sheaths. Large bundles of collagen fibers are evident.

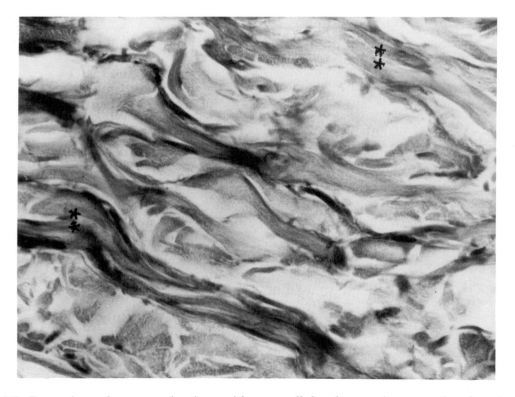

Fig. 4-5. Dense, irregular connective tissue with some cellular elements is present, but there is a large proportion of collagen fibers. Two collagen bundles are marked. ×300.

(Fig. 4-6). The collagenous bundles are arranged according to a definite plan. The particular arrangement reflects the mechanical requirements of the particular tissue. For example, in tendon, the fibers are seen to be arranged linearly, mostly paralleling the long axis of the muscle (Fig. 4-7). This arrangement is stimulated by motion; and, as with most tissues of the body, the structure is defined by functional needs.

Ligament collagen is mainly comprised of fibrillar type I collagen, with less than 10 percent being type III collagen. Ligaments are named on the basis of gross structural features.[6] Most are identified according to their bony attachment (e.g., coracoacromial ligament), their gross function (capsule), their relations to the joint (collateral), their shape (deltoid), or their arrangement with respect to another ligament (cruciate). Functional subdivision of these ligaments into separate entities has the effect of doubling the number of named discrete ligaments.

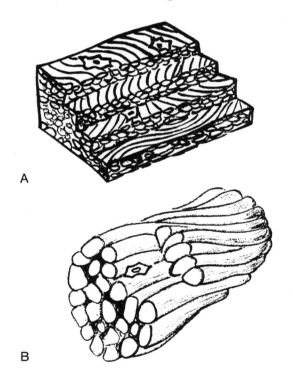

Fig. 4-6. Dense organized connective tissue. **(A)** Ligament shows bundles of densely packed collagen going in slightly different directions but primarily organized according to the main biomechanical stresses. **(B)** Tendon arranged linearly, accounting for the extremely high tensile strength. (Redrawn from Warwick and Williams.[7])

The unit of tendon is the fibril, which amalgamates into fascicles with a well defined crimp pattern.[7,8] These fascicles in turn form the gross tendon, which may or may not be enveloped with a well defined paratenon or sheath of synovium (Fig. 4-8).

> **Quick Facts**
>
> **DENSE ORGANIZED CONNECTIVE TISSUE**
>
> - Ligaments, tendons, some capsules
> - Composed of 78% water, 20% collagen, 2% GAGs
> - Collagen forms 70% of dry weight
> - Histologic arrangements reflect functional requirements

Mechanical properties of ligaments are influenced by numerous factors including age, temperature, activity, and disease.[9-11] Akeson et al. have demonstrated that the ligament substance of mature animals is superior to that of immature ones, particularly at the bone–ligament interface.[12] Activity and external physical heating modalities influence the mechanical properties of collagen. In general, ligaments become stiffer with cold and exhibit increased extensibility with heat, usually in a linear fashion.[13] Cyclic loading also allows the collagen of ligaments to stress-relax and creep, which are the desirable mechanical viscoelastic properties achieved by warming and stretching prior to vigorous activity.

Leonardo da Vinci, with his usual astute power of observation, wrote in one of his notebooks that tendons must carry out as much work as is entrusted to them. Normally the transmitted tension from muscle contraction falls well within the limits of the tendon's working capacity and its range of relative extensibility.

Despite their flexibility, collagenous fibers offer great resistance to a pulling force. Their breaking point in human tendon is several hundred kilograms per square centimeter, and their elongation at this point is only slight (Fig. 4-9).[3] The tensile strength of collagen has been estimated at 50 to 125 newtons/mm². Some studies of human collagen report a load for failure at 91 kg force (kgf); for plantar fascia it is 40 kgf.

Elliott, in a 1967 paper on the biomechanical

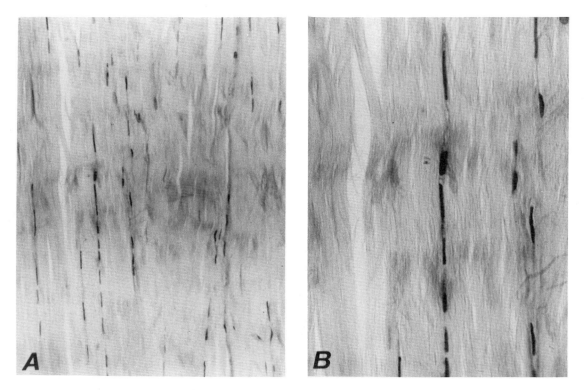

Fig. 4-7. Section of human tendon showing the regular arrangement of collagen and the tendency to a crimp pattern. **(A)** ×125. **(B)** ×300.

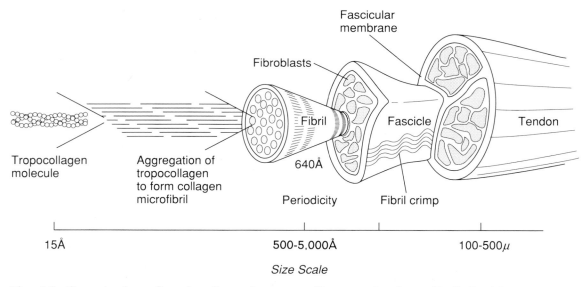

Fig. 4-8. Organization of tendon from the tropocollagen molecule to fibril, fascicles, and gross tendon structure. The presence of crimping or waveform is evident at the fascicle level. (Adapted from Bersch and Bauer,[9] with permission.)

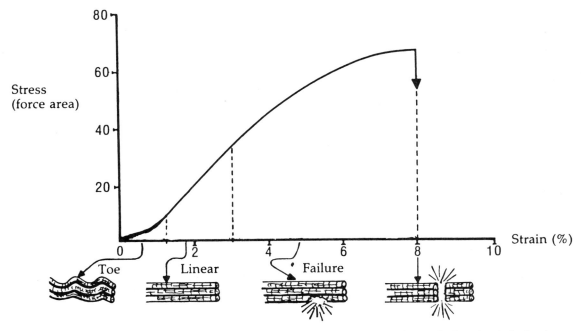

Fig. 4-9. Typical stress-strain curve for tendon. There is a transition through the elastic behavior at the toe, then plastic recoverable deformation until partial sufficient stress leads to complete failure of the tendon.

properties of tendon in relation to muscle strength, stated that the maximum contraction of a muscle may exceed the tendon's range of relative extensibility.[10] By this statement he meant the total elimination of the normal waveform a tendon assumes when not under stress.[9,11] However, even after the limit of relative extensibility, some semiplastic changes are possible owing to sliding of collagen fibers. The tensile strength of a healthy tendon is usually more than twice the strength of its muscle.

Quick Facts

FACTORS INFLUENCING LIGAMENT AND TENDONS

- Age and sex
- Skeletal maturity
- Body weight
- Activity type and duration
- Temperature
- Drugs (steroids, growth hormone)
- Trauma (micro and macro)
- Disease (collagen disorders, infection, inflammation)

Insertion of Ligaments and Tendons

Insertion of ligaments and tendons into bone commonly progresses from fibril, to fibrocartilage, to mineralized fibrocartilage, to bone. In some areas ligaments insert directly into bone via the periosteum.[14,15] Functional loading during activity maintains the strength and integrity of these transition zones.

In bone-ligament-bone preparations, ligaments are always weakest at or near their attachment to bone. The exceptions are the elderly osteoporotic person, in whom the bone tends to fail with stress, and the adolescent, in whom epiphyseal separation is common.[16] It has been established that training increases the absolute separation force, but it takes time.

This weakness may play a role in the susceptibility to ligament tears in the unconditioned athlete and the propensity to tendinitis with excessively rapid progression of intensity and duration of activity. An important clinical point is that, upon attainment of a given strength, ligaments are not readily weakened by detraining, provided some minimal stress or weight bearing is allowed. This point emphasizes the role of functional bracing and modified activity, as ligamentous weakening and bone resorption at attachment

---

Practice Points

EFFECTS OF ACTIVITY ON NORMAL TENDON AND LIGAMENTS

- Mechanical — Stress affects collagen alignment
- Hormonal — Anabolic stimulation with exercise: thyroid-stimulating hormone, testosterone, and growth hormone
- Histologic — Increased numbers of collagen fibers, larger fiber diameter
- Biochemical — Increased collagen turnover as measured by hydroxyproline assays
- Anatomic — Resorption of bony attachment sites with inactivity; changes in the mucopolysaccharides that are known to be essential for proper anchorage affected by exercise

---

sites do occur to a significant extent during 6-week cast immobilization unless specific therapy is directed at counteracting these events.[16,17]

HEALING OF COLLAGENOUS STRUCTURES

For ease of description the stages of healing are somewhat artificially divided into reaction phase, regeneration phase, and remodeling phase.[18]

Reaction Phase

The reaction phase encompasses the initial inflammatory response to trauma common to all tissues. It includes the previously described events of vasodilation, exudation of tissue fluids, extravasation of blood, secondary reactive edema, stimulation of pain fibers, chemotaxis of cells necessary for phagocytosis of debris and gearing up of the immune response, and finally the initiation of cell division and production of the elements required for early healing. These exaggerated tissue responses manifested by swelling, pain, and loss of function are minimized by the early recognition and assessment of the severity of the injury, rest, elevation, the application of cooling modalities, and the appropriate splinting and protected weight bearing. By as early as 10 minutes after injury this process is well established and peaks over the subsequent 24 hours. Well treated, this process may be minimized so there is no inhibition or delay in the early onset of the regeneration phase.[18] For ligaments, different rates of loading may influence the site of rupture, with rapid rates tending to produce tears and slower rates predisposing to avulsion from bone.[17]

Practice Point

HEALING OF CONNECTIVE TISSUE

Reaction phase

- Vasodilation, exudation, edema, and hemorrhage
- Pain and chemotaxis
- Ice, elevation, compression, NSAIDs
- Modified rest

Regeneration Phase

The regeneration phase encompasses elimination of debris, revascularization, and fibroblastic proliferation.

Elimination of Debris

The lowered oxygen tension in edematous or damaged tissue results in phagocytosis by granulocytes. Protection of the devitalized tissue from infection is also related to macrophage activity. To be effective, phagocytosis of bacteria requires opsonification by an antibody in the plasma. These antibodies combine with surface antigens to form antigen–antibody complexes, activating the complement system. The cascade of enzymic reactions that follows leads to membranolysis of bacteria, which are thus prepared for ingestion into the granulocyte by phagocytosis. The hydrolytic enzymes in the cell's lysosomes may then effectively deal with the bacteria. Similarly, these granulocytes have proteases, nucleases, and collagenases, which allow dissolution of other debris.

Whereas the granulocyte is the predominant cell in the wound for the first few days after trauma or inflammation, macrophages predominate from the fifth day. These cells are large and mobile and, like granulocytes, are capable of surviving in areas of low oxygen tension. They ingest macromolecules, converting them to amino acids and sugars. It is also probable that these cells assist in activation of endothelial cells and fibroblasts. Their numbers depend on adequate amounts of vitamin A, and their function is inhibited by corticosteriods.

Revascularization

Where inflammation is ongoing or in the presence of damaged tissue, oxygen deprivation indirectly stimulates and promotes neovascularization. Capillary buds form in the walls of functioning vessels surrounding the pathologic or damaged area. These buds grow and combine with other similar offshoots to form a capillary loop. They may form new circuits or connect with existing vessels. Initially, the basal membrane is still incomplete, and leakage occurs. Only when the new vessels are strengthened by products of the fibroblasts are they able to withstand increasing blood pressure and reduce the tendency to edema formation.

Fibroblast Proliferation

Fibroblasts are attracted to the area and often migrate along the newly formed capillaries. By day 4 after trauma an intense, irritational inflammation is established, and the fibroblasts begin to produce collagen. Hypoxia and acidosis turn on the fibroblast, but oxygen is necessary for the production of collagen.

Collagen synthesis begins with the lining up of amino acids according to the code stored in the DNA of the nucleus (Fig. 4-9). Messenger DNA provides the correct template of this sequence, and transfer RNA transports these amino acids to their place on the ribosomes in the cell's cytoplasm. Glycine is a major amino acid constituent.[3] One of the unique features of collagen is the presence of hydroxyproline and hydroxylysine, which assemble on the ribosomes, provided there is sufficient oxygen and cofactors such as vitamin C, α-ketoglutarate, and iron.[3,4] The next step involves the incorporation of two α-polypeptide chains and one right-handed α_2-helical chain into a left-handed superhelix (Fig. 4-10). This procollagen molecule undergoes glycosylation in the Golgi apparatus, separating the terminal peptides and producing the shorter tropocollagen (Table 4-1).[4]

The tropocollagen molecules, 3,000 Å (280 nm) long and 15 Å (1.4 nm) wide, are aggregated as they are extruded from the cell into bundles of overlapping molecules (one-fourth overlapped), which form collagen fibers (Fig. 4-10). This configuration gives the apparent periodicity on microscopic examination of 686 Å (64 nm).[5] Initially held together by weak hydrogen bonds, over a few days the strength increases with the stability of the intra- and intermolecule bonds.

Remodeling Phase

The remodeling phase usually lasts at least 6 months; it is initially characterized by contraction of the scar and subsequently by maturation of the collagen. It manifests as a slow increase in tensile strength as the collagen fibers become oriented and form stable mucopolysaccharide bonds. Fibroblasts apparently transform into myofibroblasts, which are capable of forming intercellular bonds by means of desmosomes. They are also able to contract owing to the presence of contractile proteins (actomyosin). The process of contraction and shrinking of the scar continues as long as the elasticity of the surrounding fibers allow. Contraction of scar is an asset in that it decreases the size of the defect in torn tissue; however, it may limit motion and cause pain, so gentle stretching is necessary throughout the healing process.

The strength and quantity of connective tissue in

Practice Points

HEALING OF CONNECTIVE TISSUE

Regeneration phase

- Minimize edema
- Protect neovascularization
- Limit duration of inflammatory response
- Stimulate protein production

Remodeling phase

- Minimize immobilization
- Balance increasing functional stresses with increasing tissue strength
- Re-establish range
- Enhance proprioception

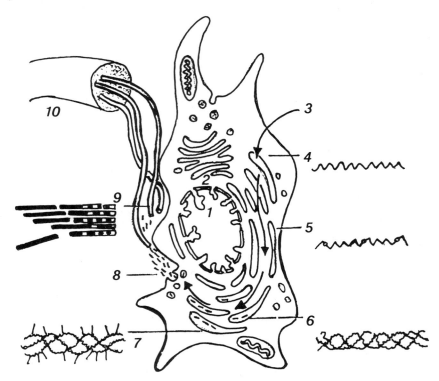

Fig. 4-10. Major steps in collagen synthesis by fibroblasts in connective tissue. (1) Encoding of DNA by mRNA. (2) Transcription into RNA molecule for protein template. (3) Amino acids enter cell. (4) Assembly of polypeptide chains on ribosomes. (5) Hydroxylation of proline and lysine on polypeptide chain. (6) Triple helix assembly into procollagen molecule. (7) Addition of carbohydrate moiety in Golgi apparatus. (8) Cleavage of terminal peptide and passage into extracellular space. (9) Aggregation of tropocollagen to form fibrils. (10) Aggregation of fibrils to form collagen bundles. (Adapted from Warwick and Williams,[7] with permission.)

TABLE 4-1. Ligament Healing Events

Event	Comment
Fibroblast proliferation	Continuing up to 5 days after injury
Amino acid chain assembly in ribosomes	Nuclear DNA switched on for collagen biosynthesis Hydroxylation of amino acid proline to hydroxyproline Requires oxygen, vitamin C, ferrous iron
Extrusion of collagen from fibroblasts	Newly formed collagen leaves fibroblast Rendered insoluble by enzymic cleavage Polymerization occurs
Cross-linking	Occurs on specific sites, giving mature collagen a recognizable structure Usually desirable, but in excess contributes to scarring and adhesions
Orientation	Occurs along lines of stress Provides high tensile strength Active over many months May be affected by activity and electrical stimulation
Binding of glycosaminoglycans	Enables formation of a stable compound of collagen as the mucopolysaccharide ground substance

the wound increases considerably over the first 3 weeks after injury. At the end of this period, the quantity of collagen tends to stabilize. On the other hand, the strength of the fibers continues to increase for several months, probably by further increases in cross-bonding and the replacement of old molecules by new ones in a more organized pattern. At 4 months after injury there is still a turnover of collagen, but the balance of lysis and production is such that the scar does not continue to thicken. The collagen is now in a state that allows maintenance of any mobility that has been achieved.

Previous studies have demonstrated that the tensile properties of the tendons and ligaments during the healing process respond to changes in physiologic stress and motion.[1,18,19] Tensile strength and stiffness are enhanced with carefully progressed exercise and decrease with prolonged immobilization.[20,21] Electrical stimulation by an implanted low amperage, direct current apparatus has produced some acceleration of initial healing of tendon as demonstrated by stiffness.[22] However, the degree of acceleration is probably not significant in the ultimate clinical functional outcome.[23,24] A more interesting finding was the decrease in relative proportion of type III collagen.[23] Type I collagen is desirable, as it is considered to contribute most effectively to the strength in ligamentous structures, whereas type III contributes to ligamentous elasticity. In the normal wound healing process, the type III to type I ratio changes dramatically with time, and electrical stimulation seems to enhance this process.

In view of some of the dramatic results reported for hydroxyproline incorporation, collagen type, and tensile strength with implanted electrodes, the possible action of electromagnetic fields generated by external sources should be an area of considerable interest to the therapist in terms of both the healing potential after rupture of a ligament and the management of tendinitis.[25-28]

Ligaments have, in the past, been viewed as passive structures. Substantial evidence exists, however, that ligaments, as well as other periarticular structures, serve important roles as signal sources for the reflex systems of the locomotor apparatus[6] (Table 4-2). If the evidence of their importance as mechanoreceptors is valid, more effort should be made to substitute for their function once this function is disrupted by trauma.[26] The introduction of significant amounts of proprioceptive training in rehabilitation programs following ligament injury or surgery is essential.

CLASSIFICATION OF SOFT TISSUE INJURY

Ligament Trauma

Ligament injury is classically divided into first (mild), second (moderate), and third (severe) degree tears (Table 4-3). In a few locations, e.g., the acromioclavicular joint, there is further classification of the degree of displacement and the amount of associated muscle trauma, but these joints are the exception.

First degree injuries entail microscopic stretching or minimal tearing of a few fibers of a ligament. It is a painful injury, but there is little loss of structural integrity. The treatment progress is guided mainly by the athlete's pain, with anticipated return to full physical activity within 10 days to 2 weeks. Indeed, controlled training may be carried out even before

TABLE 4-2. Classification of Articular Receptor Systems

Type	Morphology	Behavior
I	Fibrous capsule of joint (mainly superficial layers)	Static and dynamic receptors; low threshold; slow adapting
II	Fibrous capsule of joint (mainly deeper layers) Articular fat pads	Dynamic mechanoreceptors; high threshold; rapidly adapting
III	Joint ligaments	Dynamic mechanoreceptors; high threshold; very slowly adapting
IV	Fibrous capsule Articular fat pads Ligaments Blood vessel walls	Pain receptors, high threshold, nonadapting

(Modified from Wyke,[26] with permission.)

this point. Early protection of the joint with taping or orthoses may be desirable, and frequently little or no interruption of training is necessary.

It is the second degree injury, with moderate tearing of the ligament's collagenous fibers and some loss of structural integrity, that usually presents the most difficulty for accurate classification. In part it is because the second degree category encompasses a broad spectrum of injury. At the one extreme there is an injury similar to a first degree sprain and at the other a badly torn ligament that is bordering on complete disruption. Underestimating this second degree injury and thus allowing premature resumption of activity may lead to reinjury or possibly conversion to a third-degree situation. Conversely, overestimation of the severity gives rise to unnecessary loss of time from training. These clinical decisions are always difficult, and there is no substitution for the physician's or therapist's experience.

In general, second degree tears require 2 to 3 weeks of modified rest and rehabilitation, followed by 2 to 3 weeks of controlled introduction of increasing stress before full training is resumed. It may be as long as 2 to 3 months before full training and competition are allowed, depending on the joint involved, the magnitude of the disruption, and the requirements and stresses of the sport. The more severe second degree tears, along with the third degree injuries, may have a tendency for the healed ligaments to stretch out with time, leading to increasing functional instability, despite excellent rehabilitation and satisfactory early stability.

A third degree injury signifies complete tearing of the ligament with loss of structural integrity. In many situations, it requires complete or modified immobilization of the involved joint for a period of 3 to 6 weeks and frequently surgical intervention. Failure to treat these third-degree disruptions adequately leads to recurrent instability and possibly degenerative changes of the involved joint. This long-term implication of degenerative articular surface pathology in inadequately treated or incompletely healed major weight-bearing joints cannot be overemphasized.

It has already been stressed that each structure has an anticipated healing time, and that one cannot accelerate the normal recuperative abilities of the tissues. Therefore therapy is aimed at optimizing healing conditions. With extraarticular collagenous structures, ligamentous strength after tearing is in the region of 60 to 70 percent of normal after 6 weeks of healing. More specifically, there is often a revascularization phase during healing that is usually accompanied by a dramatic reduction of tensile strength. Because this phase usually coincides with the period during which most external supports have been removed, it is mandatory that the therapist be aware of the dangers of unduly stretching healing structures at this point. It requires considerable knowledge and skill to balance exercise progression with protection of the vulnerable tissue. It may take up to 3 months before 80 percent of the original strength is acquired. Intra-articular ligaments usually gain tensile strength more slowly. Healing times for intra-articular collagen are such that it may take up to 3 months to achieve 50 percent of the normal strength and 6 months before a functional strength of 70 percent is reached.[15,16] The reintroduction of stress to the unprotected joints must be planned with these figures in mind. Furthermore, although little is known of the effects of ligament tears on the neural protective mechanism of joints, it is likely that after significant tears there is distorted or decreased biofeedback (Table 4-2). Particularly for the major weight bearing joints, such as the knee and ankle, some specific exercises are needed to either retrain or compensate for this potential loss of sensory information.

Tendinitis and Tendon Rupture

Inflammatory conditions of the tendons may be acute or chronic. The pathologic reaction is located mainly in the tendon sheath, with tenosynovitis, tenovaginitis, or paratendinitis.

Chronic inflammation may precipitate varying degrees of degenerative change in the tendon itself, referred to as tendinosis. The latter may be associated with structural weakening and predispose to partial or complete tendon rupture. Rupture can also occur when sufficient force is applied to normal tendons.

Normal tendon is characterized by enormous tensile strength. The crimped, ultrastructural makeup of tendon means that initial stresses are accommodated by straightening out the crimped arrangement of the collagen fibers (Fig. 4-9). Greater loads stress the fibers themselves. Most day-to-day activity and even stressful sporting maneuvers are accommodated in the toe region and early in the linear phase of the stress strain curve for tendon. The linear phase represents ligamentous elasticity, and deformation is reversible. At the high ends of functional loading, plastic deformation and even microfailure may occur. Repetitive loading in this range contributes to ten-

TABLE 4-3. Ligament Injuries

Grade	Signs	Implications
First degree (mild)	Minimal loss of structural integrity No abnormal motion Little or no swelling Localized tenderness Minimal bruising	Minimal functional loss Early return to training—some protection may be necessary
Second degree (moderate)	Significant structural weakening Some abnormal motion Solid end feel to stress More bruising and swelling Often associated hemarthrosis and effusion	Tendency to recurrence Need protection from risk of further injury May need modified immobilization May stretch out further with time
Third degree (complete)	Loss of structural integrity Marked abnormal motion Significant bruising Hemarthrosis	Needs prolonged protection Surgery may be considered Often permanent functional instability

dinitis. Prolonged repetitive motion and insufficient rest may create a situation where the collagen is unable to repair the resulting microtrauma and inflammation, or there is a possible danger of major tearing. Hence tendon pathology may be classified as inflammatory lesions, degenerative changes, or structural damage rupture (Table 4-4).

The inflammatory lesions of tendons, as with bursitis, may be classified into five functional grades based mainly on the degree to which the problem interferes with activity (Table 4-5). The implication of this classification is that the tendinitis can usually be treated with modification of the duration and intensity of the training sessions in grade I, II, and III injuries. Tendinitis of a grade IV severity usually requires discontinuation of the specific aggravating factor completely and substitution with some other physical pursuit to maintain strength and fitness. Grade V tendinitis requires significant restriction of activities and in some cases, if it is resistant to prolonged nonoperative treatment, some form of surgical intervention (Table 4-5).

TABLE 4-4. Tendon Injury Classification

Pathology[a]	Degree
Inflammatory	Acute versus chronic
Degenerative	Tendinosis versus cystic degeneration
Rupture	Partial versus complete

[a] Pathologic changes are not mutually exclusive to each category.

Impending tendon rupture requires a high index of suspicion for diagnosis, and often special tests such as ultrasonography, computed tomography, and magnetic resonance imaging are necessary for confirmation. Once diagnosed, radical alteration in activity pattern is mandatory, and occasionally surgical treatment is prudent. Complete ruptures are usually associated with loss of power or of a specific active motion. Nevertheless, these injuries are frequently overlooked, making definitive treatment difficult and complex. The history of feeling or hearing a snap should alert the physician or therapist, and careful functional testing usually makes the diagnosis obvious. Treatment depends on the tendon involved, the age and goals of the patient, and the duration between rupture and diagnosis.

Pathophysiology of Tendinitis

The events of tendon healing in the case of rupture are similar to those described for ligament healing. There are some specific events occurring with tendinitis, however, that have a bearing on treatment.

The etiology of acute and chronic tendinitis can be varied, but the morphologic changes are similar. The basic feature of overuse injuries of tendons is an inflammation that causes an increase in the permeability of the cell membranes, leading to a direct connection between the intra- and extracellular spaces.[29] Release of the various mediators of inflammation leads to pain and edema. With the subsequent extracellular stasis, there is disturbance of cell metabolism.

TABLE 4-5. Staging of Tendinitis and Overuse Syndrome

Grade	Symptoms	Treatment
I	Pain only after activity Does not interfere with performance Often generalized tenderness Disappears before next exercise session	Modification of activity Assessment of training pattern Possibly NSAIDs
II	Minimal pain with activity Does not interfere with intensity or distance Usually localized tenderness	Modification of activity Physical therapy; NSAIDs; consider orthotics
III	Pain interferes with activity Usually disappears between sessions Definite local tenderness	Significant modification of activity Assess training schedule Physical therapy; NSAIDs[a]; consider orthotics
IV	Pain does not disappear between activity sessions Seriously interferes with intensity of training Significant local sign of pain, tenderness, creptitus, swelling	Usually need to temporarily discontinue aggravating motion Design alternate program May require splinting Physical therapy and NSAIDs
V	Pain interferes with sport and activities of daily living Symptoms often chronic or recurrent Signs of tissue changes and altered associated muscle function	Prolonged rest from activity NSAIDs plus other medical therapies[b] Consider splint or cast Physical therapy May require surgery

[a] In some circumstances, injection of steroids into the tendon sheath may be considered, along with other medications such as heparin.

[b] Occasionally, systemic steroids are used with appropriate reference to the benefit/risk ratio.

The residue of chronic edema leads to secondary changes in the paratendineal tissue and the tendon itself.

With acute paratenonitis (peritendinitis), modified activity, ultrasound application, and anti-inflammatory medications may rapidly resolve the problem, with relatively little residual scarring or change in the tendon. With a more intense inflammatory response, peritendinitis crepitant is a common phenomenon, often going on to chronic peritendinitis if not treated aggressively. Heparin injected into the sheath may be added to the therapeutic regimen because it counteracts the precipitation of fibrinogen to fibrin as well as having anti-inflammatory properties. Its use inhibits the formation of, and even perhaps lyses, existing adhesions.

Chronic peritendinitis occurs when the fibrin from excessive, prolonged edema organizes in the subperitenon space and forms thick, firm adhesions. The peritenon itself grossly hypertrophies, resulting in unhealthy, nonfunctional tissue. Untreated and neglected, the scarring thickens further, almost obliterating the plane between the tendon and its sheath, and making nonoperative treatment almost impossible and surgical treatment difficult or frequently unsuccessful. The tendon feels thickened, often with nodular, enlarged areas that are markedly tender.

Theories based on anecdotal medicine can be attractive, and a relation between women with tendinitis and a history of gynecologic problems related to low estrogen levels has been noted.[30] The role of low estrogen levels in osteoporosis is established, and there may be a similar mechanism in tendinitis. Estrogen has anti-inflammatory and anabolic properties. It has been reported that some patients experiencing a wide variety of tendinitis symptoms may obtain relief with estrogen therapy. Patients should be referred to a gynecologist before commencing therapy, and caution is warranted until studies support the claim that there is truly a synergic role between estrogen levels and tendinitis.

SOFT TISSUE MECHANICS, CONTRACTURES, AND STRETCHING

Poor training techniques, muscle and joint injury, and immobilization after trauma may lead to varying degrees of musculotendinous tightness and joint contractures. These problems represent either the unfavorable outcomes of treatment or insufficient therapy, albeit sometimes unavoidable. Soft tissue mechanics are discussed as a basis for the evolution of treatment regimens. Because joint contractures so frequently accompany muscle tightness, it is appropriate to outline the common principles that may be applied in both situations.

Collagen

It was demonstrated earlier in the chapter that collagen, a fibrous protein with high tensile strength, is organized into the many connective tissue structures of the body, including capsules, tendons, ligaments, and fascial sheaths. Under both normal and pathologic conditions, the range of motion in most joints is limited by connective tissue elements, which also form the principal source of passive resistance to normal motion.[31] Even in muscle there is an extensive connective tissue framework, ensheathing all of the contractile elements. Studies confirm that even for relaxed muscle the connective tissue contributes most of the resistance to passive stretching.[32] Furthermore, after trauma, healing occurs by an unspecialized form of collagen, scar tissue, which frequently causes adhesions and fibrotic contractures that must be dealt with therapeutically.

Definitions

Stretching refers to the process of elongation and may be achieved by either elastic or plastic deformation. Elastic deformation is spring-like, the stretched material recovering its pretensile dimensions after the applied load is removed. Plastic deformation refers to a putty-like behavior, where the linear deformation produced by the tensile stress remains even after the stress is removed. Plastic deformation is nonrecoverable, or permanent, elongation. Materials that have viscous properties are characterized by plastic deformation. Viscoelastic materials exhibit both viscous and elastic behavior, a point that is important to appreciate as connective tissue has viscoelastic properties when submitted to stretch or tensile stress[11] (Fig. 4-11).

When connective tissue is stretched, some of the deformation occurs in the elastic elements and some occurs as plastic deformation in the viscous elements. With withdrawal of the tensile stress, the elastic deformation recovers, but the plastic deformation remains. The deformation of connective tissue varies widely depending on the amount, duration, and speed of application of stress, as well as the tissue temperature. Attempts at gaining a permanent in-

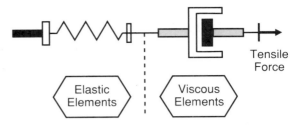

Fig. 4-11. Simplified model of collagenous tissue. Connective tissue is a viscoelastic material: When stretched, it behaves as if it has viscous and elastic elements connected in series. (After Sapega et al.[31])

crease in range of motion should make use of the conditions that are conducive to plastic deformation: (1) increased tissue temperature; (2) slow, prolonged stretching; and (3) long duration. These concepts and the data on which they are based are examined further.[27,28]

High Force Versus Low Force

The amount of stretching achieved by tensile forces is proportional to the amount of force.[27] Also, the corollary that a low force stretching technique requires more time to produce an equal amount of stretching is also true. However, the proportion of tissue lengthening that remains after tensile stress is removed is greater for the low force, long duration method, evidencing its influence on the plastic or viscous elements.[23] High force, short duration stretching favors the recoverable, elastic-type deformation. This principle does not necessarily prohibit the use of high force, prolonged duration stretching, but obviously high force application may generate pain, trigger spasm, and produce tissue rupture.

Practice Point

ELASTIC DEFORMATION	vs.	PLASTIC DEFORMATION
• High forces		• Low forces
• Short duration		• Long duration
• Normal or cold tissue temperature		• Elevated tissue temperature while stretching
		• Cool under tension

Furthermore, elongation of connective tissue is accompanied by some structural weakening, and high force stretching appears to produce more structural weakening for a given amount of stretch. Hence low force, prolonged duration stretching is usually a more comfortable, safer, and effective method.[31]

Temperature

Temperature has a significant effect on the behavior of connective tissue. Therapeutic heat is usually within the range of 102° to 110°F.[33] Using selected modalities to raise connective tissue temperature to 103°F increases the amount of permanent elongation resulting from a given amount of stretching.[32] At 104°F and above there is a thermal transition in the microstructure of collagen that significantly enhances the viscous stress relaxation of collagen tissue, allowing greater plastic deformation.[28,32] The mechanism by which it occurs is probably partial destabilization of the intermolecular bonding, allowing molecules to "creep," thereby enhancing the viscous flow properties of the tissue.[34,35]

Evidently there are also events during the cooling phase that eventually influence the permanent deformation. Tissues that are stretched under heating conditions and then allowed to cool under tensile conditions maintain a greater proportion of their plastic deformation than do structures allowed to cool in the unloaded state. Cooling under tension may allow the collagenous microstructure to stabilize at the new stretched length.[32]

A further point worthy of consideration is the fact that at temperatures within the normal therapeutic range the amount of structural weakening produced by a given amount of connective tissue elongation varies inversely with the temperature.[33] This fact is probably related to the thermal destabilization of the molecular bonds, which allows creeping of the tissue with less structural damage.[27,28,34,36]

SUMMARY

This chapter has stressed the unifying features of connective tissue throughout the body. The dense organized collagen of ligaments and tendons demonstrate clearly where structure subserves function. The replacement of collagen after injury may be strongly influenced by the manner and progression of stresses on the healing tissue. The aim of therapy is to thoroughly understand these sequences of events after trauma and skillfully apply the appropriate stimulus at the correct time so as to enhance the desirable biomechanical endpoints without jeopardizing anatomic integrity. Unfortunately, the clinical signs that reflect these microscopic changes are often vague. Careful microscopic classification of injury and a thorough knowledge of theoretic events provide the physician and therapist with the best chance of making the correct clinical judgment regarding the appropriate use of medications, modalities, and rate of progression of activity.

REFERENCES

1. Reid DC: Functional Anatomy and Joint Mobilization. University of Alberta Press, Edmonton, 1975
2. Prockop DJ, Kivirikko KI, Tiderman L et al: The biosynthesis of collagen and its disorders. N Engl J Med 301:13, 1979
3. Van der Rest M: Collagen structure and biosynthesis in the musculoskeletal system. Embryology, Biochemistry and Physiology.
4. Hardingham TE, Muir H: Binding of hyaluronic acid to proteoglycans. Biochem J 139:565, 1974
5. Bloom W, Fawcett DW: A Testbook of Histology. 9th Ed. WB Saunders, Philadelphia, 1968
6. Woo SLY, Buckwater JA: Injury and repair of the musculoskeletal soft tissues. Am Acad Orthop Surg Workshop, Savannah, GA, June 1987
7. Warwick R, Williams PL: Gray's Anatomy. 36th Ed. Churchill Livingstone, Edinburgh, 1980
8. Curwin S, Stanish WD: Tendinitis: Its Etiology and Treatment. Collamore Press, DC Heath & Co, Lexington, KY, 1984
9. Bersch DF, Bauer E: Structure and mechanical properties of rat tail tendon. Biorheology 17:84, 1980
10. Elliott DH: The biomechanical properties of tendon

Practice Point

MINIMAL STRUCTURAL WEAKENING		MAXIMAL STRUCTURAL WEAKENING
• Low forces	vs.	• High forces
• High temperatures		• Low temperatures
• Slow loading		• Rapid loading

in relation to muscular strength. Ann Phys Med 9:1, 1967

11. Stromberg D, Wiederhielm CA: Visco-elastic description of a collagenous tissue in simple elongation. J Appl Physiol 26:857, 1969

12. Akeson WH, Amsol D, Woo SLY: Cartilage and ligament. In Nicholas JA, Hershman EB (eds): Physiology and Repair Process in the Lower Extremities and Spine in Sports Medicine. CV Mosby, St. Louis, 1986

13. Woo SLY: Mechanical properties of tendons and ligaments. Biorheology 19:385, 1982

14. Laros GS, Tipton CM, Cooper RR: Influence of physical activity on ligament insertions in the knees of dogs. J Bone Joint Surg [Am] 52:257, 1971

15. Cooper RR, Misel S: Tendons and ligament insertion. J Bone Joint Surg [Am] 52:1, 1970

16. Zuckerman J, Stull GA: Ligamentous separation force in rats as influenced by training, detraining. Med Sci Sports: 5:44, 1973

17. Betsch DF, Bauer E: Structure and mechanical properties of rat tail tendon. Biorheology 17:84, 1980

18. Van der Meulen JCH: Present state of knowledge on processes of healing in collagen structures. Int J Sports Med 3:4, 1982

19. Hirsch G: Tensile properties during tendon healing: a comparative study of intact and sutured rabbit peroneus brevis tendons. Acta Orthop Scand [Suppl] 153:1, 1974

20. Noyes FR, Torvik PJ, Hyde WB et al: Biomechanics of ligament. II. An analysis of immobilization, exercise, and reconditioning effects in primates. J Bone Joint Surg [Am] 56:1406, 1974

21. Vailas AC, Tipton CM, Matthes RD et al: Physical activity and its influence on the repair process of medial collateral ligaments. Connect Tissue Res 9:25, 1981

22. Frank C, Schachas N, Dittrich D et al: Electromagnetic stimulation of ligament healing in rabbits. Clin Orthop 175:263, 1983

23. Akai M, Oda H, Shirasaki Y et al: Electrical stimulation of ligament healing: an experimental study of patellar ligament of rabbits. Clin Orthop 235:298, 1988

24. Stanish WD, Rubinovich M, Kozen J et al: The use of electricity in ligament and tendon repair. Phys Sports Med 13:109, 1985

25. Nessler JP, Mass J: Direct current stimulation of tendon in vitro. Clin Orthop 217:303, 1987

26. Wyke B: Articular neurology: a review. Physiotherapy 58:94, 1972

27. Warren CG, Lehmann JF, Koblanski JN: Elongation of rat tail tendon: effect of load and temperature. Arch Phys Med Rehabil 52:465, 1971

28. Warren CG, Lehmann JF, Koblanski JN: Heat and stretch procedures: evaluation using rat tail tendon. Arch Phys Med Rehabil 57:122, 1976

29. Kuist M, Järvinen M: Clinical, histochemical and biomechanical features in repair of muscle and tendon injuries. Int J Sports Med 3:12, 1982

30. Legwold G: Estrogen levels may affect tendinitis. Physician Sports Med 11:25, 1983

31. Sapega AA, Quedenfeld TC, Moyer RA et al: Biophysical factors in range of motion exercise. Physician Sports Med 9:57, 1981

32. Lehmann JF, Masock AJ, Warren CG et al: Effects of therapeutic temperatures on tendon extensibility. Arch Phys Med Rehabil 51:481, 1970

33. Rigby BJ, Hirai N, Spikes JD et al: The mechanical properties of rat tail tendon. J Gen Physiol 43:265, 1959

34. Mason T, Rigby BJ: Thermal transitions in collagen. Biochim Biophys Acta 66:448, 1963

35. Kottke FJ, Parly DL, Ptak KA: The rationale for prolonged stretching for correction of shortening of connective tissue. Arch Phys Med Rehabil 47:345, 1966

36. LaBan MM: Collagen tissue: implications of its response to stress in vitro. Arch Phys Med Rehabil 43:461, 1962

Muscle Injury: Classification and Healing

5

The operations of our intellect tend to geometry
— Henri-Louis Bergson

This chapter outlines the concepts behind the treatment of muscular soft tissue injuries. The principles are broad and easily applied to muscle trauma throughout the body. Because the thigh is the most frequently traumatized muscle mass, these injuries are used frequently to set out the baseline data, and the principles that apply to thigh injuries may be extrapolated in order to devise treatment programs for other muscle groups.

NORMAL MUSCLE

Most descriptions of muscle focus on the contractile elements, the muscle cell or fiber. Muscle, however, is made up of a large volume of noncontractile connective tissue, which surrounds every fiber (endomysium), each bundle of fibers (perimysium), and the whole muscle (epimysial sheath). Toward the origin and insertion, these connective tissue components blend to form tendons of insertion, allowing transmission of the muscular pull to bone. Thus although noncontractile in structure, these connective tissue elements are in reality contractile by function, and their presence and importance must be taken into account during muscle injury and recovery.

The sarcomere, which is the basic contractile unit, includes the actin and myosin myofilaments contained between two Z lines. These myofilaments are arranged in parallel bundles called myofibrils, which are the functional muscle cell or fiber. A group of muscle fibers constitutes the fasciculus, which in turn makes up the muscle contained within perimysial and epimysial sheaths (Fig. 5-1).

Contraction is achieved by successive making and breaking of the cross bridging between the actin and myosin molecules, promoting varying degrees of overlap of these fibers (Fig. 5-2), which in turn is coordinated via an adenosine triphosphate (ATP)-dependent mechanism stimulated by depolarization of the motor endplate. These basic structural considerations are presented to ensure a vocabulary for understanding the changes taking place following muscle injury.

TREATMENT OBJECTIVES

The primary treatment goals after trauma are to minimize further damage, relieve pain and spasm, reduce hemorrhage and edema, promote healing

---

Clinical Point

AIMS OF TREATMENT

- Minimize further damage
- Relieve pain and spasm
- Control hemorrhage and edema
- Promote healing
- Reduce scar formation
- Regain strength
- Regain flexibility
- Retain coordination
- Guide safe return to activity
- Avoid reinjury

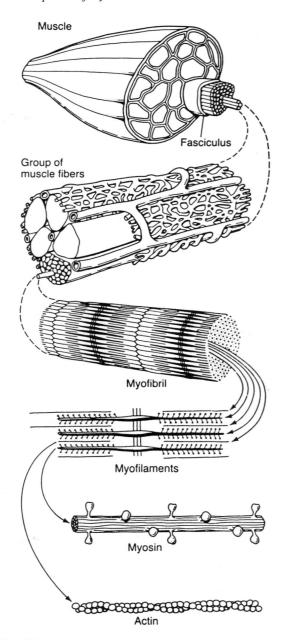

Fig. 5-1. Levels of organization within a muscle. Myofilaments form parallel bundles and constitute the muscle fiber or the cell (myofibril). Individual muscle fibers are surrounded by connective tissue, the endomycium. Groups of fibers make up a fasciculum surrounded by perimycium.

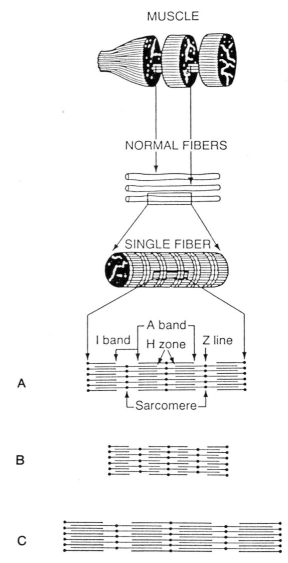

Fig. 5-2. **(A)** Contractile unit of muscle is the sarcomere, the contractile protein between two Z lines. **(B)** With contraction there is overlapping of the actin and myosin molecules. **(C)** With lengthening there is less overlap. The degree of overlap influences the ability to generate tension. (Adapted from Gossman MR, Sahrman SA, Rose S: Phys Ther 62:1800, 1982.)

with minimal scar formation, regain full flexibility, re-educate the strength and balance of power among muscle groups, and return the athlete to training and competition within the shortest possible time. The rate of progress should be such that the risks of reinjury are minimal.

To achieve these aims, a sound knowledge of muscle healing is required. It is also important to understand the events that lead to scar formation, muscle tightness and loss of range of motion, and the biomechanics of restoring normal range of motion.

CLASSIFICATION

A classification of muscle injury must at least include exercise-induced muscle injury, muscle strains, contusions, and avulsions (Table 5-1).

Exercise Induced Muscle Injury

Often referred to as delayed muscle soreness, exercise-induced muscle injury manifests as pain in muscle some 24 to 48 hours after unaccustomed or intense exercise. Excessive eccentric loading seems to magnify the response, which can vary from a mild ache to an almost disabling pain.[1] The pain is related to the breakdown of muscle cells and the associated inflammatory response (Fig. 5-3). Treatment depends on the severity of the discomfort and ranges from a light workout of graded exercises with stretching of the painful muscles to exercises in the whirlpool bath or pool. Occasionally, the reaction is severe enough to warrant rest and anti-inflammatory medications, particularly if just before an important competition.[3]

Clinical Point

RECOGNIZING COMPARTMENT SYNDROMES

- Pain—unremitting at rest
- Pain—on stretching muscle
- Pain—on palpation
- Paresthesia—distribution of involved area
- Pressure—tense to palpation
- Pulses—may be present

Confirm by compartment pressure measurements.

Acute compartment syndromes may result from excessive exercise-induced muscle damage. They occur mostly in the lower limbs, usually the anterior or deep posterior compartments, and more rarely in the upper limbs of weight lifters or body builders.[4] The syndrome of increasing pain, made worse by

TABLE 5-1. Classification of Muscle Injury

Type	Related Factors
Exercise-induced muscle injury (delayed muscle soreness)	Increased activity Unaccustomed activity Excessive eccentric work Viral infections Secondary to muscle cell damage Onset at 24–48 hours after exercise
Strains First degree (mild): minimal structural damage; minimal hemorrhage; early resolution	Sudden overstretch Sudden contraction Decelerating limb Insufficient warm-up Lack of flexibility
Second degree (moderate): partial tear; large spectrum of injury; significant early functional loss	Increasing severity of strain associated with greater muscle fiber death, more hemorrhage, and more eventual scarring
Third degree (severe): complete tear; may require aspiration; may require surgery	Steroid use or abuse Previous muscle injury Collagen disease
Contusions Mild, moderate, severe Intramuscular vs. intermuscular	Direct blow, associated with increasing muscle trauma and tearing of fiber proportionate to severity
Avulsions Bony	Specific sites vulnerable May be complication of stress fractures Osteoporosis
Apophyseal Muscle	Skeletally immature but well developed muscle strength Associated with steroid injection or generalized collagen disorders

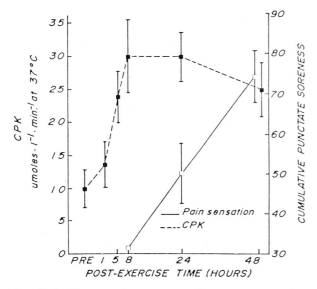

Fig. 5-3. Changes in postexercise serum creatine phosphokinase (CPK) at time intervals up to 48 hours after exercise at 90 percent of 10 repetitions maximum. Increased CPK levels correlated with muscle pain. (After Tiidins and Ianuzzo,[2] with permission.)

is minimal. In some cases, the virus-induced myalgia is associated with an inflammatory myopathy with muscle breakdown (rhabdomyolysis). Intense or even moderate exercise can magnify the effect of the muscle damage considerably, which greatly prolongs the illness; and the athlete may even run the risk of renal damage secondary to myoglobinuria. Myoglobinuria is seen to some degree with all intense exercise, but it rarely produces significant damage. By contrast, breakdown of muscle and kidney and multiple organ system failure have been reported with intense exercise in the presence of a viremia. It is unwise to allow athletes to train if they present with signs and symptoms of a significant bacterial or viral infection, particularly if associated with a fever or myalgia.

Muscle Strains

Muscular injures are classified as mild (first degree), moderate (second degree, partial tears), or severe (third degree, complete tears) (Table 5-2). They may be further subdivided according to site, as tears of the muscle belly usually heal more rapidly than do tears at the musculotendinous junction.

It is difficult to accurately assess the severity of these injuries, as they represent a broad spectrum of pathology. The better prognostic indicators include partial tears of mild to moderate severity in the muscle belly accompanied by minimal bleeding. The poorer prognostic signs include a re-tear and a severe partial or complete injury located in a closed com-

stretching the affected muscle groups and eventually sensory changes, should alert the physician or therapist. The compartment is usually tense and tender to palpation. Failure to recognize these signs and symptoms results in catastrophic permanent loss of the limb or its function. Immediate referral for compartment pressure measurements and possible surgical intervention is indicated by these signs are detected.

There is a special form of exercise-induced muscle trauma that is related to viral infections. Viral myalgia is the aching and lethargic feeling of muscles that accompanies acute viral illness. Usually it is a short-lived phenomenon, and the associated muscle injury

TABLE 5-2. Muscle Strain

Degree	Pain and Spasm	Swelling and Bruising	Defect	Loss of ROM	Loss of Function	Recovery Time (days)[a]
First (mild)	+	Minimal	0	Minimal	Minimal	2–21
Second (moderate)[b]	++	Moderate	0	Significant	Significant	20–90
Third (severe)	+++	Extensive[c]	Present[d]	Severe	Complete[e]	50–180

ROM = range of motion.
[a] Depending on anatomic site and size of muscle. Time to full training or competition.
[b] This group has the largest spectrum of injuries.
[c] May be tense with impending compartment syndrome; bleeding may track extensively.
[d] Defect may rapidly fill up with hematoma.
[e] Functional loss is always significant, but tested motions may be present owing to adjacent intact muscles.

partment with extensive bleeding (Table 5-3). Early clinical signs of significant loss of range and function and a tense, painful swelling are ominous. This degree of injury has the possibility of prolonged disability and the risk of complications of myositis ossificans, prolific scarring, slow resolution, and a danger of reinjury.

The issue of surgical repair of complete tears depends on the muscle involved, the site of the tear or avulsion, and the acuteness of the injury at presentation. For instance, a complete tear of the rectus femoris muscle treated nonoperatively is compatible with full recovery and no measurable impairment of function. By contrast, a complete tear of the triceps brachii should be surgically repaired in order to restore function. A complete rupture of the pectoralis major is usually better repaired in athletes whose sport requires maximum upper limb strength. However, if the athlete presents late, after about 6 weeks, it is possibly better to treat the tear nonoperatively.

Muscle Contusions

In contact sports muscle contusions are more common than muscle strains. With mild contusions, there may be more hematoma than a comparable mild strain. Moderate and severe contusions are difficult to distinguish from tears in that there is a significant amount of damage to muscle fibers after both injuries. Severe contusions may predispose to widespread scarring. Contusions, as with some muscle tears, may be subdivided into intermuscular and intramuscular, a subclassification that pays attention to the site and effects of the accompanying hematoma.[5,6] This grouping is particularly pertinent in the thigh (Fig. 5-4).

Intermuscular Hematomas

Intermuscular hematomas and contusions occur near the large intermuscular septa or muscle facial sheaths. Their location facilitates tracking of the hematoma with gravity and hence early dispersal of the extravasated blood, which minimizes the inflammatory response and the potential scarring; it also allows early resolution (Fig. 5-2). Clinically, the intermuscular hematoma is characterized by rapid disposal of the tense collection of blood, with early migration and tracking of the bruise, or ecchymosis, to the more distal parts of the limb. Depending on the magnitude of the damage, with this early dispersal comes more rapid recovery of range of motion and hence rapid return of function.[5,6]

Intramuscular Hematomas

Intramuscular hematomas secondary to muscle damage usually takes two to three times longer to recover than a comparable intermuscular lesion. The hemorrhage tends to be more confined, the mass often palpable, the inflammatory response greater, and the propensity for myositis ossificans higher. There is also the danger of developing a compartment syndrome in some locations. Restoration of the joint range and subsequent muscle function is proportionately slower. The residual scarring may produce pain

TABLE 5-3. Prognostic Factors for Muscle Injury

Parameter	Positive Prognostic Factors	Negative Prognostic Factors
Site	Belly tears Intermuscular contusions	Musculotendinous junction tears Intramuscular contusions
Severity	Partial tears (1st degree + mild 2nd degree) First injury	Complete tears (severe 2nd degree and 3rd degree tears) Re-tear
Clinical signs	Minimal loss of range Minimal swelling Little pain	Significant loss of range Obvious tense swelling Extreme pain
Complications	Usually preserved function	Loss of function
	Compartment syndrome rare	Compartment syndromes a distinct danger with large bleeds
	Myositis ossificans less likely Often complete resolution Early resolution expected	Myositis ossificans more prevalent Tendency for recurrent tears Prolonged disability possible

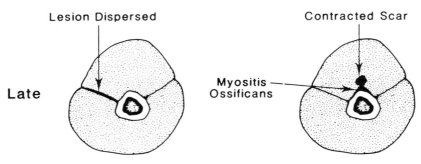

Fig. 5-4. Intermuscular hematomas tend to disperse early and easily, providing rapid resolution of symptoms. Intramuscular hematomas may predispose toward scarring, slower resolution, and protracted symptoms.

on rapid or full range of motion and increase the tendency to reinjury. Naturally, the recognition of this more severe form of muscle injury is important, so the rate of rehabilitation, progress, and return to activity can be paced accordingly (Fig. 5-4). In some situations, surgical aspiration or open drainage of a large intramuscular hematoma is indicated. Diagnostic ultrasonography or magnetic resonance imaging (MRI) facilitates planning of treatment and placement of the surgical incision in these cases. Because there is frequently difficulty in initially distinguishing intra- and intermuscular hematomas clinically, there is merit in simply assigning the injury to a mild, moderate, or severe category (Table 5-2). The most readily recognizable physical sign that correlates with increasing severity of muscle injury is the initial loss of range of motion. This obvious feature can be coupled with degree of pain and swelling to assign a severity level with reasonable accuracy.

The risk of a compartment syndrome with a large intramuscular hematoma is rare but must be stressed because of the disastrous consequences if overlooked. Recognition depends on noting the tenseness of the swelling as well as the diminishing peripheral pulses, sensation, and function. Early surgical intervention, with release of the fascia and aspiration of the clot, is necessary.

Avulsion

The commonest avulsions involve specific anatomic areas: (1) anterosuperior iliac spine with the sartorius muscle; (2) anteroinferior iliac spine with rectus femoris; (3) ischial tuberosity for the hamstring; (4) olecranon process with the triceps; and (5) patella with the quadriceps tendon. The large concentration of forces through these huge, thick tendons predispose them to mechanical failure through the bone. Occasionally in the elderly osteoporosis is a factor, whereas in the young an evolving stress fracture may be the cause of mechanical weakness. This latter situation is seen more frequently with the triceps insertion at the olecranon, but it does occur occasionally at the tibial tubercle with the ligamentum patella. In the teenage athlete, the rapid gain in strength of the muscles through hormonal change and intense training may make an open apophysis the weak mechanical site.

Musculotendinous junction ruptures may occur with normal anatomy, but all too frequently a history of local corticosteroid or systemic anabolic steroid use is implicated. Occasionally, a generalized collagen disorder is the underlying cause, and the therapist and physician must always be alert to this possibility.

HEALING OF MUSCLE TRAUMA

Muscle trauma is an enigma to many sports medicine personnel because although common and apparently straightforward there is relatively little solid information on which to base treatment decisions.

Practice Point

HEALING MUSCLE

Stage	*Goal*
Peritrauma period	Minimize initial injury
Intense inflammation	Minimize inflammation
Phagocytosis	Prevent further injury
Early healing	Re-establish range
Established healing	Increase strengthening
Restoration of function	Functional reintegration

The limited ability of muscle to fully regenerate from significant trauma without producing scar means that protection from further insult after the initial dam-

TABLE 5-4. Healing of Muscle Trauma (Moderate Severity)

Stage	Pathology	Implication for Treatment
Peritrauma period (0–6 hours)	Hemorrhage Myofibrillar retraction Disrupted cells Edema Chemotactic stimuli	*Goal: Minimize initial injury* Ice Elevation Compression Rest
Intense inflammation (6–24 hours)	Inflammation fully established Mononuclear cell invasion Release of inflammatory triggers Edema	*Goal: Minimize inflammatory response* NSAID Ice, rest Protect injured part
Phagocytosis (24–36 hours)	Intense phagocytic activity Mechanical weakening of muscle Significant edema formation	*Goal: Prevent further injury* Ultrasound (pulsed) Active range of motion No resisted work
Early healing (days 3–6)	Activated fibroblasts Fibroblast proliferation Collagen formation Satellite cells; muscle regeneration	*Goal: Re-establish range* Ultrasound Heating modalities Active range of motion Gentle resisted work
Established healing (days 7–14)	Complete muscle fiber bridging Tensile strength approx. 50% Contraction inhibited by edema and pain	*Goal: Increase strengthening* Tendency to reinjure Emphasize full ROM Heating modalities Increase resistance
Restoration of function (days 15–60)	Maturation of collagen Increased tensile strength	*Goal: Functional reintegration* Re-establish strength Re-establish full ROM Establish normal movement patterns

age is mandatory. It minimizes scarring and maximizes the potential for full functional recovery. McMaster, in 1933, demonstrated that when a normal muscle tendon unit is stretched disruption is most likely to occur at the muscle–tendon interface or the adjacent muscle.[7,8]

The description of the healing process that follows is directly from the work in our laboratory and that of Nikolaou and Garrett from Duke University.[9,10] It represents a strain and contusion of moderate severity and should be adjusted to greater or lesser injuries in regard to medication, modalities, and exercise during healing (Table 5-4).

Peritrauma Period

Gross examination of the damaged muscle immediately after injury shows localized hemorrhage, and at 6 hours the electron micrographs reveal tearing of muscle with myofibril retraction. There is rupture of small vessels and capillaries, with spillage of erythrocytes and polymorphonuclear leukocytes and some focal damage of nerve axons (Fig. 5-5). The extent of this damage would obviously be proportional to the initial trauma, and there is a proportional structural, as well as pain-inhibited, decrease in muscle strength.[10] At this stage, spilled intracellular organ-

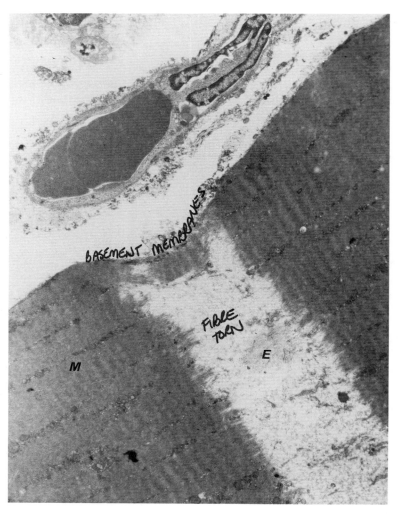

Fig. 5-5. Transmission electron micrograph of muscle 6 hours after trauma, showing retracted myofibrils at the trauma site. The intact basement membrane allows excellent regeneration. M = retracted muscle; E = edema and debris at site of tear. ×2,970.

elles, along with the escaped blood cells, generate a strong chemotaxic stimulus that attracts the cells that will be involved in the acute inflammatory process. From the clinical perspective, the main aim is to protect the muscle from further damage resulting in extension of the structural gap. Prompt removal from activity is probably the most significant aspect of protection. During these early post-trauma hours, ice, compression, and elevation serve to minimize the accompanying hematoma and rapidly accumulating, interstitial edema secondary to increased capillary permeability.[9]

Inflammation

Inflammation is fully established by 24 hours and is characterized by large numbers of mononuclear cells in the connective tissue and within the damaged muscle fibers (Fig. 5-6). These mononuclear cells may include fixed tissue macrophages, as well as monocytes that have been attracted to the area and have migrated across the vascular walls to become tissue macrophages.[9] Alternatively, the mononuclear cells may be B lymphocytes and cytotoxic lymphocytes. Mononuclear phagocytes, when stimulated, synthe-

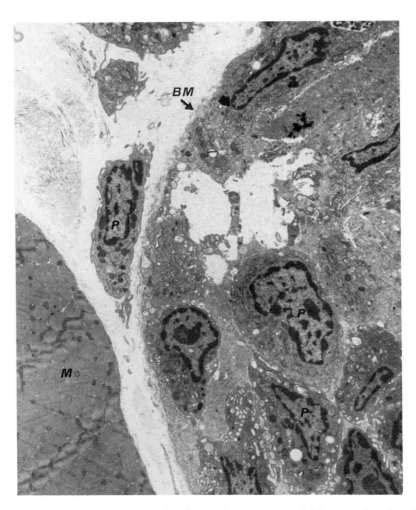

Fig. 5-6. Transmission electron micrograph of muscle trauma at 24 hours, showing invasion of a degenerating muscle cell by mononuclear phagocytes (P) within a muscle fiber and in the intercellular connective tissue. The damaged muscle possesses an intact basal lamina (BM). Transverse section of a normal muscle cell is seen (M). ×5,940.

size and release more than 80 defined molecules, which act in a highly coordinated fashion to mediate the antibacterial and anti-inflammatory activities of these cells.[11] These active substances include hydrolytic enzymes, particularly proteases, for breakdown of the protein metabolites of arachidonic acid, especially prostaglandin E_2, which is central to the inflammatory response. The catabolic aspect of the inflammatory response is a primitive vigorous response, perhaps in excess of the body's basic need for the removal of damaged tissue and initiation of healing. Indeed, an excessive inflammatory response inhibits healing.[12] It is during this phase that nonsteroidal anti-inflammatory agents (NSAIDs) may have their greatest effect, particularly when the recovery time is critical, as during sports seasons. The administration of NSAIDs after overuse injuries has been shown to significantly reduce local muscle damage during inflammation, as judged by both histochemical and biochemical criteria.[13] At the same time, the role of such substances as insulin-like growth factor-1 (IGF-1), a potent protein anabolic stimulus for skeletal muscle is not well defined in the initiation of regeneration.[14] Work by Almekinders and Gilbert showed that although piroxicam delayed the initial inflammatory reaction and the concomitant drop in passive strength of the muscle tendon unit after injury, and that it increased the maximal failure load during the late postinjury period, histologically it appeared to delay early muscle regeneration as well.[15] Our studies on NSAIDs show no interference with protein production. It is apparent that the analgesic properties of NSAIDs and modalities such as ice, ultrasound, and transcutaneous nerve stimulation (TNS) may allow resumption of movement at a time when the muscle is mechanically weak. Extreme care and good clinical judgment is needed to avoid overloading the muscle during this vulnerable period (Fig. 5-7).

Phagocytosis

By 48 hours after injury, phagocytosis of debris by mononuclear phagocytes is ongoing extracellularly and within muscle cells. Membrane-bound vacuoles, often containing amorphous material, are a prominent feature of damaged muscle cells and possibly correspond to lysosomes, representing intracellular catabolism of damaged cell constituents.[9] The muscle is weakened by this extensive invasion of macrophages. Day 2 after injury continues to be a critical period during which excessive physical activity might cause further damage, prolong the inflammatory re-

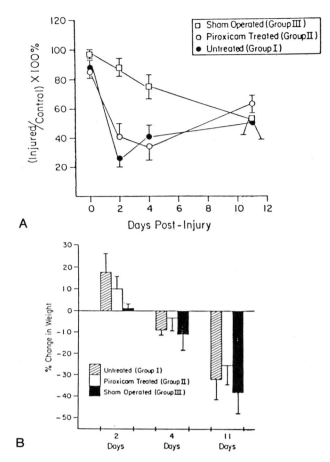

Fig. 5-7. (A) Comparison of muscle trauma in animals treated with the nonsteroidal anti-inflammatory medication piroxicam and a control group. Percentage of maximum failure load in injured muscle is compared to the uninjured side. **(B)** Percentage of wet weight of injured muscle compared to that on the uninjured side. (Adapted from Almekinders and Gilbert.[15])

sponse, and delay healing (Fig. 5-7). Gentle local therapy with active range of motion and no forced passive range of motion should be carried out. Some nonresisted isometric contractions may also be indicated at this point. With lower limb injuries, protected weight bearing is probably wise.

Early Healing

Healing is initiated with fibroplasia and early muscle regeneration. Fewer mononuclear cells are present, and numerous activated fibroblasts display elongated cytoplasmic processes and abundant rough endoplasmic reticulum, evidence of their collagen production (Fig. 5-8). Focal interstitial deposits of collagen represent early scarring and contribute to the tissue stiffness. Collagen deposition has important implications for the subsequent functional capacity of the muscle, as it replaces contractile tissue with noncontractile tissue. As the strength begins to return to the tissues, early range of motion exercises are necessary to allow lengthening of the immature plastic scar and minimize adhesion formation and orientation of collagen. Physical modalities such as ultrasound, laser, heat packs, interferential therapy, and shortwave diathermy might be used with advantage.

The muscle cells show changes characteristic of regenerating muscle. There are prominent multiple nuclei with distinct nucleoli and numerous mitochondria (Fig. 5.9). Furthermore, satellite cells are frequently seen in close approximation to the muscle cells within their basal lamina (Fig. 5-10). Satellite cells probably represent a population of myogenic cells, which appear to be central to muscle regeneration.[16,17] Factors influencing relative degrees of muscle cell regeneration compared to the amount of scarring are probably critical at this stage.

Established Healing

From days 6 to 14, established healing is evident. In our studies, fewer than 20 percent of the electron micrographic sections showed identifiable abnormal-

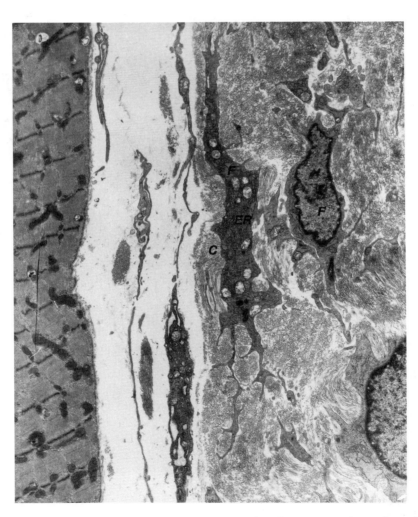

Fig. 5-8. Transmission electron micrograph of muscle 3 days after trauma. An activated fibroblast (F) with extensive endoplasmic reticulum (ER) is surrounded by newly formed collagen fibers (C) and an adjacent muscle (M). ×3,135.

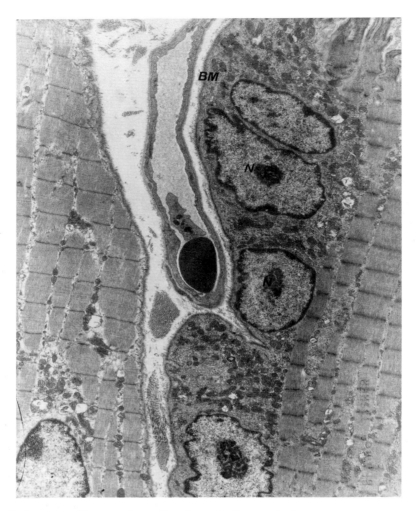

Fig. 5-9. At day 6 there is evidence of good healing. Underneath the basement membrane (BM) are multiple prominent nuclei (N). There is still some edema present. ×1,650.

ities.[9] Almekinders and Gilbert also noted regenerated muscle fibers bridging the entire defects in their studies by about day 11.[15] The tensile strength seems to be at about 50 percent of the preinjury state. Despite the decreased tensile strength, Nikolaou et al. demonstrated with isolated muscle preparations that passively strained muscle recovers its functional contractile ability as early as 48 hours after injury and is about 85 to 95 percent normal by 7 to 10 days (Fig. 5-11).[10] This finding suggests that the decreased function seen in patients in clinical situations after injury is not due to further degradation of contractile function of muscle but to edema and increased pain caused by the inflammatory nature of the healing process. Because the more severe injuries heal with greater proportions of inelastic scar tissue at a time

when pain is decreasing and function is improving, the patient is still vulnerable during this period and reinjury is frequent.

Restoration of Function

With maturation of the collagen and restoration of full volitional control of the muscle, rehabilitation efforts are directed at re-establishing strength and range of motion. Early controlled motion is desirable, as there is a decrease in protein synthesis with immobilization. Muscle regeneration is facilitated by activity.[10,14,18] Booth and Gould showed increased collagen concentration with exercise, which increased the tensile strength of the tissues.[19,20] Care and skill allow

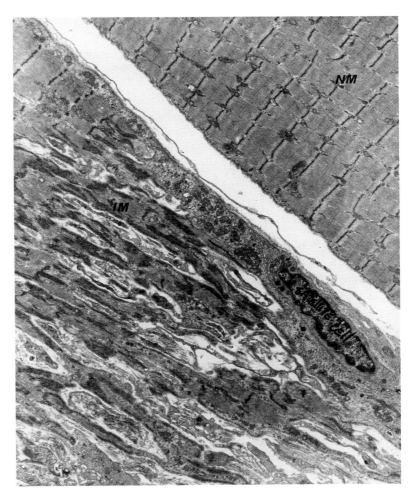

Fig. 5-10. Satellite cell is clearly seen with a double basement membrane between it and the associated injured muscle (IM). Normal muscle is also seen in this section (NM). × 1,650.

practical application of these principles without reinjury.

Comment

It should be emphasized that the direct extrapolation of animal data and laboratory information to the clinical realm is always fraught with overgeneralization. Nevertheless, the previous paragraphs provide a reasonable basic pathophysiologic framework on which to base clinical regimens. Exercise programs for mild injuries are progressed faster and those for severe injuries more slowly, but the principles remain unaltered. When the lesion is of such a magnitude that myofibrillar retraction leaves a large structural deficit in a muscle whose predictable functional loss may be unacceptable, surgical intervention is required to restore continuity. Similarly, large hematomas may result in slow healing and excessive scar, so aspiration may be considered. These clinical judgments must be made with an understanding of the abilities and limitations of the healing process and a concern for the goals of the athlete.

FLEXIBILITY, WARM-UP, STRETCHING

Classification

The basic principles of flexibility, warm-up, and stretching have been outlined in Chapter 4. Essentially there are three degrees of involvement of the

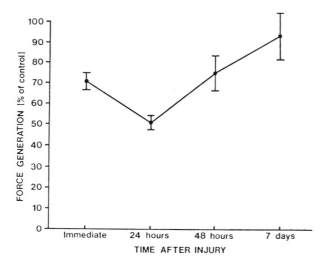

Fig. 5-11. Percent of control force generated averaged over all frequencies tested versus time after strain injury: immediate, 24 hours, 48 hours, 7 days. All values ± SEM. (From Nikolaou et al.,[10] with permission.)

musculotendinous unit in restriction of range of motion.

1. Normal physiologic tightness. This parameter is the normal amount of resistance to the extremes of motion found in all individuals, but it is more noticeable in those athletes with a tendency to tight muscles and joints. The range of motion achieved at the joint would be considered normal.
2. Excessive physiologic tightness. This condition is an exaggeration of the former condition seen in untrained individuals, athletes with normally tight muscles, or occasionally after a layoff or injury. It is also seen in many individuals as a normal accompaniment of aging. In the young individual, a measurable restriction in range would be considered unacceptable for preseason assessments and sufficient to increase the risk of injury.
3. Pathologic contracture. This degree of muscle involvement is usually seen after trauma, surgery, or immobilization. The degree of restricted range is significant and often associated with scar formation and muscle contractures. It is important to distinguish it from tight muscle secondary to bony pathology, such as a progressive spondylolisthesis or the spasm associated with central nervous system disease. Testing the reflexes should help dis-

tinguish this group, with hyper- or hyporeflexion being evident.

Treatment Implications

Normal Physiologic Tightness

The basic principle of increased tissue temperature increasing tissue plasticity is as important with normal physiologic tightness as it is with more severe decreases of limited range of motion. For this reason, the common practice of placing stretching exercises at the beginning of a warm-up routine is self-defeating. There is a higher friction force in muscles when they are cold.[21] The tissue temperatures in the extremities are relatively lower than core temperatures, particularly during the winter in cold environments. Gentle, controlled aerobic work with the addition of some controlled calisthenics, when appropriate, is usually sufficient. Indeed, more effective stretching may be carried out after at least 5 minutes of gradual progressive muscular exercise, e.g., walking, jogging, or cycling, to increase muscle vasodilation and hence local tissue temperature. There are several studies that attest to the effectiveness of this regimen.[22,23] The increased flexibility is more noticeable at the specific joints influenced by the warm-up activity. When ballistic activities are to be undertaken, stretching is advisable prior to the performance of these specific tasks. In most other situations where stretching activities are deemed desirable, particularly in individuals susceptible to muscle tightness or strains, the main bulk of the stretching is best done at the completion of the jog, cycle, or run. The implication of a stretching regimen after the main body of the workout or activity during the cool-down ensures maximum advantages from the physiologic increased plasticity generated by the activity.

Clinical Fact

INCREASING RANGE OF MOTION

- Warm-up prior to stretching
- Best results from stretching at completion of exercise
- Move slowly into stretched position
- Hold for 30 to 120 seconds
- Cool down with muscle on a stretch

Excessive Physiologic Tightness

For individuals with excessively tight muscles, e.g., tight hamstrings and gastrocnemius, a home program for stretching to ensure safe resumption of a sport is warranted. A regimen of activity, heat, stretching exercises, and a cool-down period, with the respective muscle on a stretch, is useful.[24] Indeed, the value of high repetitive motion alone or with stretching have been well demonstrated as a mechanism of gaining range.

Pathologic Contractures in Muscle and Joint

In joints with pathologic contractures, it may be necessary to add special prolonged stretching with weights and pulleys. For a flexion contracture at the knee, for example, the entire knee may be heated by hydrocollator packs wrapped in towels around the knee. A weighted cable and pulley system is used to apply a moderate but tolerable force of 3 to 15 lb in the direction of the desired motion for 30 to 60 minutes.[24] The hot packs are changed as necessary. Muscle relaxation is encouraged, and if necessary biofeedback techniques are used. This regimen suppresses reflex and voluntary motor activity by cortical inhibition of α and γ motor neurons, acting via suprasegmental pathways.[25] It is important to remember that optimal stretching can be achieved only when full reflex and voluntary muscle relaxation is achieved and all muscular resistance eliminated. There may be some initial tension in the muscles, but with adequate support and therapy it should decline. The group that initiates the myostatic reflex responds less intensely to static stretch than to rapid dynamic stretching. Furthermore, any tonic myotactic activity tends to decrease with time, as the tonic Ia afferent response shows a slow adaptation if the stretch stimulus is prolonged.[26] The weight is removed for several 30-second breaks during the stretching to relieve discomfort. When maximum stretching is achieved, strengthening and range of motion exercises may be carried out. Before termination of treatment the pulley system is applied for the cool-down time, which should start with a 5-minute application of crushed ice to the area. The stretch is always maintained to the end of the cooling period. This protocol can be used three times per week. The alternate days are used for strengthening. This technique should not be used in situations where heat is contraindicated or undesirable, particularly with the acutely inflamed, painful joint; otherwise inflammation is aggravated or perpetuated.

The technique of cryostretching is probably indicated only in limited circumstances, when the affected area is so painful that no range of motion exercises can be contemplated without the cold-induced analgesia. Several workers have demonstrated the dramatic lowering (5° to 20°F) of muscle and joint temperatures with 15 to 30 minutes of ice pack or cold water immersion.

Serial casting or spring-loaded orthosis have a role in some cases.

STRENGTH PARAMETERS

Rehabilitation of muscle should be directed at restoration of muscle strength and endurance to preinjury levels. In the case of athletes, each sport has its own normative data. Return to full training and competition presupposes that the strength has returned to within 10 percent of normal.[1,27-30] The agonist/antagonist ratios must be restored for the entire limb, not only the injured part.[31-34] To prepare athletes for the demands of their sport, muscles should also be exercised extensively in the eccentric loading mode. An analysis of the sport allows this aspect of the training to be specific and appropriate to the demands. Because injury may be associated with loss of type 1 endurance fibers, a special effort must be made to rehabilitate this component of function.

Lastly, high speed motion, with rapid development of peak torque and sudden deceleration has to be introduced with caution and certainly not until full range has been nearly restored.[35-37] It is with these explosive movements that the muscle is most vulnerable to reinjury.

SUMMARY

A simple classification of muscle trauma was outlined at the beginning of the chapter. Second degree muscle strain presents a broad spectrum of injury and therefore frequently requires a cautious approach. Understanding the structural changes at the different phases of healing allow adaptation of treatment modalities to the changing clinical picture in a logical manner. The early emphasis was on early, active range of motion. With a functional pain-free range, strengthening regimens can be put into full swing. Functional exercises start with nonballistic activities, and before high velocity work is commenced the emphasis must once more return to gaining the last few degrees of range of motion. Attention is paid to inter- and intramuscular adhesions. There are some subtle differences between contusions and muscle strains that relate to the potential for more muscle damage and hemorrhage with the former. The unusual, but significant, complication of an acute compartment syndrome was outlined, along with a guideline for early recognition. The specific regimens for individual muscle tears are dealt with in subsequent chapters.

REFERENCES

1. Cahill BR, Griffith EH: Effect of pre-season conditioning on the incidence and severity of high school football knee injuries. Am J Sports Med 6:180, 1978

2. Tiidins PM, Ianuzzo CD: Effects of intensity and duration of muscular exercise on delayed soreness and serum enzyme activities. Med Sci Sports Exerc 15:461, 1983

3. Glick JM: Muscle strains: prevention and treatment. Physician Sports Med 8:73, 1980

4. Segon DJ, Sladek JG, McCoy HJ et al: Weight lifting as a cause of bilateral upper extremity compartment syndrome. Physician Sports Med 16:73, 1988

5. Bass AL: Rehabilitation after soft tissue trauma. Proc Royal Soc Med 56:653, 1966

6. Bass AL: Injuries of the leg in football and ballet. Proc Royal Soc Med 60:527, 1967

7. McMaster RE: Tendon and muscle ruptures. J Bone Joint Surg 15:705, 1933

8. Nikolaou P, MacDonald BL, Glisson RR et al: The effect of architecture on the anatomical failure site of skeletal muscle. Trans Orthop Res Soc 11:228, 1986

9. Fisher BD, Baracos VE, Shnitka TK et al: Ultrastructural events following acute muscle trauma. In press

10. Nikolaou PK, MacDonald BL, Glisson RR et al: Biochemical and histological evaluation of muscle after controlled strain injury. Am J Sports Med 15:9, 1987

11. Adams D, Hamilton TA: The cell biology of macrophage activation. Annu Rev Immunol 2:238, 1984

12. Walters JB, Israel MJ: General Pathology. 4th Ed. Churchill Livingstone, Edinburgh, 1974

13. Salimen A, Kihlstrom M: Protective effects of indomethacin against exercise induced effects of injury in mouse skeletal muscle fibers. Int J Sports Med 8:46, 1987

14. Kvist M, Javinen M: Clinical, histochemical and biomechanical features in repair of muscle and tendon injuries. Int J Sports Med 3:12, 1982

15. Almekinders LC, Gilbert TA: Healing of experimental muscle strains and the effects of non-steroidal anti-inflammatory medications. Am J Sports Med 14:303, 1986

16. Shultz E, Jaryszak L, Gibson MC et al: Absence of exogenous satellite cell contribution to regeneration of frozen skeletal muscle. J Muscle Res Cell Motil 7:361, 1986

17. Jannische E, Skottner A, Hansson HA: Satellite cells express the trophic factor IGF-1 in regenerating skeletal muscle. Acta Physiol Scand 129:9, 1987

18. Zarins B, Ciullo JV: Acute muscle and tendon injuries in athletes. Clin Sports Med 2:167, 1983

19. Booth FW, Gould EW: Effect of training and disuse on connective tissue. p. 105. In Wilmore JH, Keough JF (eds): Exercise and Sports Sciences Review. Academic Press, Orlando, 1975

20. Coole WG: The analysis of hamstring strains and their rehabilitation. J Orthop Sport Phys Ther 9:77, 1987

21. Murphy P: Warming up before stretching advised. Physician Sports Med 14:45, 1986

22. Henricson AS, Fredriksson K, Persson I et al: The effect of heat and stretching on the range of hip motion. J Orthop Sports Phys Ther 6:110, 1984

23. Hubley CL, Kozey JW, Stanish ND: The effects of static stretching exercises and stationary cycling on range of motion at the hip joint. J Orthop Sports Phys Ther 14:316, 1986

24. Sapega AA, Quedenfeld TC, Moyer RA et al: Biophysical factors in range of motion exercise. Physician Sports Med 9:57, 1981

25. Kottke FJ, Pauly DL, Ptak KA: The rationale for prolonged stretching for correction of shortening of connective tissue. Arch Phys Med Rehabil 47:345, 1966

26. Moore MA, Hutton RS: Electromyographic investigation of muscle stretching techniques. Med Sci Sports Exerc 12:322, 1980

27. Campbell DE, Glenn W: Foot pounds of torque of the normal knee and the rehabilitation of the postmeniscectomy knee. Phys Ther 59:418, 1979

28. Grace TG: Muscle imbalance and extremity injury: a perplexing relationship. Sports Med 2:77, 1985

29. Fleck SJ, Falkel JE: Value of resistance training for the reduction of sports injuries. Sports Med 3:61, 1986

30. Grace TG, Sweetser ER, Nelson MA et al: Isokinetic muscle imbalance and knee joint injuries. J Bone Joint Surg [Am] 66:734, 1984

31. Gleim GW, Nicholas JA, Webb JN: Isokinetic evaluation following leg injuries. Physician Sports Med 6:75, 1978

32. Heiser TM, Weber J, Sullivan G et al: Prophylaxis and management of hamstring muscle injuries in in-

tercollegiate football players. Am J Sports Med 12:368, 1984

33. Knight KL: Strength imbalances and knee injury: a perplexing relationship. Sports Med 2:77, 1985

34. Merrifield HH, Cowan FJ: Groin strain injuries in ice hockey. J Sports Med 1:41, 1973

35. Hageman PA, Gillespie DM, Hill LD: Effects of speed and limb dominance on eccentric and concen-

tric testing of the knee. J Orthop Sport Phys Ther 10:59, 1988

36. Wyatt MP, Edwards AM: Comparison of quadriceps and hamstring torque values during isokinetic exercise. J Orthop Sport Phys Ther 3:48, 1981

37. Willford HN, East JB, Smith FH et al: Evaluation of warm up for improvement in flexibility. Am J Sports Med 14:316, 1986

Bone: A Specialized Connective Tissue

6

Progress is not an accident but a necessity.
— Herbert Spencer, 1882–1903

Bone is a specialized connective tissue. It provides a rigid skeleton and thus helps create recognizable shapes, protects the important viscera, and allows attachment of muscles. The expanded ends form joint surfaces and attachment sites for ligaments, and its rigid structure allows the development of levers for efficient muscle action. The normal adult bone is comprised of 30 percent organic material, mainly type I collagen, and 70 percent mineral, mainly calcium hydroxyapatite[1] (Table 6-1).

BONE AS A TISSUE

In the skeletally immature human, bone has a high organic component and therefore is more flexible. The open growth plate allows for enormous remodeling capabilities following injury. Much anabolic skeletal activity occurs during the adolescent growth spurt. The rapid longitudinal growth and endosteal apposition is offset by an increase in cortical porosity. Not until late adolescence, when longitudinal growth slows, does cortical mineral density rapidly increase.

Bone mass usually peaks during the fourth decade and serves as a mineral bank. In the older individual, bone loses some of this resiliency, as water content and organic components decrease. As age-related bone loss commences women lose about 35 to 40 percent cortical bone and 55 to 60 percent of their trabecular bone. Men lose about two-thirds of this amount. With the loss of bone volume and calcium, osteoporosis and osteopenia makes the skeleton more vulnerable, and exercise should be planned with due regard to this fact. By the same token, exercise and diet during the growing and early adult years may help establish the size and density of the bone bank

from which these involutional losses occur. Unfortunately, there is evidence that low body weight, low percent body fat, and amenorrhea or infrequent menstrual periods during early adult life may contribute to inadequate skeletal mass. Indeed, lean male distance runners may not be immune to the phenomenon of decreased axial skeletal bone mass. Furthermore, reduced bone mass over a period of years may not be easily replaced.

Quick Facts

BONE GROWTH AND CALCIUM DEPOSITION

- Most dramatic growth spurt during first two years
- Childhood longitudinal growth offset by some cortical porosity
- Childhood and adolescence: major time to accumulate skeletal mass and calcium
- Late adolescence: cortical density rapidly increases
- Bone mass peaks during fourth decade
- Bone mass sensitive to exercise and diet

Bone, like all other tissues, responds to stress. Body weight and activity stimulate bone deposition. Small, light people generally have small, light bones. The axial skeleton seems particularly affected by the type of osteoporosis seen in the athletes described above. Inasmuch as the spine is well protected from most of the stress of running, this fact should not be surpris-

TABLE 6-1.   Composition of Bone

Bone Divisions	Components
Organic (30%)	
Matrix (98%)	Collagen type I
	Noncollagenous proteins
Cells (2%)	Osteoblasts: matrix forming
	Osteocytes: resting but metabolically active
	Related to macrophage line
Mineral (70%)	
Calcium hydroxyapatite 95%:	
$(Ca_{10}PO_4)_6(OH)_2$	
Trace amounts of	
Magnesium	
Sodium	
Potassium	
Fluoride	
Chloride	

ing. Specific attention may have to be given to exercising the spine and hence stimulating calcium deposition in vertebrae. Thus well planned exercise helps build the skeleton; and properly done throughout life, activity helps maximize the strength and density of bone.

Trauma to the joint surface at any stage of life is serious. Significant joint damage is rarely repaired totally, and the specter of degenerative joint change is not a pleasant one. For this reason ligament injury, meniscal damage, and intra-articular fractures must be taken seriously, particularly in the athlete, and assessed by physicians expert in their recognition and treatment. This chapter deals specifically with injury to bone and its ability to heal.

Bone Formation

The model of the skeleton, for the most part, forms as a condensation of the mesenchyme in the embryo.[2,3] The exceptions are the bones of the vault of the skull (membranous ossification), the clavicle (mixed ossification), and the mandible (Meckel's car-

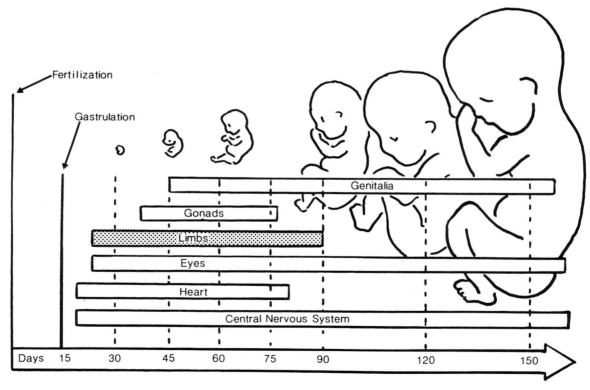

Fig. 6-1. Periods of maximum teratogenicity for the major organ systems. Days 15 to 90 comprise the most critical period. Before this time fetal death with abortion is a likely outcome.

tilage). This condensation rapidly evolves into a cartilaginous model of each bone. The future joints are represented by small clefts evolving in the interzones between the cartilaginous bone templates.

These early rapid changes occur during the first few weeks of intrauterine life and are largely completed by 12 weeks; they are obviously critical. Teratogenic materials ingested by the mother at this stage or other negative factors such as radiation can result in significant skeletal abnormalities. Completion of the joints awaits movement of the fetus[3] (Fig. 6-1). Starting as early as the fifth week of intrauterine life, a primary center of ossification gradually replaces the cartilage model with bone by a process of enchondral ossification.[1,2] In most bones, during either the late fetal stages or the first few years of life, secondary centers of ossification appear.[1,3]

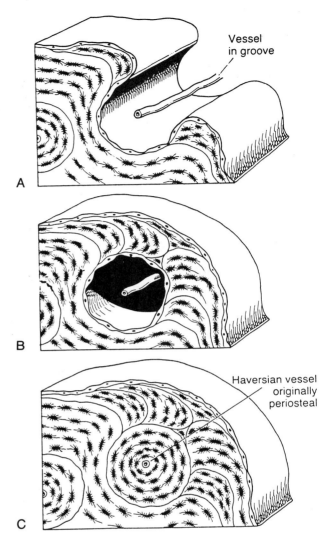

Fig. 6-2. Growth and remodeling of bone with production of haversian systems. **(A)** Resorption around a vessel. **(B)** Invagination by peripheral osteoblasts. **(C)** Generation of concentric layer of new bone. (From Ham,[4] with permission.)

Quick Facts

BONE FORMATION

- Cartilage model forms.
- First 6 weeks are critical for teratogenic effects.
- Joints start as clefts but await movement for normal formation.
- Starting at the fifth intrauterine week primary ossification centers appear to palpation.
- Most secondary centers develop after birth.

These primary and secondary centers remain separated by the growth plates until skeletal maturity. The growth plate, or physis, allows longitudinal growth. The thickened periosteum allows normal remodeling and growth in width, and it is particularly important for fracture healing. Occasionally, secondary centers of growth fail to unite to the main bone and persist as accessory ossicles, which may be a site of pathology in the athlete. The bone remodeling process begins during the fetal period, accelerates through infancy, and continues throughout life. The rate of cortical turnover and remodeling may be as high as 50 percent during the first 2 years of life in some bones but declines to about 5 percent per year in the adult.[4] (Fig. 6-2).

Osteon

The unit of bone is an osteon.[4,5] It consists of a Volkmann's canal surrounded by concentric lamellae of bone (Fig. 6-3). These lamellae have lacunae, which contain resting osteocytes. When bone remodeling is taking place, there is some transformation of cells into bone-forming osteoblasts or bone-removing osteoclasts, although the exact origin of the cells may vary (Fig. 6-4). The lacunae are connected by canalic-

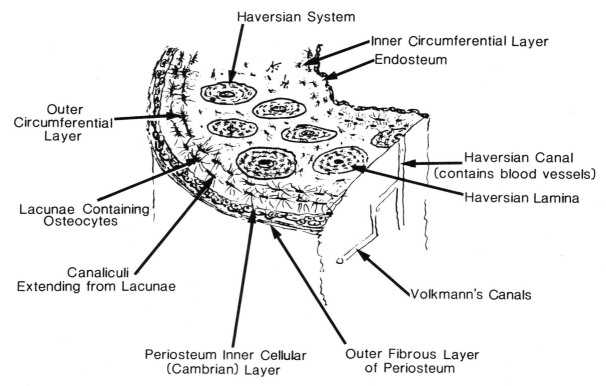

Fig. 6-3. Three-dimensional representation of the cortex of long bone. (After Ham,[4] with permission.)

uli, which are important for the transfer of nutrients and medication. Osteoblasts lay down an uncalcified matrix called osteoid, which is subsequently calcified as true bone. The various osteons amalgamate to form large haversian systems, loosely woven in medullary bone and densely packed in the cortical shell.

Medullary Bone

The medullary system has both a structural role and a storage role. The storage component is central to calcium and other mineral metabolism and is intrinsic

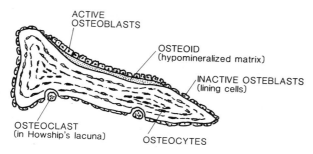

Fig. 6-4. Remodeling of trabecular bone with production osteoid by osteoblasts. Bone resorption via osteoclasts and the subsequent Howship's lacunae.

to the crystalline structure of the bone. More than 95 percent of the body's calcium is within the bone lattice and is sensitive to the controlling parathyroid hormone, vitamin D (dihydroxycholecalciferol), and calcitonin. The other large component is the marrow between the medullary bone lattice and, depending on the age of the individual, is a source of red and white blood cells. Even in the older individual this "red marrow" persists in some of the large metaphyseal regions, but large amounts are replaced by a more fatty "white marrow." Responsive to erythropoietin, red marrow is essential in the young athlete for preventing anemia and is one of the major stores of body iron. It is this latent red blood cell forming potential that is stimulated by altitude training. When bone fractures, marrow may form part of the embolizing debris that contributes to the fat embolus syndrome.

The structural role of the medullary bone is achieved by the trabecular organization along maximum lines of stress (Fig. 6-5). Clearly distinct compressive and traction trabeculae may be identified. This system evolves according to Wolfe's law of "structure subserving function" and is an incredibly efficient method of producing strength with the min-

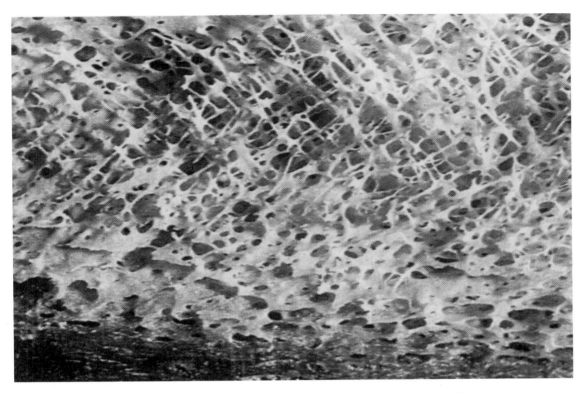

Fig. 6-5. Trabecular bone with marrow elements removed illustrating the transition to more compact bone in the periphery. The orientation of trabecular bone along lines of stress gives bone its maximum strength/weight ratio.

imal necessary bone mass.[5] In the subchondral bone, these trabeculae are arranged to augment the shock-absorbing properties of the articular cartilage (Fig. 6-6). As the articular surface properties change with osteoarthrosis, so does the nature of the subchondral bone, as it thickens (subchondral sclerosis) to take more of the load. Unfortunately, this compensatory mechanism adds rigidity to the system, further compromising the shock-absorbing properties. This rigidity, in turn, may accelerate the articular cartilage change. The reaction to exercise—ballistic, impact, and nonimpact—is individual and subtle. If symptoms are not exacerbated, it is usually considered that exercise does not adversely affect these changes.

Cortical Bone

The cortical shell gives remarkable strength to bone, particularly during compression. Its periosteal cover allows remodeling throughout life and the attachment of ligaments and tendons via a transition known as Sharpey's fibers. Hypertrophy of this cortical bone is slowly acquired in response to the stress of activity. Remarkable examples are the enormous

thickness of the second metatarsal of the ballet dancer secondary to practicing "en pointe" and the unilateral hypertrophy of the humerus of the baseball pitcher and tennis player. Indeed, in the professional

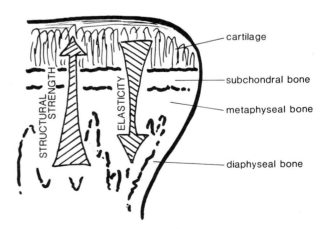

Fig. 6-6. Subchondral bone takes part in the shock-absorbing process. With articular cartilage degeneration, significant changes also occur in the supporting bone.

tennis player, the cortical thickness of the dominant side has been shown to be increased 34.9 percent and 28.4 percent in men and women, respectively, over their contralateral control arm.[5] Nilsson and Westlin showed significantly more dense bone in the distal femurs of top ranked athletes.[6] Animal studies have also confirmed this hypertrophy in response to stress.[7,8] With ill-advised, rapidly progressed activity, stress reactions may occur as the resorptive breakdown phase surpasses the bone's ability to replace itself in the remodeling process. Stress fractures may result.[9,10]

Bone retains the unique ability to regenerate without scar. Indeed, fracture healing could be called bone "regeneration." In many ways it mimics the initial formation of bone in the embryo and fetus and is an exaggeration of the normal remodeling process that occurs throughout adult life. Unfortunately, it is probably this embryonic potential that makes primary tumors of bone in the young person such disastrous neoplasms. Osteosarcoma is a tumor of children, teenagers, and young adults, and atypical skeletal pain must always be investigated with this diagnosis in mind. Although there is no evidence that trauma has any etiologic role in tumor induction, it is often the precipitating event that stimulates clinical investigation. Similarly, in the older adult and the elderly, many of the common malignant tumors metastasize to bone early. It is particularly true of breast cancer; and again in this age group, activity-induced pain of an atypical nature should raise the suspicion of neoplasia.

General Structure

The immature long bone consists of an epiphysis, an epiphyseal plate (physis or growth plate), metaphysis, and diaphysis (Fig. 6-7). The adult bone lacks the epiphyseal plate. The general structure of bone depends on function, and its size is both genetically and developmentally determined. Muscles produce ridges and tubercles secondary to their pull; ligaments develop ridges and spurs. Trauma, disease, and nutrition may leave growth arrest lines, distorted growth, deformity, and osteophytes, spurs, and cysts. Thus bone, imaged so well with radiographic techniques in the living and surviving the soft tissues in death, forms a perfect mirror of the rigors of a person's life history, life style, and health (Table 6-2).

Epiphysis

The epiphysis is the expanded bone end that, by virtue of increasing surface area, forms a support for the joint surface. The specialized nature of the subchondral bone has already been mentioned (Fig. 6-6). Hence developmental diseases of the epiphysis (epiphyseal dysplasias) are characterized by abnormally shaped joints and early degenerative change. The latter effect also may be the result of trauma and avascular necrosis (Fig. 6-8). Avascular necrosis is a condition primarily affecting very young children; and involvement of the major weight-bearing joints such as the hips must be recognized promptly in order to institute adequate therapy. A persistent, painful hip or knee in a young person must never go uninvesti-

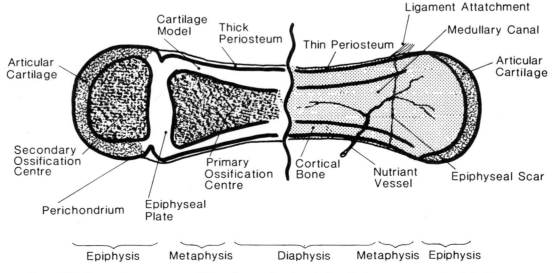

Fig. 6-7. General structure of long bones in the skeletally immature and adult human.

TABLE 6-2. General Structure of Bone

Site	Comment	Conditions	Result
Epiphysis	Mainly develops under pressure Apophysis forms under traction Forms bone ends Supports articular surface	Epiphyseal dysplasias Joint surface trauma Overuse injury Damaged blood supply	Distorted joints Degenerative changes Fragmented development Avascular necrosis
Physis	Epiphyseal or growth plate Responsive to growth and sex hormones Vulnerable prior to growth spurt Mechanically weak	Physeal dysplasia Trauma Slipped epiphysis	Short stature Deformed or angulated growth or growth arrest
Metaphysis	Remodeling expanded bone end Cancellous bone heals rapidly Vulnerable to osteomyelitis Affords ligament attachment	Osteomyelitis Tumors Metaphyseal dysplasia	Sequestrum formation Altered bone shape Distorted growth
Diaphysis	Forms shaft of bone Large surface for muscle origin Significant compact cortical bone Strong in compression	Fractures Diaphyseal dysplasias Healing slower than at metaphysis	Able to remodel angulation Cannot remodel rotation Involucrum with infection Dysplasias give altered density and shape

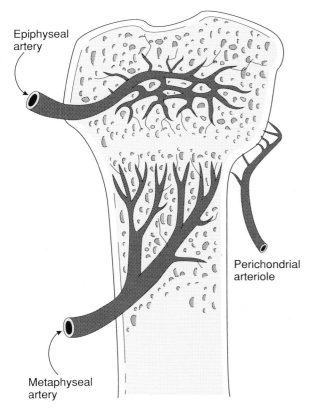

Fig. 6-8. Blood supply to the growth plate. Damage to the epiphyseal artery may give serious joint and growth deformity. (After Siffert RS, Gilbert MD: In Rang M (ed): The Growth Plate and its Disorders. Williams & Wilkins, Baltimore, 1969, with permission.)

gated. Traumatic avascular necrosis may result from the repetitive minor trauma of activity or by fractures and dislocations.

Most epiphyses form under the pressure of weight bearing, although some are partially shaped by the traction afforded by the insertion of a major tendon. In this situation they are referred to as apophyses. An example is the calcaneal apophysis developing under the pulled Achilles tendon. The every-day use of the word epiphysis is sometimes confusing, as it is frequently meant to indicate specifically the growth plate, rather than the whole unossified end of the skeletally immature bone.

Growth Plate

The growth plate, or physis, permits longitudinal growth (Fig. 6-9). Each bone closes its physis at a characteristic age. The growth plate is responsive to growth hormone, the sex hormones estrogen and testosterone, and to some degree thyroid hormone. Significant developmental disorders (physeal dysplasias) result primarily in altered growth in length, but occasionally they also affect the shapes of joints. In such cases, short stature and dwarfism are the outcome.

Traumatic disruption may result in distorted, angular growth or cessation of growth, giving a shortened or deformed limb. Inasmuch as the physeal plate is frequently the weakest mechanical portion of the bone–ligament–bone unit, growth plate disruption must be sought carefully and diligently in all apparent ligamentous disruptions in the skeletally immature patient. This mechanical weakness may

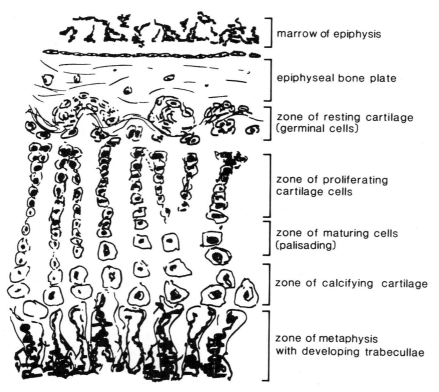

marrow of epiphysis

epiphyseal bone plate

zone of resting cartilage (germinal cells)

zone of proliferating cartilage cells

zone of maturing cells (palisading)

zone of calcifying cartilage

zone of metaphysis with developing trabecullae

Fig. 6-9. Growth plate (physis) illustrating the evolution of the proliferating cartilage cells to calcification and ingrowth of vascular buds and osteoclastic and osteoblastic cells.

manifest just prior to and during the growth spurt as a slipped epiphysis at the hip, which is another important differential diagnosis of hip and knee pain in the young athlete.

Nutritional deficiencies particularly affect the growth plate. Although rare, vitamin D deficiency rickets may occur owing to poor intake, malabsorption from the gut, or renal disease.

Metaphysis

The metaphyseal region allows for drastic remodeling of bone shape from the necessary bulbous bone end for articular surface support and ligament attachment, to a thinner, lighter more functional shaft (Fig. 6-10). Congenital disease of the metaphysis (metaphyseal dysplasia) results in abnormally shaped and thickened bones and is rare. By contrast, the circulatory microanatomy of the cancellous bone of the metaphysis makes it an important site for the initiation of osteomyelitis. It is also a frequent site of tumor, particularly for osteogenic sarcoma, where the distal femur and proximal tibia are most commonly involved.

Diaphysis

The diaphysis is the most vulnerable part for fracture in the adult athlete. Its surface forms the major site of attachment for muscle and intermuscular septa. The detailed anatomy of any specific diaphysis is dictated by its pull. The rare vitamin C and A deficiencies particularly affect the cortex, as does syphilis of the congenital and acquired variety. The frequently exposed surface of the diaphysis, e.g., the anterior tibial border in the leg and the posterior ulna ridge in the forearm, require special protection during contact and kicking sports, as well as for sports where hard, high velocity missiles predominate, e.g., cricket, hockey, and basketball.

TRAUMA TO BONE

Trauma to the Epiphysis

To understand the prognosis and rationale of treatment for fractures involving the epiphysis, it is necessary to be familiar with the histology (Fig. 6-9). The basal layer (resting cells) of the epiphyseal is a

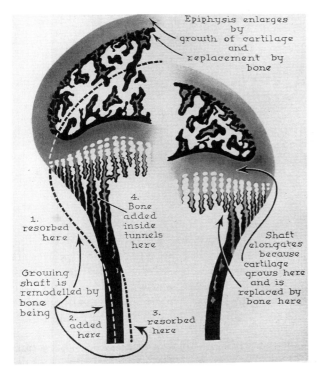

Fig. 6-10. Function of the metaphysis is to help support the joint and to allow remodeling during the process of longitudinal growth.

germinal layer that may then divide (proliferating zone) forming columns of enlarging cartilage cells (palisading). Initially storing glycogen, they are surrounded by a matrix of collagen and ground substance (hypertrophy zone). Eventually these cells start to lay down calcium in the matrix and ultimately completely surround themselves (zone of calcification). They then degenerate.

Into this zone of calcifying cartilage appear cutting cones of osteoclasts, burrowing tunnels; they are followed by neovascularization. Osteoblasts, following the same route, lay down osteoid, which is then calcified, forming immature woven bone. The immature bone subsequently remodels into mature medullary bone. This endochondral ossification process mimics the initial bone formation in the embryo as well as the ultimate process used for fracture repair. The multiplying cells obviously provide for the growth in length, and this process continues at various rates until epiphyseal closure.

Most epiphyseal fractures are associated with a strong periosteal hinge, which minimizes displacement and, provided its presence is acknowledged and utilized in reduction maneuvers, allows early stability of the separation.

The main point to recall from this discussion is that the zone of hypertrophy, which contains the least crucial cells, is the weakest layer structurally. For this reason it is the commonest area of failure with trauma (Fig. 6-9), which is fortunate because it is least likely to produce serious long-term growth changes.

Clinical Point

EPIPHYSEAL TRAUMA

Separation usually through zone of hypertrophy

- Type I — Good periosteal hinge, closed reduction, few complications
- Type II — Small metaphyseal flake, closed reduction, few complications
- Type III — May involve joint, usually open reduction, problems of joint incongruity
- Type IV — Crosses physis, open reduction, tendency to high complication rate
- Type V — Crush injury, closed treatment, high complication rate

---

Trauma to the epiphysis is best considered according to the Salter-Harris classification.[11,12] Type I fractures or separations pass directly through the zone of hypertrophy (Fig. 6-11). Type II epiphyseal separations are mainly through this same zone but usually shear off into the metaphysis and hence contain a metaphyseal spike. Both these fractures are usually held from significant displacement by a tough periosteal hinge. This periosteum is utilized as a fulcrum with closed fracture reduction, which is the treatment of choice for types I and II. Once reduced they are relatively stable and only rarely need some form of internal fixture. They heal rapidly, becoming sticky in a week and united in 3 to 4 weeks. They are usually ready for full stress by 6 to 8 weeks, depending on the site. Long-term growth problems and deformity are minimal.

The type III separations pass through the epiphyseal plate but then continue via the epiphyseal side of the physis, frequently into the joint. Type IV fractures pass from metaphysis to epiphysis by directly

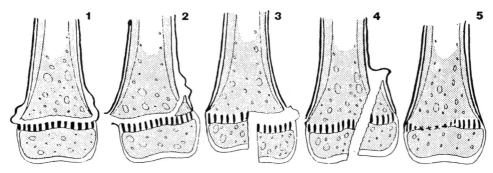

Fig. 6-11. Salter-Harris classification of growth plate injury (types I to V). The separation is usually through the zone of hypertrophy.

crossing the growth plate. These type III and IV epiphyseal plate injuries are serious on two accounts. First, the fracture line passes through the crucial germinal resting and dividing cells. Damage to these cells may result in growth arrest, angular growth, and deformity. Second, the intra-articular portion of part of the fracture may result in severe, rapid, degeneration changes if left unreduced. Absolute congruent and anatomic reduction is required with type III and IV injuries, which frequently necessitate open reduction and pin fixation.

The type V injury involves crushing of part or the whole physis. It may permanently damage the germinal layer. Unfortunately, there is little that can be done to remedy this situation. The injury is treated symptomatically, and any resultant growth arrest or disturbance is corrected when possible at the appropriate age.

There are two other injuries to the growth plate that should be mentioned. The first is frostbite to the small growth plates of the phalanges, which may result in complete growth arrest. This injury is usually seen in young skiers who do not bother to wear gloves. It may also occur in those who live in cold climates and play on the outdoor ice hockey surfaces. Education of the child, parent, and coach is necessary. The second situation is manipulation of the physis, by accident or design, via the use of anabolic steroids and growth hormones. This problem area requires a strong, honest, safe, and ethical approach by the medical team.

Fracture Healing

The high speeds and impacts of many sports make the risk of fracture an ever present concern. Thus knowledge of the first aid management of these inju-

ries is essential. Although fractures of the extremities predominate, some of the axial skeleton injuries are more dramatic. Fractured ribs jeopardize the chest and abdominal viscera, and spinal trauma threatens the spinal cord. Furthermore, the ability to protect a healing fracture and the speed at which safe reintegrating into activity is possible are all part of sports medicine. An understanding of the process of fracture healing or bone regeneration is therefore appropriate. The overall most frequent sites of fracture in sport are the hands, ankles, and feet but the injury site is very much sport-specific (Table 6-3).

Stages of Fracture Healing (Bone Regeneration)

Fracture healing traditionally has been divided into four histologically descriptive stages: (1) stage of inflammation; (2) stage of soft callus; (3) stage of hard callus; and (4) stage of bone remodeling.[13] However, it is evident that there are two other important aspects of fracture healing that are not covered in the more traditional methods of describing fracture healing: the stage of impact and the stage of induction. Bone is unique in that it may completely heal itself with tissue

TABLE 6-3. Sport-Related Fractures
(n = 840)

Sport	No.	%	Most Frequent Sites
Skiing	118	14	Hand, tibia, clavicle
Football	92	11	hand, rib, foot
Hockey	67	8	Hand, nose, clavicle
Rugby	60	7	Ankle, wrist, nose
Basketball	59	7	Foot, nose, forearm
Soccer	51	6	Tibia, hand, wrist
Volleyball	50	6	Ankle, hand, foot
Gymnastics	42	5	Foot, hand, wrist
Others	301	36	Hand, ankle, feet

that is ultimately indistinguishable from the original bone. For this reason bone healing has been referred to as bone regeneration.

Stage of Impact

The stage of impact occurs at the moment of the injury, lasting until there is complete dissipation of energy. The energy is absorbed by the bone until failure occurs. The amount of energy that can be absorbed before failure is directly proportional to the volume of bone; that is, the greater the volume of bone, the more energy that can be absorbed until fracture occurs. Simply stated, larger bones are more difficult to break than small bones. The amount of energy absorbed before failure is also inversely proportional to the modulus of elasticity, and therefore less energy is absorbed before failure with more rigid bones. Thus the elderly person with osteoporotic bones sustains fractures easily. In the very young, the greater organic component tends to allow the bone to bend, producing "greenstick," incomplete fractures.

Quick Facts

STAGES OF FRACTURE HEALING

1. Impact
2. Induction
3. Inflammation
4. Soft callus
5. Hard callus
6. Remodeling

Finally, the amount of energy absorbed before failure is directly related to the rate of the force applied; that is, the greater the rate of force applied, the more energy that is usually absorbed before failure. For instance, during skiing the tibia may be loaded so rapidly that an enormous amount of energy is stored prior to fracture and the bone seems almost to explode. The duration of the stage of impact is from the moment of trauma until complete dissipation of all energy. These factors outlined above decide the fracture pattern: a simple transverse fracture, comminution, or a segmental fracture. The type of fracture, in turn, has tremendous implication regarding the length of time required for healing.

Quick Facts

STAGE OF IMPACT

- Duration: moment of impact until complete dissipation of energy
- Energy: absorbed by all bone until moment of failure
- Amount of energy absorbed before failure depends on
  -Volume of bone: directly proportional
  -Modulus of rigidity: inversely proportional
  -Rate of loading: directly proportional

Stage of Induction

We have the least knowledge regarding the induction stage of fracture healing. It is not known when the stage of induction occurs. Cells possessing osteogenic potential are stimulated to form bone through a process of modulation. Cells that do not usually possess osteogenic potential may be induced to form bone through a process of differentiation. The progeny of these cells differentiate into bone-forming cells. Other cells that are normally bone-forming multiply and are turned on to function at their maximum potential. The stimulus that brings about induction is unknown but includes oxygen gradient, bioelectric potentials, bone morphogenic protein, and other noncollagenous proteins.

Quick Facts

STAGE OF INDUCTION

- Cells possessing osteogenic potential are activated.
- Actual stimulus is unknown but includes the following.
  -Oxygen gradient
  -Biolectric effects
  -Bone morphogenic protein (BMP)
- Duration: Stimulus decreases with time.

The duration of the stage of induction is indefinite, but it starts soon after the moment of impact and gets well under way during the stage of inflammation. It is essential to make sure that all the early clinical conditions are ideal, so the best use is made of these inductive forces while they are at their greatest, which helps to ensure sound union. With time, the influence of these inductive forces seems to lessen; and if the early opportunity for healing is lost, delayed union or nonunion becomes more likely.

Stage of Inflammation

The stage of inflammation begins shortly after impact and lasts until the major pain and discomfort begin to abate, which is probably about the time the bone ends are held together by some fibrous union. Clinically, the local swelling should be mostly subsided.

At the time of fracture there is disruption of the blood supply, hemorrhage, and the formation of a fracture hematoma. Oxygen tension and pH drop. Bone necrosis and debris cause the release of lysosomal enzymes. Inflammation sets the scene for dealing with damaged tissue and sets up the signals for repair. There is a rapid ingrowth of vasoformative elements and capillaries and an enormous increase in cellular proliferation. Furthermore, there is a change in the pattern of capillary blood distribution. In the adult at least three-fourths of the cortical blood flow is from the endosteal surface, with the remaining capillary network coming from the periosteum. With the stimulus of fracture healing this situation is reversed. Although there is tremendous hyperemic response of the endosteal circulation, there is such an enormous proliferation of periosteal vessels that a large part of the circulation is from the periosteum. It takes several days for this situation to maximize and is important for healing. Interestingly, in the child most of the cortical blood flow is already from the periosteum; thus children probably can initiate their healing response somewhat more rapidly and more efficiently than the adult. This fact, along with the thickened maximally functioning periosteal cells, may be one of the explanations of the early, rapid healing seen in children. Their normally active system needed for growth and development has to increase its intensity only slightly to cope with the needs of fracture healing.

It may seem paradoxical that there is hypoxia at the cellular level in a fracture callus that is so richly invaded with capillaries. However, the explanation is probably related to the fact that near capillaries oxygen tensions are in the range of 90 mmHg. However,

---

Quick Facts

STAGE OF INFLAMMATION

- Disruption of blood supply
  - -Hemorrhage
  - -Hematoma formation
  - -Decrease in pH
  - -Fall in oxygen tension
- Bone necrosis
  - -Release of lysosomes and chemotactic substances
- Cellular proliferation
- Ingrowth of vasoformative elements and capillaries

---

just 10 to 15 μm away from a capillary the oxygen tension measurements fall to almost zero. Thus one might conclude that despite the tremendous ingrowth of capillaries in the fracture callus seen on the microangiographic level, at the cellular level the average bone or cartilage cell is in a hypoxic environment. In essence, then, the proliferation and growth of the cells is even greater than the proliferation of the capillary circulation. This environment of low oxygen tension and decreasing pH is favorable for growth of the early fibrous or cartilaginous callus. It forms more easily than bone and functions to produce early splinting, decreasing pain and the likelihood of further fat embolus. In addition, it provides a scaffold for further circulation, cartilage production, and endosteal bone production in a rapid, efficient fashion.

Stage of Soft Callus

The stage of soft callus begins when pain and swelling subside in the extremity and lasts until the bony fragments are united by fibrous or cartilaginous tissue. This period corresponds roughly to the time clinically when the fragments are no longer movable (approximately 3 weeks for the major long bones). This period is marked by a great increase in vascularity and ingrowth of capillaries into the fracture callus. It is also marked by an even greater increase in cellularity. The PO_2 is still low, but the pH returns to normal. The hematoma between the fracture ends becomes organized with fibrous tissue, and cartilage and bone soon appear. The callus is electronegative relative to the rest of the bone during this period. Osteoclasts appear in large numbers and remove some of the dead bone fragments.

Quick Facts

STAGE OF SOFT CALLUS

- Callus electronegative
- Osteoclasts removing dead bone
- pH returning toward neutral
- Continued increase in vascularity
- Even greater increase in cellularity
- Decrease in oxygen tension

The primary callus response leads initially to external bonding callus, which is followed by medullary callus. The initial collagen is mainly type II, but ultimately this type is mostly replaced by type I in adult bone.

Pain is greatly reduced at this stage. The bone ends are now sticky and are held together by fibrous tissue. It is safe at this stage to change the cast without fear of losing position in previously unstable fractures. However, alignment may be lost, and so cast changes are done with care. By the same token, this point is probably the last chance to correct the alignment relatively easily, and so careful roentgenographic evaluation is warranted. No callus is visible on the roentgenograms.

Clinical Point

STAGE OF SOFT CALLUS

- Hematoma becomes organized with
  -Fibrous tissue
  -Cartilage
  -Woven bone
- Duration: until fragments united with fibrous or cartilaginous tissue (or both)
- Clinically: corresponds to when fragments no longer movable

---

At this stage some adaptations of the cast are permissible to allow modified training or, in some cases,

competition. It depends on the site of the fracture, its propensity to delayed or nonunion, the type of sport, and the needs of the athlete. Decisions should always aim on the cautious side, as an established delayed union or nonunion of bone is a disaster in terms of time and the need for extensive surgical therapy.

Stage of Hard Callus

The stage of hard callus begins when the fracture ends are held together with a sticky soft callus, and it is completed when the fragments are firmly united with new bone. This period corresponds to the time when the fracture is clinically and radiologically healed. The time to union varies considerably with different fractures and may be as little as 2 to 3 weeks for the small bones of the hand and as long as 3 to 4 months for fractures of the long bones, particularly the femur and tibia. This time is influenced considerably by the age of the individual inasmuch as the skeletally immature child heals much more rapidly than the adult; however, once the adult stage is reached, age has little influence. The callus converts from fibrocartilaginous tissue to fiber bone at this stage and is referred to as primary woven bone. If there is absolutely no motion present during healing, membranous bone formation may occur; but if there is abundant motion present, enchondral bone formation or primary union occurs. The amount of movement influences the amount and quality of the callus. Small amounts of movement at the fracture site seem to stimulate callus formation, but excessive movement may break down early bridging and inhibit union. The oxygen tension in the callus is still below normal, but the pH has returned to neutral by this time. The callus is still electronegative. Histologically, there may be many osteoclasts removing dead bone at this stage. New bone is abundant both subperiosteally and endosteally.

Quick Facts

STAGE OF HARD CALLUS

- Slight decrease in oxygen tension
- pH returns to neutral
- Continued removal of dead bone by osteoclasis
- Callus electronegative
- Callus converting to fiber bone

Naturally there is a great interest in how mineral is deposited in the fracture callus. In many ways, it is similar to the method of deposition of calcium and early bone formation at the growth plate or physis. In the growth plate the hypertrophic zone of cells is in a hypoxic environment, and the cells there undergo aerobic glycolysis until all of the glycogen is consumed. Mitochondria of the chondrocytes in the hypertrophic zone of the physis that had accumulated calcium begin to release the calcium as the glycogen stores are used up. In the same hypertrophic zone of the growth plate calcium released from the mitochondria begin to accumulate in the matrix vesicles. It is evident that a similar system exists in the fracture callus. The low pH and hypoxic environment stimulates calcium accumulation in the mitochondria; calcium subsequently is deposited into matrix vesicles, which then form a site for the growth of crystals. In addition, there is evidence that as soon as sufficient collagen is laid down a second site of crystal growth is available within the "hole" zones of the collagen molecules. Thus it may be that nucleation in the fracture callus occurs in matrix vesicles in the region of the chondrocytes and in collagen in other areas.

Practice Point

STAGE OF HARD CALLUS

- Duration: bone fragments firmly united by bone
- Clinical: roentgenographic evidence of bony bridging
- Effect of immobilization
  -Complete: membranous or primary bone healing
  -Incomplete: enchondral bone formation

When early callus is visualized radiologically, progressive protected weight bearing is a useful stimulus for healing. At this stage further adaptation can be made to casts or braces to allow increased training or participation in some sports. In a cyclist with a tibial fracture, for instance, a fracture brace may be used for walking and day-to-day activity, and a custom-made gaiter could be used while training on the bike. A word of caution is warranted, however, as excessive stress occasionally reverses the early callus formation.

Stage of Remodeling

Remodeling begins when the fracture, clinically and radiologically, is judged to be healed. The remodeling period ends when the bone has completely returned to normal, including restoration of the patency of the medullary canal. This process may take a few months to several years.[13,14] The fiber bone slowly converts to lamellar bone, and then the medullary canal is reconstituted. The diameter of the fracture gradually decreases to its original width. Oxygen tension is normal, and the fracture site is no longer electronegative. This stage always shows increased uptake on a technetium 99 polyphosphate scan, which indicates that remodeling is going on.

The remodeling process makes up for some deformity or malunion, but the potential for remodeling obviously depends on several factors. It can be said that clinically remodeling occurs most efficiently in the plane of the movement of the adjacent joint.[15,16] That is, anterior and posterior remodeling occurs at the elbow in the humerus much more easily than does valgus or varus malalignment. The remodeling occurs most efficiently near growth plates. The more open the growth plate, the more potential there is for remodeling. Lastly, it must be remembered that there is little if any remodeling of a rotation deformity. For this reason, during reduction of fractures one takes great care to obliterate or reduce to a minimum any residual malrotation while accepting some imperfect reduction in other planes.

One of the stimuli for bone remodeling is the stress-induced electrical charges. Such charges tend

---

Clinical Point

STAGE OF REMODELING

- Fiber bone converted to lamellar bone
- Reconstitution of medullary canal
- Callus diameter decreasing
- Fracture site no longer electronegative
- Duration: few months to several years
- More efficient remodeling
  -Open growth plates
  -Nerve bone ends
  -Deformity in plane of motion
  -Deformity minimal
- No remodeling of rotational malalignment

to be electronegative on the compression side of a deformity and cause bone deposition, whereas the opposite side, which is electropositive, is conducive to bone resorption.

Cast Disease

One of the most severe problems associated with fracture management are the adverse effects that immobilization has on body physiology. These effects, which last long after removal of the cast, include muscle wasting and atrophy, some loss of bone calcium, resorption and weakening of ligament attachment sites, and quality changes of the articular cartilage. Some of these changes are magnified by the effects of pain and effusion, particularly muscle wasting. Others, such as ligament weakening, are time dependent and totally reversible. Joint surface changes are mild up to 4 to 6 weeks and probably totally reversible; however, immobilization of longer duration may produce such significant cartilage changes that some of the effects may not be capable of healing.

An exaggeration of these immobilization induced changes is known as cast disease and includes osteoporosis, subchondral cyst formation, intra- and extra-articular adhesions, joint stiffness, articular surface softening and fibrillation, and severe muscle atrophy. It may progress so there is a significant disturbance of the autonomic nervous system control of the limb vasculature. It manifests as swelling, skin changes (e.g., hair loss and a shiny or mottled appearance), exquisite sensitivity even to light touch, and dramatic osteoporosis. In this case the immobilization induced changes merge into a reflex dystrophy.

There may be sensory dissociation in which there appears to be decreased sensation to pinprick, and even the light pressure of clothes brushing over the part are interpreted as painful. The dusky mottling of venous engorgement of venules often leads the patient to complain of bruising. However, there is no extravasation of blood, just intermittent disturbance of the local venous microcirculation.

There is definitely an intrinsic susceptibility to the evolution of this condition, but the magnitude of trauma and particularly the length of immobilization have some effect. It is therefore not surprising that methods of minimizing the need for absolute and prolonged immobilization and efforts to ensure function of the limb within a cast are central to good therapy. It is particularly true in the athlete, where the evolution of reflex dystrophy takes at least a year out of a career.

The use of dynamic splints or cast braces, muscle contraction within casts either actively or with electrical stimulation, and early motion as soon as the stage of fracture healing has progressed sufficiently are important. It is the need for early motion that makes the possibility of internal fixation attractive in some circumstances. In addition, some fractures are unstable or are intra-articular, and therefore internal fixation is the most acceptable method of ensuring a reasonable functional outcome. When a specific system of internal fixation is used, the traditional type of bone healing may not occur but, rather, a variation of bone remodeling called primary bone healing.

Primary Bone Healing (Primary Bone Repair)

When bone fragments are reduced anatomically and held rigid, primary bone repair may occur.[14] Special techniques of plates, screws, and internal fixation devices are used to achieve some compression, anatomic reduction, and the associated rigidity. Ideally, no external callus forms, and no interposing fibrous tissue or cartilage tissue appears at the fracture site. The fracture site is bridged by direct haversian remodeling, which is almost a direct osteon-to-osteon hook-up. Cutter heads form that go from one fragment across to the other fragment. Osteoclasts are in the forefront of the cutter heads to remove bone, and osteoblasts travel behind and lay down new bone. This process is a "revving up" of the normal remodeling phenomenon and is brought about by the ana-

---

Quick Facts

PRIMARY BONE HEALING

- Fracture reduced anatomically and held rigidly
- No interposing tissue
- Direct haversian remodeling (osteon-to-osteon hook-up)
- Osteoclasts tunnel from one fragment to other (cutter heads)
- Osteoblasts follow
- No external callus

tomic reduction. The surgical techniques used to achieve it are frequently referred to as A.O. techniques, developed by the Swiss Association for Osteosynthesis.

Although the advantages of this system are obvious, there are some potential drawbacks (Table 6-4). Opening a fracture site and using internal fixation devices may increase the risk of infection. Second, the actual bone healing may be slower and the quality of bone not as good or strong as healing with enchondral callus formation.[14] For this reason, there is always a race between fracture healing and the mechanical failure of the internal fixation devices. Inadequate training on the part of the surgeon and failure to observe the rules of implanting the system of internal fixation increases the rate of infection, instrument failure, and delayed union and nonunion. In contact sports, plates placed in some subcutaneous locations are uncomfortable when exposed to direct blows and may need special padding.

Lastly, the internal fixation stress shields the bone to varying degrees, which has significant implications. The bone under the plate may atrophy, remodeling in the correct lines of stress through the bone may not occur, and the bone immediately adjacent the plate may be subjected to increased forces, as the metal may form a stress riser.[15,16] For these reasons, particularly in the young athlete, it may be necessary to plan removal of the plate at some strategic point in the training cycle. This eventuality, in turn, requires a prolonged period of protection because the bone underneath the plate is mechanically weak, and screw holes form significant stress risers. The chance of refracture is high. For major long bones, internal fixation is usually removed after 12 to 18 months, after which a period of 12 to 20 weeks of protected activity may be required depending on the bone and sport concerned. There are no fast rules for these decisions, and each case must be assessed on its own merits and the experience of the surgeon. As with the initial injury care, decisions are based on the "personality of the fractures."

Factors That Influence Bone Healing

Circulation

There are several factors that may influence the rate of union, the first of which is the blood supply. Although a normal blood supply is necessary for fracture healing, anemia per se does not slow the rate of union. In other words, normal volemic anemia has no effect on union, whereas hypovolemic anemia does. By contrast, bones that have inadequate circulation heal slowly. Such bones are the distal tibia, the proximal scaphoid, and the head of the talus. Similarly, bones that are mainly articular surface and hence have little area for periosteal circulation, e.g., the femoral head and lunate, may be at risk for avascular necrosis after fracture or dislocation. Lastly, segmented fractures and badly comminuted fractures may have some avascular fragments that delay healing.

Hormones

As far as hormonal factors are concerned, there is no question that cortisone in large doses decreases or delays fracture healing. The evidence is not as clear concerning calcitonin, thyroxine, and parathyroid hormone (PTH) in regard to fracture healing. It appears these hormones merely play a passive role. Growth hormone has a stimulatory effect during the middle phase of fracture healing but probably does not result in earlier complete fracture healing. There is some question as to the negative effect of nonsteroidal anti-inflammatory medication on bone turnover; and although it is dangerous to extrapolate animal data to humans, it may be inadvisable to administer these medications for the treatment of pain associated with stress fractures.

Nutrition

Nutritional and mineral factors probably play only a passive role in fracture healing. That is, it would take marked restriction of diet to decrease fracture

TABLE 6-4.   Characteristics of Stages and Types of Bone Healing

Type of Healing	Speed of Healing	Ability to Bridge Gaps	Tolerance to Movement	Tolerance of Rigidity	Importance of External Soft Tissue
Enchondral ossification					
Primary callus response	++++	+	++++	++++	−
External bridging callus	+++	+++	+++	−	++++
Late medullary callus	++	++++ (slow)	++	+++	−
Primary cortical healing	+	−	−	++++	−

healing. It has not been shown that diet supplementation in any form increases the rate of normal fracture healing.

Bioelectric Factors

Bioelectric factors may influence bone turnover.[15,16] As early as 18 days after a fracture, significant stress-generated potentials are present. As the callus matures, the stress-generated potentials at the fracture site increase. Ultimately they decrease again at the end of healing. This pattern leads to the hypothesis that early protected weight bearing leads to the formation of stress-generated potentials in the fracture callus; which may in turn lead to orientation of the collagen fibers to form closely packed bundles. Such closely packed collagen bundles increase the callus strength and perhaps also favor mineralization. Thus the early protected weight bearing that stimulates these electrical potentials may be beneficial to the fracture callus.

Mechanical Factors

Mechanical factors affecting fracture healing have been studied incompletely. It has been shown in several studies that the effect of compression on osteogenesis does not necessarily stimulate bone formation. However, it does increase immobilization, and certainly closely approximated fragments heal more easily. Nevertheless, too much compression leads to bone resorption and certainly to cell death. In this regard, rigid internal fixation may be a good thing for fracture fixation, but one must keep in mind that it may lead to cortical osteoporosis and certainly prevents or delays remodeling. Also, because little or no callus formation occurs, one must weigh carefully the net effect of potential early mobilization versus ultimate function.

Other factors, such as induction, age, and type of bone, have already been discussed.

Electrical Activity in Bone

Electrical potentials generated in bone deserve further discussion, not only because of their role in induction but because their role and application are important to several aspects of sports medicine. Stressed bone generates electrical potentials. When bone is mechanically loaded, the area under compression becomes electronegative and the area under tension electropositive. These potentials are termed "stress generated potentials." They are not dependent on cell viability. Note also that they arise from the organic component of bone, probably from the bending of the large collagen molecules, similar to a piezoelectric effect in crystals.

> ## Quick Facts
> ### STRESS GENERATED POTENTIALS
> - Arise when bone stressed
> - Not dependent on cell viability
> - Compression electronegative
> - Tension electropositive
> - Arise from organic component

There is another type of electrical potential that arises from bone. If one measures the electrical potentials on the surface of unstressed living bone, the ends of bone tend to be electronegative in comparison to the shaft, which tends to be either electropositive or neutral. When a fracture occurs in the midshaft of the bone, the entire surface of the bone becomes electronegative. A large peak of electronegative activity appears over the fracture site that gradually diminishes as the fracture heals. Similar electronegative activity peaks can be seen opposite growth plates. These potentials are termed "bioelectric potentials." They are not dependent on stress but are dependent on cell viability. The areas of growth and repair are electronegative, whereas the inactive areas are electrically neutral or electropositive.

> ## Quick Facts
> ### BIOELECTRIC POTENTIALS
> - Not dependent on stress
> - Depend on cell viability
> - Areas of growth and repair electronegative

A study of these electrical potentials has generated an idea that electrical phenomena can be used to stimulate or increase bone healing particularly in cases where there has been delayed union or nonunion. There are several systems. One is totally invasive, where the electrodes are placed in the tissues. With the other, which is semi-invasive, only the cathode is inserted into the site of nonunion. There is a third, inductive method in which the electrodes are totally outside the skin and magnetic fields are generated within the tissues. Small electrical forces are used, and it is said that in some instances a success rate of up to 80 to 85 percent is achieved in cases of previous nonunion. Despite two decades of research, many of the applications of these electrostimulation techniques are still speculative.

Delayed Union and Nonunion

Bone union sometimes progresses more slowly than expected. Delayed union is present when fracture healing is not advancing at the average rate for the location and type of fracture under consideration. Union may be stimulated by increasing weight bearing and sometimes by externally or internally applied electrical stimulation. On occasion it is more expedient to consider open reduction and internal fixation.

Quick Facts

FACTORS IN DELAYED UNION AND NONUNION

- Poor blood supply
- Infection
- Inadequate immobilization
- Inadequate reduction
- Inadequate internal fixation
- Poor patient compliance
- Delayed diagnosis of fracture

Nonunion, on the other hand, exists when all reparative processes at the fracture site have ceased and yet bony continuity has not been restored. Sometimes nonunion takes the form of the bone ends becoming atrophic and is accompanied by a certain amount of resorption. On the other hand, the bone ends may become hypertrophic. A large wedge of bone is produced, and occasionally a synovial cavity forms between the ends of the bones. It is then referred to as a synovial pseudarthrosis. This interesting phenomenon occurs with about 12 percent of nonunions. When a fracture reaches this stage, only open treatment with excision of the synovium and internal fixation can help this bone achieve union.

Quick Facts

NONUNION

- All attempts at fracture healing cease.
- Medullary canal closes.
- Sclerotic bone ends are seen.
- Atrophic or hypertrophic changes are present.
- Pseudarthrosis may result.

Refracture

The reintroduction of unprotected physical activity always carries a risk of refracture (Table 6-5). Most refractures occur after removal of the cast or brace or after removal of internal fixation. Obviously, collision sports present the greatest risk, and the hand is particularly vulnerable. Whenever practical, prolonged protection should be used. With skiing, children and adolescents with long bone fractures, particularly of the femur and tibia, should miss the remaining season even if they sustained their fracture early and have apparently sound union. For adults, if the fracture occurs late in one season, the next season should be missed if they wish to minimize the risks. This approach is essentially conservative and safe; and most competitive skiers cannot afford such a time frame. For the noncompetitive athlete, however, the risks should be explained.

STRESS FRACTURES

When a structure is loaded repeatedly, it may break with a load that would not normally cause it to fail if it were loaded only once.[17] This situation is known as fatigue failure; and in bone it is called fatigue fracture

TABLE 6-5. Refractures[a]

Bone	Vulnerable Interval (months)	Sport Most at Risk
Tibia	12–45	Skiing
Ankle	10–20	Soccer
Metacarpal	8–31	Football
Phalanges	15–35	Volleyball
Clavicle	6–18	Hockey
Ribs	8–14	Football
Nose	5–23	Rugby
Metatarsals	8–45	Volleyball

[a] Represents series reported in the literature.

or stress fracture. It occurs in the normal bones of healthy people, the site varying according to age and activity. Stress fractures are seen in osteoporotic individuals and the elderly, as well as in healthy young athletes. Although fatigue fractures occur frequently, they are often misdiagnosed or simply overlooked because most go on to heal with an unremarkable clinical course.[18-20] Repetitive stress plays an important role in initiating many types of fracture that were once thought to be produced by a single traumatic event.

A distinction must be made between pathologic fracture and stress fracture. True pathologic fractures take place in bone with pre-existing pathology, such as fracture through a bone cyst. The subchondral bone erosion of rheumatoid arthritis may predispose to a fatigue fracture; to be more accurate, however, such breaks are pathologic fractures. Stress fractures through osteoportic bones should perhaps be considered pathologic fractures.

Spectrum of Stress Reaction

Bone is a living tissue, and its ability to respond to stress by remodeling has already been discussed. The same mechanisms used in the growth of bone and the later stages of bone healing are at play in a more subtle manner on a day to day basis.

With activity-induced stress there is accelerated adaptive turnover. Matheson et al. demonstrated that nonpainful areas of increased technetium pyrophosphate are frequently seen on scintigraphic scans.[9] These nonpainful sites are usually in the tarsal and metatarsal bones, the femur, and the tibia (Fig. 6-12).

At the other end of the spectrum is the complete defect or crack, easily visualized on plain films. Therefore it is postulated that a continuum exists, from normal remodeling through accelerated remodeling in response to exercise, weakening of trabeculae, microfracture, and if activity is not modified macrofracture.[20] It is also possible that the diffuse uptake of periostitis is a variation on this continuum (Fig. 6-13). Given sufficient time and a well planned, progressive exercise schedule, bone hypertrophy occurs.[5-8] Alternatively, accelerated, unaccustomed, intense activity with insufficient recovery period may lead to the cycle of weakened trabeculae and microfracture (Fig. 6-14).

Whether muscle fatigue makes the bone more vulnerable because of inability to facilitate shock absorbing or, alternatively, the repetitive pull of strong muscles at their origins contribute to the stress is not

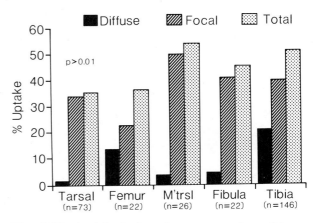

Fig. 6-12. Activity-induced stress reaction of bone. Frequency of diffuse, focal, and total uptake of scintigraphic ^{99m}Tc at nonpainful sites in the tarsus, femur, metatarsals, fibula, and tibia. (After Matheson et al.,[17] with permission.)

certain. The anatomic shape, specific stress of the activity, and local microanatomy may produce areas of stress concentrations.

These theories are not mutually exclusive, and each may play some part. What is abundantly clear is that stress fractures occur with any frequency only in greyhounds, horses, and man, and they must be taken as a sign of ill-advised and ill-conceived activity.

Some of these theoretic processes were confirmed in studies of experimentally induced excessive exercise in rabbits.[9,18,20] Vascular changes and circulatory distress within the cortical bone occur before osteoclastic resorption. Degeneration and necrosis of osteocytes due to circulatory disturbance also occurs. Periosteal new bone formation appeared at 12 days as a compensatory reaction to the osteoclastic resorption.[18] Small cracks appeared at the cement line and spread to the neighboring haversian system. At 21 days, incomplete fracture of the cortex was seen in some rabbits, and a complete fracture evolved in one rabbit.[20] Most of the tibia did not develop fracture lines, showing that it had adapted to the changes in stress by internal remodeling.[9] In short, stress fractures are a demonstration of failure on the part of the athlete or coach to judge appropriate speed and volume of activity progression.

Diagnosis

Frequently the history is helpful in the diagnosis; and if the bone is sufficiently superficial, local tenderness is palpable. (The deeply seated femur may not

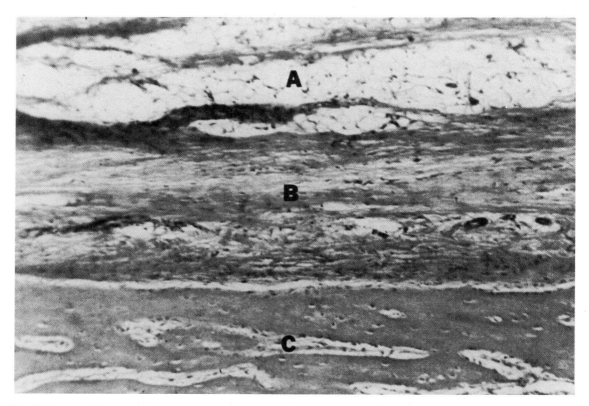

Fig. 6-13. Proliferation of periosteum in response to microfracture. **(A)** Fat. **(B)** Periosteum. **(C)** Tibial cortex.

be palpably tender.) A history of trauma may be associated with some areas, particularly the tibia and tarsal bone. Because the plain roentgenogram is usually negative initially, an index of suspicion is necessary, particularly at atypical sites. If the symptoms are severe, interfering with all activities, or if there are important activity deadlines, a bone scan allows early diagnosis and formulation of a specific treatment plan. Pain in the spine, pelvis, trunk, femur, or upper tibia is difficult to diagnose, and there is a tendency to perform scans earlier (Figure 6-15). Occasionally, negative scans are reported that become positive a few weeks later. If symptoms do not improve, repeat roentgenograms and bone scans are reasonable tests.

The average time for diagnosis of stress fractures in some series was almost 13 weeks, and the time to recovery was 2 to 96 weeks with an average of 13 weeks[7] (Fig. 6-16). Treated efficiently and early, these injuries are usually mild; but if diagnosed late, treated inadequately, or compliance by the athlete is poor, stress fractures can be a significant problem.

Clinical Point

SIGNS OF STRESS FRACTURES

- Point tenderness of bone (except well shielded femur)
- Soft tissue swelling
- Alteration of gait
- Muscular atrophy, especially anterior tibial and gastrocnemius-soleus groups
- Full and painless range of motion of adjacent joints
- Painless resisted active movement of joint
- Increased technetium 99 uptake indicating a focal lesion
- Hairline radiolucency, periosteal callus, or endosteal callus by roentgenography; associated soft tissue swelling
- Palpation of callus (with time)

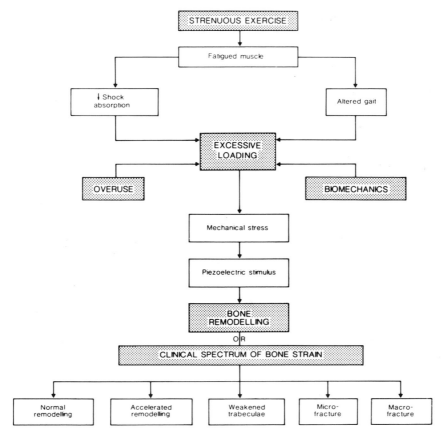

Fig. 6-14. Possible evolution of stress reaction and stress fracture of bone.

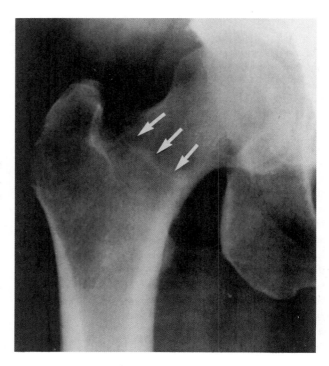

Fig. 6-15. Deeply seated femoral neck stress fracture may give pain but no obvious local tenderness and swelling. Initially, plain films may be negative; thus late diagnosis is common, as it was in this case.

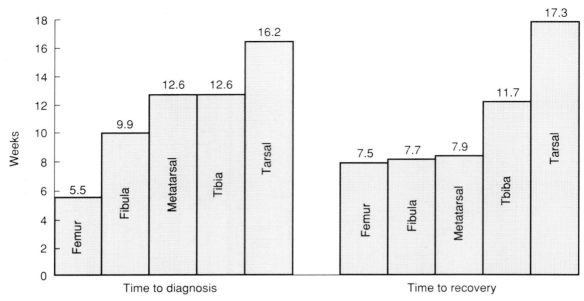

Fig. 6-16. Average time to diagnosis and healing of specific stress fracture sites. (After Matheson et al.,[17] with permission.)

Thermography may be useful for the more superficially located stress fractures. In individuals with a negative plain film and hot bone scans, an abnormal thermogram is likely in about 90 percent of the cases. It is suggested that serial thermograms may predict when resumption of activity is possible.[21]

Differential Diagnosis

Pain is usually proportional to activity and is rarely present at rest. Atypical pain and a hot scan should stimulate a diligent review and consideration of the differential diagnosis of a positive scan, i.e., neoplasia, infection, and inflammatory disorders.

Therapeutic ultrasound (US) is of potential use for detecting stress fractures.[22,23] Moss and Mowat suggested that the application of US, with a 3 cm head at 0.75 mHz sonated directly over the tibia, is frequently diagnostic.[24] If the intensity is gradually increased, to a maximum of 2.0 watts per square centimeter (W/cm^2), a positive response is defined as an unpleasant sensation (intense pressure or pain).[24] Other workers have reported pain and discomfort with 1 mHz US at 0.5 to 1.5 W applied over recent fractures.[25] They suggested it might be a valuable supplementary test for diagnosing such problems as scaphoid fractures.

Ultrasonography is a potentially inexpensive, noninvasive test with negligible side effects and few risks. Its pain-producing quality may be due to selective absorption at the fracture site or to increased reflection of the periosteum. It is known that bone and periosteum have a different acoustic impedance, and that at the bone–periosteal interface 70 percent of the energy is reflected and 30 percent is absorbed. Thus the periosteum is absorbing ultrasonic energy from both above (directly from the source) and below (reflected waves from the bone). The periosteum is poorly equipped to dispel the reflected energy. It has a rich supply of sensory receptors that become aware of a noxious stimulus if the periosteal temperature approaches 45°C.[22,23] The pain produced by US may be due to the heating effect that occurs normally at tissue interfaces but may be increased in the patient with a stress fracture. Pain on application of US may be due to the mechanical vibratory effect selectively irritating the nerve endings in the area, but Delacerda[23] found that no pain was exhibited when the US was pulsed or below 0.65 W/cm^2.

It has been suggested that the damaged periosteum over a stress fracture site may absorb continuous ultrasonic energy, converting it to heat, which causes pain. Intact periosteum or periosteum involved in significant callus formation, on the other hand, does not absorb sound energy to the same degree.

Occasionally muscle injury is visualized on radionuclide scanning. The exact mechanism of tracer uptake is not known, but it probably binds to denatured protein, other macromolecules, or the intracellular calcium that appears after muscle fiber damage or necrosis. Severe exercise-induced muscle soreness associated with elevated levels of creatine phosphokinase and myoglobin may produce transient uptake for a few days to a week.[6] Local muscle tears may be seen if more than 3 to 5 mg of local muscle necrosis ensues. Scintographic activity peaks about 3 to 4 days after the injury and decreases as phagocytic removal of the debris ensues. Similarly, myositis ossificans developing in a muscle hematoma may be visualized weeks or even months before bone is visible on the plain roentgenogram.

Distribution

The true incidence of stress fractures is not known because all centers do not have the same criteria for carrying out bone scans. Moreover, many athletes are treated successfully after only a presumptive diagnosis. Furthermore, the interest of the clinic concerned influences the common sport and pattern of athletes seen and hence the distribution of the fractures. In a review of 3,198 fatigue-induced fractures reported in the literature, 1 percent occurred in the upper limbs, 17 percent in the trunk and pelvis, and 82 percent in the lower extremities (Table 6-6). In Matheson's review of 320 stress fractures, the most common site was the tibia (49.1 percent) followed by tarsal bones (25.3 percent), metatarsals (8.8 percent), femur (7.2 percent), fibula (6.6 percent), pelvis (1.6 percent),

sesamoids (0.9 percent), and spine (0.6 percent).[17] Bilateral stress fractures occurred in 16.6 percent of cases, which comprised a large running population.

There is some association of activities with specific stress fractures (Table 6-7). In the upper extremities, clavicular fatigue fractures are associated with throwing sports; humeral fractures with tennis, basketball, cricket, and javelin; radius and ulnar fractures with wheelchair sports, weight training, and gymnastics; and scapular fractures with gymnastics. In the trunk, rib fractures are associated with lifting and rowing; vertebral fractures with football, lifting, rowing, and gymnastics; and pelvic fractures with running. In the lower extremity, hip and femoral fractures are linked to running; and tibial tarsal and metatarsal fractures are associated with running, aerobic dance, ballet, skating, walking, and hockey.

Treatment Principles

Early diagnosis is important, allowing early resolution with minimal interruption of activity (Table 6-8). An index of suspicion is therefore essential, and athletes should be treated presumptively if adequate signs and symptoms allow a clinical diagnosis, even if plain films are negative.

Activity is modified appropriately to the symptoms and physical findings. If symptoms are severe, complete rest may be required. Some alternate activity is designated to prevent loss of skill and fitness.[26] A

TABLE 6-6. Literature Review of 3,198 Stress Fractures[a]

Body Part	Incidence[b] (%)	Fractures No.	Fractures %	Frequent Activity
Upper limb		37	1	Weight training, tennis, wheelchair sports, pitching, gymnastics
Ulna	46			
Humerus	21			
Radius	12			
Scapula	2			
Other	19			
Trunk		548	17	Weight training, football, gymnastics, wrestling, diving, running (pelvis)
Vertebrae	45			
Pelvis	42			
Ribs	14			
Lower limb		2,613	82	Jogging, running, ballet, basketball, soccer, aerobic dance
Tibia	46			
Fibula	19			
Metatarsals	18			
Tarsals	10			
Femur	9			

[a] Numbers represent cases reported in the literature rather than true incidence.
[b] Percentages rounded off to whole numbers.

TABLE 6-7. Stress Fractures

Activity	Bone Involved
Running	
Sprint	Tibia
Middle distance	Fibula, tibia
Long distance	Tibia, metatarsal, tarsal
Hiking	Metatarsal, pelvis
Race walking	Pelvis, fibula
Jumping	Pelvis, femur
Tennis	Ulna, metacarpal
Baseball	
Pitching	Humerus, scapula
Batting	Rib
Catching	Patella
Basketball	Patella, tibia, os calcis
Javelin	Ulna
Soccer	Tibia, metatarsal
Swimming	Tibia, metatarsal
Skating	Fibula
Curling	Ulna
Aerobics	Fibula, tibia
Ballet dancing	Tibia
Cricket	Humerus
Fencing	Pubis
Handball	Metacarpal
Water skiing	Pars intra-articularis

careful activity history, physical examination, and biomechanical assessment allows identification of probable causes and allows education of the athlete, activity planning, footwear advice, and orthotic prescription if indicated (Fig. 6-17).[27] There is rarely a need for casting, although occasionally if the cortex has a complete defect in a major weight bearing long bone some support is necessary. The air stirrup or a brace may be appropriate. In key situations, such as significant fractures of the femoral neck, internal fixation may be considered.

At some point careful resumption of activity is necessary with a definite prescription for adding intensity or distance. If running in water is used as a method of maintaining fitness, it is essential to spend the same amount of time in the water as was spent running on land. This is an obvious but necessary statement. Furthermore, because it is primarily a relatively non-weight-bearing situation, slow reintegration into running is necessary if a reversal of the healing process is to be avoided.

Some fractures have a propensity for delayed union or nonunion, e.g., fractures of the mid tibia or fifth metatarsal, the tarsal, navicular, or sesamoid bones of the great toe, and in the upper extremity the olecranon process. These fractures may require electrical stimulation, internal fixation, bone grafting, or in the case of the sesamoid excision.

Practice Point

TREATMENT OF RUNNING-INDUCED STRESS FRACTURES

- Prescribe a rest from running.
- Relieve symptomatic inflammation with ice and possibly an anti-inflammatory agent.
- Maintain strength (especially foot dorsum and plantar flexors).
- Maintain cardiovascular fitness with swimming, biking, or both.
- Prescribe orthotics tailored to need.
- When asymptomatic, gradually reintroduce running.
- Counsel patient about training errors.

TABLE 6-8. Healing of Stress Fractures

	No. of Stress Fractures, by Healing Period		
Bone	2–4 Weeks	1–2 Months	>2 Months
Tibia			
Proximal third	—	38	51
Middle third	—	13	14
Distal third	—	35	31
Fibula	3	33	8
Metatarsals	15	42	17
Sesamoid bones	—	—	15
Femoral shaft	1	1	12
Femoral neck	—	—	9
Pelvis	—	2	5
Olecranon	—	—	5

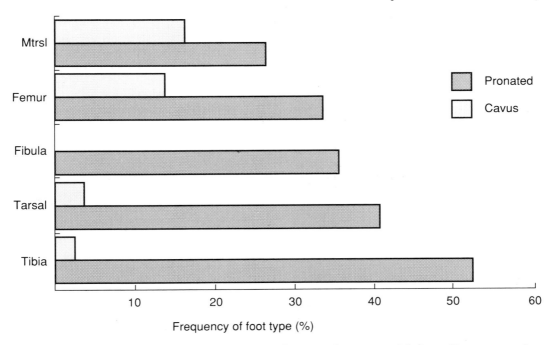

Fig. 6-17. There may be some association of specific stress fractures with foot alignment and structure. The pronated foot in runners may be significant. (After Matheson et al.,[17] with permission.)

In the long-term follow-up of 295 soldiers with stress fractures, five patterns of natural history were observed[19]: (1) uneventful recovery (47 percent); (2) protracted recovery (13.6 percent); (3) symptoms consistent with recurrent stress fractures in new sites (19.6 percent); (4) intermittent non stress-fracture bone pain (16.7 percent); and (5) chronic stress fractures (3 percent). The incidence of recurrent stress fractures was 10.6 percent. Although these military recruits were a slightly different population than the general athlete population, the principles illustrated in that report are sound. Stress fractures develop during intense, sudden increases in activity, and they may be debilitating. Some individuals seem to have a definite predisposition for their occurrence.

In summary, prevention of stress fractures should be a major concern. It involves education, early recognition, and treatment. One of the main clinical problems concerns distinguishing the potentially dangerous stress fracture, which requires complete reduction of activity or even surgical intervention, from the more usual stress reaction, which has a predictable, benign course. The differential diagnosis and pattern of hot bone scans must always be considered.

SUMMARY

Bone is a unique living tissue that is able to regenerate following fracture. In the skeletally immature patient, epiphyseal damage must always be a consideration in both traumatic and overuse injuries. Body weight and muscle contraction assist in loading the mature skeleton with calcium. Ill-advised exercise and dietary habits and regimens, as well as the lack of activity, can affect the bones negatively and predispose toward involutional osteoporosis.

The knowledge of healing times, methods of modifying activity, protection from excessive stress and reintroducing safe loading after fractures may help salvage an athlete's season. However, the danger of refracture is real, and suitable advice must be given.

Stress reaction of bone and stress fractures should always be considered as a failure of the athlete or coach to adequately progress the volume and intensity of training in a safe way. Early detection often rests on an index of suspicion, particularly at atypical sites. Early diagnosis usually allows successful therapy with only slight modification of training.

Bone is not an uncommon site of tumors in both the young and the elderly. Therefore unremitting pain must always be investigated with this unpleasant possibility in mind.

REFERENCES

1. Kaplan FS: Osteoporosis: Pathophysiology and Prevention. Ciba-Geigy Clinical Symposium No. 4. Ciba Pharmaceutical Company, Ontario, 1987
2. Reid DC: Functional Anatomy and Joint Mobilization. University of Alberta Press, Edmonton, 1970
3. Langman J: Medical Embryology. Williams & Wilkins, Baltimore, 1963
4. Ham AW: Histology. JB Lippincott, Philadelphia, 1957
5. Jones HH, Priest JD, Hayes WC et al: Humeral hypertrophy in response to exercise. J Bone Joint Surg [AM] 59:204, 1977
6. Nilsson BE, Westlin NE: Bone density in athletes. Clin Orthop 77:179, 1971
7. Saville PD, Whyte MP: Muscle and bone hypertrophy: Positive effect of running exercise in the rat. Clin Orthop Res 65:81, 1969
8. Savio L, Woo Y, Kuel SC et al: The effect of prolonged physical training on the properties of long bone: a study of Wolff's law. J Bone Joint Surg [AM] 63:780, 1981
9. Matheson GO, Clement DB, McKenzie DC et al: Scintigraphic uptake of ^{99m}Tc at non-painful sites in athletes with stress fractures: the concept of bone strain. Sports Med 4:65, 1987
10. Nagle CE, Freitas JE: Radionuclide imaging of musculoskeletal injuries in athletes with negative radiographs. Physician Sports Med 15:147, 1987
11. Ham AW: Some histophysiological problems peculiar to calcified tissues. J Bone Joint Surg [Am] 34:711, 1952
12. Salter RB, Harris WR: Injuries involving the epiphyseal plate. J Bone Joint Surg [Am] 45:587, 1963
13. Rockwood CA, Green DP (eds): Fractures. Vol. 1. JB Lippincott, Philadelphia, 1975
14. McKibben B: The biology of fracture healing in long bones. J Bone Joint Surg [Br] 60:150, 1978
15. Treharne RW: Review of Wolff's law and its proposed means of operation. Orthop Rev 10:35, 1981
16. Wolff J: Ueber die innere Architektur der Knochen und ihre Bedeutung für die Frage von Knochenwachstum. Virchow's Arch [Pathol Anat] 50:389, 1870
17. Matheson GO, Clement DB, McKenzie DC et al: Stress fractures in athletes. Am J Sports Med 15:46, 1987
18. Li G, Zhang S, Chen G et al: Radiographic and histologic analysis of stress fracture in rabbit tibias. Am J Sports Med 13:285, 1985
19. Milgrom C, Gilad M, Chisin R et al: The long term follow-up of soldiers with stress fractures. Am J Sports Med 13:398, 1985
20. Wang WG: Stress lesions of the tibia in athletes. China J Sports Sci 120:14, 1963
21. Goodman PH, Heaslet MW, Pagliano JW et al: Stress fracture diagnosis by computer-assisted thermography. Physician Sports Med 13:114, 1985
22. Cole JP, Gossman D: Ultrasonic stimulation of low lumbar nerve roots as a diagnostic procedure: a preliminary report. Clin Orthop 153:126, 1979
23. Delacerda FG: A case study: application of ultrasound to determine a stress fracture of the fibula. J Orthop Sports Phys Ther 2:134, 1981
24. Moss A, Mowat AG: Ultrasonic assessment of stress fractures. Br Med J 286:1478, 1983
25. Bedford AF, Glasgow MM, Wilson JN: Ultrasonic assessment of fractures and its use in the diagnosis of the suspected scaphoid fracture. Injury 14:180, 1985
26. Reid DC: Assessment of Treatment of the Injured Athlete. University of Alberta Press. Edmonton, 1988
27. Walter SD, Hart LE, Sutton JR et al: Training habits and injury experience in distance runners: age and sex related factors. Physician Sports Med 16:101, 1988.

Selected Conditions of the Foot

7

The Lus or Lost Souls of Ushaia

*This bone can never be burned or corrupted in all
eternity, for its ground substance is of celestial origin and,
watered with heavenly dew, wherewith God shall make
the dead rise as with yeast in a mass of dough.*
—*The Rabbi Ushaia (AD 210)*
[on the great toe sesamoids[1]]

Unaided support and bipedal locomotion are the
two main functions of the human foot, and their requirements have stimulated a high degree of anatomic specialization. The foot has evolved from a
primitive, prehensile pattern designed for grasping to
a plantigrade unit capable of bipedal weight-bearing.[1,2] These events are still reflected in the fetal development of the human foot.

Joseph has neatly summarized the necessary evolutionary adaptations of the human foot that allow efficient bipedal locomotion.[3] First, the foot has become
plantigrade, which allows most of the sole to be the
weight-bearing surface. Second, the great toe has
come to lie in apposition with the other toes and,
because of the relative immobility of the first metatarsal at the metatarsophalangeal (MTP) joint, is now
relatively nonprehensile. Third, the metatarsals and
phalanges have progressively shrunk and become
small in comparison to the hypertrophied tarsus.
Last, the medial side of the foot has become larger
and stronger than that of any other primate. Hence
the size of the functional grasping muscles has been
reduced as prehension has become subordinate to
producing a propulsive thrust.

The newborn and the young child usually have flat
feet until they begin to walk. This fact is evidence of
the dynamic, rather than the static, nature of the
arch. Tightness and adaptive shortening of the intrinsic musculature and longitudinal ligaments of the
plantar aspect of the foot gradually help produce the
characteristic arches. The extent to which it occurs is
largely determined by the osseous development.

It is probably safe to say that although the foot has
adapted well to its function in bipedal locomotion it
has not yet adapted to being encased in shoes. Foot
pain and deformity are a reflection of this fact.

To take this argument to the extreme, one could
reflect on the incredible destruction to this delicate
architecture brought about by binding of the feet.[4,5]
In some Oriental societies the toes were fixed under
the foot in a cavus position from about the age of 3 to
4 years, which resulted in deformed feet referred to
euphemistically as "golden lilies." Similar pictures
may be seen in cases of severe paralysis of the muscles
during development, e.g., due to childhood polio.
These may be contrasted with the extremely broad
feet of individuals who have never worn shoes. Muscle action, heredity, and footwear are obviously potent forces in the development of foot shape. The
examples above lend, as Gilbert and Sullivan would
say, "an air of artistic verisimilitude to what would
otherwise be a bald and unconvincing statement."

The stresses through the foot during activities of
daily living and athletic endeavors are enormous.
When they are injured, it is particularly difficult to
rest the feet adequately, thus providing a challenge to
the physicians' and therapists' ingenuity. Severe foot
pain can set up a chain of adverse compensatory
mechanisms throughout the lower limb and trunk,
giving rise to problems that may persist long after the

129

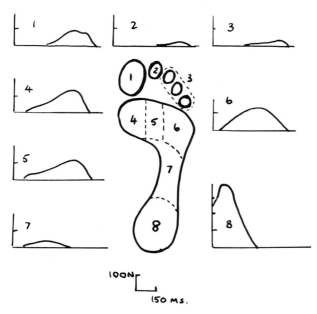

Fig. 7-1. Force through the eight areas of the foot over time caused by walking.

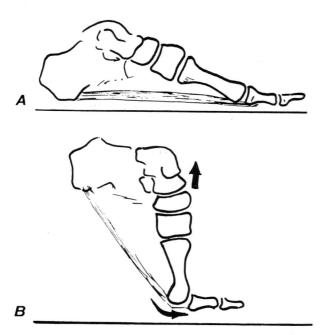

Fig. 7-2. (A) Windless effect of the plantar fascia (aponeurosis plantaris). **(B)** As the heel raises and the toes dorsiflex, the aponeurosis is wrapped around the metatarsal head, and the longitudinal arch is elevated. (After DuVries,[10] with permission.)

specific foot pathology has been resolved. Athletes should be particularly cognizant of the motto of the Roots Shoe Company: "Be Nice To Feet, They Outnumber People Two To One."

FOREFOOT

Anatomy

Functional Requirements

The forefoot has to sustain, accelerate, and balance the body's weight for at least 40 percent of the stance phase of walking.[6] During running, it further receives the impact of each touch-down; and with stopping and changing direction, it must withstand enormous shear forces.[7] Stresses absorbed on the ball of the foot must be transferred to the skeleton. The forefoot contains structures adapted for this shock-absorbing purpose, which at the same time protect the nerves and tendons. Thus encapsulated fat pads disperse pressure and protect nerves and vessels; and ligamentous structures connect the skin to the skeleton by an ingenious framework of tough bands running in vertical, transverse, and sagittal directions.[7] The shapes of the joints and their ligamentous constraints in turn accommodate both shock-absorbing requirements of weight bearing and the rigid lever needed for propulsion. With the average person taking between 10,000 to 15,000 steps per day, and the highly active athlete compounding these stresses with hours of training, it is remarkable that foot problems do not dominate all other athletic injuries. With running activities, more than 100 tons of force may have to be dissipated for every mile covered. Fortunately, foot complaints in athletes have been contained, to a large degree, by the superb advances made in sports footwear.

During walking, the maximum force acting across the first MTP joint is approximately equal to the body weight (Fig. 7-1), which is more than twice the load carried by the other toes combined. This ratio decreases to somewhat more than one-third by about age 40 to 50.[8] Thus the second to fourth metatarsal heads take proportionately greater stress at a time of life when body weight is often increased, the quality of collagen and size of the plantar fat pads deteriorating, and the mechanics of the foot frequently altered by increasing hallux valgus. This fact may account, in part, for the prevalence of foot and Achilles tendon problems in 40- to 50-year-old joggers, particularly those taking up the activity after years of a sedentary life style.

Arches and Bony Configuration

The classic description of the foot includes both medial and lateral longitudinal arches extending from the calcaneus to the first and fifth metatarsal heads, respectively. A coronal arch is derived from the shape of the cuneiform bones and can be distinguished in transverse sections throughout the metatarsal region. Anteriorly, the metatarsal heads are normally in almost the same transverse plane so they may share in the load of weight bearing.[7,9]

The tarsometatarsal and intermetatarsal joints have their close-packed position in supination. They permit a restricted range of gliding. The MTP joints are condyloid synovial articulations with a close-packed position in extension. Their acute capsular pattern, accompanying inflammation, is for more limitation of flexion than extension; however, invariably more extension is lost with prolonged joint inflammation or degenerative changes.[9] The MTP joints function mainly in flexion and extension, with some adjunct adduction and abduction. Nevertheless, joint mobilization should include rotation, a movement achieved only passively; but it is important, because the small amount of spin that represents an extra degree of freedom ensures an adequate functional range.[9]

The interphalangeal joints are synovial hinge articulations, with extension as the close-packed position. The range of motion is small and the capsular pattern inconsistent. Most people can move their toes only in gross coordinated patterns, and they have poor individual control of the digits. There are remarkable exceptions in that some individuals, born with absent upper limbs, show a latent potential for fine cortical control and muscle action. A significant amount of the functional movement of the toes in locomotion is passive, an unusual situation.

During the swing phase, there is about 30 to 40 degrees of extension at MTP joints to prevent the toes stubbing the ground. At the terminal part of the stance phase, as the heel lifts, extension is achieved at the MTP joints, depending on the individual's flexibility. The plantar aponeurosis, extending from the calcaneal tubercle, passes distally to insert into the base of each proximal phalanx via the plantar pad. Any dorsiflexion of the toes slides the plantar pads distally, placing tension on the plantar aponeurosis. The architecture of the joints allows the arch to form.[10] This "windless" mechanism creates a dynamic stable arch and hence a more rigid level for push-off (Fig. 7-2).

Muscle Action

Walking

With walking, the extensor hallucis and the extensor digitorum are active during the last 10 percent of the stance phase, throughout the swing phase, and into the initial 10 to 15 percent of the next stance phase (Fig. 7-3). They function in conjunction with the tibialis anterior to lift the toes off the ground during the swing phase and eccentrically during the initial stance phase to lower the foot, thereby preventing a slapping action. The flexor digitorum longus and flexor hallucis longus are active in midstance, just after the gastrocnemius-soleus complex clicks in, helping control and restrain the dorsiflexor movement of the tibia on the fixed foot. The posterior calf muscles cease to function at about 50 percent of the walking cycle, before most of the plantar flexion has occurred. The intrinsic foot muscles, i.e., abductor hallucis and abductor digiti minimi, are essentially active from about 30 percent of the gait cycle during stance until the end of the stance phase. These intrinsic muscles stabilize the arch along with the plantar aponeurosis and assist in keeping the toes flat on the ground until lift-off has occurred. When walking on the toes they are continuously active. It is difficult to appreciate that during normal walking there is no or little extrinsic or intrinsic plantar flexion action needed to propel the body forward during push-off.

Jogging and Running

In summary, toe motion helps stabilize the longitudinal arch passively and actively, and the action of the intrinsics further assist in maintaining floor contact until push-off. Mann and Hagy, in their classic paper, characterized jogging at approximately 6 mph and running at 12 mph.[11] The flexor hallucis longus and flexor digitorum longus act to restrain dorsiflexion during late swing and the first 50 percent of stance phase, a significant difference to walking (Fig. 7-3). The extensor digitorum and the extensor hallucis longus work with the tibialis anterior to bring about dorsiflexion of the ankle during swing and early

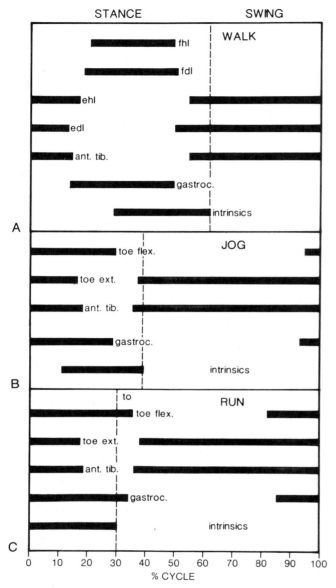

Fig. 7-3. Electromyography of the muscles about the foot and ankle. **(A)** Walking. **(B)** Jogging. **(C)** Running. The time is expressed as a percent of the cycle. fhl = flexor hallucis longus; fdl = flexor digitorum longus; ehl = extensor hallucis longus; edl = extensor digitorum longus; ant tib = tibialis anterior; gastroc = gastrocnemius; intrinsic = average activity of intrinsic toe flexors and abductor hallucis and digiti minimi. (After Mann and Hagy,[11] with permission.)

stance, similar to their function during walking. The former are active throughout most of the stance phase. The important difference for all these muscles is that the events of walking are condensed into about one-third of the time while jogging and even less

---

Practice Point

RUNNING VERSUS WALKING

- Events condensed into about one-third or less time
- Forces generated higher
- Greater whipping action on tendons
- Rest cycles shorters

---

when fast running. At the same time, the forces generated are much higher, with a proportionately greater chance of whipping action on the tendons. Moreover, the rest cycles are obviously shortened. It is the latter facts that are probably more pertinent to the development of overuse injuries when running than is the altered phasic activity.

Evaluation of the Forefoot

History

The starting point for evaluation of the forefoot is to clearly establish the chief complaint, which is usually pain but occasionally is a problem with footwear. The rest of the history frequently emanates from this point.

Pain Pattern

The location and radiation of the pain, the presence of night pain, any association with morning stiffness, and the relation to footwear are considered.[12] For instance, Morton's neuroma usually produces sharp, radiating pain between the toes that is frequently relieved by walking barefoot (whereas prominent painful metatarsal heads are often more painful when walking barefoot).

Activity History

A detailed activity history is important when determining the contributing factors as well as for planning exercise modification during treatment. Details of the athlete's plans for the current season, as well as the recreational and competitive goals, are essential. Because most athletes spend more time at their occupations than training, the stresses on the feet during this activity must be clearly defined.

Mechanism of Injury

Details of previous direct trauma, swelling, and bruising may indicate a possible mechanism of injury. In the absence of trauma, the role of overuse, alignment, or equipment must be assessed.

Past Medical History

The past medical history and family history help screen for systemic disease, including diabetes, gout, psoriasis, Reiter's syndrome, and, in the elderly, vascular phenomena.

Shoes and Terrain

The influence of shoes, terrain, slopes, speed of walking or running, and change in activity patterns may be helpful for diagnosis and treatment in the athlete.

Previous Therapy

Details of previous treatments, including drugs, orthoses, and activity modification, are usually easy to obtain. However, more important is the true compliance of the patient to these regimens in order to assess whether they were ineffective or inadequately adhered to.

Trends of Symptoms

The duration, intensity, and overall trend for improvement or deterioration give an indication of the point in the evolution of the problem at which the current intervention is going to take place. It helps to establish a realistic prognosis and time course for potential resolution of the problem. The duration of symptoms and response to previous therapy are also important factors when deciding the role and timing of surgical therapy.

Examination

The purpose of the examination is to (1) localize the symptoms to a specific anatomic location and structure; (2) identify static and dynamic structural or mechanical foot abnormalities; and (3) detect sys-

---

Practice Point

EVALUATION OF THE FOOT

History	*Examination*
Establish chief complaint	Gait
	Footwear
Pain pattern	Calluses and skin condition
Past medical history	
Family history	Tenderness
Activity history	Swelling
Mechanism of injury	Neurologic testing
Shoes and terrain	Special tests
Previous therapy	
Trend in symptoms	

---

temic conditions, e.g., collagen disease, neuropathies, radiculopathies, and vascular problems.

Gait

Gait is best assessed with the person walking barefoot. Heel–toe floor contact and varus–valgus heel alignment are carefully gauged. In the young athlete, toeing-in or toeing-out may be of concern to the parents. The magnitude and etiology of these largely self-limiting, nonpathologic alignments must be considered (Table 7-1). This examination may be supplemented by watching the patient run or walk on a treadmill or on a track. In special circumstances it may be assessed with the aid of a video or with sophisticated gait-analyzing equipment.

Static deformities are assessed with the patient prone and, when practical, standing. The relation of rear foot to forefoot alignment and the shape and mobility of the medial arch are further assessed by having the person stand on the toes.

Footwear

Footwear, sports shoes, skates, and orthoses are better examined after gait analysis in order to give a true perspective of the wear pattern.

Tenderness

Palpation of tender areas should isolate the pain to a specific anatomic structure. Subtleties in position of maximal tenderness place the problem in ligaments rather than the joint lines, bony areas rather than

TABLE 7-1. Etiology of Toeing-In and Toeing-Out in Children

Level of Affection	Toe In	Toe Out
Feet–ankles	Pronated feet (protective toeing-in)	Pes valgus due to contracture of triceps surae
	Metatarsus varus	Talipes calcaneovalgus
	Talipes varus	Congenital convex pes planovalgus
	Talipes equinovarus	
Leg–knee	Tibia vara (Blount's disease)	External tibial torsion
	Developmental genu varum	
	Abnormal internal tibial torsion	Congenital absence or hypoplasia of the fibula
	Genu valgum—developmental (protective toeing-in to shift body center of gravity medially)	
Femur–hip	Abnormal femoral anteversion	Abnormal femoral retroversion
	Spasticity of internal rotators of hip (cerebral palsy)	Flaccid paralysis of internal rotators of hip
Acetabulum	Maldirected—facing anteriorly	Maldirected—facing posteriorly

(After Tachdjian,[13] with permission.)

interdigital spaces, and tendons rather than ligaments. Certain classic findings, e.g., pain between the third and fourth metatarsal heads, give a high index of suspicion for a specific diagnosis, in this case Morton's neuroma. In the athlete the pain may be mild or vague at rest, and it is frequently helpful to have the patient go for a run or perform specific exercises to reproduce the discomfort. Such exercise, for instance, may help distinguish paresthesia of the toes due to chronic compartment pressure from that due to radicular or local causes.

Swelling

Swelling, a common phenomenon, may be due to joint effusions, a bursa, a ganglion, or a bony exostosis. Rarely, tumors are involved, e.g., fibromas in the plantar fascia, which are usually situated in the midfoot. Location and consistency, mobility, fluctuations in size, and inflammation are helpful parameters for pinpointing the cause.

Calluses and Skin Conditions

Calluses provide an index of the shear stresses applied to the foot. In adequate amounts calluses provide protection but in excess may cause pain. They clearly outline abnormal weight-bearing areas.

The overall condition of the skin mirrors the circulation, occasionally systemic disease, and nearly always the personal hygiene habits of the athlete. Excessive sweating or hyperhydrosis may cause problems, as do local conditions such as warts, corns, and intertriginous infections. The nails may be subjected to trauma by physical activity, as well as being damaged by inadequate hygiene and poor cutting and trimming techniques.

Neurologic Testing

For the athletic population, sensory testing of the foot is probably the most important neurologic test. The pattern of pain or paresthesia should be carefully mapped and any peripheral nerve areas of impairment recorded.

Special Tests

Measurements of the alignment of the foot are described later in the chapter with a detailed discussion of mid- and hindfoot conditions.

Plain roentgenograms gain in value if weight bearing views are used. Apart from structural abnormalities and the frequent accessory ossicles, it is important to gain some idea of skeletal maturation in the growing athlete (Fig. 7-4). There are also tangential views that silhouette the sesamoids. These films allow objective assessment of structural arrangement of the foot, and specific angles may be measured, recorded, and compared to known normal values. The joints

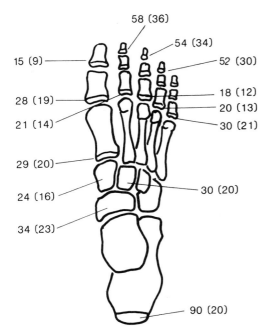

Fig. 7-4. Appearance of ossification centers of the foot recorded as months; female values are in brackets. (From Tachdjian,[13] with permission.)

and bones are closely scrutinized for clues of systemic disease and arthropathies.

Screening blood tests may help explain the onset of symptoms. The identification of parameters compatible with gout, rheumatoid arthritis, ankylosing spondylitis, and diabetes lend support to clinical impressions.

Photographs, footprint impressions, and analyses of walking and running on a treadmill or in a gait laboratory are luxuries not available to every practitioner. However, this should not be a focus of concern, as most conditions are diagnosed adequately with careful, meticulous clinical examination. Treatment success often depends more on gaining the patient's respect and cooperation than it does on the use of expensive, intricate laboratory tests.

Forefoot Conditions

The forefoot includes the metatarsals and associated phalanges. Therefore it incorporates the tarsometatarsal joints (Chopart's articulation) and the MTP and interphalangeal joints.

There is a considerable range of motion present at the MTP articulation, particularly extension. The movement of extension is used during walking and running in order to take full advantage of the subsequent contraction and thrusting power of the plantar flexors. There is relatively small range of flexion in contrast to the hand, where the dominant movement is flexion for prehension. At the MTP joint there are two degrees of freedom, as in addition to flexion and extension a certain amount of abduction and adduction may take place. These movements in two planes allow adjustment of the forefoot to different surfaces and different conditions of weight-bearing.

Nail Pathology

Trauma to the toenails may result in a change in shape and appearance of the nail plate. If it is moderate and the nail bed or root is undamaged, the nail gradually grows out. If severe, the nail may be shed, but a new, well-formed nail takes its place. If there is repetitive trauma or damage to the nail root, there is frequently permanent change and deformity of the nail plate. It should be remembered that the nails are sometimes the mirror of systemic disease and should be examined carefully.[14]

Subungual Hematoma (Black Toenail)

Etiology. Bleeding under the nail bed has been referred to by the eponyms hiker's, mountainclimber's, and runner's toe. It may be the result of a single direct blow or multiple minor contusions to the nail. Tight-fitting shoes with constant pressure or loose shoes where the momentum of the foot on decelerating or descending slopes causes repeated jamming may precipitate the problem. Stubbing the toe is another frequent mechanism.

Signs and Symptoms. The toe appears to have varying degrees of purplish or black hues as the hematoma is visible through the nail plate. The pressure of the suffused blood is painful, frequently making continuation of activity difficult. The tension under the nail may be sufficient that the toenail is ultimately lost. Prompt treatment helps to preserve the nail.

Treatment. If tense and painful, the hematoma should be decompressed by cauterizing a small hole through the nail with an electrocautery tip, if available, or a heated paper clip if it is not. Heparin from the mast cells in the nail bed usually keeps the blood liquid, and hence it is easily expressed. Relief from the symptoms is usually dramatic and immediate. It is best to place a pressure dressing on the nail to prevent reaccumulation of the blood.

In soccer players and some runners, trauma is so repetitive that the nail becomes dystrophic, thick, and unsightly. These nails may be subject to additional pressure in the toe box of the shoe and become painful. In such cases, the toenail may have to be ground down regularly to relieve symptoms.

In some individuals the nail rapidly loosens as soon as it grows, and the deformed plate is being constantly replaced with a new, equally deformed nail plate. In these instances it may be advisable to remove the nail bed and root surgically and allow the area to scar and heal.

Prevention of injury is the obvious aim by wearing properly fitting shoes and socks and by slowly breaking in new boots.

Differential Diagnosis. The differential diagnosis of a painless black spot includes malignant melanoma. Although uncommon, the nail bed is not an unusual site for it to begin. An exquisitely tender red or blue spot is likely to be a benign glomus tumor. Chronic discomfort under a dystrophic nail may be secondary to a traumatically induced subungual exostosis, which may be verified on a lateral roentgenogram.

Subungual Exostosis

Subungual exostosis is a benign outgrowth from the dorsal surface of the distal phalanx that is nearly always confined to the great toe. It is not related to the classic osteochondromas but is probably secondary to trauma or infection. Initially it may just be painful to pressure but may subsequently push the nail up from its bed, producing discoloration and longitudinal splintering of the plate in several places. It may eventually be exposed to the surface and be covered by a mass of granulation tissue. It is often confused at this point with an ingrown toenail; however, it is usually on the medial side of the great toe, whereas the ingrown toenail is more often lateral. A roentgenogram can distinguish it. Pain is variable, and it is sometimes possible to treat it by modifying the footwear or providing protective padding. If it is chronically painful or growing through the nail, surgical excision is rewarding. The differential diagnosis includes a hypertrophic dorsal distal tuft that may be associated with systemic disease, or it may just be congenital.

Onychocryptosis (Ingrowing toenail)

The normal nail plate is dense, semitransparent, cornified epithelium. The portion of the nail plate that is visible is the nail body, and the skin immediately underneath the nail is the nail bed.[6] The nail groove comprises the space between the nail fold and the nail bed (Fig. 7-5). The proximal portion of the skin covering the nail is the eponychium, or cuticle. The distal part of the skin underneath the free edge of the nail is the hyponychium. The nail matrix is part of the epidermis that forms the nail. The nail plate and nail bed grow together, going distally from the matrix.[5]

Etiology. The pressure of the nail over the nail bed retains the normal relations. Trauma to the nail, abnormal shoe pressure, and cutting the nail short and rounded near its edges may alter this relation. The nail sulcus becomes obliterated, and the soft tissue

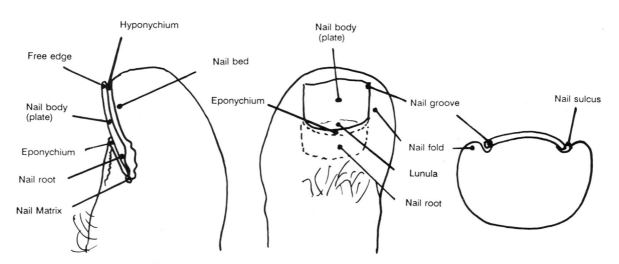

Fig. 7-5. Nail structure.

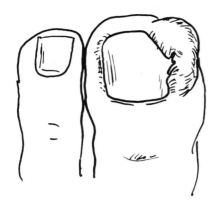

Fig. 7-6. Poorly cut nail with an absent nail sulcus, inflamed toe pulp, and an ingrowing nail spike. The normal nail sulcus depends on the integrity and pressure of the nail.

swells. The growing nail then impinges on this part of the nail bed, which becomes inflamed, more swollen, and painful. Attempts by the athlete to resect the nail only contributes to further swelling and impingement. Frequently, ragged nail spikes stick into the inflamed soft tissue, which may become secondarily infected, producing further hypertrophic granulation (Fig. 7-6).

Treatment. Initially, the treatment consists of trimming away the ingrown part of the nail. The patient is encouraged to carry out warm soaks in a solution of 1 teaspoon of Epsom salts per pan of water three times a day whenever possible. If the toe is infected, the addition of pHisoHex or povidone-iodine (Betadine) is sometimes helpful, with the application of polymycin B–neomycin–gramicidin (Neosporin G Cream) on a gauze dressing.[15] If the inflammation and cellulitis do not resolve rapidly, a systemic antibiotic is

worthwhile. Wedging of the toenail, excising any impinging spicules of nail and applying small cotton batten pledgets into the nail groove often yields satisfactory results if the condition is not too advanced. If the problem does not resolve, or if it is too far advanced on initial presentation, a series of increasingly aggressive approaches may be made.[16]

Wedge Matrix Excision. For this technique a ring block and bloodless field are required. After preparing the skin with Betadine or Savlon, a ring block of lidocaine (Xylocaine) 1 percent without epinephrine is carried out. An ellipse of tissue, including one-fourth of the nail and the surrounding hypertrophied lateral nail groove, are excised. The incision line is taken up proximal to the nail itself, toward the distal interphalangeal joint crease, to approximately 0.5 cm from the proximal nail fold (Fig. 7-7). Thorough curetting of the most proximal part of the matrix toward the interphalangeal joint down to the phalanx is necessary. Wound healing takes about 3 weeks. The advantages of wedge matrix excision are the high success rate and a less messy wound. However, postoperative pain is greater, and the operative procedure is somewhat more extensive than phenolization.

Total Nail Ablation (Zadik's Procedure). Total nail ablation is a more major procedure and may be followed by a fairly prolonged period of discomfort. It is, however, successful. Its indications are more limited, and it should be considered only if wedge matrix excision fails or the nail is markedly deformed (onychogryposis).

Ingrown toenail is probably the most common condition of the foot and is largely preventable with proper footwear and nail hygiene. When the condition exists, prompt treatment is easier than dealing

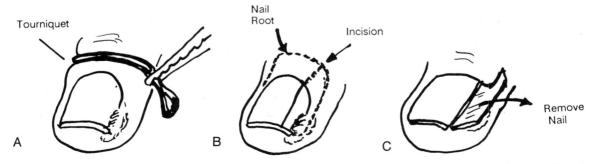

Fig. 7-7. Wedge matrix excision. **(A)** Establish a bloodless field. **(B)** Extend excision along nail and under nail fold to the nail root. **(C)** Remove offending edge of nail.

with a chronic hypertrophic granulating and deformed nail. Education of the athlete is essential.

Onychia

Onychia is an infection of the nail plate, usually on the great toe. The predisposing factors may be repetitive trauma due to footwear or activity or reactions to irritants such as nail polish or soaps. Treated promptly, there is an excellent prognosis for a normal nail. Inadequate treatment gives rise to chronic changes in the shape, thickness, and texture of the nail.

The condition is recognized by the surrounding redness or suppuration and the changes in the color and texture of the nail. The offending organism should be cultured, as the suppurative variety is usually of mixed flora with *Staphylococcus* predominating. Mild infection may be treated by soaking the foot in a foot bath of 1 to 2 tablespoons of povidone-iodine (Betadine) per liter of water for 15 minutes, up to three times a day, followed by application of an antibiotic ointment. Fungal infections, usually *Candida albicans,* may be much more resistant to therapy. Failure to gain control of the infection or any evidence of spread is an immediate indication for systemic antibiotics.

In both situations, careful débridement of the nail, treatment of any nail abnormalities such as ingrown toenail, and good foot hygiene help. Occasionally, surgical excision of the nail is appropriate or prolonged treatment with antibiotics or systemic antifungal agents. In this case, the treatment should be monitored by an expert, either a dermatologist, podiatrist, or a family physician with experience and the interest and patience to follow the foot care meticulously over several months.

Routine Nail Care

Many of the conditions affecting the nail are preventable by good nail care. The following list includes many points that require care and patient education rather than expensive and elaborate equipment.

1. Wash the feet daily with a mild soap and water.
2. Dry the feet meticulously, particularly between the toes.
3. Cut the free edge of the nail following the contour of the soft tissue.
4. Leave the nail long enough to cover all of the pulp. Do not cut too short, particularly at the edges.
5. Smooth the angles by filing with a flat file.
6. Treat any signs of inflammation promptly with antiseptic soaks and seek early professional care.
7. Do not push back the cuticle or, if necessary, only minimally.
8. Do not use sharp objects to disimpact debris under the nail or in the nail sulcus.
9. Change socks regularly.
10. Make sure shoes fit well in terms of width and length.
11. Take care with the footwear used for activities of daily living and minimize the use of high heels.

Toes

Anatomy of the First MTP Joint

The MTP joint of the great toe is condyloid and therefore allows motion in multiple planes. In practice, there is little motion other than dorsi- and plantar flexion. It is characterized by having a remarkable discrepancy between active and passive motion. Approximately 30 degrees of active plantar flexion is present and at least 50 degrees of active extension, which can be frequently increased passively to between 70° and 90° degrees.[17] The joint is stabilized dorsally by the capsule and expansion of the extensor hallucis tendon and laterally by collateral ligaments. The plantar surface of the capsule is reinforced by a fibrocartilaginous plate. This thickened capsular structure is called the plantar (accessory) ligament or plantar plate and is attached proximally to the metacarpal neck and distally to the base of the proximal phalanx (Fig. 7-8). It contains the medial and lateral sesamoid bones. The lateral edge of the plate is continuous with the deep transverse metatarsal ligament. The adductor hallucis and the lateral head of the flexor hallucis brevis attach via the lateral sesamoid to the plate and hence the base of the phalanx.[17] A similar arrangement exists with the medial head of the flexor hallucis brevis and the abductor hallucis and medial sesamoid, which tends to make the distal part of the plate stronger. The flexor pollicis longus tendon lies in the pulley formed by the two sesamoids and is covered by a fibrous digital sheath. The sesamoid bones thus serve as the weight-bearing points for the first metatarsal, with the medial sesamoid more directly under the metatarsal head.

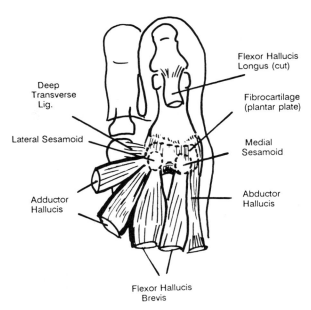

Fig. 7-8. Metatarsophalangeal joint. Tendons of flexor hallucis brevis, adductor hallucis, and abductor hallucis combine with the deep transverse metatarsal ligament to form the cartilaginous plate on the plantar aspect of the MTP joint capsule. The two sesamoids are contained within the plate.

Hallucal Sesamoids

The sesamoids of the great toe are small, seemingly insignificant bones; nevertheless, they may be the site of disabling pain in the athlete. Although largely neglected by current literature, the sesamoids have had a prominent place in myths, magic, and religion.[18]

The Rabbi Ushaia (AD 210) described a bone called the luz, probably the sesamoid, and suggested it was the repository of the soul after death. The sesamoids possibly received their modern name from Galen (AD 180) because they resemble the seeds of the plant sesamum indicum, the oil of which was used in ancient Greece as a purgative.[1,18] Versalius, in his most famous anatomic treatise (AD 1543), wrote that the sesamoid bones of the great toe were those bones that magicians and followers of occult philosophy refer to as "liable to no decay and which buried in the earth after death will produce man like a seed on the day of the Last Judgment." With such an awesome reputation, their pathology should be of some interest.[18]

They are present as early as the end of the first fetal trimester, and ossification occurs at about age 8 in girls and age 10 in boys. They are rarely congenitally absent. However, variations abound, particularly of the medial sesamoid, which is frequently bipartite or even multipartite. The incidence of these variations ranges from 2 to 20 percent. By increasing the moment arm between the flexion axis of the metatarsophalangeal (MTP) joint and the pull of the intrinsic flexors, they increase the power of flexion.[19] They may also disperse some of the impact over the metatarsal head and protect the tendon of the flexor hallucis longus.[19]

Sesamoid Pain (Sesamoiditis)

The cause of pain and tenderness underneath the first metatarsal head in athletes may be difficult to determine.[20] It is not an unusual area of pain in football and soccer players, ballet dancers, and distance joggers. Metatarsus primus varus with hallux valgus may be a predisposing factor along with excessively flexible footwear, hard or artificial turf, and repetitive traumatic loading, particularly with forced dorsiflexion of the great toe. In many cases the syndrome merges imperceptibly into that of "turf toe" (discussed at length under that heading). There is a small amount of evidence suggesting that bipartite or multipartite sesamoids may also be predisposed to injury. There are several sites of potential pain.

Bursitis

Presesamoid bursitis may produce a tender soft tissue swelling and is occasionally the manifestation of a systemic collagen disease such as rheumatoid arthritis, gout, or Reiter's syndrome. In association with a systemic disorder, the sesamoids are rarely involved as an isolated entity.

Osteochondritis

Osteochondritis of the sesamoids may give characteristic features of irregularity of the trabecular pattern, producing an almost striped appearance to the bones on the skyline roentgenographic view (Fig. 7-9). It has variously been described as "typical disease of the sesamoids," "osteitis fibrosa," "juvenile necrotic osteopathy," "traumatic osteitis," and "sesamoid insufficiency."[18] Helal believed that no such condition exists, and that the appearance is one of trauma causing a crush or stellate fracture.[18]

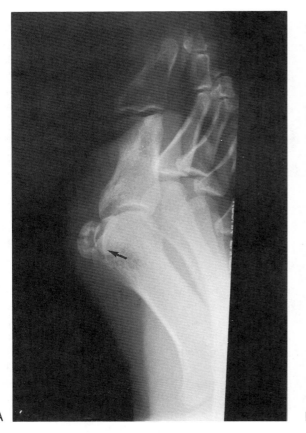
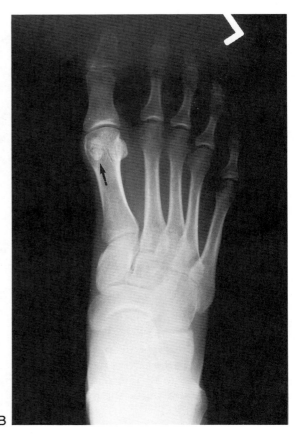

A   B

Fig. 7-9. Irregular trabecular pattern, mottling, and altered density of osteochondritis of the medial sesamoid. **(A)** Lateral view. **(B)** Anteroposterior view.

Chondromalacia

The medial sesamoid may be susceptible to chondromalacia. The diagnosis is based on pain, accurately localized to underneath the sesamoid and occurring only on weight-bearing.[18] Initially there are no obvious radiologic changes. Degeneration of the sesamometatarsal articulation is usually associated with a generalized arthropathy of the whole MTP joint.

Quick Facts

SESAMOID PAIN

- Bursitis
- Chondromalacia and osteoarthritis
- Stress fracture
- Traumatic disruption with plantar plate
- Contusion or crush fracture
- Osteochondritis
- Sesamoiditis in association with collagen diseases

Clinical Points

DIFFERENTIAL DIAGNOSIS

- Flexor hallucis longus tendinitis
- Synovitis of metatarsophalangeal (MTP) joint
- Gout
- Rheumatoid arthritis (MTP joint)
- Osteoarthritis (MTP joint)
- Tarsal tunnel syndrome

Trauma

Stress fracture or traumatic disruption of the sesamoids is difficult to distinguish from bipartite bones. Occasionally a widened gap is helpful or a progressively increasing fracture gap on serial films. The bone scan should be hot. With traumatic disruption of a large sesamoid, the absence of circumferential cortex, swelling, and hemorrhage may give a clue. Disruption of the plantar plate with separation of the sesamoid or fragments of a bipartite sesamoid is part of, and indistinguishable from, the syndrome of turf toe.

Treatment of all of these conditions revolves around stress relief by activity modification and orthotics. Nonsteroidal anti-inflammatory drugs (NSAIDs) are frequently helpful, as are warm foot baths, ultrasound, and interferential currents. Shoe modification by stiffening the sole or application of a metatarsal pad may be necessary. If a cast is used in acute conditions, a soft metatarsal pad should be applied to the area behind the metatarsal heads, and the plantar surface of the weight-bearing cast should extend out to support the toes.

If excision is indicated, it is not necessary to remove both sesamoids.[18,19] Helal has discussed fashioning a sesamoid prosthesis of silicone to replace the medial sesamoid in young, active individuals. This bone should be removed only in cases of severe, advanced pathology or intractable pain, and then only by an experienced surgeon.

Clinical Point

POTENTIAL INDICATIONS FOR SURGERY ON SESAMOIDS

- Widely displaced, painful fractured sesamoid
- Painful sesamoid not responding to 6 months of nonoperative treatment, including orthotics, shoe modification, and NSAIDs
- Recurrent, protracted sesamoid pain
- Osteomyelitis of the sesamoids
- Severe pain jeopardizing an athlete's career and not responding to alternative therapies

---

Summary

1. Sesamoid pain may occur in an otherwise normal foot placed under unusual impact stresses.
2. Radiographic changes and duration of symptoms do not always correlate with treatment success.
3. A basic diagnostic distinction depends on distinguishing fracture, inflammation, systemic disease, and nerve irritation as the primary cause of pain.
4. An orthosis may give significant relief, provided modification of the amount of toe motion is reduced during activity.
5. Occasionally, casting is required to allow the symptoms to resolve.
6. Injection is not a desirable first line therapy.
7. Establishing adequate range of motion is important in the therapy as symptoms resolve.
8. Surgical excision of the sesamoid is rarely indicated and is even disastrous in some athletes.
9. The possibility of surgical replacement with a synthetic hand-made prosthetic sesamoid may be preferable to simple excision in the highly competitive individual, but only if the overall alignment of the toe is acceptable.

First MTP Joint Sprain (Turf Toe)

Etiology

Turf toe primarily affects football, baseball, and soccer players and is caused by jamming or forced hyperextension of the hallux at the MTP joint.[21,22] The classic definition is an acute sprain of the plantar capsule and ligaments of the MTP joint of the great toe. However, because there are no established anatomic or pathologic criteria for this diagnosis, any traumatic disruption of the capsule of the first MTP joint, excluding dislocation, may be included (Fig. 7-10).[17] It thus presents a wide spectrum of injury. The incidence seems to be rising and is related to artificial turf, lightweight shoes that are too soft and flexible, and positions that require forced hyperextended position of the toes. This position is adopted frequently by linebackers and offensive linemen in football. When bearing weight over the extended toe, the MTP joint is pushed to about 100 degrees from the neutral position. This passive motion is in sharp distinction to the usual 50 to 60 degrees of active extension possible at the joint.[22] The distal first metatarsal becomes weight-bearing instead of articulating with the phalanx.[21] The sesamoids are drawn forward with this motion, allowing them to protect and bear

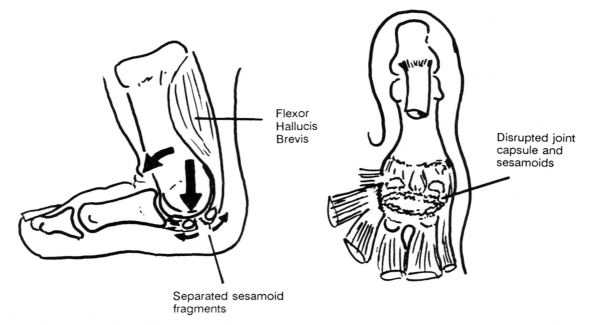

Flexor
Hallucis
Brevis

Disrupted joint
capsule and
sesamoids

Separated sesamoid
fragments

Fig. 7-10. Forced dorsiflexion with disruption of the joint capsule and sesamoid complex (turf toe). In this case multipartite sesamoid fragments split. Mostly only capsular disruption occurs and to a lesser severity than shown here.

weight underneath the metatarsal head. Injury occurs when there is overload to the toe, particularly with associated valgus stress.

Signs and Symptoms

The athlete presents with a tender, often swollen joint, usually with restricted motion secondary to the pain. If severe, the joint may be so inflamed that the overlying skin is tense and hyperemic, reminiscent of an acute attack of gout. The main area of tenderness is often over the plantar surface, particularly over the metatarsal head. Passive extension may be exquisitely painful. The injury may be the result of a single episode, but more frequently patients report that an initial injury was aggravated by repeated minor episodes. Pain and disability may not reach a maximum until 24 hours after the injury. It may also be accompanied by obvious ecchymosis. Roentgenograms usually show only swelling of the soft tissues. The spectrum of pathology includes spraining of the collateral ligaments, dorsal joint compression, plantar plate avulsion, and trauma to the sesamoids (Fig. 7-10). The long-term effects of turf toe include chronic pain and stiffness of the joint, hallux rigidus, calcification of the ligaments, and metatarsalgia. The differential

diagnosis includes dislocation or fracture of the toe, fracture of the sesamoids, inflammation of the sesamoids, flexor hallucis longus or brevis tendinitis, and gout.

Treatment

Early treatment includes attempting to reduce the amount of motion at the joint and dealing with the inflammation and edema. Ice, with either immersion therapy or via ice packs that can mold around the toe, may be combined with the systemic use of NSAIDs.

If the problem is mild, it resolves with the above regimen; more severe cases require significant reduction in activity and restriction of hyperextension by strapping the great toe (Fig. 7-11). The addition of buddy taping to the adjacent toe may help to further reduce motion. It is important to avoid pressure over the painful areas; and if the tape extends past the interphalangeal joint, a small pad should be used to prevent cuticle irritation.

If further restriction is needed and reduction of activity is impractical, the footwear should be modified. Torque-resistant shoes with stiff soles help. The proper width and length of the shoes are imperative. Occasionally, a stiff insole may be used; or a metal or

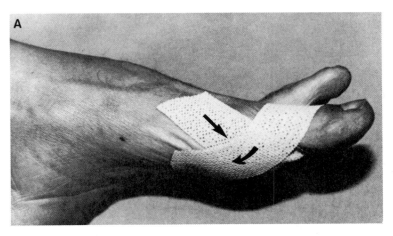

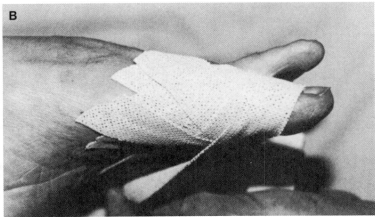

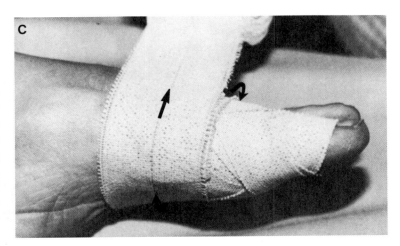

Fig. 7-11. Taping technique for minimizing the stresses of dorsiflexion for athletes with turf toe. A severely swollen toe should not be taped. **(A)** One inch tape, approximately 8 inches long is looped over the proximal phalanx, and the ends are crossed. **(B)** Several extra strips form a spica. **(C)** The ends are secured with an anchor. (From Subotnick,[15] with permission.)

plastic plate incorporated into the sole can splint the toe adequately in recalcitrant cases. This method may interfere with performance but may be the only recourse.[23]

Ideally, activity is restructured until discomfort is minimal. The therapist attempts to restore a painless active and passive range of motion. Whirlpool baths, ultrasound, and transcutaneous nerve stimulation (TNS) are helpful. Manipulations and mobilization of the joint form a major part of the therapy. It is also important to incorporate strengthening exercises. When possible, running is not resumed until 90 degrees of passive motion is restored. Before discharge, the walking and running pattern should be scrutinized to eliminate any poor substitute patterns that have been adopted during the painful period, particularly in regard to the pattern of weight-bearing and push-off through the foot. There is a tendency to roll along the lateral border of the foot and "in-toe." Failure to correct these adverse patterns rapidly results in secondary complaints of metatarsalgia, stress fractures, and stress of the tarsal ligaments.

Early aggressive care is mandatory to avoid significant loss of game or practice time. Steroid injections and local anesthesia to deaden the area to allow play or early resumption of activity rarely work and usually create significant problems. This approach is probably contraindicated, although occasionally judicious use of an injectable steroid is helpful.

This condition, first described in 1976, has become a significant factor in terms of game and practice time lost in football and soccer. Prophylaxis in the form of adequate footwear and early therapy cannot be overly stressed.

Hallux Rigidus

Hallux rigidus, a degenerative arthrosis of the first MTP joint, is characterized by limitation of range of motion and pain.[24] As the available dorsiflexion decreases below that required for normal walking or athletic activities, the gait becomes altered and the symptoms are likely to increase. The toe frequently becomes fixed in slight plantar flexion, and the athlete may be forced to bear weight on the lateral side of the foot.[11]

Quick Facts

PROPOSED ETIOLOGIC FACTORS IN HALLUX RIGIDUS

- Osteochondritis dissecans of first metatarsal head
- Trauma: single or repetitive minor events
- Primary osteoarthritis
- Prominent long first metatarsal
- Abnormal gait
- Hypermobility of first metatarsal segment

Etiologic Factors

Numerous causes of the degenerative changes in this joint have been proposed. There may be anatomic variations that predispose the second MTP joint to degenerative changes, including a prominent second metatarsal (Morton's foot), or hypermobility of the first ray. Many athletes exhibit the findings of osteochondritis dissecans at the joint, but it is not certain whether they are primary or secondary changes. Particularly, there are frequently cartilaginous or osteocartilaginous lesions of the metatarsal head.[25] Such lesions would account for the typical limited dorsiflexion and maintenance of good plantar flexion. These early lesions are difficult to visualize on roentgenograms, as they are often largely cartilaginous.[24] However, as more degenerative changes supervene, joint space is lost, subchondral sclerosis is apparent, and osteophytes appear on the dorsal margins of the joint (Fig. 7-12). The latter can become

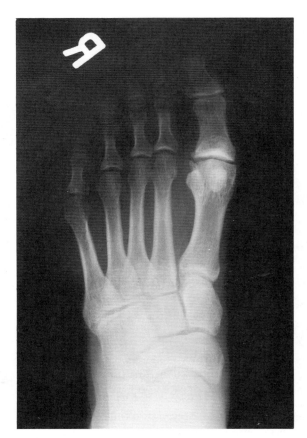

Fig. 7-12. Classic roentgenographic signs of hallux rigidus with loss of joint space, sclerosis, and large osteophytes.

huge and are out of proportion to the size of the joint. They further mechanically restrict range.

Treatment

Nonoperative treatment is directed toward decreasing the pain, maximizing the available motion at the joint, and decreasing the range of motion demanded by the patient's activities. Pain may be reduced by NSAIDs, local ultrasound, hot foot baths, and modification of activities and footwear. The shoe may be modified by applying a metatarsal bar, a rocker-bottom sole, or a stiff metal insert. The training shoes can be modified by use of a rigid plastic liner in the sole or a semirigid orthosis. The toe box must be large enough to accommodate the bony exostosis. Once pain is reduced, a significant attempt is made to correct any gait faults that have developed in order to prevent superimposition of secondary problems arising out of the altered lower limb biomechanics. Mobilization to gain all available range seems to maximize functional potential and reduces the number of acute flare-ups, particularly if the condition is not too advanced (Fig. 7-13). Surgery for hallux rigidus may involve débridement and removal of the osteophytes, osteotomy of the first ray, arthroplasty, or arthrodesis (Table 7-2).

Débridement

Arthrotomy with removal of loose fragments from within the joint and excision of the osteophytes from the joint margin (cheilectomy) gives satisfactory results, depending on the study, in as many as 85 percent of patients to as few as 60 percent[24] (Fig. 7-14). The greater the existing degenerative changes, the poorer the long-term results. Frequently, most of the articular surface is thinned and the whole dorsal half completely denuded. Intraoperatively and postoperatively it is frequently difficult to re-establish the range of extension. The plantar soft tissues are so contracted and the smooth gliding action at the joint surface so altered that even after removal of the exostosis there is mechanical impingement.

Postoperatively, intensive physiotherapy is needed to regain and establish adequate passive and active range of motion. As soon as the tissues become less sensitive, the rehabilitation program should include much passive stretching, distraction, and joint play mobilization (Fig. 7-13). Muscle strengthening and gait re-education follow as soon as pain decreases

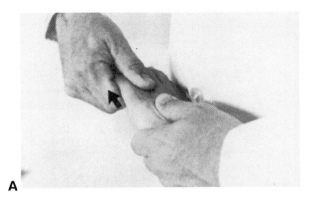

A

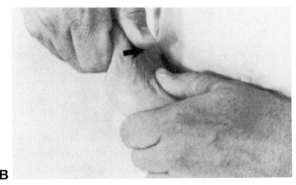

B

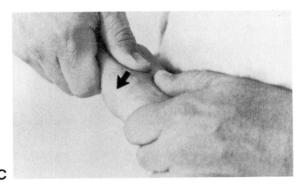

C

Fig. 7-13. Mobilization of the first MTP joint. **(A)** Distraction. Stabilize the first metatarsal head and distract along the long axis of the first ray. **(B & C)** Dorsoplantar glide. Supporting the joint as illustrated, the phalanx is glided in a dorsal **(B)** and then a plantar **(C)** direction. (From Donatelli and Wooden,[27] with permission.)

enough to reduce the risk of a flare-up in the joint, and further pain inhibition.

Osteotomy

Cheilectomy combined with osteotomy allows easier restoration of functional dorsiflexion (Fig. 7-15).

TABLE 7-2. Surgical Procedures for Hallux Rigidus

Procedure	Indications	Complications
Cheilectomy	Hallus rigidus with mild degenerative changes in the MTP-1 joint	High failure rate with more advanced degenerative changes
Dorsiflexion osteotomy of proximal phalanx	Useful adjunct to cheilectomy to gain additional dorsiflexion at MTP-1 joint	Increased healing time
Resection arhtroplasty	Relief of painful hallux rigidus in patient with low functional needs	Frequent poor functional results
Implant arthroplasty	Routine use not recommended; may allow improved function and maintain toe length after resection arthroplasty	Infection; wound inflammation; implant failure
Arthrodesis	Hallux rigidus in an active patient with more advanced degenerative changes in MTP-1 joint	Nonunion; malunion; interphalangeal joint arthritis

(After Hattrup and Johnson,[24] with permission.)

It also permits the base of the proximal phalanx to articulate with the undamaged cartilage usually found along the more plantar aspects of the metatarsal heads. This operation is more technically demanding and requires a much longer healing time than cheilectomy. Restoration of range of motion by therapy must be delayed until firm union of the osteotomy.[26]

Arthroplasty

Arthroplasties of the degenerative joint work well in the older, sedentary patient. However, in the active, young individual, they may not give the desired outcome. The resection arthroplasty (Keller), where the base of the proximal phalanx is removed, allows good initial pain relief, but more than 50 percent of patients have poor tendon function. Approximately 75 percent acquire a "cock-up" deformity with the great toe in valgus and dorsiflexion, so only about 40 percent of individuals eventually bear weight on the great toe. Subjectively, many patients are satisfied, and this procedure is probably preferable to performing an implant arthroplasty.

In an attempt to prevent the shortening and softening, various elastic spacers are available for the MTP joint. Although follow-ups results show that more than 80 percent of patients have good results, there are many complications, particularly in the young athletic population, including infection, wound inflammation, implant failure, and bony reaction to the prosthesis.

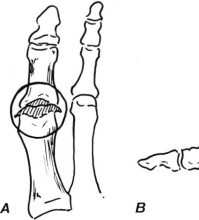
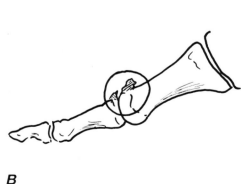

Fig. 7-14. Hallux rigidus. **(A)** Loss of joint space and lateral osteophytes. **(B)** Lateral view of dorsal osteophytes. The stippled areas must be resected to attempt to restore range.

A   B

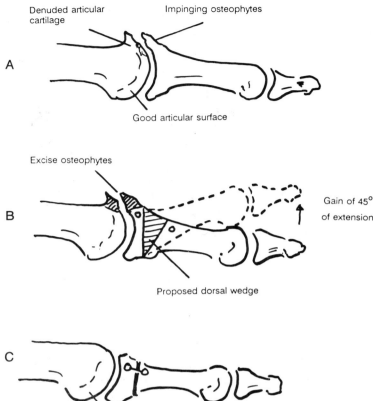

Fig. 7-15. Débridement and cheilectomy of hallux rigidus. **(A)** Osteophytic impingement. **(B)** Proposed bone débridement and wedge excision (shaded). **(C)** Osteotomy site it closed to give an increase of 45 degrees of functional dorsiflexion.

Arthrodesis

Arthrodesis of this important joint in a young athletic individual may seem a radical treatment. At least 15 to 25 degrees of dorsiflexion from the plane of the first metatarsal shaft is required for good function.[24] Insufficient dorsiflexion makes vigorous activity difficult, and excessive dorsiflexion may cause the toe to impinge on the shoe. If the perioperative complications of broken internal fixation and failed union are overcome, the late complications are remarkably few. The toe should also be fused in slight valgus to minimize shoe pressure on the interphalangeal joint. Satisfactory results are achieved in 90 percent of patients.

Hallux Valgus

Strictly speaking, the term hallux valgus refers only to lateral deviation of the great toe. However, its meaning has expanded to the point that it encompasses a progressive deformity including varying degrees of metatarsus primus varus, valgus deviation of the proximal phalanx, and bunion formation.[27] In its extreme, it includes lateral subluxation of the sesamoids, the long flexor and extensor tendons, and progressive degenerative changes of the MTP joint. It is present in 3 to 17 percent of the population, depending on age.[28]

Anatomy

The mean MTP angle is 15 degrees in adults; angles of more than 20 degrees between the long axis of the first metatarsus and phalanx are considered abnormal and constitute hallux valgus (Fig. 7-16). Nevertheless, angles as great as 30 to 35 degrees are consistently seen in series of asymptomatic patients.[29] The intermetatarsal angle is usually 7 to 8 degrees, with angles more than 10 degrees constituting metatarsus primus varus. There is a definite correlation between increasing MTP angle, forefoot width, and medial sesamoid position.[28]

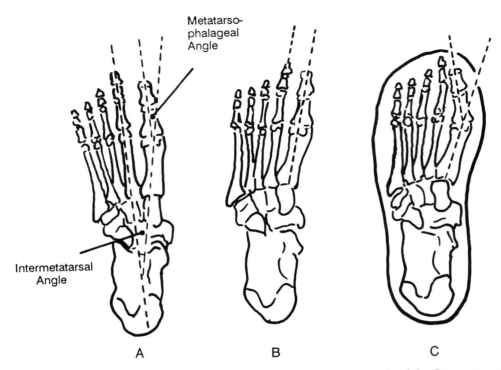

Fig. 7-16. (A) Metatarsophalangeal angle is the angle between the long axis of the first metatarsal and proximal phalanx (normal less than 20 degrees). The intermetatarsal angle is formed by lines drawn through the long axis of the first and second metatarsals (normal less than 10 degrees). **(B)** With minimal varus position of the first metatarsal shaft, the risk of bunion formation is less. **(C)** With significant metatarsus primus varus, bunion formation is common.

The joint spaces of the five MTP joints that line up in a gentle curve are seen in about 30 percent of the population. The first metatarsal is shorter than the second metatarsal shaft (index minus) in about 50 percent of the population, giving rise to the so-called Morton's, or Greek, foot. When combined with metatarsus primus varus, it is referred to as the atavistic foot. In approximately 20 percent, the first metatarsal shaft is longer than the second (index plus). When it is also combined with a long proximal first phalanx, it results in the classic Egyptian foot.

Etiology

Truslow in 1925 introduced the term "metatarsus primus varus" and considered it a predisposition to the development of hallux valgus.[30] The intermetatarsal angle usually increases with time and may not be the primary factor in the deformity, except for the fact that it predisposes the phalanx to constant lateral

pressure in poorly designed or poorly fitted shoes (Fig. 7-16). High heels and pointed toe boxes are the main offenders along with narrow forefoot fittings and contribute to the bunion. It is this factor that produces the overwhelming incidence of symptomatic hallux valgus in women.[28] There is substantial evidence pointing to footwear as the main deforming force. Sim-Fook and Hodgson, in 1958, compared "shoe-wearing" and "non-shoe-wearing" Chinese populations. Whereas metatarsus primus varus was present in 24 percent of the non-shoe-wearing population, hallux valgus was seen in only 2 percent and symptoms were nonexistent. In the "shoe-wearing" individuals, there was a 33 percent incidence of hallux valgus, many of which were symptomatic.[28,31]

Other, less significant predisposing factors include (1) pronation of the foot, imposing longitudinal rotation on the first ray, which gives additional stress as the foot rolls off it during weight bearing; (2) contractures of the Achilles tendon; (3) arthritis with loss of capsular integrity; (4) generalized ligamentous laxity; (5) variations in the shape of the MTP joint; and (6) neurologic disorders.

Whatever the etiology, the deformity tends to start off as a passively induced valgus transition of the proximal phalanx. As the MTP joint angle increases, dynamic deforming forces evolve. The adductor hallucis develops a contracture, the extensor and flexor hallucis longus generate a pull lateral to the axis of the joint, and the flexor hallucis brevis and sesamoids move laterally, producing further deforming forces (Fig. 7-17). The abductor hallucis moves under the toe, losing its ability to generate an abduction correcting vector.

Quick Facts

CONTRIBUTING FACTORS TO POSSIBLE HALLUX VALGUS

- Tight footwear
- Metatarsus primus varus
- Excessive functional pronation
- Tight Achilles tendon
- Capsular damage with osteoarthritis
- Generalized ligamentous laxity
- Associated neurologic conditions

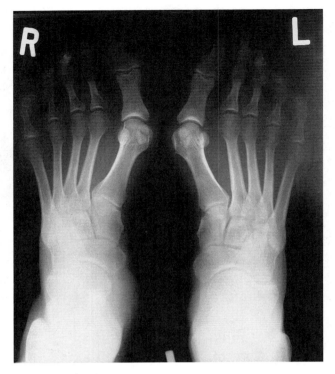

Fig. 7-17. Bilateral bunion formation with metatarsus primus varus and hallux valgus. On the left foot the deformity is sufficient to cause subluxation of the sesamoids.

Treatment

The nonoperative treatment of hallux valgus is largely preventive. The cornerstone is education and advice on footwear. For young people with a family predisposition to metatarsus primus varus, it is mandatory. Avoidance of high heels, adequate room in the toe box, and correct length and width of the shoe are the major factors in preventing or causing progressive, symptomatic disease.

With mild early hallux valgus, intrinsic foot exercises, taught carefully and often supplemented by "faradic type" foot baths for intrinsic control, may be of great assistance. It requires concern, commitment, and dedication on the part of the patient, however, and is effective only with mild deformity. Poor footwear nullifies any therapeutic effort.

Occasionally, with the athlete, it is the acute flare-up of the bunion that is so problematic. NSAIDs, foot soaks, strapping, relief padding, stretching, and molding of the footwear helps to settle these symptoms (Fig. 7-18). For skiers, figure skaters, and soccer players, a symptomatic bunion may make practice almost impossible. Prompt therapy often results in dramatic relief; it does not, however, affect the underlying etiology.

The number of surgical procedures described for this condition is phenomenal (Table 7-3). They may be summarized into categories, along with their primary indications. Whenever possible, surgery should be avoided or kept to a minimum in the young athlete. The stresses placed on this joint are enormous, and the long-term results are seldom satisfactory.

For early hallux valgus with symptomatic bunions, release of the adductor muscle with reattachment to the metatarsal head, excision of the bunion, and capsular plication may work. When the metatarsus primus varus is significant, a distal or proximal osteotomy of the first metatarsal may be warranted. If there is a large amount of joint degeneration, few procedures allow high levels of athletic performance, and fusion of the joint may have to be considered. This procedure is described in more detail in the section on hallux rigidus.

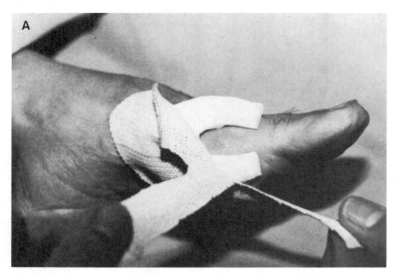

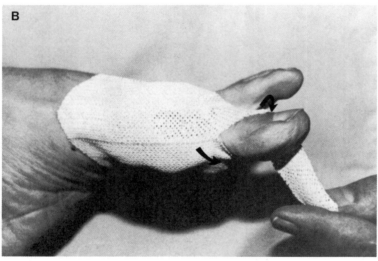

Fig. 7-18. Relief over a bunion may be achieved by relief padding. **(A)** With a horsehoe felt, although Spenco Second Skin is effective. **(B)** Padding is enhanced by varus taping of the joint. (From Subotnick,[15] with permission.)

In conclusion, this largely preventable condition, frequently based on a familial predisposition of metatarsus primus varus, may result in a situation that threatens to end a promising career, particularly for the runner, soccer player, and ballet dancer. Education is probably the most powerful tool in preventing the more serious complications of hallux valgus.

Mallet, Hammer, and Claw Toes

Contractions of the capsule of the interphalangeal or MTP joints of the toes, in association with tendon shortening, may produce a series of deformities ranging from hammer toe to mallet toe to claw toe (Fig. 7-19).

The *hammer toe* usually involves a contracture of the plantar surface of the proximal interphalangeal joint (PIP) with a mild associated dorsal contracture of the MTP joint. The plantar cushion is drawn distally, and metatarsal head pressure may be painful (Fig. 7-20). The *mallet toe* results from flexion or deformity of the distal interphalangeal joint (DIP) with plantar contracture (Fig. 7-19). The *claw toe* is a more advanced contracture of capsules and intrinsic musculature, which may also be associated with pes cavus and neurologic or primary muscle pathology. Claw toes may be the first sign of Charcot-Marie-Tooth disease (peroneal muscular atrophy). There is a significant contracture dorsally over the MTP joint with plantar contractures at the PIP and DIP joints.

TABLE 7-3. Surgical Procedures for Hallux Valgus Deformity

Procedure	Indications	Most Frequent Problems
Soft tissue plication and release of adductor hallucis (variations of McBride)	Mild to moderate hallux valgus Young person No degenerative changes in MTP joint May be combined with bunionectomy or distal osteotomy in severe cases	Hallux varus Loss of correction
Distal osteotomies (variations of chevron osteotomies)	Moderate metatarsus primus varus No or little degenerative change in MTP joint Young person Usually combined with bunionectomy and adductor release	Technical errors during osteomy Malunion Loss of correction
Proximal osteomies	Metatarsus primus varus >30 degrees Mild or no degenerative change in MTP joint Usually combined with bunionectomy and soft tissue capsular plication	Technical errors Recurrence of deformity
Resection arthroplasty (Keller)	Moderate to severe hallux valgus Elderly patient Severe MTP joint degenerative changes	Disruption of control of the great toe Shortening and soft tissue contractures leading to deformity Transverse metatarsalgia
Implant arthroplasty (Swanson)	May help pressure function of hallux Cosmetically superior (retains the length of toe)	Wound inflammation Implant failure in young
Arthrodesis	Severe degenerative joint changes Young, active person	Pseudoarthrosis Malunion Metatarsalgia Problems with footwear in fusion angle incorrect

Among the general population, it is possible that these contractures are secondary to footwear. An abnormally long digit is particularly susceptible to pressure and hence flexes up in the shoe. The main problem is the association of painful calluses and corns (clavi).

The hammer toe results in a callus over the dorsal aspect of the PIP joint, usually the fifth toe. The mallet toe frequently has a callus or corn at its distal tip due to pressure, and there is an associated pressure area over the dorsal DIP joint. Claw toes also have this distal tip lesion in association with a painful callus over the PIP joint. In addition, the athlete is likely to develop an associated plantar keratoma under the metatarsal head, particularly the second toe, which is forced plantargrade owing to the retrograde pressure on the long toe.

Mallet and hammer toes are treated nonoperatively by paring and débriding the keratomas and crest pads to relieve shoe pressure from the apex of the deformity. During the early stages mobilizing the joints and a home program taught by the therapist for the manipulation may retard the progress of the deformity and give symptomatic relief. Recalcitrant, painful hammer toes are treated surgically by shortening the toe and arthrodesis of the appropriate interphalan-

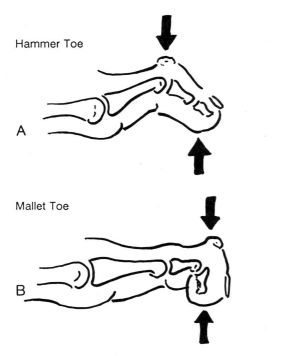

Hammer Toe

A

Mallet Toe

B

Fig. 7-19. **(A)** Hammer toe, with flexion at the proximal interphalangeal joint and an overlying corn. **(B)** Mallet toe. Flexion at the distal interphalangeal joint with potential corns over the dorsal and plantar surfaces.

geal joints (Jones procedure). Claw toes are treated by release of the MTP and interphalangeal joint capsules, extensor tendon lengthening where appropriate, and flexor tendon transfer if necessary. Severe,

---

Clinical Point

TOE DEFORMITIES

- Hammer toe
  -Significant PIP, mild MTP contractures
- Mallet toe
  -Plantar contracture DIP
- Claw toe
  -Significant DIP, PIP, plantar, and dorsal MTP contracture
- Morton's toe
  -Longest metatarsal shaft in second toe
- Morton's metatarsalgia
  -Interdigital neuroma, frequently third web space

---

recurrent, and painful corns may need to be dealt with by removing the underlying bony prominence (partial osteotomy).

Bunionettes (Tailor's Bunions)

Bunionettes are due to a combination of splaying of the fifth metatarsal (metatarsus quintus abductus) and the associated shoe pressure over the prominent MTP joint. They are common in figure skaters, skiers, soccer players, and ballet dancers. The eponym "tailor's bunion" may have stemmed from the cross-legged sitting attitude with pressure over the fifth metatarsal head or from the pressure over the lateral aspect of the foot used to work the tailor's wheel; in either case, it results from friction and pressure. Therapy consists in relieving the stresses by making an accommodation in the footwear, applying a pad around the prominence, and giving NSAIDs if there is a significant inflammatory component. Persistent problems may be dealt with by performing a proximal or distal osteotomy of the fifth metatarsal, depending on the severity and location of the deformity. Partial local osteotomy of the bump usually results in eventual recurrence of the problem.

Toe Sprains and Phalangeal Fractures

Toe sprains are common in everyday existence from stubbing the toe. In the athlete, they are even more common from kicking, landing on uneven ground, or collisions. Chronic sprains may occur secondary to running style, footwear, or the terrain. The athlete presents with the symptoms of synovitis with a hot, swollen toe that is tender to touch and to movement. Treatment consists in rest, relief of pressure, and minimizing motion. NSAIDs are useful, as are contrast baths, splinting, and taping. Rigid orthoses are rarely needed to support the sole and toe area of the shoe.

There may be an element of chronic fatigue at the insertion of the collateral ligament of the great toe, so minimal trauma produces an avulsion fracture.[32] Whatever the cause, despite considerable displacements these fractures usually have excellent functional outcomes eventually. Even nonunions and malunions do well unless complicated by the formation of corns. Occasionally when there are chronic symptoms, osteotomy or fusion solves the problem. Fractures involving the MTP joint of the great toe should be considered more carefully. Fractures of the neck of the second to fifth toes usually do well unless

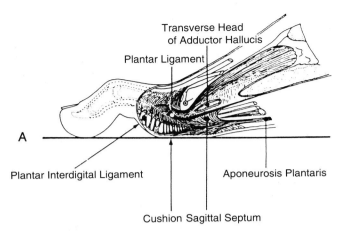

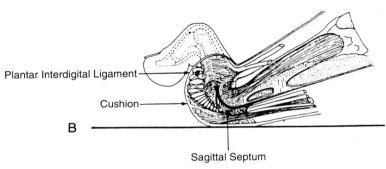

Fig. 7-20. (A) Normal toe has the fat cushion well located over the pressure area for weight-bearing. (B) With a hammer toe deformity the cushion becomes located in front of the metatarsal head, and the septa are located below it. The tendon of the interosseous muscle becomes dorsal to the axis and can no longer flex the metacarpophalangeal joint. From Bojsen-Moller,[7] with permission.)

gross displacement produces an unusual deformity or focal pressures.

Metatarsalgia

Metatarsalgia in its broadest definition includes discomfort around the metatarsal heads. However, the term "Morton's metatarsalgia" is frequently used to distinguish the pain arising from an interdigital neuroma.

Etiology

There are several possible causes of pain around the metatarsal heads. Some of these factors are better substantiated than others.

Ligamentous Factors

Chronic stretching of the transverse ligaments may result in more pressure over the central three metatarsal heads. They may be palpated on the sole and may be covered with unusual callus or even corns, particularly the second metatarsal head, where despite the apparent thickening the subcutaneous fat may be thinned. The pain is magnified by inflamma-

tion of the underlying adventitious bursa. Walking in shoes may be more comfortable than walking bare foot. This type of metatarsalgia is particularly seen in the older individual, with age-related changes in the ligaments and thinning of plantar fat pads. Excessive body weight, a valgus heel, hammer toes, pes planus, and generalized ligamentous laxity are contributing factors.[7]

Traumatic Causes

Trauma is the commonest factor in the young athlete. Landing poorly from a height, repetitive jumping, sudden increase in mileage or activity, worn or inadequate footwear, excessive training, and uneven or hard terrain may contribute to this trauma.

Mechanical Factors

Mechanical causes may be intrinsic, such as a rigid, thin cavus foot or a jogging style that entails always landing on the toes. The extrinsic factors relate to shoes that have a narrow toe box, causing compression of the metatarsal heads and subsequent intermetatarsal bursitis. It is also easy to overlook the fact that, although many athletes have superb training equipment, for their activities of daily living, which takes up the greater part of their day, their footwear is inadequate. Secretaries, receptionists, and waitresses in particular may spend many hours standing in high-heeled shoes that incline the foot and produce high stress on the metatarsal heads.

Other Causes

It is dangerous to assume all diseases in athletes are activity-acquired. Due regard to age, family history, and past medical history are important. Furthermore, it is equally fallacious to assume that athletes are necessarily healthy. To forget these last two principles is to almost certainly forget some significant condition in the differential diagnosis and perhaps to overlook some early but important sign of treatable systemic disease.

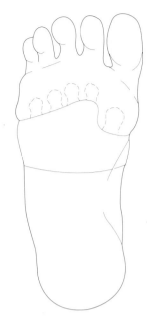

Fig. 7-21. There are several varieties of pressure relieving pads. A transverse pad, just behind the metatarsal heads and cut around the first and fifth metatarsal heads, relieves some of the weight-bearing pressure. Exact placement is crucial to decrease symptoms.

Clinical Points

- All pain in athletes is not necessarily activity-acquired.
- Activities of daily living and occupation may be more important than training in the etiology.
- Always examine the everyday footwear.
- All athletes are not necessarily healthy.
- Do not forget systemic causes of local disease.

Metatarsal pain may originate from arthritic disease that is rheumatoid, seronegative, or degenerative in nature. Metabolic factors include gout and diabetes in particular. Muscular factors, circulatory disease, and neurologic conditions may predispose to metatarsal pain.

Treatment

The key to pain relief is reducing the loading on the metatarsal heads. Methods include activity modification, footwear examination and modification, medial arch and metatarsal orthotics, and external metatarsal bars for the shoes (Fig. 7-21). Contrast baths, foot baths, and local ultrasound may be of help in selected cases. Where there is a large inflammatory component, NSAIDs or even local injection of steroid may help, but the worry of inducing fat necrosis and skin atrophy must be taken into account. Careful paring down of appropriate amounts of callus and corns is sometimes dramatic. Lastly, osteotomy of the metatarsal necks of the most prominent metatarsals assists in obtaining a more equal distribution of pressure.

Morton's Metatarsalgia

Thomas G. Morton, in 1876, presented a series of patients with a painful affliction of the fourth MTP articulation that in his opinion had not been previously described.[33] However, the first description of interdigital neuroma was by Lewis Durlacher, surgeon chiropractor to the Queen of England. He clearly outlined the condition in 1845.[34] Morton's metatarsalgia is an entrapment neuropathy, predominantly characterized by deposition of amorphous eosinophilic material followed by slow degeneration of the nerve fiber.[35] The neuroma is on the plantar surface of the intermetatarsal ligament.

Signs and Symptoms

Clinically, pain is usually at the third or second intermetatarsal space. Pressure applied axially to the metatarsal space or transverse compression with the toes extended frequently reproduces the pain.[36] However, this may also be painful in other cases of metatarsalgia. The most specific sign, not always present, is pain when the appropriate MTP and interphalangeal joints are extended; this pain is usually relieved by subsequent flexion of either of these joints. This maneuver is a neural stretch test, like the Lasegue test for sciatica, as the neuroma is stretched across the intermetatarsal ligament. Although the classic signs of pain, tingling, or numbness in the third web space are easily recognized, atypical paresthesias of the forefoot may initially confuse the diagnosis. Unlike other causes of metatarsalgia, the athlete is often more comfortable in bare feet than in shoes, at least during the early stages. Patients also report that the pain may appear consistently after a specific amount of activity.

Anatomic Considerations

No specific foot shape correlates well with the prevalence of the condition, but hallux valgus, hallux rigidus, and pes cavus are seen more frequently in some series.[36] During the last part of the stance phase, pressure is transmitted mainly to the metatarsal heads and the intermetatarsal spaces underneath the deep plantar fascia. The anterior edge of this fascia is thick and resistant, and underneath it passes the digital nerve. It is probable that during this terminal stance phase the nerve is squeezed between the plantar soft tissues and the unyielding edge of the plantar fascia. Tight shoes, anatomic considerations, and repetitive trauma are the predisposing factors.

Treatment

The footwear should be examined, making sure the forefoot and toe box are large enough and the shoe is adequate in length. The athlete should be instructed to ensure that the laces are not too tight. Injection

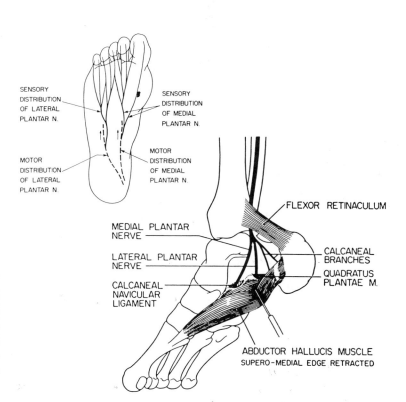

Fig. 7-22. Distribution and sensory supply on the plantar aspect of the foot of the medial and plantar terminal branches of the tibial nerve. The tibial nerve is located just behind the medial malleolus and the posterior tibial artery. (After Goodgold,[38] with permission.)

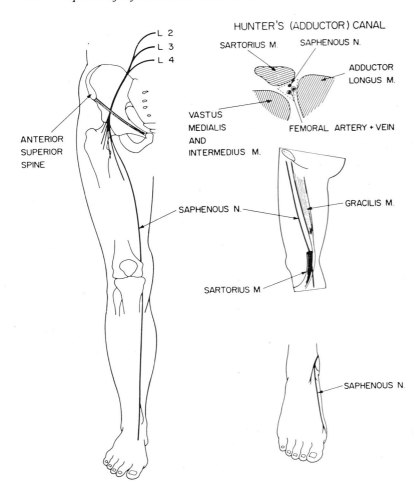

Fig. 7-23. Medial foot distribution of the saphenous nerve. It lies just anterior to the medial malleolus and lateral to the tibialis anterior tendon. (After Goodgold,[38] with permission.)

with corticosteroid followed by ultrasound, forefoot mobilization, and a temporary metatarsal pad often cures the condition.

Surgical treatment consists of division of the transverse ligament with or without excision of the neuroma. Excision has the obvious disadvantage of permanent loss of sensation of the contiguous sides of the toe. Rarely, a painful stump neuroma forms.

Local Anesthesia for Forefoot Surgery

Local nerve blocks with lidocaine (Xylocaine) 1 percent, not exceeding 4.5 mg/kg body weight, may be used.[37]

Tibial Nerve

The tibial nerve is located behind the medial malleolus by palpating the posterior tibial artery and injecting slightly posterior to it (Fig. 7-22). The tibial

nerve supplies the skin of the medial and undersurface of the great toe as far as the MTP joint and the sole of the foot from the arch to the tips of the toes.

Saphenous Nerve

The saphenous nerve is adjacent to the saphenous vein and can sometimes be palpated just anterior to the medial malleolus and lateral to the tibialis anterior tendon (Fig. 7-23). It supplies the skin of the medial ankle and the medial side of the foot.

Peroneal Nerve

The deep peroneal nerve is blocked by infiltration superficial to the ankle capsule in the interval between the tibialis anterior and the extensor hallucis longus tendon (Fig. 7-24). It innervates the web space area between the great and second toes.

The superficial peroneal nerve branches are

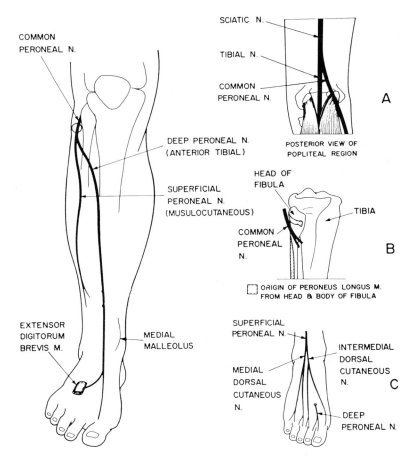

Fig. 7-24. Superficial and deep peroneal nerves supplying the dorsum of the foot. The deep peroneal nerve is located anteriorly between the tibialis anterior and extensor hallucis longus. The superficial peroneal nerve overlies the extensor digitorum longus. (After Goodgold,[38] with permission.)

blocked in a ring block fashion, as there may be several twigs crossing the anterior ankle overlying the extensor digitorum and peroneus tertius tendons (Fig. 7-24). These dorsal cutaneous branches supply the dorsum and lateral half of the foot as far as the small toe.

Sural Nerve

The sural nerve may be located adjacent to the peroneal tubercle after passing posterior to the lateral malleolus about half way between the fibula and the Achilles tendon (Fig. 7-25).

Prior to administration of an ankle block, a history of allergies and a family history of malignant hyperthermia are sought. For a complete block, a prior intravenous line should be established. Blood pressure should be monitored if a deep dissection is to be carried out and preparations made to provide for the option of converting to a general anesthetic if major foot surgery will be performed. A tourniquet at about

100 mmHg above systolic pressure may be applied just proximal to the malleoli to ensure a relatively bloodless field.

Problems of the Metatarsal Shafts

Freiberg's Infraction (Köhler's Second Disease)

In 1914 Freiberg described a series of patients in whom the second metatarsal head appeared to have been crushed or collapsed.[39] Freiberg's disease is probably an overuse injury to the cartilage or subchondral bone of the metatarsal head. Usually occurring primarily in the second and frequently in the third metatarsal, it is rarely seen in the fourth or fifth. The individual anatomy dictates the vulnerability of the specific metatarsal at risk. Hallux rigidus of the great toe may be Freiberg's infraction in that joint. The lesion is usually situated at the distal, dorsal part of the head and is consistent with aseptic subchondral cancellous bone necrosis. It may be that subchondral

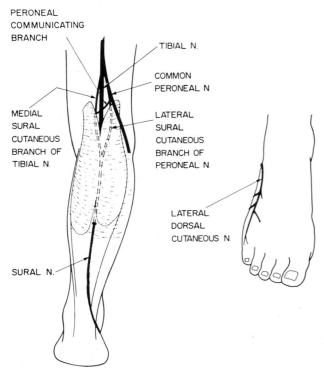

PERONEAL
COMMUNICATING
BRANCH

TIBIAL N.

COMMON
PERONEAL N

MEDIAL
SURAL
CUTANEOUS
BRANCH OF
TIBIAL N.

LATERAL
SURAL
CUTANEOUS
BRANCH OF
PERONEAL N

LATERAL
DORSAL
CUTANEOUS N.

SURAL N.

Fig. 7-25. Lateral foot distribution of the sural nerve. It may be located posterior to the lateral malleolus or over the calcaneus by the perioneal tubercle. (After Goodgold,[38] with permission.)

bone fatigue failure sets up the chain of events.[40] The onset is during adolescence (14 to 18 years of age).

The disease has been divided into stages; and early, when there is little or no deformity, rest and protection may allow symptoms to settle and bone to remodel. With more advanced disease, it may be necessary to remove any loose fragments and débride the

---

Quick Facts

STAGES OF FREIBERG'S INFRACTION

Stage 0 — Subchondral bone fracture; no deformity, roentgenogram normal
Stage I — Osteonecrosis without deformity
Stage II — Collapse and flattening of head
Stage III— Obvious separate fragment; flattened head, early arthrosis
Stage IV — Established arthrosis

---

joint (Fig. 7-26). When fully established, a dorsiflexion osteotomy of the involved metatarsal head or a wedge osteotomy of the metatarsal neck is the procedure of choice, depending on the degree of joint destruction. This condition is always suspected in cases of metatarsal pain of the second and third rays in athletes. The major differential diagnosis includes stress fractures of the shaft or neck and metatarsalgia.

Stress Fractures

The length of the second metatarsal becomes significant during push-off. Because of its length, there is no common axis for motion for all of the metatarsal heads. There is one axis through the first and second heads and another from the second through fifth heads (Fig. 7-27). When standing, there is a common sharing of the load through all of the metatarsal heads, which comes to an end as soon as the heel leaves the ground.[7] The motion then has to pass either through the axis of the medial two digits or that of the lateral four digits, depending on the mode of progression. Whichever the mode of push-off, the second metatarsal is exposed to stress. Fortunately, despite being long and slender, it is biomechanically strong with a large amount of cortical bone. Its base is wedged between the medial and lateral cuneiforms and held by strong tarsometatarsal ligaments (the short and long plantar ligaments) and by expansion of the tibialis posterior tendon insertion. It therefore forms a stable central part of the forefoot. When stresses are built up slowly, it adapts with hypertrophy, which is clearly seen in the enormously thick, corticated second metatarsal of the professional ballet dancer. When stresses are imposed too rapidly and in an unplanned manner, stress fractures frequently result. In this situation, the bone resorptive processes exceed the osteoblastic potential. The normal remodeling that occurs with functional stresses fails, and microscopic cracks rapidly become stress risers, focusing forces and perpetuating the defect. This pattern continues unless the precipitating activity is modified.

For the initial period of an evolving stress fracture, there is usually pain on weight bearing and pressure on palpation but often relatively few other signs clinically or radiologically. If activity is not modified, the pain becomes more pronounced and is frequently present all the time; there may also be associated pain and swelling of the dorsum of the foot over the injured metatarsal. Radiographic changes go from mild

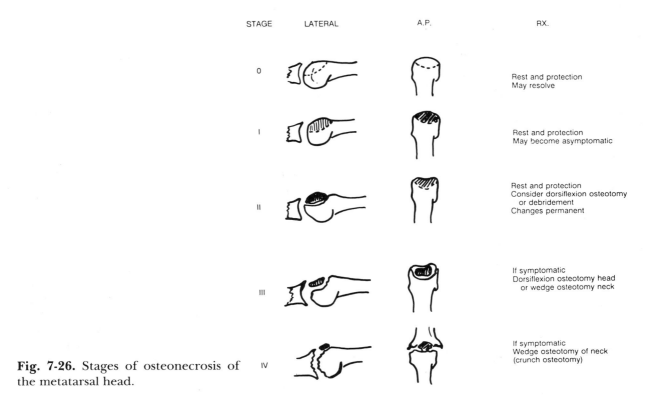

Fig. 7-26. Stages of osteonecrosis of the metatarsal head.

cortical irregularity to an obvious fracture line (Fig. 7-28). The ongoing attempts at healing produce fluffy callus. Failure to heed the increasing signs may result in displacement and prolonged healing times. The differential diagnosis is either tendinitis or metatarsalgia, depending on the location of swelling and tenderness, but a presumptive diagnosis of stress fracture should be made. If the pain persists and the plain roentgenograms remain equivocal, a bone scan is helpful.

Treatment consists in relieving stress. The magnitude of this activity modification depends on pain, the visibility of the fracture line, and the appearance of callus. A stiff shoe, a rigid orthosis, or foot cast may be considered. Usually, however, it is possible to treat these problems while allowing normal weight-bearing. Cardiovascular fitness may be maintained by pool running, the hydrolic hip flexor-extensor machines, cycling, and a rowing machine. As the fracture heals, the stair walker apparatus allows low impact aerobic activity. Before resuming full activity, the overall biomechanics of the foot should be reviewed. Healing time may be as short as 6 weeks and as long as 12.

There has been a great deal of attention given to the length of the first ray and its association with stress fracture. Drez et al. carefully documented the lack of correlation between a short first metatarsal, so-called Morton's foot, and stress fractures.[41] To be classified as short, the first metatarsal should be less than 73 percent of the second metatarsal; and to be long it should be at least 94 percent of its length (Fig. 7-29). Nevertheless, as stated at the beginning of this section, it is the offset of the mechanical axis of the medial and lateral rays that increases the loading, regardless of the relative and absolute length of the metatarsals. My findings agree with those of Drez et al.[41] and previously those of Harris and Beath[42] that stress fractures are more related to foot mechanics and activity than basic structural differences.

Fractures of the Base of the Fifth Metatarsal

There are three main fracture patterns seen in athletes. The least common is a spiral fracture of the base and diaphysis of the fifth metatarsal, and it is due to a fall from a height or a severe inversion sprain with superimposed loading. These fractures must be treated according to displacement and rotation, but they usually heal well with early weight-bearing in a below-knee cast.

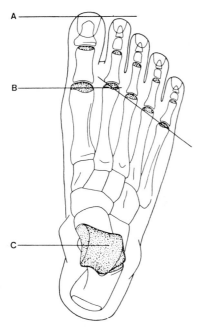

Fig. 7-27. Axes of the feet. **(A & B)** The plantar and dorsiflexion axes of the forefoot are in two different planes depending on whether weight-bearing progresses primarily through the great and second toe (transverse) **(A)** or through toes two to five (oblique axis) **(B)**. The involvement of the second metatarsal in both axes may account for the high incidence of stress fractures. **(C)** Axis through the ankle joint. This is 84° (S.D. 7°) from the long axis of the foot.

The second is the avulsion fracture of the styloid process or base of the metatarsal by the peroneus brevis tendon (Fig. 7-30). This injury, associated with an inversion sprain, is frequently seen in jumping sports. It is treated symptomatically in accordance with the associated ankle sprain unless the fragment is large and widely displaced. To ignore the latter situation usually results in an unacceptable and frequently painful bump.

The third pattern is a transverse fracture line of the proximal diaphysis described in 1902 by Sir Robert Jones, and it bears his name.[43,44] These fractures are seen in running and jumping athletes and usually represent stress reactions, although acute fractures do occur with inversion sprains. The real danger with this injury is its potential for nonunion (Fig. 7-30).

These fractures can probably be classified as: (1) acute, without pre-existing symptoms or radiologic evidence of stress reaction; (2) acute or chronic, with pre-existing symptoms or radiologic evidence of stress reaction; (3) chronic, with previous symptoms and signs of a healing stress reaction; (4) chronic, with signs of intramedullary sclerosis and little evidence of healing potential.

Despite their bad reputation, if detected before roentgenographic changes of cortical and intramedullary sclerosis are apparent, Jones' fractures heal well, provided there is not wide displacement. A short leg cast and weight-bearing as tolerated is employed.[45] The cast is removed when the patient can bear weight on the affected foot without pain, there is minimal tenderness at the fracture site, and there is radiologic evidence of progression of union. All activities except running and jumping are resumed, with some support to prevent a further inversion injury. Clinical union may occur as early as 8 weeks, but it is usually 10 to 14 weeks. Inasmuch as this delay in return to activity is 3 to 4 months, open reduction should be considered for the elite athlete. It is also appropriate in all cases with wide displacement.

When there are roentgenographic signs of delayed or potential nonunion with lucency at the fracture site, little or no callus, and evidence of intramedullary sclerosis, it may be wise to consider not only internal fixation but the possibility of a bone graft.

The key to successful treatment is careful clinical and radiologic assessment of healing potential and then a discussion with the patient of the merits and dangers of nonoperative versus operative approaches. A healing rate of more than 80 percent should be possible by nonoperative means.[44] Postcast rehabilitation of the muscles of the leg in general and the peroneal muscles specifically are necessary to avoid the catastrophe of reinjury in the athlete. It is also advisable for the jumping athlete to wear a soft ankle orthosis, of the kind prescribed for ankle sprains, for at least 6 months after fracture. This measure allows full restoration of strength and adequate bone remodeling.

Traction Apophysitis: Iselin's Disease

Iselin described traction apophysitis of the base of the fifth metatarsal in 1912.[46] This condition is seen in young individuals prior to puberty who engage in sports that put stress on the forefoot. It is a rare problem caused by recurrent microtrauma, provoking a stress reaction of the open apophysis, similar to Osgood-Schlatter's disease of the tibial tubercle.[46,47]

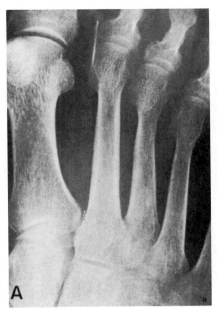 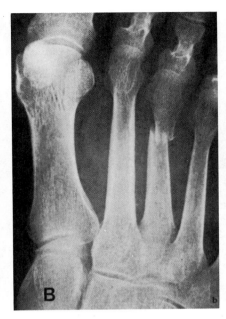 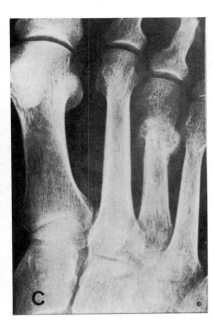

Fig. 7-28. Stress fracture of the third metatarsal shaft (march fracture). **(A)** Irregularity of cortex. **(B)** Evolution to complete disruption. **(C)** Healing with ample callus.

Ossification of the basal apophysis of the fifth metatarsal may be seen as early as age 8 years in girls and age 10 in boys, but it is seen more often between the ages of 10 and 12. Fusion is usually complete by age 15 in girls and age 17 in boys.

The athlete may present with a painful limp, inability to jump, and pain and tenderness on pressure over the bone of the fifth metatarsal due to pressure of the shoe or secondary to banging the foot against objects. Treatment depends on the severity of the symptoms and can range from ankle strapping, use of NSAIDs, and activity modification or casting. The symptoms may be persistent and tend to recur. They ultimately disappear with fusion of the apophysis. This condition is mentioned for its interest and for the sake of completeness, not because of its prevalence.

MIDFOOT, HINDFOOT, AND ARCHES

The midfoot is formed by the midtarsal bones and their articulation, i.e., the three cuneiforms, cuboid, and navicular. They form the proximal transverse arch of the foot. The calcaneus and talus form the hindfoot, and it is their position that essentially dictates the longitudinal arches of the feet.

The articulation of the midfoot with the forefoot is through Chopart's combined joint, and the junction with the hindfoot is via Lisfranc's composite articulation. Via these joints, the heel eversion combines with forefoot rotation, and sometimes in the non-weight-bearing position abduction, to produce pronation. Conversely, heel inversion with rotation, and in the non-weight-bearing position adduction, gives supination. The former (pronation) unlocks the foot, allowing adjustment of the arch and forefoot to varying terrains, and facilitates shock absorption. In the latter (supination), the close-packed position helps provide a rigid lever for propulsion.

The midfoot provides the main attachments for the dynamic control of the arch, i.e., the tibialis posterior tendon to the navicular and the medial cuneiform, the tibialis anterior tendon to the medial cuneiform, and the peroneus longus tendon to the medial cuneiform. Thus inversion and eversion at the subtalar joint in the hindfoot is controlled as a conjoint motion via the midfoot. Similarly, the ankle motion of dorsiflexion is controlled indirectly via the midfoot attachments of the tibialis anterior and posterior.

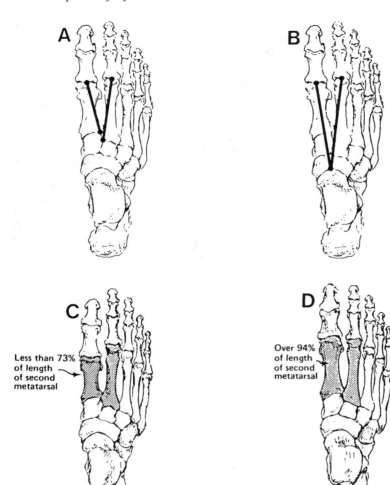

Fig. 7-29. Measurements of metatarsal lengths. **(A)** Absolute lengths. **(B)** Relative length from head of talus. **(C)** Values less than 73 percent of second metatarsal are classified as a short first ray. **(D)** Values over 94 percent of second metatarsal constitute a long first ray. (After Drez et al.,[41] with permission.)

Plantar flexion at the ankle is also produced indirectly via the pull of the triceps surae through the calcaneus. With the major weight bearing function controlled by so much indirect muscle pull and conjoined motion, it is obvious that positional changes and loss of joint play in the subtalar and midtarsal area are frequently painful and sometimes difficult to control and treat.

Examination and Alignment

There is considerable disagreement as to the value of static measurements of the foot, particularly those taken in the non-weight-bearing position. For this reason, a screening examination should probably include alignment in weight bearing positions as well as in prone lying.

Athletes are assessed by viewing them from the side while they stand in a walking position. The presence of a well formed static medial arch should be noted as well as its dynamic formation with heel raising. It should be recorded as cavus, normal, or planus and as rigid or mobile.

The heel is viewed from behind with the athlete standing, feet pointing forward, looking for valgus, neutral, or varus alignment. These factors should be reported as mild or severe.

If specific measurements of the heel alignment during weight-bearing are to be made, four points are marked on the posterior leg. The proximal two points bisect the lower one-third of the calf and Achilles tendon. The distal two are made on the calcaneus. One is at the inferior aspect and one at the superior

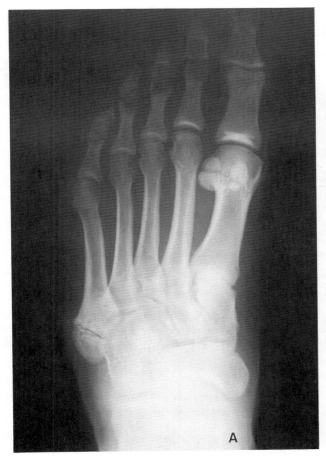

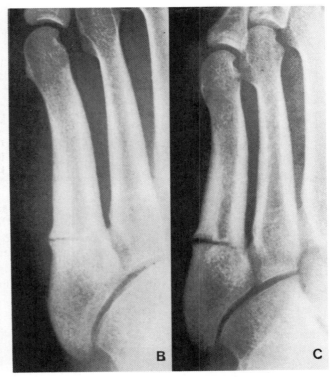

Fig. 7-30. Fractures of the base of the fifth metatarsal. **(A)** Avulsion fracture by peroneus longus. **(B)** More troublesome Jones fracture, which requires more careful attention. **(C)** In this case the fracture has extended, and nonunion is likely.

margin. These same markings may be used for assessing the non-weight-bearing foot. Five degrees either side of the neutral alignment is considered normal. In addition, from this position the presence of abnormalities such as a thickened Achilles tendon, large calcaneal exostoses, and unusual calluses should be recorded.

To assess the neutral position of the foot have the patient lie prone with the knee extended and the feet over the end of the table. Place the finger and thumb of one examining hand in the hollows over the neck of the talus on either side of the anterior portion of the ankle. Using the other examining hand, grasp the heads of the fourth and fifth metatarsals and rock back and forth until the talus lies central between the fingers, which is approximately the midposition of movement for the os calcis. Measure the number of degrees the line of the os calcis makes with the line of the tibia (Fig. 7-31). If the angle is more than 5 degrees, it is considered abnormal. While maintaining the above position, measure the angle the forefoot makes with regard to the perpendicular of the line of the os calcis. A forefoot varus or valgus more than 2 degrees is considered abnormal (Fig. 7-32).

Assessment in this unloaded position is artificial, but it does permit analysis of the main variations and makes it easier to pinpoint the source of the altered alignment. The hindfoot varus or valgus should be calculated and then recorded, along with the tibia and genu varum. The forefoot valgus, if present, has a major subtype known as the plantar-flexed first ray, in which the first metatarsal head is positioned below the plane of the lesser metatarsal heads. It is usually considered to be an acquired deformity.

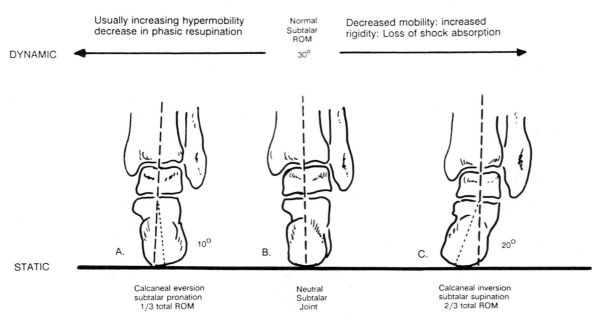

Fig. 7-31. Non-weight-bearing measurements of subtalus position. **(A)** Valgus heel (calcaneal eversion) associating with subtalar joint pronation. One-third of total range of motion is illustrated. **(B)** Neutral heel. **(C)** Varus heel (calcaneal inversion) associated with the subtalar supinated position. Approximated two-thirds of the total motion is illustrated.

There is a tendency for the clinician to be overconfident about his or her ability to measure these small variations and, more particularly, to place too much emphasis on the role of each in the etiology of specific syndromes. It has been clearly shown that tibia varum cannot be assessed well without the aid of roentgenography.[48] There are several recurring themes throughout this text.

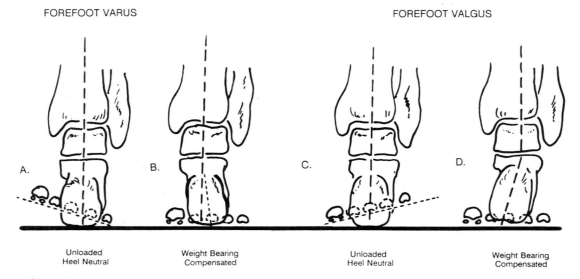

Fig. 7-32. Forefoot deformities. Non-weight-bearing forefoot varus **(A)**, which usually converts to a compensated valgus heel **(B)**. Forefoot valgus **(C)**, which usually compensates by a varus heel **(D)**. (Redrawn from Subotnick,[15] with permission.)

1. Clinicians are rarely as accurate at clinical measurements as they think they are.
2. The smaller the range of motion being measured, the greater is the inaccuracy.
3. Anatomic variations abound and most of the so-called malalignments are well within two standard deviations and therefore should be called normal variations.
4. Most overstress syndromes correlate with the degree and nature of the training.
5. Because these normal variations abound they are found in large numbers in any group who have symptoms.
6. Close scrutiny has nearly always shown that those alignments are present in equal prevalence in the nonsymptomatic population.
7. Although probably not the main etiologic factor, alteration of alignment may subtly alter biomechanics and therefore aid in destressing an injured body part and aid in the resolution of a specific syndrome.
8. Orthotics to alter alignment should be prescribed with care and usually with the understanding that it is best not to use them permanently.
9. In some cases symptoms return with discontinuation of the orthosis, or there may be definite evidence of progression of a disease process without the orthotic support; in these situations, the more permanent use of orthotics may be considered permanent.
10. Occasionally, surgery is a viable alternative to long-term orthotic use.

These broad principles have served me well over the last two decades, when the emphasis on malalignments reached its zenith during the early 1980s. With more critical surveys, more stringent requirements for publications in the better journals, and more appropriate research designs, the role of the so-called malalignment is gradually being brought into its true perspective.[41,43] These principles hold true for most of the lower limb alignments. It should also be appreciated that the incredible improvement in running shoe design and manufacture has done much to assist in reducing the incidence of repetitive impact-type injuries.

The range of motion in the subtalar joint is approximately 30 degrees (Fig. 7-31). With hypermobility in valgus, there may be dynamic decrease in the phasic resupination and hence the possibility of chronic lig-

---

Clinical Point

ALIGNMENT, MEASUREMENT, AND SYMPTOMS

- Clinicians' measurements are rarely accurate.
- The smaller the range, the greater is the inaccuracy.
- Anatomic variations abound.
- Most so-called malalignments are within 2 SD of the norm.
- Malalignments are equally present in the asymptomatic population.
- Most overstress syndromes correlate with training errors.
- Alteration of alignment may affect biomechanics.
- Alignment modification may be used as a treatment.

---

amentous or muscle stress.[49,50] With a fixed varus deformity or when the range of motion takes place mainly within the limit of the varus or valgus arc, there tends to be increasing rigidity and decreased shock-absorbing potential. It may also predispose to pathology.

McPoil et al.'s study of normal, healthy women 18 to 30 years old showed that forefoot valgus was the most common forefoot alignment; it was present in nearly half (44.8 percent) of the population. In the rear foot, subtalar varus was present in more than 80 percent of the active population[51] (Table 7-4). Furthermore, only about two-thirds of individuals had the same alignment bilaterally.

Longitudinal Arches

The true functional nature of the arches of the foot is not understood, and neither is the implication of a slightly higher or lower arch in the athlete. Feet in

TABLE 7-4. Frequency Distribution of Subtalar Varus

Site	Frequency (%), by Degree of Subtalar Varus		
	<4 Degrees	4–8 Degrees	>8 Degrees
Left	24	25	1
Right	24	22	1
Total	48	47	2

which the medial longitudinal arch is flattened are referred to as flat or pronated or are designated pes valgus or pes valgoplanus. In situations where the arch is unusually high, the condition of pes cavus or cavovarus is said to exist. The normal values are shown in Figure 7-33, but the normal variation is large.[49] The terms inversion and eversion are usually considered isolated movements of the calcaneus on the talus when the foot is non-weight-bearing.[50]

MacConaill and Basmajian conducted a study on subjects who had progressively heavier weights imposed on the supporting foot.[50] The subjects were seated with the knee flexed at 90 degrees to eliminate

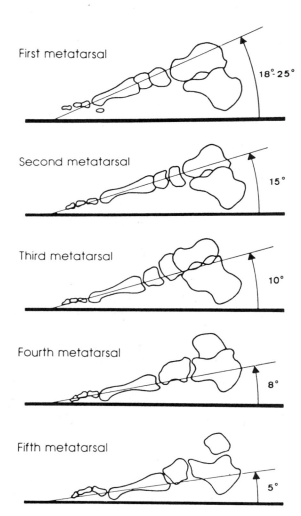

Fig. 7-33. Angles formed by each metatarsal with the floor. Normal variations are large. (After Jahss,[49] with permission.)

postural activity. The normal subjects showed little, if any, activity in the intrinsic and extrinsic foot muscles in the static posture, suggesting that the normal foot is supported mainly by passive factors (bones and ligaments). These investigators also supported the hypothesis that muscles are important in dynamic situations, e.g., push-off in gait. It was suggested that any activity displayed in these muscles is probably associated more with maintenance of the postural angle of the ankle joint than support of the arch. On the other hand, there is evidence that in people with flat feet these extrinsic muscles may be active in order to control the subtalar and transverse tarsal joints and resist further flattening of the arch and pronation of the foot.

It may become evident on further examination that this dichotomy between the flat foot and the "normal" arched foot is artificial and that the correlation of muscle activity is not with the flatness of the feet but, rather, with the amount of pain present. The foot pain that is often described may not just be a ligamentous ache but muscle fatigue brought about by abnormal posture of the feet for that particular person.

The close-packed position for all the joints of the medial arch is that of supination. In this position, with the ligaments most taut, muscular effort for supporting the body weight is obviously at a minimum. By contrast, in the pronated foot the same ligaments are more lax, and muscle activity now becomes proportionately more important in maintaining posture. The long plantar ligaments and aponeurosis form a support that prevents separation of the two ends of the arch.[50] Furthermore, as was discussed earlier, there is a windlass effect on passive dorsiflexion of the big toe that tended to increase the arch passively (Fig. 7-2), which may explain part of the mechanism for increasing the arch under dynamic situations.[10]

In summary, the following facts represent a working hypothesis, though they warrant further investigation.

1. It is impossible to define the normal arches of the feet. Variation is so considerable that the real criteria for the adjective "normal" is absence of pain.
2. The arches of the feet are usually studied, considered, and discussed in a static framework. In fact, the arches become important when walking and running and should be discussed in relation to dynamic situations — in their role as a mechanism for balance as well as for propulsion. In this light, the muscles of the leg and the intrinsic muscles of the foot become relatively more significant.

3. The intrinsic musculature is essential for walking, running, and jumping.
4. The plantar aponeurosis, long and short plantar ligaments, and "spring" ligament (plantar talocalcaneonavicular) support the apical bones.
5. Probably the real factors supporting the arches of the feet are a combination of osseous, ligamentous, and muscular components, each assuming a varying proportion of the responsibility under different conditions.
6. Usually, peroneus longus, tibialis anterior, and tibialis posterior are the extrinsic muscles that are given primary consideration in relation to formation and support of the arch. However, these muscles are responsible, along with the triceps surae, for balancing the tibia on the foot. Therefore their action on the arch is incidental in many circumstances. When these muscles contract to exert a pull on the tibia and fibula, the equal and opposite reaction at their insertion may influence the arch.
7. The longitudinal muscles are in a better position to influence the arch in dynamic situations. With the toes fixed for propulsion, the tendons of flexor digitorum longus and flexor hallucis longus tend to bowstring and form an arch.
8. The shape of the feet frequently has little to do with pathology or amount of pain. The key to painless feet is mobility. Populations who do not traditionally wear shoes have the typical pes planus. These feet are, however, mobile. The deceptively flat foot in the relaxed state may become highly arched in dynamic situations. Although these flat feet may tire easily in the older population under conditions of prolonged standing, their excellent functional capabilities are indicated by the fact that they are seen in many athletes.

Pes Planus (Flat Feet)

Radiologically the flat foot may be classified according to the degree of depression of the lateral talometatarsal angle (Fig. 7-34). However, clinically there are essentially four main classes of flat feet.[49,51,52]

Calcaneovalgus Functional Flat Foot

The first type of flat foot is simple depression of the longitudinal arch associated with varying amounts of calcaneovalgus or everted heel. It is not usually a

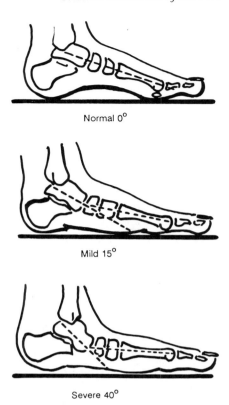

Fig. 7-34. Lateral talometatarsal angles in normal and flat feet.

cause of disability. It is, however, the type found most frequently in the active athletic population. The low arch in these cases may be considered to be the normal contour of a strong, stable foot rather than the result of weakness in foot structure or weakness in the muscles that move the foot. Occasionally, this type of foot is excessively rigid; and in this situation high levels of impact-type activities may cause symptoms. In these cases, an adequately supporting heel counter and a well-sprung, cushioned shoe give the best result. A molded flexible support may be comfortable. Attempts at imposing an arch often produces more symptoms, and a rigid orthosis is usually contraindicated. Walking and running with the hip externally rotated increases the amount of functional pronation and may aggravate symptoms. This type of movement pattern is difficult to correct and requires considerable patience on behalf of the therapist and compliance on behalf of the athlete. Treadmill running, video taping, and static running in front of a mirror are often necessary to impart a new kinesthetic sense.

Quick Facts

CLINICAL CLASSIFICATION OF FLAT FOOT

- Calcaneovalgus; usually with a normally mobile low arch
- Peroneal spastic flat foot
- Hypermobile flat foot associated with ligamentous laxity
- Tibialis posterior dysfunction
- After fracture or traumatic flat foot
- Paralytic flat foot

Spastic Flat Foot

The second type of flat foot is the peroneal spastic flat foot, which is described more fully under problems of the hindfoot. It is usually related to some structural abnormality, frequently a developmental bar between the tarsal bones (tarsal coalition). Although frequently asymptomatic for many years in the young person, it may become painful during the teens. When associated with degenerative changes, tarsal coalition may be incapacitating.

Hypermobile Flat Foot with Associated Ligamentous Laxity

The third type of flat foot may also be associated with severe and disabling symptoms. It is related to ligamentous laxity and, paradoxically, often a short Achilles tendon (Fig. 7-35). Referred to as the hypermobile flat foot, it is the commonest of the severe pes planus deformities of childhood and young adult life.[51] Typically, the heel is grossly everted with associated pronation of the forefoot. The head of the talus, navicular, and first cuneiform bones are displaced plantarward and medially. There may even be some adduction of the forefoot. Despite its flexibility, the foot does not absorb shock well, as it has used up all of the available pronation. Chronic ligament strain and subsequent discomfort is often a problem.

Treatment is directed at the tight Achilles tendon, which must be stretched without contributing to the loss of midfoot control. It is achieved by fully supporting the foot and stretching while the heel is in neutral position. An adequate medial arch orthosis (arch cookie) alone or in conjunction with some pronation (eversion) control of the heel can be used. A full foot orthosis, a heel cup, or motion control device, either built in or added to the footwear, can be effective. The more severe the alignment problem, the more important it is to make sure that everyday footwear is adequate. A semirigid or even rigid orthosis may be considered.

Tibialis Posterior Dysfunction

The fourth class of flat foot is associated with tibialis posterior tendon (TPT) dysfunction. This problem is uncommon in the young athlete and is frequently overlooked in the older individual. It is easy to confuse TPT dysfunction with the hypermobile flat foot. Johnson and Strom have reviewed the topic and presented the clinical syndrome in three stages[53] (Table 7-5).

Stage 1: Tendon Length Normal. The syndrome often remains unrecognized in this stage, because the symptoms may be only mild to moderate. The athlete may have only aching along the medial aspect of the ankle that is exacerbated by training. It is frequently difficult to localize the discomfort, but as it becomes more symptomatic, the athlete points to the course of the TPT a few centimeters proximal to the tip of the medial malleolus to its attachment on the undersurface of the navicular. The onset is usually gradual, although occasionally a twisting episode with subsequent pain is recalled. It may be useful to have the athlete go for a run or work out on the treadmill prior to examination in order to localize the site of the pathology more accurately.

On examination, tenderness is usually elicited along the TPT at the medial malleolus and distal to its insertion. Swelling may be observed when the foot is viewed from the posterior vantage point. Usually the alignment of the hindfoot and forefoot is normal at this time. The single heel raise test may unmask some weaknesses. The patient is asked to go up on the ball of the foot supporting the whole body weight. Some support may be used for balance. The sequence in the normal individual is activation of the TPT, which inverts and locks the hindfoot, followed by contraction of the triceps surae to complete the heel raise. With elongation of the TPT, the initial inversion is weak, and the patient either rises up incompletely without locking the foot or does not get up on the ball of the foot at all (Fig. 7-36). In stage 1, it should be possible to heel-raise, but it is usually done with an abnormal pattern. Roentgenograms are usually not helpful.

The pathology may be pure tendinitis with little

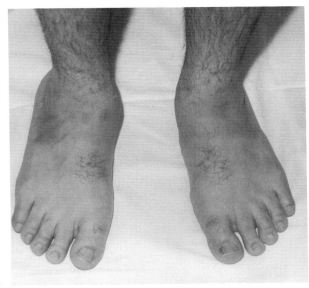

Fig. 7-35. Hypermobile flat foot with short Achilles tendon. The foot is not deformed unless the athlete is bearing weight. (**A**) Weight-bearing gives a moderate to severe pes planus. (**B**) Roentgenograms of the loaded foot.

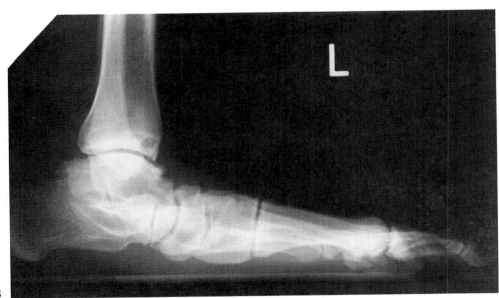

tendon change. There may be some luxuriant synovial proliferation; occasionally the tendon is grossly thickened, and sometimes degenerative changes are evident.

Treatment at this stage includes modification of activity, NSAIDs, and orthotics. If the problem becomes intractable, it may be necessary to consider surgical treatment. Surgery would include exploration of the tendon and tendon sheath with appropriate débridement. Any defect may have to be repaired. It is important to prevent stage 1 disease, an eminently treatable condition, from becoming stage 2 disease through failure of recognition or prolonged and persistent, unsuccessful, nonoperative treatment in the face of worsening symptoms. Systemic collagen disorders, particularly rheumatoid disease, must be ruled out.

Stage 2: Tendon Elongated, Hindfoot Mobile. If the condition evolves to stage 2, the symptoms have usually been present for several months to several years. The pain usually persists, even at rest. It is present along almost the whole length of the TPT. Swelling and tenderness are present posterior and inferior to the medial malleolus. The single heel raise

TABLE 7-5.   Changes Associated with Various Stages of Tibialis Posterior Tendon Dysfunction

Parameter	Stage 1	Stage 2	Stage 3
TPT condition	Peritendinitis and/or tendon degeneration	Elongation	Elongation and rupture
Hindfoot	Mobile, normal alignment	Mobile, valgus position	Fixed, valgus position
Pain	Medial: focal, mild to moderate	Medial: along TPT, moderate	Medial: possibly lateral, moderate
Single-heel-rise test	Mild weakness	Marked weakness	Marked weakness
"Too-many-toes" sign with forefoot abduction	Normal	Positive	Positive
Pathology	Synovial proliferation degeneration	Marked degeneration	Marked degeneration in joints
Treatment	Conservative: 3 months Surgical: synovectomy, tendon débridement, rest	Transfer FDL for TPT	Subtalar arthrodesis

TPT = tibialis posterior tendon; FDL = flexor digitorum longus.

test becomes markedly abnormal as the tendon weakens. As alignment changes, the "too many toes" sign may be evident. The patient is asked to assume a comfortable standing position, and the ankle and foot are viewed from the rear. From a direct midline position, the examiner counts the number of toes visible laterally on each foot. As the heel goes into increasing

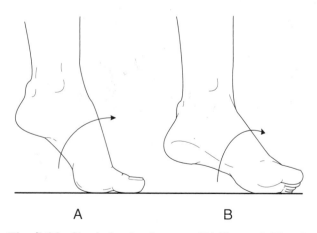

Fig. 7-36. Single heel raise test. **(A)** Normal. The tibialis posterior tendon inverts the hindfoot as the patient raises the heel. **(B)** Abnormal. With poor or absent tibialis posterior function, the patient just rolls onto the outside of the foot and has decreased ability to raise the heel.

resting eversion and the forefoot into pronation and abduction, too many toes are seen on the affected side.

Roentgenographic changes are now evident. In the anteroposterior view, the forefoot is abducted in relation to the hindfoot. The navicular subluxes from the head of the talus, and the angle between the long axis of the talus and the calcaneus increases. In the lateral view, there is sagging of the long axis of the talonavicular joint and divergence of the long axis of the talus from the calcaneus. These changes are not pathognomonic and are seen with the hypermobile flat foot. Tenograms are not useful, but magnetic resonance imaging (MRI) may demonstrate disruption of the TPT.

At this stage, there is usually marked degeneration of the tendon; it is elongated and occasionally ruptured. Treatment is usually surgical with either shortening, tenodesis, or tendon transfer being necessary. **Stage 3: Tendon Rupture, Hindfoot Deformed and Stiff.** Stage 3 is never seen in active people. The tendon has ruptured, the static supports of the foot have been damaged, and a fixed, rigid flat foot develops. The pain may transfer to the lateral aspect of the hindfoot as impingement occurs, with increasing valgus of the heel. The pain is characteristic of degenerative joint disease.[52] Deformity is the most dramatic finding. Usually some form of arthodesis is needed if the pain is severe (Table 7-5).

Other Acquired Flat Feet

There are other groups of flat feet that are not considered here; they include the acquired pes planus of trauma with fracture, the rocker bottom foot that results from ill-conceived manipulation of the child's clubfoot, and the occasional paralytic flat foot secondary to neurologic disease. Although individuals with these severe deformities are not usually successful at intensely competitive, lower limb impact sports, I have been impressed by the frequent ability of these people to engage in active recreational sports, even soccer, without special footwear or orthotics. They frequently have little or no discomfort. These motivated individuals may, however, be the exceptions that prove the rule.

Cavus Foot

The cavus, or high-arched, foot is usually stable, often has some limitation of range of motion, and frequently absorbs shock poorly. It may not be the ideal biomechanical structure for running. The anatomic variation that leads to a cavus foot may be located primarily in the hindfoot, midfoot, or forefoot. The hindfoot variants include the shape and angle of the calcaneus, the midfoot cavus is secondary to altered alignments at Lisfranc's joint, and the forefoot cavus includes the plantar-flexed first joint and other variants at Chopart's articulation. These subtleties are mainly radiologic diagnoses, but they certainly have implications where the severity of the deformity is such that surgical correction is required. For the athlete, a functional division into flexible, semiflexible, and rigid is more appropriate.

With the athlete sitting and the feet dangling, the foot drops lower than the heel and the arch is high. A flexible cavus probably exists if the arch depresses upon weight-bearing. If the arch remains high during full weight-bearing, the arch is probably semirigid or rigid.

Flexible Cavus Foot

The flexible cavus foot is frequently related to plantar flexion of the first ray. The toes may be somewhat clawed, but they are usually flexible and totally reducible.[53] If a neuromuscular disease is part of the etiology, the clawing becomes more pronounced; and with time a flexible foot may become stiff and ultimately rigid.

Treatment consists in supporting the high arch, introducing as much shock absorption as possible, attempting to keep the foot (including the first ray) in neutral, and stretching out any tight structures, including the plantar fascia and heel cords.

Semiflexible Cavus Foot

Semiflexible cavus feet usually have more advanced contracture or clawing of the toes, frequently callus formation, and a tendency to pain under the metatarsal heads. The arch flattens somewhat on weight-bearing, and the toe clawing may also improve. There appears to be an association with plantar fasciitis and other stress injuries, although these relations are not clear. Treatment of the foot is similar to that of the flexible type.[53]

Rigid Cavus Foot

In the rigid cavus foot, the relations change little from the non-weight-bearing to the weight-bearing phase. The toes frequently remain clawed, and the heel cord is usually tight. Calluses may be a problem on the metatarsal heads. Some investigators have noted an association with Achilles tendinitis and stress reaction of the tibia in distance running or endurance athletes. A well sprung shoe with adequate toe box and possibly supplementary semirigid soft orthosis is indicated if symptoms prevail. Although the Achilles tendon may be stretched, often little can be done to mobilize the foot.

Equinus Deformity

Equinus means horse-like and describes a deformity in which the foot is plantar-flexed at the ankle or within the foot. Equinus deformity is often part of the cavus foot problem, and the two conditions overlap. The more severe types are related to significant congenital deformities, the best known of which is the talipes equinovarus, or the classic clubfoot. From the athlete's point of view we are mainly dealing with heel cord tightness or post-traumatic osteophytic block to dorsiflexion.

Classification

The simplest approach is to assign categories according to the site of the major pathology; hence there are three types: ankle, midfoot, and forefoot equinus.[54] At the ankle, normal dorsiflexion may be blocked owing to osseous impingement of the tibia on the talus. In the athlete, osteophytes from the anterior lip of the tibia is the most common cause. Alternatively, there may be soft tissue restriction due to gastrocnemius or soleus tightness. Midfoot and forefoot equinus occurring at Chopart and Lisfranc's joints are often related to the cavus foot.

An equinus deformity essentially gives a relatively long leg, and abnormal stance phase biomechanics. Only mild equinus deformities are compatible with most vigorous weight-bearing activities. The more severe deformities are largely congenital and have the prefix "pes" or "talipes." An etiologic classification would include congenital, acquired, or transitional categories, which accounts for the temporary tightness frequently seen in heel cords during the growth spurt.

Quick Facts

ETIOLOGY OF EQUINUS DEFORMITY

- Congenital
  - Osseous
  - Musculotendinous
  - Neurologic
- Acquired
  - Limb length difference
  - Muscle imbalance
  - Neurogenic
  - Traumatic
- Transitional
  - Growth spurt related
  - Girls 11 to 16 years
  - Boys 12 to 18 years

Biomechanics of Equinus

When walking, plantar flexion occurs mainly from heel strike through midstance. When jogging and running, most runners have a heel-to-toe, flat foot or toe-to-heel gait pattern at initial ground contact. Dorsiflexion occurs rapidly and progresses to plantar flexion. When sprinting, which is primarily a toe-to-toe pattern, the initial dorsiflexion cushions the landing, along with hip and knee flexion. Dorsification then rapidly translates into plantar flexion (Fig. 7-37).

Approximately 10 to 25 degrees of dorsiflexion is required for these activities, and limitation of this range usually dictates some compensation in the

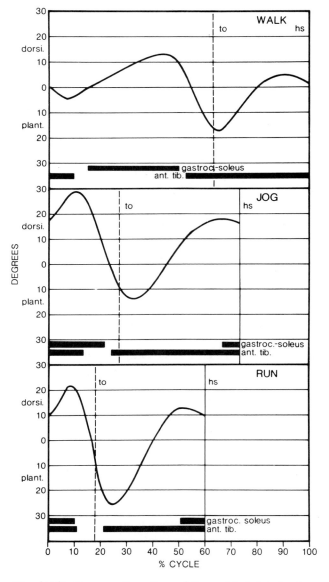

Fig. 7-37. Range of motion of the ankle joint during walking, jogging, and running. (After Mann and Hagy,[55] with permission.)

foot.[55] The compensatory mechanism of an equinus foot with significant limitation of dorsiflexion include adaption throughout the lower kinematic chain.

All of the adaptations shown in the box may be present to varying degrees. They may increase energy expenditure, decrease efficiency, and give rise to pathology, including unusual callosities, metatarsalgia, hallux valgus, neuromas, plantar fasciitis, Achilles tendinitis, and ankle sprains.

Examination

Tests for Achilles tendon tightness are described in the chapter on the hindfoot. Essentially, the test position is sitting, with the legs dangling over the examining table; dorsiflexion is measured in this position. If it is limited, it signifies possible soleus tightness, as the gastrocnemius is relaxed. If adequate dorsiflexion is present in this position and if it is limited when the knee is extended, the gastrocnemius is tight but the soleus is adequately stretched. A screening examination should rule out neurologic disease, and roentgenography helps to define bony changes, either congenital, traumatic, or adaptive. Overall, leg alignment is recorded; and observation of walking and when possible running facilitates judgment about the degree of functional adaptation.

Simple muscle tightness is the commonest factor in the athlete and is classified as mild with 6 to 9 degrees of dorsiflexion present when the knees are extended, moderate at 0 to 5 degrees, and severe at less than 0 degrees. An equinus of more than 10 degrees gives a toe-to-toe gait and most of the adaptive changes outlined.

Treatment

Treatment obviously centers around correcting the plastic deformities, e.g., muscle and tendon adaptive shortening by stretching maneuvers and compensating for the more rigid permanent osseous changes with orthosis and footwear changes. Occasionally, surgical release of the soft tissues, Achilles tendon lengthening, and osteotomy of the bones are indicated.

Accessory Ossicles and Exostosis

Numerous accessory ossicles of the feet have been described, most of which are asymptomatic (Fig. 7-38). Approximately 22 percent of children under the age of 16 have one or more accessory bones in the feet. Of these bones, only the accessory tarsal navicular and os trigonum are of sufficient clinical importance to consider further.[13]

The accessory tarsal navicular (os tibial externum) is present in about 10 percent of young people as an accessory ossification center for the navicular. In adolescents it frequently coalesces, resulting in a residual presence in 2 percent of adults. It is often bilateral and may be bifid.[15] Occasionally when it is large, it remains prominent after fusion and is referred to as a cornuate (horned) navicular. It may produce symptoms because of its prominence or because of the attachment of the tibialis posterior tendon. It may be particularly troublesome in hockey players, figure skaters, soccer players, and skiers.

The diagnosis is confirmed by visualizing the bump and frequently the overlying bursa or callus. There is tenderness on palpation and occasionally pain with resisted inversion of the foot. The clinical impression is confirmed on anteroposterior and oblique roentgenograms.

Nonoperative treatment includes the use of a medial longitudinal arch support if the symptoms are particularly related to the tibialis posterior tendon. If the prominence is the major problem, a shoemaker or orthotist can expand that portion of the skate or shoe. Occasionally a surrounding relief pad helps. NSAIDs may have a role.

When symptoms prevail and are significant, it may be necessary to remove the prominence or accessory ossicle and occasionally transpose the tibialis posterior tendon (Kidner's procedure). It is usual to rest the foot postoperatively in a cast or brace for 6 weeks if the tendon has been transposed. With a large prominence, the amount of bone that may be removed is limited by the involvement of the adjacent talonavicular joint.

Exostosis may occur wherever a joint develops significant osteophytes, but the most common site in the foot other than the prominent navicular is the area over the medial and intermediate cuneiform, the so-

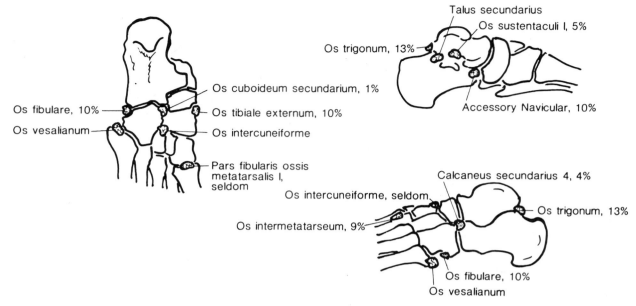

Fig. 7-38. Accessory bones of the foot. (Adapted from Tachdjian,[13] with permission.)

called dorsal exostosis, and the osteophytes that develop around the first MTP joint. Both of these areas may produce pressure with footwear and occasionally tendinitis. Adequate space in the shoe, special relief by expanding a portion of the skate or boot (by the shoemaker), a donut or sponge supplied by the therapist, and NSAIDs for the associated bursitis or tendinitis may relieve symptoms. Occasionally the osteophyte must be removed surgically.

Tendinitis

Extensor Tendinitis

The extensor tendons may be traumatized secondary to tight laces on shoes or tight foot gear over the dorsal aspects of the midtarsus. It is easily treated with local anti-inflammatory measures, changing the patterns of lacing of the shoes, or obtaining larger shoes. The bruised extensor tendons should be rested and padded with felt, sponge rubber, or Spenco Second Skin. Analgesics may be helpful.

Peroneus Longus

The peroneus longus plantar flexes, abducts, and everts the foot.[53-55] It is a plantar flexor of the first ray and may play a role in the development of a functional forefoot valgus. In the hindfoot, peroneal ten-

dinitis and subluxing peroneal tendons may be related to chronic ankle sprains. In the midfoot, pathology may be secondary to overuse, poor conditioning, or acute trauma.[15] These conditions are treated with ultrasound, NSAIDs, modification of activity, or an appropriate orthosis. Crepitating tenosynovitis may be best dealt with by an initial instillation of steroid into the tendon sheath.[54]

Cuboid Syndrome

Occasionally the uncommon peroneal cuboid syndrome (locked cuboid, calcaneal cuboid fault syndrome, subluxed cuboid) is diagnosed.[56] Following an inversion sprain, sudden forced dorsiflexion, or excessive training on uneven terrain, there may be minimal subluxation or malposition of the cuboid in a lateral and dorsal direction. Frequently, a flexible pronated foot alignment is already present, allowing the peroneus longus to exert its greatest mechanical advantage. Because the cuboid is the fulcrum for the tendon, there is a dorsal thrust on its lateral aspect tending to rock the medial cuboid down, producing the so-called locked cuboid.

Pain, which may be present even during walking, is located along the course of the peroneus longus. There may be associated peroneal tendinitis, but it is not a necessary accompaniment for the pain to exist. Maximum discomfort is elicited by pressure directed over the peroneal groove on the plantar surface of the calcaneus.

Treatment consists in manipulation of the midfoot and occasionally NSAIDs, a neutral orthosis preventing overpronation, or a cuboid plantar pad. When pain is acute, low dye strapping is considered, pulling the tape medially to counteract the pull of previous tapes.[54,55] The manipulation attempts to thrust the medial aspect of the cuboid dorsally and laterally simultaneously. The mobilizing techniques are done with the patient in a supported standing position, making sure the patient has a relaxed, flexed knee (Fig. 7-39). If the syndrome has not been present long, it usually responds to a few manipulation efforts.[56]

Tibialis Anterior

The tibialis anterior is the prime antigravity muscle functioning to decrease foot slap at ground contact. It also works as a dorsiflexor of the foot at toe-off and during the swing phase.[55] Anterior tibial as well as extensor tendinitis can occur at the midfoot level due to tight shoelaces or eyelets on shoes. Midtarsal joint dorsal hyperostosis may impinge on the tendon and surrounding soft tissue, triggering tenosynovitis. Excessive pronation elongates the anterior tibial tendon as the medial longitudinal arch drops, which may be a predisposing factor to tenosynovitis. Sudden combined plantar flexion eversion injuries may cause partial to complete rupture of the tibialis anterior tendon, which may require surgical repair. This injury is rare.

Conservative therapy for tenosynovitis of the anterior tibial tendon consists in physical therapy with ultrasound, laser, or electrogalvanic stimulation, as well as the use of oral anti-inflammatory medications. Corticosteroids can be injected judiciously into the peritendinous area but not intratendinously, as it might cause intratendinous necrosis of the tendon. Initially, resting the foot with tape using a low dye or high dye taping is helpful. A soft temporary orthosis is

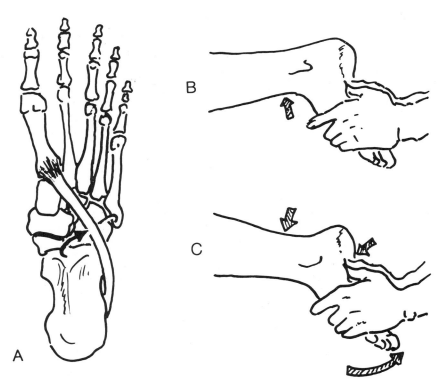

Fig. 7-39. **(A)** Left foot with peroneus longus tendon and the direction of rotation of the cuboid. **(B & C)** Thumbs are positioned over the rotated cuboid **(B),** which is manipulated with a quick thrust, applying direct pressure with the thumbs so the cuboid moves dorsally and laterally with respect to the calcaneus **(C).**

put in place to correct foot imbalances, after which a more permanent orthosis may be indicated. Appropriate rehabilitative exercises are helpful to strengthen the anterior tibial muscle and stretch the peroneals and posterior musculature. Acute partial rupture may necessitate use of a cast for 4 weeks, whereas chronic tendinosis requires physical therapy.

Chronic tenosynovitis not responsive to conservative therapy does respond to surgical tenolysis. If there is intratendinous damage, curettage of necrotic tendon is indicated with repair of the tendon using a tendon graft if necessary. If the anterior tibial tendon is repeatedly squashed between the shoe and an underlying exostosis, surgical excision may be required to eliminate the pressure.

Tibialis Posterior

The role of the tibialis posterior muscle in the evolution of foot pronation and a painful flat foot has already been discussed. Acute tenosynovitis usually responds to taping of the foot as well as physical therapy, with laser or ultrasound carried out three times a week. Ice should be used before and after light workouts. If running causes pain, substitute aerobic activities, e.g., biking and swimming is recommended. It may take 3 to 4 weeks for these problems to respond to conservative therapy. Corticosteroids should not be used for acute problems, but they may be indicated after 3 weeks for chronicity. Appropriate orthotic correction of abnormal biomechanics is indicated. Footgear must be checked and care taken to select shoes that decrease abnormal motions. A firm midsole in a shoe is necessary, especially if there is excessive pronation with a hypermobile flat foot. Strengthening exercises for the posterior tibial muscle are indicated once the acute phase is over.

All of the tendinitis syndromes, as well as the various foot pain syndromes secondary to ligamentous strains or stress reactions of bone, require careful reintegration into activity. There are several appropriate schemes, one of which is presented in Table 7-6. However the success of these programs is careful patient education and compliance.

Flexor Digitorum Longus

The flexor digitorum longus tendon may become inflamed at the plantar aspect medially in the midfoot secondary to excessive pronation or increased efforts of plantar-flexing the toes during propulsion. Dancing or jumping sports may predispose to excessive

TABLE 7-6. Resumption of Running After Lower Limb Overuse Injury

Condition	Prescription
Category I: continuous pain	Refrain from running until pain-free and no tenderness. Then begin category II.
Category II[a]: pain only on running[b]	If one has short intervals of pain with running: 1. No running for 2 weeks 2. Ten minute workout. Alternate 4 minute run and 1 minute walk. If no pain, add 5 minutes every 3 days, working up to 30 minutes, then progress to next step. If pain, cut back 5 minutes. Hold until pain-free and then progress. 3. Fifteen minute workout. Alternate 4.5 minute run and 0.5 minute walk. If no pain, add 5 minutes every 3 days, working up to 30 minutes, then progress to next step. If pain, cut back 5 minutes and work up. 4. Steady run workout, run continuously 15 minutes. Add 5 minutes every 3 days.
Category III: pain after running	1. Cut workout by 50% and progress by adding 10% a week. 2. If cutting workout 50% still causes pain, cut it by 50% again and progress by adding 10% a week.

This table is adaptable to many situations and provides a guide for activity modification with foot pain.[30,56]

[a] If pain at any step, cut back 5 minutes, hold until pain-free, then progress.

[b] Mild to moderate pain, only after a certain amount of activity.

strain of the long flexors at the mid aspect of the foot as the toes are repetitively dorsiflexed and plantar-flexed. It can be difficult to differentiate this problem from medial plantar fasciitis.

Acute flexor tendinitis is treated with rest and anti-inflammatory medication. Abnormal biomechanics must be corrected. Once the acute phase is over, rehabilitative exercises are instituted with strengthening of the flexors and balancing of the foot. Taping is most helpful and may be necessary for 6 weeks after an acute episode. Crest pads on the toes to decrease overuse of the long flexors during toe-off are helpful. Surgery is rarely indicated for flexor tendon pathology.

Flexor Hallucis Longus

The flexor hallucis longus is used for push-off. Tenosynovitis may occur secondary to overload, especially in dancing sports. Ballet dancers going en pointe may have flexor hallucis longus tenosynovitis or tendinitis at the midaspect of the foot. Supporting the foot with tape and rest, physical therapy, and anti-inflammatory medication usually corrects this problem.

For acute problems, the foot is rested, and the hallux is taped in a slightly plantar-flexed attitude with elastic tape in an effort to decrease dorsiflexion. This measure rests the long flexor and allows recovery. Activities that may cause injury or pain are eliminated from the athlete's workout, and other aerobic activities are substituted. After 3 weeks of rest and physical therapy, the athlete usually returns to competition with a hallux lock and low-dye taping of the foot for an additional 3 weeks.

Sprains of the Midfoot

The joints of the midfoot may be collectively designated Chopart's and Lisfranc's articulations. Chopart's joints are the articulations between the calca-

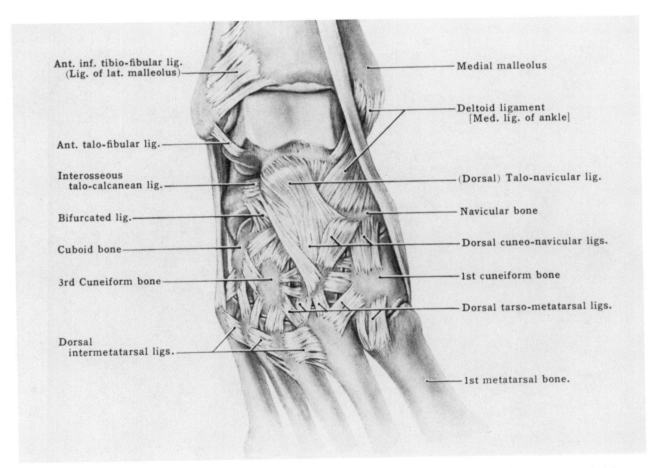

Fig. 7-40. Dorsal view of joints of the foot with major ligaments. (From Grant,[57] with permission.)

neus and talus as a unit and the midtarsal bones. Lisfranc's articulation is the articulation between the metatarsals and the three cuneiforms, and the cuboid as the proximal unit. Acute and chronic strains may cause pain in any of these articulations. Particularly in the older athlete, chronic ligamentous pain is sometimes difficult to distinguish from synovitis or degenerative arthritis of these joints. All three conditions may coexist, and diagnosis may depend on clinical examination with selected stressing of the isolated joints and diagnostic lidocaine injections to try to eliminate specific anatomic structures as the source of discomfort plus plain roentgenograms, tomograms, and computed tomography (CT) scans.

The major ligaments involved in acute or chronic stress are the dorsal calcaneocuboid and calcaneonavicular (bifurcate) ligaments as well as the dorsal talonavicular, cuneonavicular, and tarsometatarsal ligaments (Fig. 7-40).[57] The plantar structures undergoing the most stress are the calcaneocuboid (short plantar) ligament, plantar calcaneonavicular (spring) ligament, and plantar cuneonavicular and tarsometatarsal ligaments (Fig. 7-41).[57]

Prolonged or excessive pronation may predispose to chronic capsular straining of the talonavicular or naviculocuneiform joints. Acute inversion injury may produce sprains of the calcaneocuboid or the cuboid-fifth metatarsal joints. The more severe injuries may be evidenced by avulsed flakes at the ligament attachments, evident on the oblique or lateral plain films.

Depending on the severity, strapping, splints, or even a short period in a cast may be necessary. Splints are more practical for the athlete, as they may be removed for modified activity such as swimming, pool running, and daily therapy. For the chronic strain, where significant imbalance exists in the foot, a tem-

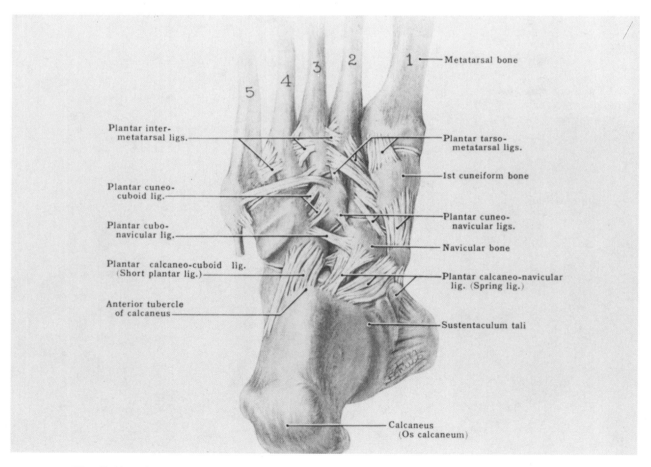

Fig. 7-41. Ligaments on the plantar aspect of the hindfoot. (From Grant,[57] with permission.)

porary orthosis is constructed. If it provides sufficient relief from symptoms, a more permanent orthotic is made. Occasionally, one or two judiciously placed corticosteroid injections are appropriate. Repeated injections into these small joints contribute to arthrosis.

With sufficient trauma, acute fractures and dislocations occur. These injuries require expert decision-making as to the adequacy of reduction and the appropriateness of internal fixation.

Osteochondrosis of the Navicular (Köhler's Disease)

The relation of Köhler's disease of the navicular to osteonecrosis is uncertain. Although some regard the condition as a normal variant or altered pattern of ossification, the predominant therapy is still one of vascular insufficiency. Köhler described the condition as a self-limiting process characterized by flattening, sclerosis, and irregular rarefaction (Fig. 7-42).[58] The average age at diagnosis is about 6 years, and frequently the child walks on the outer side of the foot with the heel in varus. Although trauma is often suggested as playing a role, the evidence is indirect.

These patients may remain symptomatic for 3 to 9 months, and the roentgenographic changes evolve over 2 to 4 years.

Treatment depends to some degree on the severity of the symptoms. Frequently an arch support reduces symptoms, and sometimes a below-knee walking cast is necessary.[59] Even with long-term follow-up of more than 30 years, degenerative joint disease does not seem to be a problem, and treatment should evolve with this fact in mind.

Stress Fractures

Joggers, walkers, sprinters, and aerobic dancers are susceptible to stress fractures, which are usually easily recognized in the neck of the second metatarsal and at the base of the fifth metatarsal. However, stress fractures of the tarsal navicular and calcaneus are radiologically more occult and associated with a long delay in diagnosis (Fig. 7-43).[60] A high index of suspicion is required in patients whose pain persists despite treatment for other diagnoses such as tendinitis, plantar fasciitis, and synovitis. In the early stages a difficult to localize and nonspecific pain is the only presenting feature. With time, if activities are not

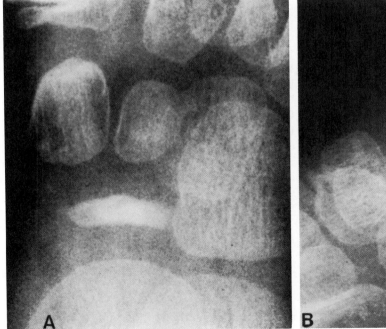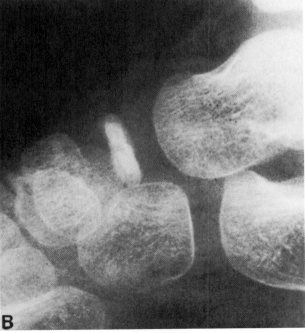

Fig. 7-42. Köhler's disease in a 4-year old child with a thick, radiodense navicular. The interosseous spaces of the tarsus are not disturbed. **(A)** Anteroposterior view. **(B)** Lateral view.

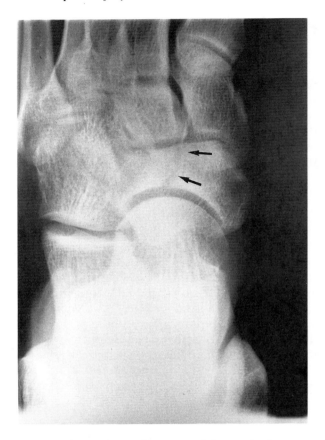

Fig. 7-43. Stress fracture of the navicular.

curtailed there may be some overlying swelling and increasing symptoms, even with walking. In the more advanced stage, the reactive bone or even a fracture line may be visible on plain films. Occasionally, CT scans are helpful, and the technetium bone scan reveals the more equivocal situations. Early treatment is activity modification and, when appropriate, an orthosis. With a symptomatic navicular fracture, internal fixation is occasionally considered. Early detection prevents wide separation and minimizes the need for surgical intervention.[61]

Peripheral Nerve Symptoms in the Foot

Proximal radiculopathies frequently lead to symptoms in the terminal branches of the nerves in the foot from the L5 and S1 roots. However, the superficial course of many of these nerves leaves them susceptible to local pressure, particularly on the dorsum of the foot. Additionally, traction neuropathies occur with ankle sprains. The diagnosis is confirmed by mapping the distribution of the discomfort, eliciting local tenderness, and producing a positive Tinel's sign to tapping.

Sural nerve neuropathy usually occurs at the lateral aspect of the foot behind the malleolus and is secondary to ankle sprains, but it also frequently occurs in connection with surgical approaches to the lateral heel, when a neuroma may be the problem.

The saphenous nerve may be compressed by tight footwear in the anteromedial midfoot. These conditions frequently respond to an adequate change in footwear but on occasion require injection of a steroid. Surgery is rarely indicated.

Compression of the anterior tibial nerve at the dorsal aspect of the midfoot is sometimes referred to as anterior tarsal tunnel syndrome. The nerve is located between the extensor digitorum tendon and the tibialis anterior tendon. The chief complaint is usually pain radiating over the dorsal aspect of the foot and frequently the first interspace or the plantar surface. Eventually this pain is replaced by numbness with some proximal radiation of symptoms.

The acute problem is treated by relieving any obvious pressure, as well as analgesics and anti-inflammatory medication. The foot is rested, and offending footgear is discarded. Chronic problems may require corticosteroid injections with long- and slow-acting cortisone every week or two followed by appropriate physical therapy to reduce inflammation. Roentgenograms are obtained to rule out underlying bone problems (hyperostosis or exostosis). When such bone problems are present, with excessive dorsal hyperostosis of the midtarsus, a partial osteotomy of the bone is indicated to form a dell, and the neurovascular bundle is decompressed. The extensor retinaculum is sectioned during this surgery and left open during closure to prevent a recurrence of the anterior tarsal tunnel. Electromyography and nerve conduction studies are sometimes helpful, but these studies are difficult in the peripheral branches of the foot.

The medial tarsal tunnel syndrome is described fully in Chapter 9.

SKIN PROBLEMS

There are some common afflictions of the skin that, although not exclusive to the feet, occur there predominantly and are specifically a nuisance to active individuals. They include blisters, corns, calluses, warts, and fungal infections.

Blisters

Blisters result when repeated friction separates superficial dead layers of the skin from the deeper epidermis and the potential space fills with a transudate of serum. Excessively loose footwear, new footwear that is stiff at pressure areas, shoes with irregularities that create their own pressure points, and unaccustomed exercise on skin that has not been stimulated to hypertrophy form a basis for developing blisters. In addition, hardwood floors or artificial turf that supplies excellent traction in sports characterized by stopping and starting also generates blisters in friction areas.

Prevention is better than treatment, and it includes adequately fitting footwear, building up time wearing new shoes slowly, properly breaking in new shoes, paring down excessive callus that may shear and allow deep blister formation, wearing socks knit of a combination of natural and synthetic fibers, and putting Vaseline or adhesive tape over developing hot spots. In individuals who sweat excessively, spraying the foot with deodorant or soaking the feet in astringent (e.g., half a cup of vinegar to a pint of water) may help. Friction may be reduced by wearing two pairs of thin socks and friction-decreasing insoles. Regular changing of socks, often half-way through training or a game, may keep the feet drier and reduce the development of blisters.

Acute blisters may be treated by simply protecting the area, or possibly by draining through a small puncture wound under sterile conditions. Healing occurs much more quickly under the biologic graft formed by the blister roof. Whenever possible leave the blister roof intact. The feet should be kept clean by soaking in antibacterial solutions, e.g., pHisoHex or povidone-iodine (Betadine), and water. Soaking may be followed by either powdering or applying Vaseline to the area, depending on the site and condition of the feet. The area is then protected with tape or moleskin. If an individual is susceptible to chronic blistering, the vulnerable area is painted with tincture of benzoin and a pad of moleskin is applied, which should reduce most of the friction. Hygiene is important, and there should be an awareness of the potential for infection with a blister.

Corns (Clavi) and Calluses (Tyloma)

The thickness of the stratum corneum varies depending on the amount of friction to which it is exposed. It varies from 0.07 to 0.12 mm over most of the body and 0.8 to 1.44 mm on the palms and soles. People who habitually walk barefoot may thicken the epidermis to 4 mm or more (Fig. 7-44). There are no blood vessels entering the epidermis. They remain in the dermis but are brought close to the epithelium by means of elevated dermal papillae, a fact worth bearing in mind while paring corns. The dermis (or corium) is a tough, flexible mixture of fibroelastic connective tissue varying in thickness from 2 to 6 mm on the palms and soles. In it lie all of the essential components of the skin, including the sweat glands, sebaceous glands, blood vessels, and nerves.

Clavi are areas of thickened skin overlying bony prominences. Keratomas are calluses, the name given to overgrowth of the epidermis. When the margins are clearly defined, they are referred to as corns or

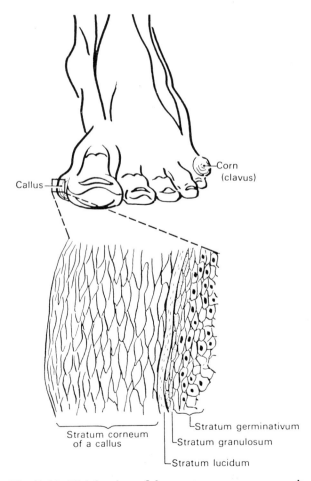

Fig. 7-44. Thickening of the stratum corneum results in callus and sometimes corn (clavus) formation.

clavi. When the margins are diffuse, the term callus suffices. The stratum corneum is compacted over the sites bearing abnormal pressure.

The pathogenesis is initially an attempt at protective bursal formation with circulatory infiltration into the site, followed by epithelial overgrowth and repeated compaction. The major sites are the metatarsal heads over hammer and mallet toes. A special callus, the bunion, forms over the medial surface of the first MTP joint.

The corns, or clavi, are of two types: the classic hard corn (heloma durum) and, in areas where maceration occurs, the soft corn (heloma molle). Corns frequently develop under the free edge of the nail (subungual clavi) and are particularly painful.

Treatment consists in sanding down small calluses with some fine abrading (Emery) paper, paring down the larger calluses and corns, making sure not to cut into the vascular dermis, and protection by means of accommodative $\frac{1}{8}$ inch adherent felt. Sometimes keeping the skin moist and supple with lanolin cream massages helps to slow re-formation of the thickened skin. If there is a particularly inflamed bursa, an injection of steroid into the base of the corn frequently allows it to settle. With persistent, painful calluses and corns, removal of the underlying bony prominence or deformity is necessary with osteotomy, arthroplasty, or arthrodesis.

Fungal and Yeast Infections

Superficial infections of the skin by fungus (principally tinea rubrum) and yeasts (usually *Candida albicans*) are common. The major area of infection is between the toes, and such infection is referred to as tinea pedis. It usually signifies a fungal infection, but mixed flora are common. Essentially these infections are slow-growing with a tendency to remain localized. Tinea pedis may be treated by soaks using a half-cup of vinegar to a pan of water. Topical antifungal agents are used to supplement this regimen.[15] The feet should be kept dry, the nails cut meticulously, and the socks changed frequently. Talcum powder or antifungal powder may be used to assist in preventing the feet from becoming moist.

If the nail or nail bed appears to be involved, or if the reddened, infected area starts to crust, produce pus, or weep, significant superinfection may be present. A physician should be consulted in this case. Nail fungal infections are difficult to eliminate.

Plantar Warts (Verruca)

The plantar wart is a viral lesion secondary to papilloma virus. When these lesions are underneath the bony prominence or weight-bearing surfaces, they are painful and interfere with activity. The key to recognizing this lesion is the way its margins may be separated or seen as being distinct from the surrounding skin. They usually have low infectivity.

Treatment consists in protecting them from weight-bearing by use of a donut pad. This measure helps relieve pain. Therapeutic ultrasound at high doses (more than 1.5 W/cm continuously) daily for 3 weeks may be effective.

Adhesive tape over the warts on a daily basis may promote resolution. This treatment is particularly effective if supplemented with some chemical compound such as Compound W, Duofilm (a combination of 15 percent lactic acid and 15 percent salicylic acid in a flexible collodion). When this form of chemical cautery is used, care must be taken to protect the surrounding normal skin. Essentially the aim of the treatment is to promote tissue desiccation. Occasionally cryotherapy with liquid nitrogen is indicated. More recently laser therapy has also been used. Excision is a decision which should be made and carried out by an experienced physician or podiatrist, since the danger of perminent painful scarring is significant.

SUMMARY

The biomechanics of the foot are complex and the stresses through the feet high. This fact in itself would lead to susceptibility to injury. However, even if nature has not produced any design errors, encompassing feet in unphysiologic and inappropriate footwear has added to the burden under which they must function. Once significant pathology exists, strict rules must be laid out for activity modification. Orthoses should be supplied only after careful analysis of alignment and biomechanics, after meticulous examination, and with a definite goal in mind. Orthotic prescription is one of the more abused aspects of sports medicine. It is fortunate that with imagination there are many ways of reducing impact, modifying footwear, and manipulating training. The advances in sports footwear has been spectacular. Nevertheless, in some instances, as in the case of the ballet dancer, treatment depends on other modalities because little modification of footwear is possible. Unfortunately, the results of surgery for many foot problems are frequently unpredictable, particularly in the young athlete, and should be undertaken only by skilled, experienced operators. Always, though, the treatment of foot pathology is a challenge.

REFERENCES

1. Garrison FD: The bone called "luz." NY Med J 92:149, 1910
2. Williams GA: Atavistic human foot: is developmental significance. Am J Phys Arthrop 16:1, 1931
3. Joseph J: Some aspects of the functional anatomy of the foot. Ann Phys Med 7:30, 1963
4. Gilula LA, Staple TW: Roentgen rounds. Orthop Rev 3:68, 1974
5. Harvey JL: Chinese bound feet. Am J Roentgenol Radium Ther Nucl Med 10:911, 1923
6. Subotnick SI: How I manage ingrown toenails. Physician Sports Med 11:65, 1983
7. Bojsen-Moller F: Anatomy of the barefoot, normal and pathologic. Clin Orthop 142:10, 1979
8. Hutton WC, Dhanendran M: The mechanics of normal and hallux valgus feet: a quantitative study. Clin Orthop 157:7, 1981
9. Reid DC: Functional Anatomy and Joint Mobilization. University of Alberta Press, Edmonton, 1970
10. DuVries HL: Surgery of the Foot. 3rd Ed. CV Mosby, St. Louis, 1973
11. Mann RA, Hagy JL: The function of the toes in walking, jogging and running. Clin Orthop 142:24, 1979
12. Smith RW: Evaluation of the adult forefoot. Clin Orthop 142:19, 1929
13. Tachdjian MO: Pediatric Orthopaedics. Vol 2. WB Saunders, Philadelphia, 1972
14. McGarvey CL: Skin and toenail problems. p. 169. In Hunt GC (ed): Physical Therapy of the Foot and Ankle. Churchill Livingstone, New York, 1988
15. Subotnick SI: Sports Medicine of the Lower Limb. Churchill Livingstone, New York, 1989
16. LeNoir JL: Onychocryptosis. Orthop Rev 6:43, 1977
17. Rodeo SA, O'Brien SJ, Warren RF et al: Turf toe: diagnosis and treatment. Physician Sports Med 17:132, 1989
18. Helal B: The great toe sesamoid bones. Clin Orthop 157:82, 1981
19. Richardson G: Injuries to the hallucal sesamoids in the athlete. Foot Ankle 7:229, 1987
20. Axe MJ, Ray RL: Orthotic treatment of sesamoid pain. Am J Sports Med 16:411, 1988
21. Sammarco GJ: How I manage turf toe. Physician Sports Med 16:113, 1988
22. Bowers KD, Martin RB: Turf-toe: a shoe-surface related football injury. Med Sci Sports 8:81, 1976
23. Couker TP, Arnold JA, Weber DL: Traumatic lesions of the metatarsophalangeal joint of the great toe in athletes. Am J Sports Med 6:326, 1978
24. Hattrup SJ, Johnson KA: Hallux rigidus: a review. Adv Orthop Surg 9:259, 1986
25. Goodfellow J: Aetiology of hallux rigidus. Proc R Soc Med 59:821, 1966
26. Moberg E: A simple operation for hallux rigidus. Clin Orthop 142:55, 1979
27. Donatelli R, Wooden MJ (eds): Orthopaedic Physical Therapy. Churchill Livingstone, New York, 1989
28. Hattrup SJ, Johnson KA: Hallux valgus: a review. Adv Orthop Surg 8:404, 1985
29. Steel MW, Johnson KA, Dewits MA et al: Radiographic measurements of the normal adult foot. Foot Ankle 1:151, 1980
30. Truslow W: Metatarsus primus varus or hallux valgus? J Bone Joint Surg 7:98, 1925
31. Sim-Fook L, Hodgson R: A comparison of foot forms among the non-shoe and shoe-wearing Chinese population. J Bone Joint Surg [Am] 40:1058, 1958
32. Jones P: Fatigue failure osteochondral fracture of the proximal phalanx of the great toe. Am J Sports Med 15:616, 1987
33. Morton TG: Peculiar and painful affection of the fourth metatarsophalangeal articulation. Am J Med Sci 71:37, 1876
34. Durlacher L: Treatise on Corns, Bunions, the Disease of Nails and General Management of the Feet. Simpkin Marshall, London, 1845, p 52
35. Lussmann G: Morton's toe: clinical, light and electron microscopic investigation in 133 cases. Clin Orthop 142:73, 1979
36. Gauthier G: Thomas Morton's disease: a nerve entrapment syndrome; a new surgical technique. Clin Orthop 142:90, 1979
37. Giachino AA: Surgeon-administered local anaesthesia for forefoot surgery. Can J Surg 31:383, 1988
38. Goodgold J: Anatomical Correlates of Clinical Electromyography. Williams & Wilkins, Baltimore, 1974
39. Frieberg AH: Infraction of the second metatarsal bone, a typical injury. Surg Gynecol Obstet 19:191, 1914
40. Resnick D, Niwayama G: Diagnosis of Bone and Joint Disorders. WB Saunders, Philadelphia, 1981
41. Drez D, Young JC, Johnson RD, Parker WD: Metatarsal stress fractures. Am J Sports Med 8:123, 1988
42. Harris RI, Beath T: The short first metatarsal. J Bone Joint Surg [Am] 31:553, 1949
43. McConkey JP: Bilateral stress fractures of the proximal diaphysis of the fifth metatarsal. Clin J Sport Med 1:44, 1991

44. Jones R: Fracture of the base of the fifth metatarsal by indirect violence. Am Surg 35:697, 1902

45. Zogby RG, Baker BE: A review of non-operative treatment of Jone's fracture. Am J Sports Med 15:304, 1987

46. Iselin H: Wachstumsbeschwerden zur zeit der Knöchern: Entwicklung der Tuberositas Metatarsi Quinti. Dtsch Z Chir 117:529, 1912

47. Lehman RC, Gregg JR, Torq E: Iselin's disease. Am J Sports Med 14:494, 1986

48. McPhoil TG, Schmit D, Knecht HG: A comparison of three positions used for evaluation of tibial varum. J Am Podiatr Assoc 78:22, 1988

49. Jahss MH: Disorders of the Foot. WB Saunders, Philadelphia, 1982

50. MacConaill MA, Basmajian JV: Muscles and Movements: A Basis for Human Kinesiology. Baltimore: Williams & Wilkins, Baltimore, 1969

51. McPoil TG, Knecht HG, Schmit D: A survey of foot types in normal females between the ages of 18 and 30 years. J Orthop Sports Phys Ther 9:406, 1988

52. Harris RI, Beath T: Hypermobile flat foot with short tendo achillis. J Bone Joint Surg [Am] 30:116, 1948

53. Johnson KA, Strom DE: Tibialis posterior tendon dysfunction. Clin Orthop 239:196, 1989

54. Subotnick SI: The cavus foot. Physician Sports Med 8:53, 1980

55. Mann RA, Hagy J: Biomechanics of walking, running and sprinting. Am J Sports Med 8:345, 1980

56. Newell SG, Woodle A: Cuboid syndrome. Physician Sports Med 9:71, 1981

57. Grant JCB: Grant's Atlas of Anatomy. 5th Ed. WB Saunders, Philadelphia, 1962

58. Köhler A: Über eine häufige bisher anscheinend unbekannte Erkrankung einzelner kindlicher Knochen. München Med Wochenschr 55:1923, 1908

59. Ippolito E, Pollini PTR, Falez F: Köhler's disease of the tarsal navicular: long term follow up of 12 cases. J Pediatr Orthop 4:416, 1984

60. Hunter LY: Stress fracture of the tarsal navicular: more frequent than we realize? Am J Sports Med 9:217, 1981

61. Alfred RH, Bergfeld JA: Diagnosis and management of stress fractures of the foot. Physician Sports Med 15:83, 1987

Heel Pain and Problems of the Hindfoot (Rearfoot)

8

In Greek mythology, Achilles was considered to be the bravest, handsomest, and swiftest in the army of Agamemnon. It is written that, his mother Thetis, dipped the child in the waters of the river Styx, rendering him invulnerable except for the part of his heel by which she had held him. In the tenth year of the war with Troy, Achilles slew Hector. The Aethiopis tells how Achilles was himself slain by Paris, whose arrow was guided to Achilles' heel by Apollo.
—Homer, Iliad

The *Iliad* clearly outlines the vulnerability of the Achilles tendon. Unfortunately, many other structures in the hindfoot are equally vulnerable. The repetitive jumping and landing inherent in many sports takes their toll on the tissues around the heel. The forces are high, and compressive and shearing stresses on the undersurface of the calcaneus are matched by traction stress around the superior and posterior surface near the attachments of the Achilles tendon (Fig. 8-1). Gaining its name from the Latin word for "spur," the internal architecture of the calcaneus makes this bone uniquely fitted to transmit all the forces imposed on it unless affected by disease processes or occasionally the unusual stresses of sport.

By linking the ankle joint with the subtalar and the midtarsal area, the calcaneus and its many articular surfaces are obviously the key to the motion in the foot. Furthermore, many structures traverse the borders of the os calcis on their way to the foot and make the diagnosis of heel pain varied and challenging.

The list of potential pathology is extensive, but plantar fasciitis and Achilles tendinitis are by far the most common problems related to activity (Table 8-1). However, for the sake of completeness, a more extensive etiologic list is discussed briefly, with emphasis on the most frequently encountered situations.[1]

Quick Facts

CLASSIFICATION OF HEEL PAIN

- Generalized conditions
- Congenital variations
- Local traumatic and overuse changes
- Conditions associated with tendons
- Nerve entrapment or trauma
- Skin problems

GENERALIZED CONDITIONS AFFECTING THE HEEL

Rheumatoid Disease

Rheumatoid arthritis often simultaneously involves many tarsal joints as well as the ankle joint and peritendinous sheaths because of the intercommunicating synovial channels. However, rheumatoid arthritis characteristically involves the small joints of the hands and feet. Early disease should be suspected in young women presenting with bilateral pain and a tendency to morning stiffness in the metatarsophalangeal joints of the feet.

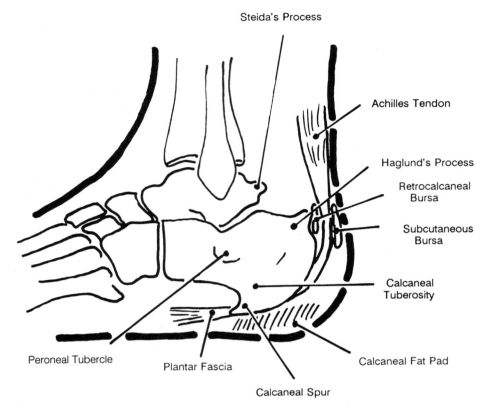

Fig. 8-1. Heel pain with potentially painful structures highlighted.

TABLE 8-1.   Heel Pain Related to Local Traumatic and Overuse Changes

Location	Condition
Plantar	Plantar fasciitis
	Calcaneal spur
	Fat pad syndrome
	Calcaneal periostitis
Medial	Tarsal tunnel syndrome
	Medial calcaneal neuritis
	Tibialis posterior tendinitis
Lateral	Lateral calcaneal neuritis
	Peroneal tendon disorders
Posterior	Retrocalcaneal bursitis
	Calcaneal apophysitis
	Haglund's deformity
	Calcaneal exostosis
Diffuse	Calcaneal stress fracture
	Neoplasm
	Calcaneal fracture

Seronegative Arthropathies

Ankylosing spondylitis, Reiter's syndrome, and gout, as well as other reactive collagen disorders, predispose the patient to synovial swelling and tendinitis. In many instances, the Achilles tendon and other tendons around the ankle are primarily involved.

Osteoarthrosis

Arthritis in the subtalar area and the midfoot is more frequently associated with trauma, either of a chronic, repetitive nature or secondary to fractures into the joint. Traumatic arthritis is difficult to treat nonoperatively and often culminates in surgical fusion of one or all of the joints of the pan-talar area.

Osteoporosis

With the increasing number of middle-aged and elderly people involved in active recreational pursuits, sports medicine has had to encompass an awareness of conditions related to these age groups. Osteoporosis, for example, affects a large percentage of elderly North Americans. Jumping activities or unaccustomed activities may precipitate crushing of the fragile architecture of the osteoporotic calcaneus, leading to fractures. These injuries range from subtle stress fractures to severely comminuted bony injuries.

Infection, Tumor, and Metaplastic Conditions

Rarely, the calcaneus is involved with tumors such as multiple myeloma, giant cell tumor, or even unicameral bone cysts, as well as infective processes of a wide variety. Pain of long duration that does not respond to usual treatment, and particularly if there is night pain, should be investigated further to rule out these unusual conditions. Furthermore, an inflammatory metaplastic condition called pigmented villonodular synovitis may involve any of the tendons around the ankle or the joints of the tarsus itself.

A careful history of the onset and nature of the pain, a general systems inquiry, plain roentgenograms of the foot, and occasionally a complete blood screen including an erythrocyte sedimentation rate (ESR) is usually sufficient to establish the presence of one of the above generalized conditions. A bone scan assists in further narrowing the diagnosis.

CONGENITAL VARIATIONS

Clubfoot

The term clubfoot encompasses a wide range of deformities, most of which involve the heel to some degree. Calcaneovarus, calcaneovalgus, pes cavus, and some pes planus deformities, if severe, may be clumped under this heading. With mild involvement there may be the usual amount of mobility of the foot, but with increasing deformity there is a tendency toward stiffness and, with excessive activity, foot pain.

Clinical Point

MAJOR CONGENITAL VARIATIONS

- Invariable associated with stiffness
- Rarely amenable to mobilization
- Orthosis to attempt to reduce impact force
- Footwear modification where necessary
- Occasionally surgery

The main clinical point is to recognize the less frequent and more subtle residual anatomic variations that are the end result of congenital problems. It is rarely possible to correct them in the adult. Management usually involves modification of footwear and activity. Symptoms frequently respond to treatment with a wide range of orthoses.

Tarsal Coalition and Peroneal Spastic Flat Foot

Tarsal coalition is a fibrous, cartilaginous, or osseous union of two or more tarsal bones that is of congenital origin. There is evidence of a hereditary component, probably autosomal dominant with nearly full penetrance.[2] Embryologically, when the primitive mesenchyme of the tarsal bones is formed, it does so in one solitary mass during the first 4 weeks of life. However, as the fetus matures and differentiates, this primitive mesenchymal tissue fragments into the various tarsal components, thus dividing into separate cartilaginous units. These cartilaginous anlages eventually start to ossify and grow into the adult form. However, if there is failure of segmentation, congenital defects with tarsal coalitions of the hindfoot and midtarsal areas may result (Fig. 8-2).

The reported incidence varies considerably with the method of investigation.[2,3] Snyder et al. found that 2.9 percent of foot skeletons had calcaneonavicular synostosis, and that if talocalcaneal coalitions were included the incidence was about 6 percent.[4] Many of these disorders are asymptomatic. When symptoms are present, they may be simply local pain or diffuse aching in the arch, sometimes is in association with intermittent peroneal muscle spasm.

Signs and Symptoms

The athlete is usually first seen during the second decade of life with mild pain deep in the subtalar area and limitation of hindfoot motion. The onset of symptoms usually occurs after some unusual activity or trauma, frequently an ankle sprain[4] (Table 8-2). Symptoms may coincide with an increase in intensity of training.

Calcaneonavicular coalitions produce poorly localized subtalar pain; but usually firm palpation over the middle talocalcaneal facet just distal to the medial malleolus reveals that tenderness is present. The slight degree of limitation of subtalar motion and mild degree of valgus deformity are not often noted in the preteen athlete. There even may be some com-

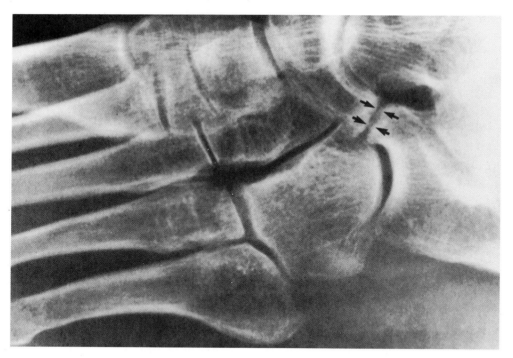

Fig. 8-2. Tarsal coalition. Oblique view of foot illustrating cartilaginous calcaneonavicular bar (coalition).

pensatory hypermobility of the talonavicular area anteriorly. With the ossification of the cartilaginous coalition, joint motion may be further restricted, which increases the chance of symptoms. Subtalar and metatarsal valgus deformity become more apparent as the coalition ossifies, resulting in pes planus of varying degrees of severity.

Talocalcaneal coalition of the middle facet is more likely to produce severe valgus deformity than any of the other coalitions.[5] Individuals whose heels remain in the neutral position seem to suffer fewer symptoms.[2] Although rare, a varus position of the heel has been reported in patients with calcaneonavicular coalition. The progressive limitation of motion of the subtalar joint may result in repeated ankle sprains and subsequent lateral ligament laxity. If not examined carefully, it may give a false impression of the amount of subtalar motion present. Furthermore, when subtalar stiffness is identified in these patients, it is important to diagnose the associated coalition, as attempts by the therapist to gain subtalar motion are counterproductive.

TABLE 8-2. Relation of Ankle Sprains and Tarsal Coalition[a]

Sport	Ankle Sprains	With Coalition	Without Coalition	Insufficient Roentgenograms
Basketball	60	32 (68%)	15 (32%)	13
Football	38	13 (57%)	10 (43%)	15
Baseball	11	2 (50%)	2 (50%)	7
Other sport	21	11 (73%)	4 (27%)	6
Total	130	58(65%)	31 (35%)	41

[a] This series gives a high percentage of coalitions, partly because all anatomic variations were included.

(Adapted from Snyder et al.,[4] with permission.)

The degree of limitation of motion varies greatly. Middle facet talocalcaneal coalition seems to eliminate or greatly restrict subtalar movement, whereas calcaneonavicular coalition usually results in only a moderate amount of restriction.[2]

Peroneal spasm may be present intermittently or continuously. Intermittent spasm is usually precipitated by activity. In severe cases the spasm may also involve the extensor digitorum longus and peroneus tertius. With normal individuals, the relaxed, dependent, non-weight-bearing foot hangs in an equinovarus position. With a peroneal spastic flat foot, it may not fall into plantar flexion and indeed may be slightly everted. The spasm in the peroneal tendons may be palpated. It should be stressed that coalitions may be asymptomatic throughout life, and the patient should be treated only according to the symptoms.

Radiology

Diagnosis may be difficult on plain roentgenograms, even with oblique views of the foot, as the bar may not be ossified. The occasional compensatory hypermobility in the talonavicular joint may result in early degenerative spurring, particularly on the talar neck. In the case of incomplete coalition, one can sometimes visualize an accessory tarsal bone referred to as the os sustentaculi, posterior to the sustentaculum tali. It may just represent incomplete bridging between the two bones. Computed tomography (CT) is probably the definitive radiologic examination for suspected bars that are not easily visualized on plain roentgenograms.

Treatment

When the condition becomes painful, it can be treated conservatively with rest, an orthosis, or immobilization in a cast for a period of time. Occasionally, a custom-made orthosis allows increased activity without symptoms. Particularly, heel wedges and an arch support seem to help those individuals with minimal symptoms. When a cast is used to settle acute but protracted symptoms, a short leg walking cast with the hindfoot molded into varus is usually most effective. It allows maximum relaxation of the peroneal muscles. However, there is a tendency for recurrence of symptoms once the resting period has ended. Excision of the bar at an early age and fusion of the area are two surgical alternatives. It should be recalled that there are other causes for peroneal spasm, especially in the older age groups, where the etiology usually can be found in inflammatory diseases of the subtalar joint, including the previously mentioned rheumatoid arthritis, degenerative arthritis, or tumor.

Accessory Ossicles

On the posterior aspect of the talus, the groove for flexor hallucis longus frequently has an elongated lateral wall called Stieda's process.[7] Between the ages of 8 and 11 years, separate ossification centers appear and usually rapidly fuse with these medial and lateral tubercles of the groove. In approximately 10 percent of the population, the lateral center persists as the os trigonum. With extreme plantar flexion, such as occurs during ballet, jumping, and bowling at cricket, the os trigonum may impinge against the posterior tibia, producing local pain. On occasion, a long Stieda's process may fracture. Local injections or nonsteroidal anti-inflammatory drugs (NSAIDs) may help, but sometimes excision is indicated. Considering the prevalence of this small bone, it is symptomatic only rarely and requires surgery infrequently.

LOCAL TRAUMATIC AND OVERUSE CHANGES

Apophysitis (Sever's Disease)

The posterior portion of the calcaneus develops as an independent center of ossification, separate from the main bone by a cartilaginous apophyseal plate. This center appears at 10 years of age and fuses with the rest of the bone at 15 years. The apophyseal plate is vertically oriented and therefore subjected to large shearing stresses by the gastrocnemius. Direct contusion to the heel by landing awkwardly or by being kicked may also precipitate symptoms. During the prepubertal growth spurt, the epiphyseal-diaphyseal junction may be mechanically weaker and vulnerable as far as the circulation is concerned. It is possible that traumatic avascular necrosis may ensue, leading to the typical roentgenographic appearances of fragmentation and altered density of the calcaneal apophysis. It may precipitate the symptoms of pain on activity and to local palpation. These symptoms frequently disappear long before the roentgenographic changes resolve. There is considerable discussion as to whether this disease actually exists, as often the normal appearance of the calcaneal apophysis is one of either density or fragmentation. In any event, a certain number of young individuals have pain in the heel with an open epiphysis, which is treated symptomatically until the discomfort resolves.

Young gymnasts are particularly susceptible to this condition because of the repetitive jumping or landing from a height, and because of the flimsy slipper used for much of their exercise. Aside from NSAIDs

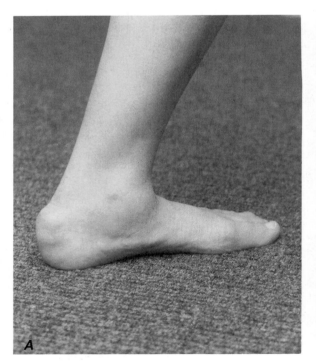
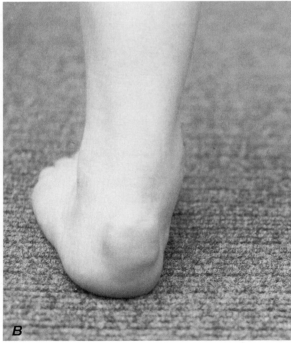

Fig. 8-3. Enlarged calcaneal process with superimposed bursa, the "pump bump." **(A)** Medial view with associated low medial arch, pes planus. **(B)** Posterior view.

and modified activity, it may be necessary for them to train in more substantial footwear whenever practical, although it greatly limits the number of activities that may be practiced.

Bony Exostosis, Calcaneal Ethesiopathy, Bursitis (Pump Bump, Runner's Bump)

The prominence of the posterosuperior lateral border of the calcaneus, or "Haglund's deformity," is probably a congenital variation but may be acquired through trauma. This prominence is susceptible to painful pressure by the heel cup of the particular sporting footwear. In association with an inflamed, overlying bursa, it produces a painful, sometimes dramatically large mass referred to as a "pump bump," or "runner's bump." The largest of these masses are usually seen in figure skaters (Fig. 8-3). The better running shoes have a small pad to reduce pressure to a minimum.

This calcaneal prominence may be related to an inflamed bursa; but like the bunion of the first metatarsophalangeal (MTP) joint, there is usually an underlying bony component. Frequently it is a bony spur. Repetitive microtrauma or microavulsions surrounding the attachments of the Achilles tendon may generate this osteophyte. A lateral roentgenogram shows this exostosis approximately 1.5 to 2.0 cm below the posterior superior tip of the os calcis, growing upward into the soft tissue shadow of the Achilles tendon (Fig. 8-4). It may be classified as an ethesiopathy, i.e., an outgrowth or tuft of cartilage

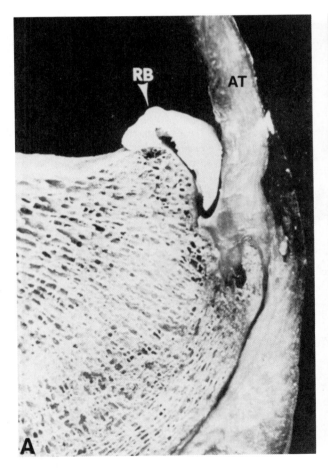
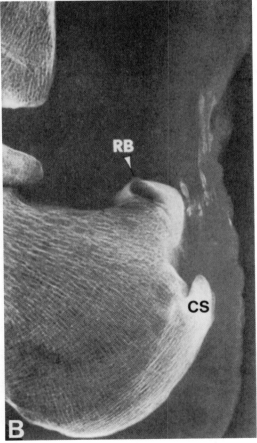

Fig. 8-4. Large retrocalcaneal bursa (RB) and spur (CS) into Achilles tendon (esthesiopathy). **(A)** Sagittal section with retrocalcaneal bursa between Achilles tendon (AT) and calcaneus. **(B)** Barium-impregnated methylmethacrylate outlines bursa on radiograph (RB). (From Resnick et al.,[8] with permission.)

or bone into the attachment site of ligament, tendon, or fascia. Although these bony spurs are frequently related to repetitive mechanical stress or local degenerative changes of the soft tissue attachments, they are often seen in relation to specific systemic diseases such as ankylosing spondylitis, gout, Reiter's disease, and rheumatoid arthritis.

A small fragment of bone has been described that is located between the Achilles tendon and the calcaneus, usually in the middle one-third of the posterior border.[8] Special oblique films may be required to outline it. It causes a painful prominence and an associated bursitis (Fig. 8-5). The etiology of the condition is uncertain, and the designation osteochondritis dissecans is probably inaccurate, although it serves the purpose of distinguishing it from the other painful protuberances. It may be mistaken for osteoid osteoma.

Whatever the etiology of these various prominences, they frequently aggravate the retrocalcaneal

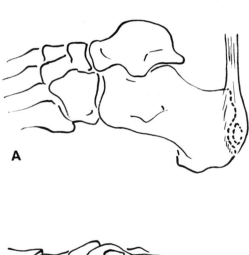

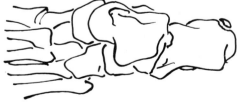

Fig. 8-5. (A) Occasionally a bony defect and fragment are visualized between the calcaneus and the Achilles tendon. **(B)** If the defect is not directly on the posterior border of the calcaneus, it may be necessary to change the angle of the x-ray beam.

> **Quick Facts**
>
> **CONDITIONS OF THE CALCANEAL APOPHYSIS**
>
> - Ethesiopathies (spur into Achilles tendon)
> - Haglund's deformity (prominent posterior superior region)
> - Sever's disease (inflamed apophysis)
> - Pump bumps (exostosis with bursitis)
> - Osteochondritis dissecans of the heel

bursa on the deep surface of the Achilles tendon or the subcutaneous bursa on the superficial surface, or they may even develop bursae of their own de novo. Occasionally, the bursa becomes inflamed without the associated exostosis. These bursae may be intrinsically painful or just uncomfortable when there is pressure of the shoe, boot, or skate.

Before embarking on treatment, the differential diagnosis must be considered, including systemic disease, Achilles tendinitis, or intrinsic conditions of the calcaneus, such as infection and tumor. A careful analysis of the roentgenogram reveals the magnitude of the bony versus the soft tissue component of the problem. Treatment includes protective padding for the area, modification of footwear, use of local modalities such as ultrasound, and either systemic NSAIDs or injectable steroid depending on the relation to the Achilles tendon (Fig. 8-6). Ultimately, if these measures are insufficient to allow resolution of the symptoms, a surgical approach may be appropriate. Depending on the lesion, this surgery ranges from excision of the bursa with the underlying exostosis or protuberance to osteotomy of the posterior calcaneus.

Contusions and Fat Pad Syndromes

Anatomy

Direct contusion to the bony calcaneus is easy to appreciate and understand; it may be a self-limiting condition relating to the immediate inflammation and resolution of the hematoma. A more difficult problem to treat is a painful heel pad involving the soft tissues. Elastic adipose tissue covers the plantar aspect of the calcaneus. Similar tissue is found in other regions subjected to pressure, e.g., over the ischial tuberosity, the fingertips, and the infrapatellar

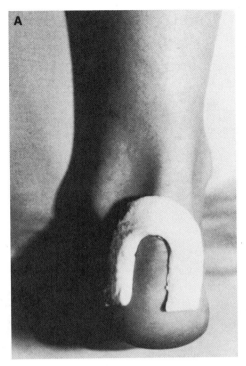 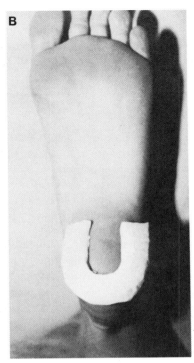

Fig. 8-6. Pressure over a painful prominence may be relieved by using viscoelastic polymers such as Spenco Second Skin, ¼ inch adhesive felt horseshoe-shaped pads or custom made orthotic device, glued directly into the shoe. **(A)** Relief around a painful retrocalcaneal bursa. **(B)** Relieving pressure over a painful plantar spur.

area. The fat cells in the heel area are compartmentalized by septa of fibrous tissue that extend from the undersurface of the calcaneus to the subcutaneous fascia. Each septum is shaped like a test tube, with the open end attached to bone and the closed end a curved loop in subcutaneous tissue.[9,10] The effect of this structure is to allow the heel pad to sustain hydraulic pressure through the fat columns. The walls bulge under pressure and then spring back promptly as the weight is relieved, ready to receive the impact of the subsequent step. With age, all collagenous structures degenerate, and the heel pad is no exception. The septum becomes less elastic and the thickness of the pad measurably decreases.[10]

Etiology

Predisposing factors are excessive body weight, poorly cushioned or worn-out running shoes, a sudden, unaccustomed amount of training, and hard, uneven training surfaces. In addition to the middle-aged runner, the thin adolescent gymnast who prac-

tices numerous vaults and landings is at risk for this condition. The heel pad may bruise or the fibrous strands rupture. Significant damage to the septal structure, with spilling of the fat cells, may result from the impact of a heavy landing from a height. Increasing pressures are then brought to bear on the calcaneus, which reacts by increasing cortical density and by

---

Clinical Point

FAT PAD SYNDROME: CONTRIBUTING FACTORS

- Thinning of fat pad with age
- Excessive body weight
- Poorly cushioned or worn-out shoes
- Single significant contusion
- Sudden increase in training
- Switch to uneven and hard terrain
- Repetitive hill work on steep inclines

bony proliferation of the margins of the tuberosity. Certainly, one of the long-standing disabilities associated with fracture of the calcaneus may be damage to this fat pad area. Bleeding into the fat pad may cause a tender scar to form.

Clinical Presentation and Treatment

The athlete complains of pain in the region of the heel pad, which increases with activity. Walking barefoot is particularly painful. These athletes usually report that at the first weight-bearing after getting out of bed in the morning the area is exquisitely sore. The process can be totally debilitating and make all attempts at running or jumping impossible.

The initial treatment consists in reducing the stresses by modifying the training schedules. Substitute activities, e.g., cycling or running in water, are important to maintain fitness levels. Attempts at relieving local stresses with donuts or shock-absorbing material are usually unsuccessful at first in severe cases, although they help in milder situations (Fig. 8-6). The footwear must be analyzed to see if it is adequate. If an orthosis is prescribed, a temporary one should be experimented with at first to ensure effectiveness. Frequently a heel cup that incorporates semirigid and soft materials is the most effective. Alternatively, basket-weave taping in a well-supported shoe may provide satisfactory relief while the acute condition resolves (Fig. 8-7). There is little place for the use of rigid orthoses in this condition. NSAIDs and local therapeutic modalities are helpful if the inflammatory component is significant. It is important to distinguish the fat pad syndrome from plantar fasciitis, as the latter may do well with steroid injections whereas the former may be made worse by such repetitive injections. Steroid atrophy, on top of fat pad thinning, predisposes to further episodes of injury to the calcaneus. It is difficult to determine how much pain originates from the fat pad itself and what proportion comes from the increased impact on the sensitive calcaneal periosteum and subchondral bone, but the treatment is similar wherever the site.

A special form of fat pad syndrome is associated with ill-advised surgical disruption of this area by poorly placed incision and dissection planes. The surgeon must bear in mind the specialized structure of the septa and fat of the heel pad during surgery, particularly in the athlete.

Whatever the treatment plan chosen for the fat pad syndrome, it should extend to the individual's every-

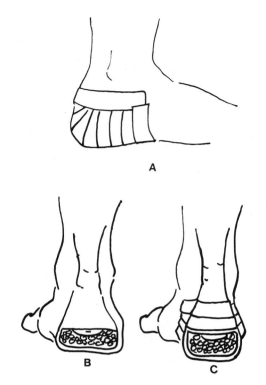

Fig. 8-7. Supportive heel taping helps to support the fat pad under the calcaneus, maintaining its height by stopping it from bulging. **(A)** Taping technique. **(B)** Splayed fat pad. **(C)** Contained fat pad.

day life as well as to the training routines and footwear. Despite excellent care, this condition may often take many months to resolve.

Fractures of the Calcaneus

Stress Fractures

Stress fractures of the calcaneus are seen in runners, ballet dancers, and jumpers. It is difficult to assess the frequency, as they are commonly overlooked and an alternative diagnosis is assigned as the cause of the athlete's heel pain. The architecture of the calcaneus is so complex that early signs are lost in the normal trabecular pattern. The commonest site is the upper posterior margin of the os calcis just anterior to the apophyseal plate and at right angles to the normal trabeculae. The other common site is adjacent to the medial tuberosity, at the point where calcaneal spurs occur. A bone scan may help in the diagnosis. The initial treatment may even include cast immobilization if the fracture line is clearly visible

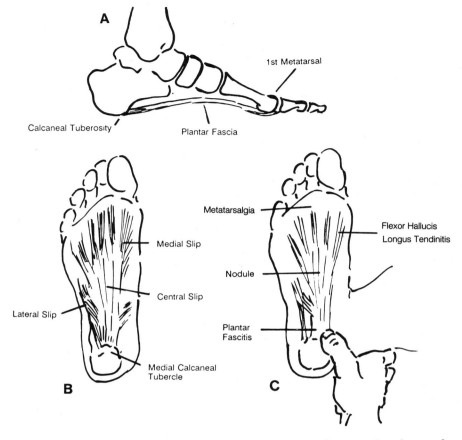

Fig. 8-8. (A) Plantar fascia (aponeurosis) is a dense fibrous band of connective tissues that extends from the calcaneus to the metatarsal heads. **(B)** Subdivisions of the plantar fascia. **(C)** Classic plantar fasciitis is located around the attachment to the medial calcaneal tuberosity. Tenderness elsewhere is usually related to other pathology, such as metatarsalgia, flexor hallucis longus tendon, and nodules, as part of the condition plantar fibromatosis.

and significant. Ultimately, therapy must include re-establishing the subtalar and midfoot range of motion, as well as heel cord and plantar fascia stretching.

Traumatic Fractures

In the older individual with osteoporosis, any awkward landing from even a minimal height may damage the trabecular structure of the calcaneus, causing fractures. Individuals who participate in motor sports or sky diving may sustain the more usual type of traumatic fractures of the calcaneus; these injuries are difficult to deal with and are associated with a high incidence of late morbidity. Much of the long-term disability is due to subtalar degenerative changes, widening of the heel, impingement of the fibula, and

damage to the fat pad. Unfortunately, none of these problems is easily dealt with, operatively or nonoperatively. Occasionally a well-constructed semirigid or soft orthosis greatly improves function.

Plantar Fasciitis and Heel Spurs

Anatomy

The plantar fascia or plantar aponeurosis connecting the calcaneal tubercles to the forefoot and spanning the longitudinal arches is intricately associated with the changes in shape, position, and shock-absorbing qualities of the foot (Fig. 8-8). Specifically, during heel strike with the toes in neutral the plantar fascia relaxes, allowing simultaneous collapse of the arch. Furthermore, during the take-off stage with rising onto the toes, the windlass effect (described in Chapter 7) on the plantar fascia helps to reconstitute the arch and generates a more rigid foot for propulsion. It therefore assists in the development of the push-off power during running and jumping. It should not be surprising that plantar fasciitis is particularly prevalent in joggers and tennis players, as well as in athletes participating in racquet sports, soccer, gymnastics, and basketball.[11]

Most athletes cannot recall exactly when the symptoms began, although the onset frequently correlates with an increase in mileage, frequency of training, or the addition of speed work or running up hills.

Clinical Presentation

The condition is usually unilateral and often noticed when getting out of bed and during initial weight-bearing in the morning. It may then ease off, only to return with activity. In severe cases, the athlete may be able only to run or even walk bearing weight mainly on the lateral border of the foot and heel. This condition frequently produces secondary problems elsewhere in the leg. Eventually these patients may limp and even have pain at rest, which includes medial arch discomfort as well as severe heel pain.

Physical Examination

The main area of tenderness is just over and distal to the medial calcaneal tubercle (Fig. 8). There may be associated diffuse discomfort to pressure over the rest of the heel and into the medial arch. Usually, however, there is one small, exquisitely painful area that is important to identify. Passive dorsiflexion of the great toe places the fascia under tension, so it may be readily palpable. There may be decreased range of motion of the first MTP joint, which should be specifically identified if present.[12] Passive dorsiflexion of the ankle may increase the discomfort, and a tight gastrocnemius–soleus complex may contribute to the symptoms. There is considerable discomfort on weight-bearing. Pain while hopping on the toes may help distinguish this entity from the fat pad syndrome, although there is considerable overlap.

Roentgenography

There is much discussion over the role of heel spurs projecting from the medial tubercle of the calcaneus in the production of pain. Various studies have re-

ported the incidence of these spurs in an asymptomatic population at between 10 and 30 percent, depending on the age group sampled. Furthermore, in individuals with symptoms, this spur may be present in about 75 percent of the painful heels and up to 63 percent on the nonpainful opposite side.[13,14] Using bone scans, approximately 60 percent of symptomatic individuals show increased uptake, either at the insertion of the plantar ligament or more diffusely over the calcaneus.[13] The formation of the calcaneal spur is the result of the mechanical stress acting through the plantar fascia onto its origin at the calcaneus. Proliferation of the traction spur may occur with or without inflammation. In the systemic conditions of ankylosing spondylitis, Reiter's syndrome, rheumatoid arthritis, and gout, the plantar fasciitis is more likely to be associated with a heel spur. In these cases the spur is sometimes large and fluffy in appearance, looking different from the usually small traction spur. A large heel spur may generate symptoms of its own.

Clinical Point

HEEL SPURS

- Frequently present in asymptomatic population (10 to 30 percent)
- Usually the result of traction
- May contribute to but usually is not the cause of pain
- When large, may be the source of pain
- May be associated with systemic disease
- Present in up to 75 percent of athletes with plantar fasciitis

---

Associated Factors

There have been numerous attempts to link the evolution of plantar fasciitis to leg length discrepancies, increased subtalar pronation, congenital pes planus, high arched foot, and height and weight based mainly on anecdotal collections of cases with poor statistical validity. There is slightly more evidence for the role of age (over 40 years), poorly constructed and ill-fitting footwear, tight Achilles tendons, and decreased range of motion of the great toe. The latter two conditions apparently prestress the plantar fascia at foot contact, so there is increased tension by take-off. Perhaps the most clearly associated factors relate to the degree of plantar flexion in the individual's gait while running, as well as the duration and type of training.[15,16] In one of the more conclusive studies, Warren noted that plantar flexion of more than 60 degrees appeared to give the runner more time to impact a backward force on the ground and stress the plantar fascia longer. Furthermore, individuals running more than 30 miles a week were more susceptible than those running less than 30 miles per week.[15]

Differential Diagnosis

Because chronic heel pain is a common manifestation of many conditions, these must be excluded before planning treatment. The fat pad syndrome, stress fractures of the calcaneus, and Sever's disease in the age group 9 to 11 years are the main conditions to rule out. More rarely, heel pain is the presenting feature of tarsal tunnel syndrome and first sacral radiculopathy. Blood tests for ESR, rheumatoid factor, HLA_{B27}, and uric acid help screen for the systemic disorders. In addition, these conditions are frequently associated with bilateral heel pain. There is a condition called plantar fibromatosis in which fibrous nodules may develop in the plantar aponeurosis in a manner similar to that seen in the hand with Dupuytren's contracture. This tumorous growth may occur at any age but frequently is seen after middle age. The causes are unknown, but histologic findings point to a chronic inflammatory process. The plantar fascia is thickened by the formation of a lobulated, firm, irregular mass of small nodules. The growth is often located in the longitudinal arch just proximal to the calcaneus. This fibrous benign tumor of the plantar fascia may be sufficiently large and painful that excision is required.

Treatment

The key to effective treatment is to establish an accurate activity history and then institute modified rest to decrease plantar impact and tension stresses. For runners, the distance should be reduced 25 to 75 percent and the time spent sprinting minimized. It may be necessary to institute a water-running program to maintain cardiovascular fitness (Fig. 8-9). Cycling is another good alternative.

Achilles tendon stretching is performed in such a way as to minimize stress on the plantar fascia, which means that unsupported stretching is not advised[17]

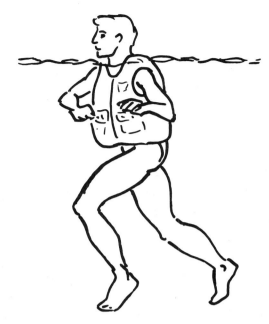

Fig. 8-9. To de-stress the lower limb, treading water with running movements with or without a flotation device may be performed. The workout should approximate the time spent normally with dry land running for a similar training effect. When land running is resumed, it must be done slowly to acclimatize to the impact of foot strike.

(Fig. 8-10). After warm-up the foot is medially rotated and supinated, which exaggerates and locks the medial longitudinal arch. It essentially puts the foot in the close packed position and allows isolation of the stretch to the Achilles tendon. With appropriately wedged boards to support the foot, the stretches may be carried out in straight dorsiflexion, as well as with the foot in the medially rotated, supinated position. The stretches are initially held for 1 minute and then progressed 3 minutes, taking advantage of the prolonged stretching effects on collagen. The rest period should entail gentle dorsi- and plantar flexion while resting the Achilles tendon and calf on a hot pack. This regimen enhances the subsequent stretch and utilizes an "active" rest period. The last stretch may be done with an ice pack strapped to the calf during the stretch to allow cool-down under tension. Some simple stretches should be taught to the patient to practice at home, as the interval between therapy sessions is usually too long. Ideally, stretches should be done twice a day. These stretches are similarly used

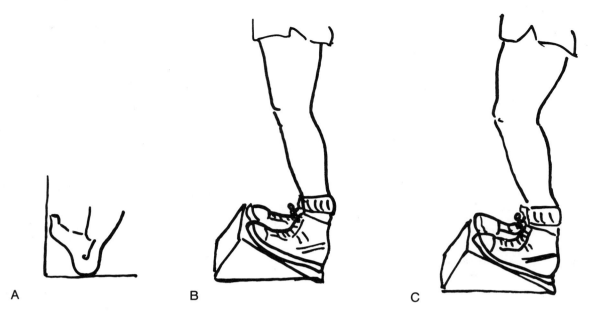

Fig. 8-10. Stretching the triceps sural. **(A)** Unsupported stretch is not ideal because it stresses the longitudinal arch and MTP joints. **(B)** Stretching with knees straight increases gastrocnemius flexibility. **(C)** Knee flexion gives a more isolated soleus stretch. The slant board forms an ideal surface.

for the treatment of Achilles tendinitis, described in the next section.

Clinical Point

ACHILLES STRETCHING PRINCIPLES

- Warm up part to be stretched.
- Give support to the part so as to isolate the stretch.
- Hold stretch for 1 minute; build up to 3 minutes.
- Use "active" rest periods.
- Rewarm when practical.
- Build up to three sets of stretching.
- Last stretch incorporates cool-down.

Specific treatment to the plantar fascia includes the use of modalities including ultrasound and electrogalvanic stimulation. Cryotherapy may relieve the discomfort both prior to specific stretching the plantar fascia and after activity. The specific plantar fascia stretching should concentrate on establishing a full range of motion at the MTP joint of the great toe.

NSAIDs are helpful, but solve the problem only when used in conjunction with a complete program. Recalcitrant cases may be helped with injections of steroid. There is a concern that the latter may lead to rupture of the plantar fascia at the heel, which has been reported. In my experience, it usually occurs in heavy linemen at football and occasionally in overweight athletes playing squash or basketball. In any event, it has not proved a disastrous complication but, rather, a blessing in disguise. All of these individuals, after a critical short period of intense discomfort followed by some bruising and swelling have become asymptomatic. Usually the symptoms of an acute rupture are resolved within 3 to 6 weeks, and there is no reasonable change in arch structure, strength, or performance. For this reason, we believe that the reported reservations about the use of cortisone injections in this situation are unwarranted. Furthermore, not to use it in severe cases removes a powerful tool from our armamentarium.

Both strapping and orthoses have a role in treatment, but only after careful examination of the footwear to ensure a firm, well-fitting heel counter, good heel cushioning, and an adequate longitudinal arch support.[11] The taping procedure of choice is the modified low dye arch support using 1-inch tape (Fig. 8-11). Prior to applying this taping, the arch should

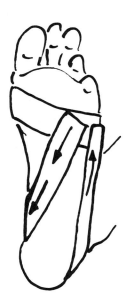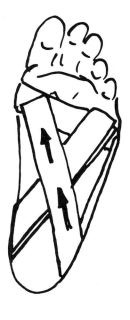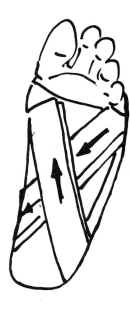

Fig. 8-11. Low dye taping for support of plantar fascia. It may be completed with a final forefoot anchor placed while the foot is bearing weight.

be relaxed and the heel and foot in neutral. Excessive tension through the strips will lead to complaints during activity. Have the athlete bear weight throughout the foot and apply final closing strips along the dorsal aspect of the foot. Care must be taken when applying tape on the medial, lateral, and dorsal aspect of the foot. Tension and tape flow are critical if skin breakdown is to be avoided with repeated taping.

For more long-term management, it is sometimes helpful to consider some form of orthotic device to keep the subtalar joint relatively neutral, support the longitudinal arch, and absorb shocks. When it is practical, some relief is built into the orthosis around the point of maximum tenderness (Table 8-3).

Cyriax recommended heel lifts to relieve the strain on the plantar fascia during early treatment. He thought that raising the heel decreased the angle between the hindfoot and forefoot, thereby shortening the distance between the attachment points of the plantar fascia.[18] Bilateral heel lifts of ¼ inch to ⅜ inch are sometimes successful, but their use should be discontinued at the earliest possible time. To achieve maximum effect from the heel lift, the heel must remain horizontal for the forefoot to drop into a plantar position. Cyriax recommended standing the pa-

tient on wooden platforms of varying heights until the minimum height that relieves symptoms is found.[18]

The timing and progression of exercises is crucial to the success of nonoperative therapy. Short and long foot flexor exercises are aggressively practiced. The athletes perform towel-gripping exercise to fatigue: three sets with a 1-minute rest between each set. Small weights are added to increase resistance.

Quick Facts

ORTHOTICS FOR HEEL PAIN

- Reduce abnormal compensation that results from pain or basic alignment of the foot.
- Increase area of plantar contact.
- Reduce point pressure over tender spots.
- Contain the calcaneal fat pad to increase shock-absorbing.
- Raise the longitudinal arch to reduce stress on it.
- Provide supplemental shock-absorbing to the shoe.

TABLE 8-3.   Calcaneal Pain: Recommendations for Orthotic Device Type by Diagnosis

Therapeutic Benefit	Type of Orthotic Device	Diagnosis
Reducing abnormal biomechanical compensation	Molded three-fourths length semi-rigid or rigid module with appropriate hindfoot and forefoot posts fabricated from a neutral position cast	Plantar fasciitis Heel spur syndrome Tarsal tunnel syndrome Calcaneal nerve entrapment Peroneal tendinitis Posterior tibial tendinitis
Reducing plantar fascial stress	Medial arch support to keep heel in neutral Relief over painful area Occasionally heel lift	Chronic plantar fasciitis
Increasing plantar contact (increases midfoot/heel weight-bearing area—total contact concept)	Semiflexible three-fourths length module or soft viscoelastic total contact orthosis	Calcaneal exostosis Calcaneal apophysitis Calcaneal bony stress syndromes and fractures
Eliminating painful plantar contact	Excavate the portion of the orthotic under the anatomically localized plantar area	Any condition with plantar tenderness during the acute stage
	Changed or alter heel counter contact	Retrocalcaneal tenderness
Soft tissue supplementation	Heel cup Cushioning materials	Fat pad syndrome Any condition as needed for altering ground reaction forces

Athletes are directed to pull with the foot into medial rotation; straight flexion and full weight-bearing arch isometrics are also prescribed. The athlete stands with the feet 12 inches apart and the knees flexed over the second toe. He or she then attempts to make the medial longitudinal arch as high as possible while keeping the head of the first metatarsal on the floor. Each isometric contraction is held for a six count. Three sets of 20 each are appropriate, although there may be some cramping initially.

Surgical treatment of severe intractable plantar fasciitis is a possible option. However, even in noncompetitive athletes, the success rate of permanent cure is in the region of 60 to 80 percent for return to activity. The procedure may involve any combination of partial plantar fascial release, removal of heel spurs, and neurolysis of the motor branch of the nerve to abductor digiti quinti as it passes underneath the abductor hallucis muscle and the medial ridge of the calcaneus.[14,19,20]

Before embarking on a surgical solution, the following considerations are important: (1) establishment of the correct diagnosis; (2) adequate nonoperative treatment; (3) supporting diagnostic data, including nerve conduction studies, a bone scan, and a blood screen for systemic disease; (4) familiarity with the detailed anatomy of the area; (5) an understanding on the part of the athlete that a full return to high performance may not be possible; and (6) the appropriate choice of incision and extent of dissection.

As with all musculoskeletal injuries, the return to activity must be graduated and planned. If surgery has been performed, cycling, swimming, and water-running can be commenced at 2 weeks, but running on land is strictly prohibited for 6 weeks. Hill work, stairs, and jumping routines have to be introduced carefully with alternate-day routines. It may be appropriate to protect the heel with strapping or a heel lift during the initial return to activity.

Plantar faciitis is one of the more common problems facing the running athlete and should be treated promptly and aggressively. Chronic heel pain is time-consuming and difficult to treat; and it is often not amenable to the usual therapies. The athlete should be made aware of this fact in order to ensure compliance with the strict progression and modification of activity.

CONDITIONS ASSOCIATED WITH TENDONS

Achilles Tendinitis

Achilles tendinitis is one of the more frequent overuse syndromes experienced in sport. It is common in recreational joggers, runners, ballet dancers, skaters, and soccer and basketball players. Achilles tendinitis may present as insidiously increasing pain and stiffness in the region of the Achilles tendon. Often the first experience is just stiffness after a long run, which gradually becomes a definite pain with further training sessions. Eventually this pain becomes persistent during the run, culminating in permanent tenderness and discomfort with walking and activities of normal daily living.

Anatomy

The Achilles tendon is covered by a thin sheath, the epitenon. Another fine sheath, the peritenon, composed of fatty areolar tissue filling the interstices of the fascial compartment in which the tendon is situated, overlies the epitenon. Hence a potential space exists between the two. A longitudinal septum carrying blood vessels runs from the deep tissues near the attachment of the peritenon to join the deep aspect of the Achilles tendon. It is rather like a mesentery and is called a mesotenon. It carries most of the blood supply to the midportion of the Achilles tendon. Inflammation frequently occurs in this sheath. The commonest site of Achilles tendinitis is about 2 cm proximal to the superior margin of the calcaneus.

Another entity is the tearing of muscular fiber from the aponeurosis, which usually involves the junction of the medial head of the gastrocnemius with its tendon. Whereas classic Achilles tendinitis has a gradual onset, the tears and associated tendinitis of the musculotendinous junction usually occur suddenly, with significant discomfort (Fig. 8-12).

The force generated through the Achilles tendon is applied to the posterior surface of the calcaneus in such a way that it always generates a vector from its point of contact and not its insertion. It is an efficient mechanism (Fig. 8-13). With the ankle dorsiflexed, this point is relatively far up on the posterior surface of the calcaneus. With the ankle plantar-flexed, the tendon moves away from the bone and its point of contact. Maximal triceps sural contraction is associated with adduction and supination of the foot. This point needs emphasizing, as the main plantar flexors can control the ankle only indirectly through the calcaneus via the subtalar joint and talus. The potential role of subtalar motion and position on Achilles tendinitis is elaborated in (Fig. 8-14).

Differential Diagnosis

The differential diagnosis includes pain and swelling of the subcutaneous or retrocalcaneal bursa. The examination should exclude contusion of the heel pad and stress fractures of the calcaneus. In addition, one must exclude tibialis posterior tendinitis behind the medial malleolus and peroneal tendinitis behind the lateral malleolus. There is occasionally inflammation of the deep fat pad lying underneath the Achilles tendon and tendinitis of the flexor hallucis longus

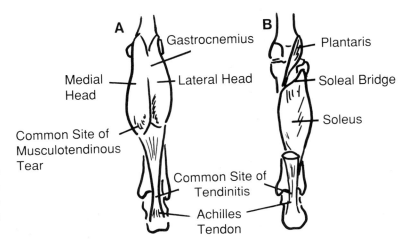

Fig. 8-12. Gastrocnemius–soleus complex (triceps sural) and plantaris. **(A)** Superficial view showing the gastrocnemius. **(B)** Deep view showing the soleus.

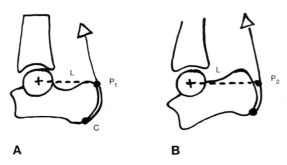

A   **B**

Fig. 8-13. Achilles tendon is inserted into the lower part of the calcaneus (C) and is separated from the upper part by a bursa. **(A)** Muscular pull is therefore transmitted to the point of contact (P_1). **(B)** This point is progressively more inferior with increasing plantar flexion (P_2). The tendon unrolls, but the level arm (L) remains horizontal and hence allows maximum efficiency of pull throughout the range.

tendon. Rarely, neurofibroma develops in relation to the tendon.

There are many systemic conditions that have been implicated in Achilles tendon disease. They include hyperuricemia and gout, pseudogout (articular chon-

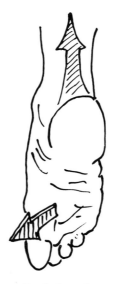

Fig. 8-14. Major pull of the triceps sural is on the medial side of the calcaneus, which means that plantar flexion is associated with adduction and supination. It emphasizes the fact that this large muscle group can work only through the ankle joint indirectly; hence the subtalar joint is always involved.

drocalcinosis), heterotopic ossification, rheumatoid arthritis, and ankylosing spondylitis.

Pathophysiology

The forces through the normal Achilles tendon can be large, amounting to several times body weight in activities such as running and jumping. Nevertheless, the Achilles tendon is well suited for these forces, having under normal circumstances a breaking strain of more than 2000 pounds per square inch (psi).

Several pathologic conditions may cause posterior heel pain, and they may occur separately or in combination. The tendon sheath or mesotenon may become inflamed in a true paratendinitis (tenosynovitis, tenovaginitis). These investing layers become inflamed and edematous; and eventually, if unresolved or recurrent, they produce a chronically inflamed, thickened, fibrotic sheath.[21] This condition may result in secondary changes in the tendon as a result of vascular embarrassment, as much of the tendinous blood supply is via its mesotenon.

The second possibility is primary pathology in the tendon. The repetitive mechanical stresses of running or other athletic endeavors result in microtears to the tendon which in turn trigger an inflammatory response.[21] It occurs primarily some 2 to 6 cm above the insertion of the tendon where the vascularity is poorest[22] and may result in areas of degeneration (tendinitis). There may be more significant tears generated in this weakened tissue and sometimes bleeding with cyst formation or mucinoid degeneration (Fig. 8-15). Occasionally in chronic situations, dystrophic calcification results.

The third situation is inflammation starting in the retrocalcaneal bursa, usually in association with direct trauma or a prominent posterior superior tuberosity of the os calcis.[21] When severe, there is frequently associated Achilles tenosynovitis or tendinitis.

Etiology

In general, the etiology can be considered as training errors, alignment factors, muscle problems such as tightness of the gastrocnemius–soleus complex, and ineffective footwear (Table 8-4). The training errors include (1) a sudden increase in mileage; (2) a single severe session; (3) sudden increase in intensity; (4) hill training; (5) switch to running as an aerobic exercise for dry land training in low impact sports, e.g., cross-country skiing and figure skating; or (6)

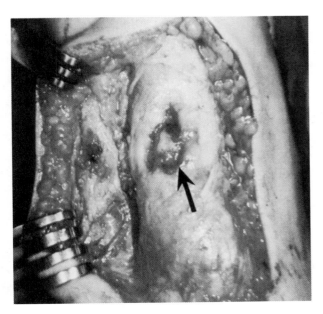

Fig. 8-15. More protracted problems may give a grossly thickened tendon, which may be complicated by partial rupture and cystic or mucinoid degeneration within the tendon, which is obviously then at risk of complete rupture.

return from a layoff. Alignment factors are related mainly to varus alignment of the heel with functional overpronation (Fig. 8-16).

In the nonathletic population, there is a normal ratio of triceps surae strength/cross-sectional area of the Achilles tendon. In the serious athlete, hypertrophy of the gastrocnemius is accompanied by an appropriate increase in the size of the tendon. This muscle power/tendon size ratio is thus maintained. Using isokinetic testing, ultrasonography, and CT evaluation of asymptomatic and symptomatic runners, it has been possible to demonstrate that this ratio is frequently not normal in the symptomatic group. Therefore failure of the tendon to hypertrophy appropriately along with the muscle may predispose it to microtrauma and subsequent tendinitis.

Jorgensen postulated that with thinning of the calcaneal fat pad the shock wave amplitude of heel strike is increased.[10] To compensate, the soleus muscle has been shown to increase its activity from 40 to 60 percent of the gait cycle, resulting in an increased load on the Achilles tendon. This situation, in association with one of the other etiologic factors, could precipitate the clinical syndrome.

TABLE 8-4. Postulated Etiologic Factors in Achilles Tendon Disease

Training errors
  Sudden increased mileage
  Single severe session
  Sudden increase in intensity
  Hill training
  Failure to warm up
  Recommencing training after period of inactivity
  Sudden change to running from other activities

Surfaces and equipment
  Repetitive jumping on hard floors
  Running on cambered roads
  Uneven terain
  Worn out shoes
  Pressure from shoe or skate on tendon
  Soft, loose-fitting heel counters
  Excessively narrow or flared heel base

Anatomic factors
  Age and tendon collagen changes
  Blood supply of tendon
  Heel pad thinning
  Rear foot valgus in flexible foot
  Rear foot varus in rigid foot
  Tibia varum
  Proximal limb and pelvic alignments
  Gastrocnemius–soleus strength to tendon size imbalance

Systemic disease
  Gout (uric acid crystal deposition)
  Pseudogout (calcium pyrophosphate crystal deposition)
  Heterotopic and dystrophic calcification
  Rheumatoid arthritis and related collagen diseases

Direct trauma
  Kick
  Blow with stick
  Laceration from skate

Clinical Examination

The Achilles tendon and heel may be examined with the patient in the sitting or the prone position with the legs over the examining table. The gastrocnemius–soleus muscle complex should be palpated to ensure that it is relaxed. Systemic palpation is carried along the tendon, over the heel, along the posterior border of the calcaneus, and down onto the heel pad (Fig. 8-17). The exact site of maximum tenderness must be meticulously elicited. The degree of swelling is noted compared to the opposite side. The extent and nodularity of the swelling is con-

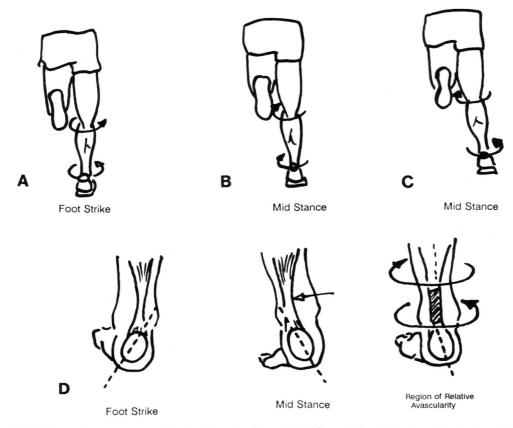

Fig. 8-16. Potential stresses on the Achilles tendon. **(A)** At foot strike the internal rotation of the limb gives functional pronation at the foot. **(B)** At midstance, tibial external rotation is linked to supination, providing an ideal situation for takeoff. **(C)** With excessive pronation the external rotation occurring in the lower limb is in conflict with the residual prolonged pronation. **(D)** Over pronation is linked to a greater whipping action, and stress on the vulnerable distal Achilles tendon. Medial arch support may modify these stresses. (Redrawn from Taunton et al.,[16] with permission.)

firmed, and by gently moving the foot passively or actively a crackling sensation may be felt. This crackling, or crepitus, is present only with a certain combination of edema and adhesions. It is referred to as "crepitating tenosynovitis."

Defects in the tendon are more difficult to feel but should be carefully recorded, as they signal impending rupture. It is possible that the more severe cases of Achilles tendinitis are secondary to rupture of a significant percentage of fibers—hence the need for careful treatment and reintroduction to activity. However, these tears are frequently intrafascicular and are rarely palpable as a defect but usually as a large fusiform swelling. Tests for Achilles tightness are performed by passively extending the knee while attempting to keep the foot dorsiflexed. Lack of 20 to 30 degrees of dorsiflexion in extension signifies gastrocnemius tightness, and inability to dorsiflex 30 to 35 degrees in flexion implicates the soleus as well (Fig. 8-18). The ability to actively resist plantar flexion may be elicited by manual testing, but it should be supplemented by alternate single leg heel raises. In addition, the ability to actively resist plantar flexion can be measured with the patient standing on the toes, alternating between the injured and healthy leg while the examiner pushes down on the patient's shoulder and tries to force the heel to the ground. The degree of pain is recorded, as is the discomfort generated by hopping. This test helps confirm the severity of the inflammation.

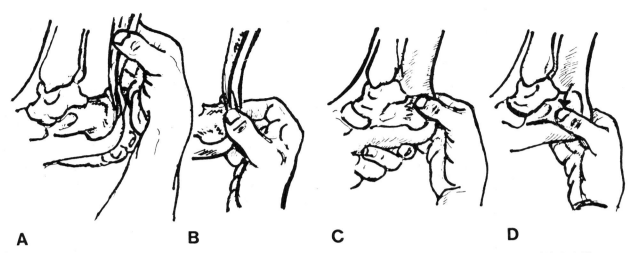

A   **B**   **C**   **D**

Fig. 8-17. Careful palpation may localize potential discrete anatomic sites of pathology. **(A)** Achilles tendon. **(B)** Retrocalcaneal and superficial calcaneal bursa. **(C)** Superior calcaneus and apophysis. **(D)** Body of calcaneus and calcaneal tubercle.

Laboratory and Radiologic Assessment

If the history and general physical examination reveal the possibility of systemic disease, and if an acute Achilles tendinitis does not respond appropriately, a blood screen and urinalysis would be indicated. Excessive fusiform swelling is also an indicator for early radiologic assessment. The plain roentgenograms may be ordered with soft tissue penetration and supplemented with a weight-bearing film. This film enables identification of dystrophic calcification, calcaneal shape, osteophytes, and ossicles, as well as measurement of the thickness of the fat pad. In recalcitrant cases, CT or magnetic resonance imaging (MRI) may assist in identifying partial tears, cystic degeneration, and early calcification (Fig. 8-15). Diagnostic ultrasonographic imaging is a noninvasive test that may yield significant information. It is capable of delineating tendon width and cross-sectional area, intertendinous necrosis, calcification, ruptures, and peritendinitis.[23]

Treatment

If the tendinitis is mild, NSAIDs, cryotherapy, and modification of activities may be sufficient to allow resolution. A careful activity history, analysis of the athlete's anatomic alignments, and scrutiny of the footwear may elicit the probable precipitating factor.

Good counseling in a cooperative patient can prevent recurrence of the problem.

When severe, acute Achilles tenosynovitis must be treated early and aggressively. Complete restriction of activities may be necessary for a period of 3 weeks, and all therapy should be started in conjunction with this rest. Therapy consists of oral anti-inflammatory medication, rest by using a shoe with a slightly high heel, and physiotherapy to the tendon in the form of ultrasound.[24] The value of the heel raise has been questioned, and undoubtedly it must be well formed, of adequate thickness, and appropriately fitted to give relief.[25] It is rarely useful for chronic tendinitis. Furthermore, reports agree that the pronated foot predisposes an athlete to Achilles tendinitis. The overpronated foot places the medial aspect of the tendon under tension, which is in agreement with the subjective finding of maximal tenderness over the medial border of the tendon.[25] Because most heel raises are wedged from posterior to anterior, they fail to compensate for a probable common etiologic factor. Therefore a more permanent orthosis should incorporate some measure of motion control for the hindfoot (Table 8-5).

In severe crepitating tenosynovitis, partial weight-bearing with crutches may be considered, along with taping the foot in equinus (Fig. 8-19). If an early response is not achieved, some physicians favor the

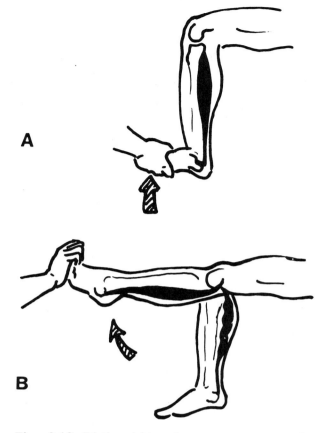

Fig. 8-18. Distinguishing between gastrocnemius and soleus tightness. (**A**) Soleus muscle. With the knee flexed the gastrocnemius is relaxed; dorsiflexion is potentially restricted by a tight soleus. (**B**) Gastrocnemius. With knee extension, the gastrocnemius is tightened behind the femoral condyles and exerts a limiting effect on dorsiflexion.

letes who have a mismatch between muscle power in the gastrocnemius–soleus complex and the size of their Achilles tendons.

Clinical Point

ACHILLES TENDINITIS ECCENTRIC LOADING ROUTINE

1. Warm up tendon by activity or modalities.
2. Achilles stretches.
   - Straight knee for gastrocnemius and bent knee for soleus.
3. Drop and stop exercises.
   - Stand on block or step so the heel is unsupported.
   - Raise up on toes.
   - Allow heel to lower as far as possible.
   - Progress to dropping (lowering rapidly).
   - Perform three sets of ten repetitions.
   - Progress as symptoms allow.
4. Repeat stretches.
5. Ice to cool down 5 to 10 minutes.

use of a resting splint or cast for 3 to 6 weeks, although this treatment has had limited success with chronic cases.

The modalities of ice, ultrasound, and laser have a role in the early management. With resolving tendinitis, heat prior to stretching routines and activity followed by ice massage at the conclusion are helpful.[24,26]

The early emphasis is on gentle stretching and isometric exercise in the pain-free range. When symptoms settle, an eccentric loading program is started. Ultimately, this eccentric stimulus is important for generating tendon hypertrophy in the group of ath-

The role of NSAIDs is well accepted, but there is some discussion over the role of injections. For early crepitating tenosynovitis, the infiltration of heparin and lidocaine may reduce the adhesion formation. There have also been promising reports with the local injection of glycosaminoglycan polysulfate (GAGPS; Anteparon, Luitpold-Werk, Munich).[27] GAGPS has been shown to inhibit the formation of thrombin and fibrin, which is considered to be an initiating mechanism in the formation of immature connective tissue, with delayed collagen formation and hypertrophic scar. In chronic cases of Achilles peritendinitis, hypertrophic scar is formed around the tendon, even up to a year.[27] It may be that these GAGP injections are more appropriate in the chronic situation.[27] There are few situations in which injections of steroid into the tendon sheath can be recommended. Many athletes with ruptured Achilles tendons have had prior injections, but it is difficult to distinguish the chronic degenerative and weakening effects of tendon degeneration from those of the injection. Certainly it is not a first-time therapy; but in skilled hands an injection

TABLE 8-5.   Treatment Strategies for Achilles Tendinitis and Peritendinitis

Stage	Control of Pain and Inflammation	Rehabilitation of Musculotendinous Unit	Control of Biomechanics
Acute	Ice massage NSAIDs	Modification of activity Water-running[a] Consider crutches[a] Cycling Stretching	Examine footwear Consider heel lift or wedge Taping of calf
Subacute	NSAIDs Ultrasound Laser	Cycling Stretching	Change running shoes Consider orthosis[a]
Resolving	Ultrasound Heating modalities prior to exercise Ice during cool-down	Eccentric loading Gastrocnemius–soleus muscle strengthening Cybex assessment Progressive return to activity	Monitoring running Consider orthosis[a]
Chronic symptomatic	Heparin with lidocaine infiltration[a] Consider cast	Stretching gastrocnemius Transverse frictions Modification of training	Orthosis
Failed therapy	Complete assessment by blood screen to rule out systemic disease. Roentgenogram to assess heel shape, fat pad thickening, and dystrophic calcification.		
Nodular or chronic significant thickening	CT or MRI to assess cystic degeneration and partial tears. Consider tenolysis or tendon exploration.		

CT = computed tomography; MRI = magnetic resonance imaging.
[a] Proportional to severity of symptoms.

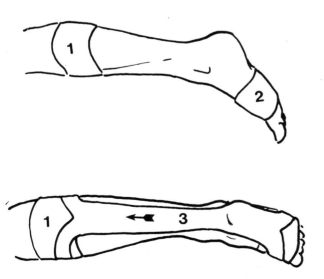

Fig. 8-19. Taping foot in equinus for relief of Achilles tendinitis.

into the sheath, may still have a limited role in the management of Achilles tendinitis. The role of transverse or cross friction, is also difficult to establish, but in the chronic situation it should help mobilize adhesions within the sheath and tendon and allow resolution with full range of motion. It is most effective when supplemented immediately with NSAIDs.

The major difficulty of treating Achilles tendinitis is evaluation of the appropriate speed and progression of activities while avoiding a flare-up of the problem. The presence of any tenderness to palpation is a sign for a very slow increase in activity. Furthermore, any residual fusiform swelling indicates an increased propensity for a flare-up of the initial problem. In these athletes a long time is required before full training can be resumed.

Surgical exploration of the tendon and decompression by longitudinally splitting the sheath may be appropriate if there is a failure of nonoperative treatment. The entire length of the tendon is exposed, dividing all adhesions by sharp dissection.[29,30] The sheath is not closed. There should not be any postoperative immobilization unless there is extensive exploration of the tendon with significant structural weakening.[30,31] Immediately postoperatively, the athlete usually requires crutches for partial weight-bearing, and the treatment aim is initially to restore the foot to neutral position and then to dorsiflexion. Strengthening is commenced at week 2 and gentle running by weeks 3 to 4. Full training is usually possible at week 6.[21,29-31]

Xanthoma of the Achilles Tendon

An indurated, indolent, nontender, slowly growing mass may develop in the Achilles tendon, particularly at its insertion. Clinically, the Achilles tendon has the appearance of being markedly hypertrophied, the mass ending abruptly at about the middle of the posterior aspect of the heel. The tumor has a lobulated feel and is not painful. It does not usually interfere with ankle motion. This tumor usually lies on and is embedded in the tendon. Microscopically, a tumor consists of groups of cells containing cholesterol fat with keratin lying in an abundant fibrous stroma. The mass is benign and grows slowly. Treatment is excision.

Achilles Tendon Rupture

Based on experimental evidence, it is generally conceded that a completely healthy tendon can withstand tremendous tensile stress without rupture. Forces of 2000 psi in the Achilles tendon have been recorded during fast running.[32] When the muscle tendon unit is tested in the laboratory, rupture does not occur through the substance of the tendon but through the muscle itself. Clinically, however, ruptures occur mainly through the substance of the Achilles tendon. Interestingly, it is often preceded by relatively minor trauma. Insight into this paradox is shown by a review of the results of biopsy specimens.

First, there is often microscopic evidence of an area of degeneration and inflammation at various stages of evolution, indicating the presence of pre-existing microtrauma or microtears within the tendon. Such tears may even be sufficient to be considered partial ruptures. They are difficult to detect, as the tendon may function normally with as little as 25 percent of its fibers in continuity. These partial tears may present as local stabbing or prickling pains associated with sudden activity and with tenderness and slight thickening upon palpation.[33]

Second, in relation to the site of tearing, there is

Quick Facts

ACHILLES TENDON RUPTURES

- Normal tendon may withstand forces of more than 2000 psi.
- Frequently microtears precede major rupture.
- Tendon can function normally with as few as 25 percent of fibers intact.
- There is probably a critical zone of circulation that correlates with the site of the tear, 2 to 6 cm above the calcaneus.

---

evidence of a local critical zone with regard to blood supply. These zones are seen with other tendons as well, e.g., the supraspinatous tendon. Particularly after the third decade of life, there is a critical area of circulation about 2 to 6 cm above the calcaneus, which coincides with the common site of rupture.

Third, at surgery after local steroid injection, small yellow deposits are seen in the tendon and its sheath. They may even be cystic areas of serosanguineous fluid near the rupture. Experiments show that following local steroid injection the tensile strength is lowered and normal healing is delayed. It is a common story to see the Achilles tendon ruptured 2 to 4 weeks after completing a course of injections.

The areas of cystic mucinoid degeneration are also seen in situations where there have not been steroid injections. They probably represent old tears, central hemorrhage, and avascular degeneration.

The clinical signs and symptoms of an Achilles tendon rupture are (1) a visible defect in the tendon; (2) inability to do heel raises on one leg; (3) swelling and bruising around the malleoli; (4) a positive Thompson test (failure of plantar flexion to occur with passive compression of the gastrocnemius on the affected side); (5) excessive passive dorsiflexion; and (6) distortion of Kager's triangle by hemorrhage or loss of continuity on roentgenogram[32,34] (Fig. 8-20). Kager's triangle is a radiolucent triangle on a lateral film of the ankle that is composed of the posterior surface of the long flexors and tibia, and of the Achilles tendon, and the superior border of the calcaneus—all bordering the fat pad. Complete ruptures of the Achilles tendon may be treated by either cast treatment or surgery. Surgical repair guarantees maximum strength of the tendon once it is healed, and it prevents overelongation of the tendon[35,36] (Fig. 8-21).

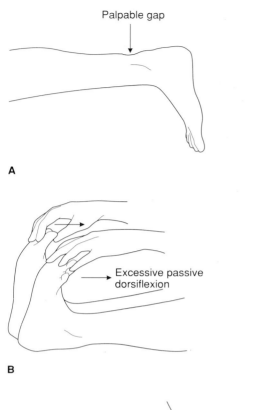

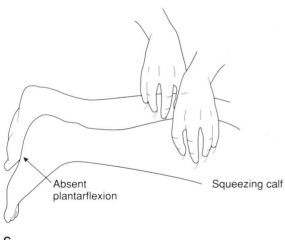

Fig. 8-20. Rupture of Achilles tendon. **(A)** Palpable and sometimes visible defect (arrow). **(B)** Excessive range of dorsiflexion. **(C)** Squeezing the calf should produce plantar flexion motion. Such motion is absent with a rupture (Thompson test).

However, nonoperative treatment offers excellent results functionally for partial tears and in the older, noncompetitive athlete. Given the risks of infection, skin slough, a painful irritated scar, and postoperative deep vein thrombosis, the nonoperative choice is a viable option for certain patient groups (Table 8-6). Delayed diagnosis of the rupture is usually better treated by surgical repair, and it occasionally requires significant dissection.

Following surgical repair, the foot is immobilized in a plaster cast with the foot in plantar flexion. At 4 weeks the foot is brought up nearer to the neutral position. At 6 weeks the cast is removed, and gentle weight-bearing is begun with crutches and slow mobilization, which should take at least 2 to 3 weeks. Rebounding activities are not allowed until 12 weeks after the surgical operation for repair. Eventually, rehabilitation should include skipping, eccentric loading, and finally jumping.

In selected complaint patients cast immobilization may not be necessary and a range of motion brace or splint limiting dorsiflexion to neutral is adequate.

Flexor Hallucis Longus Tendinitis

The flexor hallucis longus muscle lies medial to the Achilles tendon and in the groove formed by the medial and lateral posterior tubercles of the talus. Its function is integral to the smooth take-off phase of walking and running. Pain during this phase of the gait cycle points to involvement of this muscle. The manual test of flexor hallucis longus involves supporting the foot and resisting flexion of the great toe. This resisted flexion may trigger tenderness around the deep medial part of the Achilles tendon adjacent to the flexor hallucis muscle. The highest incidence of tendinitis of this particular tendon at the ankle is seen in ballet dancers and high jumpers. Runners seem to have the flexor hallucis tendinitis that more often involves the distal part of the tendon in the sole of the foot.

Tibialis Posterior Tendinitis

The tibialis posterior tendon lies just posterior to the medial malleolus. Although the muscle is difficult to isolate for testing and function, its tendon is palpable as it comes around the medial malleolus and inserts into the navicular tuberosity. A combination of plantar flexion and inversion makes the tendons stand out clearly. Tibialis posterior tendinitis is frequently seen in joggers.

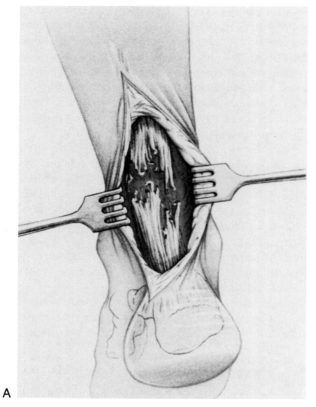
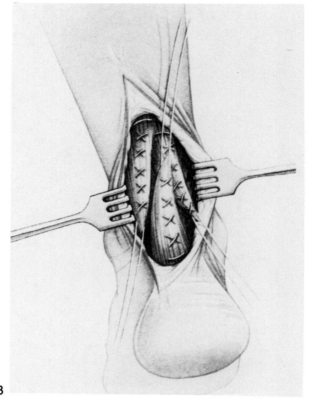

A B

Fig. 8-21. Method for resuturing a "mop end" acute Achilles tendon rupture. **(A)** Incision is made just medial to the midline to avoid the sural nerve, minimize pressure over the scar, and for best blood supply to the flap. **(B)** Disorganized fibers are gathered by Bunnell-type sutures and approximated. (From Beskin et al.,[33] with permission.)

Peroneal Tendinitis

The peroneus longus and brevis tendons are the first two tendons posterior to the lateral malleolus. After repeated inversion strain, the sheath may be stretched, and these tendons may be involved in a chronic painful tendinitis. In addition, with sufficient stretching of the sheath they may sublux or dislocate with resisted movement into plantar flexion and eversion. This uncommon tendinitis is particularly seen in figure skaters.

NERVE ENTRAPMENT

Remote Causes

Pain in the heel secondary to nerve entrapment or trauma may be either local or remote. The classic L5-S1 nerve impingement may refer pain or produce altered sensation to the lateral malleolus, adjacent heel, and lateral border of the foot. This condition is the S1 dermatome. Associated with it should be some weakness to resisted eversion on the basis of innervation to the peroneus longus and brevis. Furthermore, there may be alterations in the S1 reflex, which is the Achilles jerk. Isolated distal symptoms are not unusual as presenting signs for an acute disc. Should a proximal impingement be diagnosed, of course, the differential diagnosis of nerve root impingement must be considered.

Local Causes

Occasionally, after calcaneal fractures or in association with overuse, the medial calcaneal branch of the tibial nerve may be irritated, producing pain discretely in the area of the heel. It may occur in isolation or as part of a pronation neuritis, affecting the medial

TABLE 8-6. **Functional Strength Assessment After Treatment**[a]

Study	Year	Testing Method	Surgical Treatment (%)	Nonsurgical Treatment (%)
Gillies & Chalmers[36]	1970	Tension spring	84.0	80
		Plantar flexion, strength		
Inglis et al.[37]	1976	Cybex II	101.0	73
		Plantar flexion	88.0	62
		Strength, power	91.0	63
		Endurance		
Inglis & Sculco[38]	1981	Cybex	101.0	
		Dorsiflexion,	86.0	
		Peak strength, peak		
		torque, peak torque	91.2	
		after fatigue	71.2	
		Early repair		
		Late repair		
Jacobs et al.[39]	1978	Calibrated load cell	75.0	65
		Isometric, strength		
Nistor[40]	1981	Cybex II	83.0	79
		Plantar flexion, strength		
Persson & Wredmark[41]	1979	Isometric contraction	85.0	84
		Force, after rupture		
Shields et al.[42]	1978	Cybex II	83.5	75
		Plantar flexion	82.5	49
		Strength, power		

[a] Normal leg was used as a comparison for percentage results. (i.e., 100%.)

and lateral plantar nerves. This tarsal tunnel syndrome is dealt with in detail elsewhere (see Ch. 9).

Similarly, fractures of the calcaneus or direct trauma may damage the lateral calcaneal branch of the sural nerve, producing lateral heel pain. This condition must be distinguished from proximal nerve entrapment at the L5-S1 level. Neuritis associated with peripheral nerve entrapment is difficult to diagnose and isolate, but it may respond to anti-inflammatory treatment, systemically or locally, injection of steroid, and an orthosis. Failure to provide relief requires exploration of the nerve surgically.

SKIN PROBLEMS

Because of the repetitive loading on the heel, this area is subjected to many problems, including blisters and calluses. There is a distinct condition called "black dot heel" in which a painless, irregular, black or bluish plaque appears on the posterior or postero-lateral aspect of one or both heels. The lesion is usually horizontal but may be oval or circular, lying just above the edge of the runner's thick plantar skin. This skin is often hyperkeratotic in this region, and the plaque lies flush with the skin surface and is not palpable. Black dot heel most likely arises from a shearing stress or pinching of the heel between the counter and the sole of the shoe at heel strike during running, producing bleeding into the epidermis. When the lesion is pared down with a scalpel, reddish-brown punctate specks of dried blood are uncovered. These dark lesions may resemble a particularly dangerous form of malignant tumor called melanoma and therefore is a cause for concern. The traumatic cause should be established in order to give reassurance. This problem usually resolves spontaneously and requires no treatment or just counseling with regard to footwear.

In addition to blisters and calluses, the heel is a common site for plantar warts. These growths are discussed in Chapter 7.

SUMMARY

Conditions around the heel present a diagnostic challenge. Classic Achilles tendinitis is usually easy to distinguish; but even it has subtleties, and it is important to anticipate the early acute inflammation, which responds readily to treatment, from the more difficult chronic case and the frankly dangerous impending rupture. The unique position of the calcaneus, linking leg with foot, and its multiple articular surfaces add to the complexity of the anatomy of the area. Furthermore, its involvement with systemic disease and the changes with aging serve to make it an important area of pathology. Lastly, the heel, like the toes, suffers from the presence of confining footwear, a problem particularly noted in sports such as hockey, skiing, and figure skating.

REFERENCES

1. Doxey GE: Calcaneal pain: a review of various disorders. J Orthop Sports Phys Ther 9:25, 1987
2. Mosier KM, Asher M: Tarsal coalitions and spastic flat foot. J Bone Joint Surg [Am] 66:976, 1984
3. Simmons EH: Tibialis spastic varus foot with tarsal coalition. J Bone Joint Surg [Br] 47:533, 1965
4. Snyder RB, Lipscomb AB, Johnston RK: The relationship of tarsal coalition to ankle sprains in athletes. Am J Sports Med 9:313, 1981
5. Harris RI, Beath T: Etiology of peroneal spastic flat foot. J Bone Joint Surg [Br] 30:624, 1948
6. Cowell HR, Elener V: Rigid painful flat foot secondary to tarsal coalition. Clin Orthop 177:54, 1983
7. Tachdjian MO: Paediatric Orthopaedics. Vol. 2. WB Saunders, Philadelphia, 1972
8. Resnick D, Feingold ML, Curd J: Calcaneal abnormalities in articular disorders—rheumatoid arthritis, ankylosing-spondylitis, psoriatic-arthritis and Reiter's syndrome. Radiology 125:355, 1977
9. Miller WE: The heel pad. Am J Sports Med 10:19, 1982
10. Jorgensen U: Achillodynia and loss of heel pad shock absorbency. Am J Sports Med 13:128, 1985
11. Tanner SM, Harvey JS: How we manage plantar fasciitis. Physician Sports Med 16:39, 1988
12. Creighton DS, Olson VL: Evaluation of range of motion of the first metatarsophalangeal joint in runners with plantar fasciitis. J Orthop Sports Phys Ther 8:357, 1987
13. Williams PL, Smibert JG, Cox R et al: Imaging study of the painful heel syndrome. Foot Ankle 6:345, 1987
14. Lapidus PW, Guidotti FP: Painful heel: report of 323 patients with 364 painful heels. Clin Orthop 39:178, 1965
15. Warren BC: Anatomical factors associated with predicting plantar faciitis in long distance runners. Med Sci Sports Exerc 16:60, 1984
16. Taunton JE, Clement DB, McNicol K: Plantar fasciitis in runners. Can J Appl Sports Sci 7:41, 1982
17. Mattison R: Plantar faciitis: clinical comments. Can Sports Physiother Div Newslett 9:30, 1985
18. Cyriax J: Diagnosis of soft tissue lesions. p. 682. In: Textbook of Orthopaedic Medicine. 7th Ed., Vol. 1. Williams & Wilkins, Baltimore, 1980
19. Baxter DE, Thigpen CM: Heel pain: operative results. Foot Ankle 5:16, 1984
20. Lutter LD: Surgical decisions in athletes' subcalcaneal pain. Am J Sports Med 14:481, 1986
21. Schepsis AA, Leach RE: Surgical management of Achilles tendinitis. Am J Sports Med 15:308, 1987
22. Lagergren C, Lindholm A: Vascular distribution in the Achilles tendon: an angiographic and micro-angiographic study. Acta Chir Scand 116:491, 1958
23. Clement DB, Taunton JE, Smart GW: Achilles tendinitis and peritendinitis: etiology and treatment. Am J Sports Med 12:179, 1984
24. Frieder S, Weisberg J, Fleming B et al: A pilot study: the therapeutic effect of ultrasound following partial rupture of Achilles tendons in male rats. J Orthop Sports Physiother 10:39, 1988
25. Lowdon A, Bader DL, Mowet AG: The effect of heel pads on the treatment of Achilles tendinitis: a double blind trial. Am J Sports Med 12:431, 1984
26. Curwin SL: Force and length changes of the gastrocnemius and soleus muscle tendon unit during a therapeutic exercise program and three sport related activities. Physiother Can, suppl 3, 39:1, 1987 (abstract)
27. Sundqvist H, Forsskahl, Kvist M: A promising novel therapy for Achilles peritendinitis: double blind comparison of glycosaminoglycan polysulfate and high-dose indomethacin. Int J Sports Med 8:298, 1987
28. Sondolph-Ziuk B, Wetzel R, Trepte CT: Ultrasound diagnosis of the calcaneus tendon. Int J Sports Med 8:125, 1987
29. Kvist M, Jarvinen M: Clinical, histochemical and biomechanical features in repair of muscle and tendon injuries. Int J Sports Med 3:12, 1982
30. Williams JGP, Sperryn PN, Boardman S et al: Postoperative management of chronic Achilles tendon pain in sportsmen. Physiotherapy 62:256, 1976
31. Leach RE, James S, Wasilewski S: Achilles tendinitis. Am J Sports Med 9:93, 1981
32. DiStefano VJ, Nixon JE: Ruptures of the Achilles tendon. J Sports Med 1:34, 1973

33. Beskin JL, Sanders RA, Hunter SC et al: Surgical repair of Achilles tendon ruptures. Am J Sports Med 15:1, 1987

34. Abraham E, Pankovich AM: Neglected rupture of the Achilles tendon. J Bone Joint Surg [Am] 57:253, 1975

35. Wills CA, Washburn S, Caiozzo V et al: Achilles tendon rupture: a review of the literature comparing surgical versus non-surgical treatment. Clin Orthop 207:156, 1986

36. Gilles H, Chalmers J: The management of fresh ruptures of the tendo achillis. J Bone Joint Surg [Am] 52:337, 1970

37. Inglis AE, Scott WM, Sculco TP et al: Rupture of the tendo achillis: an objective assessment of surgical and non-surgical treatment. J Bone Joint Surg [Am] 58:990, 1976

38. Inglis AE, Sculco TP: Surgical repair of ruptures of the tendo achillis. Clin Orthop 156:160, 1981

39. Jacobs D, Martens M, Van Andekercke R: Comparison of conservative and operative treatment of Achilles tendon rupture. Am J Sports Med 6:107, 1978

40. Nistor L: Surgical and non-surgical treatment of Achilles tendon rupture. J Bone Joint Surg [Am] 63:394, 1981

41. Persson A, Wredmark T: The treatment of total ruptures of Achilles tendon by plaster immobilization. Int Orthop 3:149, 1979

42. Sheilds CL, Kerlin RK, Jobe FW et al: Cybex II evaluation of surgically repaired Achilles tendon ruptures. Am J Sports Med 6:369, 1978

Ankle Region

9

Today, the only thing that is permanent is change.
—Charles H. Mayo

ACUTELY SPRAINED ANKLE

Epidemiology

Ankle injuries in the general population are common, with inversion sprains and fractures occurring in an estimated 1 person per 10,000 per day.[1] Ankle injuries constitute up to 12 percent of the emergency room load in many centers. Ankle sprains comprise approximately 14 percent of all sports-related problems, with an injury rate of 6 per 100 participants per season; i.e., one ankle injury is anticipated for every 17 participants over a season. In the high-risk activities of jumping and running, sports ankle problems account for up to 25 percent of all time loss injuries.[2,3] In basketball they comprise more than 50 percent of major injuries and in soccer and volleyball more than 25 percent. In addition, football players, gymnasts, and team handball and field hockey players have a significant number of acute ankle injuries.

This chapter deals mainly with these acute and chronic ankle sprains and their complications, as well as ankle fractures and a group of entrapment and impingement syndromes. The latter group of conditions have the common features of a history of trauma aggravated by activity and relieved by rest. Most of these injuries are uncommon, and some are rare; all are associated with a high incidence of delayed diagnosis. Awareness of these potentially disabling conditions leads to prompt, effective treatment.[4] The commonest is the osteochondral lesion of the dome of the talus. As with the other conditions, the presence of the lesion does not always mean that it is the cause of the patient's symptoms. There may be some skepticism as to the existence of some of these syndromes as separate entities, but in the world of the highly active individual, these otherwise quiescent lesions can mitigate against success. The meniscal lesion at the ankle, the anterior impingement syndrome, and the antero-lateral corner compression syndrome produce intra-articular signs. The posterior talar compression syndrome is often specific to the ballet dancer and soccer player, and the tarsal tunnel syndrome is a neural entrapment phenomenon. Nevertheless, their proximity allows a reasonable discussion under the single heading of some selected lesions around the ankle.

Anatomy

The ankle, or talocrural joint, normally allows only the movements of dorsi- and plantar flexion; it depends for its stability on the anterior and posterior tibiofibular ligaments and the interosseous membrane, which maintain the integrity of the tibiofibular mortise (Fig. 9-1). These ligaments are strong, and their complete tearing, leading to diastasis of this joint, must be considered a serious injury. The collateral ligaments are also well designed to resist the large forces that weight-bearing and locomotion impose on them. Nevertheless, the number of traumatic injuries are easily accounted for if one considers the tremendous force generated when the whole body weight is suddenly superimposed on the inverted foot.

The functional unit of the ankle, however, must include the subtalar joint, at which the key motions of inversion and eversion take place (Fig. 9-2). The ankle and the subtalar joint work together to translate rotations occurring in the tibia about its vertical axis into rotations in the foot about a sagittal axis. These coupled motions are necessary to allow the rapid rotations that occur in the leg to be absorbed by a relatively fixed foot. The internal rotation at foot stance is linked to pronation in the foot. In the late stance, or foot contact phase, external rotation of the leg is accompanied by supination. The lateral collateral ligaments are probably involved in this torque transmission, although their role is not well delineated.[5]

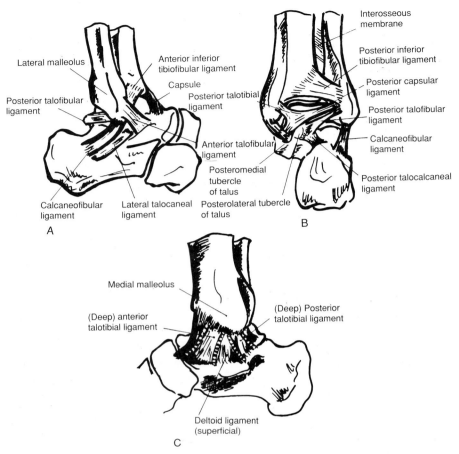

Fig. 9-1. Ligaments of the ankle. **(A)** Lateral view. **(B)** Posterior view. **(C)** Medial view. Deep portion of the deltoid ligament is dotted.

Forces

Much of the previous work on the non-weight-bearing foot is either not valid or an oversimplification of the functional anatomy. The average overall ankle joint contact pressure is 300 to 350 pounds per square inch (psi) during walking, approximately the same as the human hip.[6] The ground reaction forces are approximately 125 percent body weight during walking, 200 to 300 percent with running, and as much as 500 percent during jumping. Theoretic calculations from force platform experiments put the resultant joint forces on the talus during running (4.47 meters/s) at 9 to 13 times bodyweight (Fig. 9-3).[7]

Furthermore, the position of the fibula in relation to the tibia is crucial; and if the mortise is widened owing to disruption of the interosseous membrane

Quick Facts
FORCES AT THE ANKLE JOINT

Condition	Ground Reaction Force (Measured)	Ankle Joint Compressive Forces (Calculated)
Walking	1.0–1.2 × body weight	5 × body weight
Running	2.5–3.2 × body weight	5–10 × body weight
Jumping	Up to 5 × body weight	

Talocrural unit 300 to 330 psi while walking.

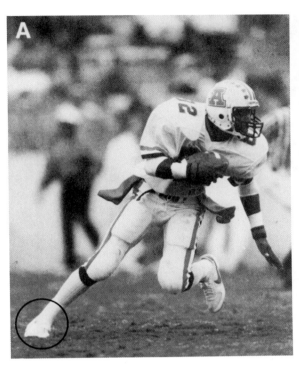
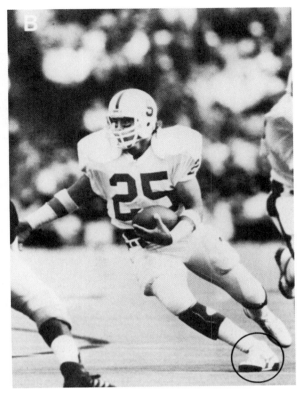

Fig. 9-2. Functional unit of the ankle must include the subtalar joint. Sudden change in direction requires considerable accommodation at the subtalar area. Stiffness in this joint throws undue stress on the ankle joint. **(A)** Inversion. **(B)** Eversion. (From Mandelbaum et al.,[16] with permission.)

and tibiofibular ligaments, degenerative changes quickly ensue. Such change is probably related to the fact that as little as 1 to 2 mm of lateral shift of the fibula may increase the joint forces by approximately 40 percent.

Lambert has shown that the fibula may support up to one-sixth of the body weight.[8] This weight-bearing role is enhanced by the fact that during the ground contact phase of running the fibula moves downward and laterally.[9] This move deepens the mortise and provides maximum stability at a time when the weight-bearing forces are highest. The movement provides tension in the interosseous membrane and tibiofibular ligament, slightly cushioning the effect of impact as well as allowing storing of energy for passive recoil as the foot unloads. The ample fibular articular surface is available for this gliding motion.[9]

At least 95 percent of isolated ankle sprains are of the lateral ligaments.[10] When the medial ligament is involved, there is more likely to be an associated lat-

eral malleolar fracture or damage to the interosseous membrane. In any event, when isolated medial collateral ligament injuries do occur, they are often associated with a prolonged recovery time.

There is question as to the exact axis of motion of

Quick Facts

LATERAL DIASTASIS

- Lateral fibula shift of 1 to 2 mm
- Approximately 40 percent decrease in weight-bearing contact
- Increases forces per unit per area proportionately
- Best detected with 20 degrees internal rotation view
- Treated aggressively — usually surgically

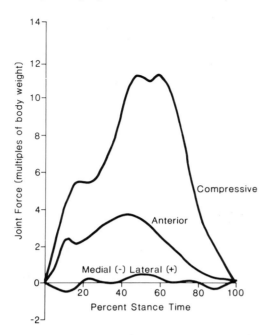

Fig. 9-3. Running at 4.47 meters/s gives peak compressive forces on the talus of 9 to 13 times body weight, anterior shear of 2.5 to 3.5 times body weight, and mediolateral shear of 0.25 to 0.33 times body weight. Achilles tendon stress is approximately 10 times body weight. (Adapted from Burdett,[7] with permission.)

the talocrural joint, but it is probably just anterior and below the tip of the lateral malleolus. The lateral collateral ligament is usually described in three bands, each having its origin at the tip of the fibular malleolus (Fig. 9-1). Under normal circumstances the bony configuration secures most physiologic motion in the fully weight-bearing position; but in full plantar flexion, in the unloaded leg, and at the extremes of traumatically induced motion, these ligaments assume a greater role (Table 9-1).

Ligaments

Anterior Talofibular Ligament

The anterior talofibular ligament passes forward as a band 2 to 5 mm thick and 10 to 12 mm long, to the neck of the talus. It is almost horizontal and relaxed in the neutral position, resisting anterior shear. During plantar flexion the ankle becomes relatively less stable because the posterior portion of the talar trochlea, being less wide than the anterior part, occupies the

ankle mortise. The anterior talofibular ligament also becomes tightened in plantar flexion and oriented almost vertically, thus being almost parallel to the long axis of the tibia. In this position it provides maximal protection against pathologic inversion movements in the ankle joint (Fig. 9-4).

Calcaneofibular Ligament

The calcaneofibular band is large and strong, about 6 mm wide, spreading out posteriorly from the tip of the fibular malleolus, at about 10 to 45 degrees, to insert on the calcaneus. It is extracapsular. It is slightly tensed in the neutral position and only moderately resists a pathologic inversion movement of the ankle. Therefore it is rarely injured alone. During plantar flexion the calcaneofibular ligament is oriented almost completely horizontally, stabilizing only the subtalar joints (Fig. 9-4). Despite this classic description of the anterior talofibular ligament resisting inversion with the foot in plantar flexion, and the calcaneofibular ligament with the ankle in neutral position, the anterior talofibular band seems to be frequently damaged during an inversion injury, regardless of the position of the ankle.

Posterior Talofibular Ligament

The posterior talofibular ligament attaches anteriorly to the digital fossa of the fibula and runs horizontally back to the tubercle of the talus. It is stressed during forced dorsiflexion trauma. In sport this band is rarely injured except during parachute jumping, in ice hockey where the player slides into the board at high speed, and on awkward landing during certain jumping activities.

Lateral Talocalcaneal Ligament

The lateral talocalcaneal ligament lies between the anterior talofibular ligament and the calcaneofibular band. It blends with these two ligaments and the capsule.

Medial Ligament

On the medial side, the ankle is stabilized by the strong, flat, fan-shaped deltoid ligament that has been described as having deep and superficial fibers. These fibers, for the most part, form a large, continuous bundle around the tip of the medial malleolus, extending to the navicular, sustentaculum tali, and posterior area of the talus.

TABLE 9-1. Change in Torque with Serial Sectioning

Foot Position and Condition	Percent Change				
	PT Ligament	CF Ligament	AT Ligament	D Ligament	Residual (articular surface)[a]
Internal rotation					
No load					
Plantar flexion	7.0	6.6	56.0	30.4	0
Neutral	2.6	5.3	17.1	75.0	0
Dorsiflexion	3.1	7.7	26.1	63.1	0
Load (670 N)					
Plantar flexion	9.8	0	45.5	44.7	28.0
Neutral	17.9	0.7	21.9	59.3	50.0
Dorsiflexion	13.9	0	35.2	50.9	27.7
External rotation					
No load					
Plantar flexion	32.5	54.3	1.3	11.9	0
Neutral	16.7	76.9	5.1	1.3	0
Dorsiflexion	0	75.0	10.0	15.0	0
Load (670 N)					
Plantar flexion	36.3	30.2	5.3	28.2	20.4
Neutral	19.1	57.1	20.5	3.2	48.7
Dorsiflexion	17.4	42.7	12.2	27.6	12.5
Inversion					
No load					
Plantar flexion	5.6	44.6	30.6	10.8	0
Neutral	15.6	49.6	30.0	1.8	0
Dorsiflexion	12.5	63.6	21.4	2.4	0
Load (670 N)					
Plantar flexion					100
Neutral	No change after cutting of any soft tissue				100
Dorsiflexion					100
Eversion					
No load					
Plantar flexion	0	13.0	13.0	74.1	0
Neutral	8.4	2.2	6.2	83.4	0
Dorsiflexion	0.6	7.4	0.6	91.5	0
Load (670 N)					
Plantar flexion					100
Neutral	No change after cutting of any soft tissue				100
Dorsiflexion					100

PT = posterior talofibular; CF = calcaneofibular; AT = anterior talofibular; D = deltoid; N = newtons.
[a] As percentage of total soft tissue contribution.
(Adapted from Stormont et al.,[10] with permission.)

Ankle Stability

With physiologic loading, the mortise formed by the articular surfaces accounts for 30 percent of the stability in rotation and 100 percent during inversion and eversion.[10] This fact means the ankle may be unstable during the process of loading or unloading but is usually stable once fully loaded (Table 9-1). Rupture of the anterior talofibular ligament results in various manifestations of instability, of which talar tilt and anterior subluxation (anterior drawer sign) are the most well known. However, rotation may be also the precipitating event in instances of instability.[11,12]

The anterior tibiofibular band works with the deltoid ligament in limiting internal rotation.[10] External rotation has the calcaneofibular ligament as a primary restraint, with the posterior talofibular band working as the primary factor in the plantar-flexed position.

With lateral ligamentous damage, the lateral part

Neutral

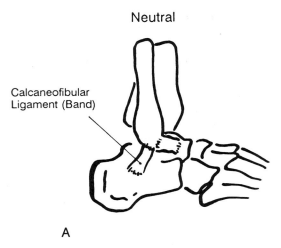

Calcaneofibular
Ligament (Band)

A

Plantar Flexion

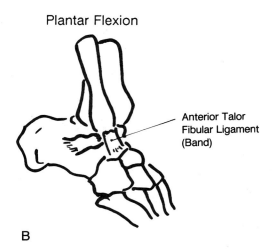

Anterior Talor
Fibular Ligament
(Band)

B

Fig. 9-4. (A) Neutral position. Anterior talofibular ligament (band) resists anterior shear. There is more tension in the calcaneofibular band. **(B)** During plantar flexion the anterior band is tightened and oriented almost vertically.

of the trochlea can slide forward in relation to its medial part, resulting in internal rotation of the talus in a horizontal plane, using the medial malleolus as a kind of axis. Anterolateral rotational instability occurs even when isolated rupture of the anterior talofibular ligament is present and is most pronounced in plantar flexion.

It is apparent that the bony configuration of the ankle joint, the movement of the fibular, and the dynamic stabilizing role of the peroneal muscles play an important synergistic role with the ligaments. These biomechanical and anatomic considerations lead to the conclusion that the anterior talofibular ligament is probably the most important stabilizing component of the lateral ligamentous apparatus; and its rupture may lead to marked chronic rotational instability. This conclusion implies that isolated rupture of the anterior talofibular ligament is not a minor injury but requires the best possible treatment in order to prevent subsequent instability leading to residual functional disabilities.

Mechanisms of Injury

The lateral ligament is damaged by excessive inversion accompanied by either plantar flexion or rotation (Fig. 9-5). A major mechanism of injury is landing from a jump. Particularly in crowded situations around the basket in basketball or the net in volleyball, severe injuries are caused by landing on another player's foot. Changing direction, particularly if associated with deceleration, may be a vulnerable movement as well. This tendency is exaggerated where there is an uneven surface with divots and ruts.

In the past, long, narrow cleats on soccer, football, or field hockey boots predisposed to injury. The adoption of synthetic molded soles, with the soccer-style pattern of multiple cleats that have diameters of 1/2 inch or more and maximum length of 3/8 inch have significantly reduced injuries.[13] This change, along with the high-top boot, particularly in combination with taping or bracing, has significantly altered the

---

Quick Facts

STABILITY OF THE ANKLE

- In weight-bearing position, the main stability is from bony structures.
- Anterior talofibular ligament is the key ligamentous structure.
- Plantar-flexed position is the most vulnerable.
- Peroneus longus and brevis are the major dynamic stabilizers.
- After rupture a rotary instability may develop as well as recurrent inversion sprains.

INVERSION   EVERSION

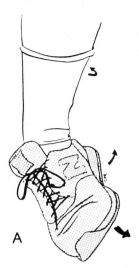
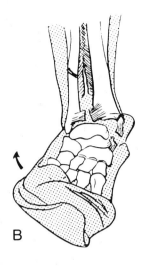

Fig. 9-5. (A) Typical inversion ankle sprain. **(B)** Isolated eversion injuries are uncommon and are usually associated with a fracture. (After Schneider and Sieber,[3] with permission.)

A   B

injury potential, particularly in athletes with chronically unstable ankles.

In contact sports, a direct blow or an opponent grabbing the foot may also precipitate a sprain. Other contributing factors to injury include a significant varus heel, weak musculature, tight heel cords, and tarsal coalition. The latter two conditions are dealt with in more detail.

Contributing Factors

Tight Achilles Tendon

During the adolescent growth spurt there may be an inequality between the rate of lengthening of the musculotendinous and osteochondral systems. Such inequality may predispose the athlete to chronic tightness in the heel cords, with the ankle not capable of dorsiflexing past neutral, even with the knees flexed to 90 degrees. This condition in turn may predispose the athlete to fibular collateral ligament strains. The mechanism relates to the fact that the gastrocnemius and soleus tendons exert their pull on the ankle joint via the calcaneus, not directly through the talus. During strong contraction or while on a stretch, their pull, along with the other flexors, tends to direct the heel into slight inversion, which increases the tendency to land on the outside of the foot during jumping maneuvers. This condition must be identified and managed as part of a preventive or treatment program.

Tarsal Coalition

Snyder et al., in a retrospective review of roentgenograms of athletes after an ankle sprain, found numerous calcaneal navicular abnormalities, of which tarsal coalition was the most frequent.[14] Tarsal coalition was seen more frequently than would be expected in the general population. The possible mechanism linking this condition to ankle sprains is unexplained. The relation is more fully discussed in Chapter 8.

Quick Facts

- *Mechanisms of Injury*
  - Landing from a jump
  - Stepping or landing on opponent's foot
  - Changing direction
  - Decelerating
  - Uneven surfaces
- *Contributing Factors*
  - Previous ankle injury
  - Low profile boots
  - Narrow, long, cleats
  - Generalized ligamentous laxity
  - Varus heel
  - Weak peronei muscles
  - Tight Achilles tendon
  - Tarsal coalition

Chronic Sprains

Chronic ankle sprain may occur during such activities as ballet, where poor postural habits and insufficient strength of the muscles controlling the subtalar joint can lead to gradual stretching of the ligaments. In some sports, e.g., football or soccer, the constant stresses and forces around the ankle can lead to chronic bone and joint changes. Indeed, in one study involving a professional football club, most of the players with an average of 10 years playing time had radiologic changes compatible with degenerative changes at the ankle joint.

Medial Ligament Sprains

Although injuries occur primarily to the lateral ligament, two circumstances seem to alter this pattern and lead to damage of the medial collateral ligament.

1. Ankle injuries may be incurred during football or wrestling from being struck (pulled or fallen on) by another player. This injury produces either an eversion sprain or a hyperplantar flexion sprain (Fig. 9-5).
2. Wrestlers appear to have a high incidence of medial ligament injuries, probably secondary to wider stance, with ankle eversion, in order to get traction on the mat.

Assessment of the Injured Ankle

History

The main points to ascertain when obtaining the patient's history include the following.

1. Previous history of an ankle injury must be determined in order to distinguish chronic functional instability from an acute injury.
2. One of the key indicators of severity is the ability to bear weight immediately after the episode and during the ensuing hours. Walking is compatible with a second degree injury, and running is sometimes possible, with pain, after a first degree injury. Inability to bear weight, except with crutches or with a significant limp, suggests a severe second or third degree injury.
3. Rapid onset of swelling frequently indicates a severe injury, although it is not a reliable sign. The amount of swelling depends on the degree of injury, the time since injury, and how the sprain has been managed since the injury. Rapidly accumulating swelling, on both sides of the joint, is usually secondary to hemarthrosis.

4. An audible sound or a sensation of popping, snapping, or cracking often accompanies a significant tear.
5. The age of the individual may influence the type of injury. Bony avulsion is more common in the older patient; and the risk of epiphyseal separation of the fibula or growth plate injuries of the tibia is present in the skeletally immature. The younger the patient, the greater is the need of oblique views or comparison roentgenograms of the uninjured side.
6. The history should uncover any systemic disease that may have some influence on ankle instability. Although uncommon in the athlete, this point may be important. Diabetic neuropathy, for instance, may be associated with a high incidence of recurrent sprains and post-traumatic arthropathy.
7. The aims, goals, and occupation of the athlete have bearing on the selection of treatment, particularly with more severe injury.

Palpation and Inspection

At the outset, it should be made clear that pain is not always proportional to the injury. Some complete disruptions are less painful than severe second degree injuries. Furthermore, there may be a short "golden" period immediately after injury and before the onset of significant pain and swelling; it is the optimal time for performing stress tests. Significant pain around the medial and lateral malleoli with a lateral ligament sprain may point to a more severe injury.

Careful assessment of the areas of swelling and the maximum areas of tenderness may help decide which bands of the ligament are affected. Furthermore, pain and tenderness elsewhere in the foot should raise a suspicion of ligamentous injury or fracture to the joints of the midfoot and metatarsal. It should be established whether the tenderness is mainly over the fibula, away from the tip, as it may indicate an ankle fracture. Surprisingly, significant malleolus fractures may be missed and treated as ankle sprains (Fig. 9-6).

Viewing the ankle from behind gives an idea of the definition of the Achilles tendon. If the definition of the Achilles tendon is lost on both the medial and lateral sides of the ankle immediately after an injury, it indicates that there is a large amount of bleeding into the joint (Fig. 9-7). This finding suggests a more serious injury that involves not only the ligament but considerable contusion of the joint surfaces. One can assume that this injury will take much longer to get better than simple stretching or tearing of the liga-

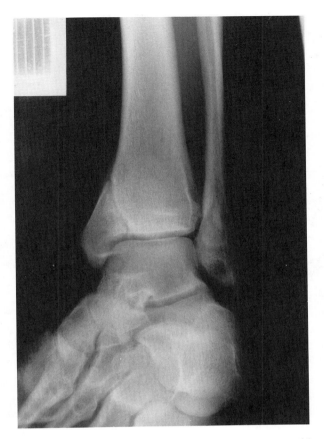

Fig. 9-6. This relatively undisplaced but severe ankle fracture of the medial malleolus was missed and treated as an ankle sprain in a hockey player. Tenderness mainly over the bone should have been the clue to the need for roentgenography, which would have prevented the delayed diagnosis.

ment without hemarthrosis and joint contusion. Similarly, excessive deformity should arouse suspicion of an ankle fracture, diastasis, or talar or subtalar dislocation. Inadequate support and therapy after injury can lead to late development of edema around the tendon, and so it does not have the same implications in terms of assessing severity.

Stress Tests

Stress tests may be performed with the athlete in the lying position with the foot hanging over the end of the bed or with the individual sitting[15] (Fig. 9-8). Comparison with the uninjured side is usually helpful. The reliability of these tests depends not only on the skill of the examiner but on the ability of the patient to relax and cooperate.

> **Practice Point**
>
> ### INDICATIONS FOR ROENTGENOGRAPHY BEFORE STRESS TESTS
>
> - Immediate significant swelling
> - Obvious deformity
> - Inability to bear weight
> - Pain mainly over bone

Anterior Drawer Sign

The anterior drawer sign is the primary test of ankle instability; fortunately it is the easiest to perform and frequently causes little pain for the patient. Therefore it is usually performed first. It specifically tests, in turn, the anterior talofibular ligament, anterior capsule, and calcaneofibular band. The positive test is frequently accompanied by a "clunking sensation." Because the anterior talofibular ligament is the one most frequently injured, it is essential to master this test (Fig. 9-8). When an anterior drawer sign is accompanied by a positive varus or inversion stress test, both the anterior talofibular and calcaneofibular ligaments are likely disrupted.[15-17]

> **Clinical Point**
>
> ### ANTERIOR DRAWER TEST
>
> - Key test for ankle instability
> - Patient often more able to relax
> - May be accompanied by a "clunk"
> - Alone signifies anterior talofibular ligament tear
> - In association with positive inversion stress means calcaneofibular tearing as well

Inversion Test

The inversion test with the ankle at 90 degrees or neutral principally stresses the calcaneofibular ligament; during plantar flexion it involves the anterior talofibular ligament more.[14] Occasionally this test is accompanied by a clunk, but this sign does not necessarily infer significant instability.

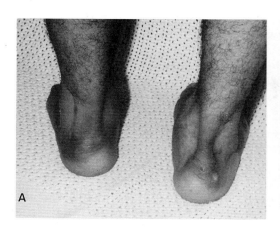
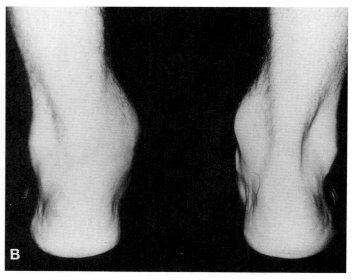

Fig. 9-7. Posterior view of sprained left ankles. **(A)** Despite swelling the Achilles tendon is relatively defined, and it is probably a second degree injury. **(B)** Immediate swelling, which obliterates the Achilles tendon contour, is probably a third degree injury.

Other Stress Tests

The eversion test is rarely positive, as it is associated with medial ligament disruption. The transverse stress is positive only with disruption of the inferior tibiofibular ligament and interosseous membrane or in association with a fracture. It is a particularly important sign to observe. Identification of this instability is usually an indication for surgery (Fig. 9-9).

Classification

For the classification of ankle ligament disruption, some investigators have associated complete tears of a single ligament, usually the anterior talofibular ligament, as a second degree injury. Tearing of both anterior talofibular and calcaneofibular ligaments, the so-called two-ligament injury, is usually considered a third degree injury (Table 9-2). However, this classification cannot cover all scenarios of combined complete and partial tearing of two bands, and thus the degree of instability to stressing must be taken into account.

Other Considerations

The examination is not complete without registering the condition of the skin, a sensory test for the sural and peroneal nerves, and confirming the presence of the tibialis posterior and dorsalis pedis pulse.

Furthermore, examination of the knee for proximal tibiofibular joint problems or a proximal fibular fracture is important. With chronic ankle instability, the knee should also be assessed for ligamentous laxity, as it may be a contributing or even the primary cause of the patient's functional instability.

As far as field tests are concerned, the absence of an anterior drawer, no significant swelling, and the ability to walking without a limp signify that it is safe to test the patient's ability to hop. If the athlete can hop without pain, tests of running and cutting are attempted on the sidelines. A satisfactory performance indicates that it is safe to attempt to return to play.[15] Attempts at hopping, running, or cutting are not allowed if the athlete is unable to walk without a limp.

Differential Diagnosis

When assessing the so-called sprained ankle, it is important to bear in mind, and rule out, fracture, dislocation, tendon injuries, and other ligamentous disruptions. The location of tenderness and swelling, obvious deformity, excessive edema, or increasing pain and swelling with weight-bearing should raise suspicions of a more complex diagnosis (Table 9-3). The commonest of these problems are fifth metatarsal fractures, cracks or avulsions of the fibular malleolus, and osteochondral lesions of the talar dome.

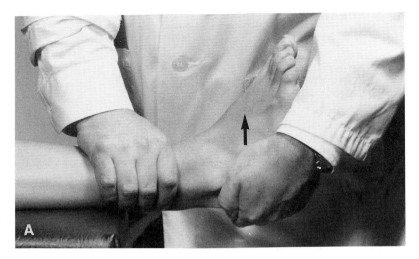

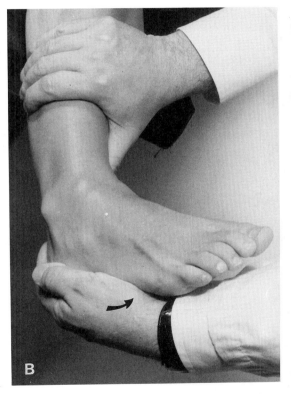
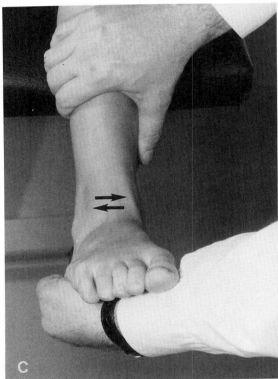

Fig. 9-8. Stress tests for ligament stability. **(A)** Anterior drawer sign. **(B)** Inversion test. **(C)** Side to side stress for tibiofibular diastasis.

Roentgenographic Evaluation

The need for roentgenography during evaluation of a recent sprain is probably summarized by De Lacey and Bradbrooke's conclusion: "no soft tissue swelling, no x-ray."[18,19] However, because swelling occasionally takes some time to evolve, a roentgeno-

gram should be considered (1) if the tenderness is mainly over the bone of the malleolus rather than the ligament; (2) if there is obvious severe deformity; or (3) if the athlete is unable to weight bear after a brief period of rest. These films prevent overlooking significant fractures.

There is a trend to consider a nonoperative ap-

TABLE 9-2.   Classification of Ankle Sprains

Severity	Pathology	Signs and Symptoms	Disability
Grade I (mild) stable	Mild stretch No instability Single ligament involved Usually anterior talofibular ligament	No hemorrhage Minimal swelling Point tenderness No anterior drawer No varus laxity	No or little limp Minimal functional loss Difficulty hopping Recovery 8 days (range 2–10)
Grade II (moderate) stable	Large spectrum of injury Mild to moderate instability Complete tearing of anterior talofibular ligament *or* Partial tearing of anterior talofibular plus calcaneofibular ligaments	Some hemorrhage Localized swelling Margins of Achilles tendon less defined May be anterior drawer No varus laxity	Limp with walking Inability to toe raise Inability to hop Unable to run Recovery 20 days (range 10–30)
Grade III (severe) two-ligament, unstable	Significant instability Complete tear of anterior capsule and talofibular ligament and associated tear of anterior talofibular and calcaneofibular ligaments	Diffuse swelling both sides of Achilles tendon, early hemorrhage May be tenderness medially and laterally Positive anterior drawer Positive varus laxity	Unable to bear weight fully Significant pain inhibition Initially almost complete loss of range of motion Recovery 40 days (range 30–90)

proach for all degrees of ankle sprain, even in the highly competitive individual. In this situation, it is often possible to establish a safe, effective treatment program on clinical examination. Stress roentgenograms or other supplementary radiographic studies are rarely necessary for the acute sprain. In situations where surgery is considered the treatment of choice for double ligament tears with associated significant capsule disruption, these tests may be helpful, particularly arthrograms or peroneal tenography. In the face of chronic functional instability of the ankle that

is not clearly due to excessive talar tilt, stress views may aid in establishing a firm diagnosis and delineate the need for late surgical reconstruction. Thus, stress films have no or little role in assessment of the acute ankle injury.

Inversion Stress Views

To clearly demonstrate the amount of instability, supplementary local anesthesia is sometimes necessary. The degree of patient cooperation is important

TABLE 9-3.   Differential Diagnosis of Ankle "Sprains"

"Sprain"	Site
Fractures	Malleolar (fibular or tibial) Fibular shaft (Maisonneuve) Talar neck Fifth metatarsal base at peroneus brevis insertion Cuboid at attachment of bifurcate ligament Osteochondral talar dome Calcaneal anterior process
Dislocations	Subtalar Talonavicular
Other ligaments	Dorsal talonavicular Bifurcate ligament (calcaneocuboid/calcaneonavicular) Talocalcaneal ligament
Tendons	Peroneal tendon subluxation Torn Achilles tendon

<table>
<tr><td>

Clinical Point

INDICATIONS FOR ROENTGENOGRAPHY

- Early, severe soft tissue swelling
- Significant bruising
- Pain mainly over malleoli
- Significant pain over fifth metatarsal base
- Athlete unable to bear weight
- Stress views mainly reserved for chronic instability

</td><td>

Clinical Point

STRESS TESTING

- *Inversion stress*
  - Abnormal: 5 to 10 degrees more than uninjured side
  - Ranges of 5 to 23 degrees reported
  - More than 90 percent of population have less than 10 degree tilt
- *Anterior drawer*
  - Test in neutral position
  - Abnormal: > 5 mm (usually)

</td></tr>
</table>

when determining the reliability of these measurements. When performing the test, care should be taken to grasp the foot only by the heel. The angle subtended by a line parallel to the subchondral bone of the distal tibia and proximal talus constitutes the talar tilt. Although angles of 5 to 23 degrees have been reported in normals, other studies have given more conservative figures.[20] For instance, in one report only 1.7 percent of the population were reported as having talar tilts of more than 5 degrees, whereas another estimated that approximately 7 percent of their sample had angles of more than 10 degrees.[21,22] Laurin and Mathieu found an average talar tilt of 7 degrees in children.[23] Most investigators agree that 5 to 10 degrees more motion on the injured side is indicative of tears to both the anterior talofibular and calcaneofibular ligaments.

Anterior Drawer Stress

The foot should be in the neutral position, as equinus tends to restrict the normal sagittal mobility of the talus, which is approximately 3.0 mm (range 2 to 10 mm).[23,24] An anterior drawer of more than 5 mm, however, is usually considered abnormal and indicative of stretching or tearing of the anterior talofibular ligament.[25,26]

Several factors detract from the validity of these measurements.

1. Degree of patient relaxation and cooperation
2. Amount of force used by the examiner
3. Normal laxity for any particular individual
4. Poor correlation of symptoms with measured instability

Arthrogram

An anteromedial injection site is used; and the extravasation pattern and the amount of dye accommodated by the joint are used to assess stability. A normal joint does not hold more than 4 to 6 ml of dye. If indicated, the test must be done early after the injury, as fibrin clot may seal tears and prevent extravasation. The incidence of extravasation of dye into the various tendon sheaths around the ankle, particularly the flexor hallucis longus and peroneal sheath, has been estimated to be as high as 25 percent,[25] which diminishes the diagnostic value of the test. Extravasation of dye proximally in front of the tibiofibular syndesmosis that covers more than 5.5 cm is indicative of a significant tear.[24]

Peroneal tenography is injection of dye into the peroneal sheath.[27] A positive test is escape of dye into the ankle joint, indicating a tear of the calcaneofibular ligament. Because it rarely occurs without associated tears of the talofibular ligament, it indicates a serious ligament disruption or double ligament tear. None of these tests should be used routinely.

Treatment Principles

My plan for treatment of moderate and severely sprained ankles is based on several assumptions generated from a literature review and past clinical experience. The premises are as follows.

1. When the large number of individuals sustaining ankle sprains are considered, the number presenting with chronic instability is not excessively high.

2. It is not always the severe tears that produce delayed instability.

3. Proponents of surgery claim good objective and subjective results.

4. Proponents of nonoperative regimens report good subjective results and variable but usually acceptable objective outcomes.

5. Long-term follow-ups of primary operative repair versus delayed reconstruction do not appear to be appreciably different.

6. There are excellent delayed reconstructive procedures available that produce good functional outcomes should chronic functional instability develop.

7. Strict immobilization is not necessary or desirable with either operative or nonsurgical approaches.

8. The key to early resolution, if nonoperative treatment is chosen, is adequate protection, minimizing edema, early motion, and early weight-bearing.

9. Inadequate protection and rehabilitation allow reinjury and eventually produce chronic instability.

10. Protection for vigorous activity may be required until full strength is regained.

11. Intra-articular fractures with loose fragments and tibiofibular diastasis must be excluded before one becomes committed to a nonoperative course (Fig. 9-9).

12. Only rarely with severe disruption in the selected, highly competitive individual are the risks of surgery balanced by a more rapid and satisfactory outcome.

13. During the treatment of chronic instability, muscle weakness, defective proprioception, and subtalar stiffness may have to be addressed.

14. Surgical treatment for chronic functional instability should be undertaken only after careful evaluation of the cause and failure of nonoperative treatment.

Using the above principles, it is possible to evolve a treatment plan for each degree of severity of ankle injury. Furthermore, like so many aspects of therapy, it is important for the patient to understand the treatment principles. The chance of a successful outcome depends on the patient carrying out instructions, adapting them to the nuances of his or her own life style, and pursuing the exercise program with determination and commitment.

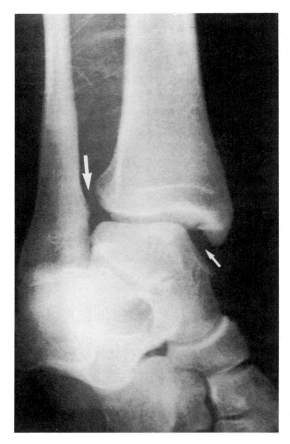

Fig. 9-9. Diastasis without fracture signifying rupture of the interosseous membrane and the anterior and posterior tibiofibular ligament. The increased width of the joint space between the talus and tibial malleolus is as important in diagnosing this injury as the space between the tibia and fibula.

Treatment of Swelling

Edema and effusion seem to play a central role in the degree of initial pain, the ability to progress weight-bearing, the rate of restoration of normal range of motion, and the duration of chronic aching and disability. Effective treatment of this problem is therefore important for ensuring the maximal return to function in a minimum time. Most investigators agree that application of ice provides excellent vasoconstriction during the first 24 hours, and that heat is contraindicated (Table 9–4). Some suggest that heat should not be used at all during the acute or subacute phase because they believe that the vasodilation created contributes to edema.[24] If relatively normal mo-

TABLE 9.4. Cold Versus Heat for Ankle Sprains

Severity of Sprain	Days to Return to Function		
	Early Cryotherapy[a]	Late Cryotherapy[b]	Heat
Moderate	6.0	11.0	14.75
Severe	13.2	30.0	33.0

[a] Application during first 24 hours.
[b] Initiated after 24 hours.

tion and weight-bearing have not been achieved, this point may have some validity.

However, provided there is adequate support during the early phases and the patient understands the importance of motion and weight-bearing, heat may have distinct advantages for the treatment of subacute and chronic swelling. The more severe the injury, however, the more important it is to institute early application of ice and compression.

Hocutt et al. in 1982 studied the effects of cryotherapy versus heat in the treatment of grade III ankle sprains.[28] Cold was applied via ice packs or an ice whirlpool bath at 40° to 50°F (5° to 10°C) for 10 to 20 minutes one to three times a day. Heat was applied using hot packs or hot soaks for 15 minutes up to three times daily. Their work suggested the use of early cryotherapy, as return to activity was, on average, 13 days for the group treated within 36 hours of injury versus 30 days when given late. Furthermore, relatively pain-free running and jumping was resumed at 6 days in the early ice group versus 15 days when heat was given early.[28] Basur et al. further stressed the need for early treatment with cold rather than late therapy with heat or cold (Table 9-5).[29]

There should be distinct reservations, however, concerning the results in these two reports because although the principle is sound the time to complete functional recovery is far too short to be representative of most clinicians' experience and probably represents an overestimation of the initial severity of the injury. Patients with true grade III injuries (with two-ligament disruption) cannot realistically be expected to have full functional recovery in less time than 6 weeks.

Sims studied ankle and leg volumes in various positions, demonstrating a significant increase in size with dependency. This point emphasizes the futility of

---

Clinical Point

ICE ROUTINE

- Apply as soon as possible after exercise sessions.
- Maximum duration should be 20 to 25 minutes.
- Reactive hyperemic redness should resolve in 15 to 20 minutes.
- Space repeated applications 20–45 minutes apart.
- With significant swelling, combine with elevation.
- Cover as much of affected area as possible.

---

treating edema in the dependent position in whirlpool baths or during electrical stimulation.[30] The effects of limb motion and activity may alleviate this tendency to some extent (Table 9-6). Indeed, dependency without motion or weight-bearing predisposes to edema and effusion.

TABLE 9-5. Cryotherapy and Ankle Sprains (Second Degree)

Treatment	Days of Therapy					
	Walk Without Pain		Climb Stairs Without Pain		Run and Jump Without Pain	
	Moderate	Severe	Moderate	Severe	Moderate	Severe
Cryotherapy early)[a]	2.6	2.7	3.7	4.2	6.0	13.2
Cryotherapy (late)[b]	5.2	9.7	6.8	13.6	11.0	30.4
Heat therapy[a]	7.8	9.7	9.0	9.7	14.8	33.3

[a] Initiated during the first 24 hours.
[b] Initiated after 48 hours.

TABLE 9-6. **Effects of Limb Position and Volume**

Parameter	Mean Volume (ml)	
	Elevated	Dependent
Before test	1094.36	1139.32
After test	1079.14	1156.46
Increase/decrease	−15.22 (−1.4%)	+17.14 (+1.5%)
Mean change	2.9% ($p > 0.001$)	

These last few paragraphs serve to reinforce the important concepts of treatment of all acute muscle and ligamentous trauma, i.e., the efficacy of early ice, elevation, and compression. Compression may be supplied by an open Gibney tape, a tensor bandage, and occasionally a cast for the more severe injuries during the acute phase. A closed Gibney tape, brace, or tensor bandage may be selected to follow. These applications are examples of compression used for support; but compression may be used for treatment as well. Massage, compression, and cryotemperature systems that combine cold with sequential pressure have been used (Fig. 9-10).

During the acute phase the Jobst Cryo-Temp System provides a range from ambient room temperatures down to 1°C (34°F). Pressure of 0 to 160 mmHg may be applied as a constant treatment or intermittently with pulses of 0 to 180 seconds on and 0 to 60 seconds off. The application may be combined

> ## Clinical Point
> ### HEATING MODALITIES FOR SOFT TISSUE SWELLING
>
> - Most heat packs: 38° to 41°C (100° to 106°F)
> - Warm whirlpool: 38° to 40°C (100° to 104°F)
> - Short wave diathermy: mild thermic × 20 minutes
> - Ultrasound: 1.5 W/cm², continuous
> - Contrast baths, whirlpool hot and cold: 38° to 40°C (100° to 104°F) × 5 minutes 8°C (47°F) × 1 minute
>   Repeat 5 times

with gentle motion. Other units, e.g., Flowtron MK2, have an air pump with an inflation–deflation cycle of 3.3 minutes, producing pressures that range from 40 to 90 mmHg. Treatment sessions usually last 20 to 30 minutes. Although most effective for early dispersal of edema, they may also have a limited role in the subacute phase. They are not effective for effusion or chronic swelling. These pressure systems are contraindicated in patients with acute thrombophlebitis, deep vein thrombosis, significant peripheral vascular

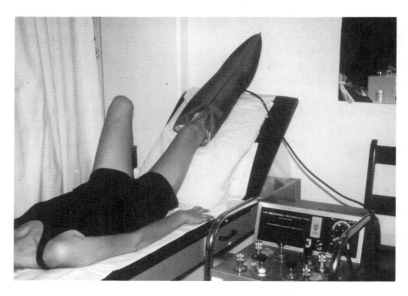

Fig. 9-10. Intermittent compression systems are available that allow elevation, pressure, and cooling for early management of sprains.

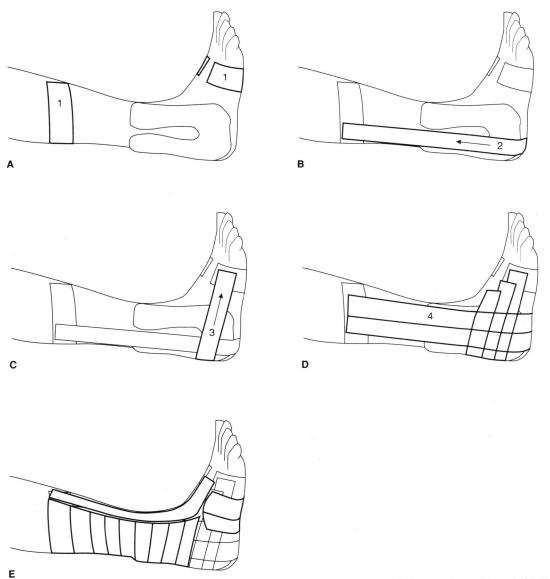

Fig. 9-11. Application of a pressure pad and open Gibney tape for acute injury and swelling. **(A)** With the ankle in neutral, adhesive felt or foam horseshoe is contoured appropriately for the individual and the location of the swelling. Then (1.5 inches) anchor tapes are placed distally and sufficiently proximal to allow good grip with the tape. **(B)** Stirrup applied pulling from medial to lateral to encourage eversion position. **(C&D)** Sequential stirrups and Gibney weaves. **(E)** Closing strips. The anterior part is left open to allow swelling. Additional support may be achieved by adding a tensor bandage.

disease, pulmonary edema, congestive heart failure, or an impending compartment syndrome.

The benefits of well planned and executed therapy may be enhanced by the judicious use of nonsteroidal anti-inflammatory drugs (NSAIDs). They are also useful for acute and chronic effusions. Tense he-marthrosis or effusion seen with acute injuries may be aspirated, which reduces the rehabilitation time. Moderate to minor effusion, however, reaccumulates; the risks of aspiration on a repeated basis are not matched by the benefits. Persistent effusions may respond to a single treatment of aspiration plus the injection of a steroidal medication, e.g., methylpred-nisolone acetate (Depo-Medrol).

Chronic soft tissue swelling responds best to heat, compression, and carefully progressed motion. For severe cases, compression stockings are appropriate. Heat may be applied as hot packs, diathermy, ultrasound, warm whirlpool, or contrast baths.

Taping

Effectiveness

Much controversy exists regarding the value of supportive strapping techniques in sport. Certainly with professional football teams it has lowered the incidence of ankle injuries. However, there is still some concern that in a few instances it has been at the expense of the knee. There is no doubt that, used intelligently, strapping has great benefits prophylactically and therapeutically.[31] The ankle joint, in particular, lends itself well to supportive strapping—and to the concomitant danger that a player may be sent back to training or competition too early.

Taping for sprained ankles is indicated in five situations.

1. The immediate postinjury phase for support, pain relief, and edema.
2. During treatment of the acute injury, when it is used mainly for support, but with the addition of a malleolar compression pad and elastic wrap; it may also contribute to reducing edema (Fig. 9-11).
3. After return to activity following an ankle injury, to prevent reinjury while continued peroneal

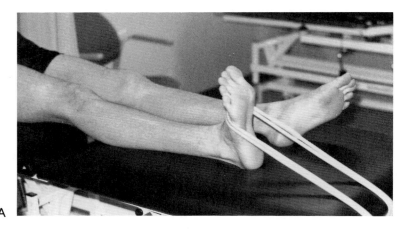

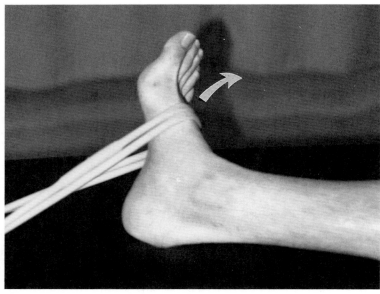

Fig. 9-12. Long-term exercise of the peronei is best carried out as a home program using surgical tubing or some other elastic commercial substitute. **(A)** Dorsiflexion. **(B)** Eversion.

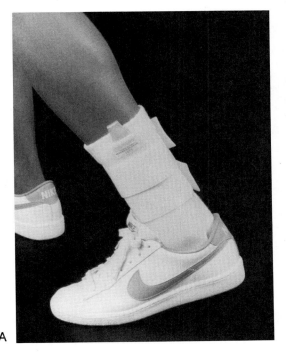 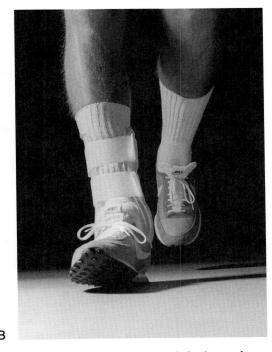

A · B

Fig. 9-13. One of the many available ankle supports (orthosis) used for both acute injuries and over the long term instead of repeated taping. (With kind permission of Aircast Inc.)

muscle strengthening is carried out for the remaining part of the competitive season (Fig. 9-12).

4. Some form of ankle support, either ankle taping or an ankle support (orthosis) to protect an individual from reinjury, to support the ankle in those athletes suffering from chronic functional ankle instability.

5. As a prophylactic measure in the uninjured competitor (Fig. 9-13).

Studies comparing the amount of support offered by four commonly used taping procedures showed that, as is expected, progressively more support is offered by the basket weave, the basket weave plus stirrups, the basket weave plus heel lock, and, best of all, the basket weave, heel lock, and stirrups.[32] Even with the last procedure, the foot–ankle complex is surprisingly mobile. An analysis of athletic trauma revealed that torques of 420 nm could be applied to the ankle joint. Only figure-of-eight lock has the strength to withstand this movement, and thus is the method recommended[33] (Fig. 9-14).

Several investigations have confirmed that although the initial range of motion may be restricted by as much as 30 to 50 percent the support is reduced by 10 minutes of vigorous exercise and by as much as 57 percent after 30 minutes[32,33] (Fig. 9-15). Nevertheless, clinical studies generally attest to the effectiveness of some form of support, not only for controlling edema but for protecting the ankle joint.

Clinical Point

ROLE OF ANKLE TAPING

- Immediate postinjury support and edema control
- Protecting the acute sprain between treatments
- Preventing reinjury with return to activity
- Supporting the chronically functional, unstable ankle
- Prophylactically on the uninjured ankle

The major variables to be considered regarding the effectiveness of taping are the type of tape used, the

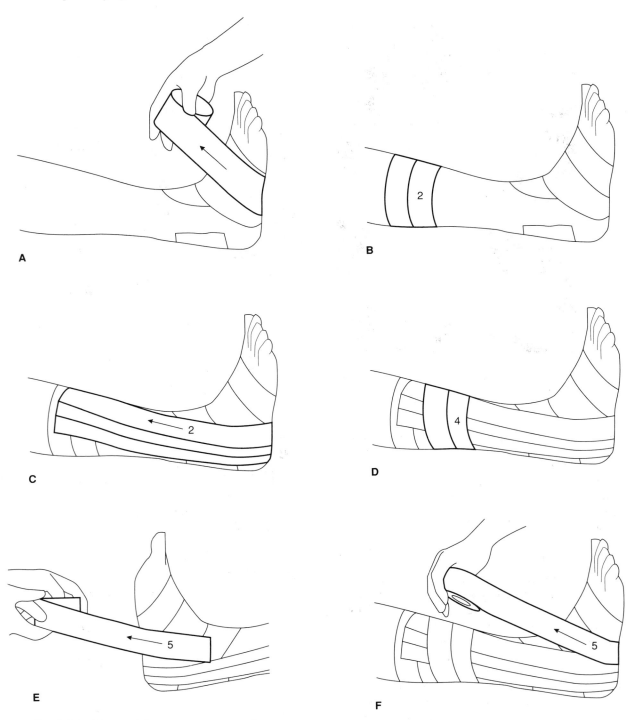

Fig. 9-14. Closed Gibney taping with figure-of-eight heel lock. **(A)** Foot positioned in neutral plantar flexion and dorsiflexion with slight eversion. Achilles and extensor pads applied with skin lubricant and wrap. Distal anchors applied (skin wrap not shown.) **(B)** Proximal anchors. **(C)** Apply stirrup from medial to lateral. **(D)** At completion of stirrup application, resecure with proximal anchor strip. **(E)** Figure-of-eight commencing medially. **(F)** Figure-of-eight passing dorsally.

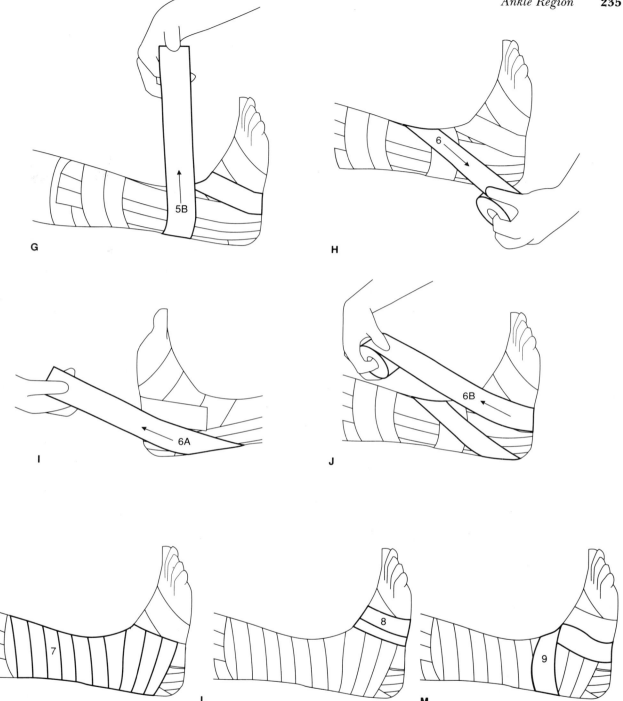

Fig. 9-14 *(Continued)*. **(G)** Figure-of-eight around ankle. **(H)** Down over distal fibula. **(I)** Wrapping around medial heel. **(J)** Completion of figure-of-eight heel lock. **(K)** Tape is filled in, and if necessary the foot component is slit along the side to the base of the fifth metatarsal with the athlete fully weight-bearing. **(L)** Distal anchor strips are then applied in this weight-bearing position to allow the forefoot to spread and for comfort. **(M)** Several reinforcing figure-of-eight strips may be used to increase support.

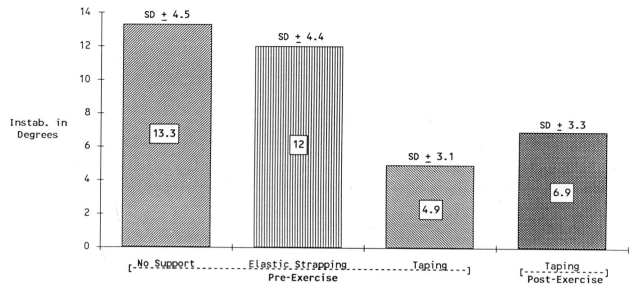

Fig. 9-15. Radiologic study of the effectiveness of taping and elastic bandage on reducing the talar tilt. The tape is shown to be most effective, with support maintained after 30 minutes of exercise. (From Vaes et al.,[32] with permission.)

height the tape is taken up the leg, and variations in individual techniques used by sports therapists.[33] One cannot overstress the role that ability, experience, and knowledge of the therapist plays in influencing the results of using taping for treatment and prophylaxis. The fact that the strapping loosens somewhat is perhaps an advantage, as it allows satisfactory range of movement but still supports at the limit of the range. Too rigid a support would lead to the same disastrous effects as the ski boot, i.e., mainly tibial fractures and knee injuries. The most common error, even with experienced therapists, is strapping too low on the leg so almost no support is achieved. The taping should be taken to midcalf in most circumstances.

Loos and Boelens, using electromyographic data, were able to support the clinical suggestion that part of the effectiveness of tape is facilitation of peroneal muscle activity, which enhances its usefulness even after it has loosened with exercise.[34]

Taping Technique

The following material outlines some important basic principles in the application of tape to the foot and ankle.

1. An accurate diagnosis of the type and severity of the injury and appropriate overall treatment

---

Clinical Point

EFFECTIVENESS OF TAPING

- Initial reduction of range of motion by 30 to 50 percent
- Decreased control by 40 percent after 10 minutes' exercise
- Effectiveness confirmed by clinical studies
- Possible enhancement of peroneal muscle activity
- Best support from basket weave, heel lock, and stirrup
- Effectiveness often proportional to skill of application

---

goals are necessary, as is an understanding of the role of taping in that plan.

2. An understanding of anatomy and biomechanics is essential so the underlying tissue damage can be put in perspective and necessary adaptations of the standard techniques made.

3. Knowledge of the specific contraindications and precautions for taping is mandatory, including known allergies to tape or other materials used

for taping. Eczema, or infection in areas of the proposed taping, inadequately protected blisters or open wounds, vascular disease with peripheral circulatory compromise, impending compartment syndromes, inadequate sensation, lack of diagnosis, and insufficient competence of the therapist at taping are contraindications.

4. Knowledge of what the athlete needs to do in the sport, the ranges of motion and forces on the specific joint, and the advisability of allowing these activities with the aid of tape is required.

5. To receive maximum support and protection from the tape, the joint must be positioned to counteract the forces that contributed to the initial injury. For example, an inversion, plantar flexion injury to the ankle requires placement of the joint in a neutral position with respect to plantar and dorsiflexion and with slight heel eversion.

6. The area to be taped must be thoroughly cleaned and shaved and be free of the possibility of skin irritation. This requirement dictates the use of protective dressing over abrasions or cuts and other highly sensitive areas. For the instance, the tape applied to the ankle can contribute to mechanical irritation of the skin, the distal aspect of the Achilles tendon, and the area anterior to the ankle joint. The use of lubricated gauze sponges helps prevent blistering of the skin in these sensitive areas.

7. The practice of strapping directly to the skin enhances the adhesive qualities of the tape. However, a pretaping underwrap is recommended if there will be repeated application and removal of the tape on the same area. The underwrap helps to decrease the possibility of skin breakdown and facilitates removal of the tape after use.

8. Continuous taping, especially over the areas where the contour and shape of the extremity change, tends to result in unequal pressure and can impede normal blood flow. Therefore it is recommended that the adhesive strapping be applied in strips. If each strip overlaps the preceding one by one-half to three-fourths, more even pressure can be attained, and separation of the tape during strenuous activity can be prevented.

9. To prevent further impairment of circulation and restriction of motion, caution should be exercised when encircling the tape around a muscle belly mass. If encircling the muscle is required, as for Achilles tendon strapping, elastic tape should be used because of its expansile properties.

10. To prevent gaping of the tape, the proper size should be selected. For areas of the foot, a width of 2.5 cm (1 inch) allows the greatest ease of application, whereas the ankle joint requires tape 3.75 cm (1.5 inch) wide.

11. Adhesive strapping should be removed promptly after a practice session or athletic contest. In all other circumstances, it should not be left on for more than 3 days. After removal of the tape, the skin should be cleansed with alcohol, powdered, and prepared for reapplication of tape, if necessary.

Braces

There are currently available several kinds of ankle brace or gaiter that may be used for acute injuries or for support with chronic ankle instability. These braces are both reasonably inexpensive and effective[35] (Fig. 9-16). Subtalar inversion has been measured by high speed cinematography on specially designed platforms that confirm the effectiveness of braces.[36] Braces have the advantage of not requiring skill to apply after selection of the correct size. It is almost impossible for athletes to apply an effective taping procedure to their own ankles, and many individuals do not have access to skilled help.[36-38] Furthermore, constant retaping of ankles over a season may be expensive. With all these considerations, an ankle brace may be an acceptable compromise.

During the initial phases after injury, particularly with the more severe second degree and third degree

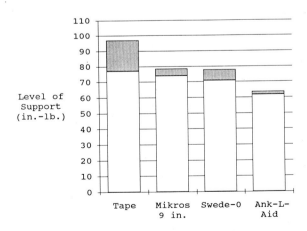

Fig. 9-16. Decrease in ankle support after 20 minutes of inversion exercise. Taping versus lace on braces. Change in support relative to freshly applied specimens indicated by the shaded portions. (From Bunch et al.,[35] with permission.)

TABLE 9-7.   Mean Ankle Range of Motion with Support

Support	Before Application		After Application		After Exercise	
	Inversion	Eversion	Inversion	Eversion	Inverstion	Eversion
Taping	53.37 ± 11.19	43.52 ± 11.00	35.20 ± 12.08	36.65 ± 9.19	40.40 ± 12.07	35.00 ± 8.69
Semirigid orthosis	53.23 ± 11.23	48.85 ± 10.00	31.88 ± 6.84	26.22 ± 8.85	32.10 ± 8.22	28.30 ± 8.18
Mean	53.00	43.69	33.54	29.94	36.25	31.87

Results are given in degrees.
(From Gross et al.,[38] with permission.)

TABLE 9-8.   Rehabilitation for Stable Ankle Sprain

Rehabilitation Steps	Treatment Aims
Stage I: immediately after injury	
Careful evaluation of injury severity	Establish accurate diagnosis
Decide need for roentgenography	Protect from further injury
Application of compression	Minimize hemorrhage
Ice in elevation	
Gentle dorsi- and plantar flexion	
Light partial weight-bearing	
Supply crutches	
NSAIDs	
Teach home ice and ROM program	
Warn of danger of tight wrap	
Stage II: acute inflammation	
Continue partial weight-bearing	Protect from further injury
Continue home ice program	Minimize edema
Compression and elevation	Maintain ROM
ROM—no inversion	Maintain fitness
Isometric resisted when 50% weight-bearing	
Set up cardiovascular program	
Stage III: subacute phase	
Cryokinetic program	Restore ROM except inversion
Consider adding other modalities	Control edema
Program weight-bearing	Resolve effusion
Increase ROM: avoid inversion	Progress strengthening
Isometric progressed to isotonic work	Gain full weight-bearing
Increased cardiovascular exercises	
Use ankle wedge and resisted exercises	
Supply with ankle orthosis	
Stage IV: rapid progression	
Add more resistance exercises	Gain full ROM and strength
Skipping and hopping	Restore "spring" in gait
Attempt to restore full ROM	Maintain fitness
Commence proprioceptive work	
Running on rebounder	
Stage V: final rehabilitation	
Modalities to resolve chronic effusion	Restore full strength and ROM
Mobilization to restore joint play	Restore proprioception
Increase strengthening	Return to activity safely
Add running forward and backward	
Starts and stops	
Figure-of-eights and wind sprints	
Functional assessment	
Establish home program	

ROM = range of motion.

injuries, the use of either a brace or a semirigid lace-up orthosis may be considered.[36,37] Off-the-shelf models and "air-inflated" splints are excellent functional substitutes for the plaster cast (Table 9-7).

Specific Treatment of Ankle Sprains

Success in the treatment of ankle injuries depends on the patient pursuing the exercise program rigorously over a long period as well as reacting appropriately to signs of overstress. The key to therapy is to get the patient to understand and respond to the treatment principles rather than to any absolute guidelines. Thus the two elements of successful therapy must be reiterated: (1) the main role of the therapist is that of teacher and educator, inspiring understanding and enthusiasm; and (2) the most potent therapeutic tool is invariably a well thought out, controlled, and faithfully adhered to exercise regimen (Table 9-8).

Grade I Sprains

Grade I sprains are mild injuries that produce pain lasting a few minutes to a few days. Frequently they do not require specific therapy and, in their mildest form, allow rapid resumption of activity with little or no detectable swelling. As they approach the severity of a second degree injury, early application of ice and pressure, protected weight-bearing, and a follow-up strengthening program assume more importance. Occasionally, NSAIDs speed recovery when rapid return to sport is required. It is wise to protect the ankle with taping or a brace for pivoting sports such as basketball, football, squash, or soccer for about 6 weeks to prevent reinjury. At the more severe end of the scale, they are treated as a grade II sprain.

Grade II Sprains

Although a moderate degree of anterior draw may be present with the severe grade II injury, these sprains may essentially be considered stable. A program is outlined in detail below for a sprain on the more severe end of this broad spectrum of injury (Table 9-8). It may be modified to suit the patient's pathology, age, occupation, and recreational needs.

Stage I: Immediately After Injury

Immediate application of ice and compression with the ankle elevated ensures minimum recovery time by minimizing edema and hemorrhage. An ice pack with a wrap may be used by the side of the playing area. It may be replaced with an open Gibney tape supple-

mented with a donut pad around the malleoli (Fig. 9-11). Within the first few hours, minimal weight-bearing using crutches is encouraged, with elevation at every opportunity. While at home, the athlete can apply bags of frozen peas for one or two 20 minute sessions in each hour, using a muslin or flannel wrap to maintain at least the neutral position or gain dorsiflexion. This step is important to allow more comfortable weight-bearing and prevent rapid heel cord tightening. This treatment may be supplemented by the early use of NSAIDs.

Stage II: Acute Phase

The acute phase of inflammation lasts several days, and continuation of the ice routine is important. Ice baths or a whirlpool bath may be used but only with continuous, gentle, active motion of the ankle to counteract the tendency for dependent edema. Pneumatic compression devices are useful, followed by active range of motion in dorsi- and plantar flexion and eversion but avoiding inversion (Fig. 9-10). Autoassisted work may be initiated. Resisted work is not started until at least 50 percent of body weight can be taken comfortably using crutches. This may be judged by pushing down on a scale. Start work on a program to maintain cardiovascular ability (Table 9-8).

Stage III: Subacute Phase

Depending on the severity, the subacute stage begins at 48 hours to 5 days after injury. The key to relieving pain is to decrease the edema and effusion and maintain or gain dorsiflexion. Some therapists may wish to continue with a cryokinetic program using ice whirlpools supplemented by a home routine using the application of frozen bags of food for 10 minutes before and after exercise (Fig. 9-17). Ultrasound, hot and cold contrast baths, and interferential current therapy may be used early during this stage and minimal thermal shortwave diathermy toward the end. NSAIDs are effective, but it is doubtful if local or systemic enzymes add to resolution.

The duration and speed of progress is often related to the degree of intra-articular contusion, hemorrhage, or effusion. Significant extra-articular edema adds to the morbidity.

The main aim during this period is to progress the weight-bearing and resisted exercises while minimizing and dispersing edema. This stage may last 5 to 14 days and terminates when the patient is able to gently hop.

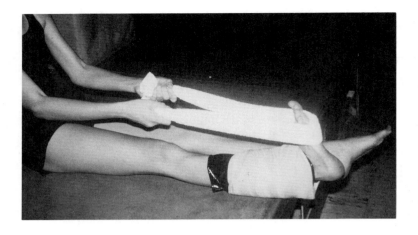

Fig. 9-17. Ice packs with autoassisted motion may be begun early and continued throughout the rehabilitation. More encircling ice bags and elevation are used during the acute stage.

Range of motion is emphasized using elastic tubing as a foot stirrup and a wedge board. The calf stretch position should be used frequently, holding for 6 to 10 seconds for 15 to 20 repetitions, at least three times daily (Fig. 9-18).[38] When there is adequate range of motion, the static cycle may be used to enhance cardiovascular fitness. Similarly, water-running without contact with the bottom is useful.

Strengthening progresses from isometric to isotonic as pain permits. At no time during this stage should inversion be mobilized, although the tibialis anterior may be exercised isometrically. For the most part, the range of motion work is given in sets of 15 to 20, with slow, steady holds at the extremes of the range.[39] The active calf and everted work are done slowly, using 10 to 15 repetitions with holds at the points of maximum contraction. The most useful equipment for evertor strengthening at this stage is rubber tubing, dental dam, or the commercially available Theraband.

At this stage some form of ankle brace should be supplied to prevent reinjury. It is useful initially for support and then for protection during the remaining season while continued strengthening work is completed (Fig. 9-13). A second sprain at this stage would set the scene for recurrent problems, so use of a brace is both cost-effective and warranted.

Stage IV: Rapid Progression

The ability to hop indicates that the athlete is capable of sustaining forces of several times body weight and hence is ready to progress both strengthening and activities[40] (Fig. 9-19). Resisted isotonic invertor work can now be done without the initial concern of stretching out the healing ligament. The use of resistance apparatus, such as the Elgin ankle exerciser,

isokinetic machines, and free weights is indicated. An important feature in rehabilitation is regaining the rebounding type of motion in the foot; skipping is one of the best activities to reestablish this ability. The emphasis on proprioceptive work using balance boards is simultaneously an excellent method of strengthening[41-43] (Fig. 9-20). Balance, proprioception and coordination are combined in a set of exercises popularized by Mattison[41] (Figs. 9-21 and 9-22).

Ultrasound and laser are important modalities for reducing chronic thickening. Gentle mobilization of the proximal and distal fibula and the subtalar joint are begun (Figs. 9-23 through 9-26). Running may be commenced, and by the end of this stage the normal "spring" should have been restored to walking, any limp eliminated, and at least 80 percent of strength returned. The "shuttle" exercises and rebounder, as

---

Clinical Point

ACTIVITY PROGRESSION

- Heel-toe walking
- Balance board work
- Rope skipping
- Jogging
- Running forward, progressing speed
- Backward running
- Running curves and circles
- Running zigzags (45 degree cuts)
- Wind sprints (90 degree cuts and decelerations)

Program rate guided by swelling, pain, ROM

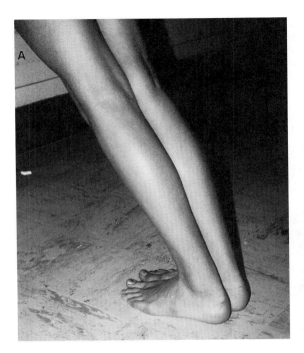
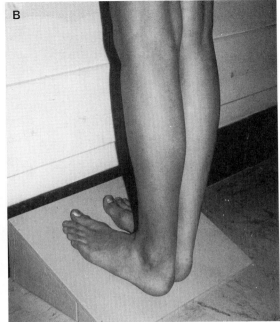
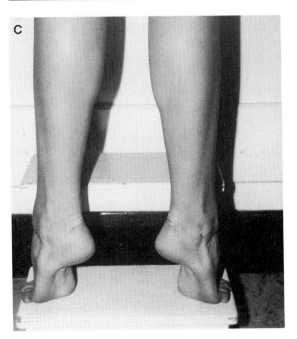

Fig. 9-18. Calf and ankle stretching progressed from **(A)** flat with or without knees bent, **(B)** on wedge, and **(C)** combined with strengthening heel raise exercises.

well as a treadmill with progressive speed and incline are useful (Fig. 9-27).

Stage V: Final Rehabilitation

Stage V may be reached as early as 2 to 3 weeks, but it usually takes longer; this period is used to prepare the athlete for return to full activity. Running is pro-

gressed to include sudden accelerations and decelerations, turning, cutting, jumping, and landing.

Talocrural and subtalar range and fibula movement are carefully assessed to ensure full establishment of joint play and normal movement patterns. Full dorsiflexion is essential before discharge. The evertor/invertor ratio should be balanced at approximately 80 percent[44] (Table 9-9). Full restoration of

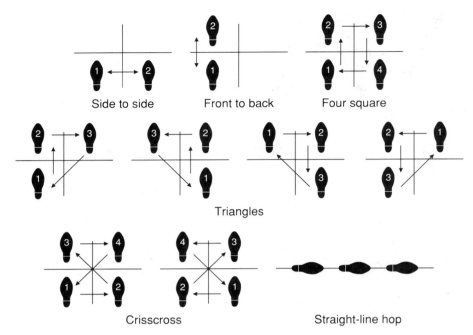

Side to side   Front to back   Four square

Triangles

Crisscross   Straight-line hop

Fig. 9-19. Eight basic hopping patterns as described by Toomey.[40] Arrow indicates the direction the athlete hops. The straight line and zig zag hops are performed forward and backwards across a 15–20 foot straight line.

power is delayed in some individuals, so the value of a good home program cannot be overstressed (Table 9-7).

Grade III Sprains

A grade III sprain is by definition an unstable one, with involvement of two ligaments. Nevertheless, there has been a gradual swing from operative to nonoperative treatment. For the average recreational athlete, there is a limited place for early surgical intervention.

The most conservative method includes 3 to 6 weeks of immobilization by a short leg (below knee) cast, progressing weight-bearing as tolerated. This step is followed by an elastic support at cast removal and gradual rehabilitation of range of motion and strength. Although this method may provide the longest interval to full recovery, it is the safest for the noncompliant patient. Long-term follow-up has shown elimination of significant talar tilt in 79 percent of patients; and 89 percent were satisfied with the functional outcomes.[44-46] Brand et al. reported slightly less encouraging figures, suggesting that 20 to 40 percent of patients have functional instability.[47]

These physicians used this finding as a rationale for early operative intervention; however, some of the poor results probably reflected inadequate therapy rather than the initial method of treatment. Evans et al. noted that at 2 years there was no significant difference between a surgically treated group and a group treated more conservatively, the results being evaluated in terms of the radiologically detectable

---

Practice Point

TREATMENT OPTIONS FOR UNSTABLE (GRADE III) ANKLE SPRAINS

- Below-knee cast for 10 to 14 days, then brace
- Taping followed by brace
- Tensor and brace from beginning
- Early surgical repair plus cast
- Early surgical repair with brace
- Below-knee cast for 3 to 6 weeks

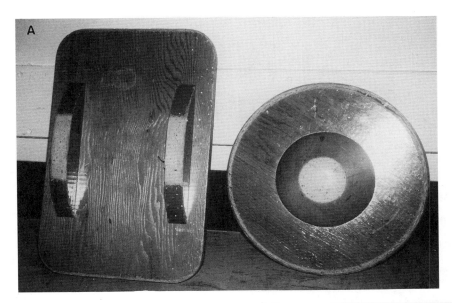

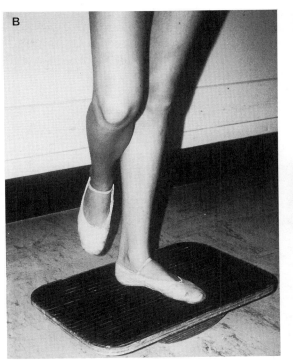

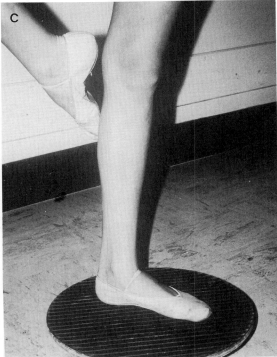

Fig. 9-20. Balance boards. **(A)** Different shapes and heights give varying stresses. **(B)** Exercises are started on the unidirectional board. The patient is progressed with double support to single leg exercises. They also stand at different angles to the axis of motion to influence different muscles. **(C)** Multidirectional board. Exercises include various positions as well as bouncing, throwing, and catching a ball. Positions may be maintained with eyes open and closed which further influence proprioception.

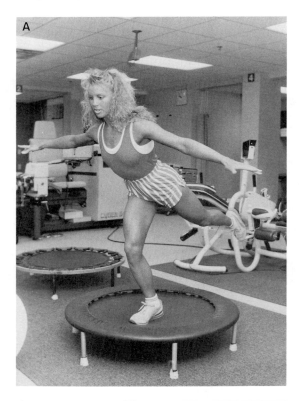

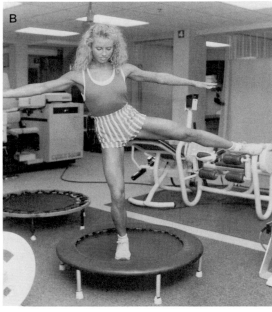

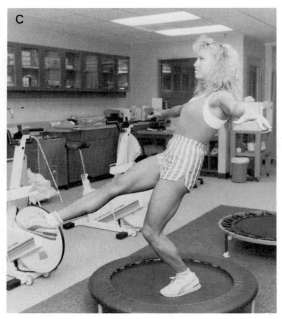

Fig. 9-21. Balance and strength exercises. They may be done directly on a firm surface or on a rebounder, which increases their complexity. **(A)** The "747" exercise. Attempt to hold trunk and arms parallel to the floor. **(B)** Spokes. Arm and leg are raised parallel to the floor. May be combined with side flexing. **(C)** Reverse "747" exercise. The leg is raised forward. An attempt is made to keep the body vertical. It is done more easily on the floor than on the rebounder. All exercises are held initially for 20 seconds on each leg and progress to 30 seconds. Concentrate on stability at the extremes of motion.

talar tilt.[48] They therefore suggested that the symptoms of late functional instability are not always due to talar tilt.

A more progressive method of treatment has been reported by Cox and Brand.[49,50] They compared a regimen that included a cast for 3 weeks followed by therapy versus taping, early weight-bearing, and aggressive therapy. Their patients had severe grade II and III injuries confirmed by arthrograms or peroneal sheath arthrography. At the end of treatment,

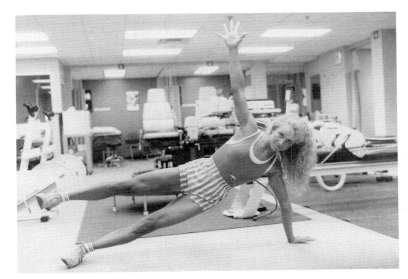

Fig. 9-22. "Devlin" exercise. Balancing on the ipsilateral foot and hand. By balancing on the lateral foot, strong evertor work is required. Keep body straight. Hold for 20 to 30 seconds.

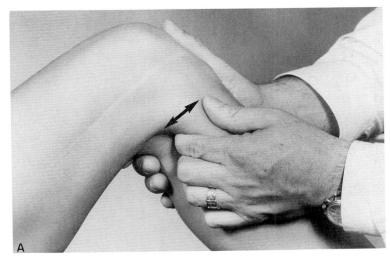

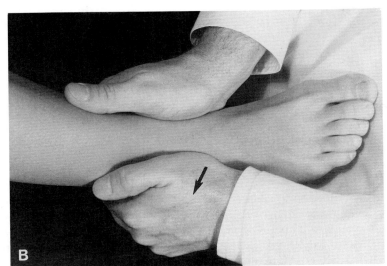

Fig. 9-23. Mobilization of fibula. **(A)** Proximal anteroposterior glide. **(B)** Distal lateral malleolar planar glide.

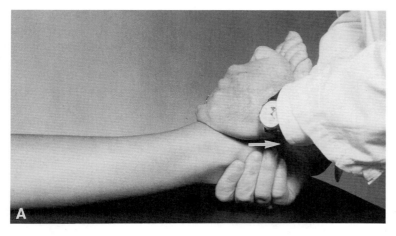

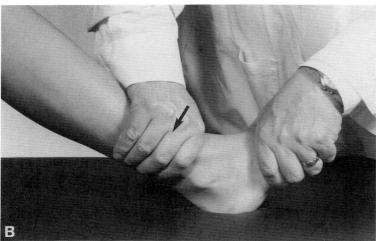

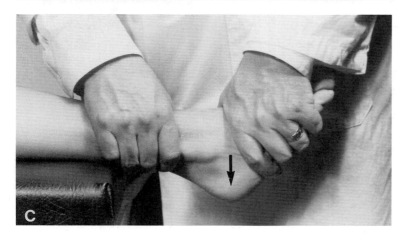

Fig. 9-24. Talocrural mobilization. **(A)** Distraction. **(B)** Posterior glide using the heel as a fulcrum. **(C)** Posterior glide of talus using the tibia as a fulcrum (supine).

the talar tilt was dramatically reduced but not normal; however, the incidence of recurrent sprains was minimal in an 8 to 24 month follow-up.[49]

The initial support may be made slightly more rigid by using an Unna Boot made of Dome-Paste bandage.

This impregnated bandage sets, providing a compromise between taping and casting. Alternatively a soft cast (3M) may be used.

Advocates of surgery suggest that only a good repair of the damaged tissue provides mechanical sta-

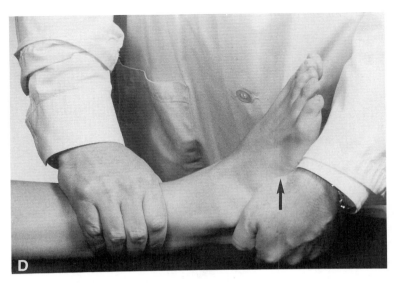

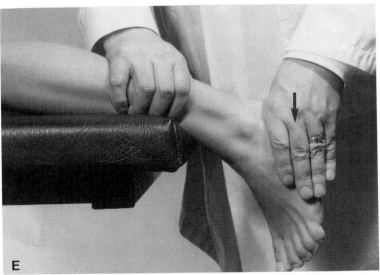

Fig. 9-24 *(Continued).* **(D)** Anterior glide of talus using tibia as a fulcrum (supine). **(E)** Anterior glide using tibia fixated (prone).

bility, and that early surgery is less extensive and more anatomic than late reconstruction. However, Freeman suggested that a comparison of surgery versus early mobilization had similar results in terms of instability, and that the overall return to activity and employment was more rapid among the nonoperative group.[51] Despite only 55 percent versus 25 percent being symptom-free at 1 year, Freeman concluded that mobilization was the treatment of choice, regardless of the severity of injury.[51]

Brostrom's work is probably that most frequently cited in the literature; he compared primary surgical repair, plaster cast immobilization, and early motion with strapping.[52] He essentially agreed with Freeman

that early motion gave the most rapid return to function, but there were likely to be more late symptoms, which he correlated with the magnitude of the anterior drawer. Nevertheless, because of the success of late reconstruction when necessary, he thought that strapping was the treatment of choice except in highly competitive individuals, whose activities required perfect ankle function. He did stress the need of at least 20 weeks for good healing and therefore the need for continued protection during activities.[52]

My approach to these severe sprains is to tape with an open Gibney supplemented with horseshoe pads initially to reduce edema. This step is followed by application of a Mikros ankle brace or Air Stirrup for

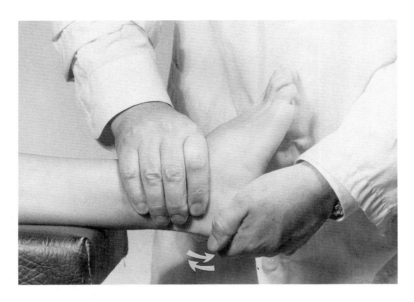

Fig. 9-25. Subtalar distraction and calcaneal rocking into inversion and eversion.

the first 7 to 10 days (Fig. 9-13). Only light partial weight-bearing is advised to allow joint damage to settle, and it is then progressed toward the end of this period as tolerated. When this regimen is not logistically possible, a plaster cast is applied for the first 2 weeks. After the initial period of strapping or casting, weight-bearing and activity are progressed using a brace over a double Tubigrip elastic stocking for another 4 weeks, at which time use of the brace is gradually discontinued except for athletic activity. The pa-

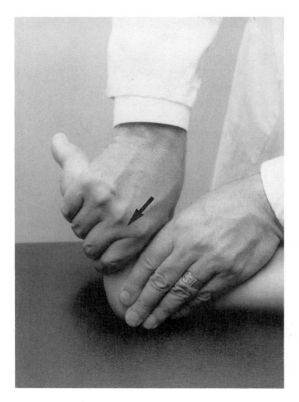

Fig. 9-26. Midtarsal joints. Dorsal and plantar talonavicular glide. Stabilize the talus and move the navicular in a dorsal and plantar direction. The hand position can be moved to grasp calcaneus and glide the cuboid.

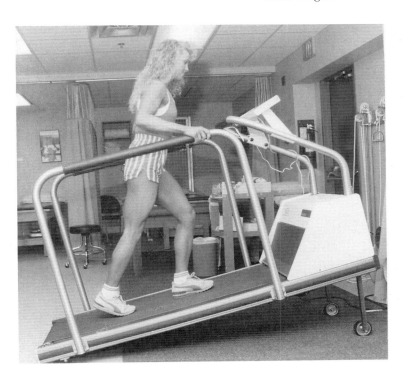

Fig. 9-27. Using the treadmill to increase running speed and introducing inclines allows a controlled method for increasing stress through the ankle.

tient is urged to use the brace for sport for the remainder of the season. The success of this program depends on excellent therapy and good patient compliance with the bracing and exercise program.

Van den Hoogenband et al., in a randomized prospective study, compared surgical repair followed by casting with casting with no repair and elastic strapping for 6 weeks.[53] There was little long-term instability in any of the groups and an early return to employment and sport in the group treated by functional means—results that support my approach outlined above. Addition of the air splint or brace allows more comfort, extra protection, and avoidance of the potential complications that accompany 6 weeks of taping.

Surgery is offered as an option but is not necessarily recommended in highly competitive individuals who have an absolute requirement for a maximally stable ankle and who have received a severe grade III injury, with obvious disruption of the whole anterior capsule as well as the anterior and lateral bands. In this case, a stress roentgenogram or arthrogram helps to delineate the magnitude of the disruption. The phase of the athlete's training or season may also influence this decision. Surgery is strongly recommended for the acute injury only if a bony ossicle is seen displaced within the joint, if a large fragment is avulsed off the lateral malleolus, or if there is a large or displaced osteochondral lesion off the talus. Even Brand et al., who recommended surgery for the above reasons, plus a severe talar tilt, operated on only 12 percent of their patients, 50 percent of whom had a talar tilt of more than 30 degrees.[50] At a mean follow-up of 11 months, Brand et al. claimed 98 percent satisfactory results with surgery. It is my experience that the best surgical results are obtained when early controlled motion is allowed. It is achieved by either a hinged cast or a rigid leg brace with a removable panel for physiotherapy. Motion must be allowed only in

TABLE 9-9. Isokinetic Evaluation of Invertors and Evertors in Adults

Degrees	Male		Female		Relative	
	In.	Ev.	In.	Ev.	In.	Ev.
30	24	20	18	14	14	12
60	20	18	15	12	12	10
120	17	14	12	10	10	8

In = invertors; Ev. = evertors.
Evertor/invertor ratio = 80 percent.
(From Wong et al.,[44] with permission.)

TABLE 9-10.   **Functional Rating Scale for Ankles**

Condition	Score
Pain	
Never hurts	5
Hurts with strenuous sports	4
Hurts with light sports	3
Hurts walking more than 5 km	2
Hurts walking less than 5 km	1
Hurts at rest or at night	0
Stability	
Never turns (no support)	5
Turns occasionally (support)	4
Turns occasionally (no support)	3
Turns frequently during daily living activities	0
Stiffness	
Never stiff	2
Stiff until warmed up	1
Stiff at all times	0
Swelling	
Never swells	2
End of day or after activity	1
Swells most of time	0
Activity	
Able to hop	2
Not as good as normal side	1
Cannot hop	0
Range of motion	
Full range of motion	4
Full plantar flexion, limited dorsiflexion	2
Limited dorsi- and plantar flexion	0

(From Seligson et al.,[55] with permission.)

dorsi- and plantar flexion until good ligament healing is achieved.[54]

The functional outcomes of these treatments may best be assessed by means of a scale modified from Seligson et al.[55] (Table 9-10).

DELAYED RECOVERY FROM ANKLE SPRAINS

Most of the continuing symptoms following a sprained ankle are directly related to ligament damage. The magnitude of the problem is difficult to assess, but Staples reported that only 59 percent of individuals were completely well at an average 9 years' follow-up.[56] However, many of the problems were minor. Incomplete or absence of rehabilitation may have played a role. The main causes are functional instability, stiffness due to loss of fibula and subtalar motion, a tight, sensitive scar, and incomplete reha-

bilitation. These factors, along with chronic synovitis, soft tissue impingement, nerve traction injury, osteochondral fracture, exostosis, and dislocating peroneal tendons, may be directly or indirectly related to ligament damage[57,58] (Table 9-11). However, there are many other causes for prolonged disability related indirectly to, or confused with, ankle sprains that must be considered. Thus nonligamentous causes for persistent symptoms should be considered if problems continue despite adequate therapy. Some of the more common conditions are discussed in detail below.

Functional Instability

One of the primary goals of treatment is the prevention of long-term functional instability. Brand et al. reviewed a large number of naval recruits with "trick" ankles that were characterized by frequent sprains and difficulty when jumping, cutting, or run-

TABLE 9-11. Conditions Causing Delayed Recovery from Ankle Sprains

Problems directly related to ligament damage
  Functional instability
  Loss of fibular and subtalar motion
  Tight sensitive scar
  Incomplete rehabilitation

Problems indirectly related to ligament damage
  Chronic synovitis
  Soft tissue impingement
  Nerve traction injury
  Exostosis from tibia and talus
  Avulsion fragments from malleoli
  Osteochondral fracture or loose body
  Interosseous membrane ossification
  Dislocating peroneal tendons
  Degenerative joint changes
  Reflex sympathetic dystrophy
  Unrecognized tibiofibular diastasis

Conditions confused with a sprain
  Ankle fracture
  Ankle dislocation
  Fracture base fifth metatarsal
  Fracture anterior process of calcaneus
  Stress fractures
  Peroneal tendinitis
  Rupture of tibialis posterior tendon
  Symptomatic os trigonum
  Posterior talar fracture

ning on uneven surfaces.[50] The most obvious cause would be post-traumatic laxity, which is certainly the cause in individuals with a talar tilt of more than 10 degrees difference between the two sides. Lesser laxity does not seem to correlate with symptoms; yet these individuals occasionally have marked instability[58] (Table 9-12). Hence other factors must come into play, the most likely being muscle weakness, poor proprioceptive control, and pain inhibition secondary to impingement or peroneal tendon subluxation. Some of these factors represent inadequate rehabili-

tation. In this regard, increasing functional instability with time may represent the seemingly incompatible coexistence of ligamentous laxity and stiffness that has been alluded to before. Subtalar stiffness and loss of motion easily ensues from post-traumatic edema, particularly when cast immobilization has been the treatment of choice. Failure to restore this subtalar motion throws increasing stress on the talocrural joint during all cutting and turning movements, gradually contributing to further stretching of already lengthened ligaments.[59]

TABLE 9-12. Relation Between Functional and Mechanical Instability*

Anterior drawer sign	No. of Patients	Functional Instability (No. of pts)	
		Absent	Present
Positive	184	118	66 (36%)
Negative	704	611	93 (13%)
Total	888	729	159 (18%)

* As indicated by the anterior drawer sign.

Although tests of lateral talar tilt may be normal, mechanical instability cannot be ruled out until the absence of an anterior drawer sign is demonstrated. Broström et al. showed that 83 percent of patients with ankle instability had a positive anterior drawer sign.[59,60]

Clinical Point

FUNCTIONAL INSTABILITY

- Symptoms
  - Frequent giving way and sprains
  - Difficulty running on uneven surfaces
  - Difficulty jumping and cutting
  - Chronic swelling
- Causes
  - Ligamentous laxity
  - Talar tilt more than 10 degrees between sides
  - Positive anterior talar drawer
  - Peroneal muscle weakness
  - Poor proprioceptive control
  - Nerve injury with initial sprain
  - Subluxing peroneal tendons
  - Pain secondary to impingement

Bosien et al. in 1955 was the first to deal with long-term problems, stating that 43 percent of patients with residual detectable instability had ankle symptoms and fully 66 percent had peroneal weakness.[61] In 1965 Freeman et al. used a modified Rhomberg test to define the possible association of a proprioceptive deficit in patients with functional instability.[43] They postulated that significant ligament trauma would damage sensory nerve endings and produce a situation where there was inadequate biofeedback from the joint. Of those individuals with functional instability, 34 percent had a positive test that was dramatically reduced to 7 percent after therapy. Following lidocaine injection to anesthetize the anterior talofibular ligament, the balance time increases, as measured by a multiaxial balance evaluator.[43]

There is also a learning curve that demonstrates some improvement with training and a tendency to delayed peroneal motor response and exaggerated angular displacement on sudden inversion stress with a modified force platform during the first few months after injury.[62] The inability to maintain postural equilibrium, as measured by computerized force plate stabilometry, correlated with functional instability but not with mechanical instability.[58,63] These studies lend some support to Freeman's postulate on altered neural responses. However, the results could also be interpreted to indicate peroneal muscle weakness instead of inadequate feedback. Indeed, improvement in all these parameters after therapy correlate well with improved strength.

Functional instability is not merely a painful, inconvenient symptom, as it increases the possibility of degenerative changes at the ankle, particularly if associated with demonstrable mechanical instability. Degenerative changes have been demonstrated on roentgenograms of at least 75 percent of individuals with significant functional instability and were confirmed at arthroscopic surgery in many.[64] Therefore these symptoms must be taken seriously, and definition of the underlying cause using physical examination, muscle testing, roentgenography, tomography, and CT scanning must be attempted so appropriate therapy may be instituted.

The mainstay of therapy is strengthening of the peroneal muscle group. With extensive use of balance routines, balance boards, and other functional apparatus, the dual requirements of training proprioceptive and increasing muscle power may be met (Figs. 9-20 and 9-21). In my opinion, however, the strengthening component is largely responsible for the overall functional improvement. This program is supplemented by the use of an ankle brace for activity, as repeated episodes of giving way and pain cause significant reflex inhibition and wasting, and they negate training efforts. Taping may be used when experienced assistance and the resources to pay for the long-term use of a tape are available.

Unfortunately, despite excellent treatment, some individuals develop severe, recurrent instability of the ankle that does not respond to exercise techniques and is too severe for treatment with an ankle orthosis. These people require reconstructive surgery of their ankle ligaments.

There are many approaches to surgical stabilization of the ankle, including direct suturing of damaged ligaments, complex rerouting of tendons to mimic the function of the anterior and lateral bands of the ligament, or simple use of the peroneus brevis to substitute for the lateral ligament (Evans repair).[65,66] The functional outcomes of the modified Evans procedure at the 5-year follow up gives "excel-

TABLE 9-13. Functional Outcomes of Late Reconstruction of Ankle Ligaments

Parameter	Evans Vainionpaa et al.[68] (n = 60)	Evans Ottosson[67] (n = 33)	Direct Suture Bronstöm[66] (n = 60)	Watson Jones Vrevc & Sirnik[69] (n = 14)
Good result (%)	87	91	85	86
Mean age	28	33	26	—
Mean follow-up (years)	5.2	5.0	2.9	—
Limitation of supination (degrees)	25	69	—	36
Swelling (%)	6.6	33.3	6.6	7.1
Subsequent sprains (%)	6.6	18.2	6.6	7.1
Discomfort with activity (%)	5.0	15.2	6.6	—

lent'' and ''good'' ratings in nearly 90 percent of individuals.[67,68] This procedure prevents talar tilt, gives good anteroposterior stability, and compares favorably with the more complicated reconstructions[69-71] (Table 9-13). The peroneus brevis has been shown to be a suitably strong substitute for the lateral ligament, and even a split-thickness graft may be adequate.[72] Furthermore, the surgical loss of the peroneus brevis muscle does not appear to result in a significant loss of eversion strength and power with isokinetic evaluation in 1 to 11 year follow-ups.[68,73] These facts, along with my experience of excellent functional outcomes, leads to a recommendation of the modified Evans procedure as the treatment of choice for late instability that does not respond to nonoperative therapy.

Peroneal Nerve and Tibial Injury

Occasionally, an ankle sprain is associated with a permanent footdrop secondary to traction or a hematoma in the epineural sheath.[74,75] Fortunately, this dramatic complication is rare. The peroneal nerve moves 5 to 8 mm during full inversion; and during forced inversion this traction is associated with a compression effect of the peroneus longus muscle closing over the nerve, pushing it against the bone. This effect is magnified by associated plantar flexion.

Bosien et al. suggested that partial peroneal nerve palsy may play a role in patients with residual symptoms from acute ankle sprains.[61] Nitz et al. demonstrated electromyographically that more than 10 percent of patients with grade II and more than 80 percent with grade III injuries had changes compatible with denervation.[74] They involved the peroneal and tibial nerve. For the most part these lesions were subclinical, but it is easy to see how they would contribute to early reinjury, peroneal muscle weakness, incomplete rehabilitation, and eventually significant long-term damage to other structures so that by the

time neural recovery is complete chronic instability has been established.

Also described is a peroneal entrapment neuropathy at the fibular neck, called the fibular tunnel syndrome, which is usually due to a direct blow.[75] Sometimes the onset of paralysis is delayed and is due to an intraneural hematoma. The diagnostic clue to this entity is often a preceding interval of intense neuritic pain.

All of these lesions have a good prognosis for full neural recovery, and surgical exploration should be reserved for atypical cases with no evidence of reinnervation. It is important to be aware of the potential for these injuries with the associated ankle sprain; if there is a significant detectable weakness or footdrop, protection with a cast, splint, or orthosis may be necessary until recovery is evident. The therapist should particularly be aware of, and look for, undue peroneal muscle weakness after resolution of the initial intense pain and swelling.

Clinical Point

NERVE INJURY WITH ANKLE SPRAINS

- Grade II
  - Peroneal nerve 17%
  - Tibial nerve 10%
- Grade III
  - Peroneal nerve 86%
  - Tibial nerve 83%

- Possibly mild traction or hematoma
- May appear clinically normal
- May prolong rehabilitation
- Contributes to functional instability
- Test carefully before return to activity

Subluxing Peroneal Tendon

Monteggia's description of a dislocating peroneal tendon in a ballet dancer in 1803 is probably the first in the literature.[76] The condition occasionally occurs spontaneously owing to anatomic variations of the bony groove and surrounding collagen, but invariably the precipitating event is an ankle sprain. It is important to try to identify this anterior subluxation of the peroneal tendons from the posterior sulcus of the fibula during the acute phases, as it is better treated nonoperatively at this stage.

The athlete may present with symptoms of pain, swelling, or a sensation of "popping" or "snapping" around the lateral malleolus. The latter is often associated with functional instability (Fig. 9-28).

Examination reveals tenderness along the peroneal sheath posterior to the fibular malleolus, with prominence of the sheath demonstrated by resisted dorsiflexion with eversion. However, there are great variations in the normal degree of laxity, and it may be difficult to confirm the dislocation clinically without the dynamics of weight-bearing motion and muscle contraction. The diagnosis is easy when a painful snapping is demonstrated. Plain films occasionally reveal a small, shell-like avulsion of the lateral malleolus. Chronic cases may be defined on computed tomography (CT) scans, where a shallow sulcus or abnormally positioned tendon are more obvious. Approximately 80 percent of normals have a definite sulcus, with the remainder being either flat or even convex.

The nonoperative treatment is directed at treating both the mechanical subluxation and the frequently associated peroneal tendinitis. Acutely inflamed tendons respond to NSAIDs and local therapy with ultrasound, laser, or interferential currents. Taping, elastic anklets, and progressive range of motion may help the mechanical problem. The greater the subluxation, the less is the chance of success with these routines. Severely dislocating tendons require surgery in approximately 40 percent of cases if a high level of activity is to be continued.[76]

There are numerous operative approaches including soft tissue reconstruction of the peroneal sheaths, transferring the lateral band of the lateral ligament with a bone block to cover the tendon, or sliding a shelf of fibula posteriorly to deepen the groove. Executed well, most of the procedures give a satisfactory outcome.

Stenosing Peroneal Tenosynovitis (Tenovaginitis)

An uncommon cause of functional lateral instability is stenosing peroneal tendinitis. The patient complains mainly of pain on the outer side of the ankle that is aggravated by exercises and relieved by rest.[76] The physical findings may be ill-defined. The tenderness is along the peroneal sheath and is made worse with active and passive motion. No mechanical instability is present. Occasionally, crepitus is felt.

Stenosing peroneal tenosynovitis has been associated with inversion injuries, fractures of the os calcis or ankle, or simply overuse. Patients with chronic, diffuse complaints related to the lateral malleolar area, sometimes associated with functional instability, should be suspected of having this syndrome. Peroneal tenography may help define the pathology.

Initial treatment is directed at mobilizing the tendon in its sheath with friction, followed by NSAIDs and ultrasound. Failure to respond to adequate modification of activity and intensive therapy may serve as an indication for surgical exploration of the sheath.

The sheath is divided, which is often thickened with constriction of the peroneal tendon and a bulbous enlargement proximal to the sheath.[76] Histologic examination of a specimen of the sheath may demonstrate some myxomatous degeneration. Postoperatively, early, gentle, active motion is encouraged, with a gradual increase in weight-bearing and intensity of exercise. An intense buildup of training should be delayed for about 6 weeks.

Tibiofibular Synostosis

Fibular motion during activity may be restricted by post-traumatic distal tibiofibular synostosis secondary to interosseous membrane damage and distal tibiofibular ligament injury[57] (Fig. 9-29). Although usually secondary to an ankle fracture, it may occur with an ankle sprain, particularly if there has been an element of diastasis.

The most frequent presenting complaints are chronic pain and swelling after activity. The discomfort is often most severe during push-off. Dorsiflexion may be limited to the neutral position. These symptoms are not surprising in view of the important

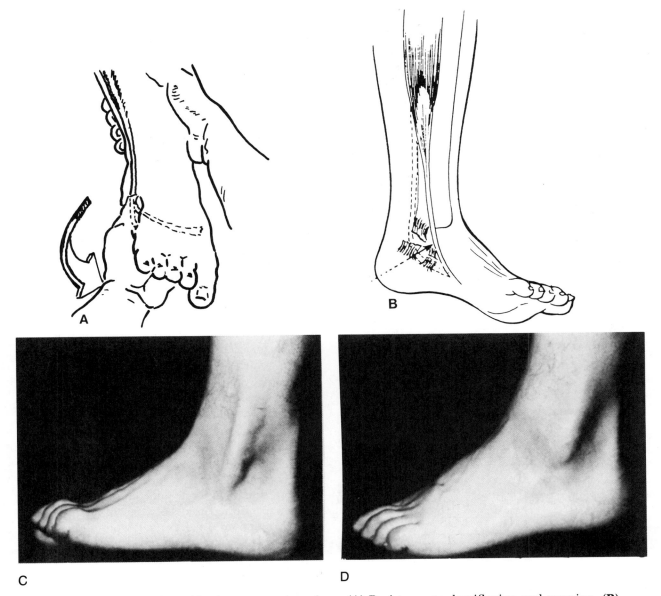

Fig. 9-28. Testing for subluxing peroneal tendons. **(A)** Resistance to dorsiflexion and eversion. **(B)** The tendon snaps over the malleolus (acute tear). **(C)** Chronic spontaneous subluxation. **(D)** Reduction.

role of the fibula in sharing up to 15 percent of the weight-bearing duties, as well as its important stabilizing function in providing dynamic control.[8–10]

The clinical differential diagnosis includes all of the impingement syndromes. The radiologic appearance of a bony mass between the two bones is conclusive so long as it is differentiated from an osteochondroma, which not infrequently is found at this site. Prolonged symptoms may require excision of the bony mass as a definitive treatment if athletes are unwilling to totally modify their activities. Occasionally, even everyday activities are a problem with this condition, so surgery still may be required when activity modification is unsuccessful.

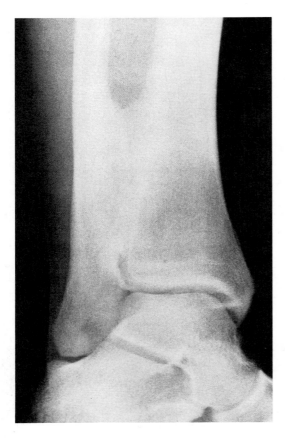

Fig. 9-29. Tibiofibular synostosis subsequent to diastasis of the tibiofibular joint and disruption of the interosseous membrane.

TRANSCHONDRAL FRACTURES OF THE TALUS (OSTEOCHONDRITIS DISSECANS)

Osteochondral lesions of the dome of the talus are uncommon, accounting for only 4 percent of all osteochondritis lesions and 0.9 percent of all fractures.[77] The true incidence, of course, is unknown because usually only symptomatic lesions are detected and, surprisingly, even they are not always revealed by standard diagnostic techniques.

Etiology

In 1959 Berndt and Hardy suggested that trauma was the only significant factor in the development of these lesions, and the term transchondral fracture has been adopted.[78] In cadaver studies they produced lateral lesions with inversion and dorsiflexion and medial lesions with inversion, plantar flexion, and lateral rotation of the tibia on the talus. Most investigators accepted this explanation.[79,80] Nevertheless, there is still support for a separate clinical entity of osteochondritis dissecans on an avascular basis.[81] Many lesions are not present on the initial films, and there is probably a spectrum of pathophysiology. At one end of the spectrum are acute shear fractures and traumatic injury, leading to damage of the subchondral vessels, which in turn causes delayed avascular collapse or separation. Perhaps at the other end of the spectrum are cases of idiopathic avascular necrosis, of which the etiology may include systemic and local factors. Inasmuch as careful scrutiny has not shown a greater propensity for any of these proposed lesions to heal differently, further speculation as to cause is not warranted, and the lesion must be dealt with "de novo" according to the symptoms of the patient. The undoubted association with trauma, in many cases, means that a high index of suspicion is important in the differential diagnosis of chronic ankle pain after injury. Such suspicion may help reduce the unacceptable delay in diagnosis of 3 to 192 months, which is frequently discussed in the literature.[77,78,80]

Signs and Symptoms

The major symptoms include a deep aching or pain aggravated by exercise, ankle swelling, occasional crepitus, clicking, true locking, or a catching sensation. The clinical signs include synovial thickening, effusion, and occasional joint line tenderness and stiffness manifested as loss of range of motion in one or both directions. In all cases, symptoms seem to be magnified by activity. With most people, there is a definite past history of an inversion sprain or ankle fracture; occasionally, the lesion is associated with true or functional instability.[80]

Radiology

Radiographically, the lesions are typically seen anterolaterally or posteromedially on the dome of the talus (Fig. 9-30).[81,82] They are classified further as to the degree of separation (Fig. 9-31). Normally, these lesions can be visualized on the routine ankle views, particularly the internal oblique projection. However, sometimes an overpenetrated view of the plantar-flexed ankle (x-ray at 1 meter with 70 kV) may facilitate visualization of the early posteromedial lesion.[81] Tomograms or CT scans allow accurate surgi-

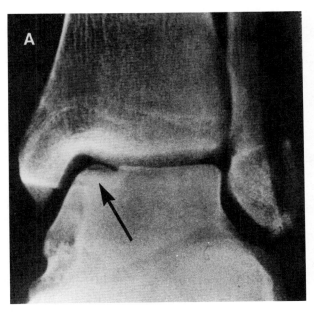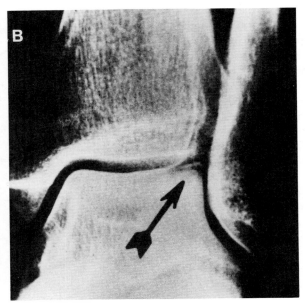

Fig. 9-30. Most frequent sites of transchondral fractures are posteromedial sites **(A)** and anterolateral sites **(B)**. (From Pavlov and Torg,[82] with permission.)

cal planning if insufficient data are obtained from the plain films.

Treatment

The silent nature of many of these lesions means that all definitive surgical treatment must be preceded by a reasonable trial of nonoperative therapy.

Grade I and II lesions may do well with some protected weight-bearing and NSAIDs. In Hagmeyer and Van der Wurff's series, stage I lesions treated nonoperatively were graded "good," whereas stage II lesions were mostly assessed "fair" to "poor"; the good results in stage II patients resulted from surgery.[77] Symptomatic (grade III) lesions are less likely to settle, but a trial of NSAIDs plus activity modifica-

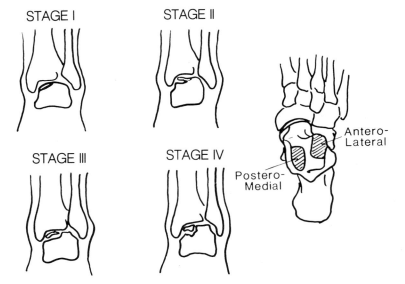

Fig. 9-31. Four stages of osteochondral lesions according to Bernt and Harty. Stage I, a small area of compression; stage II, a partially detached osteochondral fragment; stage III, a completely detached fragment but remaining in situ; and stage IV, a detached, displaced fragment. The common locations on the talar dome are shaded.

tion is worthwhile. If this regimen is unsuccessful, surgery should be recommended.[83] If the patient is reticent to undergo surgery, a patella-bearing, weight-relieving ankle brace worn for 6 weeks to 6 months usually allows the symptoms to resolve. Alternatively, a below knee, non-weight-bearing cast may be used, but it obviously has the disadvantage of allowing muscle wasting and joint stiffness in the competitive athlete. If a cast is used, the period of immobilization should not exceed 6 to 8 weeks. These symptoms may return, however, with increased activity. Canale and Belding thought that medial stage III lesions were more likely to settle with nonoperative treatment than were lateral stage III injuries.[79] The displaced type IV lesion should be operated on promptly if it is symptomatic.

When explaining the surgical options for grade I and II lesions to the patients, it is important to bear in mind the work of McCullough and Venngopal, who reported surprisingly few complications and little evidence of joint degeneration in a 10-year follow-up; their series, however, like most in the literature, was small.[84] Nevertheless, modification of activity may be a viable, preferable, acceptable option for some young athletes. The degree of symptoms, level of competition, and ultimate athletic goals obviously have an impact on the decision about if and when to operate.

Surgical treatment may be directed at removing an undisplaced loose fragment, drilling an "in situ" fragment, or removing a displaced fragment and débridement. Depending on the size and position of the lesion, arthroscopic treatment is possible.[85] The anterolateral lesion is the more amenable, and it may even be possible to drill the bed. It should be stressed, however, that a well performed procedure via arthrotomy is preferable to poorly performed arthroscopy.

In summary, most osteochondritis lesions of the talus follow a definite history of trauma, and the term transchondral fracture is probably more appropriate. Diagnosis is often unduly delayed, and suspicion of this lesion should always be entertained in the athlete complaining of undue prolongation of symptoms of swelling, stiffness, pain proportional to activity or catching and locking of the ankle after an inversion sprain. It is particularly true if these symptoms reappear after an asymptomatic period. The higher the grade of the lesion, the more active the athlete, and the greater the ankle stresses associated with the sport, the less likely is this lesion to settle with nonoperative treatment. Exposure is sometimes difficult, and adequate preoperative radiographic studies, in-

cluding tomograms or a CT scan, are often necessary. Many lesions are accessible to arthroscopic techniques, but it requires considerable experience. A well-planned, open surgical approach may be preferable.

IMPINGEMENT AND ENTRAPMENT SYNDROMES

Talar Anterior Impingement Syndrome

The talar anterior impingement syndrome is related to osteophytes on the neck of the talus or, more frequently, the anterior tibia.[85,86] Dorsiflexion causes impingement of the bony spurs, along with trapping and pinching of hypertrophied and chronically swollen synovium (Fig. 9-32).

These lesions are seen occasionally after repeated ankle inversion injuries and are particularly evident in football linemen, where chronic repeated impingement stresses of the bony surfaces during dorsiflexion play a role in the etiology. Alternatively, the osteophytes may correlate with the tibial and talar attachments of the anterior capsule and may relate to chronic traction stresses seen in runners and soccer players[86] (Fig. 9-32).

The athlete may simply complain of ankle pain and swelling proportional to activities. In mild cases, it occurs only with activities requiring sudden starts and stops or changes in direction, but in severe cases the symptoms occur with simple running or jogging.[87] The feeling of pinching can be reproduced by forced dorsiflexion, and pain is experienced with palpation along the anterior talocrural joint line. Dorsiflexion is eventually limited by bony impingement and pain. Plain lateral roentgenograms help confirm the diagnosis. Support to the theory of chronic traction or compression stresses is lent by the usual absence of degenerative changes within the joint. For this reason, removal of the anterior synovium and resection of the osteophytes is usually all that is needed to relieve symptoms, and most athletes can return to full activity. With a small spur, removal may be possible arthroscopically, but it is usually necessary to open the joint for successful excision of adequate amounts of bone.[88]

Anterolateral Impingement

Wohlin et al.[89] described a series of patients in 1950 who experienced chronic pain and swelling over the anterior and anterolateral ankle with activity.

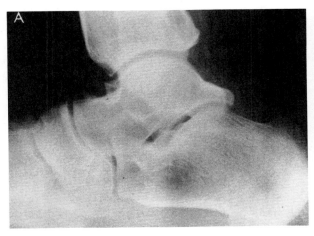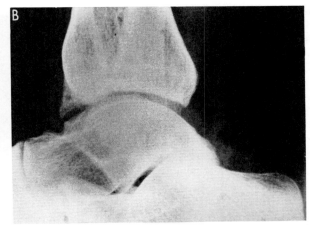

Fig. 9-32. (A) Anterior tibial spur associated with a painful limitation of dorsiflexion. **(B)** Hypertrophic spurs on the dorsal talus at the capsular insertion with normal joint space. (From Pavlov and Torg,[82] with permission.)

Often these symptoms are accompanied by a subjective feeling of instability and occasionally true giving way. There is always a history of a moderately severe ankle injury.

There are two possible etiologic explanations. First, the lesion may be secondary to traumatic synovial thickening, with incomplete resorption of the associated exudate.[89] A small portion of inflammatory infiltrate persists between the fibula and the talus; it then eventually becomes hyalinized secondary to pressure, giving rise to symptoms (Fig. 9-33).

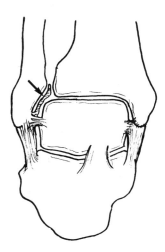

Fig. 9-33. Cross section of the talocrural joint showing a meniscoid lesion that may be related to the lateral ligament. (After McCarroll et al.,[90] with permission.)

Others have suggested that these meniscoid lesions are tears of the anterior tibiofibular ligament in which the torn fragment becomes interposed between the talus and the lateral malleolus.[90]

Although these lesions are rare, it is important to consider this possibility in athletes who have persistent pain and swelling after inversion sprains and in whom all roentgenograms and other diagnostic tests are negative. Arthroscopy reveals the lesion and the hyalinized, meniscoid-like band. Any redundant synovium may then be removed. Excision should cure the symptoms and prevent further joint irritation.

Lateral Talar Chondromalacia

Another syndrome that may be included in the spectrum of the previously described lesions of the ankle is post-traumatic chondromalacia of the lateral wall of the talus, with associated synovial reaction. The athlete complains of pain located over the anteroinferior aspect of the fibula, the associated anterolateral talus, and the joint line. There is usually a history of a single or repeated inversion injuries.

It is suggested that pain and compression at foot strike makes the athlete, usually a runner, tighten the tibialis posterior and anterior tendons and inhibits the peroneal tendons. It makes the runner susceptible to multiple inversion strains. The addition of a medial heel and inner sole wedge to the shoe may relieve impingement sufficiently to allow restoration of balanced inversion and eversion muscle action and relieve symptoms. If the condition does not settle with modified activity, orthosis, and a course of NSAIDs, arthroscopy may be warranted to rule out other causes of the pain.

Posterior Talar Compression Syndrome

Pain in the posterior ankle region may be incapacitating in ballet dancers and soccer players when due to impingement of an os trigonum or Stieda's process[91] (Fig. 9-34). This diagnosis is one of exclusion in many instances—after Achilles tendinitis, peroneal tendinitis, and flexor hallucis longus tendinitis have been ruled out.

First described in 1804, the os trigonum is present in at least 5 percent of feet, and as many as 38 percent of the adult population have an enlarged lateral process in the posterior surface of the talus.[88] It is therefore frequently present as an asymptomatic structure. Caution is warranted in oversubscribing symptoms to this normal anatomic variant. McDougall[91] proposed three mechanisms for development of the os trigonum: (1) failure of fusion of the secondary ossification center; (2) repeated minor trauma with impingement against the posterior margin of the tibia; and (3) an acute fracture due to forced plantar flexion, occasionally in association

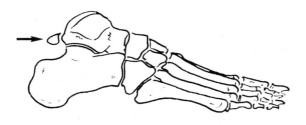

Os Trigonum

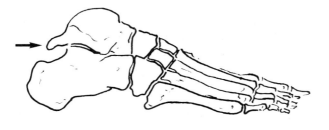

Stieda's Process

Fig. 9-34. Ostrigonum and the long lateral process of the posterior tubercle of the talus, or Stieda's process.

with avulsion of the posterior band of the lateral ligament.[92]

With the posterior talar compression syndrome, there is usually tenderness over the posterolateral aspect of the talus between the Achilles tendon and peroneals. The pain is generally reproduced by forced planar flexion. The lack of tenderness over the peroneal tendons should help exclude peroneal tendinitis.

A bone scan may be positive, but this test is not mandatory for the diagnosis. Forced plantar flexion roentgenograms confirm the painful impingement. Temporary relief should be obtained by infiltrating the area with 1 percent lidocaine. If modified activity and NSAIDs fail to relieve symptoms, excision of the os trigonum or Stieda's process and adjacent release of the tendon sheath of flexor hallucis longus usually allow resumption of activities in about 1 month.

Medial Tarsal Tunnel Syndrome

The medial tarsal tunnel syndrome is a compression neuropathy of the tibial nerve or its terminal branches, the medial and lateral plantar nerves.[93] The impingement frequently occurs in the distal two-thirds of the fibro-osseous canal, which has ill-defined limits.[94] It begins a few centimeters proximal to the tip of the medial malleolus, where the crural fascia starts to condense, forming a relatively unyielding roof, the flexor retinaculum. It ends where the medial and lateral plantar nerves enter or pass deep to the abductor hallucis. The anatomy is highly variable in regard to the site at which the tibial nerve divides into the medial calcaneal, medial plantar, and lateral plantar nerves, its terminal branches, and the method by which it exits from the canal. The medial and lateral plantar nerves leave through separate fibrous openings or, on occasion, contiguously in one canal, sometimes piercing the abductor muscle (Fig. 9-35).[94]

Etiology

There are a variety of factors that may lead to compromise of the nerve. They may present in slightly different ways, often contributing to a delay in diagnosis (Table 9-14).

Anatomic Factors

The anatomic factors include variations in the fibrous septa, areolar tissue, and retinaculum, hence limiting the capacity of the tunnel. Such variations

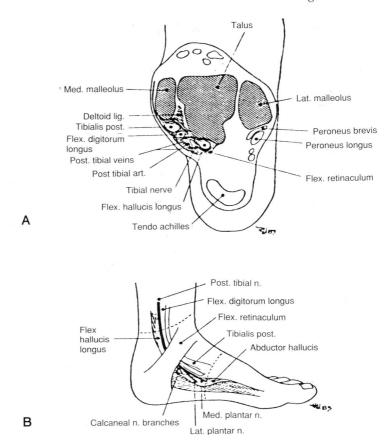

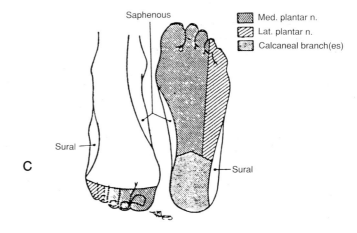

Fig. 9-35. Relation of the tendons and nerves of the tarsal tunnel in cross section (**A**) and from the medial side (**B**). (**C**) Sensory areas are supplied by the posterior tibial nerve terminal branches. (After Kushner and Reid,[93] with permission.)

may occur secondary to trauma, aging, or repeated stresses. The nerve also may be compressed by dilated and engorged veins. Occasionally, the presence of an arterial arch causes symptoms. Variations of the ab-

ductor hallucis, including an anomalous or accessory muscle, may involve the nerve distally. In athletes the repetitive stresses of running may unmask these variations, particularly in the presence of a valgus heel

TABLE 9-14. Etiology of Tarsal Tunnel Syndrome

Anatomic factors	Trauma
Septa	Fractures
Areolar tissue	Contusions
Retinaculum	Postsurgical adhesions
Vascular anomalies	Sprains
Muscular variations	Laceration
Valgus alignment	Post-traumatic edema
	Post-tramatic adhesions
Inflammatory factors	
Rheumatoid arthritis	Miscellaneous factors
Ankylosing spondylitis	Footwear
Tenosynovitis	Overuse syndrome
Thrombophlebitis	Training surfaces
	Aging
Tumor	Fluid retention
Neuroma	Pregnancy
Lipoma	Weight gain
Synovial cyst and	
ganglion	
Tendon tumors	
Neurolemmoma	

and associated pronated forefoot, which may tighten the flexor retinaculum, the arch of the abductor hallucis, and the calcaneonavicular ligament.

Trauma

The tarsal tunnel syndrome can occur as a complication of ankle, calcaneal, and metatarsal fractures. In a review of 500 os calcis fractures, 10 percent developed tarsal tunnel syndrome, more than one-fourth of which required surgical decompression. It may also occur with ankle sprains, tight casts, or post-surgically following osteotomies of the first ray or release of the Achilles tendon. All these causes may have edema and secondary fibrosis as a common factor.

Tumor

In athletes, ganglion and post-traumatic synovial cysts constitute the most common neoplasms causing pressure in the canal. The symptoms may be intermittent as they swell with activity.

Miscellaneous Factors

Chronic synovitis, ill-fitting footwear, inappropriate training surfaces, poorly graduated and planned training, fluid retention, pregnancy, and weight gain may play a role. In addition, neuropathy due to a variety of systemic causes may precipitate the problem.

Clinical Picture

There appears to be no sex predilection, and the onset is usually insidious. The commonest complaint is that of burning pain and paresthesia in the plantar aspect of the foot. Pain is exacerbated by activity and diminished by rest. The most common site of symptoms is the great toe, followed in frequency by the remaining toes and the distal sole of the foot. Occasionally, symptoms occur in the medial plantar surface of the heel. The athlete may also report that they felt a "swollen or tight" sensation, as if there is an impending cramp in the arch of the foot. For some individuals the pain may be worse at night, and they report pain relief from hanging the foot out of bed, moving it, rubbing it, or getting out of bed and walking around.

Sensory signs include hypesthesia to pinprick, diminished two-point discrimination, and a positive Tinel's sign (Fig. 9-36). Sustained direct pressure reproduces or exacerbates the symptoms. It is difficult to detect associated weakness.

The definitive test is the nerve conduction study to the abductor digiti minimi and abductor hallucis.[95] Latencies of more than one standard deviation above normal for the particular laboratory carrying out the test are considered positive, although it may be that evaluation of evoked sensory and motor potentials is a more sensitive test for pathology.[96]

Treatment

Nonoperative Therapy

Modification of Activity. The patient is given advice on intensity of training, building up mileage, and the impact of terrain, distance, and spacing of training sessions.

Modalities. Most of the physiotherapeutic modalities should be aimed at reduction of edema and scarring. They include application of ice after activity, ultrasound, interferential current therapy, laser, and shortwave diathermy. These modalities may be successful with recently acquired symptoms but rarely help an established neuropathy.

Footwear and Orthosis. In view of the highly associated valgus heel and pronated forefoot, a trial of a medial arch support or medial heel wedge may be considered. Tight lacing of shoes or skates may exacerbate the condition, as do shoes worn down at the lateral heel. Occasionally, when edema features highly in the etiology, support hose may be helpful.

Medication. Oral NSAIDs are most successful in acute-onset situations associated with tenosynovitis. Occasionally, a trial of local injectable steroid is successful, but care should be taken to avoid injection directly into the vessel and nerve. Furthermore, skin atrophy can be troublesome in this situation, and it is minimized by a deep injection of steroid with only about 1 to 2 ml of accompanying lidocaine.

Operative Therapy

Surgical release may provide rapid relief from the symptoms of the compression neuropathy, although with denervation in established cases some signs may persist. Because it is difficult to localize the exact site of compression, the entire canal is released. The flexor retinaculum is completely divided and the posterior tibial nerve freed from encompassing fibrous tissue. The branches are explored when possible in order to mobilize them as far distal as the abductor hallucis muscle. Each hiatus for the medial and lateral plantar nerves is checked and released. If there is an accessory abductor hallucis, it is excised. Care is taken not to disrupt the fine calcaneal branches, as damage produces heel numbness. If there are tortuous veins present, they should be ligated proximally and distally, and then excised. Even with careful dissection, it is impossible to identify unequivocal pathology in about 25 percent of the cases; but provided prior neurophysiologic testing has confirmed the site of compression, relief is obtained.

Partial weight-bearing or limited walking with full weight-bearing is advised for 2 weeks. By 3 weeks, more aggressive activity may be undertaken, including balance board work and running. Full return to sport usually takes 4 to 6 weeks. Recurrence of symptoms in a well decompressed nerve is rare, and the only significant, but rare, long-term complication is subluxation of the tibialis posterior tendon.[97]

Early recognition of this syndrome is not the rule, which is unfortunate, as it often resolves promptly with nonoperative treatment in its early stages. For this reason, its variation in presentation and its multitude of etiologic factors have been stressed in the hope that it will be included more frequently in the early list of differential diagnoses for medial talar, calcaneal, and medial foot pain.

Malleolar Bursitis

Repetitive friction over the malleoli, particularly the medial malleolus, may result in a protective adventitious bursa forming, which may become large and sometimes painful. It may fluctuate in size proportional to the amount of irritation. These bursa are most frequently seen in figure skaters and ice hockey players (Fig. 9-36).

Pressure-relieving pads, providing a relief area in the footwear, and NSAIDs may be effective if used early enough. Aspiration and injection with steroid must be done with care to avoid infection and skin atrophy. Invariably, the bursa recurs if long-standing or if the pressure from the boot cannot be relieved. It is tempting to excise these bursae, but this procedure is not without complications. The incision must be planned so it is away from the bony prominence. After excision, a pressure dressing should be kept on until good skin healing has been achieved and the deep tissues have become firmly adherent. Too rapid return to activity leads to recurrence of the collection of fluid, a seroma, and ultimately a bursa or (worse) a draining fistula. If this surgery is planned, it is best done in the off-season.

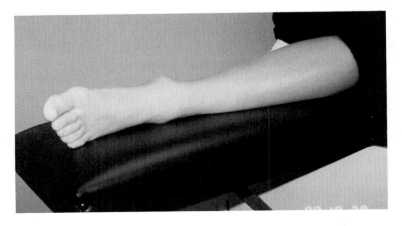

Fig. 9-36. Large malleolar bursa in a figure skater.

ANKLE FRACTURES

Ankle fractures are seen frequently in soccer, basketball, and volleyball players, occasionally in skiers and hockey players, and as a devastating injury in skydivers and rock climbers. The more protection to the ankle in the sport, the more proximal is the fracture. The association of an ankle sprain and a proximal fibular fracture (Maisonneuve fracture) should not be overlooked. In the skeletally immature, epiphysial separation and the complex Tillaux intraarticular fracture may present difficulties in diagnosis. Oblique roentgenograms and comparison with the opposite ankle are frequently necessary in the young athlete.

Classification

The simplest fracture classification is presented here. Although it does not encompass some of the more complex fracture patterns and subtle variations in biomechanics, it allows adequate description and gives an indication of the correct treatment approach (Fig. 9-37).

Fractures may be classified as single malleolar, bimalleolar, and if the posterior part of the tibial plafond is involved trimalleolar fractures. Single malleolar fractures must be screened for associated ligament injuries to the contralateral side of the ankle. Frequently, a major fracture of one side of the joint is linked to a small avulsed fragment on the opposite malleolus, indicating sparing of the ligament but signifying potential instability.

Dislocation of the ankle and tibiofibular diastasis may be easily overlooked. The former is overlooked because the joint spontaneously reduces, and the gross instability is not detected. The latter may not be evident because of the physician's failure to carefully scrutinize the width of the mortise or to obtain roentgenograms (Fig. 9-9).

The fibula is considered by many to be the key to the ankle joint because of its role in stability. Fibular fractures are usually subclassified as being (1) below the level of the joint, usually with excellent prognosis; (2) at the level of the joint, in which case anatomic reduction is imperative; and (3) above the level of the joint (Fig. 9-37). With these latter fractures the mortise is grossly unstable, malalignment of the ankle and knee joint planes frequent, and involvement of the interosseous membrane is a constant factor.

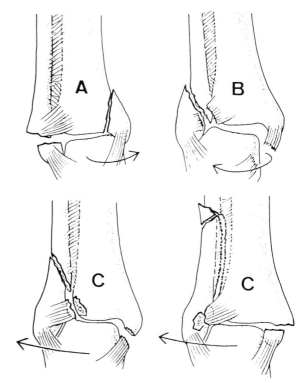

Fig. 9-37. Ankle fractures may be classified as single, bimalleolar, or trimalleolar. Special emphasis is placed on fibular fractures. **(A)** Below the level of the joint. **(B)** At the level of the joint. **(C)** Above the level of the joint involving the interosseous membrane to various degrees.

Treatment

Management of ankle fracture is based on several principles, realizing that as with all fracture care the subtleties of the fracture pattern (the "personality" of the fracture), the skills of the treating physician, and the individual requirements of the athlete dictate the final management.

Treatment guidelines include the following.

1. Open fractures of any size require immediate, thorough débridement under ideal conditions. These injuries constitute an orthopaedic emergency.
2. In order to minimize skin trauma, severely displaced or dislocated ankles should be reduced and splinted before transport of the athlete. Fail-

ure to do it may allow skin necrosis and convert a closed to an open injury.

3. Some dislocations are complex, and closed reduction is prevented by the interposition of tendons. Attempts at reduction should not be repeated without consultation with an experienced surgeon.

4. A decision should be made as to the need for surgical therapy for ankle dislocation. The more competitive the individual, the greater is the indication for open repair of ligaments and subsequent early motion.

5. Diastasis of the tibiofibular joint and widening of the mortise with a displaced fibular fracture, at or above the level of the joint, is unacceptable. Widening of 1 to 2 mm may increase joint forces by 30 to 40 percent and, in a young active individual, produce rapid degenerative changes. Open reduction and internal fixation are usually required.

6. If the posterior malleolar fragment comprises more than one-third of the joint surface on lateral roentgenograms, open reduction is indicated. Also, a significant step usually indicates fibular shortening, which must be reduced.

7. With relatively undisplaced fractures or subsequent to successful manipulation, closed cast treatment is acceptable so long as there is anatomic reduction of the joint surface and no widening of the mortise.

8. In the young athlete with dense bone that is capable of securing internal fixation devices solidly, early motion using a brace and protected weight-bearing is a good treatment option.

9. Small avulsion fragments from the tips of the malleoli are frequently extra-articular and may not be symptomatic even if they do not unite.

10. In active individuals, some protection of the ankle may be needed after cast removal in order to progress activity safely. A commercial flexible ankle brace or air cast may be suitable.

11. In many sports pressure of the footwear over the malleoli is considerable. Therefore, when possible, the incision should be placed behind the malleoli, screws used instead of plates, and the screw heads partially countersunk.

Once the cast is removed, most ankle fractures are treated as a serious sprain so far as the therapist is concerned, and rehabilitation is planned with regard to restoration of strength, endurance, range of motion, joint play, and proprioception. The protocol for ankle sprain previously outlined is appropriate in most circumstances.

SUMMARY

Ankle sprains comprise one of the more common significant injuries in sport. The tendency is to manage even severe sprains nonoperatively with early protected motion. To reduce long-term complications, particular attention must be paid to adequate mobilization of the several joints of the hindfoot, particularly the subtalar area. In addition, a prolonged strengthening protocol for the peroneal muscles is necessary to minimize the tendency to develop chronic ankle sprains. Awareness for possible weakness secondary to nerve injury is important. Chronic impingement syndromes range from the well recognized transchondral fracture of the talar dome to the more subtle entrapments of synovium, ankle meniscoid lesions, and the os trigonum. The tarsal tunnel syndrome is an entrapment problem of the posterior tibial nerve, which when recognized early may respond to nonoperative therapy. Late, resistant cases require surgical intervention. The characteristic presentation is burning or numbness in the great toe.

Ankle fractures can usually be classified according to the level of involvement of the fibula. Any widening of the mortise greatly increases the surface stresses. Because such stresses are high, even for the normal ankle, inadequate treatment leads to early degenerative changes. There is no such thing as a simple ankle fracture.

REFERENCES

1. Ruth CJ: The surgical treatment of injuries of the fibular collateral ligaments of the ankle. J Bone Joint Surg [Am] 43:229, 1961
2. Mack RP: Ankle injuries in athletics. Athletic Training 10:94, 1975
3. Schneider PG, Sieber E: Results of early mobilization with taping after primary surgical repair of lateral ligament ruptures of the ankle. Int J Sports Med 8:128, 1987 (abstract)
4. Garrick JA: The frequency of injury, mechanism of injury and epidemiology of ankle sprains. Am J Sports Med 5:241, 1977

5. Cass JA, Morrey BF: Ankle instability: current concepts, diagnosis and treatment. Mayo Clin Proc 59:165, 1984

6. Matejczyk M, Greenwald AS: A contact area study of the ankle joint. Orthop Rev 6:85, 1977

7. Burdett RG: Forces predicted at the ankle during running. Med Sci Sports Exerc 14:308, 1982

8. Lambert K: The weight bearing function of the fibula. J Bone Joint Surg [Am] 53:507, 1971

9. Weinert C, McMaster JH, Scranton PE et al: Human fibular dynamics. In Foot Science. Bateman JE (ed): WB Saunders, Toronto, 1976

10. Stormont DM, Morrey B, An K et al: Stability of the loaded ankle. Am J Sports Med 13:295, 1985

11. Rasmussen O, Kromann-Andersen C: Experimental ankle injuries. Acta Orthop Scand 54:356, 1983

12. St. Pierre RK, Velazco A, Fleming LL et al: Medial subtalar dislocation in an athlete. Am J Sports Med 10:240, 1982

13. Torg JS, Quedenfeld T: Knee and ankle injuries traced to shoe and cleats. Physician Sports Med 1:39, 1973

14. Snyder RB, Lipscomb AB, Johnston RK: The relationship of tarsal coalition to ankle sprains in athletes. Am J Sports Med 9:313, 1981

15. Roy SP: Evaluation and treatment of the stable ankle sprain. Physician Sports Med 5:60, 1977

16. Mandelbaum BR, Finerman G, Grant T et al: Collegiate football player with recurrent ankle sprains: a case conference. Physician Sports Med 15:57, 1987

17. Anderson KJ, LeCocq JF, LeCocq EA: Recurrent anterior subluxation of the ankle joint. J Bone Joint Surg [Am] 34:853, 1952

18. De Lacey G, Bradbrooke S: Rationalizing requests for x-ray examination of acute ankle injuries. Br Med J 1:1597, 1979

19. Cockshott WP, Jenkin JK, Pui M: Limiting the use of routine radiography for acute ankle injuries. Can Med Assoc J 129:129, 1983

20. Rubin G, Witten M: The talar tilt angle and the fibular collateral ligaments. J Bone Joint Surg [Am] 42:311, 1960

21. McLennan JG: Treatment of acute and chronic luxations of the peroneal tendons. Am J Sports Med 8:432, 1980

22. Cox JS, Hewes TF: Normal talar tilt angle. Clin Orthop 140:37, 1979

23. Laurin C, Mathieu J: Sagittal mobility of the normal ankle. Clin Orthop 108:99, 1975

24. Baldwin FC, Vegso J, Torg JS et al: Management and rehabilitation of ligamentous injuries to the ankle. Sports Med 4:364, 1987

25. Broström L: Sprained ankles. 1. Anatomic lesions in recent sprains. Acta Chir Scand 128:483, 1964

26. Landeros O, Frost HM, Higgins CC: Post-traumatic anterior ankle instability. Clin Orthop 56:169, 1968

27. Black HM, Brand RL, Eichelberger MR: An improved technique for evaluation of ligamentous injury in severe ankle sprains. Am J Sports Med 6:276, 1978

28. Hocutt JE, Jaffee R, Rylander CR et al: Cryotherapy in ankle sprains. Am J Sports Med 10:316, 1982

29. Basur RL, Shepherd E, Mouzas GL: A cooling method in the treatment of ankle sprains. Practitioner 216:708, 1976

30. Sims D: Effects of positioning on ankle edema. J Orthop Sports Phys Ther 8:30, 1986

31. Garrick JG, Ragna RK: Role of external support in the prevention of ankle sprains. Med Sci Sports 5:200, 1973

32. Vaes P, DeBoeck H, Handeberg F et al: Comparative radiological study of the influence of ankle joint strapping and taping on ankle stability. J Orthop Sports Phys Ther 7:110, 1985

33. Pope M, Renstrom P, Donnemeyer D et al: A comparison of ankle taping. Med Sci Sports Exerc 19:143, 1987

34. Loos T, Boelens P: The effect of ankle tape on lower limb muscle activity. Int J Sports Med 5:45, 1984

35. Bunch RP, Bednarski K, Holland D et al: Ankle joint support: a comparison of reusable lace-on braces with taping and wrapping. Physician Sports Med 13:59, 1985

36. Myburgh K, Vaughan OL, Isaacs SK: The effect of ankle quads and taping on joint motion, before, during and after a squash match. Am J Sports Med 12:441, 1984

37. Kimura IF, Nawoczenski DA, Epler M et al: Effect of air stirrup in controlling ankle inversion stress. J Orthop Sports Phys Ther 9:190, 1987

38. Gross MT, Bradshaw MK, Ventoy LC et al: Comparison of support provided by ankle taping and semi-rigid orthosis. J Orthop Sports Phys Ther 9:33, 1987

39. Torg JS, Vegso JJ, Torg E: Rehabilitation of Athletic Injuries: An Atlas of Therapeutic Exercises. Year Book Medical Publishers, Chicago, 1987

40. Toomey SJ: Four-square ankle rehabilitation exercises. Physician Sports Med 14:281, 1956

41. Mattison R: Men's volleyball prevention program for ankle injuries. CATA J Fall 1984

42. Reid DC: Ankle injuries in sports. J Sports Med 1:18, 1973

43. Freeman MAR, Dean MRE, Hanham IEF: The etiology and prevention of functional instability of the foot. J Bone Joint Surg [Br] 47:678, 1965

44. Wong DLK, Glastreen-Wray M, Andrews LF: Isokinetic evaluation of the ankle invertors and evertors. J Orthop Sports Phys Ther 5:246, 1984

45. Drez D, Young JC, Woldman D et al: Non-operative treatment of double lateral ligament tears of the ankle. Am J Sports Med 10:197, 1982

46. Cetti R: Conservative treatment of injury to fibular ligaments of the ankle. Br J Sports Med 16:47, 1982

47. Brand RL, Collins MF, Templeton T: Surgical repair of ruptured lateral ankle ligaments. Am J Sports Med 9:40, 1981

48. Evans GA, Hardcastle P, Frenyo AD: Acute rupture of the lateral ligament of the ankle: to suture or not to suture? J Bone Joint Surg [Br] 66:209, 1984

49. Cox JS, Brand RL: Evaluation and treatment of lateral ankle sprains. Physician Sports Med 5:51, 1977

50. Brand RL, Black HM, Cox JS: The natural history of inadequately treated ankle sprain. Am J Sports Med 5:248, 1977

51. Freeman MAR: Treatment of ruptures of the lateral ligaments of the ankle. J Bone Joint Surg [Br] 47:661, 1965

52. Broström L: Sprained ankles. V. Treatment and prognosis in recent ligament ruptures. Acta Chir Scand 132:537, 1966

53. Van den Hoogenband CR, Van Moppes FI, Coumans JW et al: Study on clinical diagnosis and treatment of lateral ligament lesion of the ankle joint: a prospective clinical randomized study. Int J Sports Med 5:159, 1984

54. Green TA, Wight CR: A comparative support evaluation of three ankle orthosis before, during, and after exercise. J Orthop Sports Phys Ther 11:453, 1990

55. Seligson D, Sassman J, Pope M: Ankle instability: evaluation of the lateral ligaments. Am J Sports Med 8:39, 1980

56. Staples OS: Result of study of ruptures of lateral ligaments of the ankle. Clin Orthop 85:50, 1972

57. Whiteside LA, Reynolds FC, Ellsasser JC: Tibiofibular synostosis and recurrent ankle sprains in high performance athletes. Am J Sports Med 6:204, 1978

58. Trapp H, Oderick P, Gillquist J: Stabilometry recordings in functional and mechanical instability of the ankle joint. Int J Sports Med 6:180, 1985

59. Broström L, Liljedahl SO, Lindvall N: Sprained ankles. II. Arthrographic diagnosis of recent ligament ruptures. Acta Chir Scand 129:485, 1965

60. Broström L: Sprained ankles. III. Clinical observations in recent ligament ruptures. Acta Chir Scand 130:560, 1965

61. Bosien WR, Staples OS, Russell, S: Residual disability following acute ankle sprains. J Bone Joint Surg [Am] 37:1237, 1955

62. Nawoczenski DA, Owen MG, Ecker ML et al: Objective evaluation of peroneal response to sudden inversion stress. J Orthop Sports Phys Ther 7:107, 1985

63. DeCarlo MS, Talbot RW: Evaluation of ankle joint proprioception following injection of the anterior talofibular ligament. J Orthop Sports Phys Ther 8:70, 1986

64. Harrington KD: Degenerative arthritis of the ankle secondary to long standing lateral ligament instability. J Bone Joint Surg [Am] 61:354, 1979

65. Evans DL: Recurrent instability of the ankle: a method of surgical treatment. Proc R Soc Med 46:343, 1953

66. Broström L: Sprained ankles. VI. Surgical treatment of "chronic" ligament ruptures. Acta Chir Scand 132:551, 1966

67. Ottosson L: Lateral instability of the ankle treated by a modified Evans procedure. Acta Orthop Scand 49:302, 1978

68. Vainionpaa S, Kirves P, Laike E: Lateral instability of the ankle and results when treated by Evans procedure. Am J Sports Med 8:437, 1980

69. Vrevc F, Sirnik M: Our experiernce with the Watson-Jones operation for recurrent dislocation of the ankle joint: injuries of the ligaments and their repair. p. 214. In Chapchal G (ed): Hand-Knee-Foot. Georg Thieme, Stuttgart, 1977

70. Watson-Jones R: Recurrent forward dislocation of the ankle joint. J Bone Joint Surg [Br] 34:519, 1952

71. Jackson DW: Ankle sprains in young athletes: relation of severity and disability. Clin Orthop 101:201, 1974

72. Aeearian DE, McCrackin HJ, Devito OP et al: A biomechanical study of human lateral ankle ligaments and autogenous reconstructive grafts. Am J Sports Med 13:377, 1985

73. St. Pierre RK, Andrews L, Allman F et al: The Cybex II evaluation of lateral ankle ligamentous reconstructions. Am J Sports Med 12:52, 1984

74. Nitz AJ, Dobner JJ, Kersey D: Nerve injury and grades II and III ankle sprains. Am J Sports Med 13:177, 1985

75. Clavel M, Ozain I, Laria C: Footdrop: an unusual complication of ankle sprain. Neurol Orthop 1:33, 1986

76. Anderson E: Stenosing peroneal tenosynovitis, symptomatically stimulating ankle instability. Am J Sports Med 3:258, 1987

77. Hagmeyer RHM, Van der Wurff: Transchondral fractures of the talus on an inversion injury of the ankle: a frequently overlooked diagnosis. J Orthop Sports Phys Ther 8:362, 1987

78. Berndt AL, Hardy M: Transchondral fractures (osteochondritis dissecans) of the talus. J Bone Joint Surg [Am] 41:988, 1959

79. Canale ST, Belding RH: Osteochondral lesions of the talus. J Bone Joint Surg [Am] 62:97, 1980

80. Thompson JP, Loomer RL: Osteochondral lesions of the talus in a sports medicine clinic—a new radiographic technique and surgical approach. Am J Sports Med 12:460, 1984

81. Campbell CJ, Rangwat CS: Osteochondritis dissecans: the question of etiology. J Trauma 6:201, 1986

82. Pavlov H, Torg JS: The Running Athlete. Roentgen-

ograms and Remedies. Year Book Medical Publishers, Chicago, 1987

83. Alexander AH, Lichtman DM: Surgical treatment of transchondral talar dome fractures. J Bone Joint Surg [Am] 62:646, 1980

84. McCullough CJ, Venngopal V: Osteochondritis dissecans of the talus: the natural history. Clin Orthop 144:264, 1979

85. Andrews JR, Drez DJ, McGinty JB: Symposium: arthroscopy of joints other than the knee. Contemp Orthop 9:71, 1984

86. Parks JCH, Hamilton WG, Patterson AH et al: The anterior impingement syndrome of the ankle. J Trauma 20:895, 1980

87. Hontas MJ, Haddard RJ, Schlesinger LC: Conditions of the talus in the runner. Am J Sports Med 14:486, 1986

88. Reid DC: Selected lesions around the talus. Curr Ther Sports Med 2:241, 1990

89. Wohlin I, Glassman F, Sideman S: Internal derangement of the talofibular component of the ankle. Surg Gynecol Obstet 1:193, 1950

90. McCarroll JR, Schrader JW, Shelbourne KD et al: Meniscoid lesions of the ankle in soccer players. Am J Sports Med 15:255, 1987

91. McDougall A: The os trigonum. J Bone Joint Surg [Br] 37:257, 1955

92. Cedell CA: Rupture of the posterior talotibial ligament with avulsion of a bone fragment from the talus. Acta Orthop Scand 45:454, 1974

93. Kushner S, Reid DC: Medial tarsal tunnel syndrome: a review. J Orthop Sports Phys Ther 6:39, 1984

94. Keck C: The tarsal tunnel syndrome. J Bone Joint Surg [Am] 44:180, 1962

95. Kaplan PE, Kernahan WT: Tarsal tunnel syndrome. J Bone Joint Surg [Am] 63:96, 1981

96. Fu R, Delisa JA, Kraft GH: Motor nerve latencies through the tarsal tunnel in normal adult subjects: standard determinations for corrected temperatures and distance. Arch Phys Med Rehabil 61:243, 1980

97. Langan P, Weiss CA: Subluxation of the tibialis posterior tendon: a complication of tarsal tunnel decompression. Clin Orthop 146:226, 1980

Exercise-Induced Leg Pain

10

To study the phenomena of disease without books is to sail an uncharted sea, while to study books without patients is not to go to sea at all.
— *Sir William Osler*

Injuries that occur reasonably frequently in sport and whose etiology and pathophysiology are not completely understood often acquire eponymous designations. Unfortunately, because of their lack of specificity, these terms rapidly evolve to mean different things to different clinicians and investigators. The result is a confused classification, numerous eponyms, and an unclear relation to exact pathology. Shin splints is such a term and should be used only to indicate shin soreness secondary to activity (Fig. 10-1).

The American Medical Association defines the shin splint syndrome as "pain and discomfort in the leg from repetitive activity on hard surfaces, or due to forceable, excessive use of the foot flexors. The diagnosis should be limited to musculoskeletal inflamma-

tions, excluding stress fractures or ischemic disorders."

To facilitate description and discussion, the shin splint-like syndrome is described under the following categories: (1) medial tibial stress syndrome; (2) stress fractures; and (3) compartment syndromes.[1] The differential diagnosis includes variations of the vascular, neural, and muscular systems.

These syndromes are common in activities that include running long distances, repetitive jumping or impact on hard surfaces, and inadequate footwear (Table 10-1). Therefore joggers and runners, aerobic and classical dancers, basketball and volleyball players, and sprinters comprise most of the athletes with these problems. Both the novice, who does too much too soon, and the serious competitor, who extends the duration and intensity of training out of proportion to the necessary recovery periods, may fall victim. The true incidence is difficult to assess, as the reports in the literature usually reflect the current etiologic theory of the day. Thus periostitis, stress fractures, and chronic compartment syndromes have all been featured as predominant causes. Furthermore, the patient population, the clinical bias of the investigator, and the thoroughness and aggressiveness of the diagnostic effort and sophistication of tests (e.g., bone scan and compartment pressure measurements) serve to skew the data. Nevertheless, successful treatment in the most efficient and safe manner demands a serious attempt at defining the pathology for each case. Fortunately, treatment of the less severe cases may be remarkably similar, and hence in many instances success is often ensured even for the more casual observer. In the most blatant and

---

Clinical Point

LEG PAIN (SHIN SPLINTS)

- Medial tibial stress syndrome
  - Musculotendinous strains
  - Tendinitis
  - Interosseous membrane pain
  - Periostitis
- Stress Fractures
  - Tibia
  - Fibula
- Compartment Syndromes
  - Chronic
  - Acute

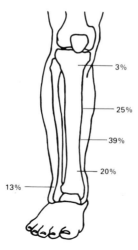

Fig. 10-1. Common sites of exercise-induced leg soreness with approximate frequency of occurrence in running sports.

painful cases, the diagnostic category is frequently apparent. These points should not be used to discredit a diligent search for the exact etiology in order to provide a key for rapid resolution in a more satisfactory way for both athlete and clinician alike. Occasionally, to overlook the correct diagnosis is the prelude to a disaster, e.g., a midtibial stress fracture progressing to a complete fracture.

Diagnosis of the exact cause of recurrent pain in the lower leg is frequently made difficult because of the lack of specific symptoms, particularly when the athlete is at rest. For these reasons, clinical investigation immediately after exercise may be useful. Such measurements can be made using a foot ergometer or treadmill or, if these tests are not available, by sending the athlete for a run. The frequency of the common shin splint syndrome should not mask the need to search for rarer and more unusual conditions in recalcitrant cases, e.g., arterial and venous anomalies.

Practice Point

LEG PAIN DIAGNOSIS

- When minimal symptoms make diagnosis difficult, send patient for a run to exaggerate findings, and examine immediately afterwards.

Finally, although compartment syndromes, stress fractures, and acute periostitis have clear diagnostic criteria, there are numerous cases that fall into the category of nonspecific shin pain. These athletes' problems are assigned labels, e.g., tendinitis, muscle strain, interosseous membrane stress, and chronic periostitis. In reality, there is no evidence that these terms add anything to our understanding any more than does the term shin splint. In fact, for these individuals, I prefer to use the term shin splint, as a reminder that I do not know the pathophysiology, or, indeed, the exact tissue that is painful. For these patients, constant review and reassessment are necessary. In most athletes the syndrome resolves, and we

TABLE 10-1.   Male/Female Distribution of 1000 Running Injuries

Injury	Male (%)	Female (%)	Total (%)
Tibial stress syndrome	6.0	8.0	6.6
Stress fracture	8.0	13.6	9.6
Compartment syndromes	0.4	1.4	0.7
Knee	32.6	30.8	32.1
Foot	18.3	14.3	17.2
Ankle	13.9	11.5	13.2
Hip	9.1	8.0	8.8
Back	7.1	8.0	7.4
Hamstring	3.2	1.8	2.8
Miscellaneous	1.3	2.4	1.6

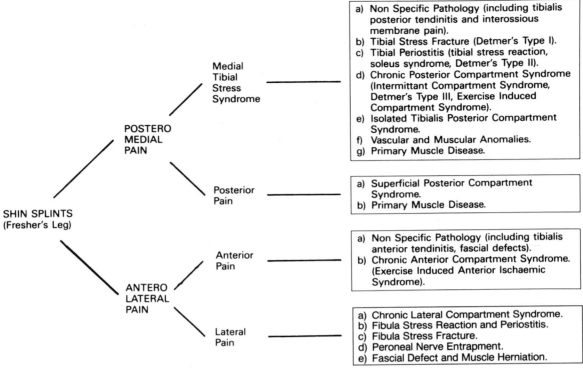

Fig. 10-2. Reasonable clinical approach to the shin splint syndrome starts with categorizing into posteromedial or anterolateral pain.

are left no wiser as to the pathophysiology. For those whose symptoms do not resolve (or get worse), usually specific tests become positive and therefore the pathology declares itself. Occasionally, shin splint syndrome remains a frustrating enigma. Classifying the symptoms by location, i.e., anterior (anterolateral) or posterior (posteromedial), is a helpful starting point, as each area has a range of known diagnostic possibilities (Fig. 10-2).

MEDIAL TIBIAL STRESS SYNDROME

Definition of Terms

Devas presented a series of tibial stress fractures (also called periostalgia, periostitis, fasciitis, soleus syndrome, Detmer's type II) in 1958, and although the fracture line was not always visible he interpreted the thickened cortex as a healed stress reaction.[1] In an attempt to explain it, a series of papers was published using different terms to describe this variety of shin splints. The pervading theory through the 1960s was

that of inflammation of the periosteum, tendon sheath, muscle belly, or interosseous membrane secondary to strain, minimal tears, or mechanical irritation.[2,3] Puranen was the first to use the term medial tibial syndrome.[4] Having excluded the possibility of stress fractures, he believed that the pain was of ischemic origin; hence fasciotomy was the treatment of choice in recalcitrant cases. Compartment pressures were not measured, and in his series only one athlete had definite ischemic muscle changes. Clement, in 1974, modified the term to "tibial stress syndrome" along with an etiologic theory based on cyclic training and stress-induced local muscle fatigue in the lower leg.[5] He postulated that this fatigue, in turn, diminishes the muscles' shock-absorbing ability; therefore Clement suggested that there is increased structural stress on bone, creating a painful periosteal reaction (Fig. 10-3), which in turn results in further muscle weakness. Hence a cycle is established that could ultimately progress to stress fracture.[5] By 1982 Mubarak et al. had amalgamated the previous terms in the appellation "medial tibial stress syndrome" and

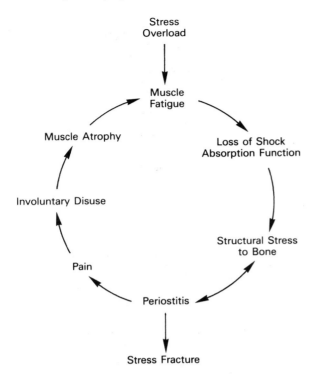

Stress Overload

Muscle Fatigue

Loss of Shock Absorption Function

Muscle Atrophy

Involuntary Disuse

Structural Stress to Bone

Pain

Periostitis

Stress Fracture

Fig. 10-3. Etiologic theory of tibial stress syndrome as originally proposed by Clement.[5]

presented arguments for the term to be reserved for the athlete suffering from periostitis.[6]

Michael and Holder, in 1985, clearly demonstrated that increased third phase scintigraphic uptake in the tibia correlated with the soleus muscle origin.[7] Biopsies demonstrated an intense inflammatory response in the periosteum at the soleus insertion, and they postulated inflammation of the adjacent fascia in those cases in which there was not increased uptake on the scan. Hence both periostitis and fasciitis are possible factors.

In an effort to clarify the previous concepts, Detmer categorized syndromes into: (1) anterolateral, which included muscular, tendinous, bony, and vascular problems in the anterior and lateral compartments, the "anterior shin splint" syndrome; and (2) posteromedial pain, which may be resolved into type I, II, and III medial tibial stress syndromes (Table 10-2).[8] The type I syndrome is bony and includes intense local stress reactions and stress fractures. Type II defects are related to the periosteum and are divided into inflammatory periostitis and painful, chronic periostalgia. Type III includes the deep posterior compartment syndromes. This section

deals specifically with the medial tibial stress syndrome type II, or periostalgia, the so-called medial tibial stress syndrome.

Clinical Presentation and Pathology

The athletes are usually runners or aerobic dancers, or they engage in other ballistic jumping-type activities. They present with a well localized area of tenderness over the posteromedial edge of the distal one-third of the tibia. There is often an area of significant, but less severe, tenderness for about 3 cm distal and 5 cm proximal to the area of maximum pain (Table 10-2). The symptoms are frequently bilateral, initially brought on by and proportional to activity. The symptoms ultimately appear with minimal exercise or even walking if athletes persist in pushing training to the limit of their ability to tolerate the pain. The symptoms usually improve rapidly with rest; but if they are of long duration or are recurrent over many cycles of attempted rest and retraining, they may not settle easily. Injection of the area with a local anesthetic may give excellent temporary relief. When mild the bone scan may be negative, but the delayed phase uptake is usually increased in a diffuse fashion in more severe cases (Fig. 10-4). The diffuse nature helps distinguish this syndrome from stress fractures. There may be some increase in exercise compartment pressures compared to those in asymptomatic individuals, but rarely to the degree seen with compartment syndromes, and the pressure always promptly returns to normal at the cessation of activity. When biopsies have been performed, it is usually possible to demonstrate inflammation in the periosteum or adjacent fascia. Eventually periosteal reaction and thickening may be evident on plain roentgenograms.

In Michael and Holder's study, the diffuse uptake on the posterior tibia correlates well with the origin of the soleus rather than the tibialis posterior muscle (Fig. 10-5). Hence with varying degrees of severity, there could be either tendinitis, fasciitis, or periostitis (Fig. 10-6).[7] Muscle stimulation of the soleus muscle shows its strong inversion action on the heel. Other investigators have confirmed its strong prime mover action in stabilizing the foot.[9,10] Furthermore, the association of pain with excessively pronated feet in the athletes in this series and the theoretic increased soleus activity to control the heel position were also cited as part of the etiology.

Detmer has distinguished a subgroup among the athletes with periostalgia.[8] He noted that some of the

TABLE 10-2. Posteromedial Leg Pain

Parameter	Medial Tibial Stress Syndrome	Tibial Stress Fracture	Chronic Compartment Syndrome
Typical location	Distal medial two-thirds of tibia	Distal or middle one-third of tibia	Posteromedial tibial border
Typical athlete	Sprinter, gymnast, aerobics	Distance runner, dancer	Distance runner, walker
Causes	Training on hard surfaces Increasing exercise intensity too rapid Poor alignment of biomechanics of running Repetitive jumping	Sudden increase in training Hard surfaces Muscle fatigue leading to increased bone loading Inadequate footwear	Sudden increase in exercise intensity Prolonged exercise bouts Muscle/fascial compartment size mismatch with exercise
Pain pattern	Only during activity May be diffuse tenderness Not aggravated by passive stretch Usually settles promptly with rest	Initially only with activity Ultimately with all weight-bearing or rest No pain on passive stretch Normally severe localized pain	Only during activity Frequently onset at set point in training May progress to pain with walking Diffuse posteromedial pain
Training surface	Often pain decreased with shock-absorbing orthosis, shoe, or training surface	Pain regardless of surface	Pain proportional to activity not surface Hill running may increase pain
Neurologic signs and symptoms	None	None	Tingling or numbness in distribution of posterior tibial nerve (sole of feet including great toe) Muscle weakness if severe
Roentgenogram	Usually negative May be diffuse cortical thickening May be diffuse uptake on bone scan	Initially negative May be visible as a crack or periosteal callus In cancellous bone as an increase in density Focal uptake on scan	None
Specific tests	None: clinical suspicion, scan	Roentgenogram and scan	Exercise compartment pressure measurements Exercise electrophysiologic studies

athletes with severe symptoms that had lasted for a protracted length of time had negative scans. To explain the pathogenesis of this problem, he hypothesized that the periosteum may be traumatically disengaged from the bone by either ballistic avulsion or subperiosteal edema or hemorrhage.[8] He also speculated that the soleus muscle is capable of generating the type of stress that would produce this pathology. Once avulsed from the bone, the disengaged periosteum remains sensitive and painful, although the inflammation may settle. Hence there may be a negative bone scan, and the biopsy may not show inflammation. With sufficient rest, the periosteum may heal firmly back to the tibia, allowing resolution of the symptoms. In those athletes with recurrent symptoms who eventually were treated surgically, Detmer claimed to have confirmed periosteal detachment and noted adipose tissue consistently between the periosteum and bone (Fig. 10-7).[8] A similar condition has been described and confirmed in race horses.

Contributing Factors

There are no pathognomonic findings among athletes developing the medial tibial stress syndrome, stress fractures, or compartment syndromes despite many attempts in the literature to identify specific alignments and body builds. Nevertheless, in an at-

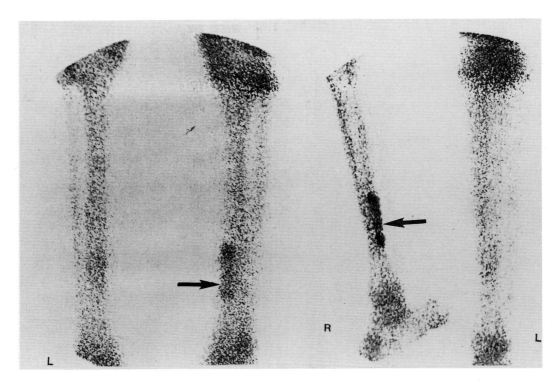

Fig. 10-4. Diffuse uptake along the right posterior tibial border in a patient with periostitis.

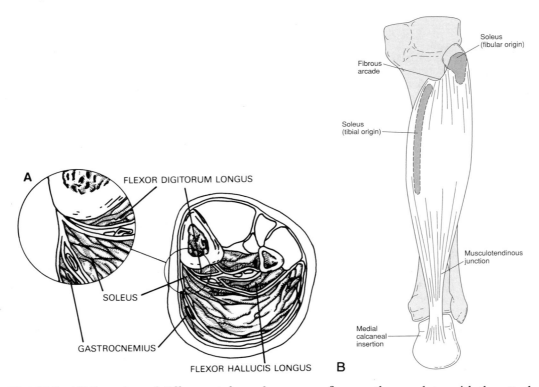

Fig. 10-5. **(A)** Location of diffuse uptake on bone scans frequently correlates with the attachment of the soleus. **(B)** Insertion of the soleus to the medial calcaneus makes it particularly important in controlling the pronation-supination subtalar motion.

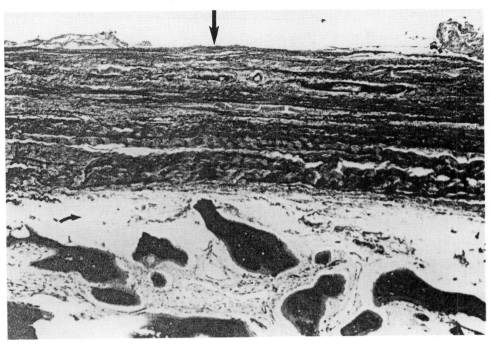

Fig. 10-6. Biopsy from shin splint patient showing markedly thickened periosteum [periostitis (straight arrow)] and new subperiosteal bone formation (curved arrow). (After Michael and Holder,[7] with permission.)

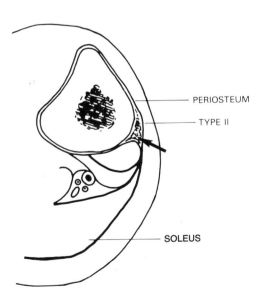

Fig. 10-7. Periosteum is elevated from the tibia with ectopic fat deposited underneath it (arrow) (Detmer type II). When this situation occurs, no ongoing inflammation or periostitis needs to be present to cause pain with exercise.

tempt to reduce stress, many of these factors must be identified and, when appropriate, modified in order to break the cycle of pain and disability. These factors, presented below, are not in any particular order of importance.

Quick Facts

CONTRIBUTING FACTORS TO EXERCISE INDUCED LEG PAIN

- Poor running mechanics
- Inappropriate footwear
- Foot shape and biomechanics
- Lower limb structural abnormalities
- Muscle tightness and imbalance
- Poor conditioning, overweight
- Inadequate warm-up and training errors
- Terrain and training surfaces
- Environment and diet

Poor Running Mechanics

According to many investigators, poor biomechanics may cause more symptomatology than any other single factor.[5,11] Leaning too hard while cornering or training on a track with excessively tight corners may force the heel into an excessive valgus position (Fig. 10-8). Similarly, an increased varus angle of the leg, producing a crossover running style, results in a valgus heel, as does running with the leg externally rotated at the hip. The net result of heel eversion or valgus is to increase pronation and perhaps throw additional stress on the tibialis posterior or soleus. Excessive pronation as a cause of the medial compartment stress syndromes is the single most common factor cited in the literature. Furthermore, in addition to the overpronation, prolongation of pronation time is important, as it reflects the length of time eccentric posterior tibial muscle control is required. Viita Sala and Kuist[12] demonstrated that in a group of shin splint patients there was greater subtalar flexibility, greater angular displacement values in inversion and eversion, and a longer time from heel strike to the maximally everted foot.

By contrast, running or jogging on the balls of the feet, with resulting delayed or no flat foot phase, may dramatically increase the work performed by the plantar flexors. This extra muscle work with these poor running mechanics may either stress the muscle origins or predispose to muscle fatigue. It is particularly true of sprinters who perform excessive rebound work and toe running early in the season.

Inappropriate Footwear

The commonest inappropriate footwear problem is wearing worn-out shoes, long past the point that they are useful for absorbing shock and for motion control.[13] Shoes that do not flex well at the metatarsophalangeal (MTP) joint may increase the magnitude of forces acting on the posterior compartment muscles. Furthermore, insufficient arch support and poor shock-absorbing qualities, to counteract the repetitive jarring of heel strike, may increase bone stress directly and indirectly through muscle action. A poorly designed or aligned heel counter, an inadequately made or shaped last, and excessive flaring of the heel may serve to increase leverage or impose poor foot biomechanics. In susceptible individuals, it may allow the development of the medial tibial stress syndromes (see Ch. 24).[5]

Pes Planus and Cavus

Because the tibialis posterior is partly responsible for supporting the medial arch, an overly flexible or flat foot may put additional stress on this muscle and its tendon.[12] By contrast, the rigid cavus foot is not set up well for absorbing shock and may throw additional stress on the tibia.

Structural Abnormalities

Skeletal variations such as excessive femoral anteversion, increased Q-angle, external tibial torsion, valgus heels, and tarsal coalition may alter biomechanics.

Muscular Imbalance

It is difficult to quantify the role of muscle imbalance in the lower leg syndromes, but it can be postulated that decreased flexibility or weakness in any of the muscle groups may predispose the individual to shin splint problems.[5,14] In one study of ballet dancers

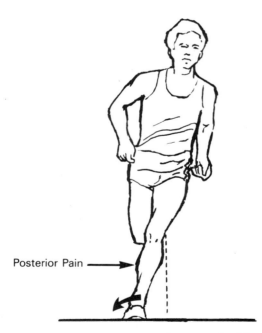

Posterior Pain →

Fig. 10-8. Excessive crossover (increased adduction angle) of the left leg increases functional pronation. Running with the hip externally rotated or excessive leaning on a curve tend to do the same thing. They increase functional pronation, thus increasing the activity of the tibialis posterior as it resists the motion. It may also stress the patellar tracking mechanism.

with shin splints, the symptomatic group tended to land with more double heel strikes than the asymptomatic group.[15] The heel seems to pop up between landing and push-off. It was thought that this represented either poor control or tight Achilles tendons. The altered technique was subtle but illustrates the need to be familiar with the subtleties of each activity.

Wallensten and Karlsson have carried out muscle biopsies on athletes with chronic shin splints and thought that the slow twitch muscle fibers covered less cross-sectional area than could be expected from the fiber composition. This situation, however, may have been an adaptation rather than a cause.[16] More recently, there has been a suggestion that mild claw toe deformity possibly with intrinsic muscle weakness produces overactivity of the flexor digitorum longus as it attempts to keep the toes flat just prior to push-off (Fig. 10-9).

Overweight

Individuals that are even as little as 10 to 15 pounds overweight may be susceptible to this syndrome, as the stresses of running are passively increased by ex-

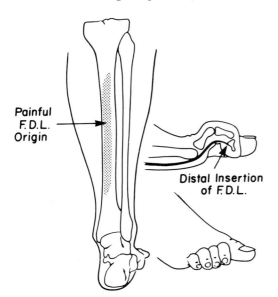

Fig. 10-9. Posteromedial, middle one-third shin pain in running athletes may be secondary to stress generated by the tibial origin of the flexor digitorum longus. This stress occurs as the muscle attempts to maintain the toe flat during push-off in athletes with subtle claw toe deformity, weakness of the foot intrinsic muscles or both. (From Garth WP, Miller ST: Am J Sports Med 17:821, 1989, with permission.)

cessive fat. Forces through the legs are multiples of body weight, and it is easy to postulate the role of these stresses in the development of an overuse syndrome particularly because many of these individuals have been previously out of shape and step up their training too rapidly. It is more reasonable to lose weight to exercise than exercise to lose weight. Overweight individuals should combine their exercise with diet and progress their activity slowly and cautiously.

Poor Conditioning and Training Loads

Poor conditioning refers to an inadequacy of bodily processes to tolerate a required workload. The lower the level of conditioning, the greater the degree of overload placed on the body for a set workload. When running, this overload is predominantly borne by the leg musculature, particularly the lateral and the posterior compartment muscles. The three most important aspects of this concept are stepping up activity too soon, a sudden increase in intense activity, or simply an excessive volume of work.

Inadequate Warm-Up

Warming up muscles before use increases the circulation to the muscles and their tendons, allowing extensibility and adequate blood flow. Failure to do so may precipitate minor tears and hence the onset of inflammation.

Uneven Terrain

Running over uneven ground or too much hill work may also place excessive stress on the various compartments of the leg, particularly if this type of activity is built up too quickly. In addition, the camber on the side of the road and the tight corners on a running track may be precipitating factors.

Hard, Unyielding Surfaces

The violent momentary impacts brought about by repetitive running on hard surfaces may produce a whipping action on the tendon and bending moments on the tibia and fibula. It has already been pointed out that stresses of running are high, being two to three times body weight at heel strike. For example, a 150 pound individual may have to dissipate as much as 110 to 120 tons of force through each leg when jogging as little distance as a mile.

The problem of a hard surface applies particularly to dancers, who frequently practice for hours on poorly sprung floors.[17] Part of this problem is circumvented by correct footwear for aerobic dancers, but for classical ballet dancers the footwear is not capable of being modified, and other adaptations must be made.

Cold Weather

Cold weather may contribute to the various shin splint syndromes by inhibiting sufficient warm-up, decreasing the compliance of the running surface, and altering running style.

Nutrition

The implication of inadequate diet is difficult to prove. Myburgh et al. carefully reviewed the food intake of athletes with shin soreness. These athletes reported a significantly lower calcium intake. Only 3 of the 25 individuals consumed the recommended dietary allowance (RDA) of calcium (800 mg).[13] Nearly 50 percent of these symptomatic athletes consumed less than half of the RDA (Table 10-3).

Treatment

Prevention is clearly the treatment of choice with respect to the medial tibial stress syndrome: careful planning of progression of activity, adjustments for climatic condition, gradual introduction of training sessions on new or different terrains, adequate warm-up for exercise, and correct spacing of training sessions. In addition, specific attention must be paid to techniques, alignment, and equipment. In essence, the treatment may be planned to: (1) reduce stress; (2) relieve pain; (3) provide alternative programs to maintain fitness; (4) correct specific etiologic factors; and (5) reintegrate the athlete into activity.

When nonoperative treatment has been carefully planned and the athlete has been compliant in follow-

---

TABLE 10-3. Daily Calcium Intake of Athletes with Shin Soreness

Calcium Intake (mg)	Injured Subjects (No.)	Controls (No.)
>800	3	15
400–799	12	8
<399	10	2
	$p < 0.005$.	

(Adapted from Myburgh et al.[13])

Practice Point

TREATMENT PLAN FOR MEDIAL TIBIAL STRESS SYNDROME

- Reduction of stress
- Relief of pain
- Alternate program for fitness
- Correction of specific etiologic factors
- Careful reintegration into activity

---

ing the program without success, surgical treatment may be considered. Although the following points of treatment are specifically for the medial tibial stress syndrome, they may be readily adapted for the treatment of stress fractures and even early chronic exercise-induced compartment syndrome.

Rest

Frequently the athlete presents with such severe symptoms and such a chronic course that an initial period of rest is necessary. Rarely, a cast or modified brace is required. More frequently a period of modified weight-bearing using crutches is adequate.

Medication

Nonsteroidal anti-inflammatory drugs (NSAIDs) are frequently helpful. A trial of NSAIDs should not be considered to have failed unless the full therapeutic dosage and course have been prescribed and taken without giving symptomatic relief. Some immediate improvement is expected if there is an inflammatory component to the problem. With good initial relief, it is permissible to continue the therapy for up to 6 weeks. Except in cases of a very mild nature, NSAIDs can never be considered adequate therapy when used alone.

Physical Modalities

The use of interferential current therapy, short-wave diathermy, and ultrasound have also been used to treat the muscular, tendinous, and periosteal type syndromes. Furthermore, it has been suggested that ultrasound accelerates bone healing. Intensities of 1 W/cm² for 6 minutes at a frequency of 1.0 to 1.5 MHz and pulsed at a 1:4 ratio have been recommended. The use of ice massage prior to, and at the cessation of, activity may be effective in relieving the symptoms of some individuals.

Other modalities that have been discussed in the literature are (1) the use of phonophoresis with a mixture of 35 mg of dexamethasone (Decadron) in 16 ml of 2 percent lidocaine gel; and (2) iontophoresis with 2 ml of 0.5 percent hydrocortisone ointment and dexamethasone sodium phosphate with 1 ml of 2 percent lidocaine ointment.[18] With the latter application, the medication is massaged into the skin of the painful area. The positive electrode and water-soaked pad are then used to drive the ions into the tissues using a low voltage direct current generator.[19] A maximum of 10 treatments may be given to avoid adverse skin changes.

Modification of Training Surface

With the transition from outdoor to indoor running, an individual can make arrangements to run alternate ways around a track on different training nights in order to avoid the problem of excessive leaning on sharp corners. Care should be taken to avoid the camber on the roads, and hill work should be eliminated while symptoms remain severe.

Modification of Activity

The distance traveled and the frequency of activity can be modified to allow a certain amount of activity within the limits of pain. In sports such as volleyball and dancing, jumping should be reduced to a minimum. The athlete can keep fit by running on a hydrogym machine, which provides a non-weight-bearing mechanism of running. Running may also be carried out in water, or cycling can be substituted. With the improvement of symptoms, distance and speed can be gradually increased. Running, jumping, or dancing techniques are carefully analyzed in order to eliminate obvious flaws in style. These points are emphasized prior to gradually increasing the intensity of training with resolution of the symptoms.

Strapping

Some individuals have received help from either strapping the leg or directly strapping the longitudinal arch.[20] This form of therapy is usually inconvenient, as it is difficult for athletes to apply the tape themselves in an efficient manner. Success with tape often indicates that an arthrosis may be helpful. Furthermore, taping may be an excellent way of limiting

motion during the early part of the treatment program. Our success with strapping has been only moderate.

Orthosis

Correction of varus heel, which may lead to overpronation and support of the medial longitudinal arch, as well as the introduction of shock-absorbing materials such as Sorbothane, may decrease symptoms. There should also be a careful distinction drawn between a temporary orthosis, made to relieve symptoms, and the need for a permanent orthosis. Many athletes needlessly wear permanent orthoses, at great expense, when a temporary support made by the therapist would have sufficed.

Occasionally, the use of a long air stirrup brace may relieve stress on the area sufficiently to allow symptoms to subside and training to continue (Fig. 10-10). This form of therapy may be contemplated in situations where certain activity deadlines are important.[21]

Footwear

Attention can be given to the footwear to make sure that the shoes are not worn out and that the wear pattern is satisfactory; when appropriate, shoes with a

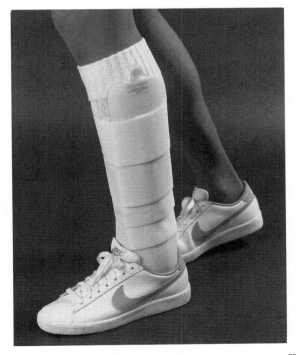

Fig. 10-10. Air splint may reduce symptoms sufficiently to allow modified training.

better support of the heel and the medial longitudinal arch are advised. The weight of the shoe, the shape of the last, and its shock-absorbing capabilities are considerations in the selection of appropriate footwear (see Ch. 24).

Exercise

Specific stretching of tight muscles and strengthening of weak muscles should be carried out in a controlled situation to overcome detectable muscle imbalance or contractures. It requires careful and complete assessment by the therapist.

Surgical Treatment

Failure to respond to rest, adequate rehabilitation, and an unwillingness to modify or change the activity pattern may lead to a consideration of surgical therapy. Because the pathology is related to the periosteum, the adjacent attachment of the posterior compartment fascia, and the investing fascia and attachment of the soleus muscle, there is some rationale for release of this fascia to relieve the stress on the area.[6,22] The addition of cauterization of the tibial periosteum may be reasonable.[8] In a report of 18 patients with symptoms lasting a mean 33 months, 78 percent described a complete cure and 14 percent reported satisfactory or significant improvement. They had resumed activity up to full competitive level, although some still experienced mild symptoms.[8] Postoperatively patients use crutches for 1 to 2 weeks, with early active range of motion of the legs. Cycling and swimming are commenced at 2 weeks, running at 3 weeks, and a goal of reaching presymptomatic levels of activity at 3 to 6 months.

Differential Diagnosis

Periostitis is not a disease but a term used to describe symptoms, and it is important to bear in mind some of the rarer causes. Acute periostitis in early acquired syphilis was first described in 1887. The involvement of the long bones is a rare manifestation in the adult.[23] Bone changes occur as early as 6 weeks after the chancre and as late as 15 months after the secondary skin eruptions.[23,24] It is possible that syphilis of the bone begins as osteomyelitis, with vascular and perivascular changes in the vessels caused by spirochetes precipitating the periostitis. Symptomatic periostitis of syphilis is characterized by nocturnal pain, exaggerated by heat and sometimes relieved by movement. At least the symptom may not be exaggerated by activity even if present. The bone scan may be uniformly hot. It is important to recall that syphilis has been called the great imitator, and a high index of suspicion is needed to consider it in the differential diagnosis.[24] Athletes are not spared from this disease.

Other, rarer causes of periosteal change include hypervitaminosis A, Paget's disease, and melorheostosis. Less rare and more significant in the young adult is parosteal and periosteal osteosarcoma.

Although not associated with periostitis, there are other unusual causes of posterior leg pain. Percy and Telep described posteromedial pain in an athlete with an anomalous muscle in the leg.[25] A soleus accessorium has been well described. It may present as cramping in the calf, aching in the posteromedial distal calf with running, painful crepitus, and swelling with activity. A definite fullness of the distal ankle is seen, and a lateral roentgenogram may show obliteration of Kager's triangle.

Primary muscle diseases such as McArdle syndrome have already been mentioned. The symptoms are usually alleviated with rest and NSAIDs; but if severe and persistent, surgical exploration or biopsy may be warranted.

STRESS FRACTURES

Stress-induced microfractures (medial tibial stress syndrome type I) are usually the result of intense, repetitive weight-bearing activities such as running, aerobic dance, or sprinting.[14] Jumping, inadequate footwear, and inappropriate training surfaces compound the problem by increasing the ground reaction forces and hence the stresses through the bone. Depending on the series and the sport concerned, tibial fractures comprise 30 to 50 percent and fibular fractures 12 to 25 percent of the lower limb stress fractures (Table 10-4).[14,26,27]

Devas was the first to clearly relate the clinical signs and plain radiologic findings in 1958, and his paper reviewed all of the key literature to that time, with special reference to the tibia.[1,27] It is interesting to note that, although the term shin splint was referred to, the terms insufficiency fracture and fatigue infraction were also used.[27,28] Two years previously, Devas had summarized the literature and presented a large number of stress fractures of the fibula in athletes.[28]

The microtrauma sustained by the bone exceeds its remodeling ability. Bone is a living tissue that accommodates to almost limitless stress if given enough time. If the stress if applied sufficiently often, and there is an inadequate period for recuperation, the bone resorption component of repair exceeds the osteoblastic element, and microscopic defects occur at the site of maximum stress risers. Stress risers are areas where mechanical stresses concentrate. With the initiation of a small crack, perpetuation of the process is likely unless some major adjustment in the training routine is made (Fig. 10-11). For some athletes it is the excessive stresses of their routine training that exceeds the bone's ability to remodel. In others it is an intense, prolonged effort on a single occasion, e.g., a race, that starts the process, which is then made worse by normal training, which was not a problem prior to this event.

There is some discussion as to whether muscle fatigue and therefore excessive bone loading is a primary factor or whether the powerful countertraction of the muscles of the leg at their origins, along with the bending moments from impact, is the major etiologic factor.

Clinical Picture

The distribution of these fractures in the tibia varies in each series, and frequently the more proximal ones are missed and classified as nonspecific knee pain (Table 10-4). The posteromedial border of the distal half of the tibia is a common site about 12 to 15 cm proximal to the medial malleolus.[29] Of these injuries, midshaft tibial stress fractures are the most difficult to manage. In the fibula they are commonly about one hand's breadth above the lateral malleolus.

There is probably a spectrum of this disorder that ranges through a diffuse stress reaction to a localized stress reaction, to a microfracture, and ultimately to a clearly visible macrofracture. Furthermore, a stress reaction evolving to a complete fracture appears differently from a healing microfracture. The radiologic picture may be confusing, not always correlating with the clinical presentation and is one reason for the confusion of terms, which include medial tibial stress syndrome (Detmer's type IB), periostitis, and medial tibial stress reaction. These describe the early response to bone overload before the obvious localized pathology of a stress microfracture has evolved (Fig. 10-11).

The tenderness may be diffuse, but usually there is one area of exquisite discomfort to palpation. As the fracture progresses, pain with activity develops to the point that even walking is symptomatic.

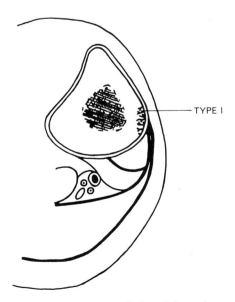

TYPE I

Fig. 10-11. Stress fracture of the tibia at its medial border (Detmer type I). Such fractures may evolve from microfractures which become macroscopic, discrete, cortical defects. They may extend over 6 to 8 cm but are usually more localized.

TABLE 10-4. Distribution of Stress Fractures[a]

Main Bone and Area	McBryde[29]	Hulkko & Orava[26]
Tibia	34	50
Upper metaphysis	7	
Upper shaft	12	25[b]
Midshaft	4	8
Lower third	11	17
Fibula	24	12
Metatarsals	19	20
Second	11	7
Third	7	8
Fourth/fifth	1	5
Femur		
Neck	7	3
Shaft	7	3
Pelvis	6	2
Others	3	10

[a] Mainly running athletes. Percentages are rounded off.
[b] Includes metaphysis and proximal third of the tibial shaft.

Specific Diagnosis

To be detected early on a plain roentgenogram, the small fracture line or the associated periosteal or medullary reaction must be caught in perfect silhouette or parallax. Later in its evolution the fracture line or callus usually becomes obvious. The decision to perform a bone scan depends on the clinical evidence, the level of participation of the athlete, activity goals, and the duration of the symptoms. It must be remembered that clinically recognizable stress fractures are part of the continuum of normal bone remodeling to physical stress. Hence at one extreme are areas of significant uptake on the scan that are clinically asymptomatic and probably represent remodeling below the clinical pain threshold. At the other extreme are cracks that are clearly apparent on plain radiographs or have even progressed to complete fracture.[30] To further complicate the picture, Milgrom et al. reported several cases of impending tibial stress fracture in which the bone scan was negative (Fig. 10-12).[31] This situation is unusual, but a highly motivated athlete with persistent and increasing bone pain may have a stress fracture despite a prior normal scan. With continued pain, either the plain film or the bone scan should be repeated. This study also illustrates the point (which has been contested by others) that in some cases the pain associated with stress fracture may occur before the radionuclide image is positive.[32] Thus the spectrum is complete.

Practice Point

INDICATIONS FOR BONE SCAN

- Magnitude of pain
- Duration of pain
- Progressive increase in symptoms
- Night pain
- Atypical location
- Unable to palpate
- Equivocal plain roentgenogram
- Unable to make a diagnosis
- Rule out infection or neoplasm

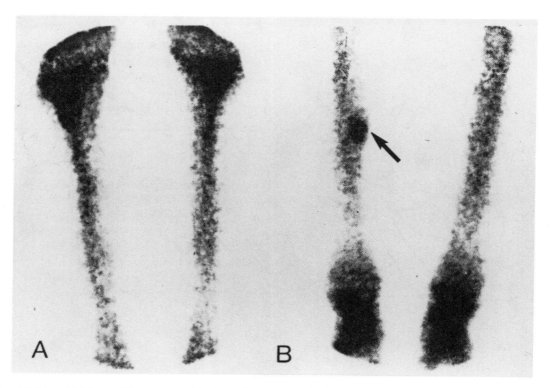

Fig. 10-12. (A) Normal bone scan 10 days after onset of bilateral tibial pain. **(B)** Bone scan 3 weeks later showing a tibial stress fracture.

Treatment

Conservative treatment is successful in most cases. The initial treatment consists of pain control, a thorough review of the training program, activity modification, footwear advice, occasionally orthotic prescription, and attention to specific strength deficits and muscle tightness.

There is some suggestion that the use of therapeutic ultrasound and pulsed electromagnetic field therapy may enhance healing, but it has yet to be proved. Attention to diet and body weight may also be considered. Overweight individuals are subjecting the skeleton to undue stress in that the impact of landing when running is about twice body weight and up to five times body weight with jumping. At the other extreme, athletes with a very low percentage of body fat, particularly amenorrheic runners, may have decreased deposition of calcium in the skeleton.

It is unusual to have to use cast immobilization. Sometimes in particularly symptomatic fractures, an air stirrup is an excellent compromise. If the fracture is progressing, particularly a midtibial fracture, an orthosis with a hinged ankle is a suitable form of protection. The period of modified, stress-relieving activity can usually be judged by the gradual resolution of symptoms (Table 10-5). However, full return to activity should await sound radiologic union in those cases in which one complete cortex was involved with a visible fracture line.

One of the aims of early therapy is to maintain cardiovascular fitness, which may be achieved by a water-running protocol, swimming, cycling, and

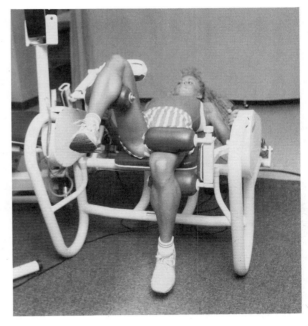

Fig. 10-13. Hydragym hip flexor and extensor omnikinetic apparatus. It allows a good cardiovascular effect and unloaded running action.

proximal muscle work on omnikinetic apparatus (Figs. 10-13 and 10-14). With healing, step machine and shuttle walking, treadmill running, and low impact aerobic work may be added (Fig. 10-15).

It has already been mentioned that midshaft tibial fractures have a tendency to become delayed or nonunion.[33-35] With patience, most of these injuries may be managed with modified immobilization or casts. Occasionally, it is more prudent to carry out an open procedure with bone grafting. This decision depends on the fracture, the athlete's sport and ambitions, and the duration of the treatment to date. A diminution of the bone scan activity, in the absence of healing, should also prompt the surgeon to consider grafting. Electromagnetic stimulation may offer some advantage in these cases.[36]

Differential Diagnosis

Pain, localized periosteal reaction on roentgenogram, and increased uptake on scan may be the hallmark of stress fractures in active individuals. However, if the plain roentgenograms do not appear typical or if the patient does not respond to therapy, new films and further investigation are warranted.

Osteoid osteomas are not rare lesions, and when

TABLE 10-5. Suggested Period of Modified Activity and Healing Times

Bone	Period of Stress-Relieved Activity (weeks)	% Healed over 2 to >8 Weeks[a]		
		2–4	5–8	>8
Tibia				
Metaphysis	4–6	—	100	—
Proximal third	8–10	—	40	60
Middle third	8–10	—	45	55
Distal third	6–8	—	55	45
Fibula	3–4	5	75	20
Metatarsals*	2–4	20	60	20
Femoral neck	12–16	—	5	95
Femoral shaft	12–16	5	5	90

[a] Healing time depends on severity and stage at which diagnosed. (Modified from Orava[33] and Hulkko and Orava[26] by supplementing with author's data.)

* Except base of 5th metatarsal.

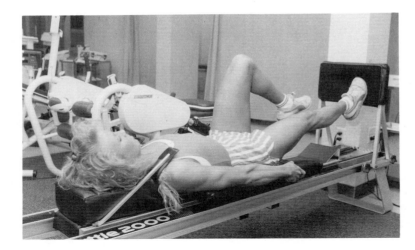

Fig. 10-14. Rebounding on the shuttle allows reintegration into training.

they occur the tibia is a frequent site. These benign tumorous or reactive lesions have a sclerotic margin and a lucent nidus that may be difficult to see. The pain may not be related to activity, and there is an element of night pain that is helped by aspirin or other NSAIDs.

Brodies abscess is another lesion that may simulate a stress reaction. It is commonly found in the distal tibia. The pain from a Brodies abscess may be intense; conversely, it may also have an asymptomatic phase.

Occasionally bone infarcts and growth arrest lines are mistaken for a stress reaction. A careful history and following the progress of the patient carefully, as well as experience in interpretation of good quality films allow the correct differential diagnosis to be made.

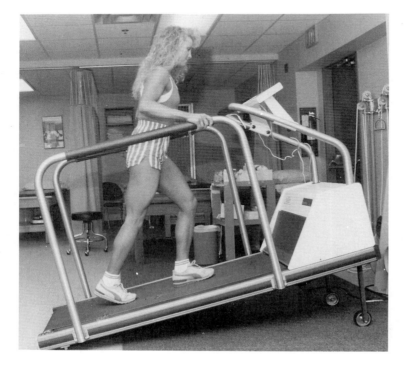

Fig. 10-15. Treadmill work can be programmed for specific progression and decreases the impact of foot contact.

COMPARTMENT SYNDROMES

Chronic Compartment Syndromes

A chronic compartment syndrome (exercise-induced ischemia, recurrent compartment syndrome, exertional compartment syndrome) exists when increased intramuscular pressure during exercise impedes the blood flow and function of the tissues within that compartment.[37] The syndrome occurs in anatomic locations that have unyielding, well defined osteofascial spaces. Although exertion and trauma play a central role, the exact etiology is not understood.

Etiology and Pathophysiology

The most common factor linking patients with chronic compartment syndromes is a high level of physical activity with repetitive dorsi- and plantar flexion motion, as characterized by walking and running (Table 10-6). Muscle hypertrophy beyond the limits of the compartment seems a plausible suggestion, but the infrequent occurrence in body builders tends to refute it. Microtrauma to muscle tissue and stress to the microcirculation and lymphatics with excessive activity may give rise to myositis and an inflammatory reaction in the capillary bed,[36] which in turn may alter capillary permeability (Fig. 10-16).

With activity there is increased blood flow to the various compartments of the leg. Such increased flow precipitates an increase in volume, which results in increased pressure within the specific muscle compartment. This physiologic situation is normal. Skeletal muscle is not well perfused during contraction, as the arterial inflow is reduced. For this reason muscle relaxation pressure during exercise, i.e., the pressure between contractions, is the most important pressure.[38] It has been shown that muscle relaxation pressure during exercise exceeding 35 mmHg impedes muscle blood flow and correlates well with the devel-

TABLE 10-6. Anterior Compartment Pressures During Selected Activities

	Pressure (mmHg)	
Condition	Group With No Symptoms	Symptomatic[a] Group
Pre-exercise		
Supine		
Resting	16 (5)	22 (9)
Max. resisted dorsiflexion	91 (32)	157 (43)
Max. resisted plantar flexion	79 (21)	89 (38)
Standing		
Relaxed	41 (9)	52 (16)
On tip toes	73 (16)	95 (29)
On heels	77 (24)	148 (49)
During exercise		
Walking (mean)	46 (12)	74 (23)
Running (mean)	66 (16)	106 (18)
Systolic	143 (32)	200 (30)
Diastolic	24 (10)	51 (18)
After exercise		
Standing		
Relaxed	66 (17)	100 (26)
On tip toes	89 (13)	138 (44)
On heels	106 (41)	183 (49)
Supine		
Max. resisted dorsiflexion	120 (47)	162 (34)
Max. resisted plantar flexion	102 (37)	138 (40)
Resting	24 (9)	44 (23)

Numbers in parentheses are standard deviations (SD).
[a] All values are significantly different from those of asymptomatic athletes.
(Adapted from data by McDermott et al.[40])

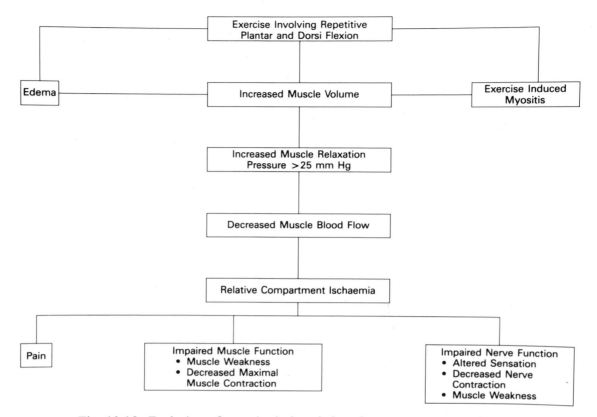

Fig. 10-16. Evolution of exercise-induced chronic compartment syndrome.

opment of pain, swelling, and impaired function.[39] In fact, compartment syndromes correlate well with the decreased difference between mean arterial pressure and muscle relaxation pressure during exercise.[37]

Under normal circumstances, resting compartment pressures are in the region of 5 to 15 mmHg and are frequently less than 10 mmHg.[40-42] Exercising pressures may rise to 60 to 70 mmHg and values of up to 150 mmHg and more have been recorded. However, the features of a healthy situation is that average pressures rarely rise above 30 mmHg, and the muscle relaxation pressures between contractions usually are in the range of 15 to 25 mmHg.[42,45] The other finding is that with the cessation of activity the pressure returns to pre-exercise levels within 5 to 10 minutes and frequently within 2 minutes (Fig. 10-17).

In summary, the characteristics of athletes with a chronic compartment syndrome are occasionally high resting pressure (20 to 30 mmHg), usually high exercising pressure (80 to 120 mmHg), and invariably a delay in return to the pre-exercise level beyond 5 to

10 minutes.[19,42] This last parameter is perhaps the most important diagnostic point (Table 10-7).

Clinical Diagnosis

Pain induced only by athletic activity, often arising at a specific point in the training session, suggests the syndrome. The pain is located along the specific muscle group involved. Depending on the severity of the syndrome, numbness or tingling may occur in the distribution of the nerve that traverses the particular compartment. If the athlete persists with the activity, despite the symptoms, muscle weakness and subsequent local tenderness ensue. The symptoms characteristically disappear fairly promptly at the cessation of exercise, although the tenderness may persist. Sometimes the pain appears at a set mileage depending on the speed and terrain, and it does not seem to worsen over a period of time. A "second day" phenomenon may be present in which strenuous activity one day leads to a decrease in exercise tolerance the

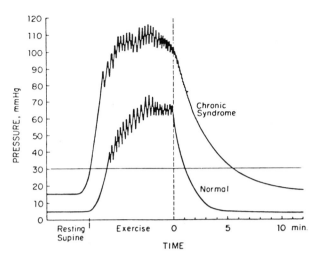

Fig. 10-17. Anterior compartment pressures recorded during exercise and rest. Typical tracing of an individual with chronic anterior compartment syndrome. The resting pressures may or may not be higher; the exercise pressures are frequently higher; and the interval to return to normal is prolonged to more than 5 minutes. (From Mubarak SJ, Hargens MA. Compartment Syndromes and Volkman's contracture. p. 218 W.B. Saunders Co., Philadelphia 1981, with permission.)

muscle weakness and impaired nerve function. Electromyographic studies and nerve conduction tests are usually normal at rest.[44] The merits of the various techniques of measuring compartment pressures are not discussed here; however, the method used, the experience of the clinician, and the measurement at rest versus exercise have significant implications.[22,36,39,40,42,44,45] Pressure measurements assist in establishing the diagnosis and confirming the extent to which each compartment is involved. Certainly no operative treatment of this condition should be undertaken without prior pressure recordings.

Practice Point

CRITERIA FOR ABNORMAL PRESSURES IN EXERCISE INDUCED COMPARTMENT SYNDROME

- Resting pressures > 30 mmHg
- Immediate (15 seconds) after exercise pressure > 60
- Two minutes after exercise pressure > 20
  – Any of the above

---

following day. In other circumstances the syndrome progresses so the athlete becomes increasingly hampered by the condition, and eventually even walking produces the discomfort. The anterior compartment muscles are more affected by skiing and walking and the posterior compartment muscles by running and jogging, although this pattern is by no means a rule.

Clinical evaluation, after exercise to the point of discomfort, is normally most fruitful with evidence of

Specific Chronic Compartment Syndromes

The anterior and deep posterior compartments are most frequently involved, but occasionally the lateral and superficial posterior compartments are implicated (Fig. 10-18). The symptoms are described for a fully developed syndrome, realizing that with a mild chronic compartment problem pain at a certain point in the activity may be the only complaint (Table 10-8).

TABLE 10-7. Intramuscular Compartment Pressures at Rest and Exercise

Patient Group	Deep Posterior Compartment Pressure (mmHg)					Anterior Tibial Compartment Pressure (mmHg)				
	Before	During	1 Min After	5 Min After	10 Min After	Before	During	1 Min After	5 Min After	10 Min After
Healthy controls	6 (3)	19 (80)	8 (5)	7 (6)	8 (6)	8 (6)	34 (32)	9 (9)	9 (8)	8 (7)
Posterior compartment syndrome	6 (3)	27 (13)	10 (7)	11 (6)	8 (4)	10 (5)	51 (31)	24 (28)	20 (26)	18 (17)
Anterior compartment syndrome	8 (7)	17 (13)	7 (7)	5 (5)	7 (6)	11 (10)	73 (48)	41 (31)	31 (30)	44 (30)

Numbers in parentheses are the SDs.
(From Wallensten and Eriksson,[22] with permission.)

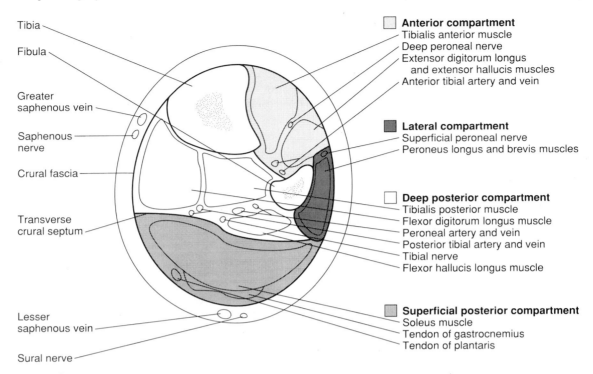

Fig. 10-18. Cross section of the leg, illustrating contents of major compartments.

Deep Posterior Compartment (Medial Tibial Stress Syndrome)

Described by Detmer as medial tibial stress syndrome type III, and as one of the two possible causes of the medial tibial syndrome by Puranen who first coined the term, the posterior medial leg pain syndrome is the most difficult to isolate from other causes of shin splints when in its mildest form.[4,8] These individuals typically describe aching or pain referable to the area adjacent to the posteromedial tibial border or deep within the distal half of the leg (Fig. 10-19). It is usually precipitated by a sudden increase in duration or intensity of exercise but then becomes persistent. Once established, the symptoms become progressive in about two-thirds of individuals, and in about one-half of the severe cases the symptoms are bilateral. When parethesias occur they are usually referred to the instep of the foot. Tenderness may appear to be along the bone, but with careful examination in a lean individual it may be possible to localize it to the muscular soft tissue posterior to the periosteal–fascial junction, deep within the leg.

In the early stages the symptoms stop promptly with the cessation of activity, but ultimately as they worsen a decline in performance brings the patient to the attention of a therapist or physician. In approximately one-third, the symptoms last up to 2 hours after exercise. Others are able to run 2 to 3 miles in pain but often regret doing so when soreness and tightness keep them awake at night.[8] In a few, the tight feeling persists from workout to workout, but it is surprising how few of these disorders develop into an acute compartment syndrome. Numbness of the toes is uncommon, but testing of muscles immediately upon cessation of exercise may reveal weakness of toe flexion and particularly inversion.

If there is pain on stretching the posterior compartment muscles into dorsiflexion, if local tenderness is significant, if plantar sensation is decreased, and if the tibialis posterior pulse is diminished, an acute compartment syndrome is likely to be developing.

Isolated Tibialis Posterior Compartment

The tibialis posterior muscle may be situated in a clearly distinct compartment of its own surrounded by the intermuscular septum and a tough muscle sheath that isolates it from the remaining deep poste-

TABLE 10-8. Signs and Symptoms of Elevated Compartment Pressures[a]

Anatomic Compartment	Initial Pain Location	Sensory Nerve	Sensory Change	Muscles Involved	Muscle Weakness	Pain on Stretch	Pulses[b]
Deep posterior	Posteromedial border tibia distal one-third of leg	Tibial nerve	Sole of foot and toes	Flexor hallucis longus Flexor digitorum Tibialis posterior	Toe flexion and inversion	Dorsiflexion toes and ankles	Posterior tibial artery
Tibialis posterior (isolated)	Posteromedial border tibia	None	None	Tibialis posterior	Inversion	Dorsiflexion ankle	None
Superficial posterior	Posterior middle one-third of leg	Sural nerve	Lateral foot	Gastrocnemius Soleus	Plantar flexion	Dorsiflexion ankle	None
Anterior	Anterior aspect of shin and leg	Deep peroneal nerve	Dorsum of foot	Tibialis anterior Ext. hallucis longus Ext. digitorum longus	Toe extension and dorsiflexion	Toe and ankle plantar flexion with inversion	Dorsalis pedis
Lateral	Middle one-third of anterolateral leg	Superficial peroneal nerve	Cleft between first and second toes	Peroneus longus Peroneus brevis	Eversion	Ankle inversion with plantar flexion	None

[a] If compartment swollen and tense and muscles tender to palpate with pain on stretch, treat as an acute syndrome unless proved otherwise.
[b] Diminished but rarely absent.

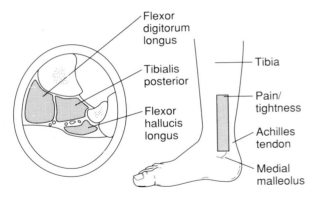

Fig. 10-19. Deep posterior compartment involvement in chronic exercise-induced syndrome.

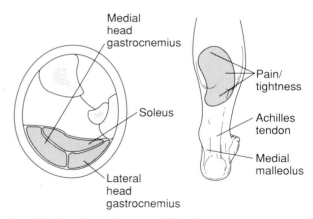

Fig. 10-21. Chronic exercise-induced compartment syndrome of the superficial posterior compartment.

rior compartment (Fig. 10-20).[46] Pain is still located along the posterior medial border of the leg, and weakness when present may be noticeable particularly at push-off. There is no associated sensory loss, although the pain may radiate to the medial arch. This muscle may be the cause of persisting symptoms in cases where operative fascial release has failed. Surgical attempts to split the fascial envelope of tibialis posterior may be necessary.

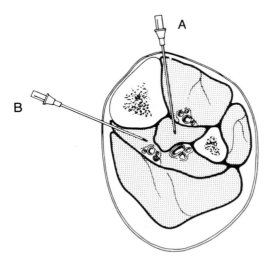

Fig. 10-20. Needle placement **(A)** for measuring the isolated tibialis posterior compartment and **(B)** the deep posterior compartment. (After Davey et al.,[46] with permission.)

Superficial Posterior Compartment

The superficial posterior compartment contains the gastrocnemius and soleus muscles and is more frequently involved in acute compartment problems secondary to muscle rupture or hemorrhage following contusion than with the chronic exercise-induced syndrome.[47,48] (Fig. 10-21). The sural nerve lies in the fascia of the compartment, and if sufficient pressure is established it may produce dysesthesia along the lateral foot, although this is rare. The usual presentation is a feeling of tightness or pain in the mid and upper calf. After exercise to the point of significant discomfort, some weakness of plantar flexion may be detected.

Anterior Compartment

The anterior compartment is the most accessible to clinical inspection and pressure measurements and therefore often the most commonly diagnosed. The aching or pain is located in the middle one-third of the anterior lateral leg, and with continued activity some weakness may be detected with active dorsiflexion—frequently experienced by race walkers, cross country skiers, joggers, and soccer players.[40,45,49] Athletes who persist in continuing their running may even report the onset of pain at a specific mileage and dysesthesia, or numbness in the first cleft of the toes. They may ultimately experience a minor footdrop due to muscle weakness before they quit (Fig. 10-22). Many of these athletes experience

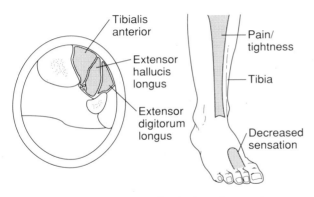

Fig. 10-22. Chronic exercise-induced anterior compartment syndrome.

tenderness over the anterior margin of the tibia; however, pain at multiple locations in the lower leg induced by running a short distance but allowing continued activity despite pain usually indicates pathology of a noncompartment syndrome nature (Table 10-9).[46] Small fascial defects with muscle herniation have been reported in 20 to 60 percent of these patients with exercise-induced ischemia and in fewer than 5 percent of athletes with anterior pain for other reasons and therefore may be a contributing factor.[44] These defects are sometimes palpable. Muscle hernias in the lower leg commonly lie over the anterior intermuscular septum between the anterior and lateral compartments. No attempt should be

TABLE 10-9. Anterolateral Leg Pain

	Musculotendinous			Anterior Tibial Syndrome		
Parameter	Periostitis	Tenosynovitis	Stress Fracture	Chronic Compartment Syndromes		Acute Compartment Syndromes
Lesion	Sterile inflammation due to strain or microtrauma to periosteum, fascial attachment or interosseous membrane	Inflammation of tendon sheath	Fibula; usually lower one-third	Anterior compartment syndrome Swelling and edema Fascial defects	Lateral compartment syndrome Swelling and edema	Usually trauma with contusion or hemorrhage
History						
Trauma	—	—	—	—	—	+
Repetitive activity	+	+	+	+	+	±
Hard surface or inadequate footwear	+	+	+	+	+	—
Pain						
At rest	Late mild	Late mild	Late moderate	Early	Early	Early severe
Non-weight-bearing	Rarely	Rarely	Rarely	Rarely	Rarely	Early sign
Walking	Late moderate	Late mild	Early sign	Early moderate	Late mild	Early sign
Running	Early	Early	Early severe	Proportional to activity	Proportional to activity	Immediate
Signs	Anterior tibial border tenderness No swelling	Tender to palpation over tendon, occasional	Local tenderness over fibula	Sensory dysesthesia and weakness Proportion to activity		Tender to palpation and stretch Swelling Sensory change Weakness
Special tests	None early Late cortical reaction on X-ray	None	Early: bone scan Late: plain film	Elevated compartment pressures After exercise Late return to normal		High resting compartment pressures

made to close these defects, as it might result in an acute compartment syndrome. Fasciotomy is the correct approach if the injury is sufficiently symptomatic. A branch of the superficial peroneal nerve is frequently located in this area and is at risk of surgical damage in an anterior compartment release.

Lateral Compartment

Only a few cases of isolated chronic and acute lateral compartment syndromes have been reported.[50] It must be distinguished from acute muscle cramping, tenosynovitis of the tibialis anterior and flexor hallucis longus, stress fracture of the fibula, periostitis, and tearing of the lateral head of the gastrocnemius (Fig. 10-23). At its extreme, the compartment may be palpated with selected swelling and stony hardness.[50] There is tenderness in the proximal half of the leg. With superficial peroneal nerve involvement there may be numbness over the dorsum of the foot and the lateral four toes as well as weakness during dorsiflexion and eversion.

The superficial peroneal nerve may be entrapped without associated compartment pressure elevation. The symptoms are pain and sometimes sensory abnormalities in the dorsum of the foot.[44,47,51,52] The causes include compression by lipoma, traction due to ankle sprains, muscle herniation through fascial defects, compression in a "peroneal tunnel" as it emerges through the fascia, and retraction of the fascia after surgical release (Fig. 10-24).[52] Sometimes nerve conduction studies are diagnostic. Treatment may be surgical exploration.

Treatment of Chronic Exercise-Induced Compartment Syndromes

It is essential to establish a firm diagnosis with chronic exercise-induced compartment syndrome because frequently nonoperative treatment is not successful. The athlete should then clearly understand the options. Particularly, the deep posterior compartment syndrome is difficult to distinguish from other conditions that produce posteromedial border tibial pain.

Differential Diagnosis

Resting discomfort and pain immediately on weight-bearing may help to distinguish stress fractures and periostitis. The diffuse pain along the ante-

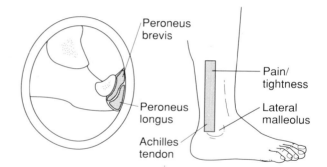

Fig. 10-23. Symptoms with lateral compartment involvement.

rior and posteromedial tibia borders associated with periostitis as well as the more local pain and sometimes swelling seen with a stress fracture, are occasionally matched by changes visible on a plain roentgenogram. Frequently, however, a bone scan is necessary to rule out bone pathology. Pain on resistance to a specific movement and palpable tenderness or crepitus help distinguish tendinitis.

Arterial entrapment syndromes, despite a history of claudication, may require a high index of suspicion for diagnosis. The commonest of these disorders in the young athlete is the popliteal artery entrapment syndrome by either the medial head of gastrocnemius or the soleal fascia (Fig. 10-25).[53] Doppler flow studies may precede the more invasive arteriogram. In the older athletic population atherosclerosis is always a possibility. Changes in peripheral pulses, atrophic skin and nail changes, and a strong family history indicate the possibility of vascular occlusive disease.

Repeated episodes of delayed muscle soreness, particularly secondary to prolonged downhill running or a sequential rapid increase in training is an obvious cause of pain and stiffness. Eccentric exercise is capable of increasing the muscle water content by 3 percent and results in high intramuscular pressures at rest.[54] There is no argument that the contractile apparatus may be damaged by eccentric exercise, but delayed muscle soreness as a prolonged cause of lower leg pain is unusual.

A rare differential includes those athletes with McArdle's syndrome, who present with weakness without pain while running. Some of them describe being able to run through the problem, the "second wind phenomenon."[55] These patients must be distinguished from athletes with a neurogenic cause of weakness. Disc disease and radiculopathy in the

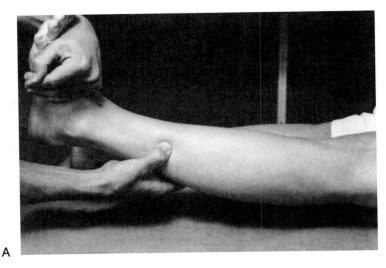

A

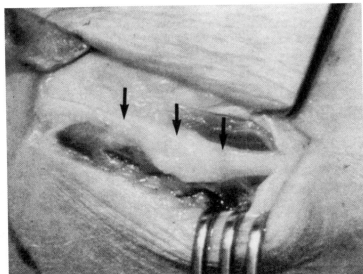

B

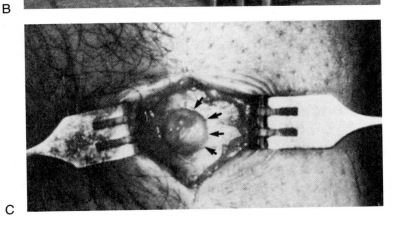

C

Fig. 10-24. Peroneal nerve compression or muscle herniation is most frequently found in the anterior or lateral compartment. **(A)** Pain over the anterior intermuscular septum while the patient actively dorsiflexes and everts the ankle may precipitate the pain. **(B)** Poststenotic swelling as the entrapped nerve emerges through the fascia. **(C)** Muscle herniation through fascial defect. (From Styf,[51] with permission.)

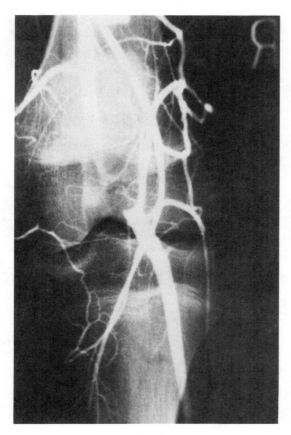

Fig. 10-25. Anomalous entrapment and occlusion of the popliteal artery secondary to pressure of fascia around the medial head of the gastrocnemius.

young patient and spinal stenosis in the older person are easy to confuse with compartment syndrome if they present with only peripheral signs. If the symptoms are more severe than those usually experienced by the athlete, or if there is an element of trauma involved, the acute compartment syndrome must always be borne in mind and ruled out (Table 10-9).

Measurement of the exercising or postexercise compartment pressure establishes the diagnosis, the magnitude of the problem, and the specific compartments involved. These measurements should be contemplated after 6 weeks of unsuccessful therapy and if there is a high clinical index of suspicion that the athlete does have exercise-induced ischemia.

Specific Treatment

Despite the fact that conservative therapy may not be successful, it is still the first step in the management of this syndrome. Extrinsic factors such as training errors, poor techniques, poor shoes, and inappropriate training surfaces are carefully elicited via the history. Intrinsic factors such as alignment, muscle imbalance, and unbalanced or inadequate flexibility are assessed. For individuals with minor complaints, education, implementation of appropriate changes, and adequate therapy may allow remission of symptoms. NSAIDs and occasionally diuretics may supplement the strengthening, stretching, orthotics, and activity modification. A well planned water-running program may be instituted in order to keep up aerobic fitness and reduce ballistic work. Dancers can perform non-bounce aerobics, and sometimes a change from running to cycling is advantageous. If this therapy is ineffective over a 4- to 6-week period and the symptoms are sufficiently disabling, surgery may be contemplated. Despite the motivation and level of participation, a change of activity in mild to moderate cases, and complete cessation of all provocative activities in severe cases may still be acceptable alternatives.

Surgical Therapy

When high compartment pressures have been confirmed and nonoperative treatment has failed, fasciotomy is the treatment of choice. Properly placed and executed surgical therapy has a success rate of close to 90 percent. Occasionally, athletes are unable to resume or progress their activity in exactly the manner they would wish. In some circumstances the failure is due to the prolonged severe nature of the preexisting syndrome with measurable changes in the function of the compartment. Some of these patients may indeed have even suffered an episode of acute compartment hypertension. In animal experiments, fascial release has been shown to decrease the muscle force that may be generated.[56] However, athletes with chronic anterior compartment syndrome usually increase their performance owing to pain relief after surgery.[37] Occasionally, after fasciotomy of the anterior compartment, the superficial peroneal nerve is entrapped. Swelling of the muscle displaces the released fascial flap, which in turn may put traction on the nerve as it emerges through the fascia.[57] It is also possible that, owing to insufficient release, there may be regeneration of the fascia or spontaneous closure of the defect. The previously mentioned isolated tibialis posterior compartment may have been insufficiently released and be a source of residual symptoms.[57]

The surgical release for exercise-induced chronic compartment syndrome may be carried out through restricted incisions and subcutaneous division of the appropriate sheaths proximally and distally. Care must be taken to avoid the sensory branches of the nerves. When there is definite evidence of involvement of the tibialis posterior muscle, a more extensive incision is required to ensure adequate release of its sheath. Furthermore, repeat surgery should be performed through the extended incision (Fig. 10-26).

Postoperatively, pressure dressings and rest for 48 hours followed by gentle partial weight-bearing and active dorsiflexion and plantar flexion are advised. The use of ice packs beginning immediately after surgery for 20 minutes of each hour is advantageous. For the first 3 weeks after surgery, the emphasis should be on range of motion and strength. Gentle running may be started at 3 weeks, supplemented by some strengthening work and a water-running program. By 6 to 9 weeks most individuals have reached or sur-

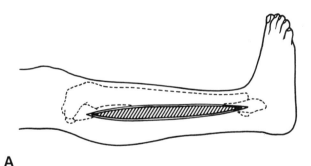

A

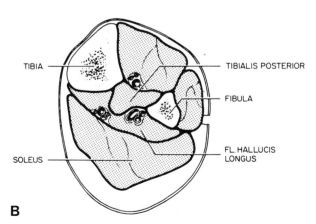

B

Fig. 10-26. (A) Degree of exposure desirable varies from case to case. This figure illustrates extensile exposure. **(B)** Location of the lateral incision, which gives access to anterior and posterior structures.

> **Clinical Point**
>
> **FASCIOTOMY POSTOPERATIVE PROGRAM**
>
> - Significant swelling and pain after surgery
>   - Ice 20 minutes during each hour
>   - Gentle range of motion
>   - Non-weight-bearing for 24 hours
>   - Partial weight-bearing until swelling reduced
>   - Range of motion (ROM) exercises
>   - Then proceed to appropriate point in program below
> - Minimal postoperative swelling and pain
>   - Ice 20 minutes every hour during day
>   - Partial weight-bearing for 48 hours
>   - Early ROM exercises
>   - Strengthening by active exercises at 48 hours
>   - Strengthening by resisted exercises at 1 week
>   - Swimming or water-running at 1 week
>   - Cycling at 2 weeks
>   - Running at 2 weeks if full ROM
>   - Resume workouts at 3 weeks
>   - Alternate-day running only initially
>   - Activity not progressed unless running and jumping are pain-free
>   - Full activity at 6 to 9 weeks

passed their preoperative levels, depending on the severity of their previous symptoms. Factors leading to the chronic syndromes are summarized in (Fig. 10-27).

Acute Compartment Syndromes

An acute compartment syndrome is a medical and surgical emergency. It must be distinguished from the chronic syndrome with respect to physiologic, diagnostic, and treatment factors if a serious, even tragic, outcome is to be avoided. (Table 10-9). An acute compartment syndrome exists when the circulation and the function of the tissues within a closed space are compromised by increased pressure within that anatomic area. The implication is that if the condition is not diagnosed and treated expeditiously, expertly, and with a due regard to the potentially serious

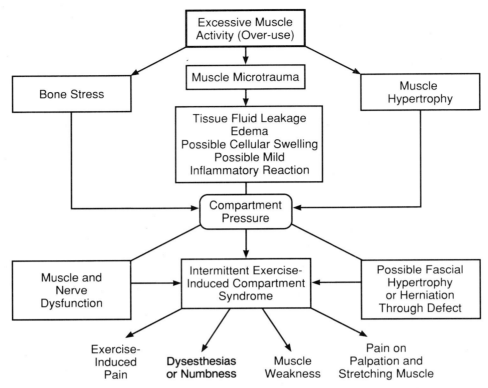

Fig. 10-27. Contributing factors to chronic exercise-induced syndromes.

outcome, permanent tissue destruction is ensured. The key, then, is recognition.

Etiology

Overall this syndrome is usually the result of significant trauma, fractures, crushing injuries, or circulatory occlusion (Fig. 10-28). However, it occasionally occurs in sports, usually subsequent to a direct blow, as in hockey, soccer, or football. There is considerable danger of initially diagnosing these situations as acute muscle strains and overlooking the more serious compartment circulatory compromise.[48,58] Other situations include excessive unaccustomed intense exercise. Surprisingly, the evolution of an acute syndrome in an individual who has a known history of chronic compartment problems is unusual. A rarer situation is contusion and bleeding in an athlete who has prolonged clotting times caused by the use of anti-inflammatory medication.[58]

Pathologic Changes

The amount of pressure required to produce a compartment syndrome depends on the duration of the increased pressure, metabolic rate of the tissues,

vascular tone, and local blood pressure. Nerve exhibits functional abnormalities within 30 minutes of the onset of ischemia, which the athlete experiences as pain paresthesia or hypesthesia. Irreversible changes are present after 12 to 24 hours but may occur sooner. Muscle exhibits functional changes within 2 to 4 hours, with irreversible changes occurring soon after. Myoglobinuria occurs after 4 hours of total ischemia, which may become maximal about 3 hours after the circulation is restored.

An acute compartment syndrome treated within 12 hours has a complication rate of less than 10 percent. After 12 hours the complication rate rises to 80 percent and the amputation rate to 40 percent!

Clinical Presentation

The signs and symptoms include increasing pain, even with the cessation of activity. The pain is out of proportion to the clinical situation. When palpable, the compartment is tense and the overlying skin may be discolored and shiny. Palpation reveals extreme tenderness. With the passage of time there is obvious sensory change in the foot depending on the compartment involved. By using two-point discrimina-

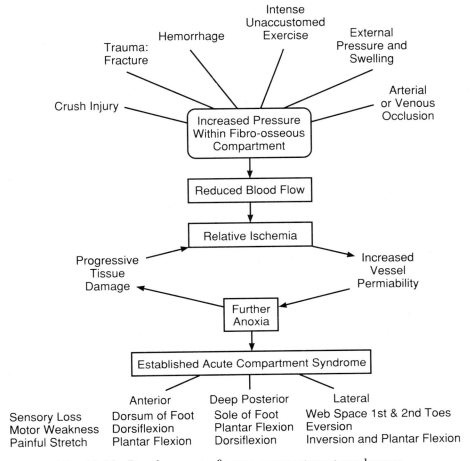

Fig. 10-28. Development of acute compartment syndromes.

tion, this sensory change may be detected early. Stretching of the muscles passively may precipitate excruciating pain, and the inability to generate a significant contraction due to pain inhibition or true pathologic changes in muscle physiology, is obvious. The pulses are usually diminished if the major vessel goes through the involved compartment, but their complete obliteration is a late sign. *A normal pulse does not rule out the syndrome.*

These signs should stimulate the need for pressure studies and frequent re-examination. In the face of normal pressure measurement but significant clinical findings, treatment is based on the clinical evidence.

Treatment

Usually compartment pressures less than 30 mmHg are acceptable; those 30 to 50 mmHg are equivocal; and those more than 50 mmHg constitute a surgical emergency. In situations where immediate definitive care is not possible or clinical signs warrant further observation, all bandages, wraps, or plaster should be completely removed. If oxygen is available it should be used to maximize the tissue PO_2. *The limb must not be elevated,* as it would decrease arterial pressure and further compromise capillary filling. Elevation of the limb by 55 cm reduces the arterial pressure by 40 mmHg without affecting local venous pressure. The early use of ice is probably acceptable.

Surgical decompression should be complete and full. There is not place for small skin incisions, and the wounds should be left open for secondary closure or skin graft. No tourniquet should be used. If the syndrome has been established for a long time or if there is extensive muscle damage, due care must be taken to monitor and treat metabolic and renal complications.

It is worth stressing again that a high index of suspicion, careful repeated examinations, and prompt surgical care may be limb-saving. The major clinical

<table>
<tr><td>

Clinical Point

ACUTE COMPARTMENT SYNDROME

- Treated within 12 hours, complication rate 10 percent
- After 12 hours, complication rate 80 percent, amputation rate 40 percent
- Need index of suspicion
- Early measurement of compartment pressures
- Believe clinical signs
- Repeated assessments
- Syndrome not ruled out by a normal pulse

</td></tr>
</table>

findings for each compartment are reviewed in Table 10-8.

Other Related Syndromes

Effort-Induced Thrombosis

Effort-induced thrombosis was first described by Sir James Paget in 1875 and Von Schroetter in 1884 —hence the term Paget-Schroetter syndrome.[59] Most of these injuries are in the upper extremities and involve throwing, pulling, swinging, batting, or pitching.[60] In the lower limbs effort-induced thrombosis has been described in joggers, skiers, marathoners, soccer players, and kick boxers.[59,61] In these situations it is frequently misdiagnosed as a Baker's cyst or an intramuscular hematoma. An index of suspicion is necessary to pick up the positive Homan sign, swelling, and calf pain. The threat of pulmonary embolism demands that deep vein thrombosis be considered in the differential diagnosis of leg pain and swelling in athletes.

In athletes an intimal tear of the vessel wall is a possibility. Other causes may be reviewed by considering the Virchow triad: decreased flow, changes in the vessel wall, and changes in the coagulation parameters of blood.[59] A flow decrease, such as that induced by long periods of sitting during travel, may increase coagulability and initiate thrombosis. Intrinsic mechanical pathology leading to repetitive trauma to the intima or violent kicking maneuvers or a blow are possibilities. Changes in viscosity may be due to hypercoagulable states, as seen with gastrointestinal malignancies, polycythemia, sickle cell disease, pa-

tients taking estrogen-containing preparations such as birth control pills, and athletes with an elevated antithrombin III level. The diagnosis is confirmed by venogram and prompt anticoagulant therapy started.

Popliteal Artery Entrapment Syndrome

Some individuals have congenital variations of their anatomy relating to the popliteal artery. In these instances the vessel is in danger of being entrapped by either a cyst that compresses the vessel, a fibrous strand that decreases the flow, or pressure due to intermittent contraction of the medial head of gastrocnemius. Sometimes it is the abnormal course taken by the vessel that predisposes it to pressure.[62] Regardless of the anatomic or embryologic anomaly, the result is episodic, and functional occlusion of the popliteal artery occurs with plantar flexion. When the syndrome persists sufficiently long, repeated internal damage may lead to thrombosis formation and complete vessel occlusion (Fig. 10-25).

The syndrome is characterized by: (1) a history of intermittent claudication in a nonatherosclerotic individual; (2) frequently unilateral occurrence in young athletes; (3) diminished pedal pulses with sustained active plantar flexion with forced passive dorsiflexion of the foot; (4) altered flow on Doppler study; and (5) confirmation with angiographic studies of occlusion and medial deviation of the popliteal artery.[63] The claudication may manifest as cramping with exercise. It is interesting that some individuals, prior to developing thrombosis of the vessel, may have the ability to run without difficulty but have classic intermittent claudication while walking.[62] Early, with only mild symptoms, a dramatic decrease in activity may be sufficient; but usually by the time the symptoms are severe enough to make an adequate diagnosis surgical treatment is required.

SUMMARY

The multifactorial nature of the problem of shin splints has led to a confusion in terms as concepts presented in the literature gradually evolved into an understanding of the various causes of leg pain induced by activity. Essentially, clinical diagnosis begins by dividing the syndromes into anterolateral and posterior medial leg pain. These categories, in turn, may be considered under (1) periosteal, fascial, and tendon problems; (2) stress reaction and stress fractures of bone; (3) exercise-induced compartment syndromes; and (4) more unusual pathology in the differential diagnosis. From the perspective of the posterior medial syndromes, they are referred to as medial tibial stress syndromes. Logical treatment requires careful observation of the athlete in order to identify the most probable cause of pain. Bone scan facilities, equipment for testing compartment pressures, and the ability to carry out sophisticated tests are sometimes required, but a specific diagnosis and specific etiology may defy the best efforts of the medical team. Ultimately, only drastic alteration in the activity level suffices to provide permanent relief of this annoying and sometimes dangerous syndrome.

REFERENCES

1. Devas MB: Stress fractures of the tibia in athletes or "shin soreness." J Bone Joint Surg [Br] 40:227, 1958

2. Slocum DB: Overuse syndromes of the lower leg and foot in athletes. Instruct Course Lect Am Acad Orthop Surg 17:359, 1960

3. Slocum DB: The shin splint syndrome: medical aspects and differential diagnosis. Am J Surg 114:875, 1967

4. Puranen J: The medial tibial syndrome: exercise ischaemia in the medial fascial compartment of the leg. J Bone Joint Surg [Br] 56:712, 1974

5. Clement DB: Tibial stress syndrome in athletes. J Sports Med 2:81, 1974

6. Mubarak SJ, Gould RN, Lee YF et al: The medial tibial stress syndrome: a cause of shin splints. Am J Sports Med 10:201, 1982

7. Michael RH, Holder LE: The soleus syndrome: a cause of medial tibial stress (shin splints). Am J Sports Med 13:87, 1985

8. Detmer DE: Chronic shin splints: classification and management of medial tibial stress syndrome. Sports Med 3:436, 1986

9. Basmajian JV: Muscles Alive. 5th Ed. Williams & Wilkins, Baltimore, 1979

10. O'Connell AL, Mortensen OA: An eletromyographic study of the leg musculature during movements of the free foot and during standing. Anat Rec 127:342, 1957

11. James SL, Bates BT, Osternig LR: Injuries to runners. Am J Sports Med 6:40, 1978

12. Viita Sala JT, Kuist M: Some biomechanical aspects of the foot and ankle in athletes with and without shin splints. Am J Sports Med 11:125, 1983

13. Myburgh KH, Srobler N, Noskes TD: Factors associated with shin soreness in athletes. Physician Sports Med 16:4, 129, 1988

14. Clement DB, Taunton JE, Smart GW et al: A survey of overuse running injuries. Physician Sports Med 9:47, 1981

15. Gans A: The relationship of heel contact in ascent and descent from jumps to the incidence of shin splints in ballet dancers. Phys Ther 65:1191, 1985

16. Wallensten R, Karlsson J: Histochemical and metabolic changes in lower leg muscles in exercise induced pain. Int J Sports Med 5:202, 1984

17. Richie DH, Kelso SF, Bellwood PA: Aerobic dance injuries: a retrospective study of instructors and participants. Physician Sports Med 13:130, 1985

18. Griffin J: Patients treated with ultrasonic driven hydrocortisone and with ultrasound alone. Phys Ther 47:70, 1966

19. Delacerda FG: Iontopheresis for treatment of shin splints. J Orthop Sports Phys Ther 3:183, 1982

20. Rasmussen W: Shin splints: definition and treatment. J Sports Med 2:111, 1974

21. Dickson TB, Kichline PD: Functional management of stress fractures in female athletes using a pneumatic leg brace. Am J Sports Med 15:86, 1987

22. Wallensten R, Eriksson E: Intramuscular pressures in exercise induced lower leg pain. Int J Sports Med 5:31, 1984

23. Lui PI: Diagnosis and treatment of syphilis. J Med Assoc State Ala 52:26, 1983

24. Meier JL, Mollet E: Acute periostitis in early acquired syphilis simulating shin splints in a jogger. Am J Sports Med 14:327, 1986

25. Percy EC, Telep GN: Anomalous muscle in the leg: soleus accessorius. Am J Sports Med 12:447, 1984

26. Hulkko A, Orava S: Stress fractures in athletes. Int J Sports Med 8:221, 1987

27. Hansson CJ: On insufficiency fractures of femur and tibia. Acta Radiol 19:554, 1938

28. Devas MB, Sweetnam R: Stress fractures of the fibula: a review of 50 cases in athletes. J Bone Joint Surg [Br] 38:818, 1956

29. McBryde A: Stress fractures in runners. Clin Sports Med 4:737, 1985

30. Martheson GO, Clement DB, McKenzie DC et al: Stress fractures in athletes, a study of 320 cases. Am J Sports Med 15:46, 1987

31. Milgrom C, Chisin R, Giladi M et al: Negative bone scans in impending tibial stress fractures: a report of three cases. Am J Sports Med 12:488, 1984

32. Roub LW, Gumerman LW, Hanley EN et al: Bone stress: a radionuclide imaging perspective. Radiology 132:430, 1979

33. Orava B: Stress fractures. Br J Sports Med 14:40, 1984

34. Green NE, Rogers RA, Lipcomb AB: Nonunions of stress fractures of the tibia. Am J Sports Med 13:171, 1985

35. Blank S: Transverse tibial stress fractures: a special problem. Am J Sports Med 15:597, 1987

36. Rettig AC, Shelbourne DK, McCarroll JR et al: The natural history and treatment of delayed union stress fractures of the anterior cortex of the tibia. Am J Sports Med 16:250, 1988

37. Styf JR: Chronic exercise-induced pain in the anterior aspect of the lower leg: an overview of diagnosis. Sports Med 7:331, 1989

38. Folkow B, Gaskell P, Waaler BA: Blood flow through limb muscle during heavy rhythmic exercise. Acta Physiol Scand 80:61, 1970

39. Styf JR, Suurkuula M, Korner L: Intramuscular pressure and muscle blood flow during exercise in chronic compartment syndrome. J Bone Joint Surg [Br] 69:301, 1987

40. Lawson S: Compartment pressures in Nordic skiers. MSc thesis, University of Alberta, Edmonton, 1989

41. Logan JG, Rorabeck CH, Castle GSP: The measurement of dynamic compartment pressure during exercise. Am J Sports Med 11:220, 1983

42. Styf JR, Korner LM: Microcapillary infusion technique for measurement of intramuscular pressure during exercise. CORR 207:253, 1986

43. McDermott AGP, Marble RH, Yabsley RH et al: Monitoring dynamic anterior compartment pressure during exercise: a new technique using the STIC catheter. Am J Sports Med 10:83, 1982

44. Styf JR: Diagnosis of exercise-induced pain in the anterior aspect of the lower leg. Am J Sports Med 16:165, 1988

45. Veith RG, Matsen FA, Newell SG: Recurrent anterior compartment syndromes. Physician Sports Med 8:80, 1980

46. Davey JR, Rorabeck CH, Fowler PJ: The tibialis posterior muscle compartment: an unrecognized cause of exertional compartment syndrome. Am J Sports Med 12:391, 1984

47. Wiley JP, Clement DB, Doyle DL et al: A primary care perspective of chronic compartment syndrome of the leg. Physician Sport Med 15:111, 1987

48. Stack C: Superficial posterior compartment syndrome of the leg with deep venous compromise. Clin Orthop 220:233, 1987

49. Sanzen L, Forsberg A, Westlin N: Anterior fibial compartment pressures during race walking. Am J Sports Med 14:136, 1986

50. Lipscombe AB, Ibrahim AA: Acute peroneal compartment syndrome in a well conditioned athlete: report of a case. Am J Sports Med 5:154, 1977

51. Styf JR, Korner LM: Chronic anterior compartment syndrome of the leg: result of treatment by fasciotomy. J Bone Joint Surg [Am] 68:1338, 1986

52. Styf J: Entrapment of the superficial peroneal nerve: diagnosis and results of decompression. J Bone Joint Surg [Br] 71:131, 1989

53. Jabre JF: The superficial peroneal sensory nerve revisted. Arch Neurol 38:666, 1981

54. Friden J, Sfakianos PN, Hargens AR et al: Residual muscular swelling after repetitive eccentric contractions. J Orthop Res 6:493, 1988

55. Slonia AE, Goans PJ: Myopathy in McArdle's syndrome. N Engl J Med 312:355, 1985

56. Garfin SR, Tipton CM, Mubarak SJ et al: Role of fascia in the maintenance of muscle tension and pressure. J Appl Physiol 51:317, 1981

57. Porabede CH, Fowler PJ, Nott L: The results of fasciotomy in the management of chronic exertional compartment syndrome. Am J Sports Med 16:3, 1988

58. Beall S, Garner T, Oxley D: Anterolateral compartment syndrome related to drug-induced bleeding: a case report. Am J Sports Med 11:454, 1983

59. Zigun JR, Schneider SM: Effort thrombosis (Paget-Schroetter's syndrome) secondary to martial arts training. Am J Sports Med 16:189, 1988

60. Kleinsasner LJ: Effort thrombosis of the axillary and subclavian veins: an analysis of 16 personal cases and 56 cases collected from the literature. Arch Surg 59:258, 1949

61. Mackie JW, Webster JA: Deep vein thrombosis in marathon runners. Physician Sports Med 9:91, 1981

62. Darling RC, Buckley CJ, Abbott WM et al: Intermittent claudication in young athletes: popliteal artery entrapment syndrome. J Trauma 14:543, 1974

63. Duwelins PJ, Kelbel MJ, Tardon OM et al: Popliteal artery entrapment in a high school athlete: a case report. Am J Sports Med 15:371, 1987

Internal Derangement and Other Selected Lesions of the Knee

11

He who hesitates is saved.
—*J. Goodfellow,* Journal of Bone and Joint Surgery, British Volume, *1980*

MENISCI AND MENISCAL–TISSUES

The semilunar cartilages of the knee, commonly referred to as medial and lateral menisci, are unique in that not all species have menisci in their knees and not all joints have menisci. They are vital for the normal function of the human knee. For centuries they were believed to be vestigial. The lack of understanding of their important mechanical role led to a prevailing "laissez faire" attitude among surgeons and unnecessary sacrifice of menisci during arthrotomy. "When in doubt, take it out" was an axiom that mostly disappeared during the 1980s but was still far too widely prevalent into the mid-1970s. Long-term follow-ups of postmeniscectomy patients and the ability to perform conservative meniscectomies via arthroscopic surgery have permitted a more thoughtful, cautious approach to the treatment of the ubiquitous meniscal pathology. Fairbank reported in 1948 that roentgenographic changes following meniscectomy included "narrowing of the joint space, flattening of the femoral condyle, and osteophyte formation," all of which he attributed to the loss of their normal weight-bearing function; since then the current belief in preserving the menisci has evolved.[1]

Anatomy

Meniscal Attachments

The shape of the menisci are to some degree related to the opposing joint surfaces. The medial tibial condyle is concave, longer from front to back, and oval.[2] The lateral tibial condyle is flatter and more circular. Similarly, the medial meniscus is C-shaped, whereas the lateral meniscus is broader and more circular. The menisci are cartilaginous and tough where compressed between femur and tibia but ligamentous and pliable at their peripheral attachments. Because the horns of the lateral meniscus are attached close together and its coronary ligament is slack, this meniscus can slide forward and backward easily on the flat lateral tibial condyle (Fig. 11-1). By contrast, the horns of the medial meniscus are attached far apart and have association with the deep fibers of the medial collateral ligament; the major portion rests on a concave surface. This configuration minimizes the motion of the medial cartilage (Figs. 11-2 and 11-3).

Structure of the Menisci

Histologically, the menisci consist mainly of a resilient white fibrous network with relatively few cartilage cells in the matrix. Triangular in cross section, the thick periphery is nourished by capillary loops at the capsular attachment and from the fringes of the synovial membrane. The thin central edge is avascular, receiving nutrition by diffusion.

On the medial side, in the region of the posterior horn, some fibers of the deep capsular part of the medial collateral ligament pass directly from femur to tibia.[3] Other fibers pass from both femur and tibia to the periphery of the meniscus (Fig. 11-4). These fibers interlace in the peripheral third of the menis-

301

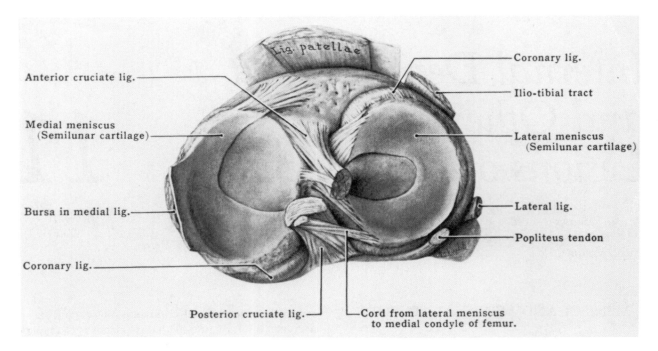

Fig. 11-1. View of the superior surface of the tibia showing the shape and main attachments of the menisci. Note the cord of ligamentous tissue from the posterior horn of the lateral meniscus (ligament of Wrisberg), which joins the posterior cruciate ligament. (From Grant,[2] with permission.)

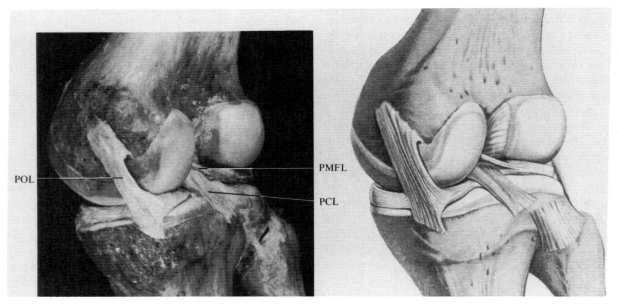

Fig. 11-2. Association of the medial meniscus and medial collateral ligament in the area of the posterior oblique fibers (POL). In other areas the meniscus is mobile, allowing it to follow the changing contours that occur during flexion and extension. The attachment of the posterior horn of the lateral meniscus is also seen where the ligament of Wrisberg (PMFL) joins the posterior cruciate (PCL). (From Müller,[4] with permission.)

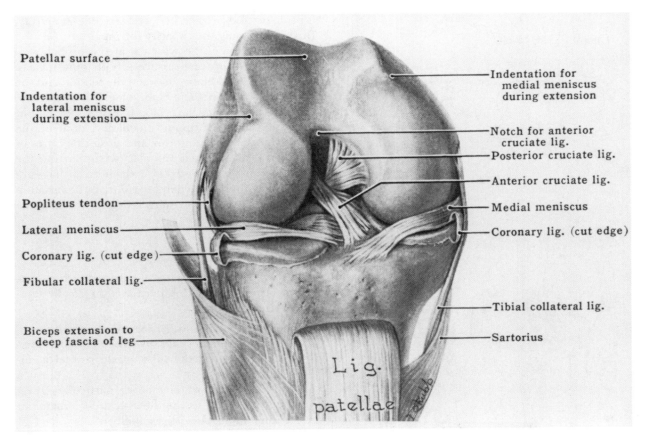

Patellar surface

Indentation for lateral meniscus during extension

Popliteus tendon

Lateral meniscus

Coronary lig. (cut edge)

Fibular collateral lig.

Biceps extension to deep fascia of leg

Indentation for medial meniscus during extension

Notch for anterior cruciate lig.

Posterior cruciate lig.

Anterior cruciate lig.

Medial meniscus

Coronary lig. (cut edge)

Tibial collateral lig.

Sartorius

Lig. patellae

Fig. 11-3. Anterior horn attachments of menisci. (From Grant,[2] with permission.)

cus, where the nutrient vessels also ramify. The meniscofemoral fibers superiorly and the meniscotibial fibers inferiorly form two layers of fibers that blend with a third middle layer formed by fibers that pass in with the blood vessels.[4] More anteriorly the same general structure exists, except that the medial collateral ligament's superficial fibers are entirely separate from both the meniscus and the deep capsular layer. The attachment of the lateral meniscus is similar except that the lateral meniscus is considerably more bulky, particularly the posterior half (Fig. 11-4).

Within the menisci, the collagenous fibers form arcades, with a large number of strands being located peripherally, giving considerable density to the peripheral one-third (Fig. 11-5). This high fiber density results in a tension-resistant ring that facilitates absorbtion of compressive forces between the tibia and femur. It also resists the deforming forces associated with motion of the knee. In the central two-thirds the fibers are more radially oriented. These architectural features probably influence the site of origin and propagation of meniscal lesions, as stresses develop where zones of different strengths adjoin.[5]

Blood Supply and Nutrition

The menisci are nourished by the blood vessels in the peripheral third, which are branches of the geniculate arteries. This perimeniscal capillary plexus, originating in the capsular and synovial tissues of the joint, supplies the peripheral 10 to 25 percent of the menisci (Fig. 11-4).[6] The anterior and posterior horns adjacent to their attachments have a particularly rich blood supply. The posterolateral corner of the lateral meniscus, adjacent to the popliteal hiatus is devoid of penetrating vessels. There is a normal variation in this peripheral vasculature that accounts for the variations in the literature, with Scapinelli reporting up to 33 percent of the meniscal substance having good vascular penetration.[7] The remaining meniscal tissue

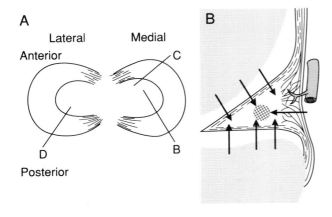

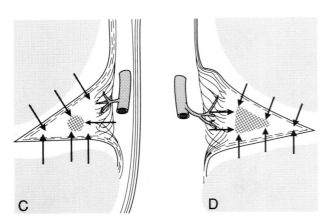

Fig. 11-4. Relations of the menisci to the ligaments and blood vessels. **(A)** Location of cross sections. **(B)** Posteromedial attachment of the medial collateral ligament to the medial meniscus. The meniscus shows three zones: a superior zone made up of femoral meniscal fibers, a basal zone of tibial meniscal fibers, and a central area. The vessels penetrate the outer third of the meniscus. Owing to inadequacy of diffusion there is relatively poor nourishment in the central area. **(C)** At the midportion the deep layer is fundamentally the same, but the superficial part of the ligament is separate from the meniscus. **(D)** Posterior horn of the lateral meniscus, which is large and has a correspondingly greater area of tenuous nutrition. This area is susceptible to mucoid degeneration and hence the greater propensity to develop ganglia (cysts) of the lateral meniscus. Arrows = diffusion ☰ = tenuous nutrition. (Modified from Müller,[4] with permission.)

is nourished by diffusion from the synovial fluid. Thus the deep central areas of both menisci are located farthest from their nutrient sources and are a site of predilection for early degenerative change.[8] It

is probably also a region of decreased cellular density, further reducing the capacity for repair.

The evolution of the avascular area is probably related to the reciprocal pressure of both joint surfaces and the popliteal hiatus between the tendon and the meniscus. Early in their embryologic development, the human menisci have blood vessels throughout their substance.[6] During postnatal development, the non-weight-bearing anterior and posterior horn attachments retain great vascularity, supporting the concept that pressure effects on the fibrocartilage are responsible for the vascular recession. Little variation in the overall vascular pattern is demonstrable in the adult.

Functions of the Menisci

The importance of normal menisci to the knee cannot be overemphasized. Their function may be summarized as follows.

1. They form mechanical spacers that contribute to the stability of the joint, evidenced by increased varus or valgus laxity subsequent to total meniscectomy.
2. The wedge shape of the menisci, particularly their posterior horns, assists the cruciate ligaments in creating anteroposterior stability.
3. They increase surface area contact across the knee by at least one-third. Indeed when the menisci are removed, the contact area drops by approximately 40 percent and the average contact stresses increase proportionately.
4. The resilience of the fibrocartilage forms a slight shock-absorbing mechanism.
5. They may assist in nutrition of the joint by promoting synovial fluid flow and distribution.
6. They take part in the locking mechanism by gliding on the surface of the tibia and by directing the movements of the femoral articular surface. The anterior aspects also fit into grooves on the femoral articular surface in the close packed extended position. (Fig. 11-3).
7. Both menisci take part in assisting and controlling the gliding and rolling motion of the knee by slight opening and closing of the anterior horns. The lateral meniscus may glide as much as a centimeter during flexion and extension.[9] These movements are discussed in greater detail later in the chapter.
8. There is controversy regarding their neural innervation; however, there is probably an important proprioceptive function for the menisci. Certainly

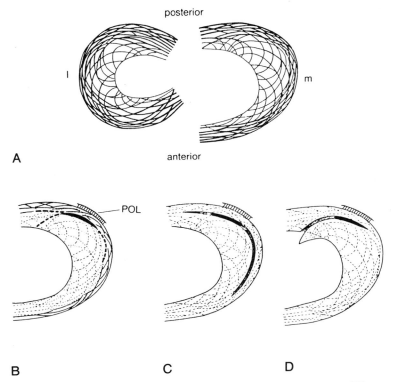

Fig. 11-5. (A) Collagenous fiber architecture of the menisci according to Wagner.[3] This fiber arrangement probably accounts for the various types of tears that are observed. **(B)** Longitudinal tear may propogate anteriorly. It then forms a potential bucket handle tear **(C)** or it may follow the curved fiber bundle to the free edge as a flap or parrot beak tear **(D)**. (After Wagner,[3] with permission.)

the neural supply is one of complex end-bulbs and Golgi type apparatus; nerves enter the menisci around the periphery from the capsule and usually supply the outer one-fourth of the meniscal substance.

Motion of the Knee

Kinematics

The most obvious movements occurring at this joint are flexion and extension; however, for normal knee function, rotation is an important component.[10] The transverse axis about which flexion and extension occurs moves posteriorly during flexion and anteriorly during extension due to a combination of rolling and gliding. This method is the only one by which the extensive femoral articular surface can be used up during flexion without rolling backward off the tibial condyles. Ligamentous stability would be mechanically impossible without these movements.

Active rotation is easily demonstrated with the knee at 90 degrees of flexion and the leg non-weight-bearing. In this position the collateral ligaments are maximally relaxed, although some rotation may occur up to the final point of extension when the joint assumes its close packed position. At this point the femur and tibia meld into a single functional unit with rotation of the leg possible only from the hip, i.e., conjoint rotation. Also, automatic axial rotation takes place inevitably with flexion-extension movements of the knee. These movements are linked and are most obvious at the completion of extension and the beginning of flexion. Lateral rotation of the tibia is associated with extension and medial rotation of the tibia with flexion.

It should be stressed that in most individuals there is no absolute extension, as the position of reference for the knee is with the leg at an angle of 180 degrees to the thigh. However, some passive hyperextension may be present; and in individuals with lax ligaments, there may be sufficient active hyperextension present to warrant the term genu recurvatum.

Locking Mechanism and Extension

The leg can be transformed into a rigid unit by means of extension. The limb may be made sufficiently stable that the quadriceps relax. Then little muscular effort is needed to maintain the standing posture, which results from a combination of knee joint position and general body balance. However, if strong contraction of the quadriceps is imposed on this already extended position, there is more rotation, and additional "screw home" movement takes place. The knee is in fact locked and has moved into its close packed position. To the layman the leg would be described as braced.

Throughout extension both menisci change shape to adapt to the increasing area of articular surface presented by the femur. Such change is achieved by spreading of the horns. In addition, during extension the menisci move forward on the tibial condyles. The lateral meniscus, traveling twice the distance of the medial meniscus, has an excursion of up to 12 mm (Fig. 11-6).

Medial rotation of the femur probably commences as early as 30 degrees short of full extension; however, it is greatest and most noticeable during the last 10 degrees. In summary, at the completion of extension:

1. The anterior edges of the menisci fit into grooves at the limits of the articular surfaces of the femur.

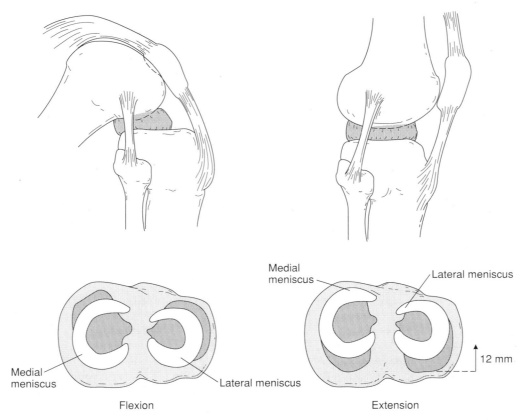

Fig. 11-6. Menisci move anteriorly during extension and posteriorly during flexion, the lateral menisci having the greater excursion, approximately 11 mm versus 5 mm for the medial. To some degree the menisci tend to move with the tibia during flexion and extension. However, when the femur is rotated on the flexed tibia, they tend to move with the femoral condyles. This motion potentially stresses the menisci and their associated coronary ligaments.

2. The anterior cruciate ligament is taut and fits into a groove in the posterior part of the intercondylar area of the femur.
3. The collateral ligaments are taut, and the joint is in the final close packed position.
4. This position is one of slight hyperextension, and the line of gravity falls anterior to the axis of movement of the knee joint.
5. The quadriceps may be relatively relaxed in the standing position.

If these five criteria are fulfilled, the joint may be considered locked. It can be seen that, without the ability to extend fully, true locking is not possible and economy of muscle work is not achieved in the standing position.

Medial and Lateral Rotation

The menisci are intimately involved in the movements of rotation at the knee. The medial meniscus, with its firm attachment to the posterior oblique ligament, has little excursion. However, the lateral meniscus moves posteriorly in internal rotation and anteriorly with external rotation of the tibia (Fig. 11-7). With the lateral popliteal corner much more freely mobile than the semimembranosis corner, there is less tendency to internal stress on the lateral meniscus. Indeed, in many series, lateral meniscal lesions are up to 10 times less frequent than medial meniscal tears (more fully discussed in the next section).

Meniscal Lesions

It is unusual to see a true, fresh, isolated avulsion of a meniscus caused by a single traumatic episode. Usually this type of injury is associated with acute ligamentous disruption. Moreover, these traumatic disruptions occur at the periphery, often in the deep capsular fibers rather than in the substance of the cartilage. They are highly vascular and suitable for repair.

Quick Facts

MECHANISMS OF INJURY

- Associated with ligamentous disruption
- Degenerative changes with age
- Repetitive abnormal stresses secondary to chronic ligamentous laxity
- Isolated or repetitive rotational stresses
- Abnormal meniscal shape or attachment

Two elements must be present in most meniscal lesions: first, attrition of the cartilage; and second, trauma to propagate the defect. Menisci become progressively more stiff as their fibrocartilage matrix changes with the normal processes of aging. As they become stiffer and less resilient, they are more sus-

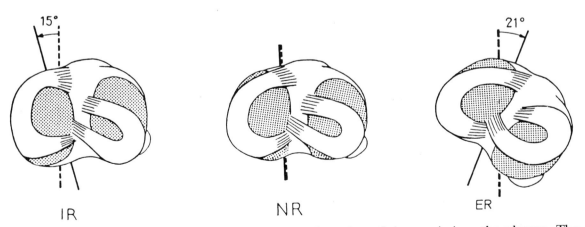

Fig. 11-7. Rotation of the right tibia with associated motion of the menisci on the plateau. The average range of internal rotation (IR) is 15 degrees, and the lateral meniscus tends to glide posteriorly while the medial meniscus moves anteriorly. The average external rotation is 21 degrees, and the glide of the meniscus is again in association with the femoral condyles, the lateral meniscus moving anterior.

ceptible to tears, which are often referred to as horizontal cleavage tears. Nevertheless, even in the young individual twisting injuries, particularly under compression, cause midsubstance tears of a horizontal, radial (vertical), or longitudinal variety. The medial edges of these tears may dislocate into the joint. These injuries are referred to as bucket handle tears. Alternatively, small tags, from the posterior or anterior horn may ultimately become symptomatic. These

injuries are called pedunculated (tag) tears or parrot beak tears (Fig. 11-8).

In the normal young North American population the medial meniscus is most susceptible to injury, being long and C-shaped. Indeed, its peripheral posteromedial attachments to the medial collateral ligament and the posterior capsule of the knee joint may make it susceptible to a special type of tear along its peripheral margins. This peripheral tear may be asso-

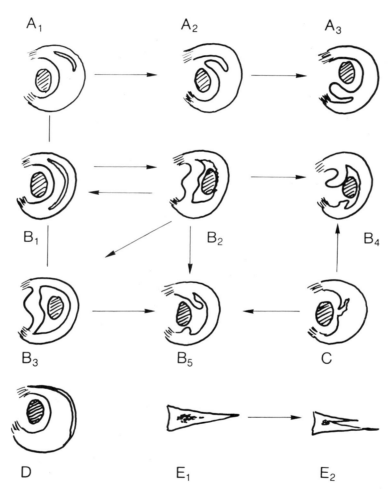

Fig. 11-8. Classification and evolution of meniscal lesions. **(A)** Longitudinal tear of the posterior horn (A_1) may progress into a posterior flap or parrot beak (A_2) or an anterior tag (A_3), which may produce locking. **(B)** If it extends forward (B_1), it may become unstable and bucket handle type (B_2). The bucket handle may continue to extend and thin out so it no longer locks the knee (B_3), or it may evolve into anterior and posterior tags (B_4). The latter may be displaced mesially or peripherally (B_5). **(C)** Some mesial tags start de novo on the edge of the meniscus. **(D)** Tears associated with ligament injuries are often peripheral longitudinal tears. **(E)** Central degeneration (E_1) may produce symptoms and are difficult to detect. These lesions (E_2) may ultimately form horizontal cleavage lesions, or the latter may start de novo.

ciated with tears of the medial ligament and capsule. The incidence of meniscal injury may be as high as 60 per 100,000 population with men being affected more often than women, in a 3:1 ratio. With the exception of perhaps wrestling, medial meniscal tears predominate in all sports.

The larger, broader, circular lateral meniscus has a high incidence of tears in the Eurasian population and is more subject to congenital variations, i.e., the broad discoid meniscus, which fills the lateral half of the joint and interferes with normal movement patterns. Lateral menisci also seem to be more prone to degenerative cysts in their peripheral margins.

In some individuals with congenitally lax ligamentous structures, the posterior horns of the menisci are highly mobile. This situation may result from anterior cruciate and capsular laxity secondary to trauma. The menisci may produce a symptomatic snap during flexion of the knee.

In summary, tears of the meniscus can be classified as follows.

1. Degenerative, horizontal cleavage tears which are seen classically in the older age group, although frequently in young individuals as well.
2. The young, active age group may tear the peripheral margin in association with ligament injuries.
3. In addition, there may be a longitudinal meniscal substance tear that eventually forms a bucket handle tear or a tag tear.

4. Traumatic anterior and posterior horn tag tears occur that may ultimately cause mechanical hindrance (tag or parrot beak tears).
5. Radial tears which may not be symptomative, but can eventually form tags.

Meniscectomy

Without the normal meniscus the knee joint suffers and is susceptible to degenerative changes. The normal meniscus carries 40 to 70 percent of the load across the knee.[11] After partial meniscectomy of bucket handle tears, contact areas decrease approximately 10 percent, and peak contact stresses increase about 50 to 60 percent.[12] After total meniscectomy, contact areas decrease approximately 75 percent, and the peak local contact stresses increase as much as 235 percent. Repair of meniscal tears tends to normalize the stress, and the increase in stress with partial meniscectomy is proportional to the amount of meniscus removed.[12]

In a series of 100 random necropsies of subjects with an average age of 65 years, 29 percent of the 400 menisci contained a horizontal cleavage lesion and 60 percent had at least one significant meniscal lesion.[13] Another postmortem investigation revealed that at least 18.6 percent had one or more horizontal cleavage lesions.[14] Because it is difficult to envisage that more than 70 percent of the elderly population suffer from symptomatic meniscal lesions, it is assumed that asymptomatic tears can and do exist.

The presence of asymptomatic lesions and knowledge of the importance of the cartilage in distributing the dynamic forces across the knee lead one to suppose that a policy of conservative meniscectomy and meniscal preservation is appropriate. Furthermore, it is difficult to show that degenerative meniscal lesions cause osteoarthritis.[15] Large lesions and bucket handle and flap tears may indent the articular surfaces and cause fissures and erosions, particularly when associated with instability. Irrespective of the relation to degenerative changes, some lesions produce sufficient mechanical or painful symptoms that operative excision is required.

A follow-up of athletes after meniscectomy revealed that complaints related to the surgery increased from 53 percent at 4.5 years to 67 percent at 14.5 years, and demonstrable knee instability increased from 10 percent to 36 percent.[16] Radiographic changes of degeneration rose from 40 percent to 89 percent. At late review, 8 percent had definite clinical osteoarthrosis. As a result of these changes, 46 percent had reduced or given up their sporting activity, and 6.5 percent had changed their occupation.[16] Radiographic changes started at about 5 years after the surgery. Most of the athletes in this series had had total meniscectomies (Table 11-1). Similar findings have been recorded by other studies, with figures for radiologic changes ranging from 18 to 80 percent at 10 years and those for significant signs and symptoms from 7 to 30 percent.[17]

Meniscal tears in children with open epiphyseal plates are relatively uncommon lesions. Early reports suggested that at 5 years after surgery children were functioning uniformly well.[18] However, subsequent studies, particularly those that have a longer follow-up, were more worrying. Ligamentous laxity, early degenerative changes, and a symptomatic joint are frequently found.[18,19] Meniscectomy in the child or adolescent is not a benign procedure, and intensive preoperative evaluation and conservative management of selected meniscal lesions in children are recommended.

Many elderly athletes have symptomatic lesions. When the classic signs of meniscal pathology are present and careful evaluation suggests that the symptoms are related to the meniscus, arthroscopy and possible meniscal débridement may allow resumption of former activity. The main complaint in athletes over age 40 is joint line pain (95 percent) followed by catching or locking (40 percent) and effusions (40 percent). Jackson and Rouse concluded that (1) typical traumatic meniscal lesions frequently occur in the older active individual; (2) age alone does not adversely affect the results of arthroscopic menis-

TABLE 11-1.   Long-Term Follow-up of Complete Meniscectomy

Parameter	Median 4.5 Years (n = 131)		Median 14.5 Years (n = 101)	
	No.	%	No.	%
Symptoms				
Swelling	25	19	29	29
Pain				
Weight-bearing	50	38	30	30
On stairs	20	15	23	23
When first walking	—	—	23	23
At rest	16	12	13	13
Needing analgesia	—	—	4	4
Sensation of instability	26	20	21	21
Signs				
Crepitus	23	18	38	38
Effusion	0	0	5	5
Quadriceps wasting	9	7	12	12
Positive anterior drawer	13	10	36	36
Joint line tenderness	13	10	12	12
Activity change				
Unchanged	69	53	19	19
Reduced unrelated	26	20	36	36
Reduced because of knee	16	12	12	12
No sport because of knee	20	15	34	34

(Data from Jørgensen et al.[16])

cectomy; and (3) the presence of degenerative changes prior to partial meniscectomy appears to be the determining factor in the eventual results.[20]

```
┌─────────────────────────────────────────┐
│                                          │
│  Practice Points                         │
│                                          │
│  TREATMENT PHILOSOPHIES                  │
│                                          │
│  • Normal meniscus is the ideal situation│
│  • Minor lesions may be better without   │
│    treatment if relatively asymptomatic  │
│  • Partial meniscectomy is better than   │
│    complete                              │
│  • Resuturing when appropriate location  │
│  • Symptomatic tears with effusions      │
│    locking or giving way may damage joint│
│  • When in doubt, observe and do not     │
│    treat                                 │
│                                          │
└─────────────────────────────────────────┘
```

The concepts described above may be summarized as follows. A normal meniscus is the ideal situation. Minor tears that cause few mechanical symptoms and only a small amount of pain on occasion, probably do not damage the joint. The knee is probably better off with a minor tear of a meniscus in situ than without a meniscus. A knee with partial removal of the meniscus lasts longer and does better than a knee that does not have a meniscus. Total meniscectomy is preferable to leaving in a large symptomatic tear, with resultant repeated giving way, locking, and effusion.

As far as meniscectomy is concerned, the younger the individual when a meniscectomy is performed, the worse are the eventual changes in the joint. Similarly, in the elderly, removing the torn meniscus from a joint that already has degenerative changes causes rapid advance of any existing osteoarthritis. Women may have worse results than men, which is related to alignment of the femurs in respect to the width of the pelvis as well as the generally slightly higher incidence of ligamentous laxity in women. Except for those with significant varus alignment, individuals do worse after a lateral meniscectomy than a medial meniscectomy. Total removal of the meniscus provides more rapid onset of degenerative changes than partial removal of the meniscus. Furthermore, those who already have some instability or degenerative changes in the knee do worse after a meniscectomy than those without degenerative changes or unstable ligaments.

Hence a healthy, normal meniscus is obviously desirable, but in the presence of a severe symptomatic tear meniscectomy is still the treatment of choice. Wherever possible, partial rather than complete meniscectomy should be carried out. Other treatment options are discussed under the section on arthroscopic surgery.

Recognition of Meniscal Lesions

Clinical Symptoms and Signs

Meniscal pathology is common; yet the clinical diagnosis is frequently difficult, even for the experienced surgeon. Indeed in some series the clinical diagnosis of meniscal lesions is accurate only in 40 percent of the cases when not supported by some other investigation. Of the large variety of tests described in the literature, the ones selected here encompass all of the main elements for stressing the menisci. Three or four well chosen and practised tests enhance clinical acumen. There is usually a need for supplementary tests if the knee is not frankly locked. Although there may be no single reliable test for meniscal tears, a combination of symptoms and signs indicate the correct diagnosis most of the time.

Symptoms

The meniscus itself has little in the way of sensory nerve supply; in fact, it is probably almost devoid of nerves except in its periphery, where it becomes confluent with the synovial lining of the joint. Therefore symptoms due to a torn meniscus are generally related to mechanical dysfunction causing traction on the periphery of the meniscus, which may produce synovitis, swelling of the synovial lining, or mechanical blocking, as is frequently seen with a bucket handle or beak tear. Additionally, the symptoms of a meniscal lesion may include the following.

1. Swelling proportional to activities
2. Pain on rotary or flexion motion, particularly near the extremes of flexion
3. Pain on the joint line
4. Feeling of weakness and insecurity
5. Giving way
6. Locking
7. Generalized aching in the knee joint itself
8. Popping, catching, or grinding

Repeated popping occurs in approximately 43 percent of patients with proven meniscal lesions, swelling in 51 percent, and pain localized to the joint line in 60 percent.[21]

Clinical Point

GIVING WAY OR BUCKLING

- Meniscal lesions
- Ligamentous instability
- Dislocation or subluxation of patella
- Loose body in joint
- Instability of superior tibiofibular joint
- Weakness of quadriceps
- Sudden pain inhibition

Signs

Effusions. Joint swelling indicates that there is a likelihood of intra-articular pathology, and it is a particularly reliable, if not specific, sign of internal derangement. Detecting a small amount of fluid requires considerable care, and the "wipe" test is probably most sensitive for this purpose (Fig. 11-9). Ballotment for a floating patella allows assessment of large volumes of fluid (Fig. 11-10).

Tenderness. Discomfort along the joint line is present in approximately 77 percent and falsely present in 11 percent of meniscal lesions. Although not specific for meniscal pathology, it is still the most

reliable sign. In the acute situation, excess pressure on the locked knee often refers pain directly to the joint line on the side of the affected meniscus (Fig. 11-11).

Locking. Inability to extend the knee may be caused by a displaced meniscal flap, a loose body, articular surface damage, or a torn anterior cruciate ligament. Pseudolocking, which may be caused by hamstring spasm, is difficult to distinguish clinically. True locking, which occurs at the time of injury, frequently prevents the terminal 20 to 30 degrees of extension and is a reasonably reliable sign. After a few hours to a few days, even if the knee remains locked it approaches extension more closely. With the chronic bucket handle tear, "locking" is usually a subtle sign and may constitute a loss of only about 5 degrees of extension. It is best visualized by lifting both of the patient's legs, keeping the malleoli together, and viewing along the length of the legs from the end of the examining table.

In a review of 272 patients with a surgically visualized bucket handle tear, 43 percent presented with a locked knee and another 37 percent had a history of locking. Fifty percent of those with a history of locking but who were clinically unlocked at the time of operation, had mobile bucket handle tears.[22] Thus unlocking of the knee joint in the presence of a

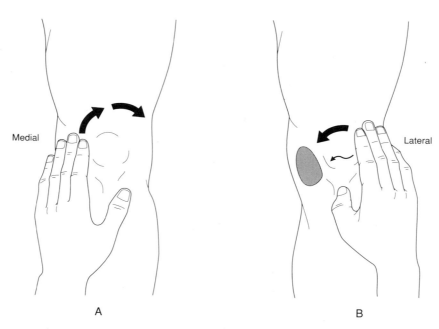

A   B

Fig. 11-9. Wipe test demonstrated on left leg. **(A)** Fluid is massaged across the suprapatellar pouch from medial to lateral. **(B)** A wiping action pushes the fluid back, and the bulge is visualized, appearing inferomedially.

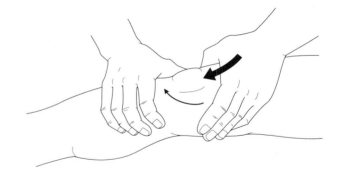

Fig. 11-10. Larger effusion may be palpated and pushed from the suprapatellar area to allow the patella to "float." A patellar tap may then be performed by balloting the top of the knee cap.

chronic tear frequently represents anterior extension of the tear, rather than relocation of the displaced fragment of the meniscus.

Manipulative Tests. Manipulative tests attempt to localize the pain to the joint line or to produce clicking secondary to the abnormal mechanics of the torn meniscus.

McMurray Test. The McMurray test is positive in about 58 percent and falsely positive in 5 percent of normal knees.[23] It is sometimes difficult to discern the "clunk" of a torn meniscal flap from other "clicks" in the joint that are secondary to patellar motion or other mechanical phenomena. The McMurray test is a forced internal and external rotary motion of the tibia that accompanies flexion and varus-valgus stress (Fig. 11-12). The key to the test is obtaining absolutely full flexion and thus it cannot be performed in the presence of significant effusion. The test may be recorded as negative, positive for joint line pain, or positive with both a pain and a clunk. This latter situation is the classic sign. Identical clicks or clunks in

both knees do not constitute a positive sign, and there should be reservation in classifying a painless "clunk" as positive.

Steinmann Test. (I and II). Starting with the knee flexed to 90° forced external rotation gives pain on the medial joint line (Fig. 11-13). Conversely internal rotation gives lateral joint line (lateral meniscal) pain. The test is performed at varying positions of the knee flexion. This test may be performed in sitting or lying. Furthermore when joint line tenderness moves posteriorly with increasing degrees of flexion it tends to distinguish meniscal pathology from injury of the capsular ligaments and osteophytes.

Helfet Sign. A positive test is dependent on a meniscal lesion mechanically affecting the conjoint lateral rotation of the tibia during extension (Fig. 11-14).

Apley Test. The Apley compression and distraction maneuvers are performed with the knee flexed to 90 degrees and the patient prone.[23] Pain only on distraction suggests possible ligamentous involvement. Pain and possible grinding on compression with forced

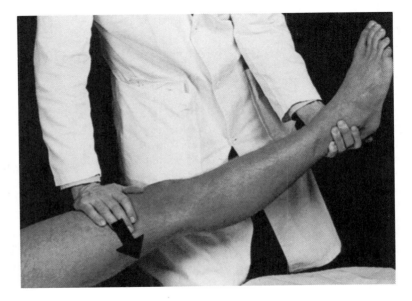

Fig. 11-11. Locking is often a subtle sign. Forced passive extension frequently produces intense discomfort at either the anteromedial or anterolateral joint line, suggesting meniscal pathology. With a more chronic locked knee, the "springy" block of a meniscal lesion is appreciated by pressure or a similar sensation experienced by letting the slightly flexed knee fall into extension, the "bounce home test."

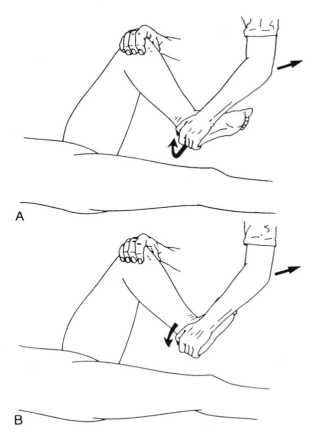

A

B

Fig. 11-12. Positive McMurray test requires both pain and a "clunk" with the forced flexion, rotary maneuver. **(A)** Internal rotation of the leg tends to stress the lateral meniscus. **(B)** External rotation tends to stress the medial meniscus.

rotation suggests meniscal pathology or articular surface changes (Fig. 11-15).

Anderson Test. Another compression maneuver is the mediolateral Anderson grind test. With the knee at 45 degrees, a valgus stress is applied as the knee is simultaneously slightly flexed followed by a varus component while the knee is extended.[21] This maneuver produces a gentle circular motion of the knee. A longitudinal or flap tear tends to give a distinct grinding sensation at the joint line (Fig. 11-16). A complex tear produces more prolonged grinding. A similar sensation may also be present with osteoarthrosis, and occasionally a pivot shift is produced if there is associated anterior cruciate insufficiency. The mediolateral grind test may be positive in up to 68 percent of cases with meniscal pathology; however, its accuracy depends on the subjective interpretation of the examiner. If the grind test is used in conjunction

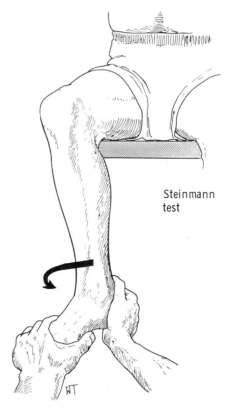

Steinmann test

Fig. 11-13. Steinman I. Meniscal pathology may be suspected if medial pain is elicited on lateral rotation (shown here) and lateral pain on medial tibial rotation. Steinmann II, the tenderness displacement test, is positive if the joint line tenderness moves anteriorly when the knee is extended and posteriorly when it is flexed. Both components of the test may be performed in lying and should be repeated in a variety of ranges.

with the McMurray and Apley maneuvers, a positive response may be elicited in up to 79 percent of meniscal lesions.

Comment. The accuracy of the McMurray, Steinmann, and Apley tests depends on relaxation of the patient, configuration of the tear, and, most importantly, the experience of the examiner.[21] The McMurray test is impossible to perform in the presence of even a moderately tense effusion because it prevents full knee flexion. This is because it is to contrast with the previous heading of manipulative tests.

Other signs.

Jump Sign. A hypermobile posterior horn of the meniscus, with or without a tissue bridge, may become incarcerated between the femoral and tibial condyles

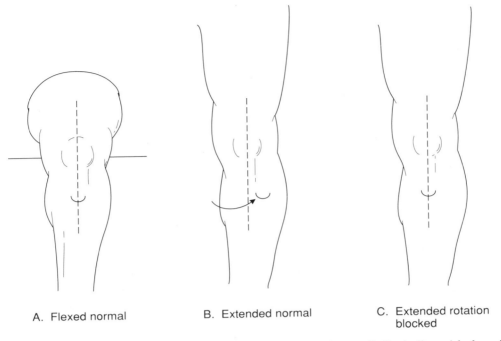

A. Flexed normal   B. Extended normal   C. Extended rotation blocked

Fig. 11-14. Helfet sign. **(A)** In the normal knee the tibial tubercle usually lies in line with the midline of the patella. **(B)** When extended, the associated lateral tibial rotation puts it in line with the lateral patellar border. **(C)** Positive sign occurs when the rotation is blocked, possibly by a torn meniscus, and the tubercle remains centered over the patella.

during the motion of flexion and extension. This situation may lead to a snapping mechanism reported by the patient or occasionally elicited by the examiner. It is usually associated with anterior cruciate insufficiency. During examination for an anterior drawer sign the femoral condyle rides up onto the posterior horn of the meniscus and then snaps back into its normal position. This "jumping" of the femur may be palpable or audible and is referred to as the "sign del salto" or the Finocchietto jump sign (Fig. 11-17). With severe ligamentous instability involving primary and secondary restraints, both condyles may do it as the tibia subluxes forward with a snap, and it has been described as the "box" sign.

Duck Waddle. In an otherwise healthy individual presenting with vague chronic symptoms suggestive of meniscal pathology, particularly if the history includes intermittent effusion, the "duck waddle" may be helpful in provoking symptoms and localizing the site of pain. It is a nonspecific test (Fig. 11-18). With even a small effusion it is often impossible for the athlete to fully flex on both knees, which is manifested by one buttock being higher than the other when viewed from behind. Significant retropatellar changes produce excessive patellar pain and prohibit completion of the test. Meniscal lesions are usually uncomfortable and refer pain to the particular joint line involved. This test is also useful when incorporated into the assessment for full recovery.

Discoid Meniscus

Described by Young on an anatomic specimen in 1889, the discoid meniscus is still the subject of much debate (Fig. 11-19). In Caucasians it is unusual, there being 467 discoid lateral menisci and 7 medial menisci involved among 10,000 meniscectomies reported by Smillie.[24] The incidence is much higher in the Oriental population. In series of athletes reported from Japan, lateral meniscal lesions were more common than medial ones, not only because the lateral discoid meniscus is more common but because it is more susceptible to trauma.[25] Kaplan, performing comparative anatomic studies of the human embryo between the fifth intrauterine week and birth, was unable to find either a lateral or a medial structure resembling a disc.[26] He postulated postnatal

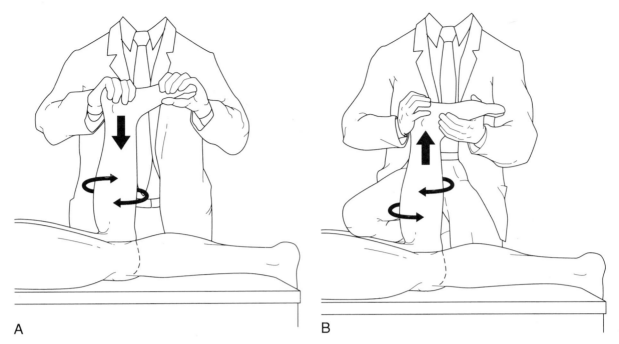

Fig. 11-15. Apley test. The patient lies prone with the knee flexed to 90 degrees and the thigh anchored by the examiner's knee or by an assistant. The leg is rotated medially and laterally, forcing the extremes of range. **(A)** Compression, which may be more uncomfortable with meniscal pathology. **(B)** Distraction, which mainly stresses the ligaments.

evolution of the discoid meniscus based on abnormal attachments and hence motion. By contrast, Tillmann demonstrated distinct discoid-shaped menisci fused to the upper tibial surface in 10-week-old embryos. Only when joint motion begins do they separate from the tibia so that they may follow the excursion of the femurs. It is suggested that further maturation and development of the characteristic crescent shape is not always complete but may be arrested at several stages, giving rise to Smillie's classification.[24]

1. Massive (primitive) disc with the early embryonic oval shape
2. Intermediate disc with a thin interposed segment between the horns
3. Infantile disc (Wrisberg ligament type) with a broadened middle segment and abnormal posterior attachment

These abnormal shapes and attachments affect the contact stresses between the tibiofemoral articulation, alter mobility, and hence change the stresses and

behavior to mechanical deformation. With sudden deformation the short, free edge may tend to tear from the center toward the periphery; however, all types of tears may be visualized. In the very young the discoid meniscus may be entirely asymptomatic. Occasionally, even in the child there is a complaint of snapping, pain or effusions. Typically, however, the symptoms due to a discoid meniscus may not be seen until the second decade, and more than 65 percent of the individuals so affected are older than 18 years at the time of onset of symptoms, particularly with the unusual medial discoid meniscus. There are no pathognomonic signs of a normal or a torn discoid meniscus. It has been suggested that the snapping knee is frequently present in the Wrisberg ligament type of lateral discoid meniscus. In some individuals a pronounced reproducible "clunk" or "thud" is felt as the knee is extended to about 20 to 30 degrees at the completion of the McMurray maneuver with the forced rotation maintained. Sometimes the clunk is present while attempting the pivot shift maneuver.

Tears of a discoid meniscus are difficult to treat

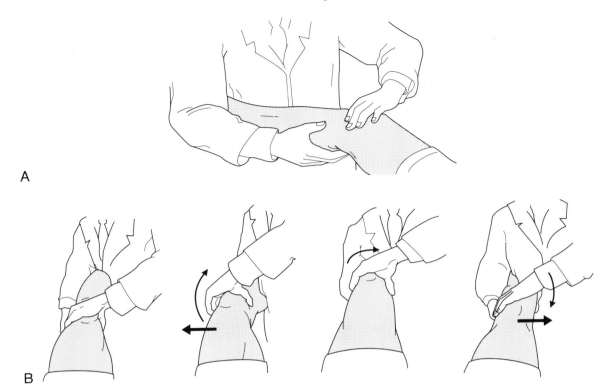

Fig. 11-16. Anderson grind test. **(A)** The patient is supine, and the leg is supported firmly with one hand while the index and finger thumb of the other hand palpate the anterior joint line. **(B)** Valgus stress is applied as the knee is flexed and varus stress as it is extended. The test is repeated with progressively increasing stress. A positive test is a painful grinding sensation.

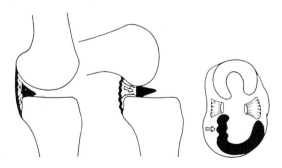

Fig. 11-17. Jump sign of Finocchietto. During an anterior drawer with the knee at 90 degrees, the posterior horn of a hypermobile medial meniscus, with or without tissue bridge, may be incarcerated between the tibial and femoral condyles. It may also occur during active flexion in the weight-bearing position, producing an audible pop or a snapping sensation. It is indicative of a hypermobile meniscus in association with anterior cruciate deficiency.

because of the young age of the individual and the large size of the cartilage. In the past they have been removed, even in the young child, when sufficiently symptomatic. Currently, the trend is to resuture where appropriate or resect the tear and even debulk or reshape them, in preference to total meniscectomy. Specifically, at arthroscopy sometimes no tear is visualized in a large discoid meniscus, but the painful snap experienced by the patient may be visualized as a buckling of the meniscal substance. A submeniscal approach and debulking and reshaping of the meniscus frequently cure the symptoms. Certain surgeons have extensive experience with these unusual meniscal lesions, and whenever practical they should be consulted about the management.

Meniscal Cyst (Meniscal Ganglia)

Central degeneration of the meniscus may give rise to ganglion formation (Fig. 11-20).[4,27] These cysts start with a small pedicle and may ultimately become

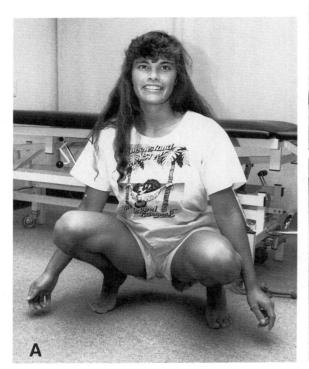 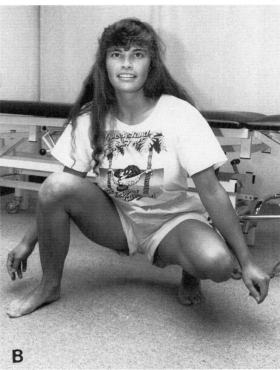

Fig. 11-18. Duck waddle. **(A)** Effusion, loss of full extension, and pain during full flexion inhibit the ability to perform a symmetric "duck waddle." **(B)** Rotation is particularly stressful on a torn meniscus.

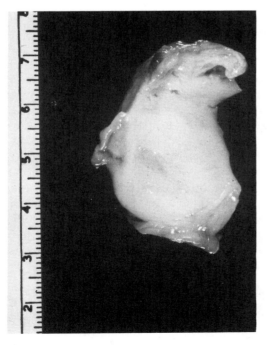

Fig. 11-19. Discoid meniscus specimen.

large. Frequently asymptomatic, they may ultimately present because of the associated pathologic changes or tears in the associated meniscus or because of the cyst itself. The commonest presenting complaint is increasing size of the cyst. The size of the cyst may fluctuate with activity. The lateral meniscus is involved more frequently than the medial meniscus, and it is usually the midportion or posterior one-third that is affected. The prominence of the cyst fre-

---

Clinical Point

MENISCAL CYST: CLASSIC PRESENTATION

- Patient age 20 to 40 years
- Dull ache on lateral side of knee
- Localized extra-articular swelling
- Swelling proportional to activity

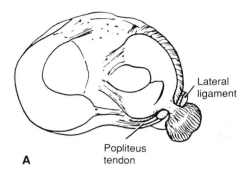

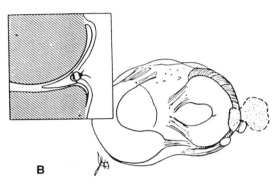

Fig. 11-20. (A) Lateral meniscal cyst and its relation at the joint line between the popliteal tendon and the lateral ligament. **(B)** Resection of a cyst anterior to the lateral ligament and resuturing of the meniscus.

quently is best visualized with the knee at 45 degrees (Fig. 11-21).

Phemister in 1923 recognized the yellowish areas of degeneration within the meniscus and the associated multiloculated character of the cyst and likened them to other cases of colloidal cystic swelling associated with a connective tissue ganglion.[28] In 1929 Barrie published a comprehensive histologic report of meniscal cysts. All of his specimens showed horizontal tears, and in most a tract could be seen connecting the tears with the cysts.[29] The concept evolved that micro- and macrotears lead to synovial fluid infiltration into the parameniscal tissue, clinically presenting as a meniscal cyst.[30]

Asymptomatic cysts should be left alone. Symptomatic cysts without mechanical symptoms sometimes respond to aspiration and injection with methylprednisolone (Depo-Medrol). Recurrent cysts or cysts with associated significant pain and mechanical symptoms, particularly if there is associated joint effusion, should be assessed by arthroscopy. Any significant meniscal lesion should be dealt with in normal fashion by arthroscopic techniques. It is then possible to decompress the cyst by multiple needle punctures and aspiration.[30] Alternatively, the cyst may be excised with scarification of the meniscal skin rim and resutured to the perimeniscal soft tissue. Routine meniscectomy and cyst excision is no longer acceptable therapy.

Common Clinical Presentations of Meniscal Lesions

In summary, there are essentially five basic clinical pictures, described in the following sections.

Clinical Point

MAIN CLINICAL PRESENTATIONS

- Lesion associated with acute ligament disruption
- Acute isolated meniscal lesion with locked knee
- Chronic meniscal tear with locked knee
- Chronic meniscal lesion, no locking
- Chronic meniscal lesion in an unstable knee

Lesion Associated with Acute Ligament Injury

The acutely injured knee associated with ligamentous disruption is difficult to assess clinically because of the pain, swelling, and altered motion secondary to the ligament tear. The index of suspicion exists when the medial collateral ligament tear is clinically apparent along the joint line. Furthermore, a complete tear of the anterior cruciate and the medial collateral ligament may be part of the "unhappy triad" and include meniscal pathology. Frequently arthroscopy is needed to confirm the diagnosis, and treatment of the meniscus depends on the overall management of the ligamentous disruption. With lesser collateral ligament injuries and peripheral meniscal tears, healing may even occur spontaneously.

Acute Isolated Meniscal Lesion

The athlete presenting with an isolated acute meniscal lesion and a locked knee may or may not have a previous history of meniscal pathology. Soon after the episode the knee is tense and swollen, frequently with a blood-tinged effusion or even frank blood at aspiration. There is considerable guarding, and many of the clinical tests are impossible to perform. The

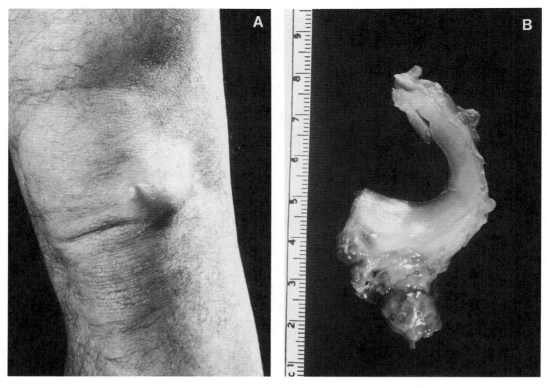

Fig. 11-21. (A) Lateral meniscal cyst (ganglion) showing bulge on joint line. **(B)** Specimen removed.

effusion and pain prohibit the McMurray test and "duck" walking. Spasm prevents the bounce test. The most useful signs are joint line tenderness, the Anderson grind test, Apley maneuvers, Steinmann test, and localization of symptoms with gentle pressure over the locked knee. If the locking is due to pain and spasm and not a displaced fragment, it will improve with time. Frequently re-examination aids in decision-making; and depending on the circumstances, arthroscopy is often indicated. A small peripheral lesion (less than 1 cm) will often heal spontaneously.

Chronic Lesion, Locked Knee

The athlete who has had previous problems of intermittent swelling, giving way, and locking may present with a subtly locked knee. This individual may even describe previous episodes of locking and be able to outline the maneuver that usually unlocks the knee. The presenting episode may be more acute than previous episodes. It is frequently possible to perform a bounce test; and provided the effusion is not excessive, all of the range of motion and rotation maneuvers may be carried out. Diagnosis is possibly easier with this type of lesion than the others, and the

usual therapy is arthroscopic surgery, which may allow both confirmation and treatment of the lesion (Fig. 11-22).

Chronic Lesion, No Locking

Chronic isolated meniscal lesions that do not produce locking are the most difficult to diagnose. Depending on the location, size, and mechanical disruption caused by the tear, the symptoms can range from mild aching or swelling (frequently in the posteromedial or posterolateral corner of the knee) or intermittent effusions with little discomfort to a disabling joint line pain with all activities. All of the tests are easy to perform, but the signs may be amazingly subtle. The "duck waddle" is useful for unmasking functional problems. Diagnosis usually depends on further tests such as arthrography, computed tomography (CT), magnetic resonance imaging (MRI) or arthroscopy.

Lesion Associated with Chronic Ligament Instability

The last common scenario is the athlete with a known anterior cruciate deficient knee who presents with a chief complaint of giving way. The diagnostic

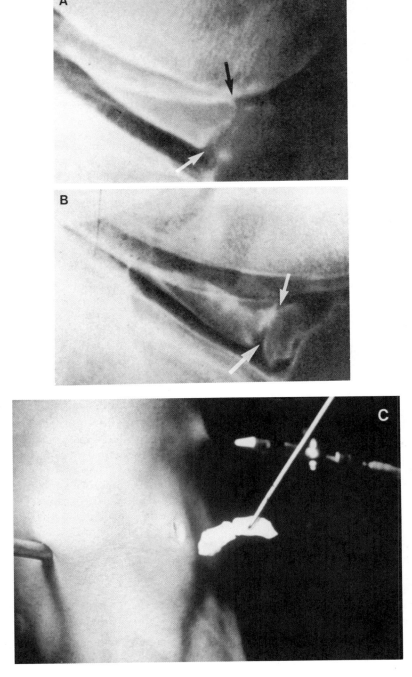

Fig. 11-22. **(A)** Arthrogram of a peripheral tear of the medial meniscus in the vascular (posterior) zone. **(B)** Mid zone. **(C)** In this case, the tear was not deemed suitable for resuturing and was removed arthroscopically.

TABLE 11-2. Accuracy of Arthrography

Parameter	Medial Arthrography[a] (%)	Lateral Arthrography[a] (%)
Sensitivity	85.6 (93.3)	53.3 (33.3)
Specificity	93.8 (93.3)	94.2 (100.0)
Predicted value of positive test	92.8 (93.3)	64.0 (100.0)
Predicted value of negative test	87.4 (93.3)	91.3 (85.7)

[a] Values in parentheses are those of the most experienced arthrographer.

dilemma involves distinguishing symptoms relating to the degree of ligament instability from the additional meniscal signs. Assessment of strength, effectiveness of bracing, and the nature and acuteness of the presenting episode are helpful. However, arthroscopy is frequently necessary to fully integrate the pathology of the joint surface, ligaments, and meniscus into a coherent clinical picture around which a definitive treatment plan may be evolved.

Comment

Although the signs of a classic tear may seem fairly straightforward, many of the meniscal tears produce more subtle signs and symptoms. Usually significant tears are accompanied by wasting of the quadriceps and hamstring muscles. However, even experienced clinicians cannot accurately rule out or diagnose meniscal lesions using only clinical tests. In addition, one must consider unusual situations such as discoid meniscus and meniscal cysts, both of which were discussed earlier in the chapter. This fact leads to a consideration of supplementary tests, e.g., plain roentgenography, arthrography, CT, and MRI.

Roentgenography and Arthrography

The plain roentgenogram has a limited but important role in the diagnosis of meniscal lesions. It is used primary to rule out loose bodies, significant degenerative joint disease, areas of osteochondritis dissecans, and, after acute trauma, fracture of the condyles or plateaus. Frequently skyline, tunnel, and oblique views are necessary to screen for these problems.

In 1975 DeHaven presented a series of patients with internal derangement of the knee.[31] The clinical diagnosis was correct in 72 percent of patients, correct but incomplete in 10 percent, and incorrect in 18 percent. Despite arthrograms, arthroscopy revealed an unexpected diagnosis in 25 percent of the patients.

Subsequently Gillies and Seligson pointed out that the clinical diagnosis was least accurate for lesions of the lateral meniscus.[32] Furthermore, Shakespeare and Rigby reported that significant meniscal tears were identified in only 77 percent of arthrograms from individuals who ultimately were shown to have bucket handle tears at surgery.[22]

In our series of 185 patients with subacute and chronic knee complaints who underwent arthrographic and arthroscopic examination, the clinical impression was completely correct in 67 percent, partially correct in another 10 percent, and in error in 23 percent.[33] Based on the arthroscopic diagnosis, arthrography of the medial meniscus had a predictive value of a positive test of 92.8 percent and a predictive value of the negative test of 87.4 percent. Arthrography of the lateral meniscus had a predictive value of a positive test of 64.0 percent and 91.3 percent for a negative test (Table 11-2).

These studies indicate that double contrast arthrography (i.e., enhancement of radiologic visualization of the structure of the knee joint by installation of air and dye) has a sensitivity of between 75 and 85 percent in some series and up to 90 to 95 percent with experienced arthrographers (Table 11-2), although there are several potential sources of error (Table 11-3). While helpful when a tear is positively identified, a negative arthrogram leads to considerable doubt about the specific diagnosis. With this point in mind, the evolution of CT scanning and MRI has

**TABLE 11-3. Arthrography:
Potential Sources of Error**

Misinterpretation of popliteal hiatus
Displaced fragment, remaining meniscus called normal
Meniscal ossicle, chondrocalcinosis
Soft tissue injection of air, mimicking peripheral separation
Contrast-coated fat pad or synovial fold simulating meniscal tear
Deep, contrast-filled synovial sulcus resembling peripheral separation
Missed tumor in fat pad
Failure to report large synovial (plical) folds

obviously heralded a new era of investigative techniques.

Computed Tomography

High resolution CT has been used successfully to visualize meniscal lesions noninvasively. When compared to arthroscopy the sensitivity of CT is 96.5 percent, the specificity 81.3 percent, and the accuracy 91.0 percent.[34] These figures improve with experience.

Clinical Point

ADVANTAGES OF COMPUTED TOMOGRAPHY

- Noninvasive
- Painless
- Requires no intra-articular injection
- Examination not impaired by effusion
- Not affected by a locked knee
- Correlates well with arthroscopy
- Popliteal tendon well visualized
- Avoids superimposition of adjacent recesses
- Picks up displaced fragment of bucket handle tears

Magnetic Resonance Imaging

There are, and have been, several limitations in the development of MRI techniques (also known as nuclear magnetic imaging, or NMR), not the least of which is the learning curve.[35] With the gradual refinement of technique, there has been an improvement in the reliability of this diagnostic test. Grade I signal intensity is globular and not adjacent to either articular surface. A Grade II is a linear signal not extending to an articular surface. Grades I and II signals are read as no tear. A Grade III signal is linear and extends to either the superior or inferior meniscal surface. It is considered a tear. Given the current number of false positives an MRI image should not be used as an indication for surgery in a patient whose history and physical examination does not seem consistent with a meniscal lesion.[35]

Its advantage is that it is a painless, noninvasive tool that does not use ionizing radiation. It provides excellent soft tissue contrast and has multiplanar imaging capabilities. Currently it is an expensive procedure but where readily available is a tempting alternative to other methods of assessing pathology.

Other Techniques

Other techniques for assisting in the diagnosis have been advocated by various groups. They include radionuclide imaging and vibration arthrography, which detects and records vibration emission from joints. The scanning techniques have made us aware of the frequent damage to the subchondral plate that is associated with tramatic meniscal pathology.[36]

Vibration arthrography helps delineate three signal types within the normal knee: physiologic patellofemoral crepitus, patellar clicks, and the lateral band signal (present in 22 percent of subjects).[37] The latter sound is probably related to the iliotibial band snapping across the femoral condyle. In symptomatic individuals lesions of the meniscus appear to produce distinct signals, which make it possible to estimate the size and location of a tear.[37] Although the present systems are somewhat cumbersome, rapid advances in computer technology may allow this experimental process to evolve into a relatively inexpensive, accessible screening instrument for knee pathology.

The noninvasive nature of some of these modern techniques make them attractive alternatives. They are judged against arthroscopy, which itself in experienced hands has a high degree of accuracy.

Arthroscopy

Evolution

The history of the arthroscope extends over nearly two centuries. Bozzini of Frankfurt am Main devised a light conductor in 1805. This instrument consisted

---

Quick Facts

ACCURACY OF MRI FOR MENISCAL TEARS

	Medial (%)	Lateral (%)
Sensitivity	97	90
Specificity	77	87
Positive Predictive Value	85	79
Negative Predictive Value	95	94
Accuracy	88	88

of a light chamber illuminated by a candle, from which a tube passed that could be introduced into body cavities. Initially, the easiest cavities to access were the urethra and bladder. Bozzini presented his findings to the Viennese Medical Society, who dismissed the instrument as a toy. In 1853 Desmoreaux published his extensive experience with this endoscopic device, and for the first time the medical profession deemed that it may be worthwhile.

The situation improved with the advent of electricity, and in 1876 Nitze introduced an instrument with a lens system, sufficient light, and a water-cooling system. It was used mainly to visualize the bladder. In 1918 in Tokyo, Kenji Takagi, Emeritous Professor of Orthopaedics, first inspected a cadavar knee through the so-called cystoscope. The remarkably clear view encouraged him to design the first arthroscope. The scope was too large in diameter for routine use, but over the next few years he perfected lens systems, made his equipment smaller, and by 1931 succeeded in producing an arthroscope with a diameter of 3.5 mm that was suitable for examining the narrow confines of the fluid-filled knee. Owing to lack of funds during the 1930s, however, it was not possible to publish all his photographs and motion pictures, a task that remained for his pupil Watanabi, who presented an atlas of superb arthroscopic photographs obtained between 1957 and 1969.

Subsequent to that time, during the 1950s to the 1970s, although many orthopaedic surgeons were enthusiastic about the arthroscope, many believed that its diagnostic and therapeutic implications were overrated. Nevertheless, with the perfected lens system, superb fibro-optics, miniaturized cameras, and array of miniaturized surgical instruments, there developed an era of arthroscopic surgery of the knee.

One might add that currently arthroscopic surgery is riding on the crest of a wave, and some of the claims have been nothing short of extravagant. However, there is a definite, clear role for arthroscopic surgery. Used wisely, it presents a significant advance in the management of problems of the knee, particularly problems related to torn cartilage. Only this aspect of the arthroscopic surgery is discussed here.

Meniscal Surgery

William Hay from Leeds described in 1803 discussed the torn semilunar cartilage, and in 1909 Robert Jones from Liverpool suggested that only the torn fragments should be removed. Subsequently, Sir Reginald Watson Jones urged that total meniscec-

tomy should be performed in cases of torn cartilage. This concept was supported as late as 1970 by Ian Smillie from Edinburgh. Their thinking was based on the concept that a meniscus may regenerate if taken back to its synovial attachment and that retained posterior horns are likely a major cause of recurrent symptoms. As a matter of fact, neither of these concepts is true. We now have evidence that a large number of individuals may have small tears in their cartilage without symptoms, and many people have small tears without evidence of related degenerative changes. By contrast, the so-called unstable tears, with major symptoms, are definitely related to the development of degenerative joint disease. The upshot is that with seriously symptomatic tears that require surgical treatment a partial meniscectomy is desirable, and this is easiest to achieve with arthroscopy surgery (Fig. 11-22). Even a small peripheral remnant, especially in the posterior horn of the medial meniscus will provide an important stabilizing factor against anterior fibial displacement.

Apart from the treatment aspect, the accuracy of intraoperative diagnosis and the potential for correcting many of these conditions makes arthroscopy an attractive tool. In our series of 185 conservative patients diagnosed as having a meniscal lesion on clinical grounds, a variety of other pathology was identified (Table 11-4).[33] A previous series by Johnson in 1982 further emphasized the potential inaccu-

TABLE 11-4. Arthroscopic Diagnosis[a]

Diagnosis	No.
Meniscal lesion	126
Medial	90
Lateral	36
Medial and lateral	16
Plical fold	33
Chondral erosion	26
Chondromalacia	25
Anterior cruciate lesion	14
Fat pad pathology	6
Loose body	5
Chronic synovitis	4
Subluxing patella	3
Pigmented villonodular synovitis	2
Foreign body (suture)	1
Synovial chondromatosis	1
Tumor, benign	2
Posterior cruciate tear	1
Normal knee	8

[a] A total of 258 diagnoses in 185 patients (double diagnosis in 67) with a clinical diagnosis of meniscal lesion.

TABLE 11-5. Importance of Diagnostic Arthroscopy

Clinical Diagnosis	% Confirmed at Arthroscopy	Usual Other Arthroscopic Diagnosis
Normal	86	Chondromalacia
Medial meniscus tear	44	Degenerative arthritis
Lateral meniscus tear	70	Anterior cruciate-tear
Chondromalacia	85	Plicae
Subluxing patellae	94	Meniscus tear
Dislocating patellae	96	Torn anterior cruciate

(From Johnson,[38] with permission.)

racy of clinical diagnosis and the revealing nature of arthroscopy (Table 11-5).[38] However, these studies should not be cited to minimize the importance and need for clinical examination. Furthermore, the simple **identification of pathology at arthroscopy does not automatically mean that the lesion is the cause of the patient's symptoms.** The more experienced surgeon is careful when ascribing symptoms to obvious pathology, and a conservative approach to all surgical procedures performed is usually eventually justified on subsequent clinical follow-up.

Postoperative Problems and Rehabilitation

Arthroscopic meniscal surgery offers several advantages, the most important of which is the enhanced ability to perform a partial meniscectomy. When sufficient facilities exist, it is easily carried out as an outpatient procedure. Although local and regional anesthetic techniques are possible, most centers use spinal, epidural, or light general anesthetic systems that provide maximal conditions for the surgeon to manipulate the joint. For patients admitted to hospital, the stay is reduced to a minimum.

Rehabilitation

Essentially, the patient's progress, resolution of effusion, re-establishment of strength, return to work and sport, and ultimate outcome, depend on the magnitude and duration of existing pathology, the associated ligament stability and articular surface changes, and the extent of the intra-articular surgery carried out. These factors influence the need for, and the rate of progression of rehabilitation. In the various reported series, the time to resolution of the postoperative effusion to just a trace amount is 10 to 14 days, number of days with walking aids 2 to 10 days, time to achieve 120 degrees of flexion 5 to 12 days, return to work or full duties 1 to 3 weeks, and return to sport 2 to 12 weeks.[39-41] There is an advan-

tage of formal postoperative physiotherapy if maximum recovery is to be achieved in the shortest possible time.

The principles of rehabilitation are the same as those used for treating open meniscectomies. They include (1) adequate control of the knee joint by effective quadriceps and hamstring contraction; (2) minimizing and dispersing effusion; (3) re-establishing range of motion; and (4) planned, slow, step-by-step reintegration into activity within the confines of pain and swelling.

Presurgically the affected leg often has a knee extensor deficit in the range of 10 to 20 percent. With open meniscectomy the effective quadriceps deficit is about 70 percent and with closed arthroscopic technique approximately 40 percent at 1 week after operation.[42]

At 6 weeks after arthroscopy there is usually still an average mean quadriceps deficit of around 10 to 20 percent and a mean hamstring deficit of around 5 percent. On this basis most activity may be resumed, but rehabilitation should still continue, even if only in the form of a home program (Table 11-6). At 8 to 12 weeks frequently there is still a small but measurable difference.[43]

Part of the delay in return to full strength may be related to minor muscle damage and denervation by tourniquet use.[44] However, in our series the time to full recovery usually reflected the patient's past experience with conditioning and strengthening techniques rather than any effect of the tourniquet (unpublished data, 1986). The rise in creatinine kinase is approximately that seen after hard physical exercise. The use of nonsteroidal anti-inflammatory drugs (NSAIDs) during the immediate postoperative period and continued for 7 to 10 days seems to minimize the postmeniscectomy synovitis and thus indirectly affects muscle wasting and perhaps allows earlier return to function. Prostaglandin inhibition after soft tissue injury is associated with enhanced recovery

TABLE 11-6. Meniscectomy Home Program[a]

Before operation
    Instruction in crutch walking
    Calf and ankle exercises
    Quadriceps setting
    Straight leg raising
    Information about the procedure, recovery room, possible complications (deep vein thrombosis, infection)

After operation

Day 1	Dorsi- and plantar flexion exercises, 10–15 repetitions (reps)[b]
	Quadriceps setting, 10–15 reps. Hold each contraction 6 seconds.
	Walking with partial weight-bearing using crutches.
	Exercises to be performed: one set every hour if possible during the day.
	Rewind tensor if feels tight.
Day 2	Increase weight bearing as tolerated.[b]
	Still use crutches.
	Quadriceps setting.
	Quadriceps extension over rolled up towel.
	Straight leg raises.
	Each exercise 10–15 reps. Hold contraction 6 seconds. Do 3–4 sets.
Day 3	Add knee exercises in sitting position.
	Add hamstring curls.
	Add abductor and adductor straight leg raises.
	Exercises 10–15 reps. Hold contractions 6 seconds. Do 3–4 sets.
	Range of motion as tolerated.[b]
Days 4–14	Continue exercises. Add resistance as tolerated.
	Remove bandage for shower.
	Discontinue crutches if can do all exercises without any problems and without quadriceps lag.
	Add calf raises.
	Cut back exercises and weights and resume crutch walking (partial weight-bearing) if effusion increases or pain increase.[b]

[a] At 10 to 14 days after operation the surgeon decides whether to progress activity or order a formal physiotherapy program.

[b] Report to physician or emergency if (1) calf gets tender, (2) leg and ankle swell, (3) the wound or knee gets red and hot, (4) pain is not relieved by the analgesics supplied, or (5) there is an onset of fever, chills, or sweats.

Clinical Point

REHABILITATION PROGRESS

1. Overcome reflex inhibition.
2. Minimize effusion.
3. Progress strengthening.
4. Re-establish range of motion.
5. Use pain and swelling as a guide to rate of progression.
6. Discontinue walking aids when effusion is minimal and there is quadriceps control.
7. Return to activity when quadriceps deficit is less than 20 percent.
8. Resume full activity when patient can duck waddle, has full range, and the strength deficit is less than 10 percent.

without causing structural weakness in healing tissues.[45] The effect of pain on reflex postoperative muscle wasting is well established, and some groups have used transcutaneous neural stimulation (TNS) to assist recovery of muscle strength and function.[45,46] Jensen et al. recorded a recovery of isokinetic muscle strength some 3 weeks earlier in the group undergoing TNS than in those in the nontreatment and placebo groups.[47] Recovery is possibly further enhanced by supplementing the regular isometric and isokinetic training programs with functional electrical stimulation.[48]

It is difficult to set hard and fast rules for rehabilitation, as every aspect of patient care is subject to the differences in philosophy and approach of the surgeon. Postsurgical support ranges from a tensor bandage, to Robert Jones compressive support, to commercial knee immobilization, to plaster casts. Weight-bearing regimes vary from unrestricted motion and walking as tolerated, to enforced bed rest or non- and light partial weight-bearing with crutches.

There is little evidence to show that rigid dressings, forced immobilization, and long-duration protected weight-bearing enhance the speed of recovery. On the other hand, support with a tensor bandage, early weight-bearing progressed rapidly as quadriceps control is ensured, and resisted exercises tailored to the resolution of effusion usually ensure maximum return to function in minimum time. This regimen also reduces postoperative complications to a minimum. Frequently the most practical approach is to arrange for the therapist to teach a comprehensive preoperative regimen, supply the patient with a well thought out information sheet, and make every provision for a dedicated home program for the first 10 days postoperatively (Table 11-6). At that time the patients may be screened as to the need for a further home program or structured physiotherapy. The more urgent and pressing the need for return to full function, the more necessary becomes intensive rehabilitation. Some surgeons insist on a completely isometric routine for the first 3 to 6 weeks; when carefully taught and diligently performed, such a program may engender excellent return to function. Part of the reason is that much of the initial strength gain is probably related to re-establishment of the neural control mechanism.[48]

Return to Activity

The program outlined in Figures 11-23 to 11-30 reflects the regimen applied to most patients undergoing arthroscopic meniscectomy. The presence of complications may slow the postoperative progress (Table 11-7). It is important during this progression to utilize the more physiologic loading weight-bearing exercises such as with the "shuttle" machine, "the stepper," and balance boards. Cardiovascular work on bicycles and treadmills must not be neglected.

The eventual return to sport may depend on pre-existing irreversible pathology and the level of participation.[25,49] In Miller's series of international or top athletes, 74 percent had an excellent result (no symptoms, full activity) at 1 year after arthroscopic meniscectomy, and another 21 percent had a good result

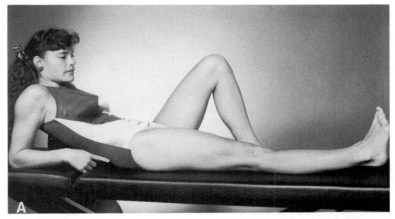

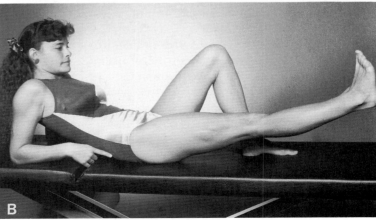

Fig. 11-23. (A) Quadriceps setting exercise. The leg is straightened as much as possible and the patella pulled proximally. **(B)** When good quadriceps control is achieved, add straight leg raising. Weights may be added.

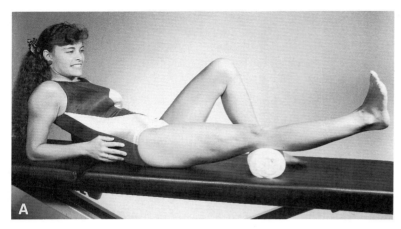

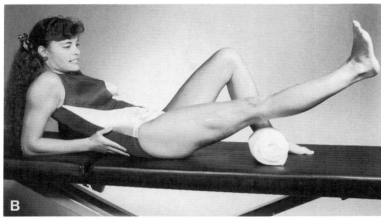

Fig. 11-24. (A) Terminal knee extension over a quads block helps to gain full extension and overcome quads inhibition. **(B)** Progress by incorporating a straight leg raise.

(full activity, minimal symptoms).[50] In a comparable series of 80 active individuals, 34 percent rated their knee as normal, 58 percent as improved, and 65 percent had returned to their sports at a 12 to 24-month follow-up.[51] Motivation, expectation, dedication, and compliance to the rehabilitation programs, as well as the stresses involved in the activity, contribute to patient satisfaction and ultimate activity potential. Lastly, the avoidance of postoperative problems is essential; however, although some of the problems can be avoided by strict adherence to a well thought out postoperative protocol, others are unavoidable consequences of surgery.

Postoperative Problems

The risk of serious complications is small. Minor problems include hemarthrosis, painful or tender scars, effusion, and fat pad pain, particularly with a central patella approach. These problems are experienced by up to 60 percent of individuals undergoing arthroscopy and for the most part are transient.

Effusion is more related to the prior condition of the knee and, along with the hemarthrosis, is proportional to the amount of surgery performed. Persistent effusion is usually due to too rapid progression of activity, poor quadriceps and hamstring control, or retained loose fragments in the joint. Pain around the patellar tendon, the fat pad syndrome, may develop up to 5 to 6 weeks postoperatively; and although it usually responds to NSAIDs, an injection of steroid may be required to relieve it. With skill, joint scuffing should be reduced to a minimum. The usual small amount of joint scratches seem to heal well within a few months, as does the retained meniscal rim. Usually most debris is irrigated from the joint, but occasional retention of a large fragment causes persistent synovitis. Rarely, small incisional cysts occur where pieces of debris have been dragged into the interior of the wound. The problems are usually easily man-

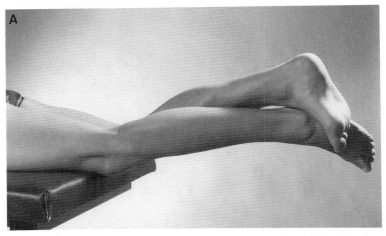

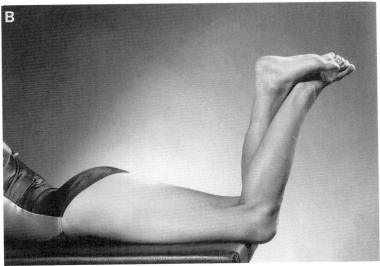

Fig. 11-25. Autoresisted hamstring curls with progressive resistance from the unaffected limb. **(A)** Starting position. **(B)** Midrange. Pressure over the patella is avoided by performing the exercise over the end of the bench.

aged by local injection of anesthetic and excision of the cyst. Some injury to small peripheral branches of the infrapatellar nerve may produce temporary or permanent dysesthesia, which is rarely as much a problem as with open meniscectomy or other knee surgery.

Infrequent but important complications include joint infection (0.04 percent), damage to the joint capsule with significant extravasation into the surrounding soft tissues (0.02 percent), synovial fistula formation (0.05 percent), compartment syndrome (0.008 percent), and instrument breakage (0.03 percent). In addition, there are some significant complications that may occur even in young healthy individuals, including damage to major nerves or vessels by the "blind" use of instruments, which is rare with simple meniscal excision but may be important with more complex surgery. Deep vein thrombosis

(DVT) is difficult to judge clinically but may be of a severity sufficient to cause pain and swelling of the leg; the incidence may be as little as 1 : 500 in patients under 40 and 4 : 100 in those over age 40 if no risk factors exist. Risk factors include smoking, obesity, use of oral contraceptives, and prolonged surgery. Minor undetected DVT is certainly more frequent. Pulmonary embolism may occur in 1 : 1000 healthy individuals, and the chance of dying from arthroscopy is approximately 1 : 50,000 in young people without increased risk factors.

When these problems and complications are combined, the list appears formidable; most complications, however, are minimal, transient, and easily treated. Even the more serious complications are usually treatable without long-term sequelae if recognized early, which is the reason the entire rehabilitation team should be familiar with their presentation.

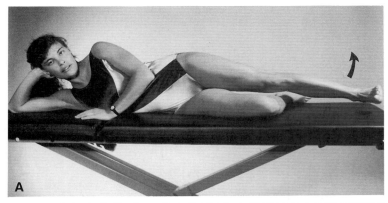

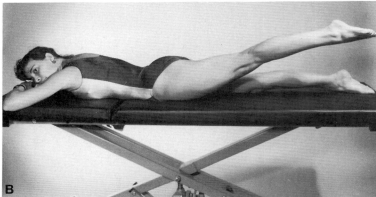

Fig. 11-26. Hip abductor and extensor work. **(A)** Starting position for abduction working gluteus medius and minimum. **(B)** Hip extension for gluteus maximus, exercised from the prone position. Take the leg as high as possible and hold. Leg weights may be added.

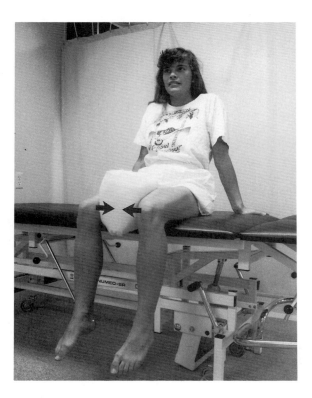

Fig. 11-27. Leg adduction using a ball or bolster as resistance. Similarly, abduction may be resisted using heavy rubber tubing.

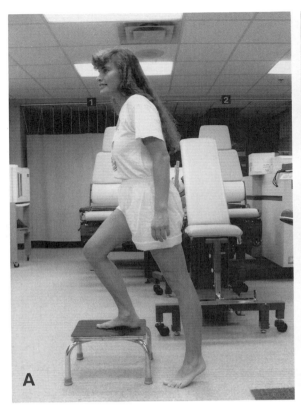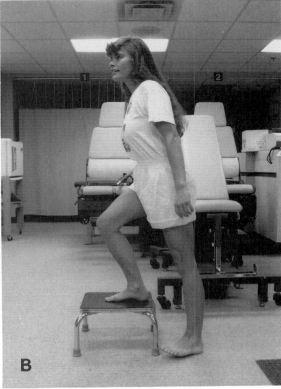

Fig. 11-28. Forward stepping or side stepups are excellent concentric and eccentric quads exercises. Forward stepping is shown here. **(A)** Starting with a low platform or telephone book, the height of the step can be raised as pain and strength allow. Initially the unaffected leg may help out by pushing off with the toe. **(B)** The progression is holding the ankle in dorsiflexion to avoid the push off. When adequate strength and range are achieved, the patient may be progressed to a stair climber machine.

Resuturing the Menisci

In 1883 Annandale carried out the first recorded repair of a human meniscus after tearing, and in 1938 Palmer advocated resuturing peripheral tears of the meniscus when associated with a torn medial collateral ligament, particularly the posteromedial corner of the knee.[52] DeHaven[53] and Cassidy and Shaffer[54] reported on the possibility of resuturing acutely torn menisci provided the tear was in the peripheral part of the meniscus itself. In 1983 Hamburg et al. outlined the success of resuturing old meniscal lesions.[55] In fact, they reported on 35 cases that were resutured up to 7 years after the injury. This historical review represents a gradual maturation of thinking. After the initial wave of enthusiasm for resuturing the meniscus during the early 1900s, it was subsequently thought to be a worthless exercise because of the poor blood supply of the menisci themselves. Subsequent studies have in fact shown that the peripheral one-third of the medial and lateral menisci of the knee have an excellent blood supply with sufficient vasculature to support healing (Fig. 11-31). Based on these data, a revival of interest in resuturing the meniscus has evolved. It has been emphasized because of the increasing awareness of the havoc that occurs in the knee following total meniscectomy, particularly in the presence of previous damage to the ligaments or joint. Although far more studies are needed, the concept of resuturing the meniscus is now accepted (Fig. 11-32). When this surgery is performed, it is essential to attempt to stabilize any existing ligamentous laxity

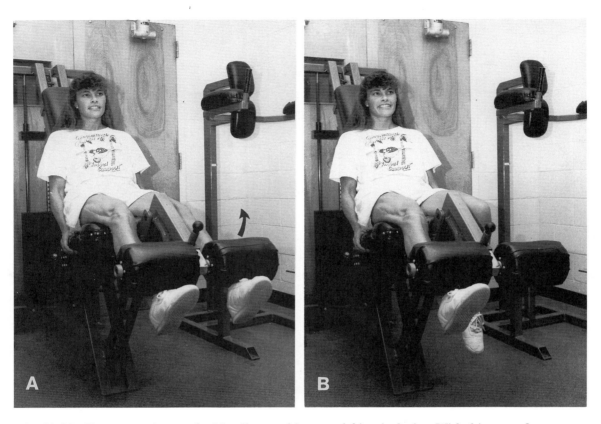

Fig. 11-29. Knee extension on the Nautilus machine, a polykinetic device. With this type of apparatus it is important that the seat and support are adjusted to align the joint with the cams. **(A)** Double leg extension using the good leg to assist the affected limb. **(B)** Isometric holds may be used at selected ranges, when this is achieved without flaring up an effusion. Single or double leg eccentric contractors are performed by lowering the bar slowly.

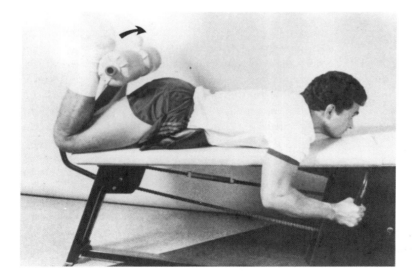

Fig. 11-30. Resisted knee flexion for hamstring work. Make sure that there is no painful pressure over the patella.

TABLE 11-7. Postmeniscectomy Protocol*

Phase	Protocol

Phase I (7–14 days post-op)	Home program as outlined
	Emphasis
	    Ankle exercise
	    Quadriceps setting
	    Straight leg raises
	Weight-bearing and range of motion as tolerated
	If supervised program may add
	    Quadriceps block work
	    Hamstring program
	    Other lower limb strengthening
	    Step-ups
	    Isometric and isokinetic resisted work
	    Possible electromyostimulation

Phase II (swelling minimal)	Commence re-establishing full range of motion
	    Quadriceps-hamstring
	    Hips-ankles
	Increase endurance work
	Increase strengthening

Phase III (no effusion, minimal discomfort)	Strengthening
	    Commence quadriceps and hamstring isokinetic work at 60 degrees per second
	Endurance
	    When 60% strength add 180 and 240 degrees per second
	    Work to 50% fatigue
	Eccentric loading
	    Shuttle machine
	    Kincom eccentric loading device
	    Half squats

Phase IV (functional training)	Criteria
	    80% Strength
	    90% Range of motion
	    Able to "duck waddle" comfortably
	Strengthening
	    Emphasis on eccentric loading
	Endurance
	    Cycling, running, skipping
	Proprioception
	    Balance boards, pro-fitter
	Function
	    Jumping
	    Sprinting
	    Cutting
	Guidelines
	    Pain decreasing
	    No recurrent effusions
	    Modify according to
	        Functional goals
	        Condition of joint surface
	        Stability of ligaments

* Guidelines for therapy progression.

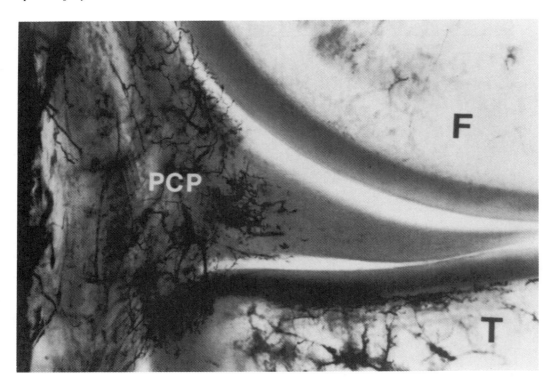

Fig. 11-31. Microvasculature of the medial meniscus. Branching radial vessels from the perimeniscal capillary plexus (PCP) penetrate the peripheral border of the meniscus. F = femur; T = tibia. This vascularity allows for possible healing with resuturing. (From Arnoczky and Warren,[6] with permission.)

in order to protect the initial repair and the long-term health of the meniscus.[50] Usually a combination of arthroscopic and open techniques is safest and most efficient. It should be emphasized that repair of the chronic meniscal lesion is neither routine, proved, nor always desirable (Fig. 11-22).

Rehabilitation protocols vary. Most include a period of immobilization at 10 to 15 degrees in a splint, brace, or cast for 2 to 6 weeks. The period of partial or non-weight-bearing parallels this time course. This period of restricted motion allows early healing of the meniscal rim. Usually protected motion from rotational torque under weight-bearing conditions continues up to 12 weeks.

A program of generalized strengthening and fitness is applied and isotonic and isokinetic work commenced when 90 degrees of flexion is achieved. Crutches are discontinued as soon as adequate quadriceps strength is gained and the athlete is ambulatory without pain. Running is begun at the return of full range of motion and when quadriceps and hamstring strength is within 5 to 10 percent of baseline. Only straight-ahead running is allowed, with no full speed sprinting or agility maneuvers until 3–6 months after operation depending on the size and location of the lesion. This regimen may seem conservative, but it is safe and provides the maximum chance of a well healed meniscal rim.[54] When more data are available it is possible that this protocol may be able to be accelerated.

Meniscal Transplant

Artificial meniscal implants have met with no success in experimental situations; however, there is a possible role for meniscal transplantation using cadaver material.[56] There are problems of harnessing, storage, and sizing as well as technical difficulties of reimplantation. Nevertheless, this procedure presents an exciting possibility for selected clinical situations. Along with the potential for joint surface allograft, it remains an avenue of salvage for the badly damaged knee in the young, active person.

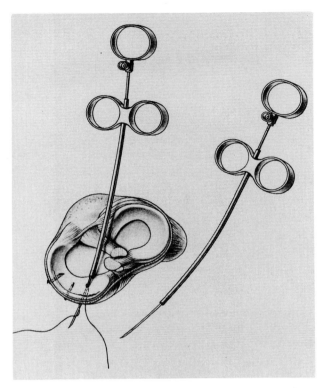

Fig. 11-32. Special instruments may be used for a combined arthroscopic and open technique.

Conclusions

In concluding this discussion on the menisci, the following points are important.

1. The menisci have vital functions in the knee, most importantly those of providing stability, absorbing shock, and distributing weight-bearing.
2. Severe, unstable tears of the meniscus lead to damage of the knee joint.
3. Many small tears are asymptomatic or intermittently symptomatic and may not cause long-standing damage to the joint if left untreated.
4. Partial meniscectomy is always preferable to complete meniscectomy when technically possible. The partial procedure is now frequently feasible owing to the emergence of excellent arthroscopic equipment and techniques.
5. Arthroscopic surgery has its major role in partial meniscectomies and seems to reduce the time spent in hospital and the time to recovery.

6. There is an evolving role for suturing selected meniscal lesions based on the concept of a good peripheral circulation, but there is still much to learn about this procedure at the present time.

OSTEOCHONDRITIS DISSECANS AND RELATED LESIONS

There are probably four distinct groups of lesions in the knee: (1) classic osteochondritis dissecans; (2) post-traumatic chondral injuries; (3) osteochondral fracture; and (4) spontaneous or idiopathic necrosis (Fig. 11-33). Unfortunately, many series have lumped these lesions together under the heading of osteochondritis dissecans, leading to confusion as to etiology, evolution, and preferred treatment. Bradley and Dandy's classic paper help resolve this issue (Table 11-8).[57]

Quick Facts

DEFECTS OF THE ARTICULAR SURFACE

- Classic osteochondritis dissecans
- Post-traumatic chondral injury
- Osteochondral fracture
- Spontaneous idiopathic necrosis

Osteochondritis Dissecans

Osteochondritis dissecans is an expanding concentric lesion that appears at the margins of an otherwise normal epiphysis, usually on the medial femoral condyle. It is seen during the second decade of life.

Etiology

Many causes have been suggested, including trauma, contact with a prominent tibial spine, abnormal ossification of the epiphyseal cartilage, pre-existing constitutional skeletal abnormalities associated with endocrine dysfunction, Fröhlich syndrome, multiple epiphyseal dysplasia, short stature, and generalized ligamentous laxity. The confusion over the role of trauma may be due to the imprecise usage of the term osteochondritis dissecans for any separation of articular cartilage from the underlying bone. Both Paget (1870), who first described the condition, and

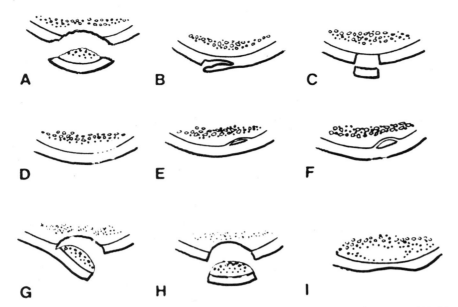

Fig. 11-33. Types of lesions of the femoral condyle. **(A)** Osteochondral fracture. **(B)** Chondral flap. **(C)** Chondral loose body. **(D–F)** Evolving osteochondritis dissecans. **(G)** Separating osteochondritis dissecans. **(H)** Osteochondral loose body. **(I)** Spontaneous osteonecrosis. (After Bradley and Dandy,[58] with permission.)

König (1887), who coined the term "osteochondritis dissecans" reported on some association with trauma, which they thought could not be the sole cause.[58,59] As Barrie pointed out, König had an ear for euphonious title, and the harmony of the words has led the profession to abuse this diagnosis.[60]

Pathology

The primary pathologic change of osteochondritis dissecans is avascular necrosis of the bone with secondary changes occurring in the overlying articular cartilage[61] that may take the form of flattening, discoloration, fissuring, or fibrillation. The lesions may separate and remain in situ and subsequently heal. Alternatively, it may become partially or completely dislodged. The fragment itself may ultimately become a loose body within the joint. The bony portion often atrophies, but the cartilaginous portion, nourished by synovial fluid, may round off and remain, sometimes even growing slightly in size. In any event, its shape soon becomes incongruent with the defect. This defect characteristically has steep sides— different from the classic traumatic chondral flap.[57,61]

Radiographic Findings

The lesion is usually a well circumscribed area in the subchondral bone with the fragment itself in varying stages of separation or union. Occasionally the fragment appears sclerotic. More than 75 percent of lesions are off the main articular area on the lateral side of the medial femoral condyle (Fig. 11-34). An-

TABLE 11-8.   Osteocartilaginous and Cartilaginous Femoral Condyle Lesions

Parameter	Osteochondritis Dissecans		Osteochondral Fracture		Chondral Injury	
	Developing	Separated	Acute	Old	Separation	Flaps
No.	16	42	7	8	64	32
Male/female	13/3	37/5	4/3	8/0	52/12	21/11
Age at arthroscopy	13 (11–18)	28 (18–41)	19 (16–22)	35 (26–49)	32 (16–47)	45 (34–67)
Hemarthrosis	0	0	7	0	0	0
Intact articular cartilage	16	2	0	0	0	0

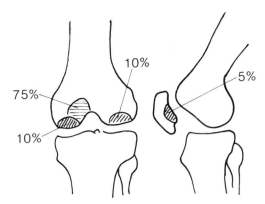

Fig. 11-34. Classic site for osteochondritis dissecans is the lateral side of the medial femoral condyle. With the extended lesion on the main articular area, it accounts for 85 percent of the lesions.

other 5 to 10 percent are extended lesions encroaching on the major weight-bearing area (Fig. 11-35). The remaining 10 to 15 percent are found on the lateral femoral condyle and patella. In fewer than 10 percent the lesion is bilateral. Frequently the roentgenograhic finding is an incidental one in a clinically asymptomatic joint. The lesion is best visualized, in most cases, on the tunnel view. The lateral view provides a second dimension. Other views help locate atypical lesions or loose bodies. Equivocal lesions are occasionally delineated with radionuclide scans, tomography, CT, or MRI.[62]

Symptoms

The signs and symptoms may reflect the evolution of the condition. With in situ lesions there may be pain, often proportional to activity, and occasionally effusions. Separating lesions may produce mechanical signs, such as catching and snapping, as well as pain and effusion. With loose bodies, effusion, intermittent locking and giving way are likely. The signs depend on the degree of separation. Other than demonstrating the presence of an effusion, meniscal tests may be positive such as a painful McMurray test and a positive Anderson grind test. Occasionally, the patient presents with the knee locked. The Wilson test has been described for detection of an early lesion; it has limited accuracy but may give adjunctive information (Fig. 11-36). Resisted extension of the knee in the sitting position is painless, and a positive test involves repeating the resisted knee extension with the patient's foot held in internal rotation. Possible im-

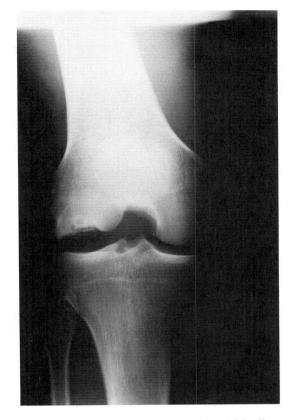

Fig. 11-35. Well advanced osteochondritis dissecans lesion on the lateral femoral condyle.

pingement of the tibial spine against the lesion gives definite pain that is relieved by allowing the tibia to come out of medial rotation.

Treatment

A logical approach to therapy depends on identifying the stage of evolution of the lesion.

Evolving Lesion In Situ (Stage I)

In the in situ lesion the articular surface is usually intact, and the chief complaint is pain. Advice regarding activity is the mainstay of treatment. Sport is reduced to the point that either pain is nonexistent or minimal discomfort is experienced. Definite painful activities are contraindicated. The more the lesion extends into the weight-bearing area, the more likely it is that the patient will be told to eliminate pivoting or torquing type activity. Any muscle wasting or mus-

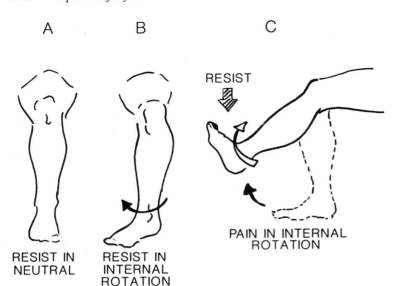

RESIST IN NEUTRAL

RESIST IN INTERNAL ROTATION

RESIST

PAIN IN INTERNAL ROTATION

Fig. 11-36. Wilson test. **(A)** Normal painless resisted extension. **(B)** Then test in forced internal rotation. **(C)** Positive test is pain during extension.

cle tightness is rehabilitated. A plan is set to roentgenograph and re-examine the patient at 3- or 6-month intervals depending on the size and evolution of the lesion. A sudden increase in discomfort or swelling should be investigated immediately. It is important to understand that this radiographic lesion may be clinically silent, and so other lesions should be sought as the potential cause of the athlete's pain. Aspirin or NSAIDs are rarely warranted unless there is significant pain or effusion. Occasionally an acute flare-up of pain requires a short period of partial (light) weight-bearing with crutches. These patients are usually 10 to 13 years of age. Essentially, treatment is proportional to the symptoms unless obvious progression of the separation occurs.

Separating or Chronically Symptomatic Lesion (Stage II)

Individuals with separating or chronically symptomatic lesions are frequently 12 to 15 years of age but may be older. Effusions are common, and the Wilson test is likely to be positive. Restriction of activity, use of crutches, and occasionally a short period of cast immobilization are reasonable approaches, although brace immobilization with motion through a predetermined range is a better option. Arthroscopy is useful if symptoms or radiologic signs progress. The articular cartilage is often soft to probing but is usually intact at surgery. If the latter is the case, it is probably best left alone. With more significant separation and demarcation, drilling or pinning may be considered.

Loose Lesion in Situ (Stage III)

Sometimes a lesion is either loose or about to become a free body within the knee. Mechanical symptoms predominate. At arthroscopy it may be seen to be almost completely separated. Depending on the stage of evolution, it is either pinned or separated enough to curet and drill the base and then pinned in situ. Its shape is nearly always congruent to the defect. Protected weight-bearing is necessary for 6 to 12 weeks, and pivoting activities are prohibited until good signs of healing are evident. Rehabilitation is designed to overcome quadriceps wasting, to restore muscle balance of power and range of motion, and to initiate alternative activities for endurance and general fitness.

Displaced Lesion or Residual Center (Stage IV)

Crepitus, effusion, pain, and possibly locking, catching, or giving way are the presenting complaints. The lesion may have been clinically silent for many years. At arthroscopy the lesion is typically steep-sided with bone exposed. When possible the loose body is retrieved and removed. It is incongruous and rarely serves as a suitable graft for reimplantation to the site of the defect. Attempts to transfer cartilage from other non-weight-bearing areas within the knee are not usually successful. Similarly, cartilage allografts and transplantation of chondrocytes are not clinically practical approaches at this time. Usually the best option is to curet the base, perhaps with associated drilling. This method may give surprisingly good results even though the metaphased cartilage that fills the defect is not normal. Usually this procedure is followed by 3 months of significantly protected weight-bearing and restricted activity. Although theoretically this period should be extended, in practice there seems to be little additional benefit from longer periods of light or non-weight-bearing, and patient compliance is a problem. Activity is slowly increased, and the therapist should attempt to titrate its progression with the symptoms. Increasing pain or effusion suggests too rapid return to activity.

Practice Point
OSTEOCHONDRITIS DISSECANS

- Evolving lesion in situ
  -Modify activity proportional to symptoms.
  -Follow carefully.
  -Roentgenograph again in 6 months.
  -Arthroscope if symptoms do not settle.
- Separating or chronically symptomatic lesion
  -Severely restrict activity.
  -Consider arthroscopy if it does not settle or roentgenographic signs progress.
- Loose lesions in situ
  -Pin via arthroscopy.
  -Depending on evolution, may need to curet crater base.
- Displaced lesions: residual crater
  -If congruous, pin in situ after curetting base.
  -If totally incongruous, drill subchondral bone of crater.

Osteochondral and Chondral Fractures

Osteochondral fractures are apparent in 6 to 10 percent of patients with acute hemarthrosis. The fragment is characteristically shaped with one surface convex and the other flat. The invariable association with trauma and hemarthrosis and the shape help distinguish this lesion from osteochondritis dissecans. It is usually seen in the adolescent and late teenager engaged in vigorous physical activity and has a high association with anterior cruciate injury. This lesion has some healing potential as bony union or production of fibrocartilage is possible.[57] Union is enhanced by reduction and fixation.

The chondral fracture is most commonly seen in the skeletally mature athlete (Table 11-8). In the older patient, calcified cartilage allows the force or injury to be transmitted across the "tide mark" or transition zone.[61] These injuries may be asymptomatic in the stable knee. In contrast, the athlete may present with symptoms of locking, catching, grating, giving way, or effusions. It is easy to confuse these injuries clinically with meniscal lesions. Diagnosis is frequently delayed. The healing potential of these lesions is much less than for osteochondral defects. Arthroscopic débridement and occasionally drilling, perhaps with fixation of the fragment, is the best solution; but the long-term prognosis for intensive activity is guarded. The therapy of these lesions postoperatively is similar to that for osteochondral fractures and includes partial weight-bearing and restricted pivoting activities for a prolonged period.

Spontaneous (Idiopathic) Osteonecrosis

The exact etiology of spontaneous osteonecrosis is unknown. Spontaneous collapse of subchondral bone and loss of support of the articular surfaces occur most frequently in association with such conditions as rheumatoid arthritis but may occur in otherwise healthy active people as well. Potentially, the process is self-limiting. The patients are usually in the fourth or fifth decade and may present with an acute onset of severe pain. The condition is more common in the tibia than the femur. There may be joint effusion. Minimal signs may be present on the plain roentgenogram, but the bone scan shows an intense focal uptake depending on the stage of the lesion. In this case, differentiation from a stress fracture is necessary. At arthroscopy the cortical plate is unstable, and the cavity contains soft amorphous material that blends with the underlying bone without a cortical plate.[62] If the lesion is large, drilling may be in order with or without curetting. Sometimes protected weight-bearing with a total contact brace with hinges prestressed to relieve some of the weight transference through the affected condyle may be of help. For most individuals, establishing the diagnosis and waiting for the resolution of symptoms is the treatment of choice. Exercise is modified accordingly.

SUPERIOR TIBIOFIBULAR JOINT

The superior tibiofibular joint has suffered from clinical and literary neglect. Although pathology of this joint is relatively uncommon, it must always be considered in the differential diagnosis of post-traumatic lateral knee pain.[63]

Anatomy

The head of the fibula articulates with the posterolateral and inferior aspects of the lateral tibial condyle, where it nestles in a sulcus. It is a phytogenetic regression from the bicondylar articulation of the distal femur, one with the tibia and one with the fibula. The joint is thus enclosed in its own capsule and does not communicate with the tibiofemoral articulation. Effusion of the knee joint therefore does not involve the proximal tibiofibular joint. There are two basic orientations, horizontal and oblique, with an arbitrary figure of 20 degrees used in the classification. The horizontal joint usually has a greater articulating area and a greater capacity for rotary mobility.[64] Anterior displacement is prevented by the bony prominence of the tibia with additional stability provided by the anterior and posterior tibiofibular ligaments, the anterior ligament being the stronger. The ligaments are reinforced by tendons — posteriorly by the popliteal tendon and anteriorly by the biceps tendon.[65] The arcuate popliteal ligament and cord-like fibular collateral ligament also insert on the fibular head and enhance stability. Because the latter two structures are relaxed during flexion, the stability of the fibular head is correspondingly less in the flexed knee posteriorly. The common peroneal nerve may be palpable subcutaneously as it winds around the fibular neck, tethered to the bone by the origin of the peroneus longus.

In some individuals the head of the fibula may be prominent, hypermobile, and laterally positioned.[64] The knee joint is a helicoid structure, and flexion and extension are accompanied by some tibial rotation. Ankle motion is not isolated but also generates some tibial rotation in addition to superior, inferior, and rotary torques to the fibula. Thus to accommodate internal and external rotary torque to the tibia, the superior tibiofibular joint allows anteroposterior, superoinferior, and rotary motion. Ogden has summarized the function of the tibiofibular joint as: (1) dissipation of torsional stresses applied to the ankle joint; (2) dissipation of lateral tibial bending movements; and (3) mainly tensile rather than compression loading during weight-bearing activities.[64] The weight-bearing function of the distal fibula with up to one-sixth of the static loads being transferred through its ligaments and articular surface were well outlined by Lambert.[66]

Mechanisms of Injury

The accepted mechanism of injury for dislocation of the fibular head is a fall on the inverted foot with the knee flexed, as the leg is violently adducted by the weight of the body. This mechanism explains the high incidence of fibular head dislocation or "silent fracture" of the upper one-third of the fibula seen in parachute jumpers. In baseball this injury may occur as the runner slides into base and lands on his trailing leg. In basketball it is seen with falls during rebounding and ball struggles.[64] Medial ligament injury or medial malleolus fracture at the ankle in association with a proximal fibular fracture is called the Maissoneuve fracture.

Whereas pure muscular contraction of biceps femoris may produce avulsion of the tip of the fibular head, sudden contraction with the knee during flexion may contribute to subluxation. Direct trauma to the fibular head may result in a contusion, sprain, subluxation, or dislocation. The commonest situation is a violent lateral blow to the weight-bearing semiflexed knee. Occasionally, subluxation and even dislocation are associated with severe generalized ligamentous laxity.

Clinical Picture

The main point in diagnosis is to be aware of the possibility of involvement of the superior tibiofibular joint during trauma. The history of the mechanism of injury is helpful. Some athletes complain of pain in the proximal joint. Many mention mild transient neuritic symptoms, e.g., shooting pain into the ankle and foot, due to associated peroneal nerve involvement. A small group complain of significant associated ankle discomfort.

With dislocation there is usually an obvious lateral bony prominence of the fibular head below the tibial plateau. The joint is tender. Although tissue swelling may be apparent, there is no knee joint effusion. Occasionally, forced dorsiflexion and plantar flexion produce lateral knee pain.

With recurrent subluxation or dislocation, particularly associated with generalized ligamentous laxity, the knee may lock when an individual squats and rotates slightly on the flexed knee. Gentle pressure over the fibular head produces spontaneous reduction with a "clunk," and the individual is able to stand again.

Sprains are sometimes difficult to assess. Stressing the joint produces local tenderness, as may "rocking" the fibular head. Activities such as toe-walking, hopping on a flexed knee, full dorsiflexion of the ankle, and resisted contraction of the biceps femoris may produce symptoms. Flexed-knee weight-bearing might help in the diagnosis (Fig. 11-37). The patient is unable to single knee bend without stabilizing the weight-bearing extremity. The leg tends to give way.

Roentgenographic Signs

The cardinal roentgenographic signs of dislocation are lateral displacement of the fibula on the anteroposterior view with proximal interosseous space widening. On the lateral view the fibula head is usually displaced anteriorly, resulting in a greater overlap of the fibula and tibial shadows (Fig. 11-38). These findings may be subtle and require comparison with the opposite uninvolved side.

Roentgenography helps detect fractures of the fibular neck and proximal shaft, avulsions, osteochondromas, and abnormal calcifications. In the skeletally immature patient, fractures through the proximal

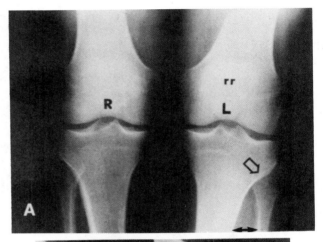

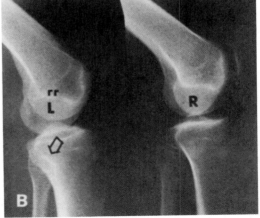

Fig. 11-38. Traumatic anterolateral dislocation of the fibular head. **(A)** Anteroposterior view. Proximal fibula is laterally displaced, increasing the interosseous distance on the left. **(B)** Lateral view. The anterior displacement results in a greater degree of overlap of the fibula on the tibia.

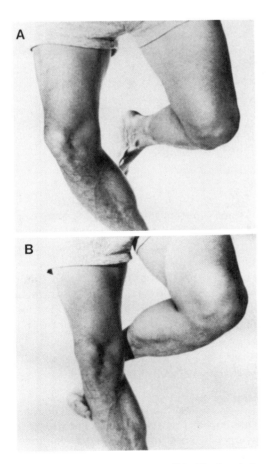

Fig. 11-37. Test for superior tibiofibular joint pathology. **(A)** Normal joint. **(B)** With tibiofibular joint pathology the individual attempts to support the joint with the uninvolved limb.

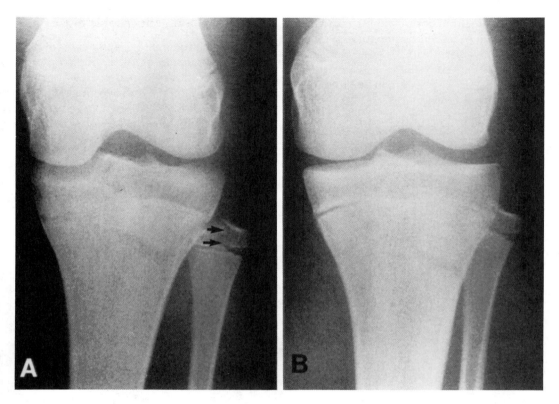

Fig. 11-39. Salter-Harris type III epiphyseal fracture of the proximal fibular. Oblique view (**A**) shows the fracture, whereas in the anteroposterior view (**B**) it is almost obscured.

fibular epiphysis, a rare injury, may also be visualized. Oblique roentgenograms help ensure that this injury is not missed. (Fig. 11-39).[67]

Treatment

Chronic pain due to local ligamentous sprain or ankle pathology is addressed by appropriate local physiotherapy modalities, NSAIDs, and gentle mobilization to ensure normal joint play. Occasionally, lidocaine and steroid injected into the joint is helpful. Care must be taken not to damage the peroneal nerve with these modalities. (See Chapter 9).

Acute dislocations are usually easily reduced by manipulation. Direct pressure may be associated with an audible "pop" and immediate dramatic pain relief. Bandaging or a cast may be helpful for allowing healing, although the joint is usually stable after reduction. Vigorous activity should await complete resolution of symptoms; and pivoting sports, may need to be avoided for up to 6 weeks.

The unstable joint may be helped by taping or support during activity and by ice and NSAIDs after exercise. Chronically symptomatic and unstable joints are possibly best treated by repair of the ligaments or reconstruction, with temporary fixation of the joint by screw or wire to allow healing. Late intractable instability and pain may be alleviated by excision of the fibular head. Fusion of the joint is not usually a good option, as it is more likely to be associated with ankle symptoms.

SUMMARY

This chapter has focused on miscellaneous lesions in and around the knee joint. The key to diagnosis is a clear, carefully elicited history followed by a specific examination using meticulous palpation techniques. No one sign is pathognomonic at the knee, and a constellation of findings is important. The most common lesion of all, the meniscal lesion, has been the subject of a revolution in diagnostic techniques and treatment approach. MRI and arthroscopy have brought to light many nuances of the normal and pathologic menisci; and long-term follow-up studies have established the importance of menisci to the health of the knee. Simple meniscectomy is no longer undertaken lightly. The adage of "when in doubt, take it out" has been replaced with a reverance reflected in Goodfellow's superb truism, "He who hesitates is saved." This chapter has emphasized diagnostic techniques and should serve to give confidence to the beginner and hopefully bring humility to the expert.

REFERENCES

1. Fairbank TJ: Knee joint changes after meniscectomy. J Bone Joint Surg [Br] 30:664, 1948
2. Grant JC: Grant's Atlas of Anatomy. 5th Ed. Williams & Wilkins, Baltimore, 1962
3. Wagner HJ: Die Kollagenfrasearchitektar der Menisken des Menschlichen Kniegelenkes. Z Mikrosk Anat Forsch 90:302, 1976
4. Müller W: The Knee: Form, Function, and Ligament Reconstruction. Springer-Verlag, New York, 1983
5. Trillat A: Lésions traumatiques du ménisque interne du genou. Rev Chir Orthop 48:551, 1962
6. Arnoczky SP, Warren RF: Microvasculature of the human meniscus. Am J Sports Med 10:90, 1982
7. Scapinelli R: Studies on the vasculature of the human knee joint. Acta Anat (Basel) 70:305, 1968
8. Gershuni DH, Hargens AR, Darzig LA: Regional nutrition and cellularity of the meniscus: implications for tear and repair. Sports Med 5:322, 1988
9. Reid DC: Functional Anatomy and Joint Mobilization. A Manual of Kinesiology. University of Alberta Press, Edmonton, 1973
10. Barnett CH: Locking at the knee joint. J Anat 87:91, 1953
11. Walker PS, Erkman PJ: The role of the menisci in force transmission across the knee. Clin Orthop 109:184, 1975
12. Baratz ME, Fu FH, Mengato R: Meniscal tears: the effect of meniscectomy and of repair on intraarticular contact areas and stress in the human knee. Am J Sports Med 14:270, 1986
13. Noble J, Hamblen DL: The pathology of the degenerate meniscal lesion. J Bone Joint Surg [Br] 57:180, 1975
14. Noble J: Lesions of the menisci. J Bone Joint Surg [Am] 59:480, 1977
15. Fahmy NRM, Williams EA, Noble J: Meniscal pathology and osteoarthritis of the knee. J Bone Joint Surg [Br] 65:24, 1983
16. Jørgensen U, Sonne-Holm S, Lauridsen F et al: Long-term follow up of meniscectomy in athletes: a prospective longitudinal study. J Bone Joint Surg [Br] 69:80, 1987
17. Allen PR, Denham RA, Swan AV: Late degenerative changes after meniscectomy: factors affecting the knee after operation. J Bone Joint Surg [Br] 66:666, 1984
18. Medlar RC, Mandiberg JJ, Lyne ED: Meniscectomies in children. Am J Sports Med 8:87, 1980
19. Manzione M, Pizzutillo PD, Peoples AB et al: Meniscectomy in children: a long term follow up. Am J Sports Med 11:111, 1983
20. Jackson RW, Rouse DW: Results of partial arthroscopic meniscectomy in patients over forty. Presented at the 49th Annual Meeting of the American Academy of Orthopaedic Surgeons, New Orleans, 1982
21. Anderson AF: Clinical diagnosis of meniscal tears: description of a new manipulation test. Am J Sports Med 14:291, 1986
22. Shakespeare DT, Rigby HS: The bucket handle tear of the meniscus: a clinical and arthrographic study. J Bone Joint Surg [Br] 65:383, 1983
23. Apley G: The diagnosis of meniscus injuries. J Bone Joint Surg [Br] 29:28, 1974
24. Smillie IS: Injuries of the Knee Joint. 5th Ed. Churchill Livingstone, New York, 1978, p. 98
25. Hoshikawa T, Kurosawa H, Fukabayashi T et al: The prognosis of meniscectomy in athletes: the simple meniscus lesions without ligamentous instability. Am J Sports Med 11:8, 1983
26. Kaplan EB: Discoid lateral meniscus of the knee joint, nature, mechanism, and operative treatment. J Bone Joint Surg [Am] 39A:77, 1957
27. Tillmann B: Zur funktionellen Morphologie der Gelenkentwicklung. Orthop Prox 1210:691, 1974
28. Phemister DB: Cysts of the external semilunar cartilages of the knee. JAMA 80:593, 1923
29. Barrie HJ: The pathogenisis and significance of meniscal cysts. J Bone Joint Surg [Br] 61B:184, 1979
30. Segar BM, Woods WG: Arthroscopic management of lateral meniscal cysts. Am J Sports Med 14:105, 1986
31. DeHaven KE: Diagnosis of internal derangement of the knee: the role of arthroscopy. J Bone Joint Surg [Am] 57:802, 1975
32. Gillies H, Seligson D: Precision in the diagnosis of meniscal lesions: a comparison of clinical evaluation, arthrography, and arthroscopy. J Bone Joint Surg [Am] 61:343, 1979
33. Allen GD, Arnett GD, Reid DC, Parkinson EG: Evaluation of subacute and chronic knee problems: a clinical, arthrographic and arthroscopic correlation. (Personal data)
34. Manco LG, Kavanaugh Jh, Lozman J et al: Diagnosis

of meniscal tears using high-resolution computed tomography: correlation with arthrosopy. J Bone Joint Surg [Am] 69:498, 1987

35. Kelly MA, Flock TJ, Kimmel JA et al: Imaging of the knee: clarification of its role. Arthroscopy 7:78, 1991

36. Mooar P, Gregg J, Jacobstein J: Radionuclide imaging in internal derangements of the knee. Am J Sports Med 15:132, 1987

37. McCoy FG, McCrea JD, Beverland DE et al: Vibration arthrography as a diagnostic aid in diseases of the knee: a preliminary report. J Bone Joint Surg [Br] 69:288, 1987

38. Johnston LL: Impact of diagnostic arthroscopy on the clinical judgement of an experienced arthroscopist. Clin Orthop 167:75, 1982

39. Petrone FA: Meniscectomy: arthrotomy versus arthroscopy. Am J Sports Med 10:355, 1982

40. Northmore-Ball MD, Dandy DJ, Jackson RW: Arthroscopic, open partial, and total meniscectomy: a comparative study. J Bone Joint Surg [Br] 65:400, 1983

41. Per Hamberg, Gillquist J, Lysholm J: A comparison between arthroscopic meniscectomy and modified open meniscectomy: a prospective randomized study with emphasis on post operative rehabilitation. J Bone Joint Surg [Br] 66:189, 1984

42. Prietto CA, Caiozzo VJ, Prietto PB et al: Closed versus open partial meniscectomy: post operative changes in the force-velocity relationship of muscle. Am J Sports Med 11:189, 1983

43. Per Hamberg, Gillquist J, Lysholm J et al: The effect of diagnostic and operative arthroscopy and open meniscectomy on muscle strength in the thigh. Am J Sports Med 11:289, 1983

44. Thorblad J, Ekstrand J, Hamberg P et al: Muscle rehabilitation after arthroscopic meniscectomy with or without tourniquet control: a preliminary randomized study. Am J Sports Med 13:133, 1985

45. Muckle DS: Open meniscectomy: enhanced recovery after synovial prostaglandin inhibition. J Bone Joint Surg [Br] 66:193, 1984

46. Smith MJ, Hutchins RD, Hehanberger D: Transcutaneous neural stimulation use in post operative rehabilitation. Am J Sports Med 11:75, 1983

47. Jensen JE, Conn RR, Hazelrigg G et al: The use of transcutaneous neural stimulation and isokinetic testing in arthroscopic knee surgery. Am J Sports Med 13:27, 1985

48. Williams RA, Morrissey MC, Brester CE: The effect of electrical stimulation on quadriceps strength and thigh circumference in meniscectomy patients. J Orthop Sports Phys Ther 8:143, 1986

49. Sherman WM, Plyley MJ, Pearson DR et al: Isokinetic rehabilitation after meniscectomy: a comparison of two methods of training. Phys Sports Med 11:121, 1983

50. Miller DB: Arthroscopic meniscal repair. Am J Sports Med 16:315, 1988

51. Cassidy RE, Shaffer AJ: A repair of peripheral meniscal tears: a preliminary report. Am J Sports Med 9:209, 1981

52. Annandale T: Excision of the internal semilunar cartilage resulting in perfect restoration of the joint movement. Br Med J 1:291, 1889

53. DeHaven KE: Commentary: repair of peripheral meniscal tears; a preliminary report. Am J Sports Med 9:213, 1981

54. Cassidy RE, Shaffer AJ: Repair of peripheral meniscal tears. Am J Sports Med 9:209, 1981

55. Hamburg P, Gillquist J, Lysholm J: Suture of new and old peripheral meniscal tears. J Bone Joint Surg [Am] 65:193, 1983

56. Canham W, Stanish W: A study of the biological behavior of the meniscus as a transplant in the medial compartment of a dog's knee. Am J Sports Med 14:376, 1986

57. Bradley J, Dandy DJ: Osteochondritis dissecans and other lesions of the femoral condyles. J Bone Joint Surg [Br] 71:518, 1989

58. Paget J: On the production of some of the loose bodies in joints. St Bartholomew Hosp Rep 6:1, 1870

59. König: Uebergreie Körper in den Gelenken. Dtsch Z Chir (Leipz) 27:90, 1887

60. Barrie HJ: Osteochondritis dissecans 1887–1989: a centennial look at König's memorable phrase. J Bone Joint Surg [Am] 69:693, 1987

61. Hopkinson WJ, Mitchell WA, Curl WW: Chondral fractures of the knee: cause for confusion. Am J Sports Med 13:309, 1985

62. Dipaola JD, Nelson DW, Colville MR: Characterizing osteochondral lesions by magnetic resonance imaging. J Arthos Related Surg 7:101, 1991

63. Radakovich M, Malone T: The superior tibiofibular joint: the forgotten joint. J Orthop Sports Phys Ther 3:129, 1982

64. Ogden JA: The anatomy and function of the proxinal tibiofibula joint. Clin Orthop 101:186, 1974

65. Turco VJ, Spinella AJ: Anteriolateral dislocation of the head of the fibula in sports. Am J Sports Med 13:209, 1985

66. Lambert KL: The weight bearing function of the fibula. J Bone Joint Surg [Am] 53:507, 1971

67. Abrams J, Bennett E, Kumar SJ et al: Salter-Harris type III fracture of the proximal fibula: a case report. Am J Sports Med 14:514, 1986

Anterior Knee Pain and the Patellofemoral Pain Syndrome

12

It is frequently better to remain uncertain about a diagnosis and feel mildly foolish than to be constantly certain and confirm that you are an absolute fool.

The patella is a unique structure that plays a central role in the normal biomechanics of the knee, although adequate function may be achieved after patellectomy. Indisputably, however, the knee functions better when the patella is present. Unfortunately, the patella remains the enigma of sports medicine and sports therapy. Across all sports and all ages, it is probably the single most common cause of pain. Its origin and development are therefore intriguing.

EVOLUTION

The bony anatomy of the hindlimbs of all tetrapods may be traced to analogous structures in the lobe-finned fish of the early Devonian Period, some 370 million years ago.[1] The earliest evidence of ambulation using limbs was found in Amphibia, where the distal femur already exhibited a bicondylar shape. The proximal part of the tibia was relatively flat and articulated with the medial condyle of the femur.[2] The lateral femoral condyle articulated with the fibula, a characteristic that remains in reptiles, birds, and some primitive mammals. During the Mesozoic Era (70 to 215 million years ago), some significant changes occurred. The head of the fibula in most mammals (except for some marsupials) receded to a point distal to the joint line. The fibula no longer articulated with the distal femur, nor did it provide support for the lateral meniscus, thus diminishing its

weight-bearing role. Furthermore, a medial offset of the femoral head and internal rotation of the femur allowed the knee to develop with its apex anterior, resulting in a more efficient gait.[1,2] The single, broad, intra-articular ligament of the now extinct Amphibia was evolving into the modern-day cruciate ligaments with their four-bar linkage system, allowing stability and the complex rolling and gliding motion of the femur on the tibia (Table 12-1).

The last two major developments occurred some 65 to 70 million years ago. The first was an obliquity of the distal femoral epiphysis in relation to the diaphyseal axis, allowing the left and right knee to approach the midline. This characteristic is considered to be associated with human bipedal gait.[2] The second was the evolution of an osseous patella (Table 12-1). This ubiquitous structure, found in birds, mammals, and a few reptiles, has become the source of one of the most frustrating problems in sports therapy. Its importance in humans is undeniable, as the patella contributes 13 percent (90 to 120 degrees) to 31 percent (0 to 5 degrees) of the entire extensor moment arm developed by the quadriceps.

Thus the complex asymmetric design of the human knee is ancient in origin. The knees of most species share similar morphologic characteristics, including bicondylar, cam-shaped distal femurs, intra-articular cruciate ligaments and menisci, and collateral ligaments with multicentric insertions. The common overall design implies a profound similarity of kinematic principles; despite this fact, no ideal animal model exists for the human knee.

TABLE 12-1. Comparative Anatomy of the Knee

Structure	Amphibians	Reptiles	Birds	Mammals
Osseous structures				
Bicondylar distal femur	Yes	Yes	Yes	Yes
Tibial plateaus	Yes	Yes	Yes	Yes
Femorofibular articulation	—	Yes	Yes	No
Osseous patella	No	Only lizards	Yes	Yes
Soft tissue				
Flat medial lig	Yes	Yes	Yes	Yes
Cord-shaped lateral ligament	Yes	Yes	Yes	Yes
Menisci	Yes	Yes	Yes	Yes
Intra-articular ligaments	Yes	Yes	Yes	Yes
Popliteus insertion on femur	No	No	No	Yes
Function				
Posterior femorotibial contact with flexion	Yes	Yes	Yes	Yes
Internal rotation of tibia with flexion	No	Yes	Yes	Yes

(Adapted from Dye,[2] with permission.)

DEVELOPMENT OF THE PATELLA

The patella is usually considered a sesamoid bone. However, it is outstanding among them because of its large size, relatively constant form, and the important part it plays in the formation of the articular capsule and biomechanics of the joint to which it belongs.[3] Its sesamoid nature and functional importance are not accepted by all, and at one time it was suggested that the patella is a part of the skeleton that is undergoing regression in man.[4] For instance, animals with the most efficient quadriceps mechanisms in terms of speed or strength may have the smallest patellae or none at all.[4] The sloth has a patella that is relatively large for its body. The fox and deer have patellae that are relatively small. The kangaroo, the animal with perhaps the largest and most well developed quadriceps mechanism for its size, is devoid of patellae. Nevertheless, subsequent biomechanical studies have quantified the patella's important functional contributions of protecting the knee from direct trauma and providing a fulcrum to augment quadriceps efficiency.[5,6]

In the 20 mm embryo (7 weeks), there is an aggregation of cells in the deep layers of the developing quadriceps mass. This early representation of the patella is present prior to any evidence of a synovial cavity.[3] By 8 weeks the patella starts to become cartilaginous, and the differentiated quadriceps is continuous at its upper and lower ends. Soon the epiphysis of the patella becomes a separate entity, and a distinct joint cavity is apparent. The patella is therefore an intramuscular element that has secondarily acquired a free articular surface. In summary, the patella started its development as a sesamoid bone and completed it in a manner similar to that of the articular surfaces of all movable joints.[3]

The medial and lateral patellar articular facets are, at first, approximately equal in size. A change in size

---

Quick Facts

PATELLA

- Found in birds, mammals, and a few reptiles
- Aggregate of cells in 20 mm embryo (7 weeks)
- Cartilaginous by 30 mm stage (8 weeks)
- Fine detail of transverse ridges await weight-bearing
- Ossifies between 3 and 5 years
- Roentgenographic appreciation of shape and position difficult until 12 years
- Contributes 13 percent of extensor moment arm at 90 to 120 degrees
- Contributes 31 degrees of extensor moment arm at 0 to 5 degrees

begins shortly after the patella has freed itself from the femur, and by about 20 weeks the patella is usually divided by a ridge into a large lateral and small medial facet. These facets are in a ratio roughly comparable to that seen in the adult. The patella, however, does not acquire the transverse ridges on its articular surface until after birth, when the knee joint is in full use, showing that the fine detail awaits function.

The patella initially ossifies at 3 to 5 years of age, commencing as multiple foci that rapidly coalesce.[7] As the coalesced ossification center enlarges, the expanding regions may be irregular and associated with accessory ossification centers.[7] The most common is located superolaterally; and, when persistent, it is described as a bipartite patella. The subchondral plate on the weight-bearing areas does not assume its actual articular shape until about 10 to 12 years. Accordingly, roentgenographic measurements of patellar alignment, shape, and position cannot be made accurately prior to this time.

PATELLA BIOMECHANICS

The patella functions to increase the mechanical advantage of the quadriceps mechanism. Ficat and Hungerford[8] suggested that throughout the range of motion the patella increases effective extension force by as much as 50 percent. They also suggested that the essential, and often overlooked, function of the patella lies in the ability of its healthy hyaline cartilage to transmit forces to subchondral and cancellous bone (Fig. 12-1). The absence of nerve endings in hyaline cartilage allows this force transmission to be done in such a way that under normal circumstances the pain threshold of the supporting bone is not surpassed.[8]

Patellofemoral joint forces vary with activity, being 0.5 times body weight during walking, 3.3 times body

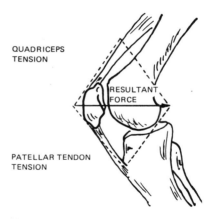

Fig. 12-1. The patella increases the overall effectiveness of the extensor moment arm by approximately 50 percent, but in doing so there is a considerable retropatellar compression force.

weight when ascending or descending stairs, and as much as 6.0 to 7.0 times body weight when squatting.[8–10] It is accepted that intermittent compression is required for adequate nutrition of hyaline cartilage. However, the question remains as to when compression becomes excessive (Table 12-2).

Several investigators[8,10,11] have documented the patellofemoral contact points from full extension to full flexion. It is generally agreed that during full extension the lower border of the patella is in contact with the suprapatellar fat pad of the distal femur and is under little or no load. If the quadriceps are isometrically set in this position, the patella moves proximally with a small lateral shift. The latter component is limited by the medial retinaculum and the patellofemoral and meniscopatellar ligaments. With flexion to 20 degrees, the tibia derotates (internal rotation), decreasing the lateral vector; and, in turn, the patella is allowed to move into the trochlea (Fig. 12-2). By 30 degrees of flexion, the patella is well seated in the deepening trochlear groove. As the knee continues on to 90 degrees of flexion, the area of contact on the patella moves upward, failing to reach the extreme medial facet (odd facet). The medial border is defined by the convex ridge separating the medial and odd facet. Ficat and Hungerford[8] suggested that this convex ridge, coming in contact with the convex femoral articular cartilage, should anatomically create a "high unit load." Further enhancement of compressive forces may occur secondary to lateral tethering by the patellofemoral and patellotibial ligaments. The contact zone widens as it proceeds proximally, facilitating

---

Quick Facts

QUADRICEPS FORCES (WEIGHT BEARING)

At 5 degrees flexion: 30 percent of body weight
At 15 degrees flexion: 1 × body weight
At 30 degrees flexion: 2 × body weight
At 45 degrees flexion: 3.0 × body weight
At 75 degrees flexion: 6.0 × body weight

TABLE 12-2. **Patellofemoral Compressive Forces**[a]

Activity	Knee Flexion Angle (degrees)	Quadriceps Extensor Moment (nm)	Patellar Compression (newtons)
Level walking	20	35–60	490–840
Cycling	29	79	880
Climbing stairs	65	54	1500
Descending stairs	60	147	4000
Jogging	50	210	5000
Rising from a chair	90	110	3800
Kicking a ball	100	180	5800
Parallel squat	120	225	7450
Rising from squat	105	70	2500
Isometric max.	60	120–225	3400–6100
Isometric max.	90	198	6900
Isokinetic knee ext.	70	284	8300

[a] Body weight approximately 65 to 80 kg.
(Adapted from McConnell,[9] with permission.)

distribution of joint reaction forces. At 90 degrees of flexion, the patella demonstrates lateral movement, tending to leave some of the medial femoral condyle uncovered. As movement continues to 135 degrees, the lateral shift continues so that at its completion the medial patellar facet lies free in the intercondylar notch, and the odd facet contacts the lateral aspect of the medial femoral condyle (Fig. 12-2).[8,11] In summary, the patella moves in a gentle curve as the knee goes from 0 to 135 degrees of flexion.

It may well be that in some individuals specific alignments exaggerate this motion, causing repetitive minor trauma to the patella and resultant peripatellar problems. This susceptibility may be unmasked by a sudden increase in intensity, increased duration, or specific types of exercise. There may even be periods of life during which symptoms are more likely to be precipitated. For instance, a vulnerable time may be during and shortly after the adolescent growth spurt, when bony architecture and muscle length–tension relation are changing. Simply stated, the pain experienced with chondromalacia may be due to an exaggeration of the normal high biomechanical forces by growth or activity, or both.

Much of this chapter is concerned with the treatment of patellofemoral pain syndromes. One is impressed that, when using an evolutionary perspective, these syndromes probably arise from the unique

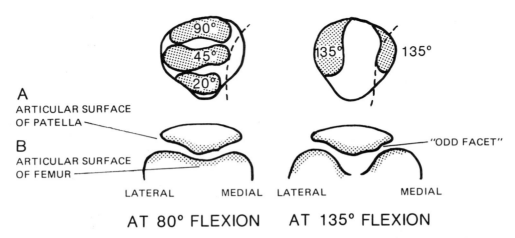

Fig. 12-2. There is no contact at full extension. **(A)** First contact is made between 10 and 20 degrees along the inferior pole. With further flexion the band of contact moves superiorly. At no stage between 10 and 90 degrees is contact made with the odd facet. **(B)** Odd facet is in contact at more than 120 degrees of flexion. (After Ficat and Hungerford,[8] with permission.)

stresses of bipedal methods of gait. By the same token, poorly controlled and badly designed activity patterns likely assume a dominant role. The challenge of treating these syndromes depends, first, on making a specific diagnosis; second, on understanding the biomechanical stresses; and lastly, on a sound knowledge of various sports so appropriate activity modification is prescribed while carrying out specific therapies.

ANTERIOR KNEE PAIN

The literature abounds with information relating to the etiology and treatment of patellofemoral pain syndrome (PFP), which may affect as many as 25 percent of the athletic population.[9] Despite its frequent occurrence, PFP remains a difficult and often frustrating condition for clinicians to treat, and permanent relief of symptoms is often not achieved. In some series, as few as 30 percent of patients have remained pain-free.[12] Consequently, many patellofemoral pain sufferers have to minimize or even abandon their leisure activities to prevent the recurrence of discomfort.

In many ways, the large volume of literature confuses rather than clarifies the issues. Currently there exists no convincing proof as to the exact etiology of the patellofemoral pain syndrome. Efforts to link what is obviously a constellation of etiologies and pathophysiologies under one all-encompassing term, chondromalacia, is not likely to further the understanding of this difficult clinical problem. For every complex the literature attempts to offer a straight forward simple solution; which is invariably wrong.

Realizing there may be some overlap, anterior knee pain may be divided into that which is always associated with articular surface damage, that which may or may not have associated cartilage damage, and that which usually manifests in the presence of normal cartilage (Table 12-3). This chapter deals with many of these problems. Frank dislocation and many conditions of the extensor apparatus, e.g., tendinitis and bursitis, however, are discussed in subsequent chapters.

PATELLOFEMORAL PAIN SYNDROME

Whereas identification of the underlying pathophysiology is difficult, the classic PFP syndrome picture is easily identified. The patient is usually young and active and complains of retropatellar or peripatellar pain precipitated by sitting for prolonged periods (movie-goer sign); the pain is proportional to the activity and is particularly evident when squatting or descending stairs. Effusion is rare, but a feeling of swelling in the infrapatellar fat pad area is frequent. Locking is absent, but clicking and a painful or painless "catching" is often a worrying symptom for the patient. Crepitus is a feature in some individuals. These symptoms have also been described under the headings patellalgia, gonalgia paresthetica, anterior knee pain syndrome, retropatellar arthralgia, the peripatellar syndrome, and patellar tracking problems.

The confounding factors are the frequent presence

TABLE 12-3. Classification of Anterior Knee Pain

Cartilage Damage	Variable Cartilage Damage	Normal Cartilage
Chondromalacia grades I–III	Plical syndrome	Overuse
Osteoarthritis grade IV	Malalignment (passive)	Retinacular pathology
Lateral facet syndrome	Quadriceps dysplasia (active)	Peripatellar tendinitis and bursitis
Osteochondral fractures	Patella variants	Fat pad syndrome
Osteochondritis dissecans	Subluxations	Sympathetic dystrophy and vascular-related syndromes

(Adapted from Insall,[13] with permission.)

of the so-called malalignments in the asymptomatic, active population and the lack of consistent correlation of retropatellar cartilage pathology with the degree of symptoms experienced. Furthermore, it is difficult to assign the source of pain with early retropatellar changes, as articular cartilage does not contain sensory nerve endings. To avoid any further confusion, the classic constellation of symptoms described above are referred to as the PFP syndrome, and the term "chondromalacia" is reserved to describe only those changes that occur in the articular cartilage, which may or may not be part of any particular anterior knee pain syndrome.

The classic PFP syndrome has been outlined with its confusing etiology; however, there are a series of other discrete anterior knee pain syndromes that are much more readily diagnosed and related to specific pathology. They include peripatellar bursitis and tendinitis, the plical syndromes, osteochondral fractures, osteochondritis dissecans, patellar subluxation and dislocation, and the vascular syndromes of reflex sympathetic dystrophy.

If it is accepted that the PFP syndrome is due to causes related to the patella itself or the peripatellar structures, and that the symptoms may be either related to changes in the patellar articular surface or occur as a result of tracking problems placing abnormal stresses on the joint surface or the surrounding soft tissue, a whole series of contributing factors may be isolated.[8,15-18] Although the earlier statements that many of these factors only loosely correlate with the pain syndrome are true and that there is little proof of their role as causative factors it is nevertheless important to attempt to identify them. Some of these factors are amenable to modification, and frequently subtle alteration of stress through the knee allows complete or partial remission of the pain (Table 12-4). It must be re-emphasized, however, that poor training habits, ill-advised progression of exercise, and too much activity are the only consistent factors that seem to characterize many of these patients. These considerations should be a starting point for all treatment planning.

Patellar Articular Surface Changes (Chondromalacia)

Normal articular cartilage is characterized by a basal layer that has most of its collagen orientation perpendicular to the joint surface and is highly effi-

cient for stress transfer and absorption. The surface layer, the laminar splendens, is largely tangential in orientation, which makes it mechanically sound for motion and reduction of friction (Fig. 12-3). Whereas the collagen bundles are effective in resisting shear, it is the highly charged proteoglycans in the ground sustance and their interaction with water molecules that provide much of the shock-absorbing qualities to articular cartilage.

Cartilage Changes

Two distinct lesions may affect the articular cartilage of the patella.[11] The first is the classic surface degeneration so commonly seen with age-dependent arthritis and, in a mild form, in many active young people. The second type of lesion appears to be initiated in the deep layers and is characterized by basal degeneration.

According to Wiberg, malacic changes may be present to a lesser or greater degree in all individuals over the age of 30 years.[19] Wiberg stressed that the etiology of surface degeneration, i.e., disuse or lack of pressure on an area of cartilage, results in the lesion being of little consequence during the athlete's activity.[8,15] This may be the same lesion that develops with cast immobilization and in the latter situations is largely reversible with up to 6 to 8 weeks of casting.

The surface degeneration depicted in Figure 12-4 is commonly seen in middle-aged individuals; when it is found in young individuals it seems to be limited to the particular portion of the medial aspect of the patella known as "the odd facet." Goodfellow et al. emphatically stated that "there is no evidence that this lesion causes patellofemoral pain" and that odd facet surface degeneration is commonly documented as a secondary finding at necropsy, arthroscopy, or arthrotomy "done for reasons unconnected with the patellofemoral articulation."[11] There have been some attempts to link these medial facet changes to prolonged periods of "hypopressure," which may not provide good chondrocyte nourishment.

A second type of articular lesion on the patella has been described as "basal degeneration" and may be related to the patellofemoral pain experienced by young, active individuals. As shown in Figure 5, it is a lesion that initially disrupts the deep layers of the articular cartilage and, if allowed to progress, then invades the surface. In many instances no visual evidence of patellar articular surface degeneration can be seen at arthroscopy performed in adolescent pa-

TABLE 12-4. Contributing Factors to the Patellofemoral Pain Syndrome

Classification and Etiology	Contributing Factors
Patellar articular surface-related	
Surface pathology	Surface fibrillation
	Basal degeneration
Biomechanical	Hypopressure (medial)
	Hyperpressure (lateral)
Trauma	Single major blow
	Multiple repetitive
Vascular	Normal patella
	Degenerative changes
	Reflex dystrophy
Dietary factors	
Patellar tracking-related	
Patellar shape	Wiberg type II
	Dystrophic
	Accessory ossification center
Patellar position	Patella Alta
	Increased Q-angle
	Associated with hyperextension
Muscular	Atrophic vastus medialis
	Dystrophic vastus medialis
	Muscle imbalance
Collagenous structures	Tight lateral retinaculum
	General ligmentous laxity
Proximal segments	
Back	Excessive lordosis/kyphosis
	L3 dysfunction
	Pelvic tilt (lateral)
Hips and thighs	Femoral anteversion
	Tight hip flexors
	Tight hamstrings
	Tight abductors
	Quadriceps/hamstring imbalance
	Growth spurt-related
	Leg length discrepancy
Distal segments	
Tibia	Excessive internal torsion
	Genu varum or valgus
Foot and ankle	Tight Achilles tendon
	Weak invertors and everters
	Hyperpronation
	Rigid cavus foot

tellofemoral pain sufferers, but palpation and probing of the same areas sometimes reveal softening that is equated to a "pitting edema."[11]

Normal articular cartilage is characterized by tangentially oriented collagen bundles at the articular surface and more vertically oriented fibers running down to subchondral bone. Goodfellow et al. suggested that when the articular cartilage is subjected to excessive compression there is disorganization of the intermediate and deep layers and incipient softening.[11] The energy-absorbing ability of the cartilage is thus diminished, which in turn leads to stimulation of nociceptive fibers in the subchondral bone. This basal layer degeneration may progress to include surface blistering and, ultimately, cartilage fragmentation indistinguishable from osteoarthrosis. What predisposes some individuals to continue on the path to degenerative joint disease is unknown.

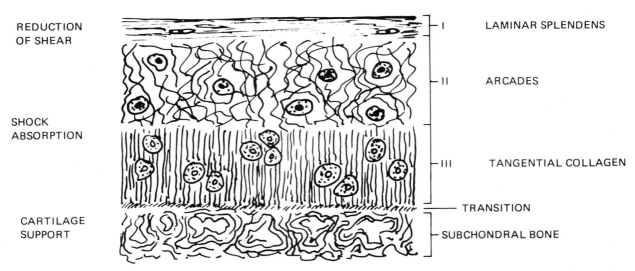

REDUCTION OF SHEAR

SHOCK ABSORPTION

CARTILAGE SUPPORT

I — LAMINAR SPLENDENS

II — ARCADES

III — TANGENTIAL COLLAGEN

— TRANSITION

— SUBCHONDRAL BONE

Fig. 12-3. Collagen fibers resist sheer stresses and are arranged in rough arcades that produce a predominance of different orientations in the different zones. The interaction with the synovial fluid on the surface minimizes friction, and the relation to the proteoglycan aggregates of the ground substance gives articular cartilage its resilience.

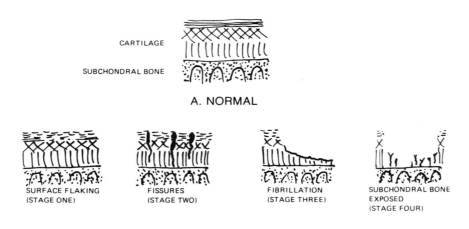

CARTILAGE

SUBCHONDRAL BONE

A. NORMAL

SURFACE FLAKING (STAGE ONE)

FISSURES (STAGE TWO)

FIBRILLATION (STAGE THREE)

SUBCHONDRAL BONE EXPOSED (STAGE FOUR)

B. PROCESS BEGINNING SUPERFICIALLY

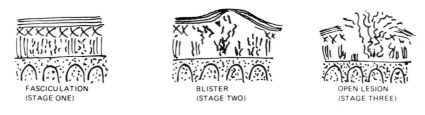

FASCICULATION (STAGE ONE)

BLISTER (STAGE TWO)

OPEN LESION (STAGE THREE)

C. PROCESS BEGINNING DEEP

Fig. 12-4. Chondromalacia may start as either a deep or a superficial process. **(A)** Normal cartilage (schematic of collagen orientation. **(B)** Surface changes, when mild, may preserve the shock-absorbing properties. **(C)** The deep process affects this property early.

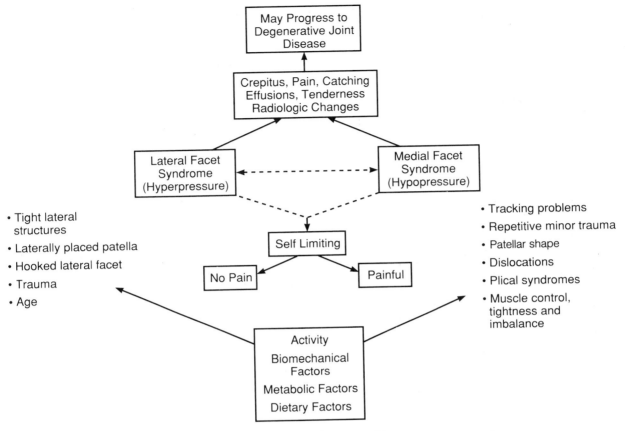

Fig. 12-5. Etiologic factors in patellar hypo- and hyperpressure syndromes.

Trabecular Orientation

The trabecular orientation of the patella is most obvious on the lateral and midcrest regions, where they are perpendicular to the articular surface. In the medial, habitual noncontact area the sheets become more oblique; and in the central portion of this zone there are few sheets and geometric organization is poor.[9,20] With significant alteration of the articular cartilage, these trabeculae are affected, a change that may be reflected in roentgenographic views of the patella.

Working Hypothesis

Summarizing, one can say that there is an area of the patella with less than optimal nutrition that bears weight only infrequently during the day (the odd facet). When it is loaded, however, it is usually under circumstances that create high forces.

Chondromalacic changes on the medial facet are usually asymptomatic until there is a sudden increase in the demands of the patellofemoral joint. The presence of a ridge that crosses the medial femoral condyle at its osteochondral junction (the odd facet ridge) causes friction of the cartilage of the medial patellar facet, as the patella rides the ridge during knee movement. It is possible that the different stiffness indices of the underlying bone causes shear stress and predisposes to degeneration of the cartilage.

It has always been difficult to correlate histologic changes with the clinical symptoms experienced by the individual. Goodfellow et al. suggested that there were two major groups of change.[11] The first type are the changes that originate primarily on the surface, which leave most of the important deep part of the articular cartilage intact to "stress-relieve" the underlying bone. Although these changes may lead to crepitus, they need not be painful. Goodfellow et al. postulated a second type of change that starts in the deepest layers of the cartilage, therefore interfering with the fibers that are "stress-protecting" the underlying bone. This change may lead to a situation where the articular surface appears grossly smooth but is not doing its job as a stress-reliever for the underlying bone.

Grading of Chondromalacia

The several systems for classifying the degree of chondromalacic changes to the patellar surface are outlined in Table 12-5, which attempts to correlate the equivalents in each system.[21-23] Each system has its merits, but the Metcalfe system has clearly defined grades and so is used throughout this chapter unless otherwise stated.

In the large group of chondromalacia patellae patients, there are many factors that may predispose the athlete to clinical problems. Trauma in the form of direct blows or increased activity may precipitate a chain of reactions, which may start a vicious cycle of pain and even surface changes. Reflex inhibition of the vastus medialis adds to the atrophy and may aggravate minor amounts of patellofemoral malalignment, which leads back into the same vicious cycle once more. Should the atrophy not be counteracted, or should the knee not be protected from the repetitive forces that are causing the chondromalacia, permanent damage may result and eventually subchondral bone may be exposed.

Lateral Facet Syndrome

The lateral facet of the normal patella is subjected to repeated high loads, which may give rise to cartilage change referred to as the lateral facet hyperpressure syndrome. Predisposing factors may include tight lateral retinacular structures, particularly the lateral patellofemoral ligament.[24]

Once established, this syndrome has a greater propensity for progression to degenerative joint disease than does medial cartilage chondromalacia. It is important to establish the presence of this syndrome because of the emphasis that must be placed on stretching the tight lateral structures[24] (Table 12-6).

In some instances, the skyline roentgenographic view reveals a well-developed hooking of the lateral border of the patella, with its obvious implications for increased surface pressure. Lateral facet syndrome in this situation has a particularly poor prognosis.

Direct Trauma

Blows to the patella may precipitate surface changes. With sufficient impact, these changes may progress to full-thickness lesions and in some cases are irreversible. Animal studies have demonstrated the relation between direct patellar impact and articular surface damage.[25] Even moderate damage may take 6 to 12 weeks to recover.

TABLE 12-5. Grading of Patellar Articular Cartilage Damage

Grade	Outerbridge[21]	Metcalf[22]	Jackson[23]
0	—	Normal. No softening, fibrillation or other evidence of chondromalacia.	—
I	Localized softening, swelling or fibrillation of cartilage.	Softening and appearance of blistering. Feels spongy when probed.	Softening of articular cartilage upon probing. Minor surface fissuring and the classic blister lesion. Closed chondrosis of Ficat.
II	Fragmentation or fissuring in an area <1.3 cm.	Fissuring and minor fibrillation, not extending down to subchondral bone when probed.	Major fasciculations of cartilage confined to the patella. Crabment appearance. Open chondrosis of Ficat.
III	Fragmentation or fissuring involving >1.3 cm.	Deep fissuring, fragmentation, and fibrillation with clefts extending down to subchondral bone when probed. Covers less than 50% of patellar surface.	Exposure of subchondral bone of the patella with surface changes in the femoral groove.
IV	Chondromalacic changes extends to expose subchondral bone.	Extensive fibrillation down to subchondral bone. More than 50% of patellar surface involved.	

TABLE 12-6. Retropatellar Syndromes

Medial Facet Syndrome	Lateral Facet Syndrome
Hypopressure	Hyperpressure
Onset usually 13–20 years	Onset usually 20–30 years
Type II–III patella	Hooked lateral facet
Rarely progresses to osteoarthritis	May progress to osteoarthritis
Sometimes mobile patella	Frequently tight lateral retinacular band
Medial pain	Lateral pain
Sometimes associated plica	Rarely associated plica
Rarely effusion	Sometimes associated effusion
Poor correlation with roentgenogram	Correlates well with roentgenogram
Variable crepitus	Often significant crepitus
Poor long-term response to lateral retinacular release	Good response to lateral retinacular release
More frequent in females	Equal frequency in males and females

Although not necessarily fitting directly into this classification, chondral or osteochondral damage may result from the shearing stress that accompanies acute or chronic ligament disruption or patellar dislocation. Frequently, the acute lesions heal. Furthermore, with severe posterior cruciate deficiency, the repetitive extra loading of the quadriceps compensatory mechanisms may result in retropatellar change.

Osteochondral Damage

Osteochondritis dissecans involves partial or total separation of an area of articular cartilage with its underlying subchondral bone due to avascular necrosis.[25,26]

A definite history of trauma is associated with about one-third of cases, although repeated minor trauma is thought to be the most common etiologic factor.[27] The patient usually presents with retropatellar pain, frequently indistinguishable from other anterior knee pain syndromes. However, a definite complaint of suprapatellar swelling and the demonstration of effusion should arouse suspicion, as these findings are infrequent in the other syndromes. Patellar crepitus is the other most consistent physical finding.

The lesion may be visualized on the lateral plain roentgenogram, but computed tomography (CT) or magnetic resonance imaging (MRI) may be necessary to clearly outline its depth and extent. Occasionally, the lesion resolves over a period of months with non-operative care, mainly with restriction of activities. Surgery is indicated for persistent pain, intra-articular loose bodies, or where there is well developed symptomatic subchondral sclerosis of the crater base. The surgery involves excision of the fragment and curettage of the crater, with or without drilling. Rarely, a large fragment may be drilled in situ and perhaps stabilized.

Untreated, this lesion may lead to extensive degenerative changes. Because the results of surgery are mainly good, prompt diagnosis and distinguishing it from the other retropatellar syndromes are important.

Plical Syndromes

Embryologically, the knee joint is formed by the fusion of three synovial compartments during the fourth fetal month. A plica exists when any portion of the embryonic synovial septa persist into adult life.[28,29] The most common, and least symptomatic, is the infrapatellar plica in the intracondylar notch, often called the ligamentum mucosum. A suprapatellar plica may separate, to varying degrees, the suprapatellar pouch from the main cavity of the knee joint. The medial patellar plica is a crescentic fold, running from the quadriceps tendon into the medial wall of the joint and ending in the infrapatellar fat pad. This medial patella plica has been given many names, including the medial synovial shelf, the ledge, plicae alares elongata, plicae synovialis mediopatellaris, and patella meniscus.[29] It is this medial plical fold that is most frequently symptomatic and is referred to in the medial plical syndrome (Fig. 12-6).

These residual rudimentary synovial folds are certainly present in more than 20 percent of knees and perhaps in as many as 60 percent. They are usually asymptomatic but may become inflamed due to either repetitive stress from activity or direct trauma. If sufficiently large, they may cause mechanical symptoms within the joint. Even relatively small plica may become symptomatic if constant inflammation and edema lead to stiffening and contracture (Fig. 12-7). In this case, the plica may bowstring with flexion, producing excess tension and perhaps an ischemic type of pain (movie-goer sign) or erosion of the adjacent articular surface. Large plical folds may cause severe articular surface erosions, metaplase to fibrocartilage, and result in protracted symptoms (Fig. 12-8).

There are no signs and symptoms that are pathognomonic. Even when a plica is visualized at arthroscopy, it is not possible to ascribe all of the patients' symptoms to this structure with certainty (Table 12-7). Symptoms are most commonly seen in the adolescent, and pain in the medial parapatellar area is the most frequent complaint. It is usually aggravated by activity, particularly running and jumping; and it is often aggravated by quadriceps exercises. In about 25 percent of individuals there is a positive movie-goer sign or pain with prolonged sitting. These two phenomena have been referred to as "shelf claudication." Other complaints include giving way, pseudolocking or catching, the sensation of cracking, snapping, or popping with activity, and pain with squatting.[30]

The most frequent clinical sign is tenderness along a line one finger's breadth medial to the patella and particularly just proximal to the inferior pole of the patella. With the knee flexed, the fold may even be palpable, or at least tender, where it is stretched across the medial femoral condyle. True effusions are rare, but there is frequently a "tight" or "swollen" sensation around the medial infrapatellar fat pad area. There is occasionally a palpable "pop" or "click" with the McMurray test, but with careful observation it can be identified as coming from proximal to the joint line.[30,31]

Nonoperative treatment consists in the usual range of therapy for peripatellar pain, including modified activity, ice application, ultrasound, hamstring stretching, patellar mobilization, vastus medialis hypertrophy, and patellar strapping. In addition, occasionally nonsteroidal anti-inflammatory drugs (NSAIDs) or injections of steroid with a long-acting

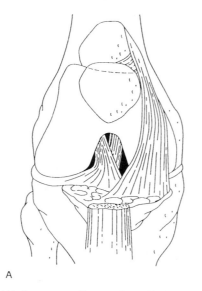
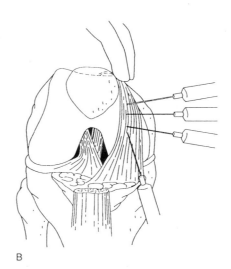

A   B

Fig. 12-6. **(A)** Suprapatellar and medial synovial plica. **(B)** In full flexion, a medial plical fold or shelf has the potential to rub on the medial condyle. The tension on the fold may produce discomfort and the "movie-goer" sign. Steroid or local anesthetic may be injected by a longitudinal stab with deposition along the needle track as it is removed or by a series of punctures.

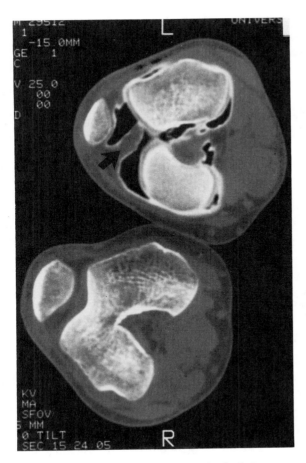

Fig. 12-7. CT scan showing a particularly large medial synovial plica in the left knee.

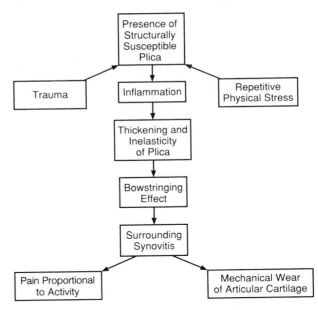

Fig. 12-8. Potential evolution of a symptomatic plical fold.

local anesthetic into the plical fold produce a dramatic response (Fig. 6).[29] If there are sufficient intractable mechanical symptoms and the plical fold has been visualized by radiographic techniques, arthroscopic resection is rewarding. Although large plicae are more likely to produce mechanical symptoms, small plicae are capable of being pathologic and generating pain.

Patellar Tracking Problems

The normal arc of patellar tracking, as the knee goes through a functional range, may be influenced by patellar shape, position, muscle power, balance and resultant line of pull, and the quality and arrangement of the noncontractile soft tissues. Any anatomic component or functional activity that disturbs the alignment from the norm may contribute to symptoms. Even if the clinician is not willing to accept

these components as proved etiologic factors, their identification allows modification in order to alter the joint mechanics and perhaps allow some resolution of the symptoms.

Patellar Shape

Wiberg attempted to classify patellae according to the shape of the articular facets[19]: Type I patellae have equal sized concave facets; type II and III have larger lateral facets, with the former associated with a concave medial articular surface and the profile of type III being more convex (Fig. 12-9). These shapes are difficult to identify, even on skyline views, and there are numerous intermediary forms.[8] Furthermore, except for dysplastic patellae, which are associated with subluxation and dislocation, and the prominently hooked lateral facet seen in some lateral hyperpressure syndromes and retropatellar arthritis, there is little correlation of patellar shape with retropatellar pathology.

Patellar Position

Patella alta, or a high-riding patella, may be associated with subluxation, possibly due to the pull of vastus lateralis producing a lateral shift of the patella before it is firmly seated in the femoral groove (Fig.

TABLE 12-7. Diagnosis of Symptomatic Plicae

Signs and Symptoms	Approx. % Present[a]
Suspicion of syndrome	
Symptoms	
Anteromedial knee pain	85
Pain aggravated by repetitive activity	85
Inferomedial tight or swollen sensation	55
Cracking, popping, snapping with activity	50
Giving way sensation	45
Pain with sitting for long periods	45
Pain with repetitive squatting	45
Signs	
Medial parapatellar pain to palpation	87
Pain or palpable band over medial condyle of flexed knee	73
Snap or grinding with McMurray test	50
Quadriceps atrophy	40
Effusion	30
Positive patellar compression test	30
More definite indicators	
Present on arthrography, CT, or MRI	100
Pain relieved by medial parapatellar local anesthetic	75
Prolonged relief with medial intracapsular cortisone	70
Large size at arthroscopy	
Mechanical impingement demonstrated at arthroscopy	60
Gritty feeling during release of metaplased shelf	60

[a] Rounded to nearest percent.

12-10).[32,33] The evidence for a relation to retropatellar chondromalacia is much more tenuous.

Patella infra, a rare condition, may contribute to tracking abnormalities and be associated with unusual patellofemoral joint loading. It is usually seen as an acquired condition in association with postoperative contractures.

Increased Q-Angle

The Q-angle represents the discrepancy between the resultant line of pull of the quadriceps muscles and the anatomic position of the ligamentum patellae. The pull of the quadriceps is represented by a vector from the middle of the patella to the anterior

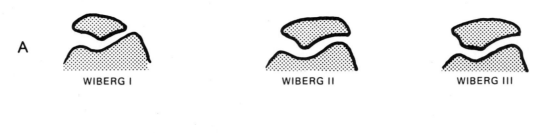

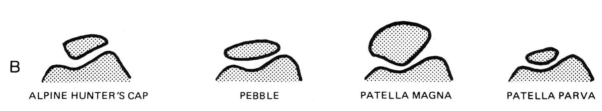

Fig. 12-9. These patellar types have been described differently by different authors. **(A)** Wiberg classic types. **(B)** A variety of dysplastic forms. (After Ficat and Hungerford,[8] with permission.)

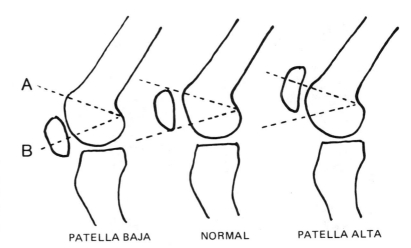

Fig. 12-10. Normal patella sits below the line of the old epiphyseal scar (**A**) and above the Bloomensaat line (**B**) in a 30 degree lateral view. The diagram shows examples of patella baja (infra), normal patella, and patella alta.

PATELLA BAJA   NORMAL   PATELLA ALTA

superior iliac spine (Fig. 12-11). It represents the result of the strong lateral pull of the huge mass of vastus lateralis and the correcting medial pull of the vastus medialis. The distal component of the Q-angle is identified by a line from the midpoint of the patella to the middle of the proximal tibial tubercle.

There is controversy surrounding every aspect of this angle. With the quadriceps relaxed, the normal Q-angle is reported to be 13 to 18 degrees.[13] In this situation, angles less than 13 degrees are associated with patella alta. Angles more than 18 degrees are associated with increased femoral anteversion. In the

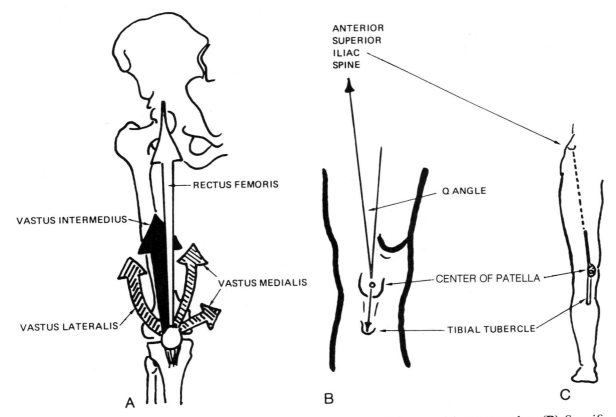

Fig. 12-11. (**A**) Line of pull of the various components of the quadriceps muscles. (**B**) Specific landmarks for measuring the Q-angle. (**C**) Goniometer placement.

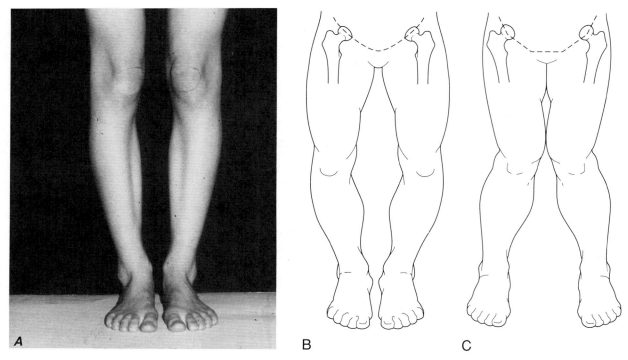

Fig. 12-12. **(A)** "Squinting" patellae. This sign potentially indicates increased femoral anteversion or femoral internal torsion. It is present to some extent in a large percentage of active young people. Other important alignments include genu varum **(B)** and genu valgum **(C)**. These latter alignments have more implication in tibiofemoral disease than patellofemoral problems.

standing position, with the feet pointing forward, the patellae face inward (referred to as squint). This so-called persistent fetal alignment is present in varying degrees in as many as 80 percent of the young, active population, usually in a mild form (Fig. 12-12). It is widely accepted, but not proved, that this alignment contributes to the patellofemoral pain syndrome. Excessive Q-angles are frequently found in individuals who have nontraumatic patellar dislocations.

Because in many ways this angle represents a dynamic situation, some investigators believe that the measurement should be made with the quadriceps contracted. In this case, the normal angle may be less than 10 degrees. It is also reported at 0 degrees, with the knees flexed to right angles.[33] Furthermore, Fairbank et al. reported an upper limit of normal for the relaxed quadriceps measurement at 20 degrees.[34] Part of the problem lies with the fact that the most crucial aspect of the measurement is the palpation of the midpoint of the patella and the upper tibial tu-

Clinical Facts

Q-ANGLE

Study	Angle (degrees)	Conditions
Hughston et al.[33]	0	Knee flexed to 90 degrees
	10	Leg extended Quadriceps contracted
Insall[13]	15 (13–20)	Lying Legs extended Muscles relaxed
Fairbank et al.[34]	20 (men) 22 (women)	Standing Muscles relaxed

bercle. Small errors in marking these points, because they are relatively close to the axis, produce large errors of measurement. It should be emphasized that this is a clinical, not a radiographic, measurement. It is my opinion that far too much has been made of this parameter for assessment of the knee.

Muscular Factors

Insufficient pull of the vastus medialis may contribute to poor tracking of the patella. The magnitude of the effect of vastus medialis pull is well illustrated by the work of Lieb and Perry.[35] Factors contributing to vastus medialis insufficiency are a congenitally atrophic or dystrophic medialis mass, reflex inhibition due to pain, and atrophy secondary to disuse.

Reflex inhibition is a powerful mechanism that not only prevents hypertrophy but contributes significantly to atrophy.[36–38] It is supported by the work of DeAndrade et al., who recorded marked inhibition of motor activity in the quadriceps when human knees were distended with plasma.[36] This finding emphasizes the futility of prescribing exercises that generate pain or effusion. Devising a rehabilitation program for knee pain that minimizes reflex inhibition of the quadriceps while promoting continued improvement in function requires skill, careful evaluation of the individual athlete, and imagination. It is this challenge that has given rise to the evolution of biofeedback techniques for knee rehabilitation.[39]

Moller et al. demonstrated a decrease in electromyographic (EMG) activity during maximal isometric quadriceps contraction in the involved limb in patients with patellar subluxation and idiopathic chondromalacia.[38] This reduction was recorded in both the vastus medialis obliquus (VMO) and the vastus lateralis (VL). Never the less, those subjects with laterally placed patellas, as measured by the congruence angle on a skyline roentgenogram, were able to centralize the patella by quadriceps contraction.[37,40] After 3 months of isometric quadriceps training, increased EMG activity could be recorded only in the group with patellar subluxation. However, the balance of activity between the VMO and VL was unchanged. Thus these investigators indicated that a more selective approach to training the vastus medialis was desirable.

There is a suggestion that a lower vastus medialis/vastus lateralis EMG ratio may be recorded by surface electrodes in patients with peripatellar pain.[41] This ratio may then be improved with specific electrostimulation of the vastus medialis over 24 sessions, with 70 Hz electrical stimulation (10 to 50 seconds on–off duty cycle, three sessions per week). This improved electrical activity is usually accompanied clinically by symptomatic improvement.

Bennett and Stauber described a unique pattern of torque production by the knee extensor musculature in patients with anterior knee pain during eccentric activity, generally during the range 30 to 60 degrees of knee flexion[41] (Fig. 12-13). They agreed that although patellar pain problems could frequently stem

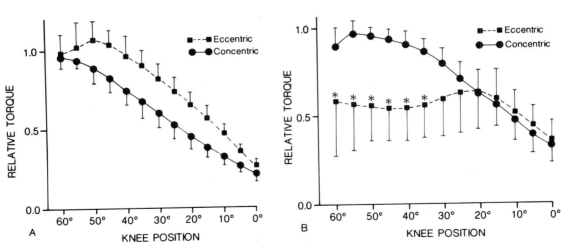

Fig. 12-13. **(A)** Relative torque for quadriceps of asymptomatic knee for concentric and eccentric contraction. **(B)** Deficit shown in the eccentric torque curve for the symptomatic limb. (* = Significant difference.) (After Bennett and Stauber,[41] with permission.)

from biomechanical disorders, there might also be a deficiency of motor control. They thought that many programs, including their own, obtained dramatic relief of symptoms with little demonstrable change in quadriceps torque. Further support for a neural component came from the fact that the major torque deficit was seen only during eccentric exercise, whereas the torque produced during concentric work was of greater magnitude.[42] Also, the rapid response to training could easily be the result of motor learning. Exactly how the training of quadriceps relieves pain remains unclear, but undoubtedly many patients report early pain relief, even after only one or two treatments.

Other investigators have noted irregular torque curves with isokinetic concentric contractions[43,44] (Fig. 12-14). Furthermore, the abnormality in the curve highly correlated with the presence of a positive dynamic compression test (Clarke sign).

These dynamic tests are most important in view of the insensitivity of simple measures of quadriceps girth. A measured difference of 2.5 cm between affected and normal limbs may be equivalent to 22 to 33 percent reduction in quadriceps cross-sectional area.[45] Thus small differences in thigh girth actually may conceal larger differences in quadriceps muscle loss. Further, Doxey reported that in subjects with patellofemoral pain small reductions in size — as little as 1 percent — could represent as much as 13.5 percent reduction in muscle bulk.[46]

Absolute, or relative, deficiency of the hamstring muscles at 60 degrees per second on isokinetic testing has been demonstrated in more than 80 percent of individuals with anterior knee pain and more than 70 percent testing at 240 degrees per second.[47] Furthermore, tightness in this group was present in more than 20 percent of athletes.

The pattern of muscle tightness frequently involves the iliotibial band, along with the rectus femoris portion of the quadriceps and the other hip flexors.[48] It is thought that tightness in these groups adversely affects the pattern of landing from jumping and indirectly affects the motion of the patella in its femoral groove. For instance, if the iliotibial band is tight, it may pull the patella laterally during knee flexion.[49] Tight hamstrings may result in increased knee flexion during running, thereby increasing the patellofemoral joint reaction forces in stance. Increased knee flexion may also result from a tight gastrocnemius, which in turn may create compensatory foot pronation because the dorsiflexion of the talus cannot be fully accommodated at the talocrural joint and so is

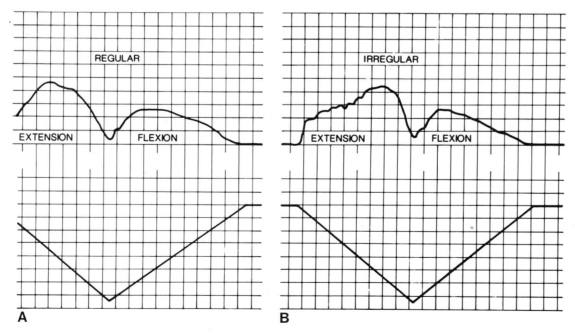

Fig. 12-14. (A) Normal isokinetic torque curve for quadriceps and hamstring. **(B)** Irregular curve when retropatellar pain affects quadriceps torque.

translated to the subtalar area.[50] The magnitude and impact of this adaptation are uncertain.

Alteration of muscle strength, contraction pattern, and flexibility may contribute to the patellofemoral pain syndrome as well as be the endpoint of prolonged discomfort. Alterations in these parameters, which can be assessed subjectively and objectively, may form a basis for diagnosis and be used to monitor progress of treatment. Furthermore, any program that does not address the problems of muscle imbalances or rely heavily on muscle rehabilitation, is doomed to failure in the treatment of the patellofemoral pain syndrome.

Patellar Subluxation

If the patellar alignment and tracking are sufficiently abnormal and the dynamic stabilizers inadequate, varying degrees of subluxation may be present, which may result in pain and sometimes a feeling of functional instability. The patient complains of a sensation of the knee feeling "weak" or "as if it will give out." However, tests for ligament laxity are negative, and internal derangement has been ruled out. The condition is diagnosed by observing the patellar position during passive and active knee flexion and extension, and occasionally by a positive apprehension test

(Fig. 12-15). Usually there is a degree of patellar laxity and hypermobility.[51] The vastus medialis may be atrophic, but it is difficult to know if it is primary or is secondary to pain. Patellar subluxation is the exaggerated functional counterpart of a constellation of static alignment factors. It lies at the severe end of the more subtle tracking problems.

Other Alignment Factors

Numerous alignment factors appear to play some role in anterior knee pain, in addition to those already discussed. They include femoral rotation, femoral neck anteversion, genu valgum, joint laxity, knee hyperextension, tibial torsion, excessive pronation, and leg length inequalities (Figs. 12-16, 12-17).[51-59]

Kujala et al., comparing young army recruits with and without a variety of knee pain syndromes, found only three significant factors in the pain group: increased height, leg length discrepancy, and patellar laxity as part of overall increased knee laxity.[51] Many reports emphasize the link between abnormal pronation of the subtalar joint and patellofemoral dysfunction, particularly in cases of the excessive lateral pressure syndrome. It is postulated that the additional internal rotation that accompanies increased pronation disturbs the normal tibiofemoral rotational rela-

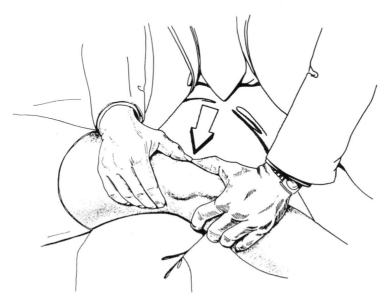

Fig. 12-15. Patellar hypermobility may be demonstrated by lateral patellar pressure with the patient's quadriceps relaxed. It may demonstrate hypermobility, apprehension, or pain, which may be manifested by the athlete contracting the quadriceps or attempting to prevent the examiner from continuing the test.

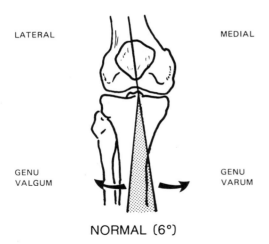

Fig. 12-16. Normal femorotibial shaft angle is 6 degrees. Clinically, genu varum exists if there is approximately 3 cm between the medial femoral condyles when the malleoli are together. Similarly, genu valgum exists if the malleoli are 3 cm apart. This measurement ensures that the shaft of the tibia is normal.

tions.[55,56] At the beginning of midstance, the flexion at the knee and pronation at the subtalar joint should have ended and started to reverse. If the subtalar joint remains pronated or continues to pronate, the tibia cannot externally rotate. Therefore increased pronation during midstance creates a biomechanical dilemma for the tibiofemoral joint.[54] Normal mechanics dictate that the tibiofemoral joint extend during midstance as the body traverses the fixed foot. Excessive pronation in magnitude or duration prevents the knee joint from acquiring the external rotation of the tibia needed for extension, which in turn may adversely affect patellofemoral tracking. The timing and magnitude of pronation may influence the propensity to cause symptoms. For instance, excessive pronation during midstance is likely to have more effect than the same amount at initial foot contact.

One of the most important studies in the area of alignment was reported by Fairbank et al.[34] Their study compared similar groups of adolescents and young adults, with and without knee pain. Several important conclusions may be drawn from their report;

1. Joint mobility, Q-angle, genu valgum, femoral neck anteversion, patellar position (patella alta),

height, and weight were not significantly different between the two groups.
2. Those individuals engaged in greater amounts of activity were more likely to have pain.
3. For the most part, the anterior knee pain syndrome appeared to be self-limiting, although it may have been a self-imposed reduction of activity in young adults, which allowed resolution of most of the symptoms.[60]
4. Retropatellar arthrosis developed rarely in this group.

These investigations concluded that chronic overloading, rather than faulty mechanics, was the dominant factor in anterior knee pain of adolescents. They postulated that the rapid medial translation of the patella as it passes into the intercondylar notch during the early stance phase may produce repeated blows of the medial facet against the medial femoral condyle. They did concede, however, that some alignments may exaggerate this tendency—hence the predisposition to symptoms. Our studies of figure skaters support this lack of specific malalignments in relation to knee pain.[58] Furthermore, our work with young, active adults whose alignments were correlated with findings at arthroscopy failed to demonstrate a relation to patellar surface pathology.[59]

Clinical Point

ANTERIOR KNEE PAIN

Chronic overloading, rather than faulty mechanics, is the dominant factor in anterior knee pain in adolescents.

As a summary to this section on alignment factors, it should be made clear that the words abnormal and malalignment cannot be assigned to parameters seen consistently in more than two-thirds of the active population and that are within two standard deviations (2 SD) of normal. Nevertheless, the degree and nature of the alignment should be recorded in each athlete complaining of these knee pain syndromes; and, when appropriate, some alteration should be made in the treatment by either active or passive means. It cannot be overstressed that careful analysis of training techniques and workload, as well as terrain and equipment, are more likely to be fruitful in the permanent resolution of symptoms.

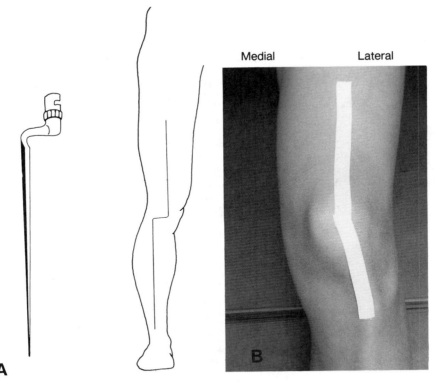

Fig. 12-17. Increased Q-angle. **(A)** Bayonet sign. Tibia vara of the proximal third causes a markedly increased Q-angle. Alignment of the quadriceps, patellar tendon, and tibial shaft resembles a French bayonet (right knee). **(B)** Q-angle with the knee in full extension is only slightly increased over normal. However, with the knee flexed at 30 degrees, there may be failure of the tibia to derotate normally and the patellar tendon to line up with the anterior crest of the tibia (left knee). This finding is not infrequent in patients with patellofemoral athralgia. (From Ficat and Hungerford,[8] with permission.)

TREATMENT PLAN FOR PATELLOFEMORAL PAIN

A careful evaluation of the patient should assist the clinician in moving from the broad chief complaint of anterior knee pain toward one of the more specific diagnostic categories outlined in Table 12-8.

Patient Assessment

History

The main points of the history are related to obtaining a specific chief complaint and a thorough outline of activity patterns, training techniques, and the footwear used, followed by details of the onset, nature, pattern, and duration of the pain. A slow spontaneous onset, with no or only minor injury suggests overuse or alignment factors. Blunt injury to the retinacular should be recorded. Past therapies are important, particularly past surgery, as are aggravating and modifying factors. The presence of definite effusions, giving way, locking, pseudolocking, and other joint problems including the back is important. With sufficient information, a pattern of joint instability, patellar instability, mechanical dysfunction, internal derangement, or peripatellar pathology may emerge. Obvious flaws or modifiable details of the activity pattern may be recorded.

Static Examination of Alignment

Examination starts with an overall assessment of alignment, with particular reference to foot position, and shape, both the static and dynamic status, genu varum or valgum, and patellar position. Pelvic obliq-

TABLE 12-8. Anterior Knee Pain

Causes	Signs and Symptoms
Anterior knee pain of adolescents	Aggravated by exercise
	Slow onset, no obvious trauma
	Often related to growth spurt
	Commonly tight muscles or muscle imbalance
	Frequently rest pain and pain while sitting
	Vague peri- and retropatellar pain
	Negative roentgenogram
Odd facet syndrome	Inferomedial pain; occasionally crepitus
	Descending stairs painful; pain proportional to activity
	Pressure over patella painful
	Negative roentgenogram
Alignment syndromes	Measurable significant increased Q-angle
	Genu varum, foot pronation or leg length discrepancy; patella and knee laxity
	Generalized peripatellar pain
	Rarely crepitus
Lateral hyperpressure syndrome	Lateral pain; stair climbing painful
	Crepitus significant
	Pressure over patella painful
	Characteristic skyline views
	May be effusion
Plical syndrome	Medial peripatellar pain
	Occasional click and pseudolocking
	May respond to injection
	Confirm on arthrogram or CT scan
Patella alta or baja	Characteristic roentgenogram
	May be associated with subluxation or dislocation
Osteochondral injury	Pain retropatellar
	May be associated with effusion
	Crepitus
	Confirm with lateral or skyline roentgenogram, or CT
Overuse syndromes of tendon	Pain located in suprapatellar pole, over inferior tip of patella or over tendon
	Responds to anti-inflammatory medication
	Pain proportional to activity
Overuse or trauma to bursa	Located over known bursal sites
	Prepatellar, infrapatellar, lateral ligament, iliotibial band, medial ligament, and under pes anserinus bursa
Fat pad syndromes	Infrapatellar pain and around fat pad
	Palpable tenderness
	Resisted extension sometimes gives sharp pain
Reflex sympathetic dystrophy	Skin changes
	Pain on all movements
	Extreme pain to palpation
	May lose range rapidly
	Atrophy may be extreme
	Positive bone scan
Osteoarthrosis	Effusion, morning stiffness; pain proportional to activity, often coming on several hours after activity
	Young patient: associated with ligament or meniscal pathology
	Middle age patient: rule out gout and pseudogout by blood and synovial fluid screen
	Confirm magnitude with weight-bearing roentgenograms
Intra-articular mechanical	Meniscal, chondral flap, osteochondritis, loose bodies
	May give anterior knee pain; catching, locking
	Frequently effusion; each need specific stress tests and radiographic view
	Index of suspicion important

No single finding is completely characteristic, but some findings are more common. The early treatment of many of these syndromes is similar, but specific therapy, medical and surgical treatment differs.

uity and leg length discrepancies are also carefully assessed. Obvious genu valgum or varum, and tibial torsion, shape are noted (Fig. 12-16).

Looking at the patient from the side reveals the degree, if any, of hyperextension and the possibility of a high-riding patella (detected by the presence of the "camel" sign) (Fig. 12-18). With one leg in front of the other, the height of the medial longitudinal arch may be easily appreciated.

Viewing from behind facilitates recording the relative positions of the posterosuperior iliac spines, the gluteal and calf bulk, and the calcaneal position. The wear pattern on the shoes and training footwear may be noted.

The laterally tilted or displaced patella may be seen best when sitting, as is patellar tracking, while the knee flexes and extends. With the knee at 90 degrees of flexion, the 90 degree tubercle-sulcus angle as described by Hughston is measured.[33,61] This measurement is defined by referencing a point at the center of the patella to a point at the center of the tibial tubercle. The angle is delineated by a line parallel to the transepicondylar axis (Fig. 12-19). With the patella well seated in the trochlea, rotational abnormalities are accounted for.[61] The normal angle is 0 degrees; more than 10 degrees is definitely considered abnormal by most investigators. The contour of

the vastus medialis is noted, particularly looking for a dystrophic outline. The Q-angle is recorded, as are the thigh and calf girths (Fig. 12-11).

At this point, special note is made of the potential for correction or biomechanical influence of an orthosis.

Specific Palpation and Stress Tests

Physical examination should be an exercise in careful, accurate anatomic identification. Each bursa, tendon, and periarticular structure is carefully palpated, with specific attention to the joint line, medial and lateral patellar facets, iliotibial band, medial retinacular area, and ligamentum patellae (Fig. 12-20). The patient should be asked to put "one" finger on "one" spot that is usually most painful, and this area is re-examined. At this juncture, some idea of the anatomic structure involved should be forming (Table 12-8). Effusion should be ruled out by the wipe test or by ballotment. It is rarely present in the classic patellofemoral pain syndrome. The suprapatellar pouch is palpated for thickness, tenderness, or nodules, which could indicate specific intraarticular pathology. The degree of laxity of the patella and the presence or absence of a positive apprehension test helps define potentially remediable problems of lat-

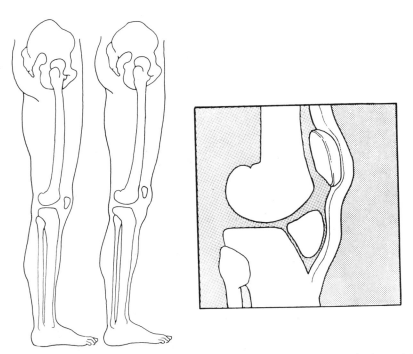

Fig. 12-18. "Camel" sign refers to the apparent double hump seen in association with a high riding patella due to uncovering of the infrapatellar fat pad. (After Hughston et al.,[33] with permission.)

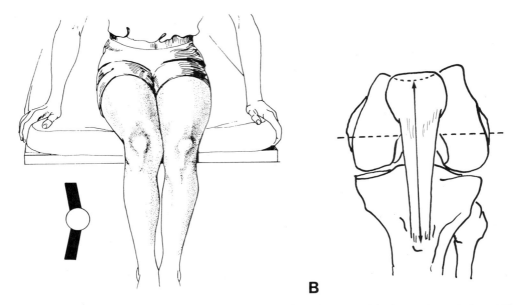

A   **B**

Fig. 12-19. Dystrophic appearance of the vastus medialis is often clearer with the patient sitting. **(A)** Q-angle in full flexion should be 0 degrees. As the patient extends the knee patella, tracking should be observed. **(B)** The extension of this examination is the tubercle–sulcus angle, which is 90 degrees at 90 degrees of knee flexion. (Adapted from Hughston et al.,[33] with permission.)

eral tightness or generalized patellar laxity and instability (Fig. 12-15).

In the supine position with the knee flexed 20 to 30 degrees and resting on a small pillow, the patella glide test may give an impression of lateral and medial retinacular tightness or integrity.[61] The lateral apprehension has been well documented, but the medial glide also gives an indication of the lateral restraints.[61] The quadriceps must be relaxed. The patella is visualized as being divided into four longitudinal quadrants, and an attempt is then made to displace the patella medially (Fig. 12-20). A medial glide of less than one quadrant is consistent with a tight lateral restraint and often correlates with a negative passive tilt. A glide of one to two quadrants is within the normal range; three and four quadrants indicates hypermobility. Similarly, a lateral glide of four quadrants signifies deficient medial restraints.[61]

With the knee fully extended, the passive patellar tilt test is documented. The examiner lifts the lateral edge of the patella from the lateral femoral condyle. The patella should remain in the trochlea and not be allowed to glide laterally as it would influence the measurement (Fig. 12-20). A tight lateral restraint is demonstrated by a negative or neutral angle to the horizontal.[61] More than 15 to 20 degrees is suggestive

of hypermobility. Females usually have about 5 degrees more tilt than males.

The knee is taken through a range of motion passively and then against resistance. Examination for a significant medial or suprapatellar plica begins with specific palpation and finishes with taking the internally rotated leg through a passive range of flexion and extension (Fig. 12-21). A locked knee is ruled out, loss of range is recorded, the degree of crepitus is assessed, and the magnitude and location of pain are determined with resistance.

The standard stress tests for ligamentous laxity help assess this component as the cause or contributing factor to the anterior knee pain. Tests for menis-

---

Clinical Point

RETROPATELLAR CARTILAGE PATHOLOGY CORRELATES WITH

- Pain on stair climbing
- Pain on patellar compression at 20 degrees
- Severity of crepitus (passive and active)

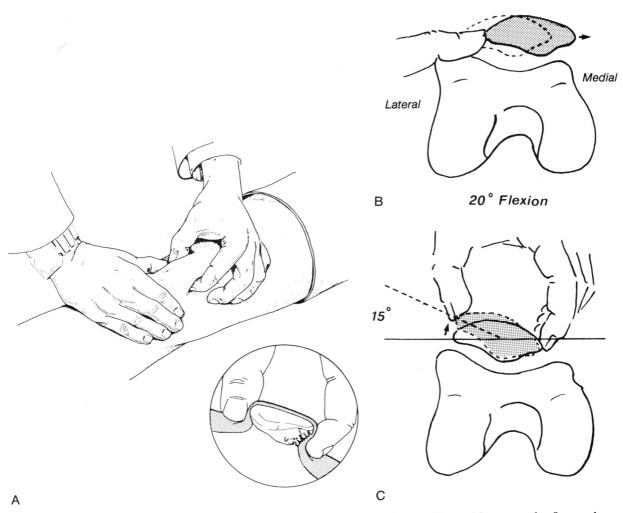

Fig. 12-20. (A) Displacement of the patella at 0 degrees allows the patella to ride up on the femoral condyle. The retinaculum may be probed with gentle palpation. Deeper palpation checks the medial and lateral facets as well as the retinaculum underneath the examiner's fingers. The suprapatellar synovium is examined for tenderness, bogginess, or nodules.[61,62] **(B)** Assessing the amount of medial and lateral glide at 20 degrees of flexion with support under the knee gives an impression of retinacular tightness. **(C)** Patellar tilt at extension with the quadriceps relaxed is usually about 15 degrees or slightly more in females.

cal pathology, including joint line pain, positive McMurray test, and a positive compression Apley test move suspicion away from patellofemoral syndromes, although these tests may be positive with a large medial plical fold.

The presence of a gross, grating sensation is compatible with significant femoral or patellar chondral defects. If significant retropatellar pathology is antic-

ipated, passive patellar compression and the active compression test (Clarke sign) are left until this point, as they may elicit so much discomfort the patient becomes unwilling or unable to cooperate further (Fig. 12-22). The examiner presses down slightly proximal to the upper pole or base of the patella with the web of the hand as the patient lies relaxed with the knee extended. The patient is then asked to contract the

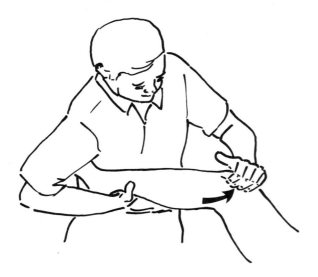

Fig. 12-21. Foot and tibia are held in internal rotation, and the patella is displaced slightly medially. The knee is passively flexed and extended, and an attempt is made to palpate the medial synovial plica.

quadriceps muscles while the examiner pushes down. If the patient can complete and maintain the contraction without pain, the test is negative. If the test causes retropatellar pain and the patient cannot hold a contraction, the test is considered positive. Note that a positive test can result in any individual if sufficient pressure is applied to the patella during contraction of the quadriceps, so the amount of pressure applied must be controlled. The best way to do it is to repeat the procedure several times, increasing the pressure each time, comparing the result with that seen on the unaffected side.[61]

Muscle tightness is carefully evaluated at the hip, knee, and ankle. Tests for hip flexor tightness (Thomas test), abduction contracture (Ober test), hamstrings (straight leg raise), knee flexors (modified Thomas test), and the soleus and gastrocnemius are recorded with regard to normal values as well as to those obtained using the opposite limbs (Fig. 12-23).

Lastly, some dynamic tests, e.g., walking, squatting, stair climbing, hopping, and duck waddle, further help assess the magnitude and location of pain.

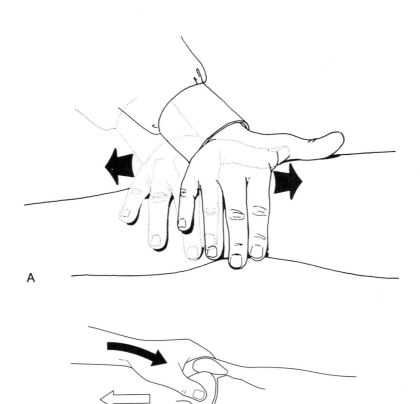

A

B

Fig. 12-22. (A) Patella is rubbed against the femoral trochlea in both transverse and longitudinal directions, making note of pain and crepitus. **(B)** Clarke sign uses the quadriceps contraction to generate retropatellar pressure. The test must be done gently initially and the results compared to those from the unaffected side.

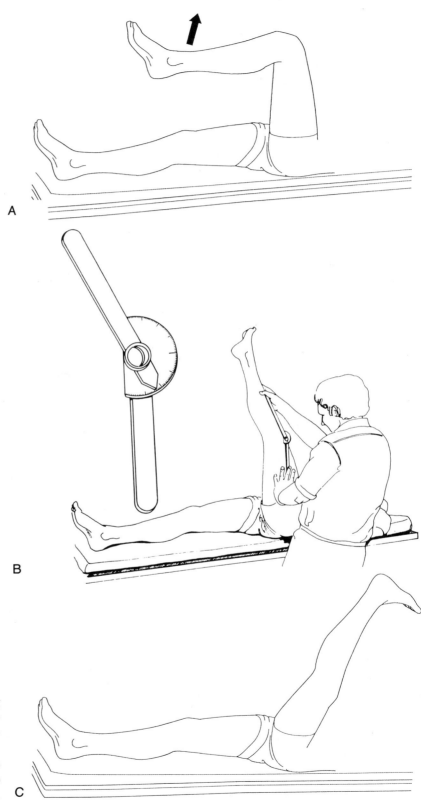

Fig. 12-23. Testing for hamstring tightness. **(A)** Hip is flexed to 90 degrees as a starting position. **(B)** Thigh is fixed and the leg extended. **(C)** In flexible individuals the knee is held straight, and the degree of hip flexion past 90 degrees is recorded.

1. Walking. The position of the foot at heel strike is noted and an impression gained regarding the magnitude of pronation, the degree of internal rotation, abnormal muscle activity, and the appropriateness of the pelvic control. In midstance, note is made of delayed supination, degree of dorsiflexion, and leg rotation. At toe-off, the presence of a heel whip and pelvic stability are recorded. A good swing phase action is also noted.
2. Walking on heels. This test allows assessment of the effect of decreasing pronation on internal rotation as well as giving a functional view of adequate gastrocnemius length.
3. Walking inverted or everted. Inversion test peronei strength and knee control. Eversion assesses available motion in the pronated foot.
4. Steps and squatting. Descending stairs and squatting are used as methods of reproducing pain, and eccentric quadriceps control. In individuals who report pain only after a significant amount of activity, repeated squats are useful to gain an insight

gain an insight into the effects of fatigue as well as the effectiveness of treatment.

The Waldron test assesses the presence of chondromalacia patellae. The examiner palpates the patella while the patient does several slow deep knee bends. As the patient goes through the range of motion, the examiner should note the amount of crepitus (significant only if accompanied by pain), where it occurs in the range of motion, the amount of pain, and if there is "catching," or poor tracking, of the patella throughout the movement. If pain and crepitus occur together during the movement, it is a sign of chrondromalacia patellae. In our study articular surface changes at arthroscopy in patients with suspected patellofemoral pain, correlated best with discomfort while ascending or descending stairs, pain with patella compression at 20 degrees of knee flexion and severe crepitus, with both passive and resisted extension.[59]

At this juncture, the broader classification of patel-

TABLE 12-9. Radiologic Contribution to Knee Pain Diagnosis

Condition	Technique and Views
Patellar position	
alta, infra (baja)	Lateral 30 degree (Blumensaat, Insall)
	Lateral 90 degree (Laurin)
	Anteroposterior (AP)
Subluxing/dislocating	Skyline (Laurin's 20 degree patellofemoral index, Merchant's congruence angle 45 degrees)
	Skyline with lateral tibial rotation
Patellar shape	Skyline 30 degrees
Wiberg I, II, III	
Dysplastic	
Magna, Parva	
Femoral sulcus angle	Skyline: Hughston's 55 degrees, Merchant's 45 degrees
Chondromalacia (cartilage wear)	Skyline 20 degrees (patellofemoral index)
	CT augmented with dye
	MRI
Osteochondritis	Lateral, AP, oblique, CT
Loose bodies	Tunnel (notch) view, oblique, AP, lateral
Meniscus	Arthrogram, CT, MRI
Plica	Arthrogram, CT, MRI
Degenerative joint disease	Weight-bearing AP, lateral, skyline
Stress fracture	Bone scan, tomogram
Reflex sympathetic dystrophy	Lateral view, bone scan
Dorsal defect of patella	Lateral view
Tumor	Routine views, CT, MRI
Infection	Bone scan, white blood cell scan
Metabolic bone disease	Routine views, bone scan, CT, MRI
Miscellaneous	Routine views, CT
Gout	
Pseudogout (chondrocalcinosis)	
Synovial chondrometaplasia	

VIEW	KNEE FLEXION	TECHNIQUE & POSITION	MEASUREMENT	IMPLICATIONS
AP	0 degrees	Standing, feet straight ahead	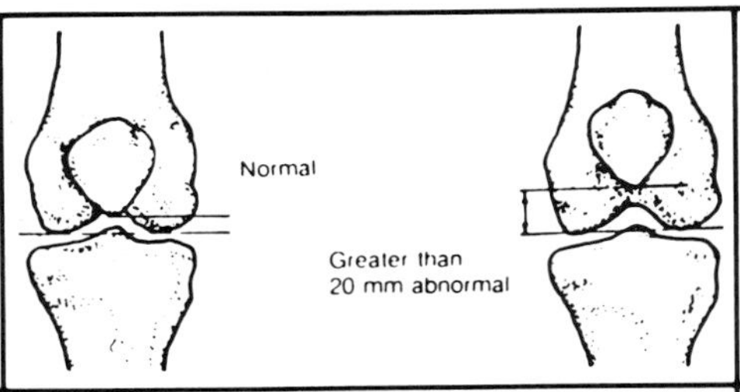 Normal — Greater than 20 mm abnormal	— Hypoplastic patella — Lateral subluxation of patella — Bipartite patella — Asymmetry of femoral condylar (abnormal femoral anteversion or femoral rotation)
Lateral	90 degrees	Supine	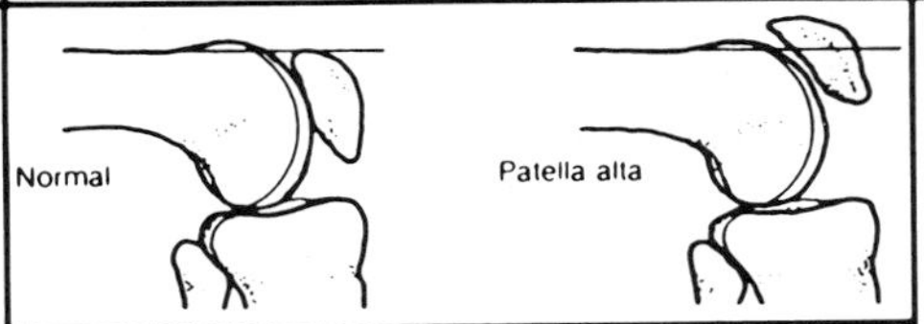 Normal — Patella alta	— Patella infera — Patellar fracture
Lateral	Approx. 30 degrees	Supine (Insali-Salvati)	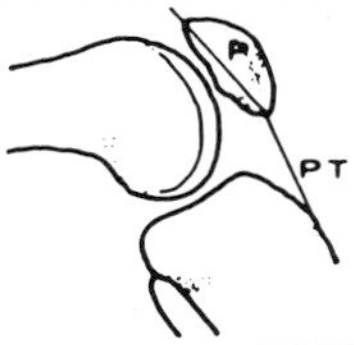 Ratio of P:PT = 1.0 More than 20% variation is abnormal	
Lateral	30 degrees	Supine	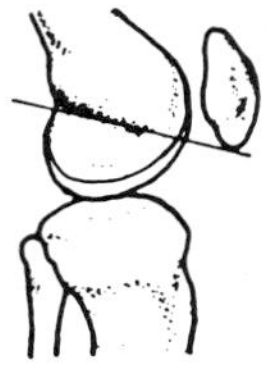 Blumensaat's line (see text)	
(Hughston) Tangential	55 degrees	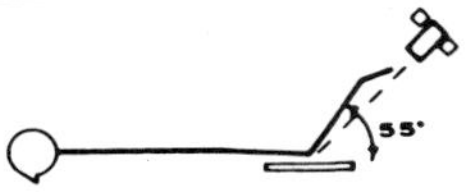 Prone position. Beam directed cephalad and inferior, 45 degrees from vertical	1) Sulcus angle: 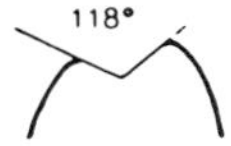 118° 2) Patella index 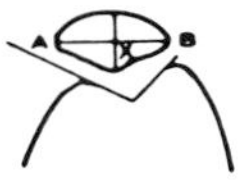 $\dfrac{AB}{XB - XA}$ NL Male 15 Female 17	— Patellar dislocation — Osteochondral fracture — Soft tissue calcification (old dislocated patella or fracture) — Patellar subluxation Patellar tilt Increased medial joint space Apex of patella lateral to apex of femoral sulcus Lateral patella edge lateral to femoral condyle Hypoplastic lateral femoral condyle (usually proximal) — Patellofemoral osteophytes — Subchondral trabeculae orientation (increase or decrease) — Patellar configuration (Wiberg-Baugartl) 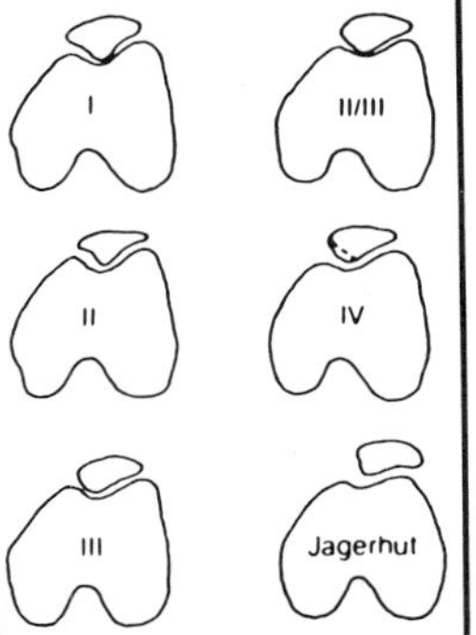
(Merchant) Tangential	45 degrees	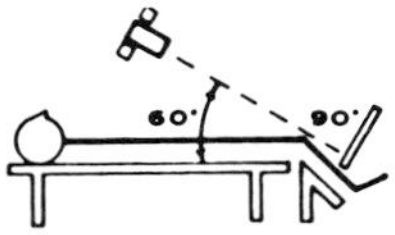 Supine position. Beam directed caudal and inferior, 30 degrees from vertical	1) Sulcus angle: 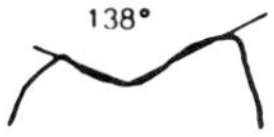 138° 2) Congruence angle: 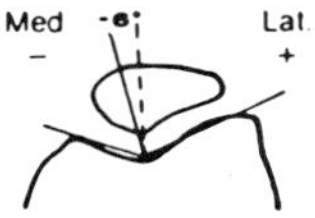 Med — Lat +	I, II/III, II, IV, III, Jagerhut
(Laurin) Tangential	20 degrees	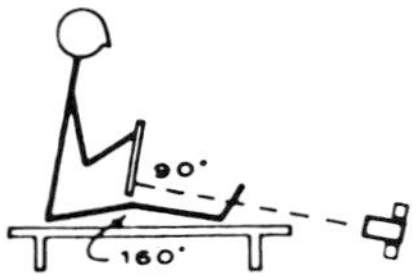 Sitting position. Beam directed cephalad and superior, 160 degrees from vertical	1) Lateral patellofemoral angle 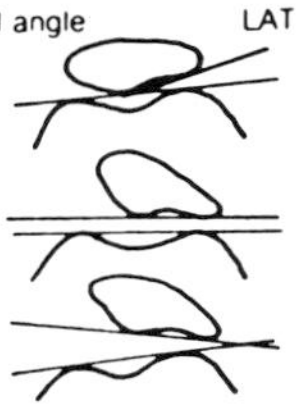 LAT — NL, ABNL, ABNL 2) Patellofemoral index Ratio A/B Med Lat Normal = 1.6 or less 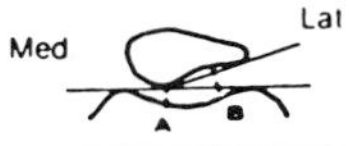	

Fig. 12-24. Summary of the radiologic views that correlate with the various published indices. (Adapted from Carson et al.,[64] with permission.)

lofemoral pain versus internal derangement, patellar instability, tendinitis or bursitis, and functional ligamentous instability should be possible.

Radiology

Attempts at defining radiologic parameters for patellofemoral pain have been largely disappointing. Nevertheless, many subsidiary diagnoses may be ruled out, as may some unusual developmental anatomic variations, such as bipartite patella and dorsal defects of the patella. In addition, certain metabolic diseases, e.g., gout and pseudogout, may be suspected. Benign tumors as well as the more serious lesions of infection and malignant tumors may be visualized. Although tumors are rare in the patella, the knee area is a particularly common site (Table 12-9). Many techniques have been described for assessing patellar position; and if these indices are used, the exact and appropriate technique described by the original author is mandatory (Fig. 12-24). These indices should never be used in isolation to make a diagnosis, only to add to the body of knowledge, supplement clinical signs, and assist in the planning of surgery. When these indices are positive in chondromalacia or patellofemoral knee pain, it usually repre-

sents some degree of hypermobility of the patella. The patellar shape and position may be assessed, and the skyline or sunrise view reveals maximum information. More than 90 percent of normal individuals and athletes with patellofemoral pain have a patellofemoral angle that opens laterally (Fig. 12-25). However, in patients with subluxation or dislocation, the patellofemoral angle is parallel or opens medially. Lateral patellar displacement is seen in up to 30 percent of individuals with patellofemoral pain associated with tracking problems (Fig. 12-26). It can also be recorded by an abnormal congruence angle (Table 12-10). The difficulty in categorizing patients into neat groups is evident in the discrepancies reported in normal and abnormal values (Table 12-11).[63-68]

Patella alta predisposes to poor tracking, subluxation, and dislocation — hence the potential for articular surface damage. It is diagnosed by an abnormal ratio of the length of the patellar tendon to the patella, an index that is normally close to 1 : 1.[63] if the patella projects above the Bloomensaat line, (the cortex of the intercondylar notch) in a 30 degree flexion lateral view, patella alta is present.[32] The patella also normally lies below a line projected from the residual distal femoral epiphysial scar.

Patalla infra, or Baja, rarely occurs as a developmental disorder, although it is seen in achondroplas-

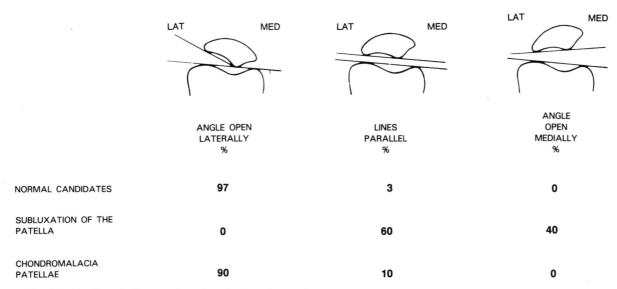

	ANGLE OPEN LATERALLY %	LINES PARALLEL %	ANGLE OPEN MEDIALLY %
NORMAL CANDIDATES	97	3	0
SUBLUXATION OF THE PATELLA	0	60	40
CHONDROMALACIA PATELLAE	90	10	0

Fig. 12-25. Patellofemoral angle. The baseline joins the summits of the femoral condyles. The second coordinate joins the limits of the lateral patella facet. They may intersect, leaving a medial or lateral patellofemoral angle, or remain as two parallel lines. Only a lateral patellofemoral angle is considered normal. (From Laurin et al.,[67] with permission.)

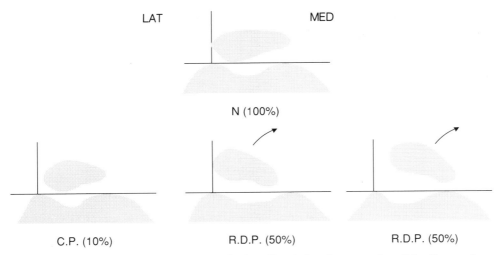

Fig. 12-26. Lateral patellar displacement. The baseline joins the summits of the femoral condyle, and a perpendicular is raised from the medial condyle. In normal individuals (N) the patella touches the vertical line or is medial to it (SD ± 2ᴍᴍ). With recurrent dislocation (RDP) 50 percent of individuals have a significant lateral shift and frequently a tilt. Most individuals with chondromalacia (CP) have normal coordinates, although 10 percent have a mild lateral shift.

tic dwarfs. The commonest etiologic factors are rupture or paralysis of the quadriceps, or after anterior cruciate reconstruction using patella tendon. Patella magna, an excessively large patella, is usually associated with the prolonged hyperemia of trauma or infection. Patella parva is sometimes also dysplastic in shape, in which case it is associated with instability. Hypoplasia of the femoral condyle, as measured by the Brattstrom sulcus angle on tangential views (skyline) of the patellofemoral articulation, is also associated with instability (Fig. 12-24).[66] There may be some indication of significant cartilage change on the 20 degrees skyline view (Fig. 12-27). However, cartilage degeneration in its early stages is difficult to visualize without the aid of arthrograms, CT scans or, better yet, MRI. Even small lesions may be visualized by the latter technique. The best overview of the role of radiology is that of Minkoff and Fein.[63]

Laboratory Data

Any indication of significant systemic inflammatory or metabolic disease requires a blood screen including an erythrocyte sedimentation rate and liver and renal function studies. These simple blood tests may be supplemented by specific antibody studies to assist in identifying rheumatoid disease, ankylosing spondylitis, and other problems. When possible, synovial fluid analysis is also an important, easy way to distinguish the disease process as noninflammatory, inflammatory, infective, or metabolic (Table 12-12).

Objective Assessment of Muscle Strength

Muscle strength may be assessed using hand-held dynamometers or isokinetic, polykinetic, or free weight systems. The main advantages of the computerized apparatus are the number of parameters that

TABLE 12-10.   Congruence Angle in Chondromalacia and Subluxating Patellae

| Study | Congruence Angle (degrees) | | |
	Mean Normal	Chondromalacics	Subluxators
Merchant et al.[68]	−6	—	+16
Aglietti[63]	−9	0	+17
Bentley[5]	—	−8.1	Normal[a]

[a] Of 33 cases, 4 were outside normal limits.

TABLE 12-11.   Roentgenographic Signs (in the 20 Degree Flexed Position)

Patellae	Patellar PFA (%)			Patellar displacement[a] (%)		PFI (%)	
	Open Laterally	Parallel	Open Medially	Medial to Touching Line "C"	Lateral to Line "C"	≤ 1.0	> 1.0
Normal (controls)	97	3	0	100	0	100	0
Subluxing	0	60	40	47	53	0	100
Chondromalacia	90	10	0	70	30	3	97

PFA = patellofemoral angle; PFI = patellofemoral index.
[a] C line is a line drawn perpendicular to the transcondylar plane in the skyline view.

may be recorded and the graphic displays. When available, they serve as a diagnostic modality, a treatment tool, and a method for ongoing assessment. Some of the abnormal patterns of contraction that are associated with retropatellar pain were discussed earlier. Eccentric muscle work assessment is also a particularly valuable parameter to record, as it reflects the functional contraction mode in many day-to-day activities. The pattern of power around a joint is as important as individual strength measurements within a group. Discrepancies between a painful and nonpainful limb may also provide some useful insights.

These tests complete the systematic and often time-consuming work-up of anterior knee pain. The importance of performing this evaluation slowly, step by step, increases with the length of time the athlete has suffered, the more medical personnel who have been consulted, and the more therapy that has been undergone without success. If the testing requires several visits to complete, it is acceptable. Individuals with protracted and resistant symptoms comprise a diagnostic and therapeutic challenge. The contributing factors are outlined in Table 12-8, from which a treatment plan may be formulated. Furthermore, a patellofemoral functional scale may assist in documenting the current status of the athlete as well as the efficacy of any treatment regimen (Fig. 12-28). Scores of more than 80 are excellent, 70 to 80 good, 50 to 70 fair, and 30 to 50 poor; scores of less than 30 indicate severe disability.

Medical Therapy

For the most part, there is relatively little place for drug therapy in the patellofemoral pain syndrome. NSAIDs are effective if there is an element of synovitis, tendinitis, or bursitis; but they rarely affect classic patellofemoral pain. Intermittent and long-term acetylsalicylic acid therapy has been suggested, particularly with reference to its cartilage-stabilizing action. However, the enthusiasm for this approach has

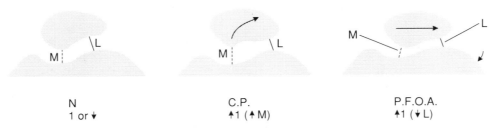

Fig. 12-27. Patellofemoral index. This index (PFI) is the relation between the relative thickness of the medial patellofemoral compartment and the lateral compartment. M is the shortest distance between the medial femoral groove and the junction between the medial and lateral facets. L is the shortest distance between the lateral facet and the lateral femoral condyle. In normal individuals the PFI is 1 : 1 or less. The index may be larger in chondromalacia (C.P.), as M may be increased, and in lateral patellofemoral arthritis (P.F.O.A.) because L is decreased. The former is due to laxity; the latter is due to articular cartilage wear.

TABLE 12-12. Synovial Fluid Analysis of the Knee

Parameter	Normal	Noninflammatory	Inflammatory	Septic
Volume	<5	Often >5	Often >5	Often >5
Color	Clear	Yellow	Yellow to opalescent	Yellow to green
Viscosity	High	High	Low	Variable
WBC/μl	<200	200–2000	2,000–100,000	>100,000
Polymorphonuclear leukocytes (%)	<25	<25	50+	75+[a]
Culture	Negative	Negative	Negative	Often positive
Crystals	Negative	Negative	May be positive	Negative
Antibodies	Negative	Occasionally few	Present	Variable
Glucose (mg/dl)	Nearly equal to blood	Nearly equal to blood	>25 lower than blood	>25 lower than blood

[a] Lower with infections with low virulence organisms or that have been partially treated.

waned. It is effective as a mild analgesic and may help in attenuating postexercise discomfort.

Intra-articular injections of steroid may assist a few individuals who have synovitis or a persistent effusion but only after mechanical derangement has been ruled out. Furthermore, in the presence of cartilage damage, recurrent steroid injection can only contribute to further cartilage atrophy. It is therefore rarely indicated. If a large, symptomatic plica is suspected, placement of steroid along the course of the plica occasionally produces dramatic relief. An intra-articular injection of lidocaine sometimes completely relieves pain; and it assists in localizing the site of pain to capsular, rather than bony, structures.

Treatment

Clinical Point

TREATMENT

- Correct training errors
- Modification of activity
- Attempts to alter biomechanics
- Muscle strengthening
- Drug therapy
- Surgery

When the pain syndrome is mild, reassuring the athlete and parent that there is little or no cartilage damage and that the injury will not progress to serious arthritis is sometimes all that is required. With this knowledge, stress is relieved and young individuals are willing to continue their activities and to handle the small amount of discomfort. This approach presupposes that the physician is satisfied that the

articular surface damage is indeed minimal and significant articular diseases have been ruled out.

Orthoses

It is preferable to commence a program of therapy without the use of an orthosis, but if progress is not made orthoses comprise a second line of supplemental therapy. Foot and knee alignment suggests the possibility and need for either a heel wedge or cup in addition to medial foot posting.

Clinical Point

FOOT ORTHOSIS

- Shock absorbtion
- Alignment correction
- Motion control
- Leg length equalization
- Heel raise
- Relief of pressure points

Knee orthoses consist of either some form of infrapatellar support or a patella-stabilizing brace. The mode of action of the infrapatellar strap is not understood, although some clinical series suggest its effectiveness (Fig. 29).[69,70] The patellar knee sleeve with various lateral stabilizing pads or straps have been well documented to relieve pain and enhance the ability to achieve quadriceps control (Fig. 12-30).[71,72] These patella braces are most effective when there is a significant tracking problem or even subluxation. They may also produce pain relief where there is minimal retropatellar chondromalacic change, but be-

Patellofemoral Function Scale

History

Pain

None	10
During vigorous activity	8
During light activity	4
At rest after activity	2
Daily pain irrespective of activity*	0

Function

Movie sign	
Absent	4
Present	0
Walking	
No restriction	5
Restricted	0
Stair climbing	
No restriction	5
Restricted	0
Jogging	
No restriction	6
Restricted	0
Sprint & cutting	
No restriction	10
Restricted	0

Orthosis**

None	4
Knee sleeve or shoe insole	2
Total contact knee orthosis	1
Walking cane	0

Examination

Effusion

None	6
Present	0

Patellar crepitus (passive)

None	6
Mild	4
Severe***	0

Patellar crepitus (resisted)

None	4
Mild	2
Severe	0

Quads atrophy

None	4
>1cm	2
>2cm	1
>3cm	0

Apprehension Test

Negative	6
Present	0

Clark's sign

In extension	
Mild or Negative	4
Severe	0
At 10° flexion	
Mild or Negative	6
Severe	0

Range of motion

Full	6
<10° limitation	4
>10° limitation	0

Pain with motion

Full and pain free	6
Mild pain with resistance***	4
Severe pain with resistance	2
Painful no resistance	0

Squatting

No problem	8
Slightly impaired	6
Not past 90°	2
Unable	0

80+	**Excellent**
70-80	**Good**
50-70	**Fair**
30-50	**Poor**
30	**Severe disability**

Needs stable knee

Only mark one in each category

*Includes night pain

**Regular use for activity

***Firm manual resistance
Compare to other knee

Fig. 12-28. Patellofemoral functional scale, which is particularly useful for assessing treatment programs.

come progressively less efficient as the degree of cartilage damage increases. It is difficult to predict which patients are likely to achieve some relief, and the prescription of these braces must always be accompanied by an exercise program for vastus medialis.

In young, active individuals who have severe protracted symptoms, there is a temptation to rest the limb by use of a cast. In conditions where theoretically there may be poor cartilage nutrition and in which muscle insufficiency may play a role, the use of cast immobilization would empirically lead only to further

deterioration of the chondromalacic process and contribute to atrophy. In practice, this fear is realized, and rarely does casting provide permanent or even temporary relief.

There is, however, an attractive alternative in patients with intractable pain who have failed other conservative therapies, who are not surgical candidates, or who are already surgical failures. It is a dynamic total contact knee orthosis with polycentric hinges locked to allow 0 to 30 degrees range of motion; it may be removed for therapy. Remarkable suc-

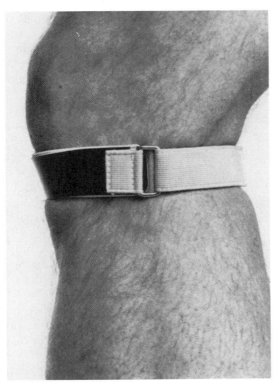
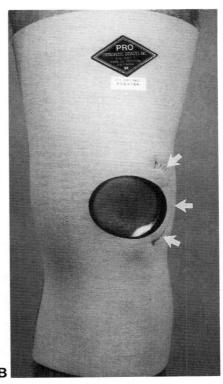

A   **B**

Fig. 12-29. (A) Infrapatellar strap as described by Levine and Splain.[69] **(B)** One variety of elastic knee sleeve with a lateral stabilizing pad.

cess has been achieved in difficult cases, but it is sometimes difficult to wean these patients from the brace, and there is a tendency to recurrence. It is, nevertheless, an important treatment technique for difficult cases. This system is most effective when used in conjunction with biofeedback training.

Exercise Modification

Exercise modification is one of the keys to successful treatment. Identification of specific triggering activities is important. For instance, the commencement of indoor track work, introduction of an intensive sprinting program, a sudden increase in mileage, or starting a running program may be modifiable factors.

The therapist should carefully explain the retropatellar forces involved in these activities, so the athlete and coach are willing to cooperate. Communication and instilling confidence are the two predictors of success for this part of the therapy. For avid runners, some form of impact reduction is necessary; and if the

syndrome is severe, water-running may be all that is tolerated.

In dancers, modification of foot position, reducing the number of jumps or pliés, practicing in more

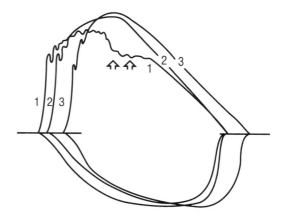

Fig. 12-30. Tracing on an isokinetic test shows a pain pattern when extension is performed without the dynamic knee support.[71,72] (1 = normal, 2 = pain, 3 = with knee support.)

Clinical Point

TRAINING ERRORS

- Sudden increase in distance
- Terrain: hills, hard surfaces, road camber
- Increased speed work
- Multiple deep knee bends
- Repetitive jumping
- Stair running routines
- Increased weight training

---

shock-absorbing footwear when practical, and "walking through" routines at rehearsals may enable continuation of activity while pain is reduced. The modification of exercise presents an excellent opportunity to complete a "patellofemoral" functional scale (Fig. 12-28). This scale, which has been modified over several research projects, is a good guide to the severity of knee pain and may be used for documenting progress.

Clinical Points

RUNNING MODIFICATIONS

- Water-running
- Simulated running on resistance apparatus
- Stair climbing machines
- Walk–run programs
- Avoid sprints with rapid stops
- Avoid extreme distances
- Cut out hills
- Build up slowly
- Consider lay off

Specific Therapy

Realizing the futility of trying to gain strength in the face of reflex inhibition and the presence of wasting due to pain or effusion, specific therapy techniques should adhere to the following principles.

1. Use appropriate modalities to reduce pain and effusion.

2. Assess joint ranges through which resistance does not generate discomfort.
3. Devise a resistance program utilizing this pain-free range.
4. Supplement strengthening with electrostimulation when appropriate.
5. When control is poor, use biofeedback training.
6. Try to include eccentric loading at some point in the program.
7. Address specific control and strength of the vastus medialis obliquus.
8. Address whole limb strength and balance of power between muscle groups.
9. Assess local hypermobility or peripatellar tightness and stretch appropriately.
10. Assess for generalized or specific muscle group tightness and correct by stretching protocols.
11. Do not ignore proximal and distal segment stretches.
12. Educate patients and promote their enthusiasm to achieve full cooperation with the program.
13. Integrate program with modification and progression of sports goals.
14. Introduce functional exercises within treatment plan.
15. Ensure that the patient has a well conceived, well taught home program to supplement therapy.
16. Do not overtreat. Get patients involved with their own care, so they fully comprehend the goals of therapy.

These principles should fit into the overall approach to the patient with patellofemoral pain outlined in Fig. 12-31.

Quadriceps Exercises

There are five basic patterns of quadriceps activity, each of which may produce a different pain response depending on the location, severity, and etiology of the anterior knee pain. Other than stressing that the exercise mode should not produce pain, the exercise approach should be tailored to the individual patient. Exercise patterns include the following.

1. Isometric straight leg quadriceps setting and leg raising
2. Isometric or isokinetic concentric knee extension
3. Extensor thrust (squatting) pattern concentric work
4. Isotonic eccentric work in a leg extension pattern
5. Eccentric quadriceps work in an extensor thrust (squatting) pattern

Treatment Plan for Patellofemoral Pain

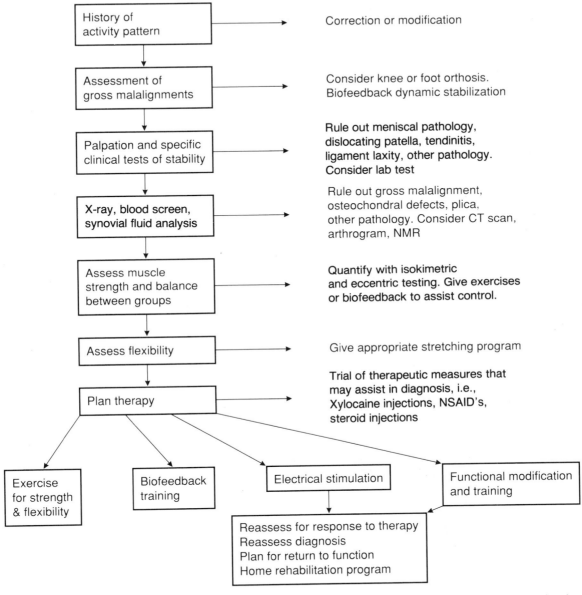

Fig. 12-31. Approach to investigation and treatment planning in patients with patellofemoral pain.

Role of Isometric Quadriceps Work in Exercise

The highest torque of the knee extensor muscles usually occurs with the knee at an angle of 60 degrees during maximum isometric contraction.[73] However, mechanical and compressive forces across the patellar and femoral articular surfaces are maximized by knee extension programs and may therefore aggravate the primary problem of retropatellar pain.[73] Furthermore, continuous and comparable electromyographic (EMG) activity is generated in all parts of the quadriceps at full extension, not just the vastus medialis.[35] Cine-EMG reveals that full extension of the knee is essential to derive maximum benefit from straight leg raising and quadriceps setting exercises.[73] Ten to twenty degrees of flexion of the knee as seen with extensor lag reduces the muscle effort in the vastus group by approximately 25 percent of the muscle effort demonstrated in full extension (Fig. 12-32).

The entire quadriceps group contracts and relaxes in unison at terminal extension and at 10 to 20 degrees of flexion. Therefore an adequate hypertrophy effect can be obtained by straight leg raising or quadriceps setting, if it is the only pain-free position for the patient.

Knight has described an isokinetic protocol utilizing a daily adjustable progressive resisted exercise (DAPRE) program.[74] It involves repeating straight-legged isometric contractions of 6 seconds followed by 4-second rest periods. The athlete lifts the weights by hand to a horizontal position; the leg is then extended freely to a position of extension, at which point the weight is lowered onto and supported by the extended leg. After a 6-second isometric hold, the weight is lifted off the leg for a 4-second rest period. On the third and fourth sets the repetitions are counted until the athlete is unable to hold the weight without bending the knee more than 5 degrees.

The first set includes 10 repetitions against 50 percent of the working weight for that day (Table 12-13). The second set is performed using 75 percent for six repetitions. On the third set, the athlete should perform as many repetitions as possible against a full working weight. The fourth set consists of maximal repetitions; however, they are performed against an adjusted working weight based on the number of repetitions performed in the third set.[74] The weight should be decreased if fewer than five were managed and increased if eight or more were performed. The working weight for the next treatment session is determined by the number of repetitions performed during the fourth set (Table 12-14).

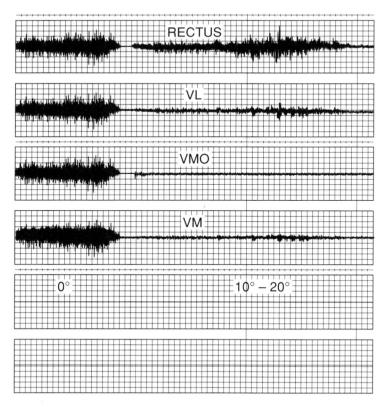

Fig. 12-32. Electromyographic recordings with maximal quadriceps contraction in full extension (quadriceps settings) versus 10 to 20 degrees of flexion. V.L. = vastus lateralis; VMO = vastus medialis obliquus; VM = vastus medialis longus (extensor portion).

TABLE 12-13. DAPRE System of Knight

Parameter	Set 1	Set 2	Set 3	Set 4
Percent of working weight	50	75	100	Adjusted[a]
No. of repetitions	10	6	Maximal	Maximal[b]

[a] Adjusted working weight for the fourth set is determined by the number of repetitions performed during the third set.

[b] The number of repetitions performed during the fourth set determines the working weight for the subsequent day's working weight.

Leg Extension Versus Extensor Thrust (Squat)

There are many discrepancies among various experimental mechanical models, cadaver studies, and in vivo calculation of quadriceps forces (Fig. 12-33). For this reason, absolute figures should be used only in general terms to help establish principles. Attempts have also been made to correlate these findings with absolute contact so the force per unit area may be expressed. There is approximately 2 cm² of contact area at 30 degrees, 3 cm² at 60 degrees, and nearly 5 cm² at 90 degrees. It is bound to modify surface pressures. Theoretically, with leg extension using 9 kg (20 lb) of resistance, a peak patellofemoral force of 120 kg occurs at 36 degrees, dropping to almost 0 at 90 degrees) of flexion. Direct experimental measurements, however, show little change in stress, through the range 10 to 50 degrees of flexion (Fig. 12-34). Pain is not necessarily related in a simple way to just compression forces. Surface shearing forces, quadriceps pull, and tension on the retinacular structure may be equally important.

The leverages involved in leg extension work magnify these forces to the point that minimal resistance may generate forces equivalent to those imposed by squatting with joint gravitational effects on body weight. Furthermore, the maximal stress is in a totally different range. Maximal loads are at 20 to 30 degrees for the leg extension motion due to decreasing quadriceps efficiency, whereas these peak forces are 60 to 90 degrees with squatting (Fig. 12-35).

Eccentric Muscle Work

Although little has been written regarding the use of eccentric muscle exercise for patellofemoral pain, some normal values have been established.[75,76] Bennet and Straube reported a rehabilitation protocol that serves as both an objective assessment of treatment progress and a therapeutic exercise plan.[41] The protocol consists in multiple sets of 10 pain-free repetitions at the constant velocity settings of 30, 60, and 90 degrees per second, for a total of 90 repetitions per session. The rest intervals are established by the patient, as is the threshold force on a computer-controlled dynamometer (KIN/COM).[41]

McConnell Regimen

An alternative approach to the nonoperative therapy of patellofemoral pain has been presented and readily accepted by a large portion of the physiotherapy community.[9] This program is based on a careful physical assessment of patellar position and overall limb alignment, the evaluation of patellar mobility or lack of it, and determination of the pain pattern in functional positions. From this information, the patellar position is optimized by judicious taping, bio-

TABLE 12-14. Working Weight Adjustment: DAPRE System

No. of Repetitions Performed During Set	Adjusted Working Weight for Fourth Set (lb)	Working Weight for Next Session (lb)
0–2	Decrease 5–10	Decrease 5–10
3–4	Decrease 0–5	Keep the same
5–7	Keep the same	Increase 2.5–7.5
8–10	Increase 2.5–5.0	Increase 5–10
>10	Increase 5–10	Increase 10–15

(After Knight,[74] with permission.)

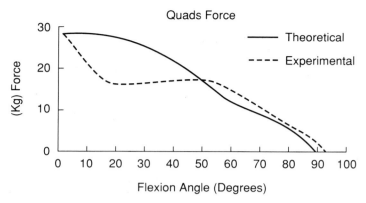

Fig. 12-33. Theoretical quadriceps force needed to produce a leg extension against 9 kg of resistance is not the same as experimentally measured values.

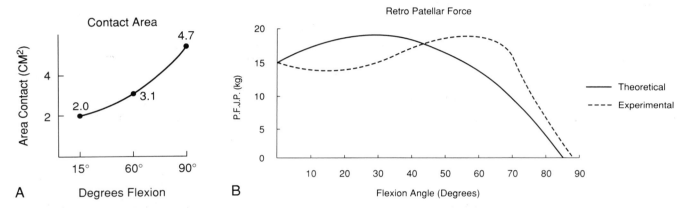

Fig. 12-34. (A) With nonresisted, active knee extension, retropatellar forces are related to the knee flexion angle. **(B)** Patellofemoral contact area also changes with knee position, which influences the theoretic versus actual forces. (P.F.J.P. = patellofemoral joint pressures.)

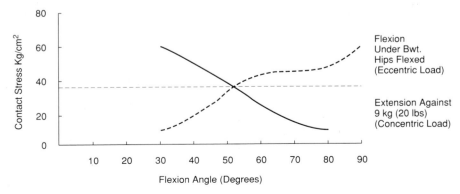

Fig. 12-35. Comparison of retropatellar contact stresses with concentric knee extension versus eccentric knee flexion illustrates contrasting loading on the patella.

feedback supplementation of vastus medialis control, stretching of tight structures on the lateral side the knee as well as generally in the limb, and instigation of a well-rehearsed home program. It should be emphasized that it is not simply a strengthening routine but a serious attempt at establishing functionally adequate control of the vastus medialis. Hence the biofeedback component is central to its success.[75–79]

Before embarking on specific evaluation of the patella, McConnell insisted on a careful assessment of all lower limb mechanics, including (1) studying all of the previously described alignment factors; (2) recording dynamic alignments when walking, walking on the heels and with feet in the inverted and everted positions, stair climbing, and squatting; (3) specific tests of muscle tightness; and (4) specific stress tests for back and knee pathology.

The glide component determines the amount of lateral deviation of the patella in the frontal plane. The normal patellar position should be approximately midway between the two femoral condyles. Almost all symptomatic individuals require a medial glide of the patella. The amount of glide possible varies depending on the elasticity of the lateral structures and, in the active situation, the strength of the vastus medialis obliquus (VMO) compared with the vastus lateralis (VL) (Fig. 12-36).

The degree of patellar tilt is detected by comparing the height of the medial patellar border with the height of the lateral patellar border. This component determines the degree of tightness in the deep retinacular fibers.

The rotation component determines if there is any deviation of the long axis of the patella from the long axis of the femur. The patella should be parallel with the long axis of the femur.

Practice Point

McCONNELL REGIMEN

- Evaluate static and dynamic alignment.
- Establish functional painful and pain-free ranges.
- Assess muscle and other soft tissue tightness.
- Carefully evaluate patellar position.
- Utilize stretching and taping to achieve corrected patellar position.
- Teach control of vastus medialis obliquus (VMO) by biofeedback.
- Progress through increasingly more difficult functional activities.
- Establish a home program.
- Reassess at intervals to make sure progress is maintained.

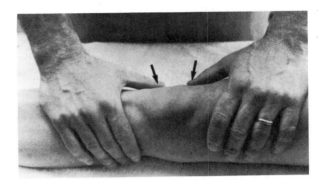

A

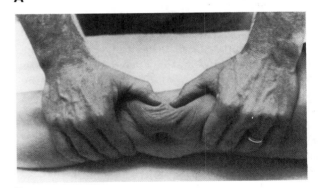

B

Fig. 12-36. Medial patellar glide assessed in the relaxed knee. The amount of glide is classified as quadrants of the patella. This maneuver also may be used to stretch the lateral retinaculum and, with slight modification of the hand position, the medial glide.

The patellofemoral joint is essentially a "soft tissue" joint, which means that regardless of the mechanical alignment, the position of the patella relative to the femur potentially can be changed. An optimal patellar position maximizes the surface area of contact and ensures an even distribution of load. To determine normal patellar orientation, three components must be examined: glide, tilt, and rotation.

Maintenance of appropriate patellar alignment is achieved by the following.

1. Stretching the tight lateral structures (a) actively, where a medial glide and a medial tilt are performed by the therapist; and (b) passively, by continuous firm taping of the patella. These maneuvers have a greater effect on stretching the lateral structures than the more traditional iliotibial band stretches, which seem to be ineffective at stretching the distal attachment of the band.
2. Specific training of the VMO to overcome any tendency of the patella to drift laterally. It attempts to maintain adequate medial pull on the patella. It cannot be done unless the patient is pain-free.

By determining which components need to be corrected, the patella can be taped into the appropriate alignment so the patient is pain-free with the knee feeling "stronger." This step also aids in distinguishing patellofemoral pain from meniscal, plical, and other pathology. If successful, with the tape in place the patient theoretically should be able to exercise and train with little or no pain, as the patellar tracking has been influenced. The major advantage of tape over the conventional straps or braces is its flexibility; that is, each individual is taught how to tape his or her own patella to change its unique alignment (Fig. 12-37).

The glide component can be corrected by firmly gliding the patella medially and taping the lateral patellar border. The tilt component can be corrected by firm taping from the middle of the patella medially, which lifts the lateral border and provides passive stretch to the lateral structures. To correct external rotation of the patella, firm taping from the middle inferior pole upward and medially is required. For correction of internal rotation, a firm tape from the middle superior pole downward and medially is needed.

A patient may have one or more of these components, and the severity varies from patient to patient. Each abnormal component must be corrected adequately if the patient is going to train and resume all activities in a pain-free manner.

The worst component is always corrected first. Three or four pieces of firm tape may be necessary to ensure that the patella is normally oriented. The tape must be a rigid, nonstretch tape, so it can effectively change patellar alignment. The tape is needed only while the VMO is being trained to actively maintain the appropriate orientation of the patella.

Once the corrected position is established, its effectiveness is tested in the various positions and readjusted if necessary (Fig. 12-38).

Preventing malalignment of the patella to affect the pressure distribution to the underlying articular cartilage may involve subtle shifts in the timing or amount of VMO activity in particular parts of the range during certain activities. **Training the VMO should be regarded as a motor skill acquisition rather** than a strengthening procedure.[77] Muscle training has been found to be specific to limb position, joint angle, velocity of contraction, contraction type, and contraction force.

Appropriate training allows the motor control system to acquire information necessary to change the length–tension properties of the agonist, in this case the VMO and its antagonist the VL. Modification of the length–tension relation changes the equilibrium point.[70] In the case of the patellofemoral joint, the new equilibrium point ideally enables appropriate alignment of the patella. It must be remembered that, as with all skill acquisition, this ability is enhanced and maintained with practice but deteriorates unless actively refreshed.[77]

It should be recalled that the vastus medialis is composed of two functional parts: the vastus medialis longus and the vastus medialis obliquus. The vastus medialis longus acts with the rest of the quadriceps muscle to extend the knee.[35] The vastus medialis obliquus, on the other hand, plays little role in extending the knee but acts to realign the patella medially during the extension maneuver. It is active throughout the whole range of extension, not just the last 10 to 15 degrees. In fact, the entire quadriceps must generate up to 60 percent more tension at this point in the range of motion. When the vastus medialis obliquus is examined anatomically, it can be seen that it arises from the adductor magnus tendon and is frequently innervated independently from the rest of the quadriceps by a branch from the femoral nerve.[35,80] These findings have significant implications for rehabilitation of the vastus medialis obliquus and the treatment of patellofemoral pain.

The normal VMO/VL ratio of EMG activity is $1:1$.[80] In patellofemoral pain sufferers, the activity in the vastus medialis decreases significantly; and instead of being tonically active, the VMO becomes phasic in action (Fig. 12-39),[38] which may explain the onset of pain further into, rather than at the beginning of, an activity.

The presence of pain, effusion, or both in the knee joint reflexively inhibits quadriceps activity, particu-

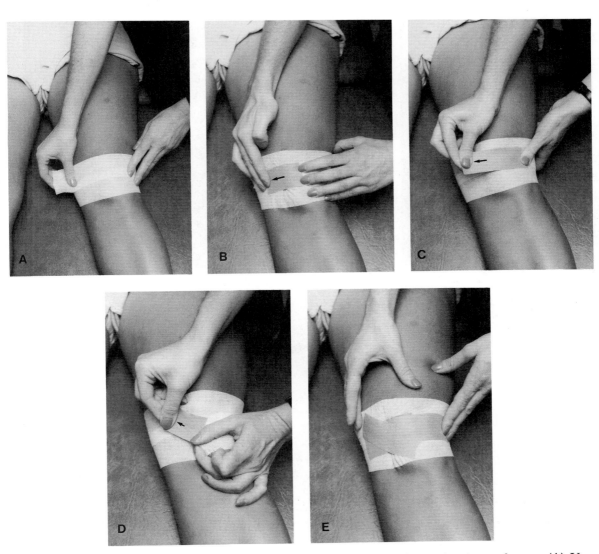

Fig. 12-37. Application of McConnell tape technique for patellofemoral pain syndrome. **(A)** Underwrap put on to protect skin (Fixomull; see design in Figure 13-10). Make sure there is enough tape medially. **(B)** Correction of patella tilt. Tape starts half-way across the patella and is then pulled medially. **(C)** Correction of glide, applied from the lateral retinacular area. Pull straight across. **(D)** Correction of a lateral rotation. **(E)** Finish tape—in this case correction of the tilt, glide, and lateral rotation is needed. The worse component is corrected first.

larly that of the VMO. **The VMO is inhibited after only 20 ml of saline is present in the knee joint,** whereas 50 to 60 ml of saline is required before the rectus femoris and vastus lateralis muscles are affected. This fact seems to be borne out clinically with the onset of patellofemoral symptoms or after a traumatic knee injury such as a ligamentous rupture and meniscal lesions. Extrapolating this concept further, unless rehabilitation is specific, many patients with early osteoarthritis with frequent episodes of low

grade effusion continue to have poor quadriceps function.

Initially, the specific training should include an isometric adduction component. This facilitates VMO contraction since many of the fibers originate from the adductor magnus. It also helps to de-emphasize the role of vastus lateralis and rectus femoris in initiating the contraction. The quality of the VMO contraction, rather than the quantity, is the primary concern. Biofeedback may be used to help augment

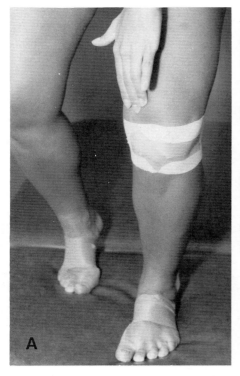

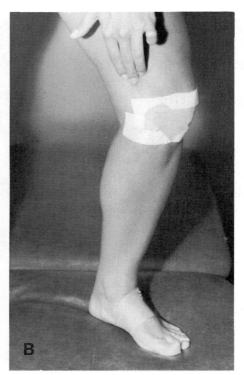

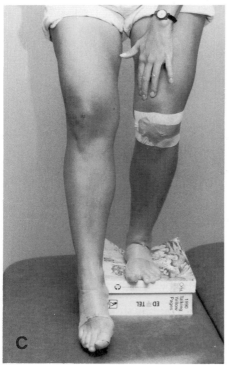

Fig. 12-38. Initially training is enhanced by tape application and biofeedback. When control is gained, a series of functional positions are adopted in this case. **(A)** Walk stance at 30 degrees of knee flexion. **(B)** Plié position facilitates contraction of the vastus medialis obliquus. **(C)** Stepping down stairs to gain eccentric control. Sport- or occupation-related position are then adopted. While the motor skill is being learnt it sometimes helps to feel the muscle contraction to facilitate biofeedback.

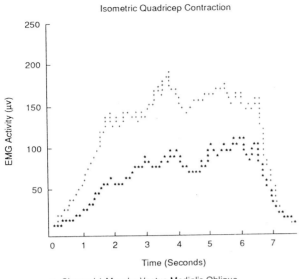

Fig. 12-39. Electromyographic activity during isometric quadriceps contraction in a patient with knee pain. Note the irregular phasic activity.

Isometric Quadricep Contraction

+ Channel 1 Muscle: Vastus Medialis Oblique

* Channel 2 Muscle: Vastus Lateralis

training. Later the adductor activity can be decreased, and isolated VMO activity should be practiced, which can be done in the sitting position to alleviate the symptoms of "movie-goer's knee" and in the walk–standing position to stimulate the support phase of running where pronation control can also be practiced.

Specific activation of the VMO can then be incorporated into the positions specific to the patient's activity or sport, e.g., a semisquat position simulating the parallel turn maneuvers for skiing or the plié for the ballet dancer. The patient is advised to practice a "little at frequent intervals," as this type of training initially requires great concentration and can cause rapid VMO fatigue. Once the VMO is fatigued, control becomes poor, training effects are decreased, and pain and effusion are likely sequelae.

To achieve patient compliance and hence long-term success, the patient must have an understanding of what the training is attempting to do. Training must never continue through pain. If pain occurs, the athlete should stop and readjust the tape before continuing the activity. The tape loosens relatively quickly if the lateral structures are extremely tight or the individual is involved in vigorous athletic pursuit. Once the tape is loose, appropriate patellar alignment is not maintained and the symptoms return. If

pain persists despite retaping, more stressful activities should not be performed until the VMO has improved sufficiently to enable pain-free activity. If the patella can be oriented correctly, and this orientation can be maintained with the tape while the VMO is specifically trained, it seems that it is possible to trigger the VMO to respond to a new length/tension ratio provided this motor program is reinforced.

McConnell reported a high rate of clinical success in returning her patients to activity free of discomfort.[9] We have also had success in our rehabilitation setting, although not to the same degree as McConnell.

Taping itself presents some problems. The 1.5-inch tape must be adherent and not possess any elastic component. The tape is important as correction of the patellar alignment gives the athlete the opportunity to train the VMO while pain-free, thereby eliminating inhibition. However, frequently the athlete must be retaped during a prolonged practice session for the particular sport. The tension placed on the skin, the chemical nature of good adhesive tape, and the frequency of skin irritation or allergies in the population may cause a high incidence of skin breakdown. The use of an adhesive-backed undercover seems to delay this problem in some patients. Applying a protective layer of OpCit or Tegaderm may permit continuation of taping without additional skin irritation.

The biofeedback component of the VMO training, without eliciting excessive contraction of the remainder of the quadriceps, is an important component; and further supplementation by electrical muscle stimulation is often helpful during the early sessions.[38] The athletes are easily discouraged if they are allowed to leave the first sessions without mastering the preferential VMO contraction.

Surgical Therapy

Surgical treatment for anterior knee pain essentially fits into five main categories.

1. Procedures that are done for major tracking problems and dislocations
2. Those done for lateral facet hyperpressure syndrome
3. Procedures to release or remove symptomatic plicae
4. Operations for patellofemoral chondromalacia of significant grades, including arthrosis
5. Procedures for patellofemoral pain of uncertain etiology, which includes many of the subtle align-

ment factors, growth, muscle imbalance, and early surface changes of chondromalacia

There is varying success with all these procedures, although most are associated with excellent early results (Table 12-15). Only reports presenting a 2-year or more follow-up are valid commentaries on the efficacy of these procedures. Surgery for vague patellofemoral pain has a poor outcome and often leads to a vicious cycle of more extensive and numerous surgical procedures. Before any surgery is attempted, there should be a concerted effort to establish a clear etiologic framework, as well as the anatomic and biomechanical goals of the procedure to be performed.[81] There should be a clearly demonstrated failure of nonoperative therapy and not simply noncompliance with therapy protocols. Although nonoperative treatment is the cornerstone of therapy for most of these patellofemoral problems, particularly those without demonstrable cartilage damage, there is the concurrent danger of waiting too long. It is equally inappropriate to delay surgery past the point where adequate intervention could delay, retard, or reverse some early articular surface damage. This protocol, then, is the art of surgery: assembling the known scientific data, carefully evaluating the athlete, projecting the consequence of continued nonoperative treatment, and picking not only the correct procedure but the optimal timing of that procedure.[82] Lastly, careful postoperative routines are essential to optimize the results of surgery and to give the best chance of extending excellent early postoperative successes into long-term or permanent improvement of function.

Arthroscopy

Arthroscopy as a diagnostic tool may be valuable in eliminating some of the more unusual intra-articular sources of pain, assessing the degree of damage to the articular surface and carrying out specific procedures such as plical release, retinacular release, or the treatment of osteochondral defects. The fat pad may be examined, and the tracking of the patella evaluated to some degree. Considerable experience along with a careful preoperative assessment is needed to place the numerous variations in anatomy in a normal knee into perspective. It is often tempting to "assign blame" just by virtue of the fact that those variations are present, when in reality they may have nothing to do with the athlete's symptoms.

Jackson and colleagues discussed the efficacy of lavage alone for obtaining pain relief of grade I idiopathic chondromalacia.[28,83] It is difficult to understand their high remission rate of 88 percent at 1 year and 82 percent at 5 years (Table 12-16). It is probable that the pain in these individuals did not stem from the patellar lesion but from the pericapsular structures. Perhaps the distention and chemical effect of the saline played a role in altering the pain pattern in these individuals.

TABLE 12-15.   Surgery for Patellofemoral Pain

Indication	Procedure
Major tracking problems (subluxation) and dislocations	Lateral retinacular release Distal or proximal realignments Goldthwaite Elmslie-Trilliat
Lateral facet hyperpressure	Lateral retinacular release Maquet procedure Lateral facetectomy
Minor tracking problems, chondromalacia grades I and II	Surgical procedures Arthroscopic assessment Distal realignment
Symptomatic plica	Arthroscopic plical release or excision
Patellofemoral chondromalacia grades III and IV and arthrosis	Arthroscopic débridement Drilling and curettage Elmslie-Trilliat distal realignment Anterior tubercle advancement Patellectomy

TABLE 12-16. Arthroscopic Lavage, Shaving, and Lateral Retinacular Release in Patients with Patellofemoral Problems and Chondromalacic Changes

Condition and Grade	Procedure	At 1 Year (% good)[a]	At 5 Years (% good)
Idiopathic chondromalacia			
I	L	88	82
II	L	63	28
	R + L	60	29
	R + S + L	63	52
	S + L	53	15
III	R + S + L	50	14
Post-traumatic chondromalacia			
I	S + L	86	83
II	S + L	79	73
III	S + L	43	20
Maltracking patella			
I	S + L + R	88	85
	S + L + R	87	65
	S + L + R	67	20
Unstable patella			
I	R + L	100	100
	S + L	35	28
II	R + S + L	55	33
III	S + L	30	25
	R + S + L	40	25

Graded according to Jackson et al.[23,83]
R = lateral retinacular release; S = shaving; L = lavage.
[a] "Good" results indicate little or no discomfort, and the patient could pursue desired activity.

Lateral Retinacular Release

With lateral retinacular release the tight retinacular structures are divided to reduce lateral pressures and centralize the patella (Fig. 12-40). This procedure is used extensively for patellofemoral pain and for patellar subluxation and dislocation. There has been some discussion as to its efficacy in redistributing retropatellar pressures, but the procedure is undoubtedly helpful for alleviating patellar subluxation or dislocation.[22,84,85] A positive apprehension test and a positive Merchant view with excessive patella overhang correlate well with success.[86] The effectiveness of this procedure is undeniable in carefully selected patients, **but by and large it is probably the most overused and abused procedure in the treatment of patellofemoral disorders.**[61,86–90] Hence there is the belief among some surgeons that it has little more than a placebo effect. Early excellent results often reverse dramatically as time elapses (Table 12-17). Kolowich and co-workers have presented some clear

indications for success with this procedure by comparing the extremes of excellent results and the failures.[61] Clearly the ideal candidate has a tight lateral tether and a normal Q-angle, or tubercle sulcus angle. Conversely, the worst results are anticipated in patients with excessive laxity of the medial and lateral retinaculum and an abnormal Q-angle if the procedure is performed simply for pain relief. There are a large number of individuals between these extremes who have no firm contraindications but who are obviously not ideal candidates; these individuals should be operated on with caution. Furthermore, inability to successfully alter the Merchant view silhouette, excessive postoperative hemorrhage, and lack of early reduction in pain correlate with poor results.

Postoperative care is essential to minimize hemorrhage and effusion. Quadriceps contractions, straight leg raising, gentle range of motion, and partial weight-bearing are keys to early success. With tense effusions or hemarthrosis, aspiration at 7 to 10 days speeds recovery. Application of the McConnell

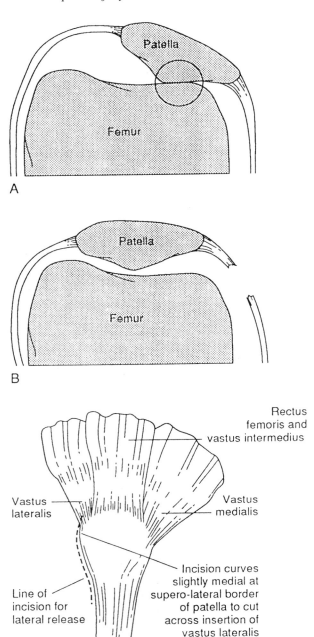

A

B

C

Fig. 12-40. (A) Lateral patellofemoral hyperpressure secondary to tight lateral reticular structures. **(B)** Theoretically, the lateral retinacular release should reduce these pressures by altering the patellar position and tracking. **(C)** Line of incision ensures some defunctioning of the vastus lateralis to add a dynamic component to the release.

techniques for vastus medialis control and patellar mobilization improves long-term results. Furthermore, it is probably wise to re-establish this program at 6 months after operation to ensure that the lateral scar is not contracting and tightening and that medialis control is maintained.

Patellar Tendon Transfers

The classic Hauser procedure for distal patellar realignment resulted in excessive tension and an unacceptable degree of long-term degenerative change. It was in part due to the distal transfer of the tibial tubercle and partly because medial transplantation generates posterior displacement due to the upper tibial configuration. The Elmslie-Trilliat procedure uses a thin wafer of bone, which in conjunction with a retinacular release is medialized to correct the Q-angle without distal displacement.[91] This procedure is excellent for correcting severe alignment and tracking problems, with particularly good long-term results in recurrent dislocation. However, there is little evidence that medialization decreases patellofemoral pressures, and it is doubtful if this procedure has any advantage over simple retinacular release for hyperpressure syndrome unless some anterior advancement of the tubercle is achieved.[92,93] Furthermore, it requires a larger incision and the use of internal fixation; hence it has a higher complication rate.

Postoperative cast immobilization for 6 weeks is common, but in athletes a cast brace, locked 0 to 20 degrees, gives adequate support along with some patellar motion and thus minimizes wasting. It is the postoperative treatment of choice. Partial to full weight-bearing is progressed as tolerated. Static quadriceps work during extension is begun immediately postoperatively, but increased resistance work is delayed until 4 weeks to allow early union of the tubercle.

Proximal Realignment

In the skeletally immature, distal bony procedures are likely to damage the tibial tubercle apophysis. Hence proximal realignment is used, combining a lateral retinacular release with advancement and plication of the vastus medialis and adjacent medial retinacular structures. With significant patellar hypoplasia, a large Q-angle, or generalized ligament laxity, these proximal procedures may be insufficient, and some form of patellar tendon realignment using only soft tissue is added (Goldthwait procedure). These procedures require 4 to 6 weeks of protection, fol-

TABLE 12-17. Lateral Retinacular Release for Patellofemoral Pain

Study	Average Follow-up (months)	Success Rate Study (%)
Harwin and Stern	30	100
Lankenner et al.[87]	25.6	79
Krompinger & Fulkerson[88]	18	79
Micheli & Stanitski[89]	18	77
Osborne & Fulford[90] (early)	12	87
Osborne and Fulford[90] (late)	36	37
Betz et al.[84] (early)	12	100
Betz et al.[84] (late)	48	67
Reid (early)[a]	14	87
Reid (late)[a]	32	68

Note: Nearly all studies with long-term follow-up report a dropping off of initial success.

[a] Personal data.

lowing which intensive therapy for the vastus medialis component of the quadriceps is mandatory to make use of the advancement of this muscle.

Tibial Tubercle Elevation

Anterior advancement of the tibial tuberosity is advocated for the relief of pain from retropatellar articular surface grade III and IV chondromalacia and arthrosis.[93–95] The operation is commonly known as the Bandi or Maquet procedure although other methods are described using an oblique osteotomy and sliding medially the wedge of tubercle.[96,97] The patella's contribution to the extension moment arm increases as the knee is extended. At full extension, the patella accounts for 31 percent of the entire extension moment arm. Between 90 and 120 degrees of flexion, the patella's contribution is as little as 13 percent.

Quick Facts

KNEE EXTENSION MOMENT ARM

Flexion Angle (degrees)	Patellar Effect (%)
0	31
30	24
60	17
90	13
120	14

Theoretically, advancement of the tibial tubercle increases the moment arm and thus the mechanical advantage of the quadriceps through the patellar ligament, which should reduce the forces acting across the patellofemoral joint. Maquet demonstrated that at 45 degrees of flexion advancement of the tubercle by 1 cm reduced the retropatellar force by 33 percent and with a 2 cm advancement by 57 percent.[96] However, anterior displacement of the tibial tuberosity must alter the contact areas of the patellofemoral articulation. Nakamura et al. suggested that a 1 cm displacement is optimal in reducing the high patellofemoral joint forces occurring at 90 and 110 degrees of flexion while causing the least reduction of the contact areas.[98] Gossling et al. confirmed that in the normal knee pressures are higher in the lateral than the medial compartments and are maximized at 0 to 30 degrees. Contact areas ranged from 0.95 to 2.30 cm², with a maximum at 45 degrees.[94] They also showed that at up to 15 mm of anterior displacement and 8 mm of medialization a decrease in force occurs with preservation of adequate contact areas. However, further elevation or medialization gives unpredictable results and increases the medial joint forces.[94]

The rehabilitation following this procedure is much the same as with the patellar tendon transfer, with modified immobilization for 6 weeks followed by intensive quadriceps rehabilitation. This procedure works well for grade III chondromalacia and moderately severe retropatellar arthrosis, with more than 65 percent of patients having excellent or good results. The more severe degrees of patella involvement do not do as well. Tubercle elevation is an excellent procedure for individuals with incapacitating pain, but the large bump formed by the advanced tubercle may be both unsightly and painful to kneeling pressures.

This fact must be taken into consideration before considering a Maquet-type operation for certain athletes with lesser involvement of their retropatellar surface.

Joint Surface Débridement

Irregular and fragmented areas of the patellar joint surface may be smoothed by shaving or débridement using either a hand-controlled rongeur or motorized shaver.[81] This procedure is often referred to as arthroscopic chondroplasty of the patella. The procedures described in this section may be done by open surgery, but they are usually performed by arthroscopy. Chondroplasty is usually reserved for Jackson's grade I or II lesions either localized or, if more extensive, still superficial. Often results as good as 78 percent are reported (Table 12-16).[23,97] These series are rarely composed of just athletes. The higher the level of competition and the more impact involved for the lower extremity, e.g., with sprinting or long-distance running, the lower is the overall ratio of success that is expected from this procedure. If débridement is restricted to small, superficial lesions, it is often a worthwhile procedure.

For deeper lesions, the sides may be defined; and using power burrs or shavers, the ragged cartilage and sclerotic bone can be abraded down to a vascular base. Occasionally, small drill holes are made into the deeper bone. This procedure is referred to as abrasion arthroplasty, fraissage, or trephining of the articular surface. The hope for these procedures is that they will prevent the shearing off of further microscopic or macroscopic fragments, which trigger joint effusions. Furthermore, it is possible that the base of the trephined lesion will fill with cells from the subchondral marrow, which metaplase into a functional fibrocartilage. By removing the large, loose flaps that are causing mechanical symptoms, the athlete may be relieved of the sensation of catching and pseudolocking.[98–100]

Like most arthroscopic procedures, the rate and progress of rehabilitation postoperatively depend to a large extent on the duration of symptoms preoperatively and the amount of articular surface damage. Simple arthroscopic chondroplasty is usually followed by rapid return to function. As soon as good quadriceps control is achieved, there is no quadriceps lag, and minimal effusion is present, crutches may be discarded. By 2 weeks postoperatively, the rate of progression can be accelerated according to the abilities of the individual patient.

Regardless of their condition, it is better to protect the joint and proceed slowly for the first 10 to 14 days. Although some patients achieve full function earlier, 6 weeks after surgery is a realistic goal. If there are large areas involved, it is sometimes prudent to extend the period of partial weight-bearing and rehabilitation before full return to activity.

The abrasion arthroplasty with exposure of subchondral bone presents a greater dilemma in regard to postoperative rehabilitation. Some of the most impressive results with this procedure are in series where the patients have had no or light partial weight-bearing for 2 months after operation. Moreoover, they have protected the joint for another 6 months to allow maturation of the newly formed fibrocartilaginous resurfacing. The athlete must fully understand this situation preoperatively. With small lesions, particularly if not on the major weight-bearing areas, some compromises may be made in this regimen so return to function may be as early as 6 weeks postoperatively. However, if the lesion is large and is situated in areas of major stress, the aims of treatment are to stop the rapid onset of degenerative joint disease, and all decisions must be made with not only the athlete's immediate goals in mind but their entire career—current as well as and subsequent competition. This procedure may therefore require careful, slowly progressed activity. The therapist plays a major role in supporting the activity restrictions decided on by the surgeon. Regimens to maintain overall fitness and exercise to the involved limb, if carefully planned, maintain the strength and minimize the time required to regain full function once all activities are resumed.

Facetectomy of Patella

In the simplest terms, the patella may be divided into medial, central, and lateral facets. Excision of all or part of the medial or lateral facets constitutes a facetectomy, which involves up to one-third of the patella. It is indicated when there is a significant lesion restricted to one of these areas, with the remaining patella in excellent condition.[101] It is occasionally necessary to combine it with a lateral retinacular release or imbrication of the vastus medialis to more centralize the remaining patella.

Postoperative care is tailored to the ability of the resutured retinaculum to become securely attached to the remaining patella. Full stress may be delayed as little as 4 weeks and as long as 8 to 12 weeks.

Patellectomy

At first thought, total excision of the patella appears a drastic solution for any retropatellar problem. Indeed, performed poorly or with any major postoperative complication such as quadriceps lag, infection, disruption of the plication, or in the presence of other major joint disease, the outcome is usually poor. Patellectomy serves as an end-stage procedure for other failed patellar surgery or when there is intractable pain associated with stages III and IV chondromalacia and a large amount of patellar surface is involved. Considering the magnitude of the underlying pathology and the fact that there is usually some associated femoral involvement when there is severe chondromalacia or arthrosis of the patella, the functional outcomes and pain relief from this procedure are remarkably good. For the treatment of chondromalacia, Duthie and Hutchinson[102] reported 68 percent satisfactory results, West 82 percent, Bentley 79 percent,[5] and Hill and Compere 75 percent.[103] The keys to success in these series were (1) mainly patellar disease; (2) adequate plication and absence of a quadriceps lag; (3) compliance of the patient; and (4) an intensive and prolonged rehabilitation program. The last factor cannot be overstressed.

Firm, consolidated healing of the plicated tendon takes time; and although early rehabilitation is aimed at gaining quadriceps control, intensive therapy is delayed for about 12 weeks. At this time, the danger of stretching out the tendon is minimal. Despite this fact, the early period after cast or brace therapy must establish a range of motion to at least 90 to 110 degrees; otherwise a full range is rarely achieved during the subsequent months. In the nonathlete this point is not as important, but even for recreation such as skiing, squash, and tennis a nearly full range is important.

Bentley pointed out that the functional results continue to improve over the first 2 years, which is in marked contrast to most surgical procedures around the knee.[5] This improvement is almost entirely due to muscle hypertrophy following intensive therapy linked with a good home program and a compliant patient. Despite these excellent outcomes, participation in recreational activities is more realistic than the pursuit of a highly competitive athletic career. Artificial resurfacing has been done in an attempt to preserve the patella, but the outcome of this procedure in young individuals is not known at this time.

SUMMARY

The frequently nebulous nature of anterior knee pain has been stressed in this chapter. However, with careful interrogation and observation, certain discrete entities emerge, including symptomatic chondromalacia, the lateral facet syndrome, osteochondral damage, and the plical syndromes. Nevertheless, there remain a large number of individuals who do not fall neatly into one or another of these categories and whom we should treat using the broad designation anterior knee pain or patellofemoral pain syndrome. Even for these patients it is possible to evolve a well planned, logical treatment approach. However, it must always be born in mind that the latter two terms are a sensible admission of diagnostic defeat. In this spirit, an open mind is maintained to evaluate the evolution of the athlete's symptoms or the acquisition of new knowledge from observation or the literature. As with all cases where symptoms are so multifactorial, patient compliance is one of the keys to success, which in turn depends on the ability of the physician and therapist to inspire confidence and to communicate.

REFERENCES

1. Herzmark MH: The evolution of the knee joint. J Bone Joint Surg 20:77, 1938
2. Dye SF: An evolutionary perspective of the knee. J Bone Joint Surg [Am] 69:976, 1987
3. Warmsley R: The development of the patella. J Anat 74:360, 1940
4. Brooke R: The treatment of fractured patella by excision. Br J Surg 24:733, 1937
5. Bentley G: Chondromalacia patellae. J Bone Joint Surg [Am] 52:221, 1970
6. Haxton H: Function of the patella and the effects of its excision. Surg Gynecol Obstet 80:389, 1945
7. Ogden JA: Radiology of postnatal skeletal development: patella and tibial tuberosity. Skel Radiol 11:246, 1984
8. Ficat RP, Hungerford DS: Disorders of the Patello-Femoral Joint. Williams & Wilkins, Baltimore, 1977
9. McConnell J: The management of chondromalacia patellae: a long term solution. Aust J Phys Ther 32:215, 1986
10. Reid DC: Chondromalacia patellae. Can Athletic Ther Assoc J 8:13, 1982
11. Goodfellow J, Hungerford DS, Zindel M: Patello-

femoral joint mechanics and pathology. J Bone Joint Surg [Br] 58:287, 1976

12. Gruber M: The conservative treatment of chondromalacia patellae. Orthop Clin North Am 10:105, 1979

13. Insall J: Patellar pain. J Bone Joint Surg [Am] 64:147, 1982

14. LeVeau B, Rogers C: Selective training of the vastus medialis muscle using EMG biofeedback. Phys Ther 60:1410, 1980

15. Soderberg G, Cook T: An electromyographic analysis of quadriceps femoris muscle settings and straight leg raising. Phys Ther 63:1434, 1983

16. Buchbinder R, Naparo N, Bizzo E: The relationship of abnormal pronation to chondromalacia patellae in distance runners. J Am Podiatr Assoc 69:159, 1979

17. Reynolds L, Levin T, Medeiros J et al: EMG activity of the vastus medialis oblique and the vastus lateralis in their role in patellar alignment. Am J Phys Med 62:61, 1983

18. Huberti H, Hayes W: Patellofemoral contact pressures. J Bone Joint Surg [Am] 66:715, 1984

19. Wiberg G: Roentgenographic and anatomic studies on the femoropatellar joint. Acta Orthop Scand 12:319, 1941

20. Fujikawa K, Seedhom BB, Wright V: Biomechanics of the patello-femoral joint. Part I. A study of the contact and the congruity of the patello-femoral compartment and movement of the patella. Eng Med 12:3, 1983

21. Outerbridge RF: The problem of chondromalacia patellae. Clin Orthop 110:177, 1975

22. Metcalf R: An arthroscopic method for lateral release of the subluxating or dislocating patella. Clin Orthop 167:9, 1982

23. Jackson RW: Surgery of the patellofemoral joint. Part III. Etiology of chondromalacia patellae. Am Acad Orthop Surg Inst Course Lect 25:36, 1976

24. Kramer PG: Patella malalignment syndrome: rationale to reduce excessive lateral pressure. J Orthop Sports Phys Ther 8:301, 1986

25. Rombold C: Osteochondritis dissecans of the patella: a case report. J Bone Joint Surg 18:230, 1936

26. Schwarz C, Blazina ME, Sisto DJ, Hirsh LC: The results of operative treatment of osteochondritis dissecans of the patella. Am J Sports Med 16:522, 1988

27. Edwards DH, Bentley G: Osteochondritis dissecans patellae. J Bone Joint Surg [Br] 59:58, 1977

28. Kinnard P, Levesque RY: The plica syndrome: a syndrome of controversy. Clin Orthop 183:141, 1984

29. Wottage WM, Sprague NF, Auerbach BJ, Shahrieree H: The medial patellar plica syndrome. Am J Sports Med 11:211, 1983

30. Hardaker WT, Whipple TL, Bassett FH: Diagnosis and treatment of the plica syndrome of the knee. J Bone Joint Surg [Br] 62:221, 1980

31. Pipkin G: Knee injuries. Clin Orthop 74:161, 1971

32. Blumensaat C: Die Lageabweichungen und Verrenkunger der Kniescheibe. Ergeb Chir Orthop 31:149, 1938

33. Hughston JC et al: Patella Subluxation and Dislocation. WB Saunders, Philadelphia, 1984

34. Fairbank J, Pynsent PB, Van Poortvliet JA, Phillips H: Mechanical factors in advance of knee pain in adolescents and young adults. J Bone Joint Surg [Br] 66:685, 1984

35. Leib F, Perry J: Quadriceps function. J Bone Joint Surg [Am] 50:1535, 1968

36. DeAndrade JR, Grant C, Dixon A et al: Joint distension and reflex muscle inhibition in the knee. J Bone Joint Surg [Am] 47:313, 1965

37. Eyring EJ, Murray WR: The effect of joint position on the pressure of intraarticular effusion. J Bone Joint Surg [Am] 46:1235, 1964

38. Moller BN, Krebs B, Tideman-Dal C, Aaris K: Isometric contractions in the patellofemoral pain syndrome. Arch Orthop Trauma Surg 105:24, 1986

39. Wise H, Fiebert IM, Kates JC: EMG biofeedback on treatment for patellofemoral pain syndrome. J Orthop Sports Phys Ther 6:95, 1984

40. Moller BN, Jurik AG, Tidermand-Dal C et al: The quadriceps function in patellofemoral disorders: a radiographic and electromyographic study. Arch Orthop Trauma Surg 106:195, 1987

41. Bennett JG, Stauber WT: Evaluation of anterior knee pain using eccentric exercise. Med Sci Sports Exerc 18:520, 1986

42. Hungerford DS, Lennox DW: Rehabilitation of the knee in disorders of the patellofemoral joints: relevant biomechanics. Orthop Clin North Am 14:397, 1983

43. Hoke B, Howell D, Stack M: The relationship between isokinetic testing and dynamic patellofemoral compression. J Orthop Sports Phys Ther 4:150, 1983

44. Winter DA: Movements of force and mechanical power in jogging. J Biomechan 16:91, 1983

45. Young A, Hughes I, Russell P, Nichols PJR: Measurement of quadriceps muscle wasting by ultrasonography. Pharmacol Rehabil 19:141, 1980

46. Doxey GE: Assessing quadriceps femoris muscle bulk with girth measurements in subjects with patellofemoral pain. J Orthop Sports Phys Ther 9:177, 1987

47. Kobler WB: Strength and flexibility findings in an-

terior knee pain syndrome in athletes. Am J Sports Med 15:410, 1987

48. Sommer HM: Patellar chondropathy and apicitis, and muscle imbalances of the lower extremity in competitive sports. Sports Med 5:381, 1988

49. McNichol K: Iliotibial tract friction syndrome in athletes. Can J Appl sports Sci 6:76, 1981

50. Root M, Orien W, Weed J: Clinical Biomechanics. Vol II. Clinical Biomechanics Corporation, Los Angeles, 1977

51. Kujala UM, Kvist M, Osterman K et al: Factors predisposing army conscripts to knee exertion injuries incurred in a physical training program. Clin Orthop 210:203, 1986

52. Percy EC, Strother RT: Patellalgia. Phys Sports Med 13:43, 1985

53. Antich TJ, Randall CC, Westbrook RA et al: Evaluation of knee extensor mechanism disorders: clinical presentation of 112 patients. J Orthop Sports Phys Ther 8:248, 1986

54. Tiberio D: The effect of excessive subtalar joint pronation on patellofemoral mechanics: a theoretical model. J Orthop Sports Phys Ther 9:160, 1987

55. Buchbinder MR, Napora NJ, Biggs EW: The relationship of abnormal pronation to chondromalacia of the patella in distance runners. J Am Podiatry Assoc 69:159, 1979

56. James SJ: Chondromalacia of the patella in the adolescent. In Kennedy JC (ed): The Injured Adolescent Knee. Williams & Wilkins, Baltimore, 1979

57. Dillon PZ, Updyke WF, Alien WC: Gait analysis with reference to chrondromalacia patellae. Am J Orthop Sports Phys Ther 5:127, 1983

58. Stott SJ: Anatomical alignment and physical characteristics of competitive female figure skaters. MS thesis, University of Alberta, 1988

59. Wilson JM: Interosseous pressures of the patella in chondromalacia. MS thesis, University of Alberta, 1985

60. Sandow MJ, Goodfellow J: The natural history of anterior knee pain in adolescents. J Bone Joint Surg [Br] 67:36, 1985

61. Kolowich PA, Paulos LE, Rosenberg TD et al: Lateral release of the patellas: indications and contraindications. Am J Sports Med 18:359, 1990

62. Faulkerson JP: Awareness of the retinaculum in evaluating patellofemoral pain. Am J Sports Med 10:142, 1982

63. Minkoff J, Fein L: The role of radiography in the evaluation and treatment of common anarthrotic disorders of the patellofemoral joint. Clin Sports Med 8:203, 1989

64. Carson WA et al: Clin Orthop 185:182, 1984

65. Insall J, Salvati E: Patella position in the normal knee joint. Radiology 101:101, 1971

66. Brattstrom H: Shape of the intercondylar groove normally and in recurrent dislocation of the patella. Acta Orthop Scand [Suppl] 68:134, 1964

67. Laurin CA, Dussault R, Levesque HP: The tangential x-ray investigation of the patellofemoral joint: x-ray technique, diagnostic criteria and their interpretation. Clin Orthop 144:16, 1979

68. Merchant AC, Mercer RL, Jacobson RH et al: Roentgenographic analysis of patella congruence. J Bone Joint Surg [Am] 56:1391, 1974

69. Levine J, Splain S: Use of the infrapatellar strap in the treatment of patellofemoral pain. Clin Orthop 139:179, 1979

70. Villar RN: Patellofemoral pain and the infrapatellar brace: a military view. Am J Sports Med 13:313, 1985

71. Lysholm J, Nordin M, Ekstrand J, Gillquist J: The effect of a patella brace on performance in a knee extension strength test in patients with patella pain. Am J Sports Med 12:110, 1984

72. Moller BN, Krebs B: Dynamic knee brace in the treatment. Arch Orthop Trauma Surg 104:377, 1986

73. Wild JJ, Franklin TD, Woods GW: Patellar pain and quadriceps rehabilitation: an EMG study. Am J Sports Med 10:12, 1982

74. Knight KL: Rehabilitating chondromalacia patellae. Phys Sports Med 7:147, 1979

75. Harding B, Black T, Braulsema A et al: Reliability of a reciprical test protocol performed on the kinetic communicator: an isokinetic test of knee extensor and flexor protocol. J Orthop Sports Phys Ther 10:218, 1988

76. Engelhorn R: Agonist and antagonist muscle EMG activity pattern changes with skill acquisition. Res Q Exerc Sports 54:315, 1983

77. Mariani P, Caruso I: An electromyographic investigation of subluxation of the patella. J Bone Joint Surg [Br] 61:169, 1979

78. Sale D, MacDougall D: Specificity in strength training: a review for coach and athlete. Can J Appl Sports Sci 6:87, 1981

79. Reid DC: Functional Anatomy and Joint Mobilization. University of Alberta Press, Edmonton, 1970

80. Spencer J, Hayes K, Alexander I: Knee joint effusion and quadriceps reflex inhibition in man. Arch Physi Med Rehabil 65:171, 1984

81. Desai SS, Patel M, Michelli LJ et al: Osteochondritis dissecans of the patella. J Bone Joint Surg [Br] 69:320, 1987

82. O'Donoghue DH: The treatment of chondral damage to the patella. Am J Sports Med 9:1, 1981

83. Ogilvie-Harris DJ, Jackson RW: The arthroscopic treatment of chondromalacia patellae. J Bone Joint Surg [Br] 66:660, 1984

84. Betz RR, Magill JT, Lonergan RP: The percutaneous lateral retinacular release. Am J Sports Med 15:477, 1987

85. Bigos S, McBride G: The isolated lateral retinacular release in the treatment of patellofemoral disorders. Clin Orthop 186:75, 1984

86. Dzioba RB: Diagnostic arthroscopy and longitudinal open lateral release: a four year follow up study to determine predictors of surgical outcomes. Am J Sports Med 18:343, 1990

87. Lankenner PA, Micheli LJ, Clancy R, Gerbino PG: Arthroscopic percutaneous lateral patellar retinacular release. Am J Sports Med 12:104, 1984

88. Krompinger WJ, Fulkerson JP: Lateral retinacular release for intractable lateral retinacular pain. Clin Orthop 179:190, 1983

89. Micheli LJ, Stanitski CL: Lateral patellar retinacular release. Am J Sports Med 9:330, 1981

90. Osborne AH, Fulford PC: Lateral release for chondromalacia patellae. J Bone Joint Surg [Br] 64:202, 1982

91. Brown DE, Alexander AH, Lichtman DM: The Elmslie-Trillat procedure: evaluation in patellar dislocation and subluxation. Am J Sports Med 12:104, 1984

92. Worrell RV: The diagnosis of disorders of the patellofemoral joint. Orthop Rev 10:23, 1981

93. Huberti HH, Hayes WC: Contact pressures in chondromalacia patellae and the effects of capsular reconstructive procedures. J Orthop Res 6:499, 1988

94. Gossling H, Fulkerson JP, Meaney JA, Becker GJ: Alteration of patellofemoral joint pressures by antero-medialization of the tibial tubercle. Am J Sports Med 15:405, 1987

95. Heatley FW, Allen PR, Patrick JH: Tibial tubercle advancement for anterior knee pain: a temporary or permanent solution. Clin Orthop 208:215, 1986

96. Maquet P: Considerations biomecaniques sur l'arthrose du genou: un traitement biomecanique de l'arthrose femoro-patellaire; l'avancement du tendon rotulieu. Rev Rhum 30:779, 1963

97. Bandi W, Brenawald J: The significance of femoropatellar pressure in the pathogenesis and treatment of chondromalacia patellae and femoropatellar arthrosis. Int Cong Ser 324:63, 1974

98. Nakamura N, Ellis M, Seedhon BB: Advancement of the tibial tuberosity: a biomechanical study. J Bone Joint Surg [Br] 67:255, 1985

99. Schonholtz GL, Ling B: Arthoscopic chondroplasty of the patella. Arthroscopy 1:92, 1985

100. Chandler EJ: Abrasion arthroplasty of the knee. Contemp Orthop 11:21, 1985

101. O'Donoghue DH: Facetectomy. South Med J 65:645, 1972

102. Duthie RL, Hutchinson JR: Results of partial and total excision of the patella. J Bone Joint Surg [Br] 40:75, 1958

103. Hill JA, Compere CL: Comparative study of patellectomy: review of procedure in chondromalacia, dislocations, subluxations, and fractures. Orthop Rev 10:41, 1981

Bursitis and Knee Extensor Mechanism Pain Syndromes

13

Ah, but a man's reach should exceed his grasp.
— Robert Browning

Among the more tangible causes of anterior knee pain, patellar dislocation, patellar tendinitis, apophysitis, and peripatellar bursitis are common. Most of these problems are associated with well recognizable signs and symptoms and hence should be ruled out before falling back on the commonly diagnosed syndromes described in the previous chapter. However, careful attention to the details of the history and meticulous palpation techniques are necessary if these often remediable conditions are to be promptly diagnosed and adequately treated and if long-term complications are to be avoided. Some of the lesions associated with the hamstring tendons and their insertions are also covered in this chapter.

PATELLAR DISLOCATION

Patellar dislocation may occur as the result of trauma to a normal knee, trauma to a knee with predisposing factors for subluxation or dislocation, and atraumatically as the result of a combination of connective tissue laxity, alignment problems, and bony or muscle dysplasia. With the exception of acute traumatic dislocation, this condition actually represents a spectrum of injury, from mild asymptomatic subluxation to a completely displaced patella. The symptoms and signs vary accordingly. (Table 13-1).

Clinical Findings

In individuals with a predisposition to dislocation, the contributing factors include passive patellar hypermobility, vastus medialis dysplasia, patella alta, patella dysplasia, increased Q-angle, genu recurvatum, and a shallow femoral groove.[1]

Acute traumatic dislocations present with pain, hemarthrosis, and a tense effusion.[2,3] Despite the fairly obvious nature of this injury, the diagnosis is frequently overlooked, or the injury is misdiagnosed as a ligament sprain. Careful palpation reveals mainly medial peripatellar pain and often slight lateral displacement of the patella, which may be masked by an effusion. A skyline view helps confirm this problem, and it may be necessary to aspirate the knee in order to obtain this film. In any event, roentgenograms are important to rule out the frequent association of a large osteochondral fragment, chipped off as the patella rides over the lateral femoral condyle. There may be avulsion of the vastus medialis from the patella

---

Practice Point

PRESENTING SYMPTOMS OF PATIENTS WITH CHRONIC PATELLAR SUBLUXATION

- Pain
- Swelling
- Feeling of instability
- Giving way
- Popping
- Trouble cutting and pivoting
- Catching
- Locking

TABLE 13-1.   Abnormal Findings in Patients with Patellar Subluxation

Finding	Incidence (%)
Passive patellar hypermobility	70
Increased Q-angle	60
Quadriceps weakness	60
Vastus medialis dysplasia	65
Patella alta	25
Retropatellar crepitus	20
Laterally placed patella	15
Positive apprehension test	30
Retropatellar tenderness	15
Knee recurvatum	15
Swelling	15
Valgus knees	10

(Fig.13-1). Occasionally the trauma is not so much a heavy blow as an impact directed laterally on the patella at a point in motion where the patella has not seated itself deeply in the femoral groove and the vastus lateralis is contracting strongly. The more prevalent and pronounced the predisposing factors, the more likely a dislocation is to occur.

After the initial dislocation, episodes may recur. In these individuals and those with congenitally predis-posing anatomy, the main complaints are pain in the retropatellar area, intermittent swelling, giving way, a feeling of instability, popping, catching, locking, and difficulty with cutting, pivoting, and twisting. There may be few or several clinical findings. They include a positive apprehension test to lateral patellar pressure with the knee flexed to 20 to 30 degrees and the quadriceps relaxed, patellar malalignment, increased Q-angle, vastus medialis atrophy or dysplasia, an ef-fusion, and crepitus (see Ch. 12). Generalized liga-mentous laxity may be detected.

Treatment

For the acute traumatic first time dislocation, in the absence of a large osteochondral fracture or a patella that does not stay reasonably centralized because of excessive tearing of the medial retinacular fibers, cast immobilization followed by intensive rehabilitation is the treatment of choice. At long-term follow-up, 75 percent have good or excellent results.[2,3] In individu-als who have several of the factors that contribute to patellar instability, first time traumatic dislocation treated nonoperatively yields about 52 percent suc-cessful results.[2]

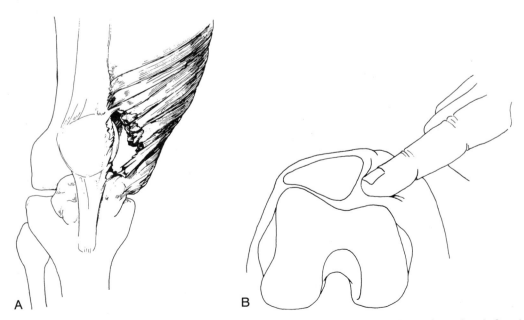

Fig. 13-1. (A) With complete disruption of the vastus medialis obliquus insertion, the defect is not always obvious because of the hemarthrosis; however, palpation may reveal the defect. **(B)** No resistance is encountered along the medial patellofemoral joint.

Practice Point

INDICATIONS FOR SURGERY

- First time dislocation, significant osteochondral fracture
- First time dislocation with inadequate or unstable reduction on skyline view
- Recurrent dislocation not responding to nonoperative treatment

---

With recurrent dislocations in athletes, an unguarded pivoting motion leads to a dynamic dislocation brought on by quadriceps imbalance. These injuries require realignment of the extensor mechanism. Such procedures are usually successful in terms of preventing further dislocation[5-7] (Table 13-2). Unfortunately, chronic subluxation, maltracking, and dislocations have often precipitated sufficient articular cartilage change that patellofemoral pain becomes a problem. It makes rehabilitation a significant challenge, as excellent extensor power and vastus medialis hypertrophy are requisites for success. Pain may restrict the rate of progress and choice of exercises.

The approach of Hawkins and his group is an effective plan for the treatment of dislocations.[2]

1. Establish the diagnosis carefully, particularly ruling out major ligamentous disruption and meniscal pathology and determine the major etiologic factors. Examination under anesthesia, and arthroscopy may be necessary.
2. Routine roentgenography, including skyline and tunnel views, is done to record patellar shape and position and the anatomy of the femoral sulcus, as well as to rule out the presence of osteochondral fragments or, if present, their size and location.
3. For patients sustaining their first patellar dislocation, in the absence of significant predisposing factors, treat by immobilization and physical therapy.
4. For patients who have a combination of predisposing factors to instability, e.g., vastus medialis dysplasia, large Q-angles, patella alta, or abnormal patellar configuration, primary surgical stabilization should be considered.
5. For patients with no predisposing factors but an obvious osteochondral fragment, arthroscopy may be helpful for documenting the size and amount of articular surface involved. Excise or reattach the fragment as indicated.
6. Patients who have a combination of predisposing factors and an osteochondral fracture probably should undergo excision or reattachment of the fragment followed by a stabilization procedure, as they are at risk of developing recurrent dislocations that may further damage the joint surfaces.
7. Patients with recurrent dislocations that have not stabilized with therapy or patellar stabilizing braces require surgical reconstruction of the extensor apparatus. Even with successful stabilization, some athletes have significant patellofemoral discomfort.[2]

JUMPER'S KNEE AND PATELLAR TENDON PROBLEMS (PATELLAR TENDINITIS)

Sports that involve sprinting, sudden starts and stops, and repetitive jumping and kicking obviously exert considerable stress on the quadriceps mechanism. Furthermore, certain trends aimed at improving athletic performance, e.g., year-round participation and intensive training, have magnified these stresses. The vulnerability of the inferior pole of the patella and the tibial tubercle, due to the apophysis in the skeletally immature athlete, is a significant factor.

TABLE 13-2.   Lateral Retinacular Release for Recurrent Patellar Dislocation

Study	Minimum Follow-Up (months)	No. of Patients	Recurrence (No.)
Betz et al.[4]	48	14	2
Metcalf[5]	48	14	0
Bigos & McBride[6]	14	13	0
Reid(personal data)	24	25	1
Average	33		3(5%)

The result of these stresses is a series of linked conditions involving the proximal and distal poles of the patella (jumper's knee), the patellar tendon, and the tibial tubercle apophysis.[7,8] These conditions may be complicated by stress fractures of the patella, avulsions of the tibial tubercle or rupture of the patellar tendon. The former conditions present as anterior knee pain that must be distinguished from the ubiquitous patellofemoral syndromes. The latter present as sudden, intense pain and frequently, sudden collapse of the knee. These situations are potential catastrophes as far as the athlete's career is concerned and they must be recognized and treated aggressively.[8] Even tendinitis may become sufficiently chronic and severe that an athletes' career is jeopardized. Prompt diagnosis and intensive early treatment often abort

the progression to chronicity. The commonest error in the management of these conditions is underestimation of their potential for prolonged, debilitating symptoms and hence inadequate early therapy on the part of the physician and noncompliance on the part of the athlete (Fig. 13-2).

Epidemiologic Features

Jumper's knee is a typical functional overload syndrome in athletes who submit their extensor mechanism to intense and repeated loading, e.g., volleyball and basketball players, high and long jumpers, weight lifters, cyclists, and soccer players. Traditionally, the term encompasses the insertional tendinopathies, but in the skeletally immature it is only logical to include

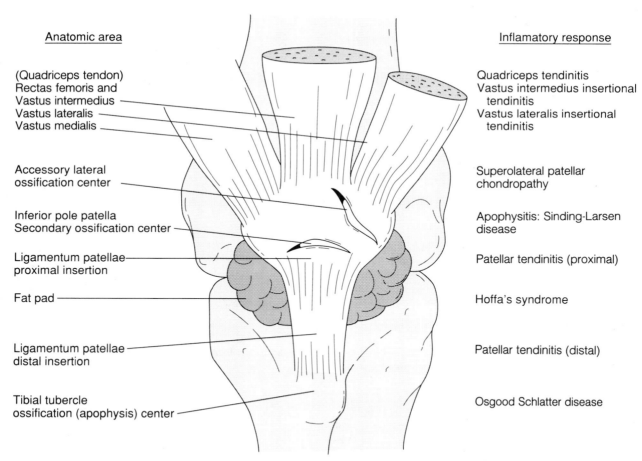

Anatomic area

(Quadriceps tendon)
Rectas femoris and
Vastus intermedius
Vastus lateralis
Vastus medialis

Accessory lateral
ossification center

Inferior pole patella
Secondary ossification center

Ligamentum patellae
proximal insertion

Fat pad

Ligamentum patellae
distal insertion

Tibial tubercle
ossification (apophysis) center

Inflamatory response

Quadriceps tendinitis
Vastus intermedius insertional
 tendinitis
Vastus lateralis insertional
 tendinitis

Superolateral patellar
chondropathy

Apophysitis: Sinding-Larsen
disease

Patellar tendinitis (proximal)

Hoffa's syndrome

Patellar tendinitis (distal)

Osgood Schlatter disease

Fig. 13-2. The term jumper's knee has been used to encompass a wide range of superior and inferior patellar pain problems including tendinitis, osteochondropathies, and irritation of the accessory superolateral ossification center. The structures involved are shown with their respective inflammatory responses.

Clinical Point

ANTERIOR KNEE PAIN RELATED TO QUADRICEPS TENDON AND LIGAMENT (Proximal to Distal)

- Superior pole quadriceps tendinitis (jumper's knee)
- Superolateral patellar chondropathy (bipartite patella)
- Inferior pole patellar tendinitis (jumper's knee, apicitis)
- Patellar tendinitis
- Inferior pole patellar chondropathy (osteochondritis, Sinding-Larsen-Johansson disease)
- Tibial tubercle chondropathy (osteochondritis, Osgood-Schlatter disease)

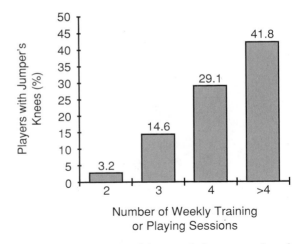

Fig. 13-3. Incidence of jumper's knee as related to frequency of training and games played. (After Ferretti,[8] with permission.)

the associated chondropathies[9] (Fig. 13-2). Insertion of the tendon into the inferior pole of the patella is involved in about 65 percent of cases. Intrinsic factors, such as the resistance, elasticity, and extensibility of the tendon, the biomechanical variation of the knee extensor mechanism, muscle strength, and overall limb alignments, have been implicated. However, it is the extrinsic factors that probably play the greatest role. In particular, the number, duration, and intensity of training sessions are important (Fig. 13-3). The playing surface is also significant. Ferretti reporting in a survey of volleyball players an incidence of 37.5 percent in the athletes playing or training regularly on concrete versus 4.7 percent in those practicing on wooden (parquet) floors[8] (Fig. 13-4).

Whereas Ferretti was unable to identify consistent alignment problems at the knee or foot, Sommer made some interesting observations on lower limb movement patterns in basketball and volleyball players.[9] In addition to hip flexor shortening, and relative or absolute weakness of the glutei abdominals and hamstrings, the upper leg tends to adduct and internally rotate during take-off at the drawback stage, where a semicouched position is adopted. The knee joint assumes a characteristic valgus and internally torqued position (Fig. 13-5). This sequence is again adopted when landing, frequently with abnormal distribution of weight across the forefoot. This observation has also been made in dancers. It is possi-

ble that this movement pattern, which becomes exaggerated with fatigue, is responsible for increased stress and strain behavior on the tendon, particularly during the eccentric loading phase of landing. If this hypothesis is true, attention to the appropriate muscle groups, as well as analysis and correction of jumping patterns, must be part of the treatment program. In addition, individuals who are engaged in vigorous activities may develop symptoms related to the patellar ossification centers. Whereas the bipartite patella is relatively common, it is usually asymptomatic. However occasionally this epiphyseal plate is painful (Fig. 13-2). Palpation of a particularly painful area at the superolateral pole of the patella should always lead to a consideration of this condition. For the most part it is treated in a manner similar to that for other inflammatory lesions of the extensor apparatus. It usually responds well to rest or modified activity but on occasion requires surgical excision to resolve the symptoms. The apophysis separates on rare occasions; an injury that is usually missed during the acute phase and has to be dealt with subsequently, either by lateral retinacular release or, if significantly displaced, by facetectomy (Fig. 13-6).

Signs and Symptoms

The key to diagnosis is exact localization of the point of maximum tenderness and, in the skeletally immature, the location of the apophysis (Fig. 13-2). The history is one of gradual increasing pain until

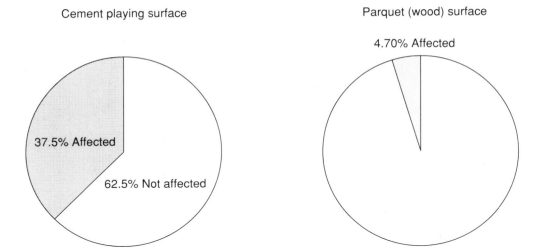

Cement playing surface

37.5% Affected

62.5% Not affected

Parquet (wood) surface

4.70% Affected

Fig. 13-4. Hard playing surfaces increase the prevalence of symptomatic extensor tendon problems. (After Ferretti,[8] with permission.)

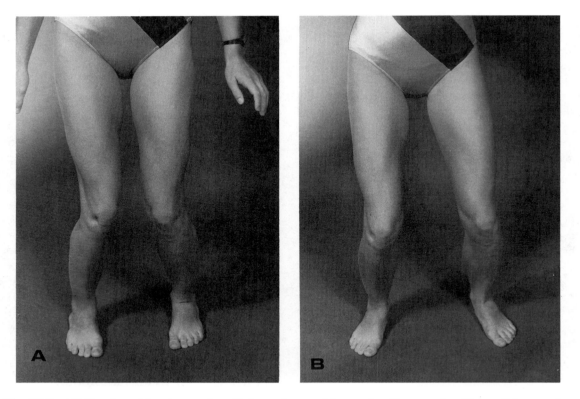

Fig. 13-5. **(A)** Evasive adduction and medial rotation position on landing or takeoff, possibly stressing the extensor apparatus. **(B)** Corrected landing and takeoff positions, with the lower limb alignment allowing flexion and extension over one movement plane.

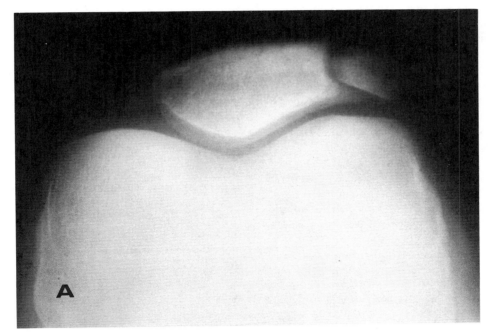

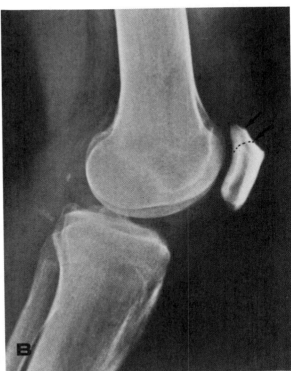

Fig. 13-6. **(A)** Bipartite patella with the superolateral fragment displaced. **(B)** Elongation of the proximal pole of the patella with chronic hyperemia of quadriceps tendinitis.

eventually all activity is precluded and even walking may be difficult. During jumping activities the pain may initially occur only after the activity or during repetitive jumping. There may be a phase when the discomfort decreases as the tendon warms up with activity. Although all of the variations of alignment and patellar position should be noted, none is pathognomonic in the diagnosis of the condition.

With Osgood-Schlatter disease, obvious enlargement of the tubercle or even separate ossicles may be present, which may be prominant (Fig. 13-7). Occasionally it is of sufficient magnitude as to give problems with kneeling.[10,11]

The diagnosis of Sinding-Larsen-Johansson disease (inferior pole patellar chondropathy) is embraced by remembering its usual mild nature, its greater incidence among boys and girls aged 10 to 14 years, and the point tenderness over the inferior pole of the patella.[12,13]

It has already been stressed that it is traditionally

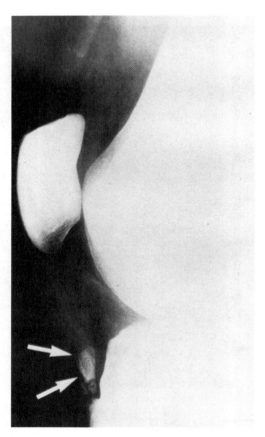

Fig. 13-7. Osgood-Schlatter disease with separate ossicles formed in the patellar tendon.

thought that the commonest accessory ossification center (bipartite patellae), in the superolateral pole, is mostly asymptomatic. This ossification center is usually present by 12 years of age and is present into adult life in approximately 2 percent of the population. It is approximately nine times more common in boys than girls and occurs bilaterally in 40 percent of the cases.

Pathology

In the supra- and infrapatellar junctions of tendon with bone, the histology of classic jumper's knee may include pseudocystic cavities at the borderline between mineralized fibrocartilage and bone, increased thickness of the insertional fibrocartilage by myxomatous and hyaline metaplasia, and mineralization of the fibrocartilage nearest the bone. It represents significant change from the normal orderly transition of tendon insertion from tendon collagen, to fibrocartilage, to mineralized fibrocartilage, to bone. The tendon itself is rarely involved in this process unless corticosteroid injections have been used. These changes described above are compatible with focal degeneration and microtearing as the result of an overload situation.[12-14]

With Osgood-Schlatter disease, there is evidence of inflammation or necrotic zones and calcification in the marginal zones of what appears like fresh tears in the tendon interface. There is evidence of callus and varying degrees of bone formation in areas where the ossicles are forming (Fig. 13-7).

Roentgenographic Examination

In the adolescent, plain roentgenograms establish the degree of maturation of the epiphysis. Occasionally there is radiolucency of the involved pole. Rarely, with advanced tendinitis, there may be some speckled degenerative calcification of the tendon.

With Sinding-Larsen-Johansson disease, irregularity of the inferior patellar pole is seen frequently. Occasionally with protracted symptoms, there is elongation of the involved pole (Fig. 13-8). This elongated pole has been recorded as developing a stress fracture, and whenever there are protracted symptoms repeat roentgenograms should be obtained to rule out this injury. Failure to do so may result in an avulsion fracture. With Osgood-Schlatter disease there may be fragmentation of the tibial tubercle apophysis, and occasionally an extremely large ossicle develops within the tendon.

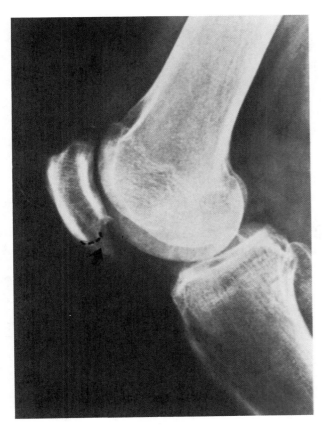

Fig. 13-8. Sinding-Larsen disease may produce sufficient hyperemic and inflammatory stimulus, causing elongation of the inferior pole of the patella.

Practice Point

COMPLICATIONS OF JUMPER'S KNEE

- Stress reaction patella
- Stress fracture patella
- Avulsion apophysis
- Patellar tendon rupture
- Formation of accessory ossicles
- Growth acceleration
  — Large tubercle
  — Patella magna
- Growth arrest
  — Knee hyperextension (genu recurvatum)

Treatment of Jumper's Knee and Patellar Tendinitis

Treatment for insertional tendinitis and for patellar tendinitis in the remaining portion of the tendon is similar and based on severity (see p. 425 for grading system). Apophysitis of the inferior pole of the patella and the tibial tubercle are dealt with separately because of the different treatment approaches and natural histories.

Tendinitis

Patients with pain only after activity (grade I) and no undue functional impairment are advised to make sure they warm up well before training and to use ice packs or ice massage after activity. It may be wise to add a regimen of nonsteroidal anti-inflammatory drugs (NSAIDs). If the pain seems to return after discontinuing the medication, further modification of activity is required and perhaps consideration of a knee sleeve made of some elastic material. We have had some experience with using a patellar tendon taping technique that may be used to supplement the rest of the treatment approach. Patients may be taught to tape their own knees (Fig 13-9). Consultation with the coach is the best way to reduce the amount of jumping and rebounding during practice.

If the pain is more significant (grades II and III) and is beginning to interfere with activity, greater modification of training is required. Before activity, the effects of heat on tendon plasticity should be utilized. A hot pack or hot water heating pad may be applied for 10 to 15 minutes followed by stretching. After activity, cooling-down on a stretch using ice massage is also helpful. There is a limited role for steroid injection, and it is used only in conjunction with a significant period of rest.

The exercise approach at this point should be via an eccentric-concentric program for the anterior tibial muscle group while pain is severe, moving into an eccentric loading program for the quadriceps as pain decreases. Simultaneously, careful re-education of take-off and landing patterns must be undertaken to prevent the tendency for recurrence. Assessment of hip flexor tightness, hamstring and gluteal strength, and abdominal muscle power indicates the amount of time that must be devoted to these groups.

The anterior tibia program may stretch the infrapatellar ligament, change the quadriceps/foreleg strength ratio, or alter the biomechanics of take-off and landing. Whatever the mechanism, this program

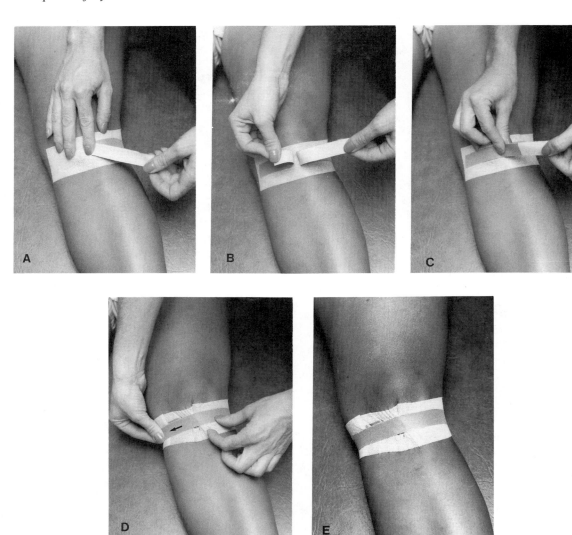

Fig. 13-9. After assessment of patellar tendon alignment, this taping protocol may be used along the same principles as "tennis elbow" taping. After applying a self-adhesive base (Fixomull Stretch, BDF Beiersdorf, AG Hamburg), the following steps are taken. **(A)** A long 0.75 inch wide strip is taped over the area of maximum tenderness (Leukosport). **(B)** A short strip is placed opposite to meet exactly at the tender spot. **(C)** The tapes are pinched together over the tender area, with the skin almost raised. **(D)** Folded back on itself, it is either pulled medially or laterally depending on alignment factors. **(E)** Completed taping technique. (Jenny McConnell Course 1984, Edmonton.)

seems to be effective and does not require extensive equipment.[14] The athlete starts with the foot in full plantar flexion, and the therapist then produces some overpressure on the dorsum of the foot, stretching the anterior tibialis (Fig. 13-10). A resisted concentric contraction follows as the foot goes into full dorsiflexion. The therapist then provides the resistance for a maximum eccentric contraction as the athlete

slowly allows full plantar flexion once more. This exercise may be done during practice sessions as well as therapy sessions. Usually three sets of 10 to 15 repetitions are desirable, but in any event the muscle is worked to fatigue.[14]

As soon as possible an eccentric loading program for the quadriceps is added. As this eccentric strengthening program progresses, the Curwin and

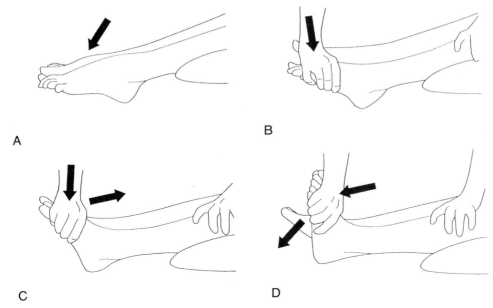

Fig. 13-10. Sequence of exercises for symptomatic patellar tendinitis. (**A**) Athlete starts with foot in full plantar flexion. (**B**) Therapist exerts pressure on the dorsum of the foot and toes to stretch the pretibial muscles. (**C**) Patient is told to dorsiflex the foot against resistance at a steady rate (concentric). (**D**) Patient then allows the therapist to slowly plantarflex against resistance (eccentric). The patient may be taught to use the opposite foot for resistance.

Stanish routine of "drop and stop" is integrated into the program.[15] After the warm-up, the hamstrings and quadriceps are stretched using a static or hold–relax proprioceptive neuromuscular technique. The specific antigravity "drop, stretch, and stop", is carried out with small, squatting maneuvers that are progressed to a larger range (Fig. 13-11). The stretching is then repeated with associated ice massage.

With unremitting, protracted symptoms, surgery may be considered. The following principles are relevant.

1. For disorders of the proximal patella, the tendon is elevated from the patella, the proximal pole drilled, and the tendon reattached through selected drill anchor holes. This procedure is rarely needed. Occasionally when symptoms are related to a painful or displaced accessory ossification center, the latter must be removed surgically (Fig. 13-6).

2. For disorders of the distal patella, the tendon is elevated from the patellar apex, the periosteum scraped, and the bone multiply drilled. Osteotomy is seldom required (Fig. 13-8). If there has been considerable pain along the length of the tendon, it should be split longitudinally to search for degenerative or atrophic areas. Where there is gross malalignment, associated retinacular release may improve the results considerably.

3. For disorders of the distal tendon, where there is dystrophic calcification or an old ossicle from previous Osgood-Schlatter disease, the tendon is split longitudinally and any bony fragment present is removed (Fig. 13-7).

Postoperative management depends on the extensiveness of the surgery. Some time is needed for secure tendon reattachment, which may delay full stress with activities for 2 to 6 weeks.

Osgood-Schlatter Disease

The aim of treatment of Osgood-Schlatter disease patients is to balance activity levels with symptoms. Continued pain and inflammation may result in an excessively large tibial tubercle, large intrapatellar tendon ossicles, or even tendon rupture. Essentially, however, despite these complications, the disease is fairly benign, and the treatment is matched to the main symptom, which is pain.[10,11]

The condition presents between the ages of 8 and

Step 1. Warm up. • Cycling, step machine, etc.
            • Passive warm up – hot packs.

Step 2. Stretch quadriceps.

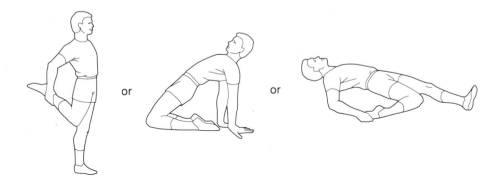

• May give static
  or hold-relax
  stretch.
• Repeat 3 times.

Step 3. Specific exercises.

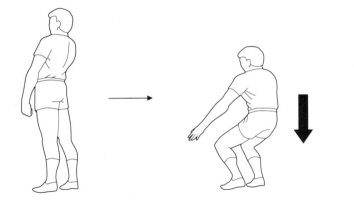

• Stand with feet apart.
• Lower body to crouch.
• May do slow or rapid
  depending on pain.
• Return quickly to upright.
• 3 sets of 10 repetitions.

Step 4. Repeat stretch.
            • as per step 2.

Step 5. Cool down
            • Preferably put tendon on stretch.
            • Lying, knee flexed.
            • Ice pack or ice massage.
            • Approximately 5 minutes.

Fig. 13-11. Eccentric loading program includes a warm-up, hold–relax–stretch routine, drop and stop exercise, repeat stretch, and then an ice cool-down.

13 in females and 10 and 15 in males, who are affected about three times as often. In 25 to 33 percent of the cases, there is bilateral involvement.[10] The tuberosity does not appear as a discrete structure until 12 to 15 weeks of fetal life. In the newborn the proximal epiphysis of the tibia consists of a cartilaginous plate (Henke's disk), which persists until about age 11 years in girls and 13 years in boys. It projects downward, similar to a tongue, over the diaphysis. In this projection, one or more ossification centers appear

between the ages of 8 and 12 in girls and 9 and 14 in boys. These centers eventually form the tuberosity, with closure and disappearance of the epiphyseal cartilaginous plate occurring at about 18 to 19 years at the latest.

The pain is treated by modifying activity. Occasionally a knee sleeve helps. The athlete is instructed to reduce sprinting, jumping, and kicking. If simple modalities such as ice, aspirin, and short courses of NSAIDs fail, it is occasionally worth immobilizing the knee in a long-leg cast in extension or a cast brace locked at 0 to 30 degrees for 6 to 8 weeks.

If these measures do not help, the athlete and parent should be instructed that they have a choice of significant activity restriction or tolerating the discomfort. The possibilities of an elongated tubercle and possible surgery for a painful ossicle should be explained. They should be warned that minor discomfort on a continuing basis is acceptable, but that severe pain resulting in a limp or loss of sleep is not. Furthermore, protracted symptoms must be reinvestigated to rule out tumor. No surgery is appropriate until the apophysis is closed, at which time the problem has usually resolved. Sometimes a soft, painful ossicle must be removed (Fig. 13-7). Occasionally, prior to cessation of growth, a large, custom-made protective pad or donut may be helpful in sports where there is much contact, e.g., volleyball. Having stated the need for delaying surgery, King and Blundell-Jones presented a series of 77 patients (mean age 13.5 years) who were operated on for removal of a painful ossicle.[16] Their success rate was good, and there were no serious complications, i.e., there was not growth arrest with genu recurvatum. It is therefore possible that in carefully selected cases surgery is warranted before growth ceases.

CATASTROPHIC MECHANICAL FAILURE OF EXTENSOR APPARATUS

Complete mechanical failure of a portion of the extensor apparatus may be termed catastrophic because in many cases it signals the end of a career in top level competition, although there are a number of reports of athletes returning to preinjury level of competition. These cases may be unilateral, but there are a significant number of bilateral ruptures reported in the literature.

Patellar Tendon

The usual site of rupture in the adult is the patellar tendon, frequently near the tibial tubercle (Fig. 13-12). This may be associated with prior treatment using local injections of steroid, which represents the greatest risk factor in the athlete.[16–18] In the general population, rheumatoid arthritis with and without systemic steroid use, systemic lupus erythematosus with steroid use, renal failure, and (probably) anabolic steroid use may make the tendon susceptible to rupture. The prevalence of anabolic steroids abuse may explain some of the unusual musculotendinous junction ruptures seen in athletes known to be on these drugs.[19,20] There are repeated cases reported in gymnasts free of known systemic disease, as well as in a variety of other athletes who have had protracted tendinitis or Osgood-Schlatter disease with associated tendon degeneration.[14,15,21,22] The small verticle projection from the surface of the patella into tendon, the so-called tooth sign, described by Greenspan et al.,[23] is sometimes present with ruptures of the

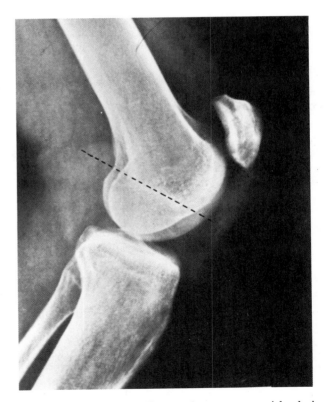

Fig. 13-12. After patellar tendon rupture with obvious patella alta. The patella is well above Bleumenstaat's line.

TABLE 13-3. Catastrophic Disruption of the Extensor Apparatus

Site	Predisposing Factors[a]
Avulsion of tibial tubercle	Skeletally immature Osgood-Schlatter disease; trauma Histologic changes during preclosure period
Patellar tendon rupture (Ligamentum patellae)	Ossicle in the patellar tendon Elongated proximal attachment site Anabolic steroid, corticosteroid (oral or injected) Trauma in association with ligament rupture Tooth sign Old Osgood-Schlatter disease
Avulsion of distal pole patella	Recurrent patellar dislocation or subluxation Stress fracture patella; direct blow Sinding-Larsen syndrome Sudden quadriceps contraction with slipping
Sleeve fractures of the patella	Skeletally immature Ages 8–12 years
Quadriceps tendon rupture (superior pole patella)	Sudden violent contraction with slip or fall Tooth sign; steroid injection Rheumatoid arthritis; systemic lupus Systemic corticosteroids Prolonged tendinitis; direct trauma Elongated proximal pole patellar

[a] Repetitive jumping, sprinting activities, and kicking sports are common risk factors.

patellar tendon and the quadriceps tendon. This sign probably represents reactive bone formation in the degenerating quadriceps tendon near the proximal patellar pole. Other risk factors are listed in Table 13-3 and include ossicles in the patellar tendon, direct trauma, and an elongated distal patellar pole, probably due to an old epiphyseal injury or Sinding-Larsen disease.[17–19,23,24]

Treatment involves recognizing the impending or partial rupture and adequately reducing the activity level, particularly jumping and sprinting, or surgical repair of the complete rupture. Occasionally with a shredded tendon, wiring is necessary through the patella to keep tension off the healing tendon. Rehabilitation is tailored to the degree of trauma, adequacy of repair, and compliance of the athlete.

Quadriceps Tendon

Complete rupture of the quadriceps apparatus from the superior pole of the patella is usually seen in conjunction with severe ligamentous disruption of the medial or lateral side of the knee and the cruciates.[21] It is treated by direct surgical repair, and these athletes do well. The rehabilitation challenge is usually to establish a full range of flexion while giving adequate time for healing of the primary repair of the quadriceps apparatus and associated ligament injury.

Avulsion of Tubercle

The third group consists of individuals who have a long history of Osgood-Schlatter disease and who experience avulsion of the tendon, with a small portion of tubercle (or more, usually) in skeletally immature athletes who have active disease. They avulse the tubercle through the apophysis. These injuries are usually type I fractures, i.e., a small flake of bone avulsed from the distal apophysis (Fig. 13-13). Occasionally, the tibial tubercle is fractured owing to the forceful contraction of the quadriceps with associated passive knee flexion or through sudden deceleration of the foot, even with nonpathologic predisposing factors.

Frequently the athlete describes landing from a jump, experiencing sudden pain, and the knee collapsing. The initial clinical impression is that the individual has torn a meniscus, sustained an anterior cruciate tear, or dislocated the patella. Careful examination reveals an inability to generate a quadriceps contraction, the alta position of the patella, and ten-

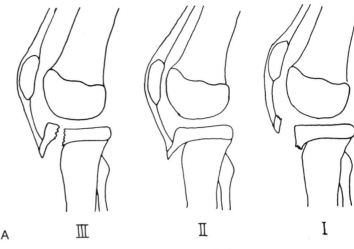

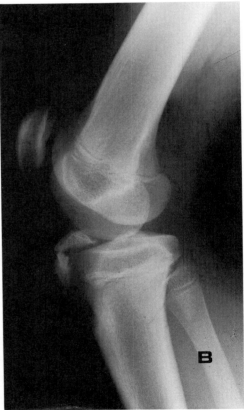

Fig. 13-13. (A) Watson-Jones classification of fractures of the tibial tubercle. **(B)** Skeletally immature athlete with avulsion of the tubercle apophysis and intra-articular fracture of the tibial plateau. The injury was a violent deceleration maneuver (grade III).

derness over the tubercle. These avulsions usually occur in males between the ages of 14 and 16, when the quadriceps muscles are gaining in strength but the growth plates are still open. The growth plate of the tibial tuberosity has a unique histologic structure that is adapted to stress generated by the patellar tendon.[18,23,24] It is largely composed of fibrocartilage, rather than the classically described multiple cell columns, and is well adapted to withstand tensile forces. Endochondral ossification of the tibial tuberosity growth plate is similar to all epiphyseal cartilage, and closure usually occurs between 17 and 18 years of age in boys and 15 to 16 years in girls. During the period prior to closure, there is some structural modification in which columnated cells replace most of the fibro-cartilaginous elements, and therefore there may be less ability to resist severe tensile forces,[25] which explains its vulnerability during the preclosure period (Fig. 13-13).

Treatment consists in cast or brace immobilization of impending avulsions or undisplaced fractures for 3 to 4 weeks, followed by slowly increased activity with restriction of jumping and sprinting. Displaced fractures require open reduction and internal fixation to allow restoration of adequate mechanics. Growth retardation and recurvatum have not been a problem with this regimen.

Avulsion of Distal Pole of the Patella

The fourth group are athletes who sustain an avulsion of the distal pole of the patella (Fig. 13-14). This distraction force is usually accompanied by a direct blow. The most common configurations are transverse or comminuted fractures (80 to 85 percent) and longitudinal fractures (12 to 27 percent). Avulsion fractures of the superior or inferior pole are rare, accounting for fewer than 5 percent of all patellar fractures.[25] Some of them are possibly stress reactions with subsequent overuse or fatigue fractures occurring.[26]

The treatment initially depends on the size of the fragment and the degree of displacement. Small fragments in situ may be reattached surgically. Intra-articular fractures require anatomic reduction. Occasionally, small fragments are best excised. Attention may have to be paid to the predisposing factor (subluxation or dislocation), and the combination of excision and fixation plus retinacular release is worth considering.[26,27]

There is a special variation of this avulsion injury to the inferior pole, designated a sleeve fracture of the patella.[27] It occurs in a much younger age group, usually 8 to 12 years. Here an extensive sleeve of cartilage is pulled off the patella, usually on the take-off leg during jumping (Fig. 13-14). The diagnosis may initially be difficult owing to pain and a tense hemarthrosis. Because the small bony fragment has a large sleeve of cartilage, anatomic reduction is important. Tension band wiring and relatively early controlled motion, usually at 2 weeks, is a good approach.[27] A satisfactory outcome is anticipated.

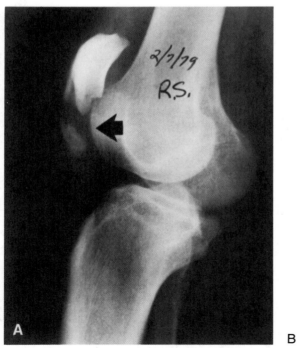
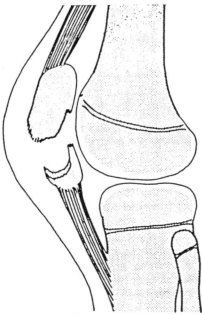

Fig. 13-14. **(A)** Avulsion of the patellar tendon with a flake of bone from the inferior pole. **(B)** In the skeletally immature patient the avulsion may represent a "sleeve" fracture with a substantial amount of articular surface.

OTHER TENDINITIS

With the numerous tendons passing across the knee it is surprising that inflammation associated with repetitive use is not more common. Patellar tendinitis is certainly the most prevalent condition. Clinically, it is difficult to distinguish the tendinitis from the associated bursitis. Three specific syndromes are described here that are related: semimembranosus tendinitis, popliteal tendinitis, and biceps femoris tendinitis.

Semimembranosus Tendinitis

The semimembranosus is a powerful flexor and medial rotator of the knee and its complex insertion on the proximal tibia makes diagnosis of insertional tendinitis difficult. The tendon is comprised of five, almost indistinguishable slips fanning out on the posterior medial corner of the knee that reinforce (1) the medial expansion of the capsule and (2) the posterior medial capsule where, in conjunction with the posteromedial oblique fibers of the superficial part of the medial collateral ligament, it constitutes the posterior oblique ligament; (3) slips that may pass to the posterior part of the medial meniscus or (4) the posterior capsule; and (5) the main insertion lying in a groove just below the joint line and going directly into bone. This combination of capsular and bony attachment makes it easy to understand why this muscle plays such a key role in dynamic knee stability, both in the normal and the anterior cruciate-deficient knee.

When the tendinitis involves the part of the tendon proximal to its insertion, the diagnosis is based on palpable tenderness. The more distal insertional tendinitis is a diagnosis of exclusion. Occasionally it is associated with a hot bone scan showing that the inflammatory response involves all layers of the insertion into bone (Fig. 13-15). The pattern of distribution and intensity of uptake help distinguish it from stress fractures or avascular necrosis of the medial tibial plateau.[28] Furthermore, negative arthroscopy for posteromedial knee pain and the absence of effusion should lead to consideration of semimembranosus tendinitis.

The treatment is similar to that of other tendinitis: reduction of the precipitating activity, substitution of exercises to maintain fitness and strength, and local therapy. Local treatment includes physical agents such as ultrasound, laser, interferential current, and medications such as NSAIDs or even occasionally

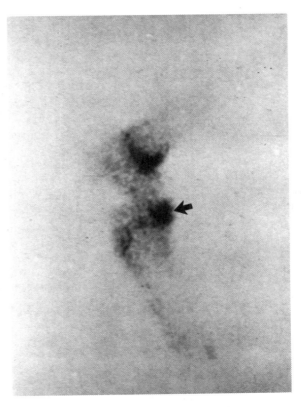

Fig. 13-15. Occasionally the bone scan at the insertion of chronically inflamed tendons is hot. This patient shows increased uptake at the semimembranosus insertion. (From Ray et al.,[28] with permission.)

local infiltration with lidocaine (Xylocaine) and corticosteroid. Because injection may weaken the tendon, considerable activity modification is appropriate as well as carefully infiltrating around rather than into the tendon.

Occasionally the semimembranosus becomes mobile in its surrounding fascia as it crosses the tip of the posterior tibial condyle. A painful snapping tendon results. This entity, as with protracted, recalcitrant tendinitis, warrants exploration and either débridement or resuturing of the tendon or its sheath.[28]

Popliteal Tendinitis

Popliteal tendinitis is an uncommon overuse injury found in runners and even when present is frequently misdiagnosed as iliotibial band syndrome. Inasmuch as the treatment is almost identical, for these entities, misdiagnosis is not a great cause for alarm unless surgical exploration was planned for a recalcitrant syndrome. Furthermore, as with iliotibial band syndrome, the differential diagnosis is important.

Anatomy

The popliteus muscle has three slips of origin, the main tendon being thick and strong and arising from the lateral femoral condyle in a groove just inferior to the lateral epicondyle.[29] As the popliteus tendon goes through the recess of the capsule adjacent to the lateral meniscus, it is ensheathed in synovium to varying degrees. It then passes the juxtaposed biceps femoris tendon running deep to the lateral collateral ligament. At the posterolateral corner there is reinforcement from the posterior capsule and fibula, sometimes called the arcuate ligament. The third set of fibers have their origin at the lateral meniscus, the posterior cruciate ligament, the posterior capsule, and the ligaments of Winslow (frequently called Humphrey) and Wrisberg. These capsule reinforcements partially constitute the oblique popliteal ligament.[29,30] The fibers of origin merge into a thick muscle belly, which insert into the posterosuperior part of the tibial condyle (Fig. 13-16).

Function

These diverse femoral, capsular, and meniscal fibers point to the four possible functions of the popliteus. The first is internal rotation of the tibia or lateral rotation of the femur, which may be a key motion in unlocking the extended knee in the unloaded or loaded position, respectively. Second, the slips from the lateral meniscus allow retraction of the posterior horn during flexion and internal rotation of the knee, which serves to protect the meniscus from the receding lateral femoral condyle.[31] Third, it may work synergistically with the posterior cruciate ligament in preventing forward displacement of the femur during deceleration and downhill running, although there are no dynamic studies of the popliteus during running (Fig. 13-17). Fourth, it dynamically reinforces what may be an anatomically weak posterolateral capsule.

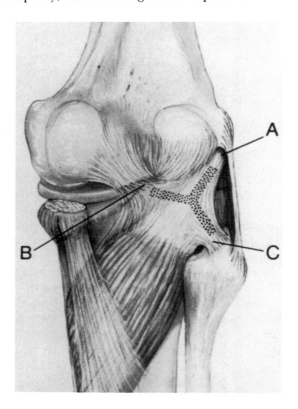

Fig. 13-16. Popliteus muscle. **(A)** Lateral fermoral condylar origin. **(B)** Combined oblique popliteal fibers with origin from the lateral meniscus, posterior cruciate, posterior capsule, and ligaments of Winslow and Wrisberg, **(C)** Fibers from the fibular head contribute to the arcuate ligament.

Quick Facts

FUNCTIONS OF THE POPLITEUS

- Assists unlocking mechanisms of the knee
- Prevents impingement of the posterior horn of the lateral meniscus
- Synergically with posterior cruciate preventing posterior glide of tibia
- Reinforces posterolateral capsule

Pathology and Etiology

Acute tears and avulsions of the popliteus tendon are seen in conjunction with lateral ligament and posterior cruciate injuries. These injuries are noted during surgical reconstruction. More rarely, isolated avulsion occurs and may go undetected. Occasionally these injuries are sufficiently symptomatic that arthroscopic evaluation has allowed identification of the lesion, and repair may be considered.

Acute and chronic popliteal tendinitis is generated by much the same mechanisms as the iliotibial band syndrome (discussed in detail p. 424). They include increased mileage, downhill running, overstriding,

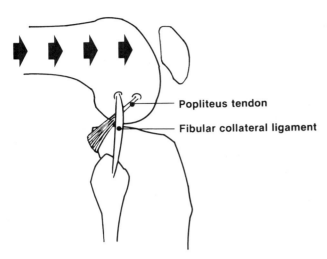

Fig. 13-17. Popliteus may work synergistically with the posterior cruciate ligament to prevent anterior displacement of the femur.

some alignment problems, and improper shoes. In essence, training errors predominate. Occasionally a slip or fall during running precipitates the inflammation.

Clinical Presentation

The athlete complains of late knee pain aggravated by running, particularly on hills, and occasionally descending stairs. Initially, the pain may occur only during activity but ultimately may appear with walking. There may be a specific knee position that produces a sharp pain, frequently at about 30 degrees of flexion.

Clinical Point

LATERAL KNEE PAIN

- Iliotibial band syndrome
- Lateral meniscal pathology
- Lateral meniscal cyst
- Lateral joint arthrosis
- Lateral patellar facet syndrome
- Chronic lateral ligament insufficiency
- Biceps femoris tendinitis
- Fabella syndrome (sesamoiditis)
- Proximal tibiofibula-fibular joint problems
- Popliteal tendinitis
- Popliteus muscle compartment syndrome

Walking stiff-legged may eliminate the symptoms. Some athletes report a sudden onset of pain in the middle of a run, or a mild background ache, which may become severe enough to stop them from running.[30] There is a suggestion that the pain may be related to swelling of the popliteus muscle belly in its fascia, giving a compartment-like syndrome rather than tendinitis, but this proposal is speculative.

Consideration of the anatomy reveals the list of potential structures that may produce lateral knee pain (Fig. 13-18). Careful, meticulous palpation is usually the key to clinical diagnosis, supplemented by specific stress tests and correlated with the patient's history. Palpation may be best carried out with the patient's leg resting on the examiner's shoulder, which leaves both of the examiner's hands free to explore each structure during relaxation as well as with hamstring contraction. Because there is some evidence that internal rotation of the tibia at 90 degrees of knee flexion gives strong electromyographic output from the popliteus, the source of the pain may be partially isolated by this maneuver (Fig. 13-19).

Treatment

Treatment obviously is based on identifying training errors, reducing the stress on the tendon, using appropriate modalities, and supplying NSAIDs and occasionally orthoses. The same principles are applied as outlined in the section on the iliotibial band syndrome. Rarely, surgical exploration is indicated. If it can be established that the discomfort is associated with elevated compartment pressures, the popliteal fascia may be released.

Biceps Femoris Tendinitis

Biceps femoris tendinitis presents in a fashion similar to that of the two previously described tendinitis syndromes. It is diagnosed by its location along the course of the tendon. The most common site of inflammation is near the insertion of the tendon, but it may be more proximal when it is associated with crepitation of the sheath. Attention to style and training techniques usually allow prompt resolution.

DISEASES OF THE BURSA

Bursae are synovial sacs that are fluid-filled, which decrease the friction generated by the motion of one tissue over another. Frequently found protecting tendons from an underlying bony prominence, they

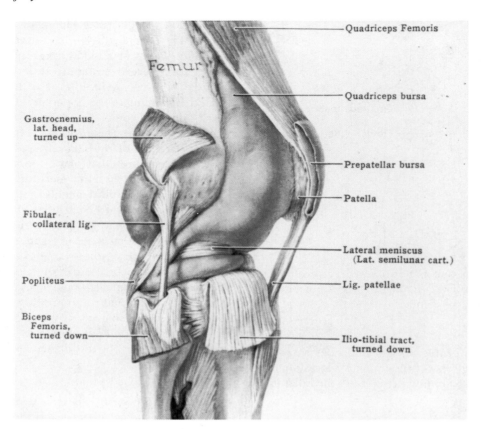

Fig. 13-18.   Lateral view of the knee showing structures that may be a source of pain. Biceps tendon and iliotibial band have been reflected down to show the popliteus tendon and lateral ligament. (From Anderson,[32] with permission.)

are also seen between tendons and between bone and the overlying skin. They are subject to inflammation secondary to trauma or athletic and occupational overuse. This may be involved secondary to an extension of a joint effusion, infection, metabolic or degenerative disease, arthritis, or neoplasms.[33] The bursae around the knees, shoulders, elbows, hips, and heels are those most frequently affected in athletes.

General Signs and Symptoms

Bursal syndromes associated with overuse classically present as a burning or aching pain that initially comes on at a certain point during activity but ultimately persists from one activity session to another. A detailed knowledge of anatomy allows careful, specific palpation and localization of the individual bursa concerned (Figs. 13-20 and Fig. 13-23). By probing deeply along the course of the adjacent ligament and tendons, the localized nature of the inflamed bursa may be verified. Other bursae, particularly the large,

anteriorly placed prepatellar bursa (housemaid's knee) and superficial infrapatellar bursa (parson's knee), are obvious because of the swelling (Fig. 13-21). Localizing the swelling as extra-articular confirms the diagnosis. When the inflammation is associated with a direct blow (e.g., a kick, hitting the boards in hockey, or landing heavily in volleyball), there may be associated hemorrhage in the bursa. In these circumstances there is considerable heat and redness of the overlying skin.

General Treatment Principles

It is important to distinguish a sterile inflammation from an infected bursa. Local signs of spreading erythema, exquisite pain, inguinal nodes, and systemic fever should be treated promptly. If antibiotics are not immediately successful in reducing all systemic and local signs, open drainage or excision of the bursa is mandatory. Aspiration to confirm the presence of organisms is always prudent prior to commencing

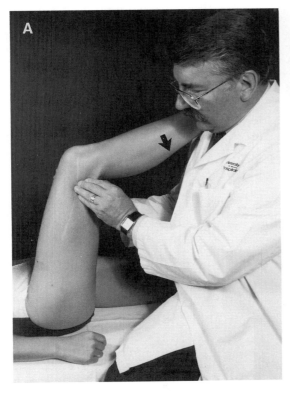
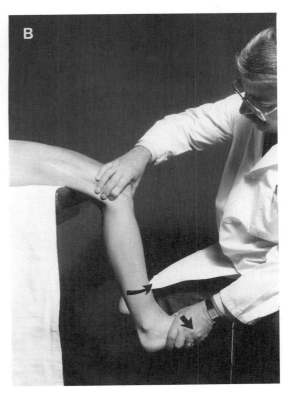

Fig. 13-19. Lateral joint structures may be palpated. **(A)** In conjunction with dynamic contraction of the hamstring muscles, with the leg resting or pushing down on the examiner's shoulder. **(B)** In association with resisted internal tibial rotation to activate the popliteus.

antibiotic treatment. If not infected, these large inflamed bursae may be treated by application of ice, interferential currents, NSAIDs, and when necessary a protective pad may be fabricated to prevent further trauma. If the problem persists or rapid resolution is necessary, aspiration and injection with cortisone are appropriate, but great care to ensure sterility is mandatory. A pressure dressing after aspiration is helpful.

For smaller painful bursae, ice, ultrasound, and NSAIDs are usually effective. When persistent, a careful analysis of the movement involved, modification of training, and local steroid injection usually prove effective. Sometimes persistent recurrent bursitis requires surgical excision of the offending thickened tissue in order to effect resolution.

Classification

Traumatic Bursitis

Acute traumatic bursitis usually involves the superficially situated bursae over the olecranon processes, greater trochanter, and the prepatellar area. They

may be complicated by bleeding which generates a hemobursa.

Chronic bursitis is either an extension of the acute bursitis due to multiple repetitive small blows, such as is seen in the olecranon bursitis of wrestlers, or as part of an overuse syndrome, e.g., the repeated rubbing of the malleolar bursa in figure skaters, the calcaneal bursa in runners, and the iliopsoas bursa of jumpers. In other situations with adjacent tendons, the condition merges imperceptibly into tendinitis. This subject is not discussed here.

Infected Bursitis

Infected bursitis is seen as an extension of an overlying skin lesion, secondary to a penetrating wound, or frequently in sport secondary to contamination after aspiration, particularly when a corticosteroid injection has been used in conjunction with the aspiration. These prolems may evolve quickly, spread rapidly, and cause the athlete to be very sick. Early detection is essential to ensure rapid resolution

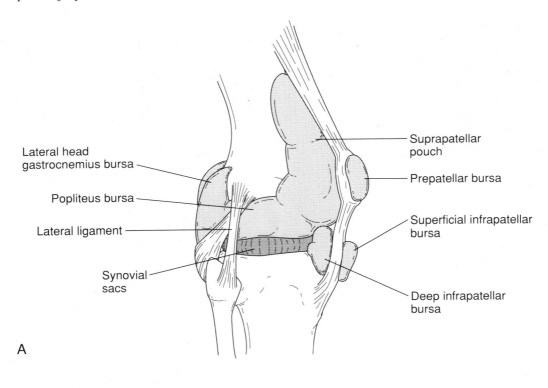

A

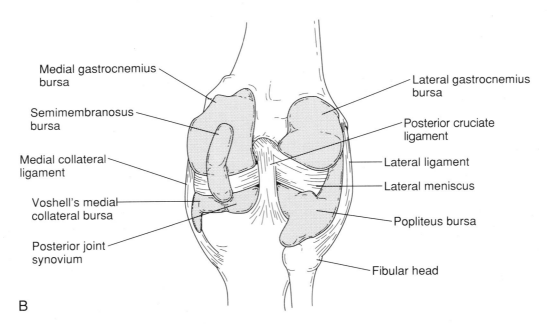

B

Fig. 13-20. (A) Bursa and synovial reflections on the lateral side of the knee. **(B)** Bursa and synovial reflections on the posterior aspect of the knee.

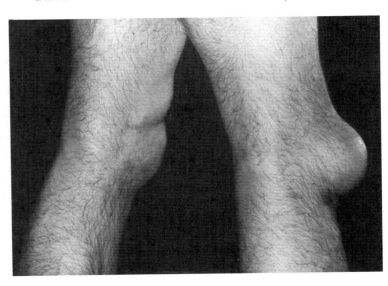

Fig. 13-21. Extra-articular swelling of severe prepatellar bursitis.

with minimal protracted complications. The prepatellar, olecranon, and malleolar bursae are most frequently involved. Intense redness, increasing pain, uncomfortable palpable regional nodes, and spreading cellulitis are local signs. Aspiration may reveal a serosanguineous exudate with streptococcal infection and purulent drainage with staphylococcal infection. With increasing infection, all motion is painful, there is associated muscle spasm, and systemic signs of fever occur.

Treatment includes appropriate blood work (erythrocyte sedimentation rate and white blood cell count), antibiotics, aspiration or drainage, culture and sensitivities of the pus, and occasionally excision and drainage. This condition should not be taken lightly or undertreated. Failure to resolve on an adequate antibiotic regime should raise the suspicion of unusual organisms. Prepatellar bursitis has been well described in the tertiary stage of syphilis, where usually the swelling develops slowly and is doughy to palpation. The pain is less, and there is a propensity to sinus formation. True Baker's cyst, uncommon today, is a tuberculous abscess involving the knee and popliteal bursa.

Bursitis Associated with Arthritis

Bursae that communicate with a joint are essentially subject to the same pathologic processes as the joint. Therefore, frequently, acute symptoms of rheumatoid arthritis are associated with concomitant symptoms in the communicating bursa. At the knee it includes synovial extension around the coronary fibers, and frequently the gastrocnemius and semimembranosus bursae.

With osteoarthritis the latter two bursae are often distended simply because the intra-articular effusion is being pumped into the bursae. They may enlarge to the point of causing symptoms of aching and pain, frequently proportional to the activity, by pressing on other sensitive structures or occasionally because of rupture and extravasation of their content into the surrounding tissues.

With gout, urate deposits in the bursal wall may produce symptoms and signs that are similar to those seen with an acute infective process. Treatment, like all of the associated bursitis in this group, is directed mainly at the underlying disease process.

Neoplasia and Metaplasia

Neoplasia of bursae, osteochondromatosis, pigmented villonodular synovitis, and synovioma are unusual conditions. When they do occur, it is frequently in the popliteal bursa and in association with involvement of the knee joint.

Specific Bursae

Patellar Bursitis

The bursae associated with the patella and patellar tendon include the prepatellar bursa, the superficial infrapatellar bursa, and the deep infrapatellar bursa (Fig. 13-20).

Prepatellar Bursitis (Housemaid's Knee)

The prepatellar bursa is most vulnerable to traumatic damage. Contusions may occur when landing heavily on a hard surface (as with football or rugby), when protective pads slip (e.g., during a volleyball game), from direct blows, or kicks in soccer, and from hitting the boards in ice hockey.

The swelling may occur almost immediately or over a period of 24 to 28 hours. Occasionally, the fluid is largely blood, constituting a hemobursa. The swelling may vary from a slight fluctuance to the size of a small orange (Fig. 13-21). There may be immediate pain relating to the contusion and bruising of the underlying soft tissue and patella. Thereafter pain is usually proportion to the amount of swelling and activity. With chronic bursitis, the area may be almost asymptomatic other than for the swelling and discomfort on firm pressure over the bursa. There may be significant warmth and inflammation, and careful observation of its evolution of symptoms, occasionally with appropriate blood tests or aspiration, enables differentiation between a sterile and an infective situation.

Treatment consists in protection from further trauma by activity modification and appropriate padding. Relief of pressure with a foam, donut-shaped dressing may help. Therapy with interferential currents, NSAIDs, and aspiration (if large) usually allow resolution. It is tempting to use corticosteroid infiltration, which works well. However, absolute sterile technique is mandatory.

If the bursal swelling fails to resolve, the bursal walls become chronically thickened adhesions and septa develop, and the condition becomes self-perpetuating. In these situations small fragments of bursal wall or fibrin deposits may float free in the bursa, occasionally becoming firm, loose bodies; they are referred to as "rice" bodies and contribute to the ongoing bursitis. Direct pressure over these fragments may produce exquisite pain. This type of painful, self-sustaining bursitis is best treated by bursal excision. Adequate postoperative pressure dressings and healing time are necessary if recurrence is to be avoided.

Infrapatellar Bursitis (Parson's Knee, Carpet-Layer's Knee)

There are two infrapatellar bursae, one lying deep to the quadriceps tendon. They are superficial, and unless there is significant swelling it is difficult to distinguish which bursa is involved. Essentially the treatment is the same as for any other bursa with a choice of heat or ice before and after exercise depending on acuteness and symptoms.

Other physical modalities and NSAIDs are helpful, as is molded stress relieving padding if repetitive pressure is a perpetuating factor. Judicious cortisone injection may be warranted, but care must be taken to avoid the tendon.

The differential diagnosis includes Osgood-Schlatter disease in the skeletally immature athlete and patellar tendinitis and fat pad syndrome in the older athlete. It is only rarely necessary to excise this bursa.

Tibial Collateral and Pes Anserinus Bursae

Tibial Collateral Ligament Bursa

In 1943 Brantigan and Voshell described in detail the bursa lying deep to the superficial fibers of the medial collateral ligament.[34,35] This bursa is variable in extent and location, lying between the capsule and the ligament, the medial meniscus and ligament, or the tibia and ligament (Fig. 13-22). Its function is obviously to facilitate gliding of the superficial medial collateral fibers over the tibia and meniscus during flexion and extension. It is important to include this bursitis in the differential diagnosis of patients presenting with medial joint line pain at the level of the medial collateral ligament. Its anatomic proximity to the medial meniscus makes the misdiagnosis of meniscal pathology frequent, with the result that unnecessary and unproductive surgery, and occasionally even unwarranted meniscectomy, may be performed. The differential diagnosis must also include a meniscal cyst.

Injection of lidocaine into the bursa with immediate relief of symptoms usually means that a corticosteroid injection will cure the condition (Fig. 13-23). Considerable care is necessary not to allow significant extravasation of steroid, which may produce some unsightly fat and skin atrophy or even depigmentation of the area.

Anserine Bursa

The pes anserine bursa lies superficial to the distal part of the medial collateral ligament, separating it from overlying semitendinosus and gracilis tendons (Fig. 13-24). Careful palpation allows localization and recognition of this entity. It is somewhat easier to distinguish from meniscal pathology than is tibial collateral ligament bursitis, as it is further from the joint

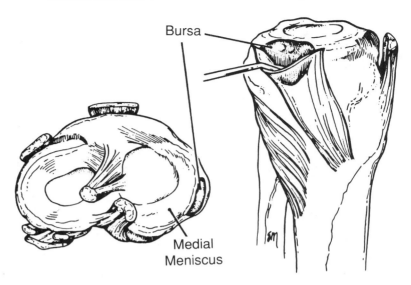

Fig. 13-22. Tibial collateral ligament (Voshell's) bursa.

line. It may be confused with semitendinosus or semimembranosus tendinitis. The anserine bursa may communicate with another bursa lying deep to the sartorius. It is often inflamed as part of the overuse complex called "swimmer's" knee, which involves overstress of the medial collateral ligament. If the usual ice or heat, transverse friction, or NSAIDs do not effect resolution, injection of steroid frequency settles the condition.

Bursae Around the Lateral Ligament

Lateral Ligament and Popliteus Tendon Sheaths

There are no specifically named bursae around the lateral ligament, but there is bursal tissue deep to the ligament (Fig. 13-20). In addition, synovial extensions from the joint follow the lateral meniscus and the popliteus tendon. Popliteal bursitis and popliteal tendinitis merge imperceptibly into one and clinically are usually indistinguishable. It is difficult to distinguish separate inflammatory involvement of these

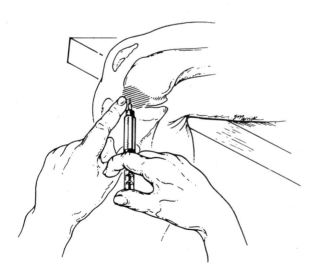

Fig. 13-23. Injection of lidocaine or cortisone into the tibial collateral ligament bursa may serve either to confirm the diagnosis or as treatment.

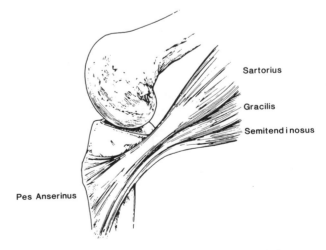

Fig. 13-24. Muscles of the pes anserinus on the medial proximal tibia glide smoothly because of the associated bursal tissue.

specific lateral structures. Only careful palpation, response to modification of activity, and treatment directed at reducing inflammation help establish the specific diagnosis. Cysts of the lateral meniscus, degenerative meniscal pathology, and meniscal tears must be considered in the differential diagnosis.

Iliotibial Band Syndrome

There is a sheet of bursal tissue deep to the iliotibial band where it crosses the prominence of the femoral condyle (Fig. 13-24). Inflammation of this bursa gives rise to the iliotibial band syndrome. This is a particularly common syndrome in running sports.

Anatomy. The iliotibial band, or tract, is a condensation in the fascia lata, representing the major line of pull of the tensor fascia lata muscle and the gluteus maximus muscle. On its deep surface, it is associated with the lateral intermuscular septum. The vertically oriented collagen fibers become thicker as they approach Gerdy's tubercle adjacent to the tibial tubercle on the lateral proximal tibia (Fig. 13-25). At no point is the band totally discrete.[36,37] The action of the proximal muscles serves to tense the band during supporting actions, particularly when bearing weight on one leg. In addition, the tensor fascia lata pulls the band anteriorly during hip extension. However, the amount of motion is small. More importantly, the internal and external rotation of the hip during running, skating, and cross country skiing produce a friction point at the greater trochanter, producing the potential for trochanteric bursitis. The second point

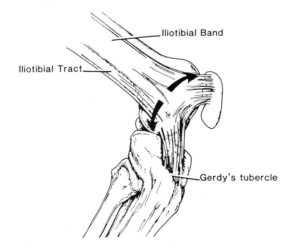

Fig. 13-25. Iliotibial band as a condensation of the fascia lata. Distally the band slips forward and backward over the femoral condyle.

of friction is caused by the flexion and extension movements of the knee, which bring the thickest portion of the band, which is adjacent to the lateral femoral condyle, anterior to the axis of motion in the last 30 degrees of extension. The band moves posterior to the axis of knee motion and the condylar prominence during flexion movements past this 30-degree point. Orăva noted a reddish brown bursal thickening under the iliotibial band adjacent to the prominence of the lateral condyle (the femoral epicondyle).[38] Apart from the pathology generated by friction, this movement of the band across the axis of motion at the knee is intrinsic to the lateral pivot shift phenomenon in unstable anterior cruciate-deficient knees.[39]

Characteristics of the Syndrome. Iliotibial band friction syndrome is an overuse injury induced by friction in the bursa overlying the lateral femoral condyle, iliotibial band, or underlying periosteum.[57] It is more frequently seen in lean individuals, who have a minimum of loose connective tissue and fat in the plane between the band and the prominence of the condyle. It may be associated with varus alignment of the knee, but there has been difficulty linking this syndrome with any specific foot alignment. It may be precipitated by a contusion but it is usually seen during activities that require continuous running, not activities that permit rest between flexion–extension bursts. It may be aggravated by training errors, e.g., excessive distance in a single run, stepping up mileage too quickly, and inadequate warm-up. In addition, running consistently on the same side of a cambered road precipitates the syndrome, usually in the leg on the down side. It is particularly painful during downhill running.[40]

In runners the symptoms usually start as a mild aching sensation on the lateral side of the knee, which increases as the athlete increases the mileage. Initially the pain is present only while running, and the athlete may be unable to locate the source of the discomfort at rest. In some individuals the pain comes on at a remarkably constant point in their workout, but if athletes persist in pushing themselves further, the pain progresses to being present even with walking and ultimately persists between training sessions. The syndrome presents as pain over the condyle, sometimes radiating distally to the tibial attachment or even to the calf or proximally up to the lateral thigh. There is usually localized tenderness to pressure about 2 to 4 cm and proximal to the lateral joint line over the prominence of the lateral condyle.[40,41]

The pain is usually most intense when the leg comes into contact with the ground at foot strike through to midstance. Walking with the knee extended may provide relief. Walking down stairs may be particularly painful. The degree of pain on movement can be categorized on a 1 to 5 severity scale.

Practice Point

SEVERITY OF OVERUSE SYNDROMES

Grade I -Pain comes on after running but does not restrict distance or speed

Grade II -Pain comes on during a run but does not restrict distance or speed

Grade III-Pain comes on during a run and restricts distance or speed

Grade IV-Pain is so severe it prevents running

Grade V -Pain is continuous during activities of daily living

---

Diagnostic Tests. In many individuals there is some associated tightness in the iliotibial band that is elicited by the Ober test (Fig. 13-26). In the normal individual the upper medial femoral condyle should drop level with the lower medial condyle. Tightness in the band is demonstrated by failure to achieve this position and points to a definite avenue of treatment, namely a specific stretching protocol.

Etiology. The following factors may be used in designing treatment.

1. Biomechanical malalignments. Genu and tibia varum may cause excessive tightness of the band at the knee, as might leg length discrepancies. Both varus and valgus heel alignment have been suggested, but these relations are not conclusive. Valgus heel alignment goes with varus knees, whereas the varus heel may be a separate cause.
2. Training errors. Sudden increases in distance or inadequate warm-up may be a cause.
3. Terrain. Excessive hill work, running on a cambered road, or suddenly switching to indoor running on a poorly sprung track or concrete surfaces may precipitate an attack.
4. Anatomic variations. Thin individuals with large prominent femoral condyles and tight iliotibial bands are susceptible.
5. Sex. The condition has been reported more often in men, which may be related to the greater number of men participating in running activities, but might also be related to decreased body fat. Alternatively in women less distinct iliotibial band, greater valgus at the knee, and less connective tissue tightness, may be a factor.

Renne described a maneuver in which the athlete stands on the affected leg with the knee flexed 30 to 40 degrees. This position brings the iliotibial band into tight contact with the prominence of the lateral femoral condyle and may precipate the pain,[41] which may be further accentuated by having the patient hop in this knee-flexed position.[39]

Noble described the compression test for the iliotibial band syndrome.

The athlete is supine with the affected knee flexed to 90 degrees.[40] Pressure is placed over the proximal prominent part of the lateral femoral condyle. The knee is gradually extended, and at 30 to 40 degrees the athlete complains of pain similar to that experienced while running.

Treatment. A thorough activity history should point to the possibilities of altering distance, terrain, running shoes, pattern of training, and warm-up habits. Running or training should be reduced to the point of little or minimal pain and a graduated schedule of activity planned. In particular, hill running should be avoided until the athlete has been asymptomatic for at least 4 weeks. Anti-inflammatory medication and local therapy with modalities such as ultrasound, ice, or microwaves may be effective. Local application of ice using the ice massage technique is often effective before and after running in mild cases or upon resumption of running activities in severe cases.

Passive stretching exercises for the iliotibial band are important. Initially, gravity stretches can be performed associated with hot packs applied to the iliotibial band and lateral thigh. With this maneuver, patients lie on their side with their back near the edge of the plinth, affected side facing up. The unaffected leg is flexed to reduce lumbar lordosis. The painful leg is held in extension at the hip, and the knee is allowed to hang over the edge of the plinth and passively adduct under the influence of gravity. It may be necessary to stabilize the pelvis. This position is held for 15 minutes with a rest periodically to prevent discomfort. Further active stretching may be performed following the initial passive stretch, and it may be added to the athlete's warm-up routine on a regular basis.

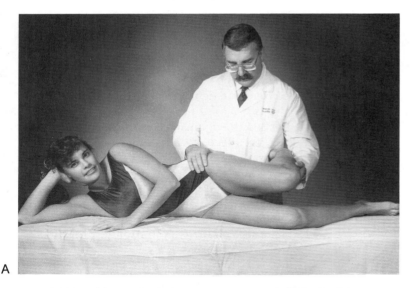

A

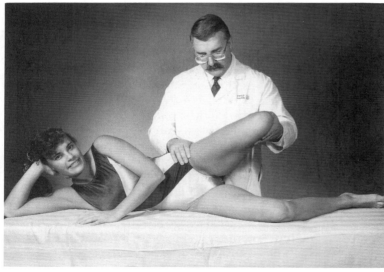

B

Fig. 13-26. Ober test. The patient lies on the side, the affected side uppermost. The unaffected limb is either straight or more classically held flexed toward the abdomen. **(A)** The examiner grasps the ankle of the affected side and flexes, and **(B)** circumducts the hip, bringing it back into full abduction and extension. *(Figure continues.)*

The first exercise is done standing with legs extended and crossed at the ankle. The affected leg is the leg that is adducted. With the knees locked, the athlete side-flexes laterally as far as possible. The stretched position is held for a count of 30 seconds. This exercise is repeated five times (Fig. 13-27).

A variation on this exercise, using the same starting position, is to rotate the waist away from the affected side, flex the trunk, and attempt to touch the heel of the affected leg (Fig. 13-27). This position is maintained for a count of 10 seconds and is repeated five

times. It stretches both the iliotibial band and the hamstrings.

Another exercise is done while lying on the side, the normal leg uppermost and the knees and hips extended in a straight line with the trunk (Fig. 13-28). Patients flex at the waist, pushing themselves up into a resting position on the hip of the affected side, placing their hand directly under the shoulder, and bearing weight on the extended arm and hand. It is essential to maintain back extension to maximize tension on the iliotibial band. It is important to not substitute

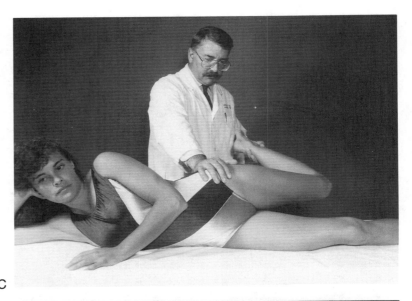

C

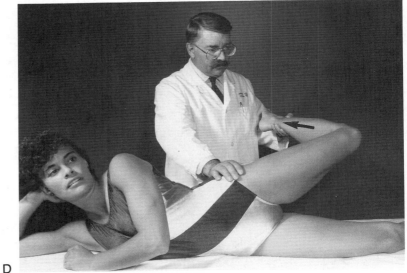

D

Fig. 13-26 *(Continued).* **(C)** A normal test when the knee falls past neutral into adduction, and **(D)** a tight iliotibial band prevents the knee falling past the neutral position.

lateral flexion of the trunk for adduction of the hip. It is sometimes necessary to place the opposite foot on the floor to stabilize the pelvis. The position is held for 10 seconds and repeated five to ten times. These exercises should be repeated at least twice a day.

Any leg length discrepancy should be corrected and orthotics may be considered, including a lateral shoe wedge. Soft running shoes with less motion control or shock-absorbing insoles may also be tried. The concept is to encourage a slightly more pronated position of the foot.

For resistant cases, hydrocortisone injection may be tried. Rarely, surgical release of the posterior fibers of the iliotibial tract is undertaken.

Differential Diagnosis. The pain of iliotibial band syndrome is discrete and well above the joint line. More diffuse pain or pain nearer the joint line should lead to a consideration of lateral meniscal pathology and meniscal cysts, lateral ligamentous strains, popliteal tendinitis, degenerative joint disease, and related metabolic joint conditions (e.g., gout).

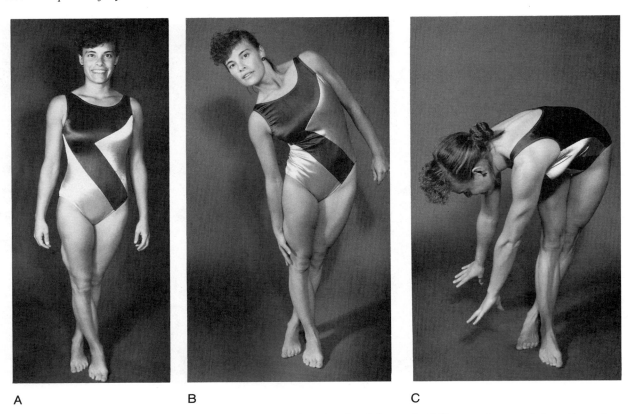

Fig. 13-27. Iliotibial band stretch. **(A)** The patient has both knees in full extension, and the affected leg is extended at the hip and adducted as far as possible. **(B)** Athlete then side-flexes the trunk maximally to the unaffected side. **(C)** Alternatively, the patient may rotate at the waist away from the affected side, flexing trunk and attempting to touch the heel of the unaffected leg.

Bursa of Popliteal Fossa

Numerous and variable bursae have been described in the popliteal fossa in relation to the hamstring tendons (Fig. 13-29). The degree of communication with the knee joint is variable. On the lateral side there is bursal tissue around the biceps femoris as well as extension of the popliteal bursa posteriorly. On the medial side, the joint may communicate with the bursa under the medial head of the gastrocnemius. More superficially there is the important bursa between the medial head of the gastrocnemius and the semimembranosus. This bursal sac is the one most frequently considered when the term semimembranosus bursa is used, although the designation has been used to describe several other bursal extensions including the one between the semimembranosus and the semitendinosus.

These bursae are usually symptomatic in relation to

an extension of knee joint pathology directly or as the result of distention secondary to knee joint effusion. This popliteal swelling is commonly referred to as a Baker's cyst. There is frequently a palpable mass that is sometimes tense and sometimes fluctuant. It is usually not tender. The chief complaint is aching in the fossa. Aspiration usually reveals a jelly-like substance or clear synovial fluid. Occasionally, the semimembranosus bursa enlarges anterior to the tendon, and so the mass is visible medially instead of posteriorly in the fossa (Fig. 13-29).

Therapy is usually directed at the primary knee pathology. However, if the knee is sufficiently symptomatic, bursal injection with steroid, or excision, may produce dramatic relief.

Although other conditions are rare, the differential diagnosis is important as it includes aneurysm and tumor. Aneurysm of the popliteal vessels may be distinguished by recognizing the pulsation and detecting

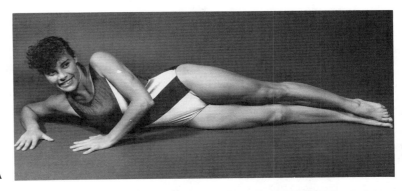

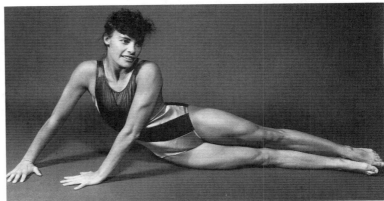

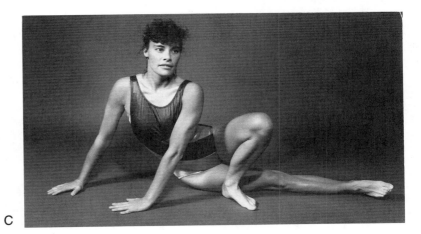

Fig. 13-28. Iliotibial band stretch. **(A)** Athlete lies on the affected side, hips and knees extended. **(B)** Using the arms, the patient side-flexes. **(C)** Opposite foot may be used to assist stabilization and maximize the stretch.

a bruit. Such findings indicate the need for arteriography. A hemangioma presents as a painful, tender, soft swelling, increased local temperature, dilation of superficial vessels, and frequently calcification seen by plain roentgenography. Neoplasms seen in this area include fibrosarcoma; depending on the stage, this diagnosis is usually made only at surgical exploration.

DORSAL DEFECT OF THE PATELLA AND DIFFERENTIAL DIAGNOSIS

There is a benign dorsal defect of the patella originally described by Caffey in 1972 and frequently referred to as Haswell's lesion.[42,43] It is seen typically in

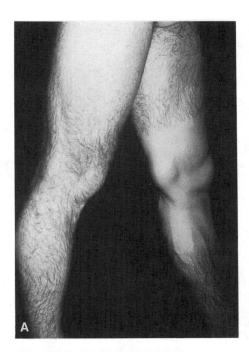

Fig. 13-29. Occasionally the semimembranosus bursa expands anterior to the tendon. **(A)** It then becomes visible and palpable medially. **(B)** Cyst at surgical dissection. *(Figure continues.)*

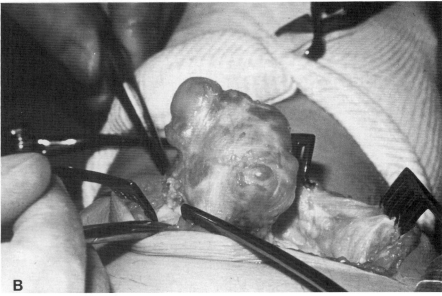

the superolateral quadrant of the patella, and it appears as a lucent area surrounded by sclerosis (Fig. 13-30).[44] Histologically, these lesions are composed of either necrotic bone or vascular fibrous connective tissue. They have been followed in individuals over many years and do not seem to change in appearance. They are occasionally symptomatic in athletes and may display increased uptake on a bone scan. The differential diagnosis includes osteochondritis dissecans, osteomyelitis (Brodie's abscess), chondroblastoma, giant cell tumor, eosinophilic granuloma, aneurysmal bone cyst, intraosseous ganglion, hemangioma, and enchondroma.[44] These defects should be observed and followed if asymptomatic; however, they should be biopsied if they appear hot on a bone scan and the patient presents with symptoms.

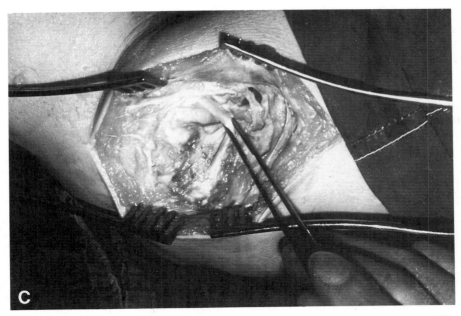

Fig. 13-29 *(Continued).* **(C)** Cyst removed, revealing semimembranosus tendon (indicated by forceps).

PERIPATELLAR NEURITIS

Pain from direct involvement of the nerve root may result from disc protrusion, or via peripheral irritation of the infrapatellar branch of the saphenous nerve or the lateral retinacular nerves.

The peripatellar region is mainly innervated from the L4 root, along with some lateral and medial contribution from L3 and L4. L2 is involved superiorly and S2 posteriorly. Therefore a wide variety of nerve

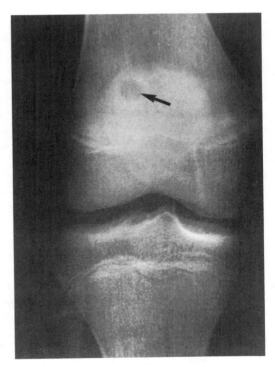

Fig. 13-30. Dorsal defect of the patella seen as a lucency in the superolateral patella.

Practice Point

NEURAL PAIN REFERRED TO KNEE

- Proximal nerve root irritation, from L2, L3, or L4 (radicular)
- Femoral nerve entrapment at pelvis
- Surgical neuromas of infrapatellar branches of the saphenous nerve or lateral retinacular nerves
- Post-traumatic neuromas or neuritis of the peripatellar nerve endings
- Referred pain from hip pathology

root and peripheral nerve entrapments can produce pain in the knee. Pain due to pathology of the hip is frequently referred to the medial thigh or knee, particularly in the young individual where early slipped capital epiphysis may present as a limp and knee and thigh pain. Often painful, limited hip rotation is the only localizing sign. Fortunately, there is usually sufficient clinical evidence that disc pathology and hip disease are rarely confused with primary knee complaints.

Entrapment neuropathy of the infrapatellar branch of the saphenous nerve may occur after surgery, with a neuroma being a complicating feature. Nevertheless, isolated neuritis of this nerve has been reported under several names, including infrapatellar neuritis, retinacular nerve neuroma, gonyalgia paresthetica, and influenza knee.[45,46] This condition may occur bilaterally and present as a "tickling" or "sore" sensation in the affected area, occasionally transient pins and needles, or just a numbness to touch. The extent of involvement varies. Hyperesthesia is another method of presentation. Usually it is possible to treat these patients with local methods of desensitization, injection of steroid, or just waiting out the symptoms. Very painful neuromas complete with the Tinel sign, may require exploration and removal.

Many investigators have pointed out the difficulty of trying to isolate the source of peripatellar pain to the patellar articular surface and bone, and thus have directed their attention to the retinacular nerve fibers. Fulkerson has particularly noted the frequent dramatic relief of pain with retinacular release that does not seem to be the result of realignment.[45] It has been postulated that neural fibrosis and loss of myelinated fibers in the lateral peripatellar retinaculum may be the source of pain. This is conceivably secondary to chronic straining, or stressing of the retinaculum, particularly where there is gross alteration in the patellar alignment and tracking. Fulkerson called this disorder localized retinacular degenerative neuropathy.[45] It is difficult to determine to what extent these demonstrated changes in the peripheral nerves contribute to the symptom complex and, more importantly, to what degree they can be influenced by (1) physical modalities such as ice and heat; (2) medication such as NSAIDs or intracapsular steroid injection; (3) realignment endeavors such as exercises for vastus medialis hypertrophy; (4) retinacular taping; (5) stretching, and (6) surgical release.

VASCULAR PROBLEMS AND REFLEX DYSTROPHY

It has been suggested that there is a constellation of vascular disturbances that may produce patellar pain. A venous engorgement syndrome was proposed in which abnormal venous channels and high intraosseous venous pressures resulted as a response to articular surface pathology. In our study of intraosseous venous pressures in patients with knee pain, previously reported relations could not be confirmed, and the syndrome of high intraosseous venous pressures leading to knee pain in a young, active population is probably rare.[47] It may be a more important syndrome in individuals with established retropatellar arthrosis.

There is an uncommon phenomenon of patellar reflex dystrophy.[48] This syndrome usually arises in response to direct trauma, cast immobilization or as a surgical complication. It is characterized by extreme generalized peripatellar sensitivity, skin changes, inability to generate a significant quadriceps contraction, and classic roentgenographic osteopenic changes involving mainly the patella. There is often a strong disassociation between various sensations in the limb, with a mixture of hypersensitivity to light touch and yet decreased response to pinprick testing. One of the significant findings is a painful loss of joint range not responding to careful, skillfully coordinated physical therapy. A bone scan is usually positive. It is important to identify this condition early, and it requires intensive, prolonged care for a favorable outcome.[49]

Clinical Point

SIGNS SUSPICIOUS OF REFLEX DYSTROPHY

- Night pain
- Pain not related to activity
- Disassociation of pain and touch
- Atrophic skin changes
- Generalized swelling
- Loss of range of motion
- Poor quadriceps control
- Roentgenographic signs of osteopenia
- Increased uptake on bone scan
- Good response to guanethidine block

Treatment

Physical Therapy

Early in the evolution of the syndrome, gentleness and persistence are the key factors. Mobilization in a warm pool with active and active-assisted exercises is often tolerated the best. Frequent, active flexion and extension of the knee within the range of comfort carried on as a home program is important. Stimulation of the autonomic control of the arteriole and capillary bed, by alternating hot and cold at 5-to 10-minute intervals, may have a positive effect on interrupting the vascular spasms.

Manipulation under general anesthesia is generally not recommended, although sometimes it is difficult, particularly in postoperative cases, to distinguish between intra-articular adhesions and reflex sympathetic dystrophy. Any gain from manipulation is usually quickly lost, and the fibrous reaction to the trauma of manipulation makes the situation worse than before. If manipulation is contemplated, it may be done as part of an overall treatment approach in which an indwelling epidural catheter is used initially to instill lidocaine or morphine. Continuous passive motion and electrical stimulation are applied with gradual introduction of active motion as tolerated. Subsequently, the analgesic is changed to the intravenous form and then the oral form, and the patient is able to assist in the range of active exercises. The epidural catheter may have to remain in place for 4 to 5 days, which requires a well coordinated team approach headed by an experienced anesthetist.

Medical Treatment

It is important that the patient receive sufficient analgesia, and frequently an NSAID is adequate. Timing of dosage can be arranged to assist the therapist.

Drugs that have been used include (1) vasodilators; (2) curarizing agents; (3) ganglionic blockers; (4) local anesthetics;(5) antihistamines; (6) anabolic hormones; (7) vitamins; and (8) steroids. There are, however, few large series that have assessed their efficacy.

Sympathetic ganglionic block with local anesthetic or with guanethidine has been one of the most consistently beneficial therapies. It may be helpful for establishing the diagnosis, as often a dramatic improvement is evidenced for the duration of the block. With a good initial response, long-acting agents and repetitive blocks may be used to interrupt the cycle. The relief obtained from the blocks allows the patient to participate in a rehabilitation program.

Permanent Sympathetic Ganglion Block

Sympathectomy should be considered only after serious and concentrated efforts have been made to ameliorate the disorder through medication and physical therapy. A result similar to that seen with a sympathetic block can be expected. There tends to be an inverse correlation between the length of the disease and the success of sympathectomy. When medical means fail and symptoms are sufficiently debilitating, one should not delay a long time before sympathectomy.

Bone Core Decompression

Core decompression is complex and possibly operates at several levels. When elevated intraosseous venous pressure exists, there is a measurable reduction after the coring. There is often an immediate and dramatic reduction of pain postoperatively. Creation of the trough in the bone cuts across many vascular channels and thereby stimulates revascularization as part of the process of reossification.

Results from the core decompression are variable, and it should not be used as the sole treatment modality. There is probably an optimal time for this intervention. Sudeck described three phases through which the classic syndrome passes: hypertrophy, dystrophy, atrophy. Ficat and Hungerford believed the best time for core decompression is after the first phase and before the establishment of permanent tissue changes.[48]

FAT PAD SYNDROMES

Hoffa's Disease

There is an ill-defined syndrome that involves pain and swelling of the infrapatellar fat pad, frequently referred to as Hoffa's disease.[50] Point tenderness over the anteromedial or anterolateral joint line—with or without symptoms of clicking, pain on forced extension, catching, and discomfort on sitting for long periods—may be related to inflammation of the fat pad. On examination, the tender, puffy, fat pad bulges out on either side of the patellar tendon. This syndrome merges into and is difficult to distinguish from the other patellofemoral pain syndromes, patellar tendinitis, and superficial and deep infrapatellar bursitis and plical pathology. Although usually precipitated by trauma in football, soccer, and volleyball players, it may also be seen as a complication of arthroscopy caused by irritation of the probes or the arthroscope in anterior portals. In this case, it may present as late as 2 to 3 weeks after surgery and delays recovery unless treated aggressively.

The treatment consists in protecting the fat pad in sports where repetitive contusion is a problem and local therapy with ice, ultrasound, or interferential currents. Systemic therapy includes the use of aspirin or NSAIDs. Occasionally steroid injection into the fat pad is effective. Rarely, operative resection of the fat pad is required.

Entrapment of the Fat Pad

Occasionally, a large fat pad is entrapped between the articular surfaces. This syndrome is impossible to distinguish clinically from anterior horn and bucket handle meniscal lesions. Pain on palpation of the anterior joint lines, effusion, locking, catching, giving way, and extreme pain on forced extension are the common presenting findings. At arthroscopy an engorged, beefy-looking fat pad nodule is seen to be entrapped during motion of the knee. It is sometimes difficult to visualize, as it may block the arthroscope. Other variants are a tough, white, fibrotic, metaplased tongue of the fat pad secondary to prolonged and repeated entrapment. Rarely, a blackened, necrosed protuberance, often with associated hemorrhage, may be seen that leaves little doubt as to the diagnosis.

INFRAPATELLAR CONTRACTURE SYNDROME

A syndrome has been described by Paulos and his colleagues that incorporates some of the elements of both the previously described clinical pictures.[50,51] This syndrome is frequently seen after anterior cruciate reconstruction and occasionally as the result of arthroscopy or direct trauma.[52] It results in loss of range of motion, both extension and flexion. Flexion exceeding 125 degrees is usually adequate for many activities, although the athlete may complain of an inability to squat. By contrast, lack of extension of more than 10 degrees may cause problems in all activities, including a limp when walking, retropatellar

pain, and possibly even late arthrosis.[53] This condition is described more fully with the complications of ligament reconstructive surgery (see Ch. 15).

SUMMARY

This chapter has encompassed a collection of discrete entities presenting as anterior, medial, and lateral knee pain. Together they form a major portion of the overuse syndromes at the knee. Generally, they are easily treated, but unfortunately delayed presentation for therapy can lead to disabling, intractable problems. Furthermore, if neglected, they are associated with uncommon but catastrophic ruptures of the extensor apparatus.

Patellar dislocation should be easily recognized, but because the practitioner treating the athlete frequently does not see the patient at the time the patella is actually out of joint it is often overlooked and the symptoms are attributed to ligamentous laxity, chondromalacia, or meniscal pathology. So long as awareness is maintained, the history carefully elicited, and the specific tests diligently carried out, this entity can usually be dealt with effectively.

Lastly, some uncommon diagnoses have been given more space here than they deserve, mainly because they are infrequently covered in many sports medicine texts. They include popliteal tendinitis, dorsal defects of the patella, reflex dystrophy, and the infrapatellar contracture syndrome.

The syndromes in this chapter are anatomically discrete entities. Treatment regimens should have a strong functional and biomechanical basis if the dual purpose of successful resolution is to be accomplished while maintaining adequate levels of strength and fitness.

REFERENCES

1. Cash JD, Hughston JC: Treatment of acute patellar dislocation. Am J Sports Med 16:244, 1988
2. Hawkins RJ, Bell RH, Anisette G: Acute patellar dislocations: the natural history. Am J Sports Med 14:117, 1986
3. Henry JH, Craven PR: Surgical treatment for patellar instability: indications and results. Am J Sports Med 9:82, 1981
4. Betz RR, Magill JT, Lonegram RP: The percutaneous lateral retinacular release. Am J Sports Med 15:477, 1987
5. Metcalf R: An arthroscopic method for lateral re-

lease of the subluxation or dislocating patella. Clin Orthop 167:9, 1982

6. Bigos S, McBride G: The isolated lateral retinacular release in the treatment of patellofemoral disorders. Clin Orthop 186:75, 1984

7. Blazina ME, Kerlan RK, Jobe FW et al: Jumper's knee. Orthop Clin North Am 4:665, 1973

8. Ferretti A: Epidemiology of jumper's knee. Sports Med 3:289, 1986

9. Sommer HM: Patellar chondropathy and apicitis and muscle imbalances of the lower extremities in competitive sports. Sports Med 5:386, 1988

10. Mital MA, Matza RA: Osgood-Schlatter disease: the painful puzzler. Physician Sports Med 5:60, 1977

11. Osgood RB: Lesions of the tibial tubercle occurring during adolescence. Boston Med J Surg 148:114, 1903

12. Martens M, Wouters P, Burssens A, Mulier JC: Patellar tendinitis pathology and results of treatment. Acta Orthop Scand 53:445, 1982

13. Sinding-Larsen MF: A hitherto unknown affection of the patella in children. Acta Radiol 1:171, 1921

14. Black JE, Alten SR: How I manage infrapatellar tendinitis. Physician Sports Med 12:86, 1984

15. Curwin S, Stanish WD: Tendinitis: Its Etiology and Treatment. Callamore Press, DC Health, Lexington, 1984

16. King AG, Blundell-Jones G: A surgical procedure for the Osgood-Schlatter lesion. Am J Sports Med 9:250, 1981

17. Donati RB, Cox S, Echo BS, Powell CE: Bilateral simultaneous patellar tendon rupture in a female collegiate gymnast: a case report. Am J Sports Med 14:231, 1986

18. Mirbey J, Besancenot J, Chambers RT et al: Avulsion fractures of the tibial tuberosity in the adolescent athlete. Am J Sports Med 16:336, 1988

19. Michia H, Stang-Voss C: The predisposition to tendon rupture after doping with anabolic steroids. Int J Sports Med 4:59, 1983

20. Wood TO, Cooke PH, Goodship AE: The effect of exercise and anabolic steroids on the mechanical properties and crimp morphology of the rat tendon. Am J Sports Med 16:153, 1988

21. Bowers KD: Patellar tendon avulsion as a complication of Osgood-Schlatter disease. Am J Sports Med 9:356, 1981

22. Kelly DW, Carter VS, Jobe FW, Kerlan RK: Patellar and quadriceps tendon ruptures—jumper's knee. Am J Sports Med 12:375, 1984

23. Greenspan A, Norman A, Tchang FKM: "Tooth" sign in patella degeneration disease. J Bone Joint Surg [Am] 59:483, 1977

24. Ogden JA, Southwick WO: Osgood-Schlatter disease and tibial tubercle development. Clin Orthop 116:180, 1976

25. Heckman JD, Alkire CC: Distal patellar pole fractures: a proposed common mechanism of injury. Am J Sports Med 12:424, 1984

26. Dickoff SA: A case report: longitudinal stress fractures of the patella—a cause of peripatella pain in a runner. J Orthop Sports Phys Ther 9:194, 1987

27. Houghton GR, Ackroyd CE: Severe fractures of the patella in children: a report of three cases. J Bone Joint Surg [Br] 61:165, 1979

28. Ray JM, Clancy WG, Lemon RA: Semimembranosus tendinitis: an overlooked cause of medial knee pain. Am J Sports Med 16:347, 1988

29. Basmajian JY, Lovejoy JF: Functions of the popliteus muscle in man. J Bone Joint Surg [Am] 53:557, 1971

30. Allen M, Ray G: Popliteus tendinitis: a new perspective. Sports Train Med Rehabil 1:219, 1989

31. Lovejob JF, Harden TP: Popliteus muscle in man. Anat Rec 169:727, 1971

32. Anderson JE (ed): Grant's Atlas of Anatomy. Williams & Wilkins, Baltimore, 1983

33. Turek SL: Orthopaedics Principles and their Application. p. 1237. In: Bursae Around the Knee. 3rd Ed. JB Lippincott, Philadelphia, 1977

34. Brantigan OC, Voshell AF: The tibial collateral ligament: its function, its bursae and its relationship to the medial meniscus. J Bone Joint Surg 25:121, 1943

35. Keslan RK, Glousman RE: Tibial collateral ligament bursitis. Am J Sports Med 16:344, 1988

36. Terry GC, Hughston JC, Norwood LA: The anatomy of the iliopatellar band and iliotibial tract. Am J Sports Med 14:39, 1986

37. Sutker AN, Barber FA, Jackson DW et al: Iliotibial band syndrome in distance runners. Sports Med 2:447, 1985

38. Orava S: The iliotibial tract friction syndrome in athletes—an uncommon exertion syndrome on the lateral side of the knee. Br J Sports Med 12:69, 1978

39. Reid, DC: Assessment and Treatment of the Injured Athlete. University of Alberta, Edmonton, 1984

40. Noble CA: Iliotibial band friction syndrome in runners. Am J Sports Med 9:232, 1980

41. Renne J: The iliotibial band friction syndrome. J Bone Joint Surg 57:1110, 1975

42. Denham RH: Dorsal defect of the patella. J Bone Joint Surg [Am] 66:116, 1984

43. Haswell DM, Berne AS, Graham CB: The dorsal defect of the patella. Pediatr Radiol 4:238, 1976

44. Gamble JG: Symptomatic dorsal defect of the patella in a runner. Am J Sports Med 14:425, 1986

45. Fulkerson JP: The etiology of patellofemoral pain in young active patients: a prospective study. Clin Orthop 179:129, 1983

46. Massey JW: Entrapment neuropathy of the infrapatellar branch of the saphenous nerve. Am J Sports Med 8:456, 1980 (letter to the editor)

47. Reid DC, Wilson J, Magee D, Vargo J: Interosseous venous pressures in the patello-femoral pain syndrome. Am J Knee Surg 3:1, 1990

48. Ficat RP, Hungerford DS: Disorders of the Patello-Femoral Joint. Williams & Wilkins, Baltimore, 1979

49. Tietjen R: Reflex sympathetic dystrophy of the knee. Clin Orthop 209:234, 1986

50. Paulos LE, Rosenberg TD, Drawbert J et al: Infrapatellar contracture syndrome: an unrecognized cause of knee stiffness with patellar entrapment and patella infera. Am J Sports Med 15:331, 1987

51. Payr E: Zür operativen Behandlung der Kniegelenksteife. Zentralbl Chir 44:809, 1917

52. McConkey JP, Leung P, Li D: Magnetic resonance imaging in knee stiffness syndrome after anterior cruciate ligament surgery. Clin J Sports Med 1:176, 1991

53. Sprague N, O'Conner R, Fox J: Arthroscopic treatment of postoperative knee fibroarthrosis. Clin Orthop 166:165, 1982

Knee Ligament Injuries: Anatomy, Classification, and Examination

14

The knee is a joint, not an entertainment.
—J. Noble, Journal of Bone and Joint Surgery. British
Volume, 1986

Injuries to the knee ligaments are common in sports and recreation, which is not surprising in view of the lack of bony structural integrity, the long levers afforded by the femur and tibia, the huge muscular torques, and the impacts at high velocities. Indeed, Johnson reported that anterior cruciate injuries could be recorded in 1.2 percent of freshmen attending the University of Vermont.[1]

Before knee instabilities can be described and understood, a review of the surgical anatomy is necessary, as it differs somewhat from the basic anatomic textbook descriptions. The structures around the knee can be divided, for purpose of description, into four main groups: medial ligamentous complex, lateral ligamentous complex, posterior capsular structures, and internal structures of the knee. It must be realized that although gross repairs or substitutions for these structures are frequently performed with apparent ease, the subtle spiral arrangements of the fibers, the changing axis of motion, and the critical nature of the points of insertion of these ligaments make successful reconstruction a difficult task.

To discuss the function of each component of the static and dynamic structures around the knee as isolated entities is to fail to appreciate their important and intricate interrelations during normal motion. Nevertheless, for the sake of clarity with this already complex subject, that is what must be done. For most clinicians, it is sufficient to recognize acute ligamentous disruptions and have some idea of their severity so that those requiring surgery are appropriately referred. They must also be able to distinguish ligamentous laxity as a cause of functional instability from patellar subluxation, loose bodies, and meniscal pathology. Many diagnostic tests are presented, and each clinician must select those that seem to work best. Experience and practice are prerequisites for detecting some of the more subtle abnormal motions. No single test is pathognomonic, although some (e.g., a positive pivot shift test) invariably indicate that one ligament (in this case the anterior cruciate) is nonfunctional. The degree of involvement of other structures, which is important in surgical decisions, requires a constellation of signs to allow logical decisions. After years of increasing complexity, the central role of the anterior and posterior cruciate ligaments has become more obvious and concepts of reconstruction simpler. Nevertheless, each patient and each injured knee presents a challenge that has frequently led the experienced knee surgeon to realize that, in many ways, the more we know the less sure we are in many clinical situations.

ANATOMY

Bony Structure

The knee joint is characterized by large, incongruent articular surfaces and the presence of menisci. It is designed to transmit the forces of walking and standing and is capable of withstanding the stresses and heavy thrusts of jumping and running. It is incredible that the two apparently incompatible properties of stability and mobility have been amalgamated so well at this joint. The stability is most obvious during complete extension, whereas mobility is possible during flexion. Phylogenically, the knee is a three-joint system that has evolved with the upright posture into a single joint with one capsule. It may be said that the knee works essentially by axial compression under the influence of gravity and muscle action.

The femoral shafts slope from the wide human pelvis to almost midline at the knee joints. The articular surfaces are set in such a way that the tibia is nearly vertical, which is achieved by the medial femoral condyle being larger and projecting more than the lateral condyle (Fig. 14-1). This configuration creates a normal angle of about 10 to 12 degrees, which if increased is referred to as knock-knees, or genu valgum. The opposite condition, genu varum, occurs if the lateral femoral condyle projects too far. In the condition of bowlegs the knee joints are usually normal and the deformity is frequently the product of an abnormal tibia.[2] The normal angle at the knee has the effect of predisposing the patella to lateral displace-ment. The anterior projection of the lateral condyle and the low insertion of the vastus medialis counter-act this tendency.[3,4]

Medial Ligamentous Complex

The ligamentous support of the medial side of the knee is formed by the medial capsule and reinforced by the overlying ligamentous structures. These layers may be separated by bursal tissue, which facilitates independent movement.[3] For descriptive purposes this medial ligamentous complex is divided into thirds.

Anterior Third

The anterior portion is formed by the anterior capsule and reinforced by the extensor retinaculum, which is an expansion of the vastus medialis aponeurosis. It extends anteriorly from the medial border of the patella and patellar tendon to the leading edge of the superficial tibial collateral ligament. Contraction

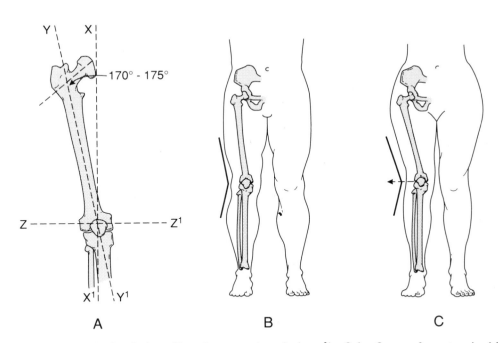

Fig. 14-1. **(A)** Mechanical axis (x–x¹) and anatomic axis (y–y¹) of the femur do not coincide. The femora slope inward, placing the knee nearer to the line of gravity and requiring an offset of the femoral condyles. Because the transverse axis of the knee (z–z¹) is almost horizontal, in full flexion the leg does not align with the femoral shaft but approaches the buttock in line with the ischial tuberosity. **(B)** Normal male alignment. **(C)** The wider female pelvis tends to increase the varus of the femur and hence increase the Q-angle. It therefore produces a greater tendency to lateral displacement of the patella with quadriceps contraction.

of the vastus medialis helps tighten this portion of the medial ligamentous complex and thereby contributes a dynamic component to the stability of the knee.

Middle Third

The middle section is composed of the medial portion of the capsule reinforced by the tibial collateral ligament, which is itself arranged into two layers. The deep layer, referred to as the coronary ligament or deep capsular ligament, is comprised of an upper meniscofemoral portion and a lower meniscotibial portion. It has also been referred to as the middle capsular ligament of Slocum and Larsen.[5,6] It is the intimate association of this layer with the medial meniscus, particularly toward the posterior corner, that accounts for the high incidence of meniscal pathology with tears of the medial collateral ligament. (Fig. 14-2).

The superficial layer, the so-called superficial medial ligament or long fibers of the medial collateral ligament, has an arc-like insertion proximally into the medial femoral condyle. Distally these fibers insert into the tibial condyle at a considerable distance from the joint surface and deep to the tendons of the pes anserinus. For the sake of completion, the most posterior oblique fibers of the superficial medial collateral ligament blend with the posteromedial corner of the capsule, and combined they are referred to as the posterior oblique ligament. This structure is part of the posteromedial corner of the knee described below. As the knee is extended, the posterior fibers of the superficial collateral ligament are tightened, and the anterior fibers come under less tension. The reverse is seen during knee flexion. A mechanism is thus provided by which part of the ligament is always under tension, giving a significant static stabilizing force to this side of the joint. The distal insertion of the superficial medial collateral ligament is designed in such a way that it enables the condyles of the tibia to rotate freely during flexion and extension, with the proximal insertion of the ligament serving as part of

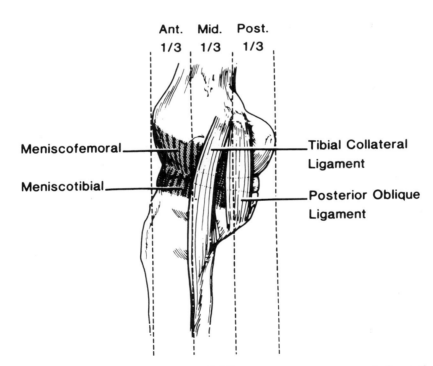

Fig. 14-2. Anterior, middle, and posterior medial ligamentous structures reinforce the capsule. The anterior third is dynamic owing to the quadriceps expansion; the middle third is enhanced by the superficial and deep fibers of the medial collateral ligament and the posterior third by the posterior oblique fibers of the medial collateral, which is further reenforced by fibers from the medial hamstrings.

the axis of motion. Surgical interference with the insertion of these ligaments during repairs for chronic instability is critical. There is slightly more margin for error of placement with distal advancements than with proximal advancements.

Posterior Third

The posterior portion of the medial ligamentous complex, or posteromedial corner, as it is referred to, is formed by the posteromedial capsule reinforced by several structures. It is taut during extension and lax during flexion, and it forms a sling around the medial femoral condyle. The reinforcing structures are numerous, consisting of the posteriormost fibers of the superficial collateral ligament sweeping inferiorly from the femur, forming, as previously mentioned, a thick structure known as the posterior oblique ligament (Fig. 14-2).

Clinical Point

POSTEROMEDIAL CORNER OF KNEE

- Deep medial collateral ligament in association with medial meniscus
- Posterior superficial fibers blend with capsule
- Expansions from semitendinosis also reinforce capsule
- Combined structure called posterior oblique ligament
- Torn with significant valgus or rotary stresses

In addition, the multiple insertions of the semimembranosis reinforce this posteromedial corner while further dynamic support is provided by the sartorius, gracilis, and semimembranosis (Fig. 14-3). Their tendons of insertion are known collectively as the pes anserinus.

In summary, the multicentric origin, the fan-like arrangement of the fibers, and the changing radius of curvature of the femoral condyles allow some portion of the superficial tibial collateral ligament to remain taut throughout the range as it slides posteriorly as much as a centimeter from extension to flexion.

Quick Facts

MEDIAL CAPSULAR COMPLEX

- During flexion the anterior fibers of the superficial medial ligament are tense.
- During partial extension the posterior fibers and adjacent posteromedial capsule take up the strain.
- During full extension the whole ligament is taut owing to associated rotation.
- Quadriceps and hamstring expansion lend dynamic support.
- Several bursa are associated with the ligament and hamstring tendons, and their inflammation may mimic meniscal or ligament pathology.

Lateral Ligamentous Complex

The lateral ligamentous complex may be divided into anterior, middle, and posterior portions.

The anterior portion is formed by the capsular ligament, which extends from the lateral border of the patellar tendon and patella to the anterior aspect of the iliotibial band (Fig. 14-4). This part of the capsule is reinforced by the lateral expansions of the quadriceps tendon, also known as the lateral quadriceps retinaculum. There are several reinforcing fibers in this portion of the lateral retinaculum, originating from the iliotibial band (patellofemoral ligament). They provide a dynamic stabilizing force to the side of the knee and the patella.

The middle portion of the lateral capsule of the knee is supplemented by the iliotibial band, which also provides an important dynamic support.[7,8] The posterior portion of the lateral complex of the knee is formed by ligaments that blend into a single functional unit called the arcuate complex (Fig. 14-5). The components of this complex are the fibular collateral ligament and one of the aponeurotic slips from the insertion of the popliteus muscle.[9] Unlike the medial side of the knee, these ligaments are usually not considered to be in direct contact with the meniscus. However, this concept is not entirely true, as the popliteus muscle attaches to both the femoral condyle and the lateral meniscus.[3,10] The popliteus muscle serves an important role by helping to initiate flexion by

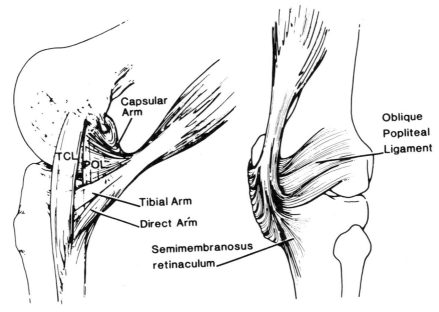

Fig. 14-3. Dynamic reinforcements to the posteromedial corner of the knee, with five components to the semimembranosis insertion. TCL = tibial collateral ligament; POL = posterior oblique fibers.

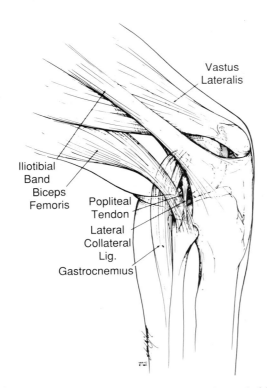

Fig. 14-4. Anatomic structures on the lateral side of the knee.

unscrewing the locked extended knee. It also enables withdrawal of the lateral meniscus to prevent its impingement during flexion. It is facilitated by the fact that the lateral tibial plateau is slightly convex in profile and curves back over the posterior margin of the tibial condyle. This posteromedial corner of the knee is further reinforced by the dynamic action of the biceps femoris, the popliteus muscle (as mentioned), and the lateral head of the gastrocnemius muscle.

Posterior Capsule Structures

The most significant static and dynamic stabilizing structures posteriorly are the posterior capsule reinforced by the arcuate complex, the oblique popliteal ligament and the expansions of the semimembranosis medially and the biceps femoris laterally (Fig. 14-5). More remotely, it is reinforced by the medial and lateral heads of the gastrocnemius.

The oblique popliteal ligament is a dense thickening in the posterior capsule made up of a continuation of the popliteal fascia and part of the insertion of the semimembranosis. It is particularly influenced by the contraction of the latter muscle.

Posterolaterally, the popliteal fascia and expansions of the biceps and femoris form dynamic sup-

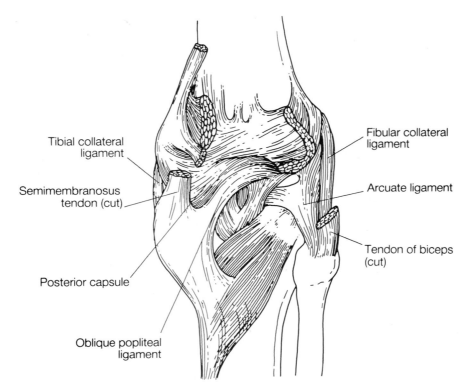

Fig. 14-5. Posterior ligamentous structures.

ports and, together with the lateral ligament, form the arcuate complex. This arcuate complex is an essential component of some of the lateral reconstructive procedures on the knee.

Quick Facts

STABILITY OF THE KNEE

- Structural — bony
  - Intercondylar eminences
  - Expanded condyles
- Static — capsular
  - Menisci
  - Primary restraints (anterior and posterior cruciate ligaments)
  - Secondary restraints (capsule, collateral ligament)
- Dynamic — muscular
  - Hamstrings
  - Quadriceps

Cruciate Ligaments

The structure of the cruciate ligaments is exceedingly complex from an architectural and a functional viewpoint.[11] Their integrity influences the axis of the motion of the knee, and they are the primary stabilizers in the anteroposterior plane. Both ligaments are taut in the first 20 degrees of knee flexion. The ligaments are surrounded by synovium, which makes them difficult to visualize fully at open surgery or with the arthroscope, and their blood supply is dependent on this synovial covering. Ligaments appearing grossly intact may in fact have considerable interstitial tearing and attenuation masked by this synovial sleeve. In addition, some groups of fibers may be torn, whereas others are intact, causing functional instability in only certain parts of the range of motion.

Anterior Cruciate Ligament

The anterior cruciate ligament (ACL) may be damaged in as many as 72 percent of knee injuries presenting with an acute hemarthrosis.[12] It is recognized as the main restraint to anterior gliding of the tibia on the femur, accounting for 87 percent of the restraining forces.

The ACL has been described as consisting of two main functional components, an anteromedial band and the larger posterolateral fibers. Although somewhat artificially separated for the purpose of analytic description, they are in reality intimately connected. Spiraling around each other through a full 90 degrees, they finally insert not as distinct cords but splayed out over a broad, flattened area in close relation to the upper posterior limit of the lateral femoral condylar articular surface (Fig. 14-6). The insertional arrangement, together with their spiral configuration, enables sufficient tension from the various groups of fibers to give support throughout the whole range of flexion.[10,13] The posterolateral fibers supply most protection during extension and the anteromedial fibers during flexion, although both sets of fibers are more relaxed in the range of 60 to 90 degrees. At full extension of the knee, both cruciates are taut; however, the ACL develops significantly more tension and is an important stabilizer of the fully extended knee, resisting hyperextension.[10,14,15] It is surgical or artificial reduplication of this highly efficient and ingenious arrangement that has defied orthopaedic surgeons since the days of Hey-Groves.

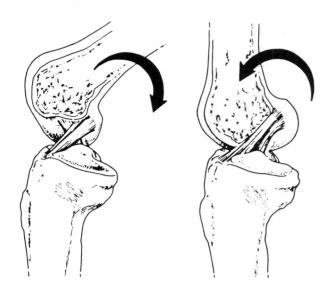

Fig. 14-6. Anterior cruciate ligament with changing tension in the different ranges: anteromedial during flexion and posterolateral during extension.

Quick Facts

ANTERIOR CRUCIATE LIGAMENT

- Damaged in 72 percent of knees presenting with hemarthrosis
- Posterolateral bundle supports best in extension
- Anteromedial bundle supports best in flexion
- At full extension both are taut
- Main resistance to anterior tibial glide

Posterior Cruciate Ligament

The posterior cruciate ligament (PCL) is thicker and approximately twice as strong as either the ACL or the medial collateral ligament (Fig. 14-7). The PCL consists of two parts, although they are inseparable. The anterior part comprises the bulk of the ligament. The fanning out of the insertion and spiral configuration ensure that this ligament is perfectly located to have some of its fibers under tension throughout the whole range of motion of the knee. The range of least tension is 25 to 40 degrees. The importance of the PCL in controlling tibial posterior subluxation and normal motion cannot be overemphasized (Fig. 14-8).

In association with the ACL, the PCL guides the "screw home movement."

Quick Facts

POSTERIOR CRUCIATE LIGAMENT

- Main restraint to posterior tibial glide
- Least tension at 25 to 40 degrees flexion
- Approximately twice the strength of the anterior cruciate ligament

---

The screw home movement, or internal rotation of the femur on the tibia during terminal extension, is due to the contour and longer weight-bearing area of the medial femoral condyle. It is guided primarily by the posterior cruciate ligament, especially the shorter medially positioned fibers, and is aided by the taut

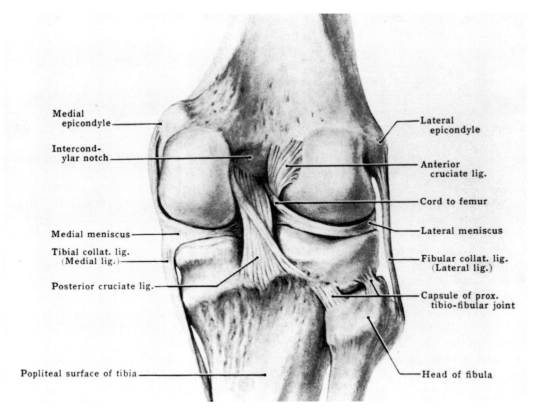

Fig. 14-7. Posterior insertion of the posterior cruciate ligament with the slip from the lateral meniscus (ligament of Humphrey). (From Anderson Grants Atlas of Anatomy, with permission.)

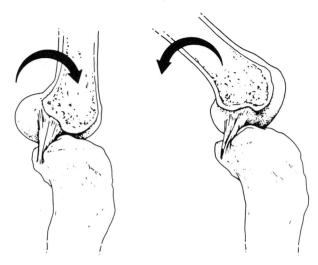

Fig. 14-8. Changing tension on the posterior cruciate ligament.

ACL which stabilizes the lateral femoral condyle. It is therefore no wonder that if the ligamentous elements of the knee become stretched, it is almot impossible to restore normal mechanics by ligamentous reconstruction. Unfortunately, once the subtleties of these changing axes of motion are lost, the surface forces generated on the articular cartilage are such that accelerated degenerative changes are the rule.

Role of the Menisci

Over the years the menisci have enjoyed roles that have ranged from one of serving no significant function to the current concepts of their importance. The freedom at which they have been removed and discarded for questionable pathologies has followed the anatomic literature pari passu. These concepts are outlined in detail in Chapter 11 along with a discusion of meniscal pathology.

Certain meniscal functions are ill-defined, such as

their role in the nutrition of the joint and their function in controlling motion. Other roles, however, are more definite. Pope, for instance, has emphasized the large increase in articulating surface area offered by these menisci and their dramatic effect on reducing the force per square inch through the knee joint surfaces by approximately one-third.[16]

The medial meniscus is connected at its anterior and posterior horns to the tibia. However, throughout most of its circumference it has a femoral attachment in the form of a strong, deep, capsular ligament, or the medial meniscofemoral ligament. The lateral meniscus is also secured to the tibia at both of its horns and more tenuously to the femur by the lateral meniscofemoral ligaments.

Concept of Isometricity

The subtle anatomic arrangement of the natural cruciate ligaments allows a perfect length–tension arrangement through the full range of motion. Because surgeons are unable to duplicate the multifiber, broad insertional arrangement, a special effort is made to place grafts or reconstructions along isometric points. This effort allows a fairly constant distance to be maintained between the two ends of the graft, which lessens in the presence of either articular surface pressure or laxity throughout the functional range. Although no absolute isometric point exists, usually a fixation point, or fulcrum, can be achieved that allows no more than 2 to 5 mm of length change throughout the range, which is functionally acceptable.

The femoral attachment is at the back of the notch adjacent to the lateral condylar articular surface (Fig. 14-9). The point moves forward with increasing flexion. Because it is so far posterior in the functional range of 0 to 60 degrees, the "over the top" position, slightly posterior to the isometric point, is an acceptable functional position.[14–16] This compromise is frequently adopted in surgical reconstructions.

INSTABILITIES OF THE KNEE

There has been an increasing effort on the part of clinicians and researchers to delineate more clearly some of the complex instabilities of the knee. It has become apparent that clinical tests and descriptive terms limiting themselves to instability in one plane are inadequate to describe the complex pathology that occurs at the knee. It is now also clear that the pattern of instability may change over a period of time from that detectable in the acute stage to one of the currently recognizable forms of rotary instability.

There has also been some confusion because of the attempts at oversimplification. It is partly because various combinations of anatomic injury may give rise to the same clinical instability. Instead of recognizing this fact, various schools of thought have developed, each with its own interpretation of the exact etiology underlying any one specific instability. Many of these theories are not mutually exclusive, which must be taken into account when reviewing the literature. Even for the expert, it is becoming difficult to understand the multitude of tests for instability of the knee and the implications and validity of the many studies on the mechanisms of injuries.

Clinical point
- Various combinations of anatomic disruption may give rise to the same clinical instability.

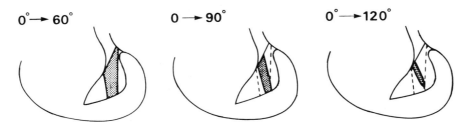

$0° \rightarrow 60°$ $0 \rightarrow 90°$ $0° \rightarrow 120°$

Fig. 14-9. Absolute isometric placement of the anterior cruciate ligament is a goal that probably cannot be obtained. The area of application of force is affected by the knee position and is more anterior in greater angles of flexion. The over-the-top position is close to the isometric point.

With the acutely injured knee it is important to identify the main structures that are disrupted as well as the magnitude of the injury so that logical decisions may be made concerning the possible need for bracing or surgery. To some degree this task is made easier by the precise location of the pain and tenderness as well as the presence of a hemarthrosis. By the same token, protective spasm and fear may complicate the task of accurately assessing the degree of injury.

In the chronically unstable knee, the subtleties of rotary instability are readily appreciated with experi-ence and careful examination. The classification of the instability may be important when planning sur-gery and evaluating treatment outcomes. When there is considerable involvement of the secondary re-straints, it helps establish the need for a more global surgical techniques. For the most part, however, di-rect surgical reconstruction of the ACL and PCL overcomes the functional instability. Hence the em-phasis on complex classification and specific correla-tion with anatomic disruption of the secondary re-straints has been de-emphasized. Nevertheless, the

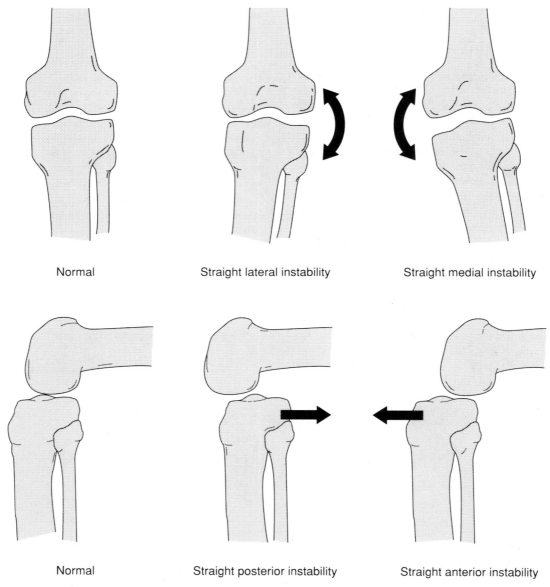

| Normal | Straight lateral instability | Straight medial instability |

| Normal | Straight posterior instability | Straight anterior instability |

Fig. 14-10. Simple one-plane instabilities.

classification of rotary instabilities and the newer conceptualization of a bumper model are presented.

Classification

Examination of the knee involving the application of varus, valgus, anterior, and posterior directional forces is well established. These tests elucidate the component of the instability occurring in one plane (Fig. 14-10).

Rotary or complex instabilities occur when the abnormal or pathologic movement is present in two or more planes.[22] The basic rotary instabilities about the knee can be divided into four groups (Fig. 14-11).

1. *Anteromedial instability.* With this entity the me-

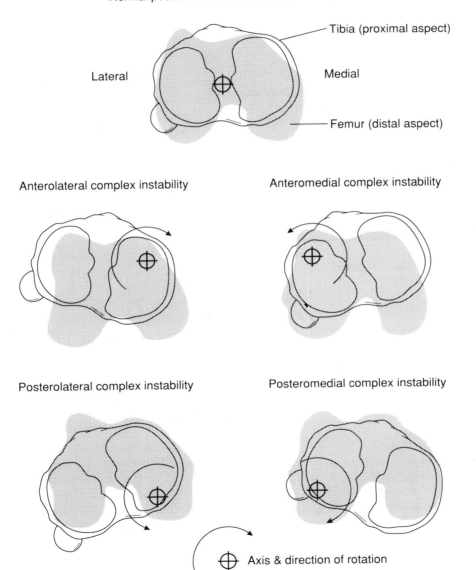

Normal position of the left knee, no rotation

Lateral — Medial

Tibia (proximal aspect)

Femur (distal aspect)

Anterolateral complex instability

Anteromedial complex instability

Posterolateral complex instability

Posteromedial complex instability

Axis & direction of rotation

Fig. 14-11. With rotary instabilities, the ligamentous laxity induces displacement of the axis of rotation, and the instability is named according to the abnormal displacement of the respective medial or lateral tibial condyle. (After Nicholas and Hershman,[22] with permission.)

dial tibial plateau subluxates anteriorly on the femur. The axis shifts anteriorly and laterally.

2. *Anterolateral instability.* This problem is more recently appreciated and the most common pathologic motion in which the lateral tibial plateau subluxates anteriorly on the femur. The axis in this case shifts anteriorly and medially. (This chapter emphasizes mainly the anteromedial and anterolateral instabilities.)

3. *Posterolateral instability.* This instability is one in which the lateral tibial plateau subluxates posteriorly on the femur, with the axis shifting posteriorly and medially.

4. *Posteromedial instability.* Here the medial tibial plateau subluxates posteriorly on the femur. The axis in this case naturally shifts posteriorly and laterally.

5. *Combined complex.* If the above instabilities are present in combination, they are referred to as complex combined rotary instabilities. They are difficult to assess, even more difficult to treat, and carry a significant long-term morbidity even in the most experienced hands.

Naturally, as with any classification, there are advantages and disadvantages to these groupings. Certainly these definitions accurately describe the abnormal movements present both functionally and during clinical examination. However, there is considerable disagreement as to the exact cause of the instability from the anatomic point of view. It has been emphasized that this is partly because different combinations of anatomic injury can lead to the same clinical instability as their endpoint. In addition, the instabil-ity pattern may change with time. It is well recognized that a simple acute valgus instability frequently, over a period of time, evolves into a more complex rotary instability. Subsequent surgical intervention, e.g., meniscectomy, may contribute to the laxity.

"Bumper" Model

Noyes and Grood developed a model of ligament instability by substituting rubber bumpers for capsular and ligamentous restraints to tibial motion.[21,23] The tibia is represented by a line. The two central bumpers are the ACL and PCL. The remaining bumpers are the four corners of the knee in which the combined capsular and ligamentous restraints may be subdivided to make a more complex model (Fig. 14-12). The positions of the bumpers are determined by the slack length of the ligaments. In effect, the tethering effect of the ligament and the restraining force they apply when stretched is represented by the restraining force of the bumpers when they are compressed. The bumpers are placed in the same position the ligament would reach at its "just-taut" length. Thus the cruciate bumpers and extra-articular bumpers change their position with normal flexion and extension allowing for the increased normal anteroposterior translation at 30 degrees of flexion and maximal rotations at 80 to 90 degrees of flexion (Figs. 14-13 and 14-14).

With tearing of any particular restraint, the natural looseness, or the acutely and chronically acquired laxity, obviously affect the eventual instability. How-

---

Clinical Point
LAXITY TESTS

- There is no consensus on the significance of all abnormal joint motions.
- Isolating a ligament for stress testing requires a joint position that allows other supporting structures to be lax.
- The increased laxity with a ligament injury reflects the additional joint motion required to tighten the remaining restraints.
- Final diagnosis is not based on the laxity present but if the final subluxation position is abnormal comparing it to that of the uninjured knee.

Quick Facts
BUMPER MODEL RULES

1. Tibia is represented by a moving line.
2. Bumpers are defined as tension stops.
3. Bumpers may represent combined or single structures.
4. Bumper compressibility represents ligament stiffness.
5. Distance between bumpers represents "just-taut" length where resistance begins.
6. Loss of a bumper represents ligament injury and motion resisted by the remaining primary or secondary restraints.

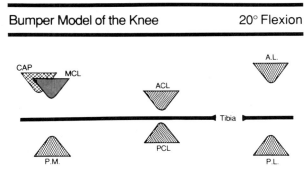

Fig. 14-12. "Bumper" model of the knee. The primary restraints are the anterior cruciate ligament (ACL) and posterior cruciate ligament (PCL). Secondary restraints are the medial collateral ligament (MCL), capsule (CAP), posteromedial corner including the posterior oblique ligament (PM) on the medial side; on the lateral side are the anterolateral capsule (AL) and posterolateral capsule (PL), including the lateral ligament, iliotibial tract, and expansion from the biceps femoris (PL). The tibia is represented as a solid line.

ever, it must be again emphasized that functional instability is a more subtle phenomenon, not solely related to specific ligamentous laxity or any single test; hence it cannot be totally represented by this "bumper" model or the preceding classification of instability.

RECOGNIZING THE UNSTABLE KNEE

Functional instability is usually the result of acute ligament disruption or chronic attenuation superimposed on an acute injury. Nevertheless, the patient assessment must rule out the other causes of instability that either contribute to the athlete's problem or may be the sole cause. They include meniscal lesions, chondral damage, osteochondral fragments, loose bodies, and patellar subluxation and dislocation. Acute and chronic injuries are discussed together here, but it must be realized that the acute injury is complicated by pain and the chronic injury by internal derangement and attenuation of multiple secondary restraints.

History

A history of pain is not always a good guide to these injuries. Some of the more serious injuries may be no more painful than some of the minor injuries. Indeed

there are circumstances where partial ligament tears may produce more pain than complete third degree tears.

With acute injuries the key points are the feeling or hearing of something "pop" or rip, the sensation of the knee going out of joint, and the subsequent inability to weight bear. The report that the knee felt wobbly when attempting to walk or run is also ominous. Eighty percent of individuals experiencing a painful significant "pop" as their knee gives way have an anterior or posterior cruciate injury or a meniscal lesion.

In the presence of trauma, the main thrust of the history should be establishing whether the person complains of an effusion or hemarthrosis. An effusion is the method by which the joint reacts to all stress and usually takes several hours to accumulate. By contrast, an acute hemarthrosis is usually well formed after 1 to 2 hours, leaving a tense, inflamed knee. It has been shown that more than 80 percent of individuals presenting with an acute hemarthrosis have surgically treatable lesions, the most common of which is partial or complete tear of the ACL. Two-thirds of these ligamentous lesions are associated with meniscal damage. The other diagnoses compatible with acute hemarthrosis are peripheral meniscal tears, osteochondral fractures, or posterior cruciate injuries. It is important to stress that, whereas a hemarthrosis usually accumulates rapidly, the absence of tense swelling after the first few hours does not necessarily rule out significant injury. Occasionally the hemorrhage is contained within the synovial sheath surrounding the cruciate ligaments, particularly with partial tears. Furthermore, the main vessels of the cruciates may bleed slowly owing to vessel constriction followed by clotting. Hence the report of swelling delayed for 12 to 24 hours must still be taken seriously. Furthermore, associated chondral fractures and midsubstance mensical tears may produce

---

Clinical Point

POST-TRAUMATIC SWELLING

- Acute hemarthrosis is an indication of significant intra-articular pathology
- Mostly accumulates in first few hours
- However delayed effusion does not rule out hemorrhage

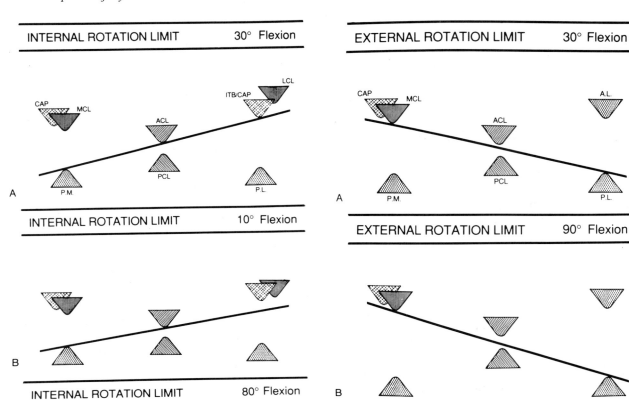

Fig. 14-13. Limits to internal rotation. **(A)** At 30 degrees of flexion, internal rotation is limited by the anterior cruciate ligament (ACL) centrally and the anterolateral restraints. Posterior translation of the medial plateau is limited by the posteromedial restraints. **(B)** At 10 degrees of flexion, the posterior bumpers move in closer toward the posterior cruciate ligament (PCL) owing to a reduction in the slack present in the posterior capsule. In addition, the ACL bumper moves posteriorly as a result of tightening the ACL–PCL complex. Therefore, internal rotation of the tibia is now limited by the ACL centrally and the posteromedial restraints alone. The tibia can no longer rotate far enough to engage the anterolateral restraints. **(C)** At 80 degrees flexion, the posterior

Fig. 14-14. Limits to external rotation. **(A)** At 30 degrees flexion the external rotation of the tibia is limited by the bumpers, which stop anterior translation of the medial plateau and posterior translation of the lateral plateau. Because of the position of the structures there is no direct involvement of either the anterior (ACL) or posterior (PCL) cruciate ligaments in limiting external rotation. **(B)** At 90 degrees flexion the posterior bumpers are moved posteriorly, reflecting the increased slack in the posterior capsule. As a result, the PCL is nearly taut at the limit of external rotation. Removing the posterolateral restraints would only give a small increase in external rotation at this flexion angle.

bumpers move farther posteriorly, reflecting the increased slack in the posterior capsule. In addition, the distance between the ACL and PCL bumpers has increased slightly to reflect the increased laxity of these structures. The anteromedial–anterolateral structures are now moved posteriorly owing to tightening of the extra-articular restraints with knee flexion. Internal rotation is limited by the anterolateral and posteromedial restraints without direct involvement with the ACL.

slowly accumulating effusions rather than tense hemarthrosis.

For the chronically unstable knee the ease of giving way should be established, as it provides a clue as to the possible success of rehabilitation and bracing. The amount of pain and swelling accompanying each episode, as well as the degree of effusion after activity, may indicate the degree of potential for joint damage. Any suggestion of locking or catching is also important, it may be related to the magnitude of the instability or the associated pathology, e.g., meniscal lesions, loose bodies, or chondral flaps.

Observation

With the acute knee, the ease of weight-bearing and motion, the location of the swelling and bruising, and the presence of a deformity may give an initial impression of severity. With severe tearing, the initial hemorrhage may extravasate and cause considerable pitting edema all around the knee after 24 to 48 hours. The inability of the athlete to control the quadriceps by bracing the knee and lifting it straight may indicate the severity of the reflex muscle inhibition.

With recurrent chronic instability, general alignment and the presence of obvious swelling and muscle wasting are important observations. The presence and extent of previous surgical scars are also significant.

Palpation

With the large number of specific ligament stressing tests available, and the ability to utilize expensive technology such as MRI for diagnosis, it is tempting to overlook the important role of a detailed history and careful precise palpation. Particularly in the acute situation, meticulous palpation may reveal the site of pathology. This examination is begun by methodically going over all the structures around the joint including the ligaments along their entire length as well as the medial and lateral joint lines. It is important to ascertain if the major area of tenderness is all along the medial border of the patella. If present it may signify a subluxing or previously dislocated patella, an injury frequently misdiagnosed as a ligament tear. If this lesion is overlooked, it leads to incorrect treatment. Even in the chronically unstable knee, patellar dislocation must be ruled out by palpation and attempts at patellar displacement.

It may help to isolate the collateral ligaments even more by testing the knee in 90 degrees of flexion for the medial ligament and in the figure-of-four position for the lateral ligament[24] (Fig. 14-15). Effusion is ascertained by ballottement or the wipe test depending on the magnitude of the swelling.

Specific Tests for Ligament Instability

One-Plane Instabilities

The term one-plane instabilities is confusing in that, although an isolated tear of the medial or lateral collateral ligaments does result in a one-plane abnormal motion, a tear of the primary restraint (i.e., the anterior and posterior cruciate ligaments) rarely produces a simple instability. In reality this section describes one-plane tests, but even isolated rupture of the ACL nearly always produces anterolateral rotary instability, and isolated PCL tests frequently cause posterolateral instability. Thus these one-plane tests are useful for distinguishing injuries to the primary restraint, but the rotary tests are needed to describe the actual complex abnormal motions that evolve from damage to these structures.

Practice Point

CLINICAL TESTS

- One-plane tests help define the ligaments injured.
- Isolated collateral ligament tears may produce one-plane instabilities.
- Rupture of the cruciate ligaments invariably produces a rotary instability.

One-Plane Medial (Valgus) Instability

In normal clinical practice, minor simple medial instabilities are a frequent occurrence. The diagnosis is based on a valgus or abduction strain placed on the knee in either 30 degrees of flexion or in full extension (Fig. 14-16). With a normally hyperextending knee, three positions should be tested.

One-plane valgus instability in 30 degrees of flexion usually denotes a tear of at least second degree severity of the middle third of the capsular ligament and the parallel fibers of the medial collateral liga-

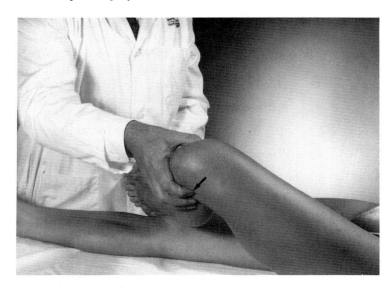

Fig. 14-15. Adapting the figure-of-four position puts the lateral ligament under tension and makes it easier to palpate.

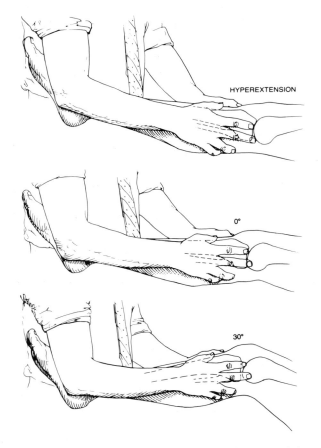

HYPEREXTENSION

0°

30°

Fig. 14-16. Collateral ligaments may be tested in neutral position and 30 degrees of flexion, as well as in hyperextension for the naturally lax knee.

ment. With the leg tested during flexion, the key to an accurate test is sufficient muscular relaxation on the part of the patient. Sometimes it is helpful to have the thigh resting on the examining surface with the leg flexed over the edge, the support from the table aiding the relaxation. (Fig. 14-17). On occasion, local infiltration of anesthetic into the ligament or the joint may be necessary to ensure relaxation. Even this measure, however, sometimes fails to provide the necessary information, and an examination under anesthesia is then required. This situation is frequently the case, when assessing an acute knee injury, and it may form a valuable part of the work-up when considering surgical reconstruction of a complex, chronic instability.

With the knee tested in full extension, any demonstrable instability is a major one in that it signifies posteromedial capsular laxity as well as damage to the medial capsular ligament and the collateral ligament. Most investigators would agree that a certain amount of attenuation or tearing of the ACL or PCL is necessary if the laxity is gross. When performing this test, it must be remembered that the normal extended position for many patients is hyperextension. This point is confirmed by assessing the normal knee and then the valgus stress carried out in hyperextension, at zero degrees (neutral position), and at 30 degrees of flexion to avoid an erroneous conclusion regarding the state of the posteromedial capsular structures (see Fig. 14-16).

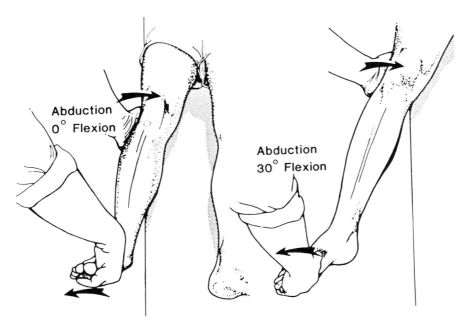

Fig. 14-17. Abduction stress (valgus) test for medial structures with the thigh supported to enhance relaxation.

One-Plane Lateral (Varus) Instability

Varus or adduction stress placed on the knee in 30 degrees is positive when there has been disruption of the middle third of the lateral capsule ligament (Fig. 14-18). According to the degree of instability, the fibular collateral ligament may or may not be disrupted. A roentenogram of the knee may reveal "the lateral capsular" (Segond's) sign, which is the identification of a flake of bone that has been avulsed

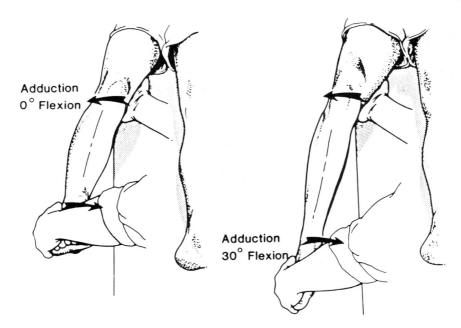

Fig. 14-18. Adduction (varus) stress test for the lateral ligament.

by the capsular attachment from the tibia (Fig. 14-19).

With the knee fully extended, demonstrable instability denotes considerable disruption. According to the severity of the injury, the structures potentially torn or stretched are as follows: middle third of the lateral capsular ligament, fibular collateral ligament, and posterolateral corner including the arcuate popliteal complex. In addition, if the instability is gross, one or both cruciate ligaments may be involved as well as occasionally the biceps femoris tendon and the iliotibial band. Generally, however, this amount of damage produces rotary instability, if not in the short term certainly over a period of time.

One-Plane Anterior Instability

The anterior drawer sign is generally accepted as a test of the integrity of the ACL. If the instability is gross, there must be associated capsular disruption. **Anterior Drawer Test at 90 Degrees of Flexion.** The drawer test — performed with the hamstrings relaxed, the hip flexed to 45 degrees, and the knee at 80 to 90 degrees — is the most commonly used test for one-plane anterior instability (Fig. 14-20). The examiner stabilizes the patient's foot by sitting on it. The examiner's hands are cupped around the proximal aspect of the tibia and fibula in the region of the hamstring insertion. Relaxation of the hamstrings should be ensured by palpation prior to administering a drawer. A positive test is displacement of the injured knee by 6 mm or more. The test is graded 1+, 2+, or 3+ (keeping in mind that this judgment is subjective). As with all ligament stress tests, the quality of the end feel is also important, and a minimal drawer with a soft end feel can still be considered positive. A positive anterior drawer is a useful finding; when negative, however, one must consider several possibilities. The pain may be making relaxation of the hamstrings and muscles difficult or impossible, or an associated tear of the meniscus may be preventing forward gliding of the tibia. In addition, a large effusion may make flexion to 90 degrees impossible, so the test cannot be effectively carried out.

If the athlete is able to flex relatively comfortably to 80 to 90 degrees but cannot relax enough for an adequate examination, the suggestion of a positive anterior drawer is sometimes confirmed by letting the patient sit with the leg dangling over the edge of the examining table (Fig. 14-21). This gravity-assisted relaxation may allow the examiner to demonstrate an unequivocally positive sign. However, as with all of

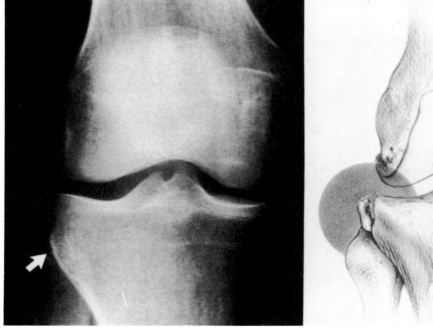
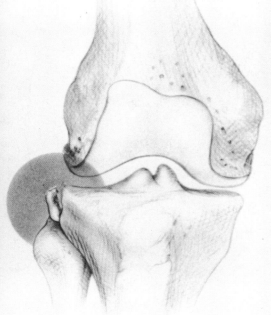

Fig. 14-19. Lateral capsular avulsion fracture (Segond's sign).

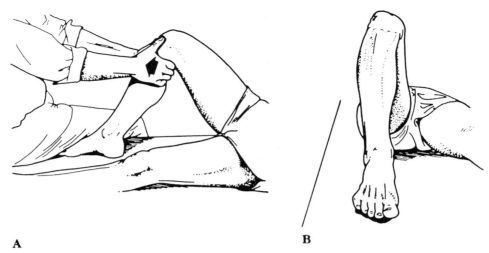

A   **B**

Fig. 14-20. Anterior drawer test. **(A)** Examiner's hands cup the proximal tibia, and the foot is stabilized by sitting across it. Relaxation is essential. The drawer may be blocked by hamstring spasm or a meniscal tear, or the position may be difficult to adopt because of effusion. **(B)** Foot is in neutral position.

the anterior drawer tests at 80 to 90 degrees of flexion, the correlation with surgical findings is not always good. Tears of the anterior cruciate ligament proved at arthroscopy may often have gone undetected clinically.[25]

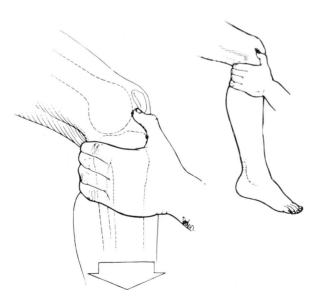

Fig. 14-21. With the thigh supported and the leg dangling, gravity may assist the patient to relax while performing a gentle anterior drawer test. This test may clarify an equivocal drawer test done in the prone position.

Anterior Drawer at 20 to 30 Degrees of Flexion (Lachman Test). The anterior drawer test done at 20 to 30 degrees of flexion is considered the best indicator of ACL injury[25] (Fig. 14-22). This test was originally described by Torg.[26] The patient's femur is stabilized by grasping the lateral distal thigh while the medial proximal tibia is drawn forward (Fig. 14-23). A positive test is indicated by a soft end feel and disappearance of the infrapatellar hollow. To perform the Lachman test effectively, the anterior tibial force must be applied posteromedially, which is best achieved by the examiner being on the same side of the bed as the leg under examination. *Reaching across to examine or compare legs alters tibial rotation introduces significant error to the test.*[27]

There are several advantages of the Lachman test over the anterior drawer test at 90 degrees of flexion.

1. It can often be done adequately in the presence of an effusion.
2. It does not require knee flexion and therefore does not produce as much pain.
3. The hamstrings do not block the forward glide easily.
4. It is not blocked readily by a torn meniscus.
5. Relaxation may be enhanced by placing a pillow under the injured knee so the leg rests with the knee flexed 20 to 30 degrees. The Lachman maneuver may then be performed without needing to lift or support the leg, which sometimes permits

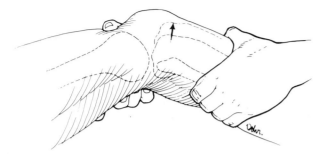

Fig. 14-22. Lachman test, viewed from the medial aspect.

more relaxation in athletes who are tense, nervous, or in a great deal of pain.

Quick Facts

GRADING THE LACHMAN TEST[28]

Grade I	Proprioceptive appreciation of a positive test (end feel)
Grade II	Visible anterior translation of tibia
Grade III	Gross anterior tibial translation (subluxation)

---

6. It may be specific for the posterolateral fibers of the ACL. It is definitely a more sensitive test for the cruciate-deficient knee, the magnitude of displacement being greater than with the anterior drawer test for any given cruciate deficiency.

Practice Point

SIGNIFICANCE OF ACL STRESS TESTS

Fibers damaged	90 Degrees Ant. Drawer	20 Degrees Lachman	Pivot Shift
Anteromedial	+	−	−
Posterolateral	−	+	+
Complete	+	+	+

When internal rotation is added to the anterior glide at 20 degrees, maximum displacement of the lateral tibial plateau may be visualized (Fig. 14-22).

The test may be difficult to perform if the examiner has small hands or if it is done on athletes with large thighs. However, there are several variations of the test that allow the examiner to circumvent these difficulties.[28,29]

Lachman Test with Patient Prone. The patient is prone, and the leg is supported with the knee flexed 20 to 30 degrees. Both hands grasp the tibia, and the fingers and thumbs palpate the joint line and are the sensors of abnormal motion.[29] Anteroposterior tibiofemoral movement is attempted; its interpretation and the quality of the endpoint are no different from that when the patient is supine. However it does require practice to be able to do the test effectively. The uninjured leg is tested first in the same position (Fig. 14-24).

Apart from ease of performance, the prone position offers other advantages: Gravity assists the forward movement of the tibia, so small hands can perform the test effectively; hip extension stabilizes the femur; the fingers provide a sensitive "arthrometer"; and, for some curious reason, relaxation seems to be enhanced. The test can be used just as effectively to test posterior laxity and for this seems more sensitive than the routine Lachman test.[29,30]

Modified Lachman Test. To allow more leverage with one hand, a series of modifications of the Lachman test may be considered (Fig. 14-25): (1) supporting the thigh on the examiner's knee, which may be useful for in-the-field assessment; (2) using an assistant to stabilize the thigh, which has the disadvantages of needing two people to perform the test and some loss of sensitivity, as the main examiner does not have control of the femur and tibia; (3) using a strap to support the thigh while the examiner grasps the proximal tibia with two hands. If the examiner sits at the end of the bench, the leg may be supported at 20 to 30 degrees by resting the leg on the lap.

Dynamic Extension. With the "no touch technique" the patient lies supine with a firm pillow under the thigh and the injured knee flexed 30 to 40 degrees.[31] The patient is encouraged to relax, being reassured that the examiner will not touch the knee. Alternatively, the examiner may use the closed fist as a firm bolster. While the examiner closely observes the lateral aspect of the knee, the patient is asked to raise the heel off the examination table by extending the knee and then to replace the heel on the table and relax the quadriceps. The test is then performed on the contralateral knee. When there is "isolated" rupture of the ACL, the lateral tibial plateau gently subluxates

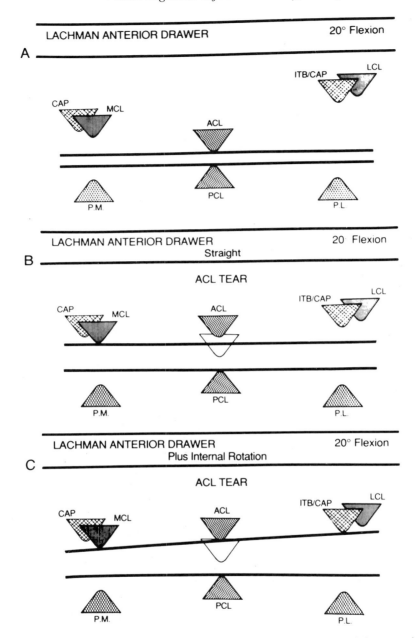

Fig. 14-23. The Lachman anterior drawer test (Bumper model). **(A)** Straight anterior drawer alone tests the anterior cruciate ligament (ACL). **(B)** After ACL rupture, a straight anterior drawer tests the medial ligamentous structures that control the amount of subluxation. **(C)** After ACL rupture an anterior drawer plus internal rotation is required to reach the maximum anterior subluxation to the lateral tibial plateau.

or slides forward on the femoral condyle as extension is initiated (Fig. 14-26). Even more noticeable is the slide back into a reduced position when the knee relaxes into the flexed position. This test is particularly valuable for acute ACL disruptions, but accurate assessment of the subluxation requires clinical expertise and experience.[30,32] Excessive lateral tibial plateau gliding defines a positive test.

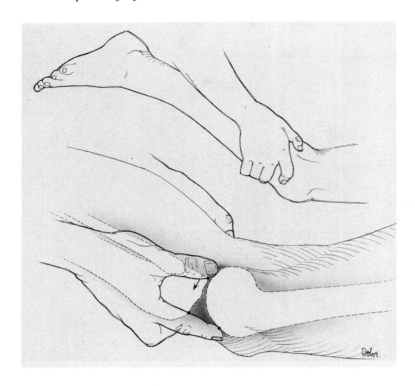

Fig. 14-24. For the individual with small hands, the prone Lachman test has some advantages. It also allows visualization and palpation of the posterior joint.

During active extension and flexion, a false-positive subluxation and relocation may be elicited in patients with rupture of the PCL or with posterolateral rotatory instability. In these patients, the lateral tibial plateau is subluxated in 30 to 40 degrees of flexion (posterior sag). Initiation of extension pulls the tibia back into a reduced position. This anterior gliding simulates a positive test but represents movement from a subluxated position to a reduced position. It can be augmented by placing a hand on the leg just above the ankle joint and gently resisting the active extension (described later).

One-Plane Posterior Instability

Pure posterior instability is rare in that the mechanism of injury is often violent and frequently produces a combined type of instability. Isolated PCL tears have been described with forced internal rotation just short of full extension. It correlates with tension in the ligament at that point.

Posterior Sag Sign During Extension. With the examiner at the end of the table, both heels are supported and raised so the legs may be viewed in profile. If an obvious posterior sag is seen on the injured side, there is usually a combined injury of the PCL and some involvement of the secondary restraints—

either the medial or lateral collateral ligament. With a significant sag, some posterior capsular stretching is necessary as well.[33] Many individuals with excessive normal hyperextending knees sag in a bilaterally symmetric fashion. In these individuals damage to the PCL alone may cause a positive sag during extension.

Posterior Sag (Godfrey Test) and Drawer During Flexion. Careful visual inspection of the profiles of the knee, particularly the tibial tubercles at 80 to 90 degrees of flexion, frequently detects a posterior sag of the tibia. This maneuver is sometimes called the Godfrey test. A positive test denotes considerable PCL damage (Fig. 14-27). This visualization is essential for a baseline from which to judge if subsequent anterior and posterior drawer stresses are positive. If the knee is already posteriorly subluxed, only a subtle "end feel" change is noted with the posterior drawer, and the anterior drawer gives a false positive result as it restores the tibia to its normal alignment.

90-Degree Quadriceps Active Test. PCL deficiency may be further confirmed with the 90-degree quadriceps active test.[34] With the patient supine and the knee flexed to 90 degrees, the posterior sag of the tibia is visualized in silhouette. The examiner supports the thigh with one hand, which may also monitor the state of relaxation of the quadriceps muscle. The other hand stabilizes the foot, and the patient is

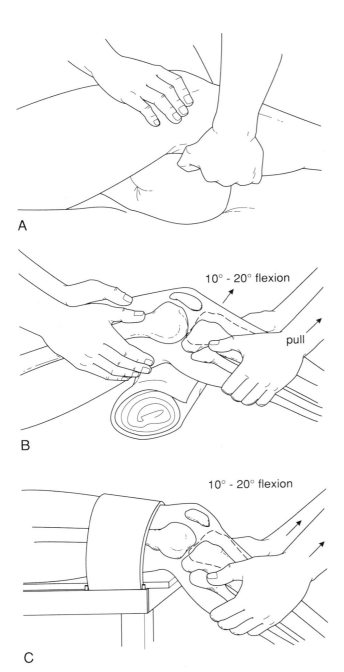

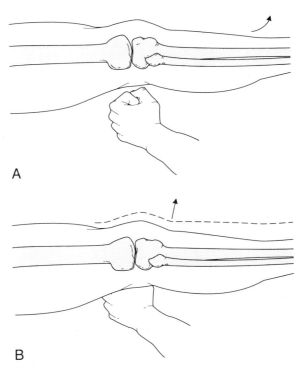

Fig. 14-26. Dynamic extension test demonstrates the anterior shear developed by the quadriceps during the last 20 to 30 degrees of extension. The examiner's fist is placed under the knee. **(A)** After relaxing completely, the patient is instructed to raise the heel (normal knee). **(B)** With anterior cruciate ligament deficiency the anterior drawer of the tibia is visualized as the patient lets the leg relax; the tibia may be seen to drop back. This test may be done as a no-touch technique using a pillow or by using the examiner's fist.

Fig. 14-25. Three modifications of the Lachman test. **(A)** Examiner's thigh and hand is used to stabilize the femur. This test is useful for field adaptation. **(B)** An assistant aids stabilization, allowing the use of both of the examiner's hands on the tibia. **(C)** Using a strap on an exercise bench.

asked to gently attempt to slide the foot down the table while the motion is resisted (Fig. 14-28). A test is positive when the quadriceps contraction restores the tibia from its "sag" position to an equal contour with the unaffected knee.

Dynamic Posterior Shift Test. The dynamic posterior shift test is a clinical method for evaluating straight posterior instability and posterolateral rotary instability. It is a simple test that serves as an adjuvant to other tests of insufficiency of the posterior structures of the knee.[35] The prerequisite for a positive test is posterior sagging or subluxation of the tibia. The examiner maintains the hip at near 90 degrees of flexion and controls rotation of the femur. The hamstrings are placed on a stretch, and their tightness

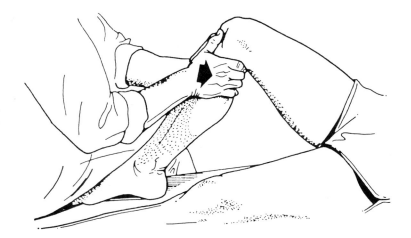

Fig. 14-27. Posterior cruciate ligament deficiency. Note the silhouettes of the tibial tubercles for a posterior sag. The abnormal motion may be enhanced with a posteior drawer.

assists gravity in generating subluxation of the tibia posteriorly. They also provide dynamic loading as the knee is gradually extended from the 30 degrees flexed position by simultaneous anterior pressure on the patient's foot and posterior pressure on the thigh (Fig. 14-29). In knees with posterior instability, the posteriorly subluxated tibia suddenly reduces as the knee joint nears full extension. A jerk or "clunk" is often felt by both the examiner and the patient. This test is particularly easy to perform and is reliable for detecting posterior instability of the knee.

Rotary Instabilities (Complex)

In the normal knee the ACL and PCL contribute to functional instability and keep the axis of rotation near the center of the joint. Internal and external rotations of the flexed knee are accompanied by tightening of the secondary restraints and, particularly internal rotation, by increased tension on the cruciate ligaments. Thus the anterior drawer is maximal at approximately 90 degrees with the foot slightly externally rotated (approximately 10 to 15 degrees); this position constitutes the functional neutral rotation position (Fig. 14-30). All further external and internal rotation tightens the knee and reduces the drawer. Despite this functional position, the neutral position in most tests, and in common usage, is the midposition, or zero position; hence this position is used for the remainder of this chapter.

Anteromedial Rotary Instability

Patients who demonstrate excessive anterior displacement of the medial tibial condyle are exhibiting anteromedial instability. The axis of motion has moved to the lateral joint compartment. With the anterior drawer test performed at 90 degrees of flexion and the tibia in neutral rotation, the medial tibial condyle moves anteriorly in excess of the lateral condyle.

Slocum Test. Significant anteromedial rotary instability is demonstrated by performing the drawer test in at least 25 to 30 degrees of external rotation (Fig. 14-31). If this or greater external rotation fails to decrease the drawer and the medial tibial condyle still translates anteriorly, it is considered a positive medial rotatory instability test of Slocum.[6] This test is not specific for one ligament but implies disruption of the posteromedial joint structures as well as the ACL. The pathology may involve the medial collateral ligament, the posterior oblique fibers, and the ACL. In the presence of this instability, a medial meniscectomy greatly increases the functional disability. Meniscal pathology is indeed common, as this abnormal motion is frequently the late outcome of "O'Donaghue's unhappy triad" of medial meniscus disruption, medial ligament damage, and an ACL tear.[4]

Anterolateral Drawer Test in 20 Degrees of Flexion. This test is a variation of the Lachman test, with a medial rotation bias to the anterior drawer on the tibia. It serves to confirm an already positive Slocum test and is definitely easier to perform in the acute knee. It demonstrates the same combination of deficiencies as described above (Table 14-1).

Anterolateral Rotary Instability

In the normal knee, the ACL prevents the sudden tendency toward forward gliding of the tibia as the knee approaches extension. This tendency is particularly pronounced on the lateral side. A powerful an-

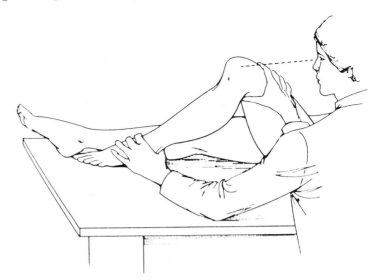

Fig. 14-28. Ninety-degree quadriceps active test. As the patient tries gently to slide the foot down the table against the examiner's resistance, anterior translation of the tibia occurs in the posteriorly subluxed tibia secondary to posterior cruciate ligament deficiency.

terior shear is developed by the quadriceps during the last 30 degrees of extension and the transition of the line of pull of the iliotibial band from posterior to the knee flexion axis to a position anterior to this axis.

The normal ACL resists this tendency, along with additional supports from the secondary medial and lateral restraints.

In the ACL-deficient knee, the shearing forces are

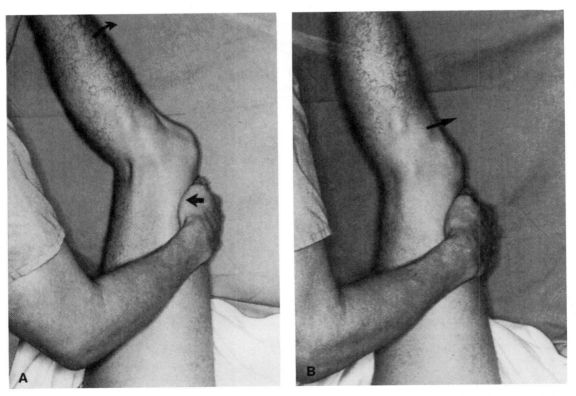

Fig. 14-29. Dynamic posterior shift test. **(A)** Subluxated tibia due to gravity and pull of hamstrings. **(B)** Dynamically reduced as knee nears full extension.

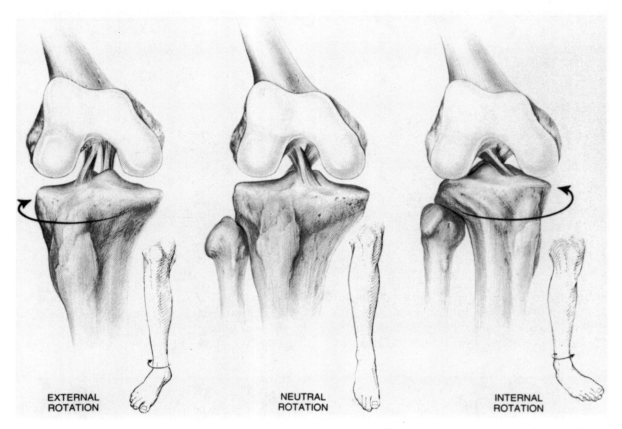

Fig. 14-30. With the knee flexed to 90 degrees the cruciate ligaments become successively tighter with internal rotation. The secondary restraints contribute more during external rotation.

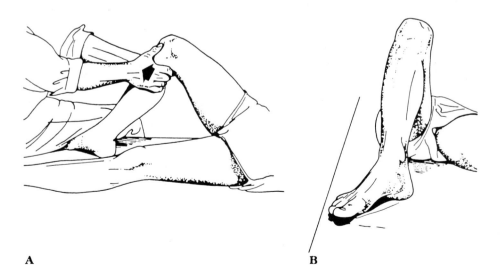

A **B**

Fig. 14-31. Slocum test. **(A)** Positive anterior drawer **(B)**, which fails to tighten in 25 degrees of external rotation of the leg.

TABLE 14-1.　Laxity Tests

Test	Degrees of Flexion	Primary Restraint			Secondary Restraint		
		Medial	Central	Lateral	Medial	Central	Lateral
Anterior drawer	20/90	—	ACL	—	TCL + MM	—	ALS
Ant. drawer + int. rotation	20/90	—	ACL	ALS	—	—	FCL + PLS
Ant. drawer + ext. rotation	20/90	TCL + MM	ACL	—	PMS	—	—
Pivot shift	15	—	ACL	—	MM + TCL + PMS	—	ALS + CL
Posterior drawer	20/90	—	PCL	—	PMS + TCL	—	FCL + PLS
Post. drawer + ext. rotation	30	—	—	FCL + PLS	—	PCL	—
	90	—	PCL	FCL + PLS	—	—	—
Post. drawer + int. rotation	20	TCL + PMS	—	—	—	ACL + PCL	—
	90	TCL + POL	PCL	—	—	ACL	—
Valgus	5	TCL + PMS	—	Bone	—	PCL + ACL	—
	20	TCL	—	Bone	PMS	PCL	—
Varus	5	Bone	—	FCl + PLS	—	ACL + PCL	—
	20	Bone	—	FCL	—	ACL	PLS
Ext. rotation	30	PMS + TCL	—	FCL + PLS	MM	PCL	—
	90	MM + TCL	PCL	FCL + PLS	PMS	—	—
Int. rotation	20	TCL + PMS	ACL	ALS	—	PCL	FCL
	90	TCL + POL	ACL + PCL	ALS	—	—	FCL

ACL, PCL + anterior and posterior cruciate ligaments; ALS = iliotibial band + anterior + mid. lateral capsule; PLS = popliteus, posterolateral capsule; PMS = posterior oblique ligament + posteromedial capsule; MM = medial meniscus; POL = posterior oblique ligament; TCL = tibial collateral ligament; FCL = fibular collateral ligament.

particularly high when an athlete is decelerating or changing direction. As the knee approaches extension during these maneuvers, the increasing valgus stress and axial loading exaggerates the speed at which this "pivot shift" occurs (Fig. 14-32). The convex surface of the lateral tibial plateau enhances this tendency to "skid" anteriorly.

The sudden shift of the lateral compartment is experienced as a "giving way" sensation, often associated with significant pain and subsequent swelling. In the past there has existed considerable disagreement as to the underlying pathology that accompanies a positive anterolateral pivot shift, but there is now a uniformity of opinion that the basic constant lesion is one of ACL functional instability.

Although this abnormal motion was alluded to by Palmer in 1938, it was MacIntosh and Galway who went against the tide of modern opinion and empha-

sized the nature of the common ACL-deficient functional instability and popularized the "pivot shift" concept.[11,36] Many variations on the MacIntosh pivot shift test have been described, but all are based on the same basic principle (Table 14-2).

MacIntosh Lateral Pivot Shift Test. The patient lies supine, and significant effort is made to ensure relaxation of the affected limb.[38] The internally rotated foot is lifted from the examination table with the knee allowed to sag into extension. The examiner pushes with the heel of the hand on the proximal tibia while applying a strong valgus stress with slight compression. As the leg is flexed from full extension, the posterior capsule relaxes; and by 5 to 10 degrees the tibia partially dislocates. With the internal rotation, any subluxation of the lateral tibial plateau with ACL deficiency is exaggerated. Further flexion gives a sudden relocation at approximately 30 to 40 degrees,

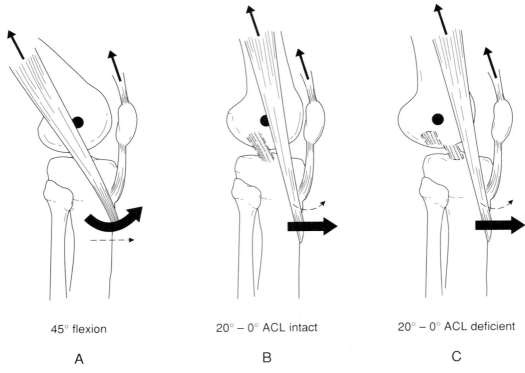

45° flexion   20° – 0° ACL intact   20° – 0° ACL deficient

A   B   C

Fig. 14-32. Anterolateral pivot shift. **(A)** Knee in 45 degrees flexion. The quadriceps anterior shear is small, and the iliotibial band (ITB) lies behind the axis of rotation. **(B)** Nearer to extension the quadriceps shear increases, and the ITB lies anterior to the axis. Anterior shift is resisted by an intact pivot shift. **(C)** Pivot shift with anterior cruciate ligament deficiency.

usually in a dramatic fashion (Fig. 14-33). There may be a false-negative test with failure of the patient to relax, hamstring spasm, or a locked knee. Painful impingement with the pivot shift may impair further testing.

This *classic pivot shift test* may be modified either to increase the sensitivity or to grade the magnitude of the abnormal motion. By performing the classic test in three different rotations, the amount of pivot for any degree of ACL laxity changes. Neutral rotation decreases the magnitude of the shift, and lateral rotation of the tibia decreases it further. Hence if a significant pivot shift is still present with the tibia laterally rotated, the instability is of major proportions[39] (Fig. 14-34).

Grade I Pivot Shift. There are abnormal movements only when the tibia is held in maximal medial rotation; they are absent in neutral or lateral rotation (Fig. 14-35). The shift may be felt as a gentle sliding reduction, barely palpable in the awake patient but slightly

---

Practice Point

CLASSIC PIVOT SHIFT AND LACHMAN TESTS

Grade I (trace)   -Abnormal movement only when tibia is held in medial rotation
                     -Lachman test usually is less than 10 mm

Grade II (moderate)-Positive test with foot neutral
                     -Lachman test is usually 10 to 15 mm in magnitude

Grade III (severe)   -Abnormal motion even when tibia is held in lateral rotation
                     -Lachman test is greater than 15 mm

TABLE 14-2. Tests for Detecting Anterior Subluxation of the Lateral Tibial Plateau

Test	Steps in Testing	What Happens During Testing	Advantages	Disadvantages
Lateral pivot-shift test[37] (MacIntosh)	Patient supine and relaxed. Lift internally rotated foot off the examining table with knee extended. Flex the knee while applying valgus stress.	Reduction in full extension, then subluxation with impingement followed by sudden relocation.	Differentiates between insignificant looseness and disabling subluxation. Use as indication for surgery.	False-negative tests in presence of locked knee and hamstring spasm. Painful impingement in full extension may impair further testing.
Test for anterior subluxation of the lateral tibial plateau[44] (Losee)	Patient supine and relaxed. Flex knee and hip 45 degrees. Externally rotate tibia. Let knee slowly extend while applying a valgus stress.	Reduction in flexion, then sudden subluxation without impingement followed by relocation at full extension.	Reproduces what happens when knee gives away. Demonstrates efficacy of repair when used during surgery.	False-negative tests in presence of locked knee and hamstring spasm. Shows insignificant looseness as well as disabling subluxation.
Jerk test[40] (Hughston)	Patient supine. Flex knee 90 degrees and hip 45 degrees. Internally rotate tibia. Let knee slowly extend while applying valgus stress.	Reduction in flexion, less noticeable subluxation followed by relocation.	None.	Too many false-negative tests because subluxation may not be recognized.
Anterolateral rotary instability test[6] (Slocum)	Patient lies on sound side with unstable knee up and extended and medial aspect of ipsilateral foot resting on table. Patient maintains ipsilateral pelvis rotated posteriorly 30–50 degrees. Knee pushed into flexion.	Subluxation at 10 degrees flexion, then impingement with further flexion, followed by sudden relocation.	Easier to do in heavy or tense patients.	False-negative tests in presence of locked knee and hamstring spasm (test under anesthesia). Not always sensitive.

more obvious in patients under general anesthesia. It corresponds with the American "trace" pivot shift and the French *ressaut en bâtard*.[39–41] In a knee showing a grade I pivot shift, the medial plateau moves, on average 5 mm and the lateral plateau 12 mm (Fig. 14-36). The Lachman test is less than 10 mm of anterior drawer.[38]

Grade II Pivot Shift. The test is positive in the neutral position as well as in medial rotation but negative when the tibia is held in a position of definite tibial lateral rotation (Fig. 14-36). Movement on the lateral tibial condyle is easily appreciated, and a less obvious shift of the medial side may be seen or felt by the examiner's fingers. When the tibia is medialy rotated, there is now a definite "clunk." The distinction between grade I and II pivot shifts is based on the presence of the abnormal movement in neutral rotation and by the different nature of the shift in medial rotation. The test is regarded as grade II even if only one of these two distinctions is present.[42] Grade II pivot shift is associated with an average of 10 mm medial and 18 mm lateral plateau movement, which corresponds to about 10 to 15 mm subluxation during a Lachman test. It is often the amount seen in a fresh isolated complete ACL rupture or chronic instability of moderate degree.

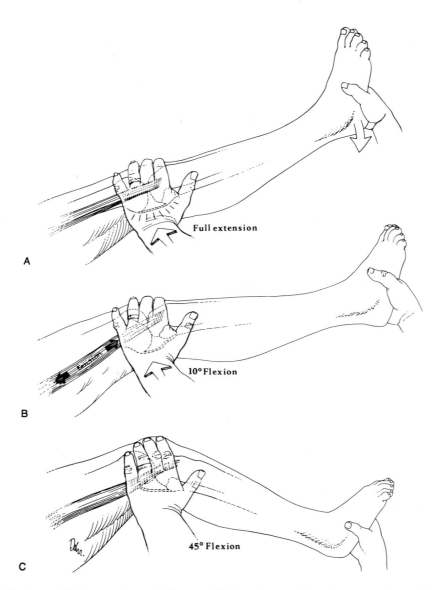

Fig. 14-33. MacIntosh's lateral pivot shift test. **(A)** Starting position in extension with stress valgus and internal rotation. **(B)** With slight flexion the lateral tibial plateau subluxes. **(C)** Pivot shift is felt as a reduction phenomenon in further flexion.

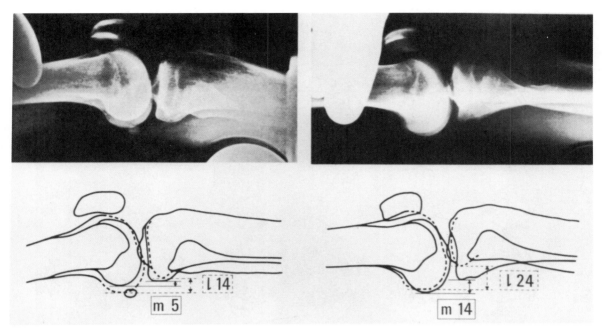

Fig. 14-34. Lateral stress roentgenograms and diagrams showing grade II **(left)** and grade III **(right)** pivot shifts. L = lateral tibial condyle, M = medial tibial condyle.

Grade III Pivot Shift. Abnormal motion with a pronounced "clunk" can be produced when the tibia is in either neutral or lateral rotation (Fig. 14-36). In medial rotation, the shift is definitely present but less obvious. This degree of shift is seen in the acutely injured knee when there is some associated damage to the posteromedial or posterolateal corner as well as a complete ACL injury. It is also present in knees with chronic ACL instability with significantly stretched secondary restraints.[41]

The grade III pivot shift corresponds to 15 mm medial and 22 mm lateral subluxation. This shift is equivalent to a Lachman test of more than 15 mm drawer (Table 14-3).

There is another refinement to the classic pivot shift test of MacIntosh that may enhance an equivocal result, it is the abduction position of the hip.[42] When relaxing the iliotibial band, the secondary restraints on the lateral side are further relaxed. The pivot shift score may be enhanced as much as one grade in 90 percent of patients by this maneuver.

Other factors that influence the grade of the pivot shift include rupture of the iliotibial band and pre-existing natural ligament laxity, which may be seen in the noninjured knee.

The effect of the shift is frequently diminished by: (1) complete rupture of the medial collateral ligament, which may paradoxically prevent a valgus load being placed through the lateral compartment and hence obviate the fulcrum for the test; (2) a displaced bucket handle tear that is blocking or maintaining reduction; and (3) advanced osteoarthritic changes with formation of osteophytes and disappearance of the convexity of the lateral plateau[43] (Fig. 14-37). There should be a word of caution when comparing different systems of grading the pivot shift test. Some systems call gentle gliding of the lateral tibial plateau occasionally seen in normal knees as grade I. In these systems all grades of abnormal shift are advanced one grade.

Losee's Anterolateral Subluxation Test. In Losee's variation of the pivot shift test the patient is supine and relaxed, and the hip and knee are flexed to 45 degrees at the starting position (Fig. 14-38). The tibia is externally rotated. The knee is allowed to extend slowly while maintaining a valgus stress. The tibia goes from a reduced position in flexion, to sudden subluxation as the knee approaches extension, and then finally to reduction in full extension. The examiner sees and feels the subluxation.[44] In many ways this test

Grade Medial Neutral Lateral

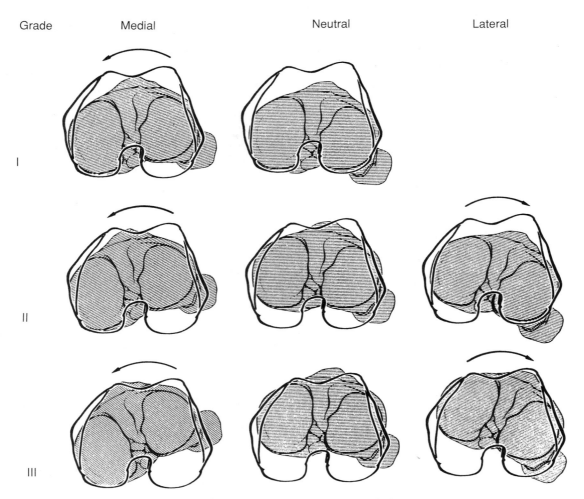

Fig. 14-35. Anterior translation of the tibia during the pivot shift (magnitude illustrated by clear space at the back of the femoral condyles). The test is performed with medial, neutral, and lateral rotation of the leg. Shift present (grade I) in medial rotation, (grade II) medial and neutral and (Grade III) even in lateral rotation.

reproduces what happens when the knee gives way during sports and is useful intraoperatively to judge the efficacy of the repair. It demonstrates all grades of pivot shift when done carefully, as the fully reduced starting position during external rotation allows visualization of even minor pivot shifts as it partially dislocates. This test is the mirror image of the classic MacIntosh test.

Hughston's Jerk Test. The patient should be relaxed and lying supine. The starting position for the leg is 45 degrees flexion of the hip and 90 degrees flexion of the knee. The tibia is held internally rotated (Fig. 14-39). The knee is allowed to extend slowly while valgus stress is maintained. With a positive test subluxation of the lateral tibial condyle on the femur occurs at about 20 degrees of flexion. With further extension spontaneous relocation occurs. This abnormal motion is described in engineering terms as a "jerk," which is a sudden change in the rate of acceleration between anterolateral rotary instability, but this test often fails to show up the lesser subluxation.

Slocum's Anterolateral Subluxation Test. This test is useful in patients who have large or heavy legs or who are finding it particularly difficult to relax. The patient lies on the sound side with the unstable knee uppermost and extended. The medial side of the foot

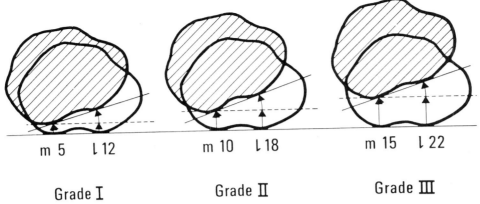

Fig. 14-36. Correlation of maximal tibial subluxation with the three grades of pivot shift: average, medial (M), and lateral (L) shifts, in millimeters. M = medial condyle, L = lateral condyle.

rests on the examining table as a fulcrum. The pelvis tilts posteriorly 30 to 50 degrees. The examiner pushes down on the knee, allowing it to move into flexion while maintaining a valgus stress. The tibia moves from the reduced position to a subluxated one as the knee approaches extension. This test is rarely as sensitive as the previously described tests.

Noyes' Flexion-Rotation Drawer Test. At the start of the test the tibia is supported as the femur drops back and rotates externally, leaving the tibia subluxated and internally rotated. The knee is held in about 5 to 10 degrees of flexion (Fig. 14-40). Slight internal

rotation pressure and anterior drawer enhances the test. A flexion rotation drawer is produced by gentle but firm posterior and lateral pressure on the tibia to reduce the subluxation.[12] This test assesses the function of the ACL in control of both translation and rotation, and is an excellent way to test the apprehensive subject. This is potentially the gentlest of the pivot shift tests.

Anterior Drawer in 90 Degrees of Flexion and Internal Rotation. A modification of the original Slocum and Larson anterior drawer at 90 degrees of flexion may test anterolateral subluxation. In the

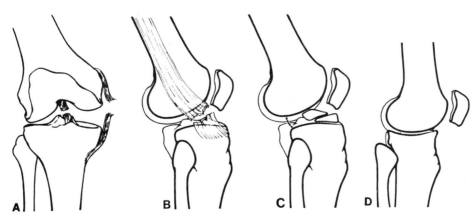

Fig. 14-37. Factors that influence the pivot shift. **(A)** Complete medial collateral ligament rupture prevents a valgus load from being established through the lateral compartment. **(B)** Associated rupture of the iliotibial band enhances the shift but delays reduction until further flexion. **(C)** Displaced bucket handle may block reduction. **(D)** Osteoarthrosis with osteophytes may flatten the normal convexity of the lateral plateau and obliterate the pivot shift.

TABLE 14-3. **Classification of Pivot-Shift Type Tests**[a]

Laxity Grade	Structures Involved			Positive Test	Comments
	ACL	Iliotibial Band, Lateral Capsule	Medial Ligaments, Capsule		
Moderate (grade I)	+	−	−	Lachman test Flexion-rotation drawer Losee test, ALRI Pivot shift "slip" but not "jerk" (internal rotation)	Subtle subluxation-reduction phenomenon. Secondary ligamentous restraints limit the amount of joint subluxation but may stretch out later with repeated injury. Pivot shift and jerk tests do not show obvious jump, thud, or jerk, although the subluxation may be detected as a "slip" with experience.
Severe (grade II)	+	+	−	All tests positive Pivot shift (internal rotation and neutral)	Hallmark is an obvious jump, thud, or jerk with gross subluxation-reduction during the test. It indicates laxity of other ligamentous restraints, either a normal physiologic laxity (lateral capsule, iliotibial band) or injured secondary restraints.
Gross (grade III)	+	++	++	All tests positive (pivot shift in all positions)	Hallmark is a gross subluxation with impingement of the posterior aspect of the lateral tibial plateau against the femoral condyle. The examiner must effect reduction to allow further knee flexion.

[a] ALRI = frequently in individuals with hyperextension at the knee and with some generalized ligament laxity on a congenital, not traumatic, basis, a soft pivot shift sensation is present. It is physiologic. In some classifications it is graded I instead of 0. In that case all of the above grades go up one. (ALRI is anterolateral rotory instability.)

normal knee medial rotation of the foot should tighten up the cruciate ligaments and the posterolateral secondary restraints.[5,31] With severe injury to both sets of ligaments and capsular structure, the medial rotation fails to control the drawer and the test is positive (Fig. 14-41).

Active Pivot Shift. Some patients with sufficient ACL deficits may be able to actively induce an anterolateral subluxation of the tibia. The mechanism is probably different from the dynamic pivot shift that occurs with functional instability and has a separate mechanism from the standard passive pivot shift tests.

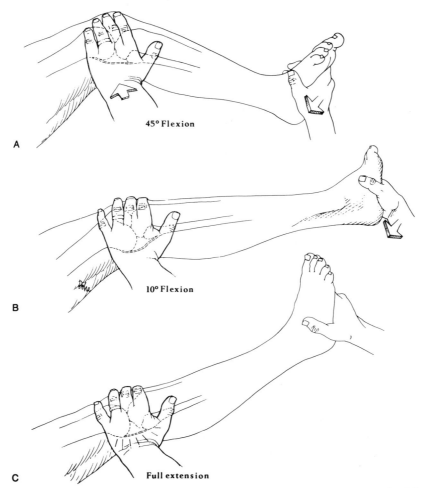

Fig. 14-38. Losee pivot shift test **(A)** The 45 degrees flexed knee is reduced with external tibial rotation. **(B)** Knee is allowed to extend with strong valgus pressure. A positive test is a definite "thud" as the tibia becomes subluxated and internally rotates between 20 and 10 degrees. **(C)** Complete extension reduces the knee as the posterior capsule tightens.

With the patient seated and the foot of the affected leg firmly planted as a fulcrum, the tibia is actively subluxated anteriorly by muscle action. It is probable that the popliteus muscle, by inducing an internal rotation movement on the tibia, spins the lateral plateau anteriorly in the face of the altered axis in the ACL-deficient knee. Electromyographic data tend to substantiate this theory.[45]

Posterolateral and Posteromedial Rotary Instabilities

Posterolateral and posteromedial rotary instabilities are complex and require significant damage to the PCL. At one point PCL injuries were consid-

ered rare, with only sporadic reports appearing until about 1920 when an information explosion occurred.[40,46–48] Athletes constitute a large percentage of patients who develop these injuries.[48] In Kennedy and Grainger's series, 41 percent sustained their injury at sports, with football and hockey accounting for half[13]; in Cross and Powell's series, 47 percent were sport-related and nearly half of these were due to rugby.[49] These data represent the difference in popularity between these sports on different continents.

There are three classic mechanisms of injury. The most prevalent is an anteroposterior force applied to the flexed knee (dashboard-type injury), as well as

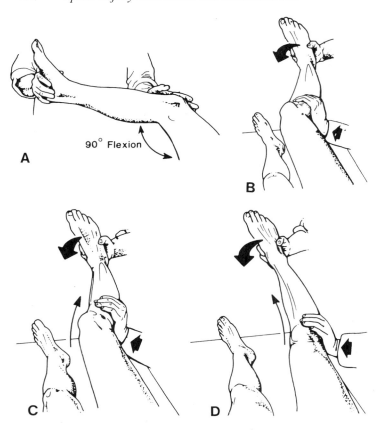

A 90° Flexion

B

C   **D**

Fig. 14-39. Hughston jerk test. **(A)** Starting position. **(B)** Foot internally rotated and a valgus stress at the knee. **(C)** As knee extends, subluxation occurs at about 20 degrees. **(D)** With reduction in full extension.

hyperflexion and hyperextension injuries involving the posterior capsule, or the posterior cruciate. Kennedy and Grainger reported that 45 percent of patients sustained the dashboard type,[13] and Cross and Powell reported 31 percent by this mechanism in their series, many of which occurred at sport.[49,50] Severe twists with varus or valgus force and deceleration rotation may also rupture the PCL.[13] However, the most common reported clinical experience is PCL disruption associated with multiple ligament injuries. Loos et al. reported that 46 percent had associated medial collateral tears, 64 percent posterior oblique capsular ligament damage, 31 percent lateral compartment damage, 44 percent ACL tears, and 29 percent meniscal tears.[47] Moore and Larson reported no isolated PCL but associated ACL tears in 77 percent, often with either medial or lateral ligament injuries.[51] Hughston et al. agreed that isolated tears are uncommon and that ACL (86 percent) and medial compartment injury as well as meniscal damage are frequently associated.[40] The importance of distinguishing the

"isolated" injury from that associated with obvious significant associated ligament disruptions is that the prognosis for the former injury, even without surgery, is much better.

With selected cutting of the PCL, the knee becomes progressively more unstable as it moves into flexion.[15] The degree of posterior excursion increased from an average of 1.2 mm in the extended position to 9.6 mm at 90 degrees of flexion. *The PCL is the primary restraint for the posterior drawer at both 30 and 90 degree angles flexion.*[52] It accounts for 95 percent of the restraining force independent of rate of loading and position of the knee. The secondary restraints to posterior displacement of the tibia are the posterolateral capsule, the popliteal tendon, and the medial collateral ligament (Table 14-4). Thus although increased posterior laxity has been associated with medial collateral ligament and posterior capsular injury, a significant drawer cannot occur without PCL disruption.[38,49,50]

Posterior Sag and Posterior Drawer. The posterior

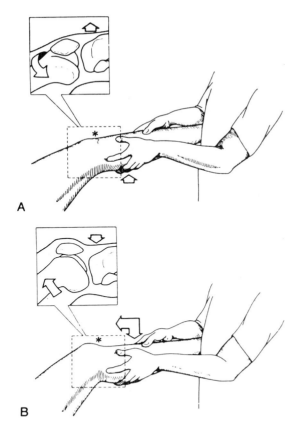

A

B

Fig. 14-40. Flexion-rotation drawer test. **(A)** With the leg supported, the weight of the thigh causes the femur to drop back posteriorly and, more importantly, to rotate externally thus leaving the lateral tibial condyle subluxated. **(B)** Gentle flexion with compression and downward pressure over the proximal leg reduces the subluxation. This move is a gentle pivot shift maneuver. (From Jonsson et al.,[25] with permission.)

sag sign during extension and flexion has been discussed in the section on one-plane posterior instability. This sag is reversed by quadriceps contraction, and in functional situations it may be the cause of excessive patellar pressures, which would explain the high incidence and distinctive pattern of anterior knee pain in athletes with PCL insufficiency. Indeed, in many cases the initial injury may have been overlooked, and it is the patellar pain that causes the patient to seek treatment. Furthermore, it is worth reemphasizing that the posterior sag sign is pathognomonic of PCL damage, and failure to recognize it

leads to an erroneous conclusion that the abnormal anteroposterior motion results from ACL laxity. Both posterior drawer and posterior sag are present with posterior rotary instabilities.

External Rotation Recurvatum Test. Slight modification of the gravity-assisted posterior sag emphasizes posterior subluxation of the lateral tibia plateau. With the patient lying supine and relaxed, one or both legs are lifted by grasping the toes. A positive test is the recurvatum with the subtle addition of posterolateral sagging of the lateral tibia (Fig. 14-42).

Reverse Pivot Shift. In the reverse pivot shift test the foot is held in external rotation and the knee is extended from its position while pressure is applied to the lateral aspect of the proximal part of the tibia.[53] A "jump," which is analogous to the pivot shift, occurs at 30 degrees of flexion[46] (Fig. 14-43). It represents reduction of the posterior subluxation of the lateral tibial plateau and hence is indicative of posterolateral rotary instability.

Posterolateral Drawer Test in 90 Degrees of Flexion. Classically this test is positive in the presence of both acute and chronic PCL and posterolateral rotary instability.[54] A positive response to the posterolateral drawer test, particularly if associated with the previously described external rotation recurvatum test, is diagnositc of an acute tear of the PCL and the arcuate ligament complex[55] (Table 14-5) This point is particularly true if it is also associated with a positive varus stress at 30 degrees of flexion.

The posterolateral drawer test may be best performed with the leg flexed over the end of the table, although it can also be done in the classic drawer position (Fig. 14-44).[54,55] When the secondary posterolateral restraints are torn, particularly the arcuate complex, the tibia rotates posteriorly and laterally about the axis of the PCL. With a combined arcuate and PCL tear, the tibia is subluxated posteriorly, and there is substantial posterolateral subluxation with rotation.

Reverse Prone Lachman Test. The knee joint is tested with the patient in the prone position for the reverse prone Lachman test. The tibia is grasped as for the classic prone Lachman test so the fingers may appreciate any abnormal glide of the tibia. A posterior glide is attempted, and the posteromedial and posterolateal corners are carefully observed (Fig. 14-45). This position also provides the opportunity to observe swelling and to palpate for tenderness in the acute injury.

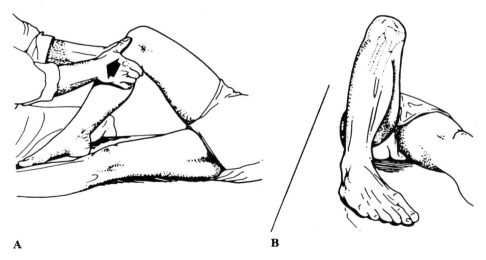

A   **B**

Fig. 14-41. **(A)** Anterior drawer test with tibia in internal rotation. **(B)** Position of foot. This test is positive only when there is significant damage to the anterior cruciate ligament and the posterolateal secondary restraints.

Varus and Valgus Stress in Full Extension. The exact implication of positive varus and valgus laxity in full extension is a contentious issue. Loos et al. summarized the physical findings reported with acute ACL injuries.[47] They concluded that the presence of a posterior drawer sign in association with varus or valgus laxity in full extension was the most reliable indicator of PCL disruption. It is obvious that the appropriate secondary restraints must also be torn.

Hughston et al. elaborated on the significance of the valgus stress.[40] They concluded that if the abduction stress test on a patient with an acute knee injury is 2+ or 3+ at 30 degrees of flexion, but negative at 0 degrees, there is a tear of the medial compartment ligaments but the PCL is intact. On the other hand, a 3+ abduction stress test at 0 degrees indicates the presence of an associated rupture of the PCL.[46]

Complex (Combined) Rotary Instabilities

Complex (combined) rotary instabilities are secondary to major ligamentous disruption of the joint. Most are chronic injuries—often complex rotatory instabilities that have progressed over a period of time. The functional status of the knee is poor, and high levels of physical activity are impossible without customized bracing. Even with derotation braces there are many situations in which performance is not satisfactory. Although many of the lesser instabilities sometimes lead to fairly rapid onset of post-traumatic arthritis, the combined problems inevitably lead to deterioration of the joint. The knee is unreliable and unstable, and pain is a common feature. The kinematics of the knee are severely distorted.

These complex instabilities are not discussed in de-

TABLE 14-4.   Rotatory Subluxations

Grade	Position of Test (Degrees)	Position of Rotation Axis	Lateral Tibial Subluxation	Medial Tibial Subluxation
I (FCL, TCL)	30 or 90	Center	↓Post	↑Ant.
II (FCL, PLC)	30	Med.	↓	—
III (FCL, PLC, partial PCL)	30 and 90	Far med.	↓↓	↓
IV (FCL, PLC, PCL)	30 and 90	Far med.	↓↓↓	↓↓

FCL = fibular or lateral collateral ligament; TCL = tibial or medial collateral ligament; PCL = posterior cruciate ligament. PLC = posterolateral complex (arcuate structures.)

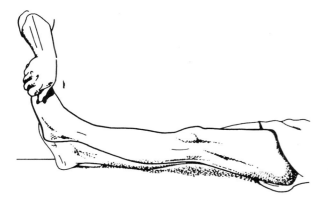

Fig. 14-42. External rotation recurvature test for posterolateral instability. A positive test is posterolateral sagging and is indicative of posterior cruciate ligament injury. Both legs may be lifted simultaneously for comparison.

tail. They require careful assessment, often over several occasions, and frequently under anesthesia. Determining the exact pathology leading to the instability requires experience, and the surgical repair is even more challenging. Rarely are reconstructions compatible with top level performance, and the rehabilitation of these knees is time-consuming and demanding.

ROLE OF RADIOLOGY

Plain Roentgenography

The standard anteroposterior roentgenographic view allows visualization of tibial spine fractures that suggest ACL avulsion and reveal the lateral capsular sign, or Segond's fracture (Figs. 14-23 and 14-52). As its name implies, this sign suggests tearing of the posterolateral capsule. Avulsion of the apex of the fibula by the lateral collateral ligament may also be seen as may other osteochondral fractures of the femur or tibia.

Depressed plateau fractures are usually obvious, but undisplaced ones are better outlined with oblique films. The classic osteochondritis dissecans fragments from the intercondylar notch of the medial femoral condyle are better visualized on the oblique film. The lateral view best shows posterior tibial margin fractures which may indicate avulsions by the PCL.

A skyline view outlines patellar fractures when pa-

tellar dislocation is suspected to be the cause of an acute hemarthrosis.

Skeletally Immature Patients

The presence of the epiphyseal plate in the adolescent child represents a weak link in the chain. Tenderness over the sites of the growth plates should always raise suspicion that an epiphyseal injury has occurred and the ligaments remain relatively undamaged. A roentgenogram is advisable before stress testing in these cases (Fig. 14-46). Furthermore, there is a tendency for avulsion of the tibial spine in stress injuries to the ACL, which requires immobilization in extension or open reduction, depending on the displacement[57] (see Fig. 14-47, below).

Special Studies

Should arthrography be indicated for any specific clinical, economic, or geographic reason, the status of the cruciate ligaments is sometimes revealed by double contrast studies. Tomograms or computed tomography (CT) scans more accurately delineate plateau fractures and avulsions of the tibial spines, and the presence of occult subchondral fractures are often revealed. Magnetic resonance imaging (MRI) adds a further dimension. The accuracy of all these studies often depends on the interest and care with which they are done. Orthogonal views accurately delineate cruciate ligament injuries. As with arthroscopy, meticulous, thoughtful physical examination of the knee should dictate the need and role of these supplemental examinations.

TRAUMATIC DISLOCATION OF THE KNEE

Severe disruption of the knee is uncommon in sport, and it is possible that team physicians and therapists may encounter only one during a career.[38-60] Nevertheless, there are some significant considerations that make early recognition and prompt therapy mandatory. It seems that these injuries should be obvious, and indeed if the knee stays grossly subluxated or dislocated they are. However, many immediately reduce spontaneously (occult dislocation), making recognition and distinction from simple ligament disruption more difficult unless the clinician is aware of the possibility.[58] The major concern is the associa-

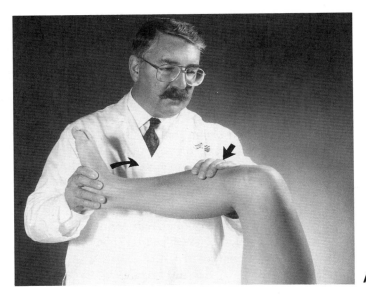

A

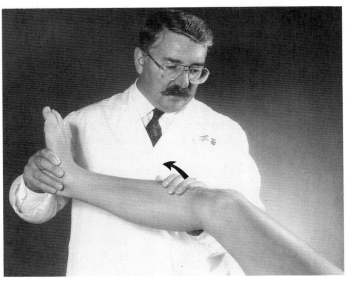

B

Fig. 14-43. Reverse pivot shift. **(A)** Starting at 90 degrees of flexion. **(B)** Reduction of the posterolateral subluxation occurs at about 30 degrees.

tion of popliteal artery damage. If popliteal artery flow is lost and not restored within 6 to 8 hours, amputation is a usual outcome.[58]

Total dislocation is not always necessary for such damage; disruption of the normal articulation is sufficient to significantly stress and stretch the neurovascular structures that may create this problem. Hence the precaution of checking circulation in all major ligament disruptions must never be overlooked.

Classification

Dislocations have been classified according to the direction in which the tibia is displaced in relation to the femur (Fig. 14-48). The anterior and posterior displacements are the ones most likely to result in disruption of popliteal artery flow. The artery is tethered proximally as it comes through the adductor magnus hiatus, distally at the soleal bridge, and in between by the geniculate vessels (Fig. 14-49). The

TABLE 14–5. Operative Findings in Patients with Posterolateral Rotary Instability[a]

Patient	FCL[a]	Arcuate Ligament	Popliteus	Biceps	ITB	ACL	Mid One-Third Lateral Capsule	Lateral Meniscus
1	+	+	+	+	−	−	−	−
2	+	+	+	+	−	−	+ (Segond's fracture)	−
3	+	+	+	+	−	−	−	Peripheral tear
4	+	+	+	−	−		−	
5	+	+	+	+	−	Hemorrhage but intact	+ (Partial tear)	Tear in body
6	+	+	+	+	Partial		+ (Partial tear)	−
7	+	+	+	−	−	−	−	−
8	+	+	+	+	−	−	−	−
9	+	+	+	−	−	−	−	−
10	+	+	+	+	Partial	−	−	−
11	+	+	+	+	−	−	+ (Partial tear)	
12	+	+	+	+	−	−	−	Peripheral tear

FCL = fibular collateral ligament; ITB = iliotibial band; ACL = anterior cruciate ligament; + = ligament disruption; − = normal appearing ligament.

[a] Consistent findings were tears of the arcuate ligament complex consisting of the fibular collateral ligament, arcuate ligament, and popliteal musculotendinous unit.

risk of vessel disruption may be as high as 40 percent of dislocations in the anteroposterior plane and 33 percent with all other dislocations.[58] Frequently it is not possible to infer the direction with occult (reduced) dislocations.

Management

The following rules are safe and have served me well, bearing in mind the potentially disastrous outcome of undetected vascular damage.

1. If both cruciate ligaments and a collateral ligament are disrupted, assume that the knee was dislocated.
2. If both medial and lateral collaterals are torn with one cruciate ligament, assume dislocation.
3. If the valgus or varus stress in full extension has absolutely no "end feel" and relatively little pain, assume dislocation.
4. If there is lateral collateral ligament disruption, a cruciate injury, and damage to the common peroneal nerve, assume dislocation.
5. If dislocation is suspected, do not place the limb in an encircling cast or restrictive bandage; use a posterior support.
6. Always admit the patient to hospital.
7. If the distal pulses are present, monitor for the evolution of a compartment syndrome.
8. Consider anteriography if surgical reconstruction of the multiple ligaments is a possibility in an acutely dislocated knee.
9. Early athroscopy with significant disruption of the ligaments and capsular structures of the knee may be dangerous. The high flow and positive pressure may cause extravasation of the irrigating fluid into the popliteal space, further compromising the circulation.
10. Assess circulation with reference to the seven *P's*.
    a. *Pulselessness.* Absence of ankle or foot pulses indicates the need for arteriography. Do not rely on Doppler studies, or fasciotomy. Do not accept a diagnosis of arterial spasm. The state of the artery must be determined. Usually there is an intimal tear, and exploration of the vessel is indicated.
    b. *Pain.* It is difficult to distinguish the pain of the trauma from the pain of vascular insufficiency. However, leg and foot pain in excess of knee pain is suggestive.
    c. *Pallor.* This sign is difficult to evaluate alone; but in association with other signs, particu-

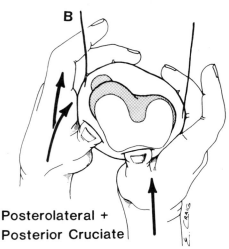

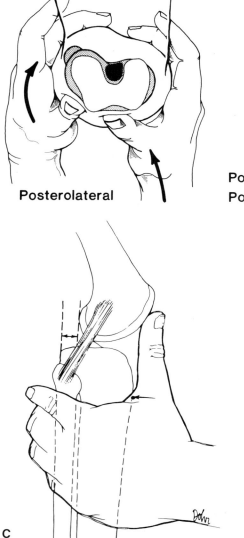

A

Posterolateral

B

**Posterolateral +
Posterior Cruciate**

C

Fig. 14-44. Posterolateral drawer test performed to detect posterolateral instability. **(A)** Tibia rotates posteriorly and laterally around the posterior cruciate ligament (PCL) if it is intact. **(B)** With combined PCL and posterolateral instability there is posterior translation, and the joint demonstrates an increase in posterolateral subluxation. **(C)** Position of the hands in the lateral view.

larly a cold foot, pallor may indicate arterial insufficiency.

d. *Paresthesia.* The importance here is to assess increasing signs of nerve damage. Whereas the peroneal nerve may be involved in the initial injury, increasing signs, particularly involving more than one peripheral nerve, should not be attributed to the initial trauma or swelling.

e. *Paralysis.* This sign is difficult to distinguish from the initial injury unless it is progressive.

f. *Popliteal evaluation.* A note is made of rapid, tense swelling in the popliteal fossa, which may signify a hematoma from the popliteal artery.

g. *Prompt arteriography and surgery.* Any suspicion of arterial damage should stimulate rapid assessment by arteriography and an expedited trip to the operating room. The long-term prognosis starts to deteriorate at 4 hours and rapidly becomes poor at 8 hours. In our series of popliteal artery damage, the amputa-

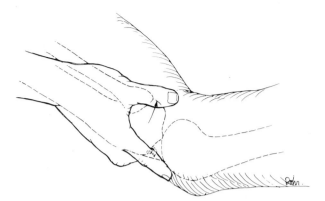

Fig. 14-45. Reverse prone Lachman test. Posteromedial and posterolateal corners may be palpated and visualized while the posterior glide is performed.

tion rate was seen to be twice as high at one city hospital as at another. The cause could be directly related to the delay in getting the patient to the operating room.

In conclusion, maintain a high level of suspicion that dislocation may have occurred when there is sig-

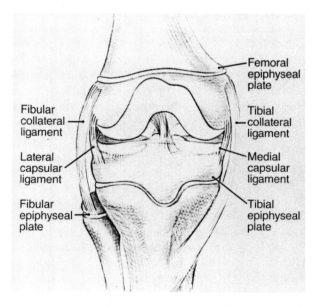

Fig. 14-46. Neither capsule nor cruciates cross the femoral epiphyseal plate, and only the tibial insertion of the superficial medial collateral is distal on the tibia. Thus with relatively strong ligaments, there is significant stress concentration on the physeal plate. It frequently results in physeal separation instead of ligament disruption.

> **Clinical Point**
> **DISLOCATED KNEE**
>
> - Major ligament disruption may be associated with dislocation.
> - Approximately one-third of dislocations are associated with popliteal artery damage.
> - After 8 hours the amputation rate is high
> - Do not use an encircling dressing or cast.
> - Do not procrastinate; consider arteriography.
> - Arthroscopy with insignificant ligament disruption may be dangerous.
> - Amputation rate correlates with delay in diagnosis and definitive surgery.

nificant ligament injury, particularly if both cruciate ligaments are torn and if the peroneal nerve is involved. Once a diagnosis of dislocated knee is suspected, arterial injury must be assumed and every effort to carefully monitor the vascular status of the limb carried out. Do not procrastinate; obtain an arteriogram and a vascular consultation at an early time. If facilities are not available for these, transfer the patient as soon as possible to a location where they are. Arthroscopy may be dangerous, further adding to the extravasated blood and fluid and further compromising circulation. Prompt surgical attention may save the limb.

KNEE ARTHROMETERS AND FUNCTIONAL TESTS

The ability to quantify instability in any specific direction at the knee is obviously an attractive concept. Unfortunately, most arthrometers are limited to one-plane analysis, and usually the anteroposterior drawer is recorded in millimeters. However, the latter measurement does not always bear a direct relation to rotary instability. Furthermore, the magnitude of the drawer and even the degree of measured rotary instability, should it be possible to measure it, do not hold a simple relation to true functional instability.

Thus a person with a large drawer may have a functionally stable knee; and, conversely, a barely percep-

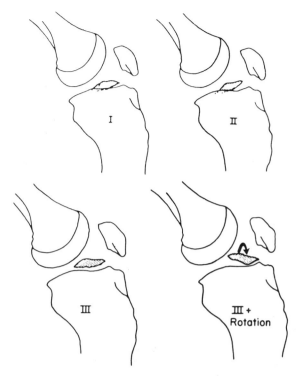

Fig. 14-47. Adaptation of the Meyers and McKeever classification of intercondylar eminence fractures. Type I, slight elevation; type II, anterior portion hinged out of its bed; type III, entire fragment is free; type III+, fragment is elevated and rotated.

tible drawer may be associated with significant disability. There is, however, a fair correlation for many individuals, and attempts at objectivity when assessing pre- and postsurgical stability are important; and they are an improvement on purely subjective impressions alone. The confounding factors are obviously muscle strength, proprioception, reflexes, and many more subtle influences. Indeed, these unloaded 15 to 20-lb pulls offered by most the machines can in no way be expected to mimic the rapidly changing high torques experienced under the conditions of significant joint loading that occur in sport.

Knee Arthrometers

The commonest devices available are the Stryker Knee Laxity Tester, the MEDmetric KT-1000, and the Genucom Knee Analysis System. The Stryker system is operationally the least complex. It includes a patient positioning seat, a force applicator, and a measuring instrument for recording the millimeters of displacement resulting from an anteroposterior drawer test.[61] At 20 degrees of flexion and with 89 newtons (N) of applied force, normal knees have a mean displacement of around 2.5 mm and ACL-deficient knees about 8.2 mm.[62]

The KT-1000 knee arthrometer also measures anteroposterior displacements resulting from the anteior or posterior drawer or by the quadriceps active method (Fig. 14-50). At 20 degrees of flexion and 89 N force, the mean anterior displacement values were 5.65 mm for normals and 13.0 mm for ACL-injured knees. A compliance index, which is the difference between the laxity measured at 67 N (15 lb) and 89 N (20 lb), of more than 2 mm is considered abnormal, as is a difference of more than 2 mm between the two sides (Fig. 14-51). The first of these indices is usually reliable, but the latter may not be.[63]

The Genucom system is a computerized tool that allows description of several ligament laxities. It is a complicated device and utilizes an electrogoniometer and a dynamometer. The normal values for the anterior drawer of 93.45 N at 30 degrees flexion is 5.67 mm with this system.

These instruments all have high test and retest reliability in normal knees, but they become less accurate in the cruciate ligament-deficient knee. In addition, at least for the noncomputerized models, intraobserver error may be significant. There is a considerable learning curve. Certainly, data collected with one device cannot be directly compared with those from another.

Computerized Muscle Tests

Various computerized dynamometers are available for evaluating muscle strength and endurance, including isokinetic apparatus such as Cybex, polykinetic machines such as Hydragym, and eccentric loading devices such as KinCom. The information achieved from one device is not easily transferable to another; nevertheless, they may all be valuable for assessing (1) muscle weakness as a possible contributing factor to the magnitude of a functional instability; (2) the need for, or efficacy of, a specific rehabilitation program; and (3) the progress of retraining power and endurance after injury or surgery. Their results may be used as guidelines regarding the need for further rehabilitation and to assist in the discussion with regard to returning to training and sport.

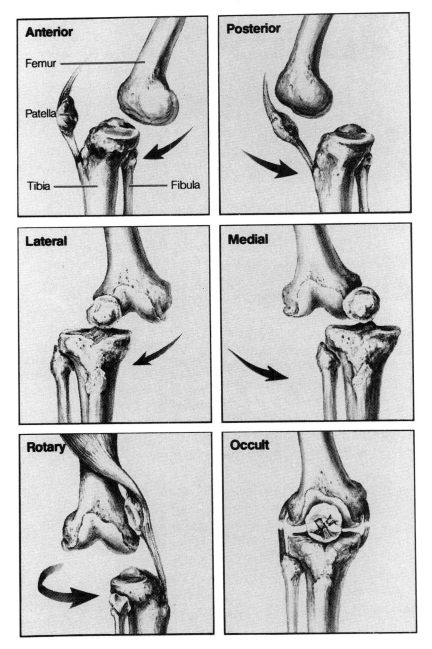

Fig. 14-48. Classification of dislocation. Arrow indicates the direction in which the tibia is displaced on the femur.

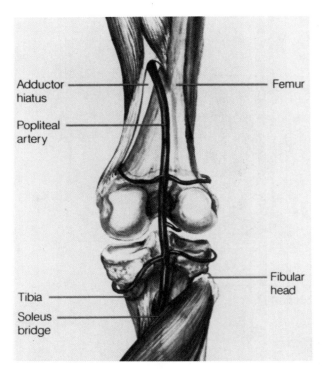

Adductor hiatus

Popliteal artery

Tibia

Soleus bridge

Femur

Fibular head

Fig. 14-49. Popliteal artery is tethered at the adductor hiatus and soleus bridge. Hence significance tibial displacement is liable to produce vascular damage.

Functional Tests

There are a series of activities that require control, strength, and stability around the knee in order to perform at an optimal level. They also reproduce some of the components of sport. It is natural that these activities should have been adapted as functional tests in order to assess the magnitude of functional instability at the knee. They include the crossover test, the hop index, the figure-of-eight circuit, and the slalom circuit. The first two have the advantage of requiring little space and hence are practical in a clinic setting. The latter two must be set up in an open area and are suitable as rehabilitation field tests.

Crossover Test

For the crossover test the athlete stands with feet on a level about 8 inches apart. The examiner stabilizes the foot of the ACL-deficient knee. The athlete steps quickly over to the side using a crossover movement of the leg (Fig. 14-52). With the foot fixed, there is a differential rotation of the tibia relative to the femur, which may give the patient a sensation of uneasiness or even a functional pivot shift with subluxation of the anterolateral tibia. This test is not particularly sensitive or specific.

Hop Index

For the hop index a standing or broad jump is performed three times on each limb (Fig. 14-53). The average distance on the affected side is divided by the average distance on the normal side.[64] This test is obviously affected by pain, the strength of the quadriceps and calf muscles, confidence in the knee, and laxity. There is some question as to the sensitivity of this test. In our series the hop index distinguished the moderate and severe ACL-deficient patients from

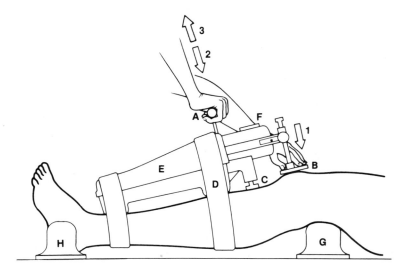

Fig. 14-50. KT-1000 knee arthrometer.

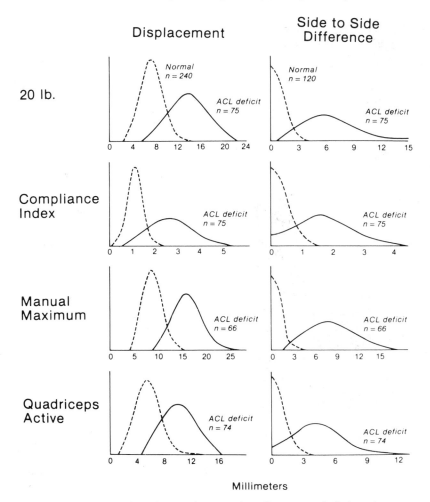

Fig. 14-51. Parameters for normal and anterior cruciate ligament deficient knees on the KT-1000 with a 20 lb pull. Compliance index, maximum manual drawer at 20 degrees, and the quadriceps active test are shown. Side-to-side differences are given.

normals, and it correlated well with the KT-1000 series and the Lysholm scale.[64] The distance hopped in a set time may be a better test.

Figure-of-Eight and Slalom Circuit

The figure-of-eight and slalom circuit tests have the distinct disadvantage that they require significant space and must be set up accurately to be reproducible (14-54). Both tests are sensitive to muscle weakness, pain, and swelling around the knee. Nevertheless, they are useful tools and can be used alone on a timed basis for rehabilitation or expressed as a ratio of a set sprint, such as 10 to 20-meter straight run. In

our series we compared all data to a 10-meter dash, which measures mainly acceleration ability in a straight line. The time for the figure-of-eight run and the ratio to the straight run were able to distinguish the ACL-deficient from normal athletes; in the ACL-deficient group it also distinguished between patients wearing two different types of knee orthosies from nonbraced patients (Fig. 14-55).

The timed slalom circuit distinguished the ACL-deficient athletes from normal athletes. This test did not seem to be able to distinguish the braced from the nonbraced ACL group. This finding surprised us, and it is possible that a greater learning curve is required for the slalom, as the test was not distinguishing ACL deficiency but some other parameter.[65]

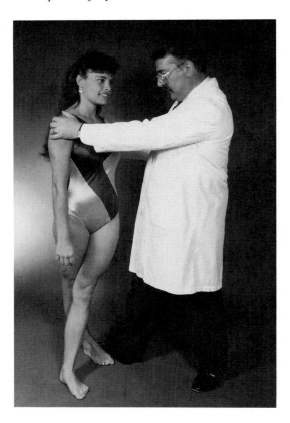

Fig. 14-52. Cross-over test unmasks a significant anterior cruciate ligament deficiency but is not sensitive. It tests the stance leg (here the patient's left leg).

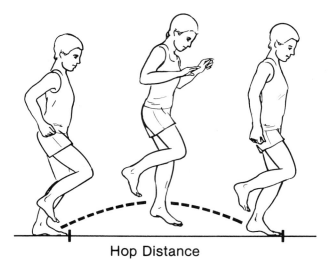

Hop Distance

Fig. 14-53. Standing one-leg hop is performed three times on each limb. The average distance on the affected side divided by the average distance on the normal side is called the hop index.

Knee Scoring Scales

A large number of knee scoring scales are available resulting in difficulty when comparing disability and results of treatment. The Activity Rating Score, Lysholm Scoring Scale, and Knee Function form from Cincinnati are three of the more common scales.[66,67] Of them, the Cincinnati rating scale is the most detailed and complex.

Cincinnati Rating System

The series of questions in the Cincinnati Rating System ascribe 50 points for symptoms and 50 points for function.[66] It is an excellent method of looking at the many parameters that influence function and the ability to perform and compete at sport (Table 14-6).

Lysholm Scoring Scale

Lysholm Scoring Scale is not complex and is perhaps the most widely used scale (Table 14-7). In our series it correlated well with the hop index and the KT-1000 knee arthrometer tests. Nevertheless, it is an inadequate scale from which to monitor rehabilitation. There is a tendency for athletes to overrate their ability on this scale.

Activity Rating Score

The Activity Rating Score is a broad but useful scale that is easy to apply before and after therapy or surgery in order to place an individual in an activity group. In this scale, "light sports" refers to nonpivoting activities and little sudden acceleration and deceleration. At 2 years, postsurgical scores of 5, 6, and 7 are usually considered satisfactory outcomes, depending on the severity of the preoperative condition.

"Limited sports without brace" usually means that the individual can run, is able to accelerate and decelerate satisfactorily, but does not have full confidence in rapid cutting movements even though the knee may not acually give way with these activities. By con-

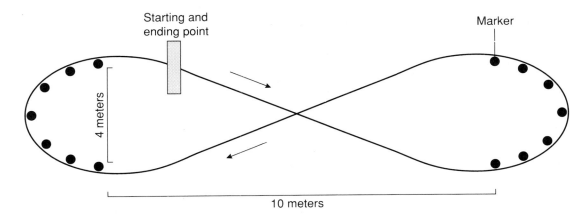

A

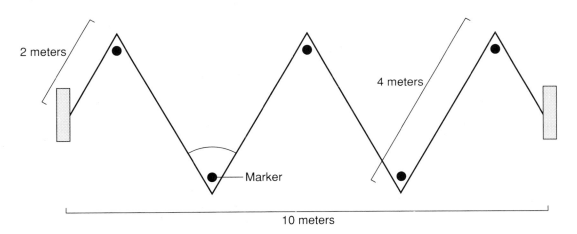

B

Fig. 14-54. Figure-of-eights (**A**) and Slalom circuits (**B**) may be adjusted so they are sport-specific.

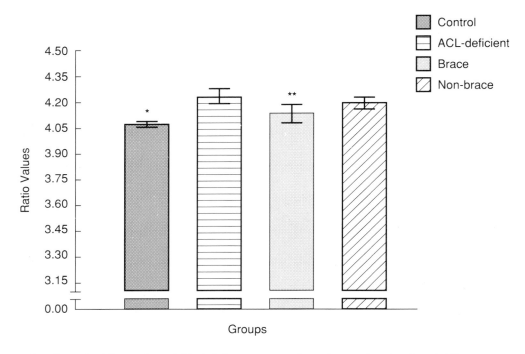

*Significantly different from ACL-deficient group and non-brace situation (p < 0.05)
**Significantly different from non-brace situation (p = 0.04).

Fig. 14-55. Figure-of-eight versus straight-running-without-a-brace ratio for a control group and an anterior cruciate ligament (ACL)-deficient group. Also shown is an ACL-deficient group with and without a brace. This test is able to differentiate ACL deficiency patients from normals and braced individuals from those who are not braced.

trast "vigorous sports with brace" indicates that individuals may experience instability with high-velocity pivoting maneuvers and may develop effusions and pain if they participate in aggressive sports without a brace.

Quick Facts

ACTIVITY RATING SCORE

Score	Criterion
1	Nonambulatory
2	Interferes with daily activity
3	No sports
4	Light sports with brace
5	Vigorous sports with brace
6	Limited sports without brace
7	Unlimited sports without brace

SUMMARY

Serious knee ligament disruption is a common, devastating injury in some sports. The development of functional instability has serious implications for performance in the short haul and the unpleasant possibility of degenerative joint disease in the long term. Hence careful early assessment and appropriate therapy are essential. In essence, any person sustaining an injury to the knee that leads to an acute hemarthrosis should be examined by an expert in order to reduce the possibility of a serious injury being overlooked. Often a clinical examination is not adequate. It is sometimes necessary to apply a local or intra-articular injection of some analgesic agent or even place the person under general anesthetic to complete the examination. Furthermore, some people need an arthroscopic examination to delineate the extent of the injury.

TABLE 14-6.   Cincinnati Rating System

Symptoms (50 points)

Left	Right			Left	Right	
			1. Pain			*Location of Pain*
___	___	20	No pain, normal knee, performs 100%	___	___	Medial (inner side)
___	___	16	Occasional pain with strenuous sports or heavy work, knee not entirely normal, some limitations but minor and tolerable	___	___	Lateral (outer side)
				___	___	Anterior-patellar (front/knee cap)
				___	___	Posterior (back of knee)
___	___	12	Occasional pain with light recreational sports or moderate work activities, frequently brought on by vigorous activities, running, heavy labor, strenuous sports.	___	___	Diffuse (all over)
						Pain Occurs On
				___	___	Sitting
				___	___	Kneeling
___	___	8	Pain, usually brought on by sports, light recreational activities or moderate work. Occasionally occurs with walking, standing, or light work.	___	___	Standing
						Type of Pain
				___	___	Sharp
				___	___	Aching
___	___	4	Pain is a significant problem with activities as simple as walking. Relieved by rest. Unable to do sports.	___	___	Throbbing
				___	___	Burning
___	___	0	Pain present all the time, occurs with walking, standing, and at night. Not relieved with rest.			
___	___		I do not know what my pain level is. I have not tested my knee.			

Intensity of pain: ___Mild ___Moderate ___Severe
Frequency: ___Intermittent ___Constant

2. Swelling

Left	Right		
___	___	10	No swelling, normal knee, 100% activity
___	___	8	Occasional swelling with strenuous sports or heavy work. Some limitations but minor and tolerable.
___	___	6	Occasional swelling with light recreational sports or moderate work activities, frequently brought on by vigorous activities, running, heavy labor, strenuous sports.
___	___	4	Swelling limits sports and moderate work. Occurs infrequently with simple walking activities or light work (about 3 times/year).
___	___	2	Swelling brought on by simple walking activities and light work. Relieved with rest.
___	___	0	Severe problem all of the time, with simple walking activities.
			I do not know what my swelling level is. I have not tested my knee.

If swelling occurs it is: (check one box on each line)
Intensity: ___Mild ___Moderate ___Severe
Frequency: ___ Intermittent ___ Constant

3. Giving Way

Left	Right		
___	___	20	No giving way, normal knee, performs 100%.
___	___	16	Occasional giving way with strenuous sports or heavy work. Can participate in all sports but some guarding or limitation is still present.
___	___	12	Occasional giving way with light recreational or moderate work. Able to compensate but limits vigorous activities, sports, or heavy work; not able to cut or twist suddenly.
___	___	8	Giving way limits sports and moderate work, occurs infrequently with walking or light work (about 3 times/year).
___	___	4	Giving way with simple walking activities and light work. Occurs once per month. Requires guarding.
___	___	0	Severe problem, with simple walking activities, cannot turn or twist while walking without giving way.
			I do not know my level of giving way. I have not tested my knee.

(Continued)

TABLE 14-6. *(continued)* **Cincinnati Rating System**

4. Other Symptoms (unscored)

	Knee Stiffness			Kneecap Grinding			Knee Stiffness
_____ _____	None		_____ _____	None		_____ _____	None
_____ _____	Occasional		_____ _____	Mild		_____ _____	Occasional
_____ _____	Frequent		_____ _____	Moderate		_____ _____	Frequent
			_____ _____	Severe			

Function (50 points):

Left	Right		
			5. Overall Activity Level
_____	_____	20	No limitation, normal knee, able to do everything including strenuous sports or heavy labor.
_____	_____	16	Perform sports including vigorous activities but at a lower performance level; involves guarding or some limits to heavy labor.
_____	_____	12	Light recreational activities possible with rare symptoms, more strenuous activities cause problems. Active but in different sports; limited to moderate work.
_____	_____	8	No sports or recreational activities possible. Walking activities with rare symptoms; limited to light work.
_____	_____	4	Walking, activities of daily living cause moderate symptoms, frequent limitations.
_____	_____	0	Walking, activities of daily living cause severe problems, persistent symptoms.
_____	_____		I do not know what my real activity level is. I have not tested my knee, or I have given up strenuous sports.
			6. Walking
_____	_____	10	Normal, unlimited.
_____	_____	8	Slight/mild problem.
_____	_____	6	Moderate problem: smooth surface possible up to about 800 yards (800 m).
_____	_____	4	Severe problem: only 2–3 blocks possible.
_____	_____	2	Severe problem: requires cane, crutches.
			7. Stairs
_____	_____	10	Normal, unlimited.
_____	_____	8	Slight/mild problem.
_____	_____	6	Moderate problem: only 10–15 steps possible.
_____	_____	4	Severe problem: requires bannister, support.
_____	_____	2	Severe problem: only 1–5 steps possible.
			8. Running Activity
_____	_____	5	Normal, unlimited: fully competitive, strenuous.
_____	_____	4	Slight/mild problem: run half-speed.
_____	_____	3	Moderate problem: only 1¼ to 2½ miles (2–4 km).
_____	_____	2	Severe problem: only 1–2 blocks possible.
_____	_____	1	Severe problem: only a few steps.
			9. Jumping or Twisting Activities
_____	_____	5	Normal, unlimited, fully competitive, strenuous.
_____	_____	4	Slight to mild problem: some guarding, but sports possible.
_____	_____	3	Moderate problem: gave up strenuous sports; recreational sports possible.
_____	_____	2	Severe problem: affects all sports; must constantly guard.
_____	_____	1	Severe problem: only light activity possible (golf, swimming).

Total: Left_____ Right_____

(After Noyes et al,[66] with permission.)

Variations of the Lachman test are the easiest to perform and are the keys to detecting anteroposterior instability, particularly ACL damage. The pivot shift test reflects ACL damage, and the posterior pivot shift is positive in the presence of PCL damage, but these tests are not always easy to do during the acute phase.

A classification of the various rotary instabilities helps the surgeon analyze the potential magnitude of involvement of secondary restraints and hence the

TABLE 14-7. Lysholm Knee Scoring Scale

Limp (5 points)	
None	5 _____
Slight or periodic	3 _____
Severe and constant	0 _____
Support (5 points)	
Full support	5 _____
Cane or crutch	3 _____
Weight-bearing impossible	0 _____
Stair climbing (10 points)	
No problems	10 _____
Slightly impaired	6 _____
One step at a time	2 _____
Unable	0 _____
Squatting (5 points)	
No problems	5 _____
Slightly impaired	4 _____
Not past 90 degrees	2 _____
Unable	0 _____
Total	_____
Walking, running, jumping (70 points)	
Instability	
Never giving way	30 _____
Rarely during athletic or other severe exertion	25 _____
Frequently during athletic or other severe exertion (or unable to participate)	20 _____
Occasionally in daily activities	10 _____
Often in daily activities	5 _____
Every step	0 _____
Pain	
None	30 _____
Inconstant and slight during severe exertion	25 _____
Marked on giving way	20 _____
Marked during severe exertion	15 _____
Marked on or after walking more than 1¼ miles (2 km)	10 _____
Marked on or after walking less than 1¼ miles (2 km)	5 _____
Constant and severe	0 _____
Swelling	
None	10 _____
With giving way	7 _____
On severe exertion	5 _____
On ordinary exertion	2 _____
Constant	0 _____
Atrophy of thigh (5 points)	
None	5 _____
1–2 cm	3 _____
>2 cm	9 _____
Total	_____

need for, and suitability of, various surgical procedures.

There is still much work to be done to evaluate and develop functional tests that accurately reflect the effects of cruciate ligament deficiency or performance. One of the difficulties is that the degree and magnitude of the anterior drawer does not always correlate with functional instability. Most knee arthrometers measure only simple one-plane abnormal motion.

Even the experienced clinician makes errors of diagnosis and misses associated injuries. Patience and practice are the key, but as confidence is gained it is important to keep in mind the ever-present misdiagnosis. The wise clinician learns to distinguish a negative examination from one that is inadequate. When in doubt, a repeat assessment at an early date is mandatory. Also exciting is the development of computed tomography and magnetic resonance imaging. These noninvasive studies are expensive at present, but as technology advances they will become more commonplace.

Lastly, a word of caution must be included regarding the vulnerable epiphysis in the skeletally immature athlete and the possibility of overlooking a knee dislocation with associated popliteal artery damage in the adult. Some guidelines have been outlined that can minimize the potential catastropohic outcome of these injuries.

REFERENCES

1. Johnson LL: Lateral capsular ligament complex: anatomical and surgical considerations. Am J Sports Med 7:156, 1979
2. Reid DC: Functional Anatomy and Joint Mobilization. 2nd Ed. University of Alberta Press, Edmonton, 1975
3. Brantigan OC, Voshell AF: The mechanics of the ligaments and menisci of the knee joint. J Bone Joint Surg [Am] 23a:44, 1941
4. O'Donaghue DH: Analysis of end results of surgical treatment of major injuries to the ligaments of the knee. J Bone Joint Surg [Am] 37a:1, 1955
5. Nicholas JA: The five-one reconstruction for anteromedial instability of the knee. J Bone Joint Surg [Am] 55a:899, 1973
6. Slocum DB, James SL, Larson RL et al: Clinical test for anterolateral rotary instability of the knee. Clin Orthop 118:63, 1976

7. Terry GC, Hughston JC, Norwood LA: The anatomy of the iliopatellar band and iliotibial tract. Am J Sports Med 14:39, 1986

8. Gerdy PN: Troisiere Monographie Maladies des Organes du Movement Os Muscles. Chez Victor Masson, Paris, 1855

9. Kaplan EB: The iliotibial tract: clinical and morphological significance. J Bone Joint Surg [Am] 40a:817, 1958

10. Van Domelen BA, Fowler PJ: Anatomy of the posterior cruciate ligament: a review. Am J Sports Med 17:24, 1989

11. Palmer I: On injuries to ligaments of knee joint: clinical study. Acta Chir Scand [Suppl 53] 81:3, 1938

12. Noyes FR, Bassett RW, Grood ES et al: Arthroscopy in acute traumatic hemarthrosis of the knee. J Bone Joint Surg [Am] 62a:687, 1980

13. Kennedy JC, Grainger RW: The posterior cruciate ligament. J Trauma 7:367, 1967

14. Hetzy MS, Grood ES, Noyes FR: Factors affecting the region of most isometric femoral attachment. Part II. The anterior cruciate. Am J Sports Med 17:208, 1989

15. Girgis FG, Marshall JL, Monajem ARS: The cruciate ligaments of the knee joint; anatomic functional and experimental analysis. Clin Orthop 106:216, 1975

16. Crowninshield R, Pope MH, Johnson RJ: An analytical model of the knee. J Biomech 9:397, 1976

17. Edwards RG, Lafferty JF, Lange KO: Ligament strain in the human knee. J Basic Eng 92:131, 1970

18. Kennedy JC, Hawkins RJ, Willis RB: Strain gauge analysis of knee ligaments. Clin Orthop 129:225, 1977

19. Trent PS, Walker PS, Wolf B: Ligament length patterns; strength, and rotational axes of the knee joint. Clin Orthop 117:263, 1976

20. Van Dijk R: The behaviour of the cruciate ligaments in the human knee. Dissertation, Department of Orthopaedic Surgery, Catholic University, Nijmegen, The Netherlands, Rodop, Amsterdam, 1983

21. Noyes FR, Grood ES: Classification of ligament injuries: why an anterolateral laxity or anteromedial laxity is not a diagnostic entity. p. 185. In Griffin PP (ed): Instructional Course Lectures. American Academy of Orthopedic Surgeons, Park Ridge, IL, 1987

22. Nicholas JA, Hershman EB: The lower Extremity and Spine in Sports Medicine. Vol. 1. CV Mosby, St. Louis, 1986

23. Feagin JA: The Crucial Ligament. Churchill Livingston, New York, 1988

24. Magee DJ: Orthopaedic Physical Assessment. WB Saunders, Philadelphia, 1987

25. Jonsson T, Althoff B, Peterson L et al: Clinical diagnosis of ruptures of the anterior cruciate ligament: a comparative study of the Lachman test and the anterior drawer sign. Am J Sports Med 10:100, 1982

26. Torq JS, Conrad W, Kalen V: Clinical diagnosis of anterior cruciate ligament instability in the athlete. Am J Sports Med 4:84, 1976

27. Frank C: Accurate interpretation of the Lachman test. Clin Orthop 213:163, 1986

28. Draper DO: A comparison of stress tests used to evaluate the anterior cruciate ligament. Physician Sports Med 18:93, 1990

29. Rebman LW: Lachman's test: an alternate method. J Orthop Sports Phys Ther 9:381, 1988

30. Feagin JA, Cooke TD: Prone examination for anterior cruciate ligament insufficiency. J Bone Joint Surg [Br] 71b:863, 1989

31. Cross MJ, Schmidt DR, Mackie IG: A no touch test for the anterior cruciate ligament. J Bone Joint Surg [Br] 69b:300, 1987

32. Katz JW, Fingeroth RJ: The diagnostic accuracy of ruptures of the anterior cruciate ligament comparing the Lachman test, the anterior drawer sign, and the pivot shift test in chronic knee injuries. Am J Sports Med 14:88, 1986

33. Ogata K, McCarthy JA, Dunlap J et al: Pathomechanics of posterior sag of the tibia in posterior cruciate deficient knees: an experimental study. Am J Sports Med 16:630, 1988

34. Daniel DM, Lawler J, Malcolm L et al: The quadriceps anterior cruciate interaction. Orthop Trans 6:199, 1982

35. Shelbourne KD, Benedict F, McCarroll JF et al: Dynamic posterior shift test: an adjuvant in evaluation of posterior tibial subluxation. Am J Sports Med 17:275, 1989

36. Galway RD: The pivot shift syndrome. J Bone Joint Surg [Br] 54b:558, 1972 (abstract)

37. Galway RD, Beaupré A, MacIntosh DL: Pivot shift: a clinical sign of symptomatic anterior cruciate ligament insufficiency. J Bone Joint Surg [Br] 54b:763, 1973

38. Gurthler RA, Stine R, Torq JS: Lachman test evaluation: quantification of a clinical observation. Clin Orthop 216:141, 1987

39. Jakob RP, Staubli HU, Deland JT: Grading the pivot shift: objective tests with implication for treatment. J Bone Joint Surg [Br] 69b:294, 1987

40. Hughston JC, Andrews JR, Cross MJ et al: Classification of knee ligament instability. Part I. The medial compartment and cruciate ligaments. Part II. The lateral compartment. J Bone Joint Surg [Am] 58a:159, 1976

41. Lamaire M, Miremad C: Les instabilities chroniques anterieures et internes du genou: étude théorique, diagnostic clinique et radiographique. Rev Chir Orthop 69:3, 1983

42. Bach BR, Warren RF, Wickiewicz TL: The pivot shift phenomenon: results and description of a modified clinical test for anterior cruciate ligament insufficiency. Am J Sports Med 16:571, 1988
43. Jakob RP: Pathomechanical and clinical concepts of the pivot shift sign. Semin Orthop 2:9, 1987
44. Losee RE, Johnson TR, Southwick WP: Anterior subluxation of the lateral tibial plateau: a diagnostic test and operative repair. J Bone Joint Surg [Am] 60a:1015, 1978
45. Peterson L, Pitman MI, Gold J: The acute pivot shift: the role of the popliteus muscle. Am J Sports Med 12:313, 1984
46. Barton TM, Torq JS, Das M: Posterior cruciate ligament insufficiency: a review of the literature. Sports Med 1:419, 1984
47. Loos WC, Fox JM, Blazina MF et al: Acute posterior cruciate ligament injuries. Am J Sports Med 9:86, 1981
48. Torisa T: Isolated avulsion fracture of the tibial attachment of the posterior cruciate ligament. J Bone Joint Surg [Am] 59a:68, 1977
49. Cross MJ, Powell JF: Long term follow up of posterior cruciate rupture: a study of 116 cases. Am J Sports Med 12:191, 1984
50. Trickey EL: Rupture of the posterior cruciate ligament of the knee. J Bone Joint Surg [Br] 50b:334, 1968
51. Moore HA, Larson RL: Posterior cruciate ligament injuries: results of early surgical repair. Am J Sports Med 8:68, 1980
52. Butler DL, Noyes FR, Grood ES: Ligamentous restraints to the anterior-posterior drawer in the human knee: a biomechanical study. J Bone Joint Surg [Am] 62:259, 1980
53. Insall JN, Hood RW: Bone-block transfer of the medial head of the gastrocnemius for posterior cruciate insufficiency. J Bone Joint Surg [Am] 64a:691, 1982
54. Baker CL, Norwood LA, Hughston JC: Acute combined posterior cruciate and posterolateral instability of the knee. Am J Sports Med 12:204, 1984
55. DeLee JC, Riley MB, Rockwood CA: Acute posterolateral rotary instability of the knee. Am J Sports Med 11:199, 1983
56. Shino K, Shuji H, Keiro O: The voluntary evoked posterolateral drawer sign in the knee with posterolateral instability. Clin Orthop 215:179, 1987
57. Crawford AH: Fractures about the knee in children. Orthop Clin North Am 7:639, 1976
58. Bloom MH: Traumatic knee dislocation and popliteal artery occlusion. Phys Sports Med 15:143, 1987
59. Green NE, Allen BL: Vascular injuries associated with dislocation of the knee. J Bone Joint Surg [Am] 59a:236, 1977
60. Kennedy JC: Complete dislocation of the knee joint. J Bone Joint Surg [Am] 45a:889, 1963
61. Highgenboten CL, Jackson A, Meske NB: Genacom, KT-1000, and Stryker knee laxity measuring device comparisons: device reproducibility and interdevice comparison in asymptomatic subjects. Am J Sports Med 17:743, 1988
62. Boniface JR, Fu FH, Ilkhanipour K: Objective anterior cruciate ligament testing. Orthop Rev 9:391, 1986
63. Daniel DM, Malcom LL, Losse G et al: Instrumented measurement of anterior laxity of the knee. J Bone Joint Surg [Am] 67a:720, 1985
64. Daniel DM, Malcom LL, Stone ML et al: Quantification of knee stability and function. Contemp Orthop 5:83, 1982
65. Fonseca ST: Validation of a performance test for outcome evaluation of knee function. Thesis, master of science, University of Alberta, 1989
66. Noyes FR, McGinniss GH, Grood ES: The variable functional disability of the anterior cruciate ligament deficient knee. Orthop Clin North Am 16:47, 1985
67. Lysholm J, Gillquist J: Evaluation of knee ligament surgery results with special emphasis on use of scoring scale. Am J Sports Med 10:150, 1982

Figures 14-2, 14-3, 14-6, 14-8, 14-17, 14-18, 14-20, 14-27, 14-31, 14-39, 14-41, and 14-42 are from Poole RM, Blackburn TA, Jr: Dysfunction, evaluation, and treatment of the knee. p. 493. In Donatelli R, Wooden MJ (eds): Orthopaedic Physical Therapy. Churchill Livingstone, New York, 1989, with permission.

Knee Ligament Injuries: Treatment

15

Though we seem to be progressing in circles, A.C.L. reconstructions do provide a functional improvement in the majority of patients with disabling instability.
—R. Larson, 1990

The operation is but one incident, no doubt the most dramatic, yet still only one in the long series of events which must stretch between illness and recovery.
—Sir Birkley Moynihan, 1926

Significant injury to the major ligaments of the knee is an unfortunate and sometimes catastrophic outcome of sport. The ubiquitous nature of these injuries is illustrated by Johnston's claim that 1.2 percent of 18-year-olds arriving at the University of Vermont had evidence of prior anterior cruciate ligament (ACL) damage.[1] Although we envision contact and collision sports as being the major threat to these ligaments, there is now ample evidence that internal torques generated by the quadriceps and fulcrums provided by the femoral condyles are frequently sufficient to produce ligament disruption during deceleration and pivoting, without additional external body contact.

Injuries to the collateral ligaments can be unpredictable in their healing capabilities and functional outcomes, but for the most part as isolated trauma their management is well established. Posterior cruciate ligament (PCL) injuries are discussed separately. The problem of managing the more common ACL injury is discussed at length. About 60 percent of these injuries are partial or complete ACL tears in association with significant damage to the secondary restraints. Isolated partial or complete ACL tears make up the remainder. The problem of the ACL-deficient knee is that it may interfere with activity, or make it impossible, owing to functional instability. Furthermore, the altered biomechanics and stresses on the knee predispose to early meniscal damage and

subsequent onset of degenerative changes within the joint. The appropriate choice of therapy is not always easy to establish, and every case must be individualized according to the magnitude of the injury, the potential or existing functional instability, and the age, needs, and goals of the athlete. An understanding of the treatment options is better accomplished be reviewing the evolution of the major concepts with respect to the cruciate ligament-deficient knee.

Quick Facts

ACL-DEFICIENT KNEE

- Common in active young people
- May interfere with activity
- May make activity impossible
- May predispose to meniscal lesions
- May predispose to degenerative joint changes

HISTORICAL PERSPECTIVES

Pioneering Concepts

Acute ACL disruption was first recognized in 1850 by Stork. The first acute repair was reported by Robson in 1885, followed by Hey-Groves who discussed reconstruction in 1917.[2,3] Alwyn Smith, that same year, stated that: "When the tibia can be brought forward in full extension, the anterior cruciate is definitely ruptured" and thus set the foundation for the Lachman test.[4] He also suggested electrical stimulation to prevent muscle atrophy. A year later Hey-Groves hinted at the presence of a pivot shift when he stated: "Sometimes this forward slipping of the tibia occurs abruptly with a jerk."[3] Publications during the next two decades concentrated on developing an understanding of the role of the various ligaments and the evolution of several basic surgical techniques.[5-8]

Refining Concepts of Instability

Larson and colleagues outlined a sequence of evolving concepts they termed "the modern era of ACL awakening," beginning during the 1960s.[2,9] Rotational instabilities started to be identified as the primary cause of disability in the active individual, although undue emphasis was still placed on the medial side of the knee, as evidenced by the gaining popularity of the pes anserinus transfer and the Nicholas five-in-one procedure.[9-11] An important switch occurred during the mid-1960s when McIntosh, and independently Lamaire, defined more carefully the mechanics of the "pivot shift" and suggested extra-articular repairs to prevent it.[12] With the more frequent use of the Lachman and pivot shift tests and the introduction of arthroscopy as a clinical tool, the diagnosis of ACL injury and deficiency became more reliable and consistent, setting the scene for a better understanding of surgical objectives.

Metamorphosis of Surgical Techniques

As the extra-articular repairs of Lamaire, McIntosh, Ellison, and Losee gained popularity and as studies began to have long-term follow-ups, the ability of these procedures to produce functional stability was put into perspective.[13,14] Two concepts thus became apparent.

1. Dynamic procedures such as the Ellison iliotibial band transfer and the biceps femoris tendon transfer rarely remain dynamic but may continue to provide tenodesis action.[15]
2. Extra-articular procedures are probably best reserved for augmenting acute repairs and, in the chronic situation, for individuals with less func-

tional demands on their knees. There is a tendency to show return of laxity with these repairs at long-term follow-up.

During the 1970s various intra-articular procedures using many different autogenous tissues were developed, and the results were carefully evaluated during the 1980s. These studies provided a framework within which most knee surgeons work.

1. Simple attempts at repairing acute ACL tears did not provide satisfactory results, as the damage to the internal architecture of the whole ligament is usually disrupted, and significant stretching occurs during revascularization.[16] Repair plus augmentation significantly improved the results of these acute ACL injuries.
2. Various tissues were tested for their initial strength and compared to the normal ACL. The patellar tendon gained popularity as a graft subsequent to claims that a 14-mm, full-thickness, central one-third strip tested in vitro at 175 percent, and the medial one-third at 160 percent, of the ACL.[16] However, its strength is probably overestimated, as a full 14-mm strip is rarely taken, and the tendon itself is weaker if not taken as a bone–tendon–bone preparation. There is also considerable weakening during the revascularization phase. Thus distal fascia lata at approximately 100 percent of the ACL, semitendinosus at 75 percent, and gracilis at 49 percent may be suitable substitutes. It has not been possible to show that the type of collagen used appreciably alters results.
3. There evolved an increasing awareness of the importance of preserving the menisci because of their protective effect on the joint surface and their contribution to joint stability.
4. During the mid-1980s several improvements in surgical techniques developed from a better understanding of isometricity of graft placement and proper tensioning of the substituted ligament. Arthroscopically assisted placement and better fixation techniques have both had a considerable influence on rehabilitation. The use of braces instead of casts during the postoperative period has also revolutionized the timing and approach to rehabilitation. The stimulus for their use was a better comprehension of the deleterious effects of prolonged immobilization on the joint surface and bone mass, as well as the impact on muscle wasting. Newer materials, improved design, and greater accessibility to functional

braces during the later stages of rehabilitation have allowed some protection and increased patient confidence in the use of their knee upon return to activity.

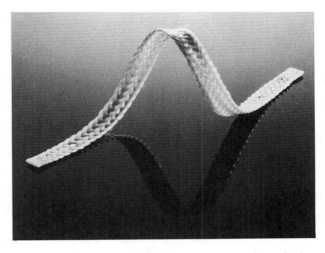

Fig. 15-1. Kennedy ligament augmentation device (LAD, 3M Company) is an example of a synthetic augmentation device that may serve as a splint during the revascularization phase.

with both technical and biologic problems. They still have to go through the revascularization phase, and the biologic response of the joint is not fully elucidated. Harvesting, storage, sizing, ensuring sterility and avoidance of disease transmission, and reimplantation with adequate fixation are formidable challenges for the 1990s.

Synthetic Materials and Allografts

The end of the 1980s led to an acceptance of many synthetic materials and a revived interest in the role of allografts and xenografts. The synthetic materials may be used to augment autograft material while it revascularizes and strengthens or may simply be used as a prosthetic replacement (Fig. 15-1).

Although there is no clear indication that augmentation of biologic material with synthetic grafts improves the long-term results, it is probable that certain ligament augmentation devices may allow early weight-bearing and motion and more rapid progression of rehabilitation.

Prosthetic replacements currently have limited but definite indications for use, usually in the multiply operated knee (Fig. 15-2). It is accepted that eventually all replacements will probably fail, but they may provide adequate stability during their period of functional integrity.

Allografts are an attractive concept but are replete

Factors Yet To Be Resolved

1. Measurement of instability is an inexact science. There is still a need to develop systems for reliably comparing results of different treatment approaches. It has become clear that clinical findings and functional results do not always correlate well with each other.

2. There are many mysteries that need to be resolved relating to the biochemical and enzymic changes that occur within joints after injury.

3. The gradual emergence of early motion, rapid progression of weight-bearing, the emphasis on eccentric and functional loading, and the speedy transition from brace support to free activity has revolutionized the approach to rehabilitation. Although these obvious benefits have generated considerable enthusiasm, there must still be some concern as to their impact on eventual clinical and functional stability.

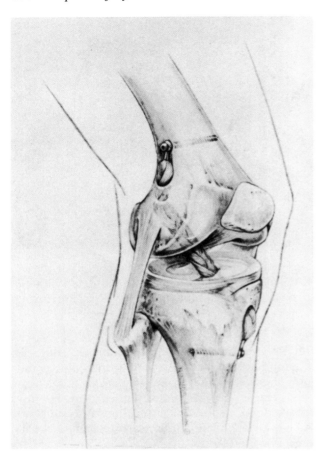

Fig. 15-2. Totally synthetic ligament used as a complete replacement. These ligaments have a definite but limited place in knee ligament surgery. (From Feagin,[15] with permission.)

TREATMENT OPTIONS

Acutely Injured Knee

The management options for the acutely injured knee depend on establishing an accurate diagnosis, making a judgment with regard to the potential functional outcomes, appreciating the needs and circumstances of the injured athlete, and then recommending and carrying out a specific treatment plan.

It is essential to believe that an accurate diagnosis has been made. If a history of significant trauma exists and the patient presents with an acutely swollen knee and the clinical tests outlined in Chapter 14 do not yield sufficient evidence of the magnitude and

specificity of the ligament injury, examination under anesthesia and possibly arthroscopy should be considered. In some situations, computed tomography (CT) scans and magnetic resonance imaging (MRI) may provide a more noninvasive avenue of diagnostic help. Clearly, several points must be established.

1. Involvement of the primary restraints, the ACL, and the PCL, and the magnitude of their damage if present. It is important to ascertain if there is partial or complete tearing, whether it is isolated or is present in combination with other ligament injuries, and the presence or absence of avulsed bone from the origins or insertions.
2. Magnitude and combinations of damage to the secondary restraints including the collateral ligaments and the expansions from the dynamic stabilizers, e.g., the medial and lateral hamstrings to the posteromedial corner, the iliotibial band laterally, and the vastus medialis anteromedially.
3. Possibility of associated meniscal injury.
4. Presence of overt fractures and osteochondral fragments and the presence of more covert transchondral cartilage defects and subchondral trabecular injury.
5. Pre-existing condition of the knee.
6. Activity goals of the athlete.

Practice Point

DECISION MATRIX: ACUTELY INJURED KNEE

- Magnitude of damage to primary restraints
- Associated injury to secondary restraints
- Meniscal tears: magnitude and possibility of repair
- Chondral and osteochondral fractures
- Pre-existing stability of knee
- Activity goals, age, occupation

Further advice must be based on some generalized outcome measures, which suggest that nonoperative management of isolated ACL and PCL tears may produce acceptable results. This figure may overemphasize the potential of the intensely competitive individual. It is suggested that combined tears of the ACL and secondary restraints have an acceptable nonoperative outcome in one-third of patients; one-third need to wear a brace for activity; and one-third ultimately require surgery. These figures take into account that many individuals are willing to modify their life styles as an option to surgical intervention. The results of PCL damage plus associated secondary restraint injury are less promising with nonsurgical therapy.

Chronic Functional Instability

The solution to functional instability includes rehabilitation, use of knee orthoses, activity modification, or surgical reconstruction.

Atrophy and weakness of the quadriceps and hamstring muscles are frequent clinical findings in patients with long-standing ligamentous instability of the knee.[17] This atrophy may persist despite the athlete's ability to return to a relatively good level of function. Usually return to endurance sports is achieved more readily than the ability to perform activities that require explosive maximal contractile efforts of the quadriceps or decelerating pivoting activities. Unless the rehabilitation program emphasizes explosive push-off activities, and if the athlete does not engage in a self-administered or therapist-controlled refresher rehabilitation program periodically, there is a tendency to either not correct, or to develop, type II (fast twitch) fiber atrophy. This development contrasts with the early type I fiber atrophy seen with cast immobilization[18] (Fig. 15-3). With rapid running speeds, individuals with ACL-deficient knees have been shown to have a significant increase in tibiofemoral rotation compared to that in their normal knees (Fig. 15-4). Additional hamstring control is required at high velocities to compensate for this motion.[17] This abnormal rotation in the loaded limb may be one of the factors in the evolution of meniscal pathology.

Thus rehabilitation must be based on functional deficits of the hamstrings and quadriceps muscles, with attention to both power and endurance. Sufficient attention to proprioceptive training and functional drills is necessary. The needs of the patient are established by interrogation, muscle testing, and functional assessment. The rehabilitation may constitute the whole treatment or be augmented by a knee orthosis or surgical reconstruction.

If surgery is to be undertaken on the chronic ACL-deficient knee, the decision must be made about whether to reconstruct by extra- or intra-articular means. If intra-articular routes are chosen, either an isometric bone tunnel or an over-the-top technique may be used.

The over-the-top position is not entirely isometric, but its posterior position tends to make the knee tighter at 20 to 30 degrees of flexion, which is a position of function for pivoting activities. The over-the-top method is technically easier, as errors of judgment about graft position are less critical than with the bone tunnel technique. Incorrect isometry in the bone tunnel technique results in the knee being tighter at the 90 degrees of flexion position and slightly looser in the position of function nearer full extension.

Practice Point

MANAGEMENT PROGRAM FOR CHRONIC LIGAMENT LAXITY

1. Identify and correct strength, power, and endurance deficits and promote neuromuscular coordination in all lower extremity muscle groups.
2. Establish a maintenance exercise program to prevent recurrence of muscle deficits.
3. Modify or substitute specific types of activity or sports.
4. Counsel on the risk of future arthritis when activities are pursued or continued despite symptoms, particularly chronic swelling or recurrent giving way.
5. Recommend an appropriate knee brace to be used during recreational and sports activities.
6. Assess the functional knee disability after successful completion of the previous five steps. These steps usually require a minimum of 3 to 6 months.
7. Consider arthroscopy for knees resistant to this program to define the true extent of joint deterioration, for counseling purposes, and for potential treatment of meniscal pathology that appear to be preventing rehabilitation.
8. Perform periodic examinations and closely follow up to detect subtle joint deterioration before it is too late to modify activities or intercede surgically.

(After Noyes et al.[19])

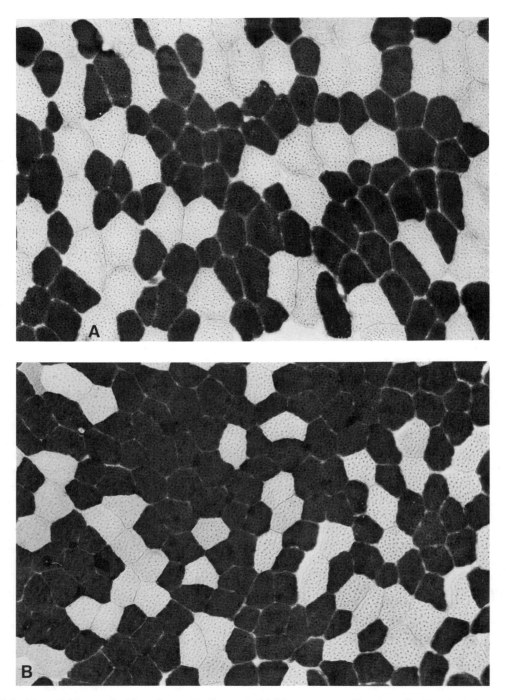

Fig. 15-3. Type I (slow twitch) and type II (fast twitch) fibers are readily identified by their histochemical staining characteristics. Examples of human quadriceps femoris stained for alkaline triphosphatase at pH 4.55. **(A)** Predominantly type I (light). **(B)** Predominantly type II (dark).

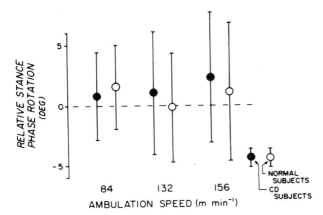

Fig. 15-4. Comparison of relative stance phase tibial rotation (RSTROT) at increasing speeds in normal and anterior cruciate ligament-deficient knees. (After Czerniecki et al.,[17] with permission.)

Further decisions include selecting the appropriate tendon for replacement; the semitendinosus and gracilis, fascia lata, and partial width quadriceps tendon are popular choices. These tendons may be used alone or augmented with synthetic material. The final surgical decision concerns the possible use of totally synthetic ligaments or a ligament transplant of autograft, allograft, or xenograft material.

SPECIFIC INJURIES

Accurate diagnosis of the specific ligamentous involvement is essential if logical treatment regimens are to be planned; perhaps just as importantly, these regimens must be evaluated stringently and honestly after a suitable follow-up period. It may require repeated examination, and in some circumstances examination under anesthesia, or arthroscopy. The specific tests have been clearly outlined in Chapter 20 (Table 15-1). Associated pathology such as meniscal tears and chondral fractures must be dealt with.

The following suggestions relate to the advisability of surgery, what type of surgery, the potential of nonoperative treatment, and the nature of this treatment. Treatment decisions must be surgeon-, patient-, and ligament-specific. It should be appreciated that there is a discrepancy of opinion among experts regarding all critical decisions within the treatment matrix.

Bony avulsion with instability is nearly always an indication for surgery, as bone heals well. Incomplete

lesions can probably be safely treated nonoperatively, assuming the diagnosis is accurate. Combined ligament injuries may be a reasonable indication for surgical repair. Isolated ligamentous injuries are probably treated as effectively nonoperatively as operatively, depending on the circumstances. Furthermore, simple repair of cruciate ligaments is rarely

TABLE 15-1. Tests for Ligamentous Instability About the Knee

Tests Used to Determine Instability	Structures Injured to Some Degree if Test Is Positive[a]	Comments
One-plane medial (straight medial) instability		
Abduction (valgus) stress with knees in full extension	Medial collateral ligament (superficial and deep fibers) Posterior oblique ligament Posteromedial capsule	When significant opening may involve ACL or PCL. Severe trauma may tear medial quadriceps expansion or semimembranosus
Abduction (valgus) stress with knee flexed (20–30) degrees	Medial collateral ligament (superficial and deep fibers)	Opening of 12–15 degrees may signify injury to PCL. If tibia externally rotated, stress is taken off PCL. If tibia internally rotated, stress is increased on PCL cruciate ligaments.
One-plane lateral (straight lateral) instability		
Adduction (varus) stress with knee in full extension	Lateral collateral ligament Posterolateral capsule Arcuate-popliteal complex Biceps femoris tendon Posterior cruciate ligament	If either cruciate ligament is torn (third degree sprain) or stretched, rotary instability is also evident and the magnitude of opening greater.
Adduction (varus) stress with knee slightly flexed (20–30 degrees) and tibia externally rotated	Lateral collateral ligament Iliotibial band	External rotation of tibia results in relaxation of both cruciate ligaments. With flexion the iliotibial band lies over the center of the lateral joint line. If tibia is internally rotated, stress is increased on both cruciate ligaments.
One-plane anterior instability		
Lachman test (20–30 degrees knee flexion)	Anterior cruciate ligament Posterior oblique ligament Arcuate-popliteal complex	Medial collateral ligament and iliotibial band lax in this position. Tests primarily posterolateral bundle of ACL in some individuals.
Anterior drawer sign (90 degrees knee flexion)	Anterior cruciate ligament Posterolateral capsule Posteromedial capsule Medial collateral ligament	May test primarily anteromedial bundle of ACL. If ACL and medial or lateral structures are stretched, rotary instability is also evident. Increasing drawer with damage to secondary restraints.
One-plane posterior instability		
Posterior drawer sign (90 degrees flexion) Posterior sag sign	Posterior cruciate ligament Arcuate-popliteal complex Posterior oblique ligament	If PCL and medial or lateral structures torn or stretched, rotary instability is also evident.
Anteromedial rotary instability		
Slocum's test (foot laterally rotated 15–20 degrees)	Medial collateral ligament (superficial and deep fibers) Posterior oblique ligament Posteromedial capsule Anterior cruciate ligament	Test must not be done in extreme lateral rotation of tibia, as passive stabilizing results from "coiling" to maximum rotation.
Anterolateral rotary instability		
MacIntosh's lateral pivot shift test Slocum's "ALRI" test Crossover test Flexion-rotation drawer test	Anterior cruciate ligament Posterolateral capsule Arcuate-popliteal complex	Tests cause reduction of subluxed tibia on femur. Greater with stretching of secondary restraints.

(continued)

TABLE 15-1. *(continued)* **Tests for Ligamentous Instability About the Knee**

Tests Used to Determine Instability	Structures Injured to Some Degree if Test Is Positive[a]	Comments
Slocum's test (foot medially rotated 30 degrees) Losee's test Hughston's jerk test	Anterior cruciate ligament Posterolateral capsule Arcuate-popliteus complex Lateral collateral ligament Iliotibial band	Tests bring about anterior subluxation of tibia on femur, causing patient to experience "giving way" sensation. Slocum's test must not be done in extreme medial rotation of tibia, as passive stabilization results from "coiling" to maximum rotation.

Posteromedial rotary instability
    Hughston's posteromedial drawer sign
Posterolateral rotary instability
    Hughston's posterolateral drawer sign
    Jakob's test (reverse pivot shift maneuver)
    External rotation recurvatum test
    Passive leg extension with hip flexed to 90 degrees
	Posterior cruciate ligament
	Arcuate-popliteus ligament
	Lateral collateral ligament
	Biceps femoris tendon
	Posterolateral capsule
	Anterior cruciate ligament
		Posterior cruciate ligament
		Posterior oblique ligament
		Medial collateral ligament
		Semimembranosus muscle
		Posteromedial capsule
		Anterior cruciate ligament

[a] The amount of displacement gives an indication of how severely and how many of the structures are injured. The first structure listed in the primary restraint and is damaged even with a mild to moderately positive test. A significant degree of abnormal motion may involve all of the structures listed.

(Data from Magee,[20] with permission.)

acceptable, and augmentation with another tissue is usually necessary for acceptable results. We must admit that our knowledge of the natural history of ligament disruption is still incomplete. Whatever treatment option is chosen, it should be with due regard to the ability of the patient and the particular center to carry out all facets of the treatment in an exemplary manner.

Nonoperative treatment must not be confused with neglect. Such treatment depends on specific knowledge of the amount or need for immobilization and the use of a variety of orthoses coupled with intensive physical therapy. The following section outlines a possible approach to specific ligament injuries.

Medial Collateral Ligament

The medial collateral ligament is subject to an infinite variety of tears (Fig. 15-5). O'Donoghue's works are frequently cited in defense of operative intervention for the treatment of acute medial collateral ligament (MCL) injury.[11] However, his remarks are usually taken out of context, as his attention was directed primarily toward the severe mixed type of injury. Indeed, although he did report on surgically treated

---

Practice Point

MEDIAL COLLATERAL LIGAMENT TEARS

- First degree tear (mild)
  - No significant instability
  - Localized pain
  - Minimal bruising
  - Pain inhibition
- Second degree tear (moderate)
  - Stable in extension
  - Mild to moderate instability in flexion
  - Possible hemarthrosis
  - Inability to fully extend
  - Firm end feel
- Third degree tear (severe)
  - Instability in flexion and extension
  - Soft end feel
  - Early hemarthrosis or effusion
  - Later edema and ecchymosis

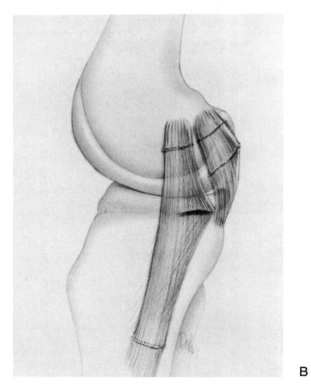
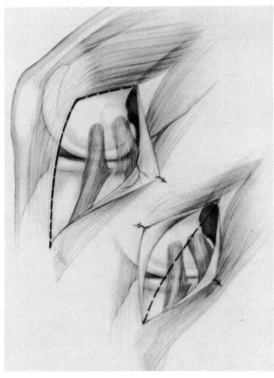

A   B

Fig. 15-5. (A) Medial collateral ligament is subject to an infinite variety of tears. **(B)** Careful dissection along the line of the vastus medialis and extension distally parallel to the retinacular fibers allows a search for tears of the individual parts without disrupting the anatomy. Alternatively, a simple linear incision may be made with equal flaps. (From Feagin,[15] with permission.)

complete MCL ruptues, he left the possibility of non-operative treatment open.

First Degree MCL Injury

Nonoperative treatment of isolated MCL injuries can produce excellent results. The key to this treatment is an accurate diagnosis of severity and the exclusion of associated injuries. There is little doubt that first degree MCL injuries are best treated by early mobilization and strengthening exercises. Pain and joint efffusion are the key to the speed at which treatment is progressed. Some protection against valgus stress may be necessary for early return to pivoting and contact sports. It may take the form of short-term taping in sports where braces are prohibited (Figs. 15-6 and 15-7). Where desirable and permissible, a knee orthosis worn for a more protracted period of time — 6 months with contact sports during contact drills and games (Fig. 15-8).

Second Degree MCL Injury

Second degree injuries are best managed nonoperatively.[13] They comprise a broad spectrum of injury and frequently require some degree of immobilization. The latter may be a brace with "stops" to allow limited range of motion while protecting from undue valgus stressing. The more severe the injury, the more important it is to recognize the changing length and tension in the collateral ligament throughout the range of motion. Restriction of extension into the last 20 to 30 degrees for 4 to 6 weeks is usually sufficient depending on the severity of the injury (Table 15-2).

In an attempt to make the clinical decision more objective Hastings outlined some parameters that may be used to supplement clinical tests.[21] For first degree injuries with no associated cruciate damage, valgus stress roentgenograms at 20 degrees of flexion performed under general anesthesia reveal less than 4 mm of opening, as measured at the edge of the

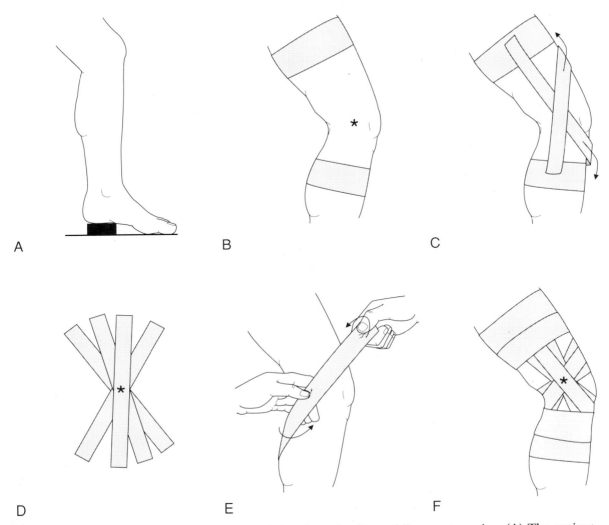

Fig. 15-6. Cross (X) taping for either medial or lateral collateral ligament sprains. **(A)** The patient stands with the heel supported on a small block to induce slight knee flexion. **(B)** Anchors are applied. **(C)** Initial cross straps are applied. **(D & E)** Several reinforcing straps are applied next. **(F)** Final anchors.

condyles. Knees with evidence of an intact cruciate ligament and valgus opening of between 5 and 12 mm are usually second degree injuries.

Third Degree MCL Injury

Approximately 80 percent of third degree MCL injuries have associated cruciate ligament damage or meniscal pathology, and it is on that basis that many investigators advise surgical intervention[12,21] (Fig. 15-9). These knees usually open more than 12 mm in excess of the uninjured knee with valgus stressing at

30 degrees. The end feel is soft. However, if the Lachman test is negative or minimal and the pivot shift is absent, nonoperative treatment is the method of choice for most individuals.[22,23]

Some investigators insist that if a castbrace, or orthosis is to be used, the third degree injury should be immobilized, with motion limited to 30 to 90 degrees of flexion for 4 to 6 weeks to allow adaptive shortening during healing.[21] This degree of restriction of range may not be necessary.

Behrens and Templeton reported on long-term results of operatively and nonoperatively treated MCL

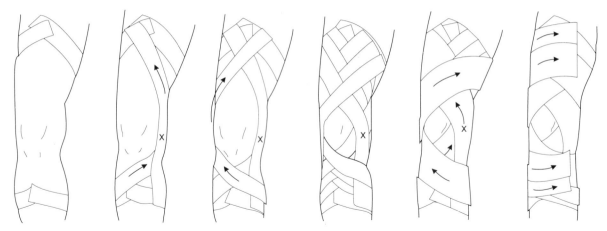

Fig. 15-7. Heavy supportive taping for an unstable knee. Such taping may be used alone or in conjunction with bracing.

Practice Point

CRITERIA FOR NONOPERATIVE TREATMENT OF MCL INJURY

- All first and second degree injuries
- Third degree injuries
  — Relatively stable in extension
  — Firm end feel in extension
  — Absent pivot shift
  — Willing to cooperate with treatment
  — Availability of therapy
- Absence of indication for surgical intervention, such as
  — No bony or cartilage fragment
  — No bony avulsion
  — No significant peripheral meniscal lesion

---

injuries. Half the conservatively treated and 95.6 percent of the operatively treated patients had some complaints.[23] Operative intervention prolonged the rehabilitation and generally produced significantly worse results with respect to overall satisfaction, frequency of pain, and residual laxity.[23] They found little difference between those with lesions isolated to the superficial medial collateral ligament or in combination with posterior oblique ligament damage.

When surgical repair of the MCL injury is warranted, meniscal resuturing is often required, and careful attention should be paid to minimally disrupt-

ing the already damaged structures (Figs. 15-5 and 15-9). Depending on the site and nature of the tear, either plication of the ligament substance is required, or proximal or distal stapling is indicated. Optimal postoperative therapy includes a limited range of motion brace and intensive rehabilitation. With contact

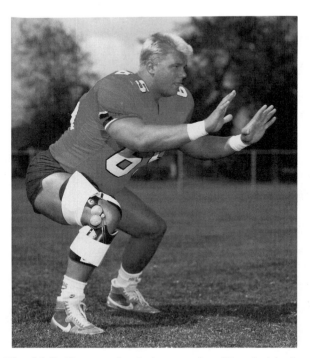

Fig. 15-8. Knee orthosis (generation II) suitable for additional support for a healing ligament injury during contact drills. The device should obviously be covered to protect other players from injury.

TABLE 15-2. Knee Rehabilitation for First and Second Degree MCL Injury

(Phase I) First week
    At time of injury
        Ice, elevation, compression
        Adequate examination
        Determine need to examine under anesthesia
        Determine need for arthoscopy
        Possible roentgenogram
        Knee immobilizer; protected weight-bearing
        Consider need for restricted range of motion brace
    Days 2–7[c]
        Maintain general cardiovascular fitness
        Maintain general strength
        Range of motion in whirlpool (ice versus heat)
        Overcome reflex inhibition
        Ambulation progressed as tolerated
        Tensor or Neoprene knee sleeve
        Avoid valgus stress
        Quadriceps and hamstring work
(Phase II) Commencing second week
    Continue cardiovascular work

    Progression of quadriceps and hamstring work
        Range of motion within pain
        Attempt to reduce edema and effusion
        Local therapy to tender area over ligament (ultrasound)
        Progress eccentric loading
        One-fourth to one-half squats; cycling
        Step-up exercises
        As pain and swelling resolve, commence jogging

    Criteria for progression to phase III
        No effusion
        Minimal or absent femoral or tibial condyle tenderness
        Full range of motion[a]
        No sudden increase in laxity
Phase III[b]
    Continue cardiovascular and general strengthening
        Specific terminal quadriceps control
        Proprioceptive exercises
        Increase acceleration–deceleration work
        Commence agility drills (specific to sport)

    Assess need for continued bracing
    Evaluate for return to training of sport
        Full range of motion
        Nontender over MCL
        No effusion
        Muscle strength > 90% normal

    Rule out need for further investigation such as
        Increasing instability
        Persistent effusion
        Giving way, locking, or catching
        Increasing pain

---

[a] Depending on the severity of the second degree MCL injury, it may be necessary to restrict full extension longer.

[b] With third degree MCL injuries this regimen may be delayed to accommodate the initial restriction of range, although many clinicians believe this delay is not necessary.

[c] Alternatively, this program is commenced during the postsurgical period at the discretion of the surgeon.

(After Czerniecki et al.,[17] with permission.)

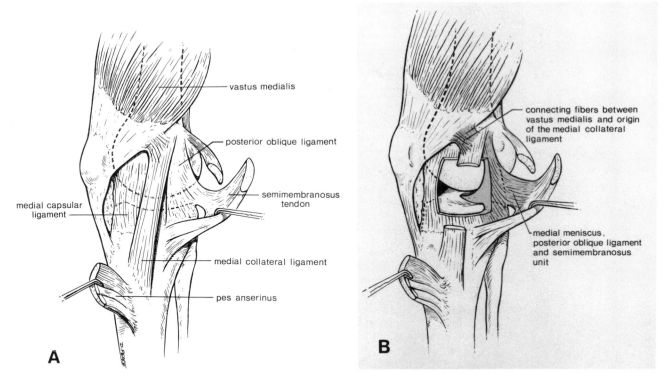

Fig. 15-9. (A) Medial ligamentous complex with the semimembranosus and its capsular reflections turned back. **(B)** Association of the posteromedial corner and the deep fibers of the medial collateral ligament with the medial meniscus, make it vulnerable to associated pathology. According to Müller, the superficial anterior medial collateral ligament is dynamized by the vastus medialis expansions and the posterior oblique portion of the semimembranosus. (From Feagin,[15] with permission.)

sports and repetitive pivoting activities, it may be advisable to wear a knee orthosis for as long as 1 year after the injury.

Laboratory studies on ligament healing indicate the following.[24,25]

1. MCL healing is probably by distinct scar formation rather than true ligament regeneration.
2. The sequence of hemorrhage, inflammation, and proliferation of fibroblasts is rapid, but the subsequent remodeling is slow, taking many months.
3. Some degree of laxity may improve spontaneously with scar contraction; however, scar may ultimately stretch out again when placed under stress.
4. When primary restraints are significantly damaged, the secondary stretching of the other capsular restraints with time is more likely to be significant.

Chronic Valgus Laxity

The chronically stretched medial collateral ligament may give little trouble when the recreational activity requires minimal sudden directional changes. However, pain or swelling following activity, on a consistent basis, suggests undue functional instability. It may be improved by rehabilitation, bracing, or both. The evolution of medial meniscal lesions must be suspected if the above complaints are accompanied by either giving way or locking. Occasionally, isolated chronic medial collateral ligament laxity requires ligament reconstruction. The latter should be planned carefully and is usually best achieved with posteromedial plication in association with distal or proximal transplantation of the tibial or femoral origins, respctively, often with a sliver of bone. The postoperative regimen is similar to that of the acute repair (Table 15-2).

Lateral Collateral Ligament Injuries

Isolated injuries to the lateral ligamentous structures are relatively uncommon, and few clinicians have a large experience. Invariably, the more severe lateral ligament tears are associated with rotary instability. DeLee et al. classified lateral instability as 1+ with 0.5 mm of joint opening, 2+ with 5 to 10 mm, and 3+ with more than 10 mm of joint opening over the contralateral side, with the knee in extension and with adequate relaxation or general anesthesia.[26]

Nonoperative treatment of grade I and II injuries produces acceptable results, much along the lines of the previously described medial collateral ligament sprains. Grade III injuries usually require operative repair to ensure the maximal chance of functional recovery.[26,27] The possibility of peroneal nerve injury must always be borne in mind, as it complicates rehabilitation.

Grade II and III lateral cruciate ligament (LCL) injuries treated conservatively result in some varus laxity, but the dynamic supports provided by the quadriceps and iliotibial band are largely able to compensate particularly with the grade II damage. With significant residual laxity and functional instability, bracing or ligamentous reconstruction is possible. When surgery is considered, careful assessment of PCL and ACL function is mandatory if reasonable success is to be achieved.

Acute ACL Tear

Partial Tears

Partial tears of the ACL are probably best handled nonoperatively. However, several facts are known.

1. By and large, the progression of partial tears to complete ACL deficiency is related to the degree of tearing, the presence of any increase in anterior tibial translation, and the occurrence of any subsequent reinjury.[28]
2. Partial tears involving one-fourth or less of the ligament infrequently progress (12 percent), whereas tears involving one-half or three-fourths of the ligament do so in 50 percent and 86 percent of the cases, respectively.[29]
3. The ability to return to former levels of activity is not as good as some of the literature suggests. The most optimistic reports rarely looked at functional parameters in a stringent way. Although two-thirds of patients continue to function at sport, they often do so in the presence of moderate to significant problems.[30] These individuals require education to reduce the risk of future degenerative changes.
4. A giving-way type of reinjury is experienced with more than half of the partial tears, showing a potential increased risk for reinjury.

Based on these facts it is possible that selected patients from this group may be better treated initially with surgery, but for most individuals a wait and see policy is probably appropriate. The standard exercise regimen for quadriceps and hamstring strengthening must be supplemented by a carefully chosen functional rehabilitation program if any measure of success is to be achieved. It is important to be aware that even the isolated cruciate ligament injury may be associated with chondral fractures, subchondral damage, and the possibility of loose fragments within the joints. The timing of acute repairs is also subject to some change in philosophy, with many surgeons feeling that waiting 10 days to three weeks will allow a decrease in edema and restoration of motion which will reduce the tendency to postoperative stiffness and not detract from the surgical and functional outcome.

Complete Isolated ACL Tears

Essentially, complete isolated tears are an extension of the latter group and are associated with slightly increased morbidity. The prognosis of complete tears in highly active and competitive individuals is poor, with only a few athletes returning to unlimited sports.[31,32] Nevertheless, many individuals are satisfied with their decreased functional level.

If the patient's goals and situation suggest that operative treatment is best, simple repair is not sufficient as it results in a functionally normal joint in only about 50 percent of knees,[33,34] which represents little advantage over the nonoperative approach. For individuals not wishing to pursue the nonoperative route, surgical repair of the cruciate ligament stump, when practical, accompanied by some secondary procedure is advisable. The minimal additional re-enforcement is extra-articular tubulation of a strip of fascia lata that is stapled to the lateral femoral condyle at its junction with the shaft. This repair allows approximately 90 percent of patients to return to sport; and of these individuals, about 70 percent return to preinjury levels. This type of augmentation has the disadvantage of stretching a little with time. However, the procedure is easy to perform, is associated with little morbidity, and leaves most structures intact for any subsequent procedures that may ultimately be necessary. I recommend this approach only for those patients electing to undergo acute repair who have good collagen, a relatively tight knee due to intact secondary restraints, and a minimal to moderate pivot shift. For the highly competitive athlete this repair may not be enough.

My preference for augmenting an acute repair utilizes the semitendinosus tendon and occasionally the gracilis if additional tendon is required. The operative technique involves passing the semitendinosus tendon through a proximal tibial drill hole, through the stump of the ACL, and over the top in what is considered to be an acceptably isometric position (Fig. 15-10). This approach assumes that the semitendinosus graft acts as an internal splint that may metaplase to a functional ligament. It may also act as a direction finder for the ACL stump fragments and form a framework around which the torn ACL may heal. The ACL stump may provide some vascularity

and improvement in the remaining proprioception. There are many surgeons who believe that maintaining and repairing the ACL stump adds little or nothing to the final results. There are two basic criticisms against the use of the semitendinosus graft. The first relates to the weakening effect of removing a hamstring muscle, which is an important agonist to ACL function; and the second relates to the insufficient strength of the graft. McConkey has reported on a large series of patients followed for 2 to 8 years (P. McConkey, personal communication, 1990). The graft was as strong as partial width patellar tendon grafts in most cases and stronger than fascia lata. Furthermore, isokinetic testing at 2 years showed that the hamstring recovers full strength, as measured by peak torque and the fatique index. The KT-1000 with a 20-lb pull produced on average a 1.7 mm side-to-side difference, which is well within the acceptable limits. Excellent functional levels have been achieved by this technique. Postoperative rehabilitation closely followed the protocol that is outlined elsewhere for chronic reconstruction procedures. Indeed, there is a trend to treat all ACL injuries in a similar way, whether acute or chronic.

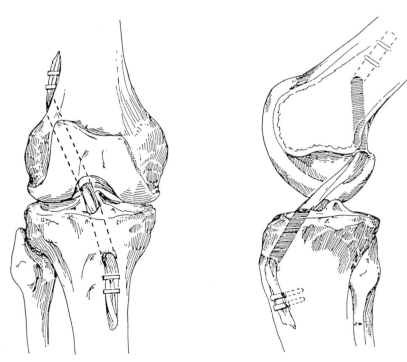

Fig. 15-10. Intra-articular repair using semitendinosus and gracilis. In this case a small flake of cortex on the posterior aspect of the bone tunnel is left intact and thus is slightly anterior to the top position. (After Schaefer RK and Jackson DW. In McGinty JB (ed): Operative Arthroscopy. Raven Press, New York, 1989.)

Combined ACL Injuries

When the acute ligament disruption involves secondary restraints, along with the ACL injury, somewhat better results are usually achieved by repairing the damaged tissues operatively while augmenting the ACL repair. The higher the competitive level of the athletes, the more likely they are to require operative repair for acceptable functional results.

Chronic ACL-Deficient Knee

Individuals with chronic ACL deficiency present with multiple episodes of giving way and recurrent pain and effusions. Physical examination reveals a positive Lachman test and a marked pivot shift. It is essential that the muscle strength is assessed and a failure to respond to adequate rehabilitation established. Individuals who do not have the enthusiasm and drive to carry out a full and determined exercise program are poor candidates for surgery, as they are unlikely to cooperate and execute the necessary postoperative regimen that is essential for maximizing the functional potential. The use of a brace should be considered and discussed. For some this method is neither practical nor efficacious. Wherever possible, the status of the articular surfaces, menisci, and secondary restraints must be carefully documented. This may require arthroscopic assessment.

The surgical choices are numerous but ideally should minimize morbidity, allow for rapid rehabilitation, and produce reliable functional results.[35-37] I have had considerable experience and success with two intra-articular techniques but have reservations concerning the use of extra-articular procedures.

Extra-articular Procedures

Extra-articular procedures usually employ a tubulated strip of fascia lata. The distal insertion onto Gerdy's tubercle is left intact. This 9 to 12 cm strip may be passed under the lateral ligament and secured to the lateral femur adjacent to the distal lateral intermuscular septum and femoral condyle. This technique is a modification of the Ellison procedure. I have performed this surgical approach with and without augmentation using the Kennedy ligament augmentation device (LAD). The 2- to 5-year follow-up showed a tendency to the development of an unacceptable amount of anterior drawer at 30 degrees of flexion with objective testing, as well as a disconcerting varus laxity at late follow-up in some individuals. A few showed a return of a mild to moderate pivot shift. Nevertheless, most of the patients were satisfied, probably because they had returned to sport and had completed intensive rehabilitation; most could even resume high speed pivoting activities, frequently with a knee brace. (Fig. 15-11). Even those who had a return of some pivot shift seemed to be functionally improved for the most part, which is difficult to explain. The addition of the LAD improved the objective testing of this procedure and may allow more rapid rehabilitation. I reserve the extra-articular procedure for augmenting other repairs when indicated or for selected cases in which intra-articular intervention is thought not to be advisable.

Intra-Articular Reconstruction

Of the many intra-articular techniques, I prefer the substitution using either the central one-third of the patellar tendon (bone-patella tendon-bone) or the

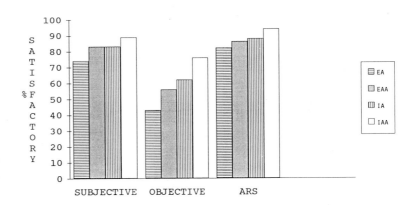

Fig. 15-11. Subjective results of anterior cruciate ligament substitution are inevitably better than stringent objective testing suggests. It probably reflects the athletes' increased ability to carry out their sport and recreational objectives, as noted in the excellent activity rating scores (ARS). A Kennedy LAD was used for augmentation. EA = extra-articular; EAA = augmented extra-articular; IA = intra-articular; IAA = augmented intra-articular.

semitendinosus, with the addition of gracilis tendon when required. The over-the-top position provides an acceptably near-isometric placement, for the latter tendons and it may be combined with grooving the lateral femoral condyle to achieve an even more theoretic isometric point. In practice, this step is probably not necessary and seems to add little if anything to the functional outcome. Whichever tendon is used the tibial tunnel is directed toward the ACL stump or sightly medial to the midline adjacent to the anterior horn of the lateral meniscus. Absolute isometry is not possible, but careful placement of the drill holes allows early motion with minimal stretching of the graft. Although a tight knee is desirable, excessive tightness leads to either restricted range of motion or undue stretching of the graft. Proper tension allows maximum use of the viscoelastic properties of the tissues. The aim is to mimic normal knee laxity. A notchplasty to increase the space in the intercondylar area is rarely necessary. Any meniscal pathology is corrected, preserving as much meniscus as possible, or repairing and resuturing where practical.

Restitution of a functioning ACL frequently obviates the need to carry out further surgery on the stretched secondary restraints. However, careful preoperative assessment reveals those individuals in whom more extensive plication and reconstruction are necessary. These procedures may be done as open surgery or by arthroscopically assisted techniques. In addition, augmentation with an LAD is possible. At 2- to 5-year follow-ups of the intra-articular over-the-top technique using the central one-third patellar tendon graft (unaugmented) or augmented with an LAD, produced excellent functional results (Fig. 15-11). Similarly, KT-1000 knee arthrometer measurements and isokinetic testing showed excellent return to a highly satisfactory status (Table 15-3). Similar results have been obtained using the nonaugmented and augmented semitendinosus and gracilis graft.

TABLE 15-3.   Anterior Laxity: KT-1000 Arthrometer (20 lb Drawer[a])

Surgery	Normal Leg	Preop. (Inj.)	Postop.[b] (Inj.)
Extra-artic. (LAD)	7.2 ± 2.8	13.9 ± 4.5	11.5 ± 4.4
Intra-artic. (OTT)	7.7 ± 2.7	13.8 ± 3.8	9.8 ± 3.6
Intra-artic. (LAD)	7.5 ± 2.4	14.2 ± 3.9	8.8 ± 2.8

[a] An 89 newton pull.
[b] Two to five year followup.
LAD = ligament augmentation device; OTT = over the top repair.

Ligament Augmentation Devices

The purpose of synthetic augmentation in ACL substitution is to provide a temporary splint that carries the load while maintaining joint stability until the autogenous tissue is biologically able to assume that function (Fig. 15-12). During the revascularization phase of autogenous tissue, the tensile strength drops dramatically. Initially a transplanted tendon may elongate only 3 mm under a 500 newton (N) load, but after 6 weeks that working load range elongates the tendon 13.0 mm. Whereas totally synthetic ligaments are ultimately plagued with material failure, the augmentation concept allows gradual hypertrophy, maturation, and strengthening of the patient's own tissue. In fact, it forms a load-sharing splint, initially taking the bulk of the stresses; ultimately much less of the patient's graft tissue takes over. Nevertheless, the ultimate function of groups with and without augmentation may be similar. The existing potential advantage of the LAD is that, accompanied by adequate fixation, it probably allows an accelerated rehabilitation process with early weight-bearing, good range of motion, and limited need for external support and bracing.

PCL Disruption

Isolated PCL injury may occur without significant damage to other structures, but it is an unusual injury.[38] The most common clinical experience is reflected in Loos et al.'s series in which 46 percent had associated medial collateral ligament tears, 64 percent posterior oblique capsular ligamentous damage, 31 percent lateral compartment damage, 46 percent ACL tears, and 29 percent meniscal tears.[39]

Acute PCL Injuries

When acute tears are associated with bony avulsion, operative fixation of the fragment is nearly always indicated and the chances of a successful functional recovery are excellent.[39,40] The need for repair of the acute midsubstance PCL disruption is more controversial. It is possible that an isolated lesion without associated internal derangement may be successfully managed nonoperatively. However, in some highly active individual, particularly if there is disruption of other structures, surgical repair is warranted.[38] If repair is selected, augmentation with a bone–patella–bone graft, or the semitendinosus is necessary to make the functional outcomes clearly

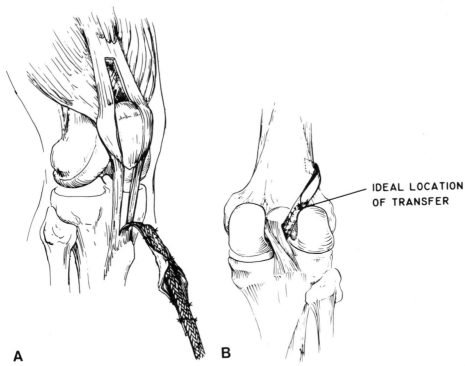

IDEAL LOCATION OF TRANSFER

A   **B**

Fig. 15-12. **(A)** Augmented reconstruction using the central one-third of the patellar tendon. In this case it is augmented with a Kennedy LAD. **(B)** "Over-the-top" position. Usually the LAD is sandwiched between an tubulated in the graft. (After Kennedy and Galpin,[43] with permission.)

superior to those achieved with nonsurgical treatment. Patients returning to sport without surgical treatment have usually rehabilitated their quadriceps to a high level of efficiency and some supplement this with bracing[41] (Table 15-4). Cain and Schwab demonstrated earlier quadriceps contraction to increase dynamic stability in the PCL-deficient patient.[42] They determined that in the PCL-deficient knee the quadriceps contracted approximately 9 percent of the gait cycle prior to heel strike during jogging, versus 12 percent after heel strike in normals, a difference of 21 percent.[34] This increased activity may be related to the reduced mechanical advantage of the quadriceps that occurs with posterior sagging of the tibia. (Fig. 15-13).

Chronic Posterior Deficiency

Many individuals with a PCL-deficient knee are unable to perform as well as they wish. The first stages of treatment are to rule out meniscal pathology, make sure that the quadriceps and hamstrings have been rehabilitated to their full capability, and, where suitable, supply a knee orthosis. Should this regimen still not result in a satisfactory level of function, the nature of the instability must be clearly defined utilizing the tests outlined in Chapter 14. Simple posterior sag is easier to deal with than that associated with excessive posterolateral drawer or varus and valgus opening. Whatever the repair chosen, consideration must be given to associated advancements and plication of

TABLE 15-4. Cybex Evaluation of Posterior Cruciate Disruption Treated Nonoperatively[a]

Patient Status	Injured/Uninjured Knees, Mean Ratio (%)		
	45 degrees	90 degrees	180 degrees
All patients	97.7	99.9	100.4
Dissatisfied	89.6	91.2	95.2
Satisfied	100.6	100.3	102.3
Same sport, decreased level	89.2	91.3	95.0
Full return to same sport	103.0	104.5	103.0

[a] Quadriceps function.
There were 25 patients with a follow-up 2.2 to 16.0 years (mean 6.2 years).
(After Parole and Bergfeld,[41] with permission.)

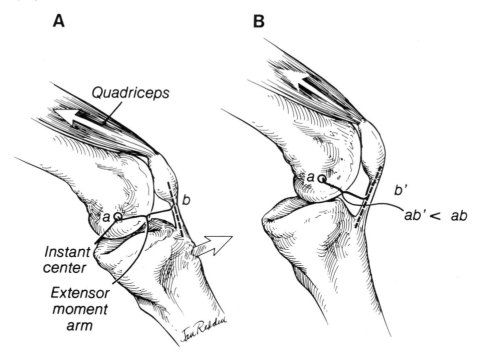

Fig. 15-13. (A) Normal knee. As the knee nears full extension the resultant force of the quadriceps produces a vector that tends to force the tibia anteriorly with respect to the femur. It may assist in eliminating the posterior sag in a PCL-deficient knee. **(B)** PCL-deficient. The full effectiveness of this dynamic mechanism is reduced by a decreasing moment arm (ab' < ab) around the instant center of rotation when there is posterior subluxation. (From Cain and Schwab.[42] Baylor College of Medicine, with permission.)

the medial and lateral structures, as appropriate. All follow-ups of late PCL reconstruction have noted a discrepancy between the measured posterior sag and the functional improvement.[39,40,43] Bone-patellar-bone, the semitendinosus, and sometimes the medial head of the gastrocnemius are suitable substitutions. Occasionally enhancement with an LAD is appropriate to gain either additional support or length.[43,44] Late reconstruction does not produce as good results as acute repairs, possibly because of the increasing stretching of the secondary restraints and the potential articular surface damage and meniscal pathology.

Evaluation of Outcomes

Many issues regarding the need for timing and selection of surgical procedures are still unsettled. It is incumbent on each surgeon and therapist treating patients with ligament problems to carefully evaluate the preoperative status as well as the therapy outcomes. Many of the tools for such evaluation were discussed in Chapter 14. The experience of the surgeon and therapy team greatly influences results. A questionnaire evolved by Noyes and his group helps to establish the patient's goals and expectation of surgery and to what extent that has been achieved (Table 15-5). Furthermore, Noyes' scale for grading the functional level as it relates to varying intensity of participation in sports can be adapted to evaluate nonoperative therapy as well as surgery (Table 15-6).

REHABILITATION

After some surgical procedures, the rehabilitation process contributes to reducing complications and perhaps minimizing recovery time. However, after reconstructive surgery to the knee, rehabilitation is as important as the surgical procedure itself. During long-term follow-ups of surgically treated patients, approximately 80 percent of individuals have at least a mildly positive Lachman test. Fortunately, functional recovery does not correlate well with the ultimate tightness of the knee. However, by contrast,

TABLE 15-5. **Patient Goals and Perception of Results of Surgery**

1. **How does your current level of activity compare with that before surgery/injury?**
   a. I have increased my level of activity.
   b. I am fully competitive. I have returned to the full level of work or sport as before injury.
   c. I have returned to previous work or sport but have limitation of activity.
   d. I am able to participate in light recreational or moderate work activities. I participate in different sports, limited return.
   e. I have not been able to return to sports or moderate work, but I have no problems with daily activities.
   f. I have difficulty with daily activities or light work.

2. **Why have you limited your activities?**
   a. I do not limit my activities.
   b. I have decreased my activity level in order to decrease wear and tear on my knee.
   c. I have no desire to participate in activities at a higher level, although I believe my knee would tolerate them without significant problems.
   d. I am in a rehabilitation program that limits my activities.
   e. I have significant symptoms whenever I increase my activity level.
   f. I have another injury or problem not related to my knee injury that does not allow me to increase my activity level.

3. **Why did you have surgery/go through the rehabilitation program?**
   a. I wished to return to full competitive athletics or heavy work.
   b. I wished to return to an active athletic life style involving recreational activities including twisting, turning, and jumping or moderate work.
   c. I wished to return to light recreational sports (golf, swimming, bowling) and activities of daily living (shopping, stairs, walking).
   d. My goal was to diminish my symptoms, which occurred with activities of daily living (shopping, walking, stairs).

4. **Did you achieve your goal?**
   a. Yes.
   b. No, due to:
      i. Pain.
      ii. Swelling.
      iii. Giving-way.
      iv. I have changed my goal. I no longer have the same desire to participate in that activity.

5. **The overall condition of my knee compared to that before surgery or since injury:**
   a. Has improved.
   b. Has stayed the same.
   c. Is gradually getting worse but is still tolerable.
   d. Is much, much worse.

6. **Regarding future surgery on the ligaments of your knee to provide better stability:**
   a. Under no circumstances would I consider major surgery on my knee joint as I have learned my deficits and have adjusted accordingly.
   b. I would undergo an operation if it was guaranteed to be successful in relieving my symptoms and increasing my activity level.
   c. I would undergo surgery if it gave me a 50% chance of decreasing my symptoms and increasing my activity level.
   d. I may need surgery, as my knee condition is getting worse during any activity.

(From Noyes et al.[19] with permission.)

increased quadriceps and hamstring strength does seem to be related to the ability to participate in sports.[45]

This section focuses on a detailed progression of rehabilitation for the postoperative period after ACL reconstruction. Extrapolating the principles outlined within this section, however, the protocol may be adjusted for most ligamentous injuries of the knee, provided certain key points are taken into consideration: (1) patient factors, such as age, occupation, activity

---

Clinical Point

KNEE REHABILITATION

- Without it, full function is rarely achieved.
- Ill-timed, it may prevent optimal results.
- Badly administered after surgery, it may reduce the patient to pre-operative levels of function.

TABLE 15-6. Evaluation of Pre- and Post-treatment Sport Participation and Intensity Level of Play[a]

Activity	Before Therapy or Surgery			After Therapy or Surgery		
	Intensity[b]		Participation[c]	Intensity[b]		Participation[c]
Baseball and/or softball	Full	Light	1 2 3 4 DK DD	Full	Light	1 2 3 4 DK DD
Basketball, netball, and/or volleyball	Full	Light	1 2 3 4 DK DD	Full	Light	1 2 3 4 DK DD
Bowling and/or golf	Full	Light	1 2 3 4 DK DD	Full	Light	1 2 3 4 DK DD
Cycling	Full	Light	1 2 3 4 DK DD	Full	Light	1 2 3 4 DK DD
Dancing (vigorous)	Full	Light	1 2 3 4 DK DD	Full	Light	1 2 3 4 DK DD
Football	Full	Light	1 2 3 4 DK DD	Full	Light	1 2 3 4 DK DD
Gymnastics	Full	Light	1 2 3 4 DK DD	Full	Light	1 2 3 4 DK DD
Hockey	Full	Light	1 2 3 4 DK DD	Full	Light	1 2 3 4 DK DD
Jogging and/or running	Full	Light	1 2 3 4 DK DD	Full	Light	1 2 3 4 DK DD
Martial arts	Full	Light	1 2 3 4 DK DD	Full	Light	1 2 3 4 DK DD
Soccer and/or field hockey	Full	Light	1 2 3 4 DK DD	Full	Light	1 2 3 4 DK DD
Swimming	Full	Light	1 2 3 4 DK DD	Full	Light	1 2 3 4 DK DD
Tennis	Full	Light	1 2 3 4 DK DD	Full	Light	1 2 3 4 DK DD
Other (specify)	Full	Light	1 2 3 4 DK DD	Full	Light	1 2 3 4 DK DD

[a] Patients circle one entry in each column.
[b] Full = high intensity level; light = light intensity level.
[c] 1 = normal activity (no symptoms); 2 = normal activity (occasional symptoms); 3 = limited activity (discomfort and instability); 4 = no activity (severe symptoms); DK = no attempt at activities (do not know); DD = not interested in sport participation (do not do).
(From Noyes et al,[19] with permission.)

goals, and the ultimate life style the individual wishes to pursue; (2) surgery-related factors, such as the experience of the surgeon, the type of procedure performed (whether intra- or extra-articular, augmented or nonaugmented), the nature of the graft, and the method of fixation; (3) joint factors, such as the general nature of the patient's collagen, the condition of the menisci, the joint, and the involvement of secondary restraints; (4) supporting scientific data on histology and pathophysiology of ligament healing, the articular surface response to immobilization, biomechanical principles of stresses on the joints, and (5) knowledge of exercise physiology and muscle biochemistry in order to relate functional goals to the proposed rehabilitation program.

Currently, rehabilitation techniques appear to have evolved through two stages and to be entering a third. Up until 1970, most rehabilitation techniques were based on resisted unloaded knee extension work. They emphasized strength, with little attention paid to endurance work and always followed a period of casting. During the late 1970s and early 1980s there was an explosion of rehabilitation and orthopaedic literature emphasizing the changing stresses on the cruciate ligaments at different parts of the range, the production of anterior shear by quad-

---

Practice Point

KEY FACTORS IN REHABILITATION DECISIONS

- Type of surgery performed
- Strength of fixation
- Initial strength of graft
- Anticipated changes during revascularization
- Condition of secondary restraints
- Condition of joint surface and menisci
- Secondary procedures performed to supplement repair
- Characteristics of patient's collagen
- Need and type of external support
- Postoperative complications
- Age, occupation, and resources of patient
- Recreational and competitive sports goals
- Condition of other joints
- Changing knowledge of tissue biomechanics
- Surgeon's specific concerns and guidelines

riceps work in the last 30 degrees of extension, the need for protracted protection of the repair during the revascularization phase, as well as the evolution of electrical stimulation techniques, continuous passive motion, and the development of postoperative bracing. Nevertheless, most patients were till treated with an initial period of casting.

Currently, with better isometricity of grafts obtained during surgical procedures, secure methods of graft fixation, and the knowledge that an absolutely tight knee is not as important as elimination of the pivot shift, has allowed the evolution of an increasingly aggressive approach to rehabilitation. This rehabilitation approach is based on early motion, early protected weight-bearing, and quadriceps and hamstring work through the loaded joint. Braces are utilized to allow comfort and protection from sudden unguarded motion and in many instances are not supplied at all. The rate of progression is not based as much on rigid timing as on the absence of effusion, the lack of pain, and the ability to gain muscle control. The traditionally unloaded leg extension is rarely used, and emphasis is on functional exercises that incorporate a strong element of endurance training and proprioception work. The late phases are characterized by an analysis of the functional components of the sport, which are then incorporated into the rehabilitation program.

The subsequent concepts are based heavily on the work of Paulos, Eriksson, Costill, Solomonow, and their colleagues.[45-49] From a study of these investigators' work it is apparent that the normal guidelines for judging progression, i.e., swelling, pain, and range of motion, must be supplemented by a careful consideration of tissue biomechanics, including the type of fixation, the nature of the graft, and the anticipated healing reactions.

Rehabilitation Objectives

Preoperative Objectives

1. Carefully assess the preoperative status.
2. Document patient's goals.
3. Maximize preoperative joint and muscle condition.
4. Provide patient education material and teach pre- and postoperative routines.

Postoperative Objectives

1. Protect ligaments while healing to allow maximum long-term stability.

2. Restore normal pain-free mobility to the knee in order to allow progression of activity.
3. Train muscular power in order to provide secondary restraints when ligament stability is lost.
4. Retrain muscular endurance and functional training in order to allow gradual return to activities.
5. Retrain normal coordination, including co-contractions, balance, and biofeedback in order to prevent reinjury.
6. Perform functional testing, and explain to the patient about setting rehabilitation and activity goals as well as a lifelong exercise program.
7. Consider the role of an orthosis in long-term management.

Specific Rehabilitation

Preoperative Period

The preoperative period should be used to maximize the condition of the patient's muscles in preparation for surgery. The patient's goals should be carefully elucidated and the degree of laxity to the primary and secondary restraints documented. Where available, an isokinetic muscle test, an activity rating score, and knee arthrometer measurements are performed. Just prior to the surgery the patient should be educated on what to expect and what to attempt during the immediate postoperative period (Table 15-7).

Early Rehabilitation Phase (Surgery to 6 Weeks)

The early rehabilitation period is divided into the perioperative period, the early postoperative period, and the protected motion period. The aim during this time is to allow safe, early healing; and it usually lasts about 6 weeks. There are two basic philosophies, and it is the second of these two approaches that is emphasized and discussed at length in this chapter. Nevertheless, there are still many adherents to a more conservative approach, and so the rationales for both are outlined (Fig. 15-14).

Maximum Protection Approach

The first approach is concerned with disruption of the suture line, fixation, and early stretching of the cruciate ligament repair or substitution. It also is concerned with the rapid reduction of the strength of the repair as revascularization occurs. Paulos et al.[45]

TABLE 15-7.   ACL Reconstruction: Intra-articular Over-the-Top Technique

Time Period[a]	Program	Goals or Criteria for Progression
Preoperative phase	Administer protocol questionnaire Physical assessment Activity rating score KT-1000 Cybex Preop. education material	Preparation for surgery Establish baselines Review short- and long-term goals
Early rehabilitation phase (surgery to 6 weeks)		
Perioperative period (1–4 days)	Incision care Brace applied in OR 15 degrees extension block[b] Encourage quadriceps-hamstring co-contraction Teach transfer techniques CPM optional Brace may be off at night[c] Discharge partial weight-bearing Teach home program	Deal with pain Watch for complications[d] Gain muscle control Ensure safe crutch walking
Early postoperative period (5–14 days)	Progressive weight-bearing Brace worn for walking Tubing drills, hip adduct, flex, ext. Wall slides Isometric hamstrings/quadriceps co-contraction Active isotonic hamstring work Sitting calf raises Well leg cycling Functional electrical stimulation optional May shower if wound okay	Allow wound healing Wean out of brace at night Encourage active ROM Need quadriceps control to progress W/B Absence of complications
Protected motion (2–6 weeks)	Review with surgeon Brace off PRN during therapy Upgrade hip abduct/adduct. (surgical tubing—Hydrogym) Resisted isotonic hamstring Slow, controlled eccentric, two-legged squats (to 60 degrees) Resisted leg press (sport cord or shuttle) Patella mobilizing Walking PWB to FWB Swimming with upper extremity emphasis (flutter kick) Begin cycling if 110–115 degrees flexion present Well-leg work for cross-over effect General aerobic work	Protect from unguarded stress Establish active ROM Gain quadriceps/hamstring control Observe for postop. complication Stress axial loaded exercises D/C crutches when FWB and symmetric gait Maintain general fitness Maintain general strength
Intermediate rehabilitation phase (6–12 weeks)	Follow-up by surgeon Leg press for strength and endurance Hamstring strength and endurance Double-leg squats to 60 degrees Linear proprioceptive drills (AP progress to side/side) Tube walk, tube run Step machine Cycle, minimal tension, build up speed	Needs 110 degrees flexion to enter this phase May D/C brace except isolated stress situations If knee stiff start vigorous ROM work Make sure hip, patella, second toe are in alignment Emphasize strength of hamstrings Maintain cardiovascular endurance

(continued)

TABLE 15-7. *(continued)*   **ACL Reconstruction: Intra-articular Over-the-Top Technique**

Time Period[a]	Program	Goals or Criteria for Progression
	Run in pool Power walk on level Retrowalking	Gradually move into terminal extension with all exercises Do not flare up synovitis
Preparation for activity (12–24 weeks)	Follow-up by surgeon Single-leg squats to 60 degrees Power walk program to run High speed retrowalk Multidirectional high speed balance drills Low and high speed strength and endurance activities in all ranges Cycle, swim-flutter kick Cross-country ski, skate, wearing brace No high impact work	Progress to running depends on functional control, absence of synovitis, and patient's confidence Emphasis on strength and proprioception Increase high speed drills Try to avoid unloaded resisted knee extension in 0–45 degrees However, make sure has full active range by the end of this phase

Return to activity (24+ weeks)	Follow-up by surgeon
	Running drills, straight runs, figure-of-eights, circles, shuttle run
	Functional drills, hopping, back-peddling, jumping
	Caricoa, lunging
	Consider fitting orthosis for high risk activity
	Sport specific reintegration drills
	Patient education re
	   Long-term exercise program
	   Activity selection
	   Adverse signs (locking, swelling, giving way)
	Consider Cybex, KT-1000 before discharge
		With running program, acceleration and speed as tolerated
		Control distance and intensity; add deceleration maneuvers last
		Orthosis when sufficient muscle bulk and functional need
		Activity assessment and advice
		Look for adverse signs such as locking, swelling, or giving way, which may indicate evolution of meniscal pathology or failure of repair

Follow-up (1, 2, 5 years)	Clinical examination Activity rating score Cybex, KT-1000	To evaluate efficacy of treatment protocols

[a] Guidelines only. These periods may be shortened or lengthened at surgeon or therapist discretion.
[b] Hinged soft brace is worn to provide comfortable support for weight-bearing.
[c] If patient is more comfortable with brace off.
[d] Hemorrhage, deep vein thrombosis, wound, or deep infection.

pointed out that the data for tensile strength of healing tendon and extra-articular ligaments underestimates that required for intra-articular structures. Extra-articular collagen shows a return to values approximately 75 percent of the original strength at 6 to 12 weeks. By contrast, after intra-articular ligament repairs and substitution, because of the weakening during revascularization, the ligament probably reaches only 25 to 50 percent of its ultimate strength during the same time period. Furthermore, there is minimal tension on the graft in the range 30 to 90 degrees of flexion (Fig. 15-15). The use of a cast for this first 6 weeks may assist in maximally protecting the healing structures. However, with this duration of restricted motion there is concern about the amount of muscle wasting, the effect on the health of the articular surfaces, and the possibility of late stiffness and joint contractures. There is even a question about whether cast immobilization significantly protects the repair, which is probably going through its most vulnerable phase after 6 weeks, which is still subsequent to cast removal. If a cast is applied, the use of electrical stimulation should be considered, either by utilizing the technique of a pad over the lumbar spine and the femoral nerve or by cutting a window in the cast to stimulate the vastus medialis. The effectiveness of electrical stimulation of muscle is still open to some debate, although the work of Eriksson and Haggmark

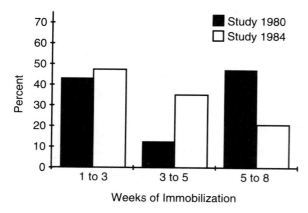

Fig. 15-14. Survey of knee surgeon's routines for length of immobilization after anterior cruciate ligament reconstruction in 1980 and 1984. The trend toward shorter periods of restricted motion is apparent. (Adapted from Bilko et al,[68] with permission.)

is impressive.[46,47] They demonstrated a reverse in the normal trend of muscle wasting with daily electrical stimulation (Fig. 15-16). Because of the concerns mentioned above a second philosophy of treatment has evolved.

Early Function Approach

The second approach, outlined in detail below, is the one I favor. It stresses that excessive immobilization of the knee is accompanied by articular surface changes, some of which are irreversible. Particularly, there may be retropatellar changes that subsequently

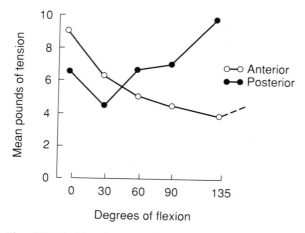

Fig. 15-15. Tension on the anterior and posterior cruciate ligaments during knee range of motion.

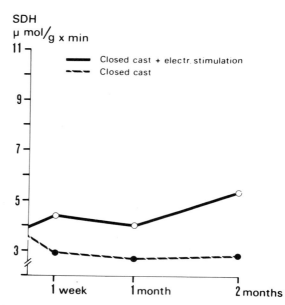

Fig. 15-16. Activity of succinyl dehydrogenase (SDH) in a group of patients with a closed cast versus those with a closed cast plus electrical stimulation after anterior cruciate ligament reconstruction. The electrical stimulation appears to prevent some of the fall in SDH. (From Eriksson and Haggmark,[46] with permission.)

cause retropatellar pain or arthralgia. In addition, the usefulness of gently applied stress in aligning collagen structures, secondary to the mechanical stimulus, has also been thought to be important. Furthermore, even gentle movement may decrease the speed of muscle atrophy (Fig. 15-17). These arguments have led to the concept that it might be possible to use a cast brace or orthosis within a limited range of motion beginning at the early postsurgical period. There is also evidence that, at long-term follow-up, early motion and isokinetic training do not produce an increased incidence of late instability.[50] The reconstructed ligament takes up to 1 year to resemble the normal ACL in regard to vascularity, histology, and strength. It is important to distinguish stress on the graft due to the simple length – tension relation of taking the knee into full extension or flexion, from stress due to the anterior shearing forces developed by either unloaded quadriceps contraction in the last 40 degrees or acceleration-deceleration motions (Figs. 15-18 and 15-19).[57] The former is usually addressed at surgery, with attempts at accurately plac-

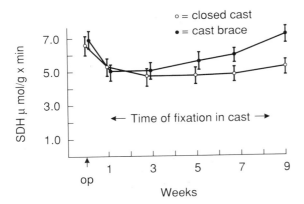

Fig. 15-17. Activity of the oxidative enzyme succinyl dehydrogenase (SDH) in vastus lateralis following cast brace versus cast immobilization after anterior cruciate ligament reconstruction. The patient with a cast brace returned to normal values faster. (From Eriksson,[47] with permission.)

Practice Point

RECONSTRUCTION PROTOCOL

1. Preoperative phase
2. Early rehabilitation phase
   a. Perioperative period (1–4 days)
   b. Early postoperative period (5–14 days)
   c. Protected motion period (2–6 weeks)
3. Intermediate rehabilitation phase (6–12 weeks)
4. Preparation for activity (12–24 weeks)
5. Return to activity
6. Late follow-up

---

ing the graft in the isometric position and ensuring unrestricted range of motion. The second feature, anterior shear, must be protected against for the first few months postoperatively. Thus there is the apparent paradox of allowing early full range of motion to stimulate a healthy joint and ensure an early functional arc of motion while restricting unloaded resisted extension movements in the last 40 or 30 degrees of motion. As is discussed later, axial loading and quadriceps-hamstring co-contraction minimize the adverse anterior shearing phenomenon, allowing a much more aggressive, yet safe, approach.[53,54]

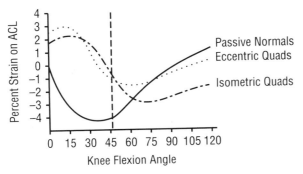

Fig. 15-18. Simulated eccentric and isometric quadriceps tests. Quadriceps activity significantly increases anterior cruciate ligament strain in the 0 to 45 degree range. (From Krakow and Vetter,[51] with permission.)

Hence if early motion and exercise are to be commenced, there are several important principles that must be followed while progressing to advanced stages of the rehabilitation process.

1. Early motion limits the adverse affects of surgery and immobilization of the joint surface, capsule, ligaments, muscle, and bone.
2. The reconstruction must be protected to some degree from single episodes of excessive loading or cyclic shearing stresses.
3. Active knee extension in the range 0 to 40 degrees, including straight-leg raising and unloaded knee extension in the terminal phases, may involve an undesirable anterior shearing force and translation of the tibia on the femur (Table 15-8).
4. Loading the tibiofemoral joint reduces the anterior translation from quadriceps shearing forces and hence permits functional quadriceps strengthening early in the program.
5. Exercise activities that allow valgus or varus and internal and external tibial rotation stresses should be avoided. A safe posture to assume when changing positions is to have the knees flexed to 60 to 90 degrees and the legs squeezed together.
6. *The progress of the rehabilitation phases is not based on rigid time limits.* Acquisition of muscle control and strength, adequate range of motion, absence of pain and swelling, balance, and confidence are key features in guiding the rate of progression.
7. Progression of weight-bearing requires adequate range of motion and control of muscles. The knee

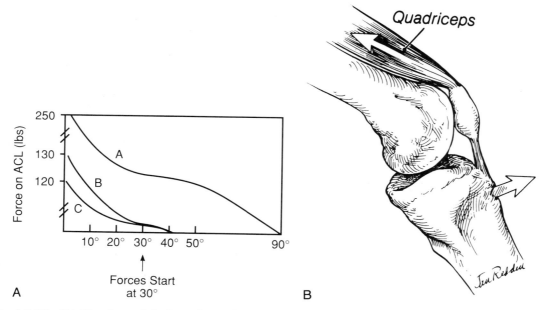

Fig. 15-19. **(A)** Classic straight leg raise with and without resistance throws undue stress on a recovering and revascularizing anterior cruciate ligament (ACL) reconstruction. Curve A = quadriceps force; curve B = ACL force, 7 lb on foot; curve C = ACL force, no weight on foot. **(B)** Similarly unweighted knee extension produce an undesirable anterior shear. (After Krakow and Vetter,[51] with permission.)

is aligned carefully over the foot in the stance phase. Crutches are initially used to allow a comfortable progression of weight-bearing and then to practice walking in a normal symmetric heel-toe fashion. Their use may be prolonged for safety reasons, such as uneven ground or slippery icy surfaces, walking long distances, or when the muscles are fatigued.

8. Intensive exercise every day is neither necessary nor desirable. A complete rest for 2 days each week allows recuperation and decreases the early tendency to effusion and tenderness.

Perioperative Period (1 to 4 Days)

The perioperative period is usually spent in hospital, although it is possible with the use of arthroscopically assisted techniques, adequate oral analgesics, and a protected environment to discharge the patient on the day of surgery. The more standard therapy is 1 to 4 days of hospital care. The emphasis during the perioperative period is on dealing with pain, making sure postoperative complications such as atelectasis, deep vein thrombosis, wound infection, hemorrhage,

wound dehiscence, and compartment syndrome either do not occur or are detected and treated promptly. It is imperative to gain early quadriceps control and quadriceps-hamstring co-contraction to protect the joint and allow early progression of weight-bearing. The brace is worn until this control is gained, with locks to prevent the last 15 degrees of extension. This limited extension is comfortable for the patient. The soft brace with side hinges usually allows about 10 degrees more than is set, so the patient has almost full extension.

Continuous passive motion and functional electrical stimulation are optional, and their value assumes less significance when an aggressive program of range of motion, weight-bearing, and early functional exercises are planned within the protocol. Pain, immobilization, and effusion are the three most potent stimuli to muscle wasting and reflex inhibition.[54–56] The amount of muscle wasting is minimized by restricting surgical exposure, particularly of the joint capsule and synovium, and reducing pain. The former is often aided by arthroscopically assisted techniques. Pain may be controlled by adequate analgesics, support, occasional aspiration of painful tense effusions, and

TABLE 15-8.   Maximum Isometric Concentration of Quadriceps and Hamstrings

Angle (degrees)	Maximum Extension Force (kg)	Maximum Shear Force (kg)	Maximum Compression Force (kg)
Quadriceps			
5	14.5 ± 2.5	12.2 ± 2.1	80.9 ± 14.1
15	21.3 ± 2.7	12.2 ± 1.5	131.4 ± 16.5
30	28.1 ± 2.8	7.3 ± 1.4	177.2 ± 17.5
45	33.5 ± 3.0	0.0 ± 1.6	228.1 ± 20.4
60	32.9 ± 2.7	-7.2 ± 1.5	235.4 ± 19.3
75	30.5 ± 2.9	$-214. \pm 2.0$	233.1 ± 22.1
90	28.2 ± 2.7	-36.5 ± 2.9	226.1 ± 21.8
Hamstrings			
5	14.1 ± 2.2	-7.3 ± 4.4	139.4 ± 2.1
15	12.3 ± 2.1	-28.7 ± 7.9	121.3 ± 2.0
30	12.1 ± 1.9	-42.8 ± 9.7	91.1 ± 1.5
45	11.5 ± 1.9	-55.7 ± 9.3	70.4 ± 1.4
60	11.1 ± 1.5	-62.3 ± 9.5	49.1 ± 1.6
75	9.9 ± 1.2	-74.0 ± 9.0	37.9 ± 1.5
90	7.1 ± 1.0	-80.1 ± 11.0	9.4 ± 1.0

Negative values are posterior shear; positive values are anterior shear.
(After Yasuda and Sasaki,[53] with permission.)

allowing range of motion and weight-bearing within the tolerance and comfort of the patient for a few days.[56] It is possible to further reduce wasting by leaving an indwelling catheter in the spinal canal with an epidural anesthesia system that may be maintained on the ward for the first 24 to 36 hours.[55] This measure, combined with continuous passive motion and electrical stimulation, is efficacious; but during a rehabilitation process that, in any event, takes several months, the significance of the epidural anesthesia protocol may be outweighed by its potential risks and the cost.

Practice Point

PERIOPERATIVE PHASE: GOALS

- Deal with pain
- Be alert to complications
- Gain muscle control
- Encourage partial weight-bearing

The brace may be removed while the patient is in bed or while the leg is supported if it is more comfortable. If there are no postoperative complications and the wound is healing well, the patient may be discharged with instructions for a home exercise pro-gram; the brace may be removed at night and for showering. Straight-leg raises are not performed during these early stages of rehabilitation because of the potential stresses on the graft by unloaded isolated quadriceps contraction. The patient is instructed to use either the sound leg or upper limbs to support the affected side when necessary (e.g., transferring out of or into bed). Furthermore, by internally or externally rotating the limb, the abductors or adductors of the hip assist in raising the limb.[57]

Early Postoperative Period (5 to 14 Days)

During the 2 weeks of the early postoperative period, wound healing progresses, and the emphasis is on active range of motion and gaining further quadriceps and hamstring control. Wall slides are an excellent method of passively increasing knee range of motion. The patient lies supine with the foot of the affected knee against the wall (Fig. 15-20). The leg is initially in extension and is allowed to slowly go into flexion. A towel is used to minimize friction. The sound leg may be used to provide support if there is insufficient muscle control to lower the leg slowly. Similarly, the sound leg may assist the return to extension. The idea is to eliminate most of the quadriceps activity. About 20 repetitions are performed, with an attempt to increase the range of flexion as the set progresses. This exercise should not be done in

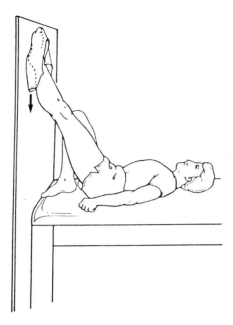

Fig. 15-20. Wall slides.

the presence of a tense effusion. Although progression of weight-bearing is encouraged, good alignment of the hip, knee, and foot are more important, with a symmetric pattern and good control while walking. Shifting of weight from one leg to the other is practiced. Exercises are begun for the hips using rubber tubing (sport cord) for resistance. Adduction work may have the added advantage of stimulating the vastus medialis and assisting patellar tracking. Undesirable shear on the knee during leg extension work is minimized by performing loaded (weight-bearing) exercises. Sitting calf raises and active isotonic hamstring work are initiated; and gentle, controlled, one-fourth or one-half squats are begun (Table 15-7). General cardiovascular work is best done with well-leg cycling.

With the over-the-top technique and solid screw and washer or staple fixation, there is little to fear from loss of continuity of the graft with bone. However, with a bone–patellar tendon–bone graft and the use of screw fixation in a bone tunnel, solid union may occur as early as 3 weeks and as late as 3 to 4 months. With this type of repair the fixation site may be the weakest link in resisting tensile forces, not the graft itself.[30] Thus the surgeon may elect slower initial progression and greater protection than outlined in this protocol. Techniques to improve bone fixation should allow earlier motion without compromising the fixation site.

Protected Motion Period (2 to 6 Weeks)

The emphasis during the next time period is to encourage active range of motion, progress functional loading, and protect the repair from sudden or repetitive undesirable shearing forces. The therapist and physician must still be alert to the evolution of postoperative complications, particularly infection and deep vein thrombosis.

Heel slides are used to encourage motion. They may be progressed by having the patient sit on a bench or mat with the back supported. A towel is placed under the involved foot to decrease friction and allow an easy sliding motion. The patient actively flexes the knee until it is possible to grasp the distal tibia and perform a gentle autoactive assisted movement. This progression on the wall slide allows less chance of the patient compensating for decreased knee range of motion by hip hiking.[57] Progression depends to a large extent on the resolution of pain and effusion. Hip work is up-graded, and cycling is begun with no resistance and within the comfortable range of motion (Figs. 15-21 and 15-22). Normally 110 to 115 degrees of flexion are necessary. Isometric hamstring work is a particularly important exercise at this stage, as knee flexion may be difficult owing to pain and therefore decreases the ability to

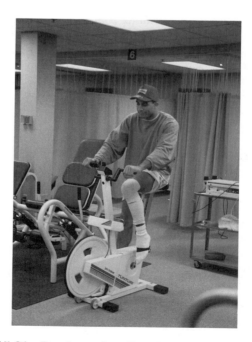

Fig. 15-21. One-legged cycling for a cardiovascular effect may be progressed to two-legged cycling when about 110 to 115 degrees of flexion are possible.

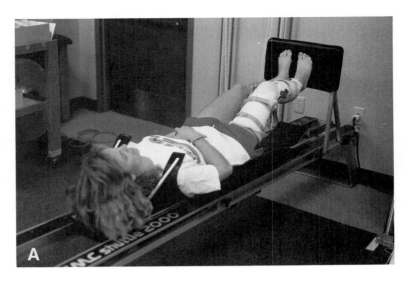

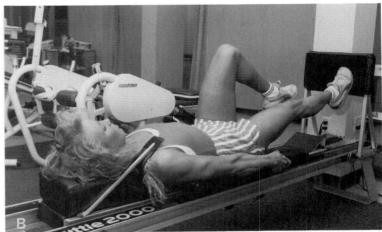

Fig. 15-22. (A) Initially the "shuttle" provides an excellent mechanism for early axial loading. **(B)** As soon as good quadriceps control is ensured the brace may be removed.

do isotonic work. If equipment is used for resisted isokinetic hamstring work, care must be taken to avoid undesirable shear when returning to the extended position. Machines that provide alternate concentric and eccentric work are best. Swimming using the flutter kick is encouraged for cardiovascular work. General strengthening and well-leg work for the crossover effect are stressed. Sport (rubber, surgical) tubing is the ideal light, portable exercise device for performing multiple loaded quadriceps exercises. Starting these early activities does not appear to increase joint effusion, hemarthrosis, or soft tissue swelling, which resolves to a great extent by about 14 to 20 days. Furthermore, there is little evidence that controlled early motion will stretch the ligamentous reconstruction.[58]

There is always a significant decrease in thigh cir-

cumference within the first few weeks after knee ligament reconstruction. It starts early and progresses despite any closely supervised rehabilitation program. Noyes et al. pointed out that it was related to the type of procedure, and that it may be that the degree of capsular and synovial disruption dictates the magnitude of this reflex atrophy within the initial few postoperative days.[58] Arthroscopically assisted reconstructions cause only about 25 to 38 percent of the loss of thigh girth that is found with open operative procedures. By the seventh postoperative day thigh girth is diminished about 4 cm on average for open techniques versus 1 cm for arthroscopic surgery. By 3 weeks after surgery the open-surgery patients have lost about 6.5 cm of thigh circumference compared to approximately 2.0 to 3.5 after arthroscopically assisted ligament repairs.[58]

The focus of this muscle atrophy is to some extent specific. For instance, the work of Spencer et al. showed that the threshold for reflex inhibition for vastus medialis to effusion alone is approximately 30 cm of fluid, whereas for rectus femoris and vastus lateralis it is 50 to 60 ml[59] (Fig. 15-23). It is apparent that traditional therapeutic regimens are ineffective in preventing this reflexively generated atrophy, although early motion and weight-bearing does minimize it to some degree.[60-63]

The emphasis on quadriceps rehabilitation is based on their preferential wasting after knee injury and specifically on the data that have shown that this initial atrophy tends to be maintained, even in chronic ACL-deficient knees.[64] However, isolated quadriceps contraction results in an increased strain on the ACL up to fivefold, particularly over the last 40 degrees before full extension (Fig. 15-22).[65] This point raises a dilemma when outlining the precise role of quadriceps exercises in ACL rehabilitation, particularly in situations where new reconstructions may be going through a period of relative weakening. It highlights the potential importance of the hamstrings as an ACL agonist possibly counteracting shearing forces and thus effecting strain reduction within the ligament. This forms the rationale for the application of hamstring co-activation as a potential rehabilitation modality.

One of the first reports demonstrating co-contraction by the agonist and antagonist muscles was by Sherington in 1909.[61] His data indicated that this agonist-antagonist co-activation originated from the motor cortex as a general command to perform a specific motion rather than isolated triggering of single muscles.[61] More recently DeLuca confirmed that agonist and antagonist are jointly contracted during performance of some specific tasks.[66] They named this phenomenon the "direct common drive", alluding to the fact that activation of the antagonist was simultaneous with the agonist and that control probably originated in the motor cortex. Additional sources of excitation of the antagonist muscles are afferent impulses generated via the muscle spindle. The muscle spindle, a stretch receptor, has powerful monosynaptic connections to the motor units of the muscle in which it resides.[65] As the knee extends, for example, muscle spindle receptors within the elongating hamstring become stretched and hence active, exciting the hamstring to mild co-contraction, opposing or controlling the extension movement.[49] Antagonist muscle is also sensitive to joint angle, to the force level developed by the agonist muscle, and to the orientation of the joint to the gravity vector.[67] Furthermore, electromyographic (EMG) recordings from quadriceps and hamstring muscles reveal that direct stress on the ACL has a moderate inhibitory effect on the quadriceps but simultaneously excites the hamstring.[67] In patients with ACL-deficient knees, similar recordings may be obtained in the loaded knee. This finding has led to the following conclusions.

1. A primary, quick-to-respond reflex arc from the mechanoreceptors in the ACL to the hamstring

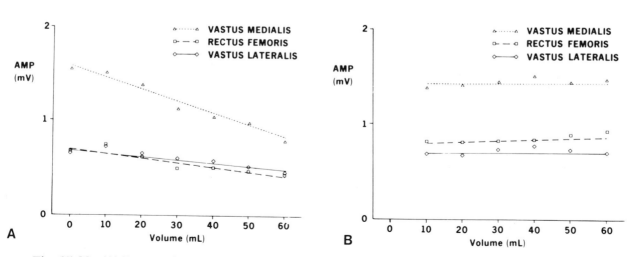

Fig. 15-23. **(A)** Intra-articular saline infusion reduces the quadriceps H-reflex amplitude. **(B)** It may be modified by an infusion of local anesthesia (lidocaine 1 percent). (After Spencer et al,[59] with permission.)

groups may exist and such a reflex arc may allow dynamic torque regulation on demand during ligament overloading.

2. A secondary reflex arc from mechanoreceptors in muscles and joint capsules exists that provides hamstring stimulation and activation in the presence of knee instability.

These facts lend support to the important dynamic role of the hamstring in both ACL-intact and ACL-deficient knees. The co-contraction effect combined with, and enhanced, by loaded knee exercises should provide sufficient attenuation of the potential anterior shearing action of the quadriceps contraction, thereby allowing early institution of weight-bearing and other specific axial-loaded knee exercises. Correct alignment during these early exercises is essential.

Practice Point

EARLY WEIGHT-BEARING

- Unloaded quadriceps work in the last 40 degrees of extension may produce an undesirable anterior shear.
- The hamstrings are able to counteract this tendency.
- Weight-bearing and axial-loaded exercises enhance hamstring co-contraction.
- Hamstring co-contraction is stimulated by stretch receptors in the muscle spindle and by capsular structures in the knee.
- Motion is controlled in patterns by the cortex.
- Early protected weight-bearing and axial-loaded knee extension are probably safe.

It is possible that progression during the first few weeks and the subsequent phase may be safely accelerated when an LAD is incorporated into the surgical repair. Indeed, this point may be the single most important advantage of these devices. Furthermore, consultation with the surgeon regarding the type and adequacy of fixation of the reconstructed ligament greatly influences the rate at which stresses may be applied to the knee. The duration of bracing and the timing of resisted or loaded work through a full range must be clarified.

Intermediate Rehabilitation (6 to 12 Weeks)

There has been some doubt as to the efficacy of quadriceps and hamstrings co-contraction in reducing the undesirable anterior shear. However, Yasuda and Sasaki have demonstrated in some elegant experiments that, at 5 degrees of knee flexion and with co-contraction, an anterior force of 15 percent of the tension of the quadriceps is exerted on the tibia[53] (Fig. 15-24) At about 7 to 10 degrees, this anterior shear becomes zero; and as the angle of flexion increases further, a posterior drawer is exerted on the tibia. Tension of the quadriceps or hamstrings during maximum simultaneous isometric contraction is 30 to 60 percent of that achieved during separated isometric contraction of each muscle. Thus if carefully taught and supervised, these co-contraction exercises could probably be safely introduced even earlier than during this intermediate phase.

Most of the athletes are able to fully weight-bear and have been weaned from the brace, except for isolated situations that particularly stress the knee (Fig. 15-25). If the knee is stiff, it is important to place greater emphasis on those exercises that promote knee extension. However, there is a distinct difference between treatments that encourage extension and those that irritate the joint and stress the surgical repair (Fig. 15-26). As weight-bearing is incorporated into power walking, maintenance of correct hip, knee, and foot alignment is essential. Hamstring strength and endurance feature strongly during this phase. As the resisted exercises gradually move into terminal extension, it is important not to exacerbate a synovitis. Short arc quadriceps exercises may be used, provided they are performed in such a way that hamstring co-contraction is ensured. If the patient is seated with the involved knee flexed and supported over a bolster to 45 degrees, each leg extension is preceded by hip extension that triggers the hamstring contraction.[57] The patient maintains this extension effort at the hip while holding the leg extension for about 10 seconds, followed by 5 seconds of relaxation. This exercise, like many of the specific drills are done in sets of 10 repetitions at this stage.

Toe raises are usually begun once the patient is fully weight-bearing comfortably. They may be done with surgical or rubber tubing or in the standing position, raising up onto the balls of the feet and slowly lowering. Usually sets of 20 repitions are used for this exercise.

Resisted tube walking, the step machine, reto-walking, running in the pool, and cycling stress endur-

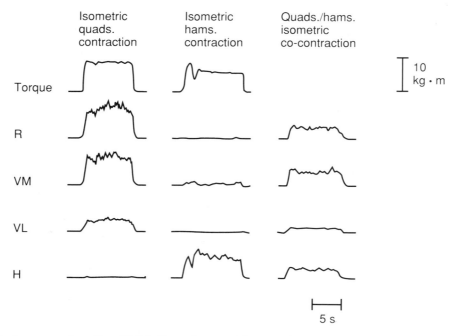

Fig. 15-24. Integrated surface EMGs from the quadriceps. Three conditions are illustrated: isometric quadriceps contraction, isometric hamstring contractions, and isometric co-contraction. The torque component is reduced with co-contraction. R = rectus femoris; VM = vastus medialis; VL = vastus lateralis; H = hamstrings. After Yasuda and Sasaki.[53]

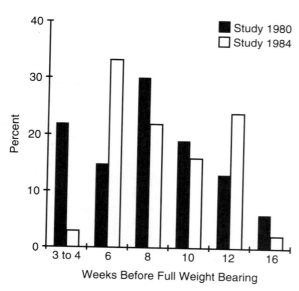

Fig. 15-25. Trend toward increasingly aggressive rehabilitation is illustrated by the earlier full weight-bearing permitted by the same group of surgeons surveyed in 1980 and 1984.

ance. Squats to 60 degrees with double legs, progressing to some single-leg squatting, utilize strong controlled eccentric and concentric weight-bearing quadriceps work. This exercise can be dangerous, and immaculate alignment and control are mandatory. Running on a minitrampoline is a good progression for endurance and balance (Fig. 15-27). For many individuals the therapist can set up a detailed pro-

---

Practice Point

INTERMEDIATE REHABILITATION PHASE (6 to 12 WEEKS)

- Encourage extension
- Emphasize hamstring co-contraction
- Only loaded knee extension 0 to 30 degrees
- Commence balance work
- Progress weight-bearing activities
- Power walking
- Intense, nonresisted cycling
- Water-running

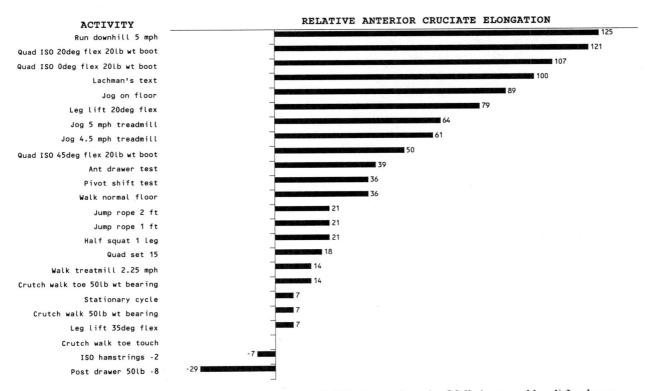

ACTIVITY — **RELATIVE ANTERIOR CRUCIATE ELONGATION**

Activity	Value
Run downhill 5 mph	125
Quad ISO 20deg flex 20lb wt boot	121
Quad ISO 0deg flex 20lb wt boot	107
Lachman's text	100
Jog on floor	89
Leg lift 20deg flex	79
Jog 5 mph treadmill	64
Jog 4.5 mph treadmill	61
Quad ISO 45deg flex 20lb wt boot	50
Ant drawer test	39
Pivot shift test	36
Walk normal floor	36
Jump rope 2 ft	21
Jump rope 1 ft	21
Half squat 1 leg	21
Quad set 15	18
Walk treatmill 2.25 mph	14
Crutch walk toe 50lb wt bearing	14
Stationary cycle	7
Crutch walk 50lb wt bearing	7
Leg lift 35deg flex	7
Crutch walk toe touch	
ISO hamstrings -2	-7
Post drawer 50lb -8	-29

Fig. 15-26. Relative anterior cruciate ligament (ACL) elongation. An 80-lb (external load) Lachman test equals 110 units of ACL anteromedial fiber elongation. All other values are illustrated relative to this figure.

gram the patient may practice at home or in the local gymnasium. Adequate rest is also part of this phase, and a 2-day break should be built into each week. Progression to the next phase depends on achieving the necessary criteria, which include nearly a full range of motion, good quadriceps and hamstring control, satisfactory single leg balance, and the ability to power walk, maintain satisfactory alignment, and perform intense nonresisted cycling. The effusion should be resolving, and pain should be absent, although there may be mild discomfort with some activities.

Preparation for Activity (12 to 24 Weeks)

The objectives during the phase at 12 to 24 weeks is to progress strength and balance to the point that the athlete is ready to reintegrate into activity and commence sport-specific training. The rate of progression depends on attaining functional control of the quadriceps and hamstrings through a nearly normal range of motion and the ability to increase resistance and speed without producing a synovitis.[68-70]

The presence of tension and mechanoreceptors in the synovium, capsule, menisci, and cruciates was emphasized by Kennedy et al.[71] They further emphasized the possible role of injury to these structures in regard to functional instability in what he called the "neurogenic contribution" (Fig. 15-28). This altered proprioceptive feedback was measured and quantified by recording the treshold value for detection of passive motion. In normal knees there is less than 2 percent variation in the threshold values between the two sides. In ACL-deficient knees there may be a variation of more than 25 percent between the injured and normal knees.[71] *There should be a particular emphasis on proprioception* through multiple balance exercises (Fig. 15-29). During the first half of this period there is considerable revascularization activity of the graft, with associated weakness and plasticity; hence unloaded resistance in the range 0 to 45 degrees is stillminimized. Although the earlier phases of rehabilitation emphasized hamstring work, it is of the utmost importance at this stage to correct any existing quadriceps deficits. In most studies the quadriceps muscle mass is more sensitive to knee pathology,

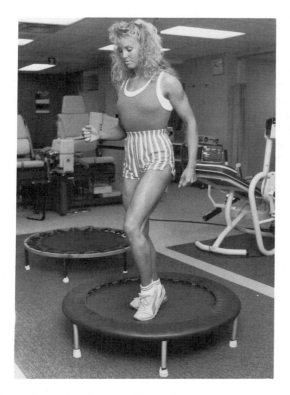

Fig. 15-27. Minitrampoline allows reduced impact while providing a good endurance and balance exercise.

specifically ACL deficiency, than are the hamstrings.[54,71] Hence progressive increased quadriceps work aimed at both eccentric and concentric contraction are pursued until adequate torque profiles are achieved. (Figs. 15-30 and 15-31).

Hip strengthening, water-running, swimming, and cycling are progressed at will. Running in the pool is increased in intensity, and jogging may be attempted either on a treadmill or a level terrain. It is important that the athlete feels confident in the ability to run. There should be no competition between patients at this stage of their rehabilitation, and they should be progressed according to their own parameters of recovery of strength, range, and control. Skipping is an excellent method of developing endurance and progressing weight-bearing in a controlled, dynamic fashion. It stimulates rebounding and push-off.

During this phase of rehabilitation, one must consider the resumption of running activities (Fig. 15-32). There is a large discrepancy among experts as to when it is advisable; about one-fifth of knee experts allow running at 2 months, whereas 50 percent prefer to wait until 6 months. The mean value is about 4.7 months. While the forces involved, even with jogging, are multiples of body weight, anterior sheer may be maintained. However, no sudden starts and stops should be allowed at this stage.

If running is attempted, good style and alignment are more important than speed and distance. Usually the first run should be restricted to about one-fourth to one-half mile to establish the reaction of the joint. Distance is built up at one-fourth mile at a time every two or three sessions so long as no deleterious reactions occur.[70]

Special emphasis should also be placed on the endurance component. The principle of specificity of training is important. Costill et al., in a study of patients after knee surgery, showed that although patients were able to restore their quadriceps power by

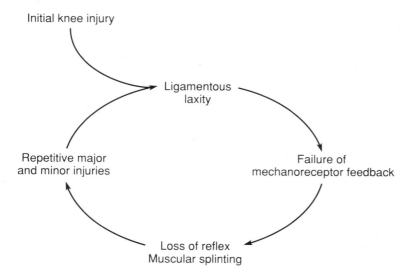

Fig. 15-28. Neurogenic contribution to progressive knee instability as hypothesized by Kennedy et al.[71]

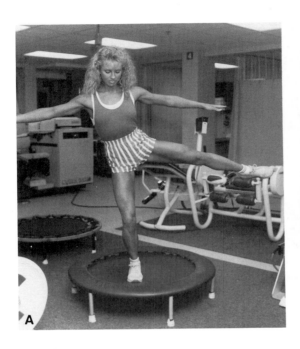

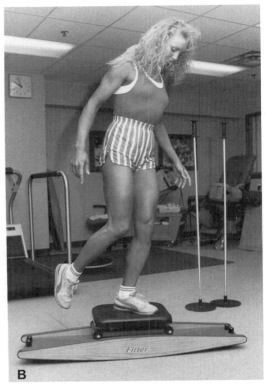

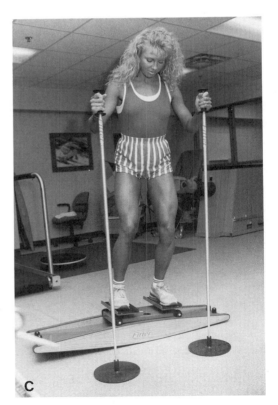

Fig. 15-29. Balance exercises to enhance proprioception and strength on the minitrampoline (**A**) and using a profitter (**B&C**).

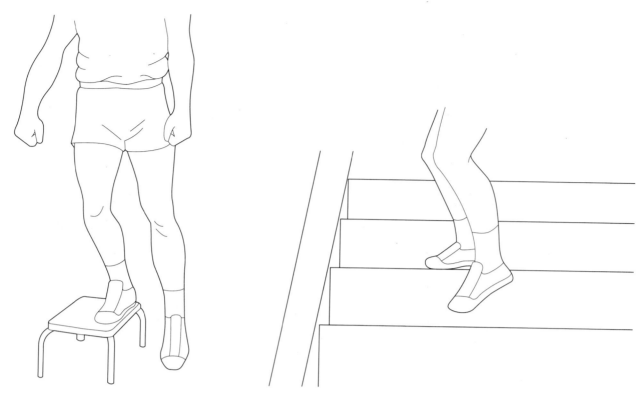

Fig. 15-30. Lateral step-ups. The height and number of steps are progressed as tolerated.

Practice Point

RUNNING PROGRESSION

1. Should be able to power walk without synovitis flaring up.
2. Commence jogging on flat terrain.
3. Initially alternate with pool running and power walking.
4. Control distance and intensity.
5. Make sure good style is maintained.
6. Introduce deceleration last.
7. When comfortable in straight runs, add the following.
   — Figure-of-eights
   — Planting and changing directions
   — Shuttle runs
   — Running backward

---

6 weeks after surgery using a knee extension table, when they were tested for endurance on a leg press machine with rapid repetition work they were still 20 percent weaker on the operated leg (Fig. 15-33).[48] This work shows that although the patients were able to normalize knee extension strength through weight training their ability to generate maximum tension during the more complex task of leg press was far from restored. This finding suggests that patients should be trained doing a variety of activities, and the rehabilitation should ultimately include exercises that require tension development throughout the range of motion.

It should be recalled that there is selective atrophy of endurance fibers (Fig. 15-34); which are referred to as type I, or oxidative, fibers (also called slow twitch or red fibers). These fibers are resistant to fatigue and develop small tension at a slow rate. They have a large Ia afferent input with a built-in bias for early recruitment. They have also been referred to as postural fibers. Costill et al.'s work illustrates the inability to

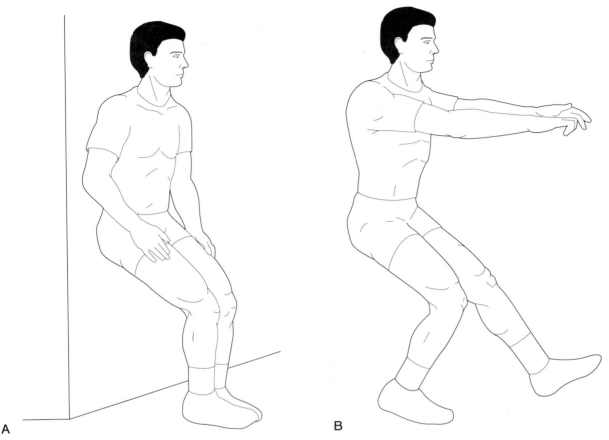

A   B

Fig. 15-31. (A) Wallsliding. **(B)** Single-legged one-fourth knee bends. There is usually automatic co-contraction of the hamstrings and quadriceps. It is imperative that this exercise is done with perfect alignment and control. Initiative and caution should be used when prescribing these exercises.

influence this type of fiber with low repetition/high resistance work. Succinyl dehydrogenase activity, which represents type I fiber activity, is reduced by 26 to 42 percent with cast immobilization; and even after 6 weeks of strength training, retesting for this enzyme reveals low values. However, when high repetition work in the form of cycling is added to the program, it can be seen that there is a rapid recovery of the endurance potential. High repetition work, then, is essential in order to hypertrophy these type I fibers (Fig. 15-33).

If athletes are mainly working on their own, it is essential that they receive adequate, specific instructions. Carefully planned review visits are used to assess the reaction of the joint and ensure safe progression.

Return to Activity (Final Rehabilitation: 6+ Months)

At the end of 6 months it is time to progress the running activities. Patients should now have good muscle control, have full or nearly full active range of motion at the knee, be able to power or fast walk without or with a barely perceptible limp, and have confidence in their ability to run. Distance is build up independently of speed. Attention to good running style is important. If there are no adverse signs, acceleration and speed are progressed. The figure-of-eight circuit and sport special drills gently introduce turning and deceleration components (Figs. 15-35 and 15-36).

At approximately 6 months it is probably safe for

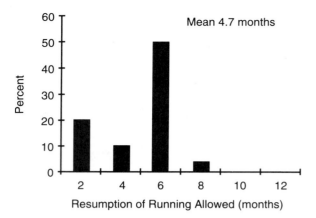

Fig. 15-32. Approximately 50 percent of surgeons surveyed allow resumption of running activities at 6 months after anteior cruciate ligament reconstruction. (Data from Paulos and Noyes.[45])

an all-out effort to establish some baseline of strength and endurance from both the concentric and eccentric points of view. Each clinic should develop its own set of normals, and it must be noted that the results of testing on one of the many computerized testing devices are not necessarily the same on others. Some figures are given in Table 15-9[72] as a rough guide.

Consideration of a custom-made orthosis is important at this time. For individuals who have previously worn a knee brace, some modifications of the original

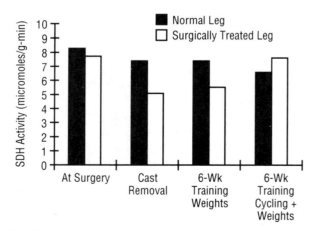

Fig. 15-33. Succinyl dehydrogenase (SDH) activity in the vastus lateralis muscle of the surgically treated and untreated legs of the men who weight trained only and those who did some endurance work (cycling) as well. (Data from Costill et al.[48])

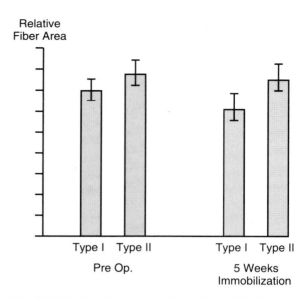

Fig. 15-34. Relative area of type I and II fibers immediately before and 5 weeks after anterior cruciate ligament reconstruction. Atrophy is largely restricted to type I fibers (means and SD). (Data from Eriksson.[47])

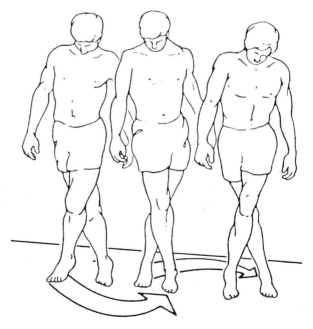

Fig. 15-35. Carioca crossover drills produce increasing torque.

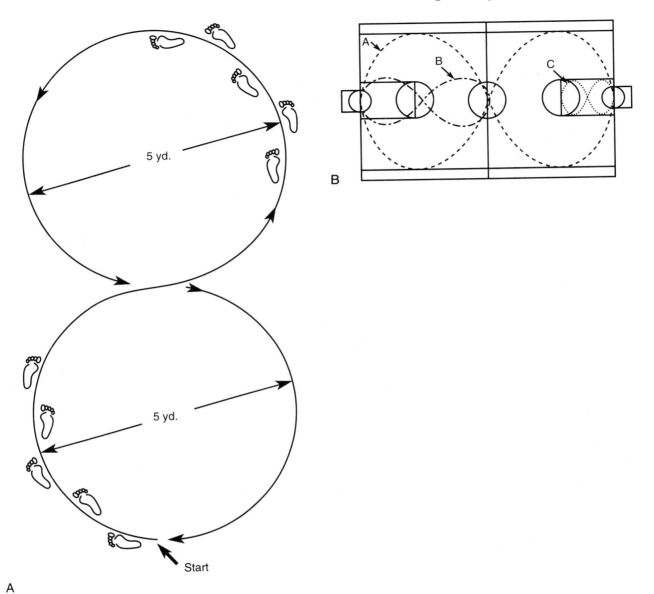

A

Fig. 15-36. (A) Figure-of-eight running allows excellent controlled progression by either (i) jogging or sprinting, (ii) sprinting on straight section versus curves, or (iii) changing the size of the "eight." **(B)** Drill is made sport-specific by fitting the patterns to the specific playing surface, in this case a basketball court. A, B, and C show shorter and narrow patterns.

brace may allow a reasonable fit. For others who have dramatic wasting or change in thigh contour, or for athletes who have not worn a brace, usually the size of the leg has stabilized sufficiently to make construction of a custom-made orthosis cost-effective. The need for such a brace depends on the activity goals of the athlete and the stability of the knee.

Circuits and wind sprints are valuable particularly because of their emphasis on endurance. The adage that the athlete goes as far as his good leg can take him should be remembered. It is difficult to accurately assess the progress of the patient without good testing facilities. The work of Young with ultrasound and that of Ericksson with CT scanning have indicated

TABLE 15-9. **Concentric and Eccentric Peak Torque with Hamstring-Quadriceps Ratios**

Patient Group	Concentric Peak Torque		Eccentric Peak Torque		Concentric Ratio	Eccentric Ratio
	Hamstrings	Quadriceps	Hamstrings	Quadriceps		
Males aged 15–24	1.21 (0.24)	2.98 (0.57)	1.44 (0.33)	3.09 (0.88)	0.42 (0.10)	0.49 (0.12)
Males aged 25–34	1.08 (0.28)	2.49 (0.66)	1.37 (0.32)	2.67 (0.82)	0.45 (0.11)	0.55 (0.19)
Males All	1.16 (0.26)	2.76 (0.66)	1.40 (0.33)	2.88 (0.86)	0.43 (0.10)	0.51 (0.15)
Females aged 15–24	0.87 (0.16)	2.19 (0.51)	1.06 (0.26)	2.37 (0.90)	0.41 (0.08)	0.49 (0.16)
Females aged 25–34	0.85 (0.18)	1.98 (0.49)	1.11 (0.28)	2.36 (0.77)	0.44 (0.08)	0.49 (0.12)
Females All	0.85 (0.17)	2.12 (0.51)	1.06 (0.26)	2.36 (0.85)	0.42 (0.08)	0.49 (0.14)

All values are newton meters per kilogram of body weight (mean and SD, in parentheses).
(Data from KinCom [Kinetic-Communicator].[72])

that a simple tape measure and recordings of thigh girth are poor indicators of muscle ability and strength.[55,56] Indeed, much of what we measure of a rapidly hypertrophied muscle may be the noncontractile connective tissue or neural control (Fig. 15-37).

Although some individuals show good muscle bulk and almost equal strength betwen the two sides, integrated electromyographic (EMG) studies have shown that often the vastus medialis has not kept up with the hypertrophy of the rest of the quadriceps muscles. During this period of time, it may be worthwhile adding a period of electrical stimulation, with an emphasis on biofeedback techniques for vastus medialis control.

A careful examination of range is important; and although flexion contraction of up to 5 degrees more than the normal side may be acceptable and compatible with excellent functional results, excessive loss of range generally produces symptoms and inhibits full return to activity (Fig. 15-38). A decision must be made as to whether adequate range may be achieved by rehabilitation techniques or whether manipulation or arthroscopic surgery is indicated.[73] CT scans and, when available, MRI are particularly valuable for assessing the potential cause of the loss of range and which structures may need either resection or debulking.

The rehabilitation techniques for the stiff area should promote range of motion without causing a reactive synovitis. Adequate preconditioning, e.g., hot packs or high speed light resistance cycling, is important. This phase may be followed by prolonged stretching techniques and mobilization of the patella and tibia, particularly into external rotation.[74] Hamstring and calf muscle stretching is emphasized. Walking on the heels and striding backward promote extension. Active and resisted exercise and electrical

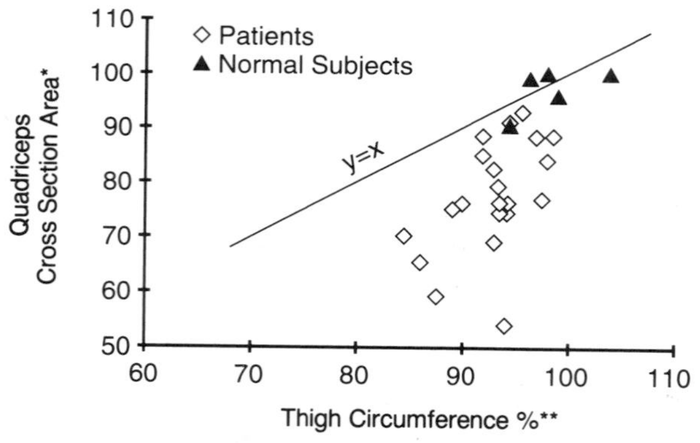

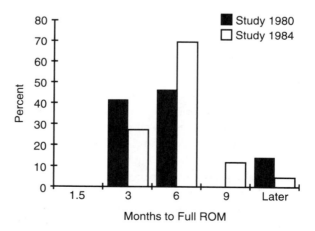

Fig. 15-37. Injured/uninjured limb ratio for quadriceps cross-sectional area plotted against the equivalent ratio for thigh circumference squared. *, Quadriceps cross-sectional area = injured/uninjured percent; **, thigh circumference² = injured/uninjured percent. (Data from Young et al.[56])

Fig. 15-38. With more aggressive rehabilitation techniques, full range of motion is anticipated by about 14 to 20 weeks in most patients. (Data from Paulos and Noyes.[45])

stimulation supplementation of terminal extension over a roll are important techniques. There is a limited, but sometimes effective, role for the application of a specially modified cylinder cast to gain the remaining knee extension down to −5 degrees. This cast is applied in the maximum extension allowed; the anterior portion is cut out to allow further extension, and sequential wedges of felt are placed in the back of the cast. The cast passively and slowly stretches out some of the remaining flexion contracture[72-74] (Fig. 15-39).

In some instances postsurgical knee stiffness can be progressive and constitute a considerable treatment dilemma. This problem is described more fully in the section on the infrapatellar contraction syndrome.

During this period of final rehabilitation it is essential to distinguish the functional elements from the specific activity goals (Table 15-10). The former may then be tentatively and safely progressed under ideal situations before the athlete is allowed to return to unsupervised full training and competition. The functional drills include hopping, figure-of-eights, shuttle run, back-peddling, single-leg squats, carioca, stair-running, lunges, and kicking (Fig. 15-36, 15-37, 15-40). Deceleration with pivoting and direction change is particularly difficult to control and is introduced cautiously.[47,70] Similarly, running on uneven terrain, running fast downhill, and running downstairs are activities that require considerable control.

At the end of rehabilitation there should be a gradual resumption of competitive sports, and most individuals should be warned that they must still wear the knee brace. Even at 9 months the strength of an unaugmented cruciate ligament substitution/or repair may still be only 60 to 70 percent of its ultimate strength. Educating the patient on the basics of knee mechanics and function are important, as a lifelong exercise program should be established. For many competitive athletes, the best advice at this time might

be to consider giving up contact sports. Participation in pivoting sports may also have to be modified. Indeed, superficial surveys report a high percentage of return to activity with ACL injury whatever the treatment regimen. However, more specific studies show that the greater the degree of cutting and pivoting, the more likely it is that athletes will modify their participation[75] (Fig. 15-41).

Some athletes become depressed at this point and believe that they are falling behind schedule. It is important to encourage them and to let them know that the average time to return to full activity following this type of surgery is approximately 9.5 months and that as many as one-fifth of such patients do not return to full activity until 1 year or more (Fig. 15-42).

An honest, thorough assessment of the knee is in order at this time so that realistic goals may be set. Often, even with the best repairs, there is some laxity compared to the good knee. Dynamic supports are of permanent importance in stabilizing this type of knee during activities. It is well to remember that if the ligament's protective reflexes are to be initiated solely by pain, no tendon stretch reflex could act in time to protect the ligament complex. This point has been illustrated by Pope et al., who noted that ligament rupture occurs at about 73 milliseconds but a sustained protective contraction may not be developed until about 330 milliseconds (Fig. 15-43).[75,76] Of course the application of loading may be slightly slower in many sports, but it is not slow enough always to allow time for reflex protection. In this regard, visual clues are important so that sufficient time is given to enhance for muscular protection. One must also consider the work on articular mechanoreceptors. The kinesthetic sense or feedback may be inadequate from the knee after rupture of the cruciate ligaments and may not fully redevelop with repair.[76] This problem would further impede thigh protective reflexes and thus leave the individual more suscepti-

Fig. 15-39. Dropout cast (MacIntosh). With control of the upper thigh, the tibia can be wedged into extension by placing pads below the ankle and above the patella. Extension is more easily achieved with a low force over a long period of time. Undue pressure must be avoided, and the technique requires meticulous attention. (From Highgenboten et al,[72] with permission.)

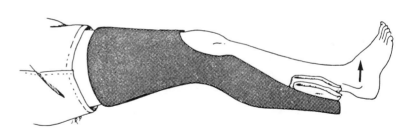

TABLE 15-10.   Summary of Eight Epidemiologic Studies Using Prophylactic Knee Braces

Reference	Subjects	Type of Knee Brace	Outcome
Anderson et al.[81]	Nine professional players with knee injuries	Anderson Knee Stabler	Subjects played nine games over two seasons without reinjury to the knee
Grace et al.[96]	Albuquerque and Santa Fe high school players: 250 nonbraced; 83 double-hinged brace		Knee injury rates: Nonbraced 4% Single-hinged braces 15% Double-hinged braces 6%
Hansen et al.[99]	University of South California (1980–1984); 329 nonbraced; 148 braced	Anderson Knee Stabler	Injury rate for nonbraced players: 11% Injury rate for braced players: 5%
Hewson et al.[95]	University of Arizona: exposures to injury: nonbraced (1977–1981) = 28,191; braced (1983–1984) = 29,293	Anderson Knee Stabler	No statistical difference in MCL injuries between nonbraced and braced periods
Rovere et al.[100]	Wake Forest University: nonbraced (1981–1982); braced (1983–1984)	Anderson Knee Stabler	Knee injuries: 16.1/100 players during nonbraced period; 7.5/100 players during braced period
Schriner[101]	High school players (n = 1,246) from 25 schools in Michigan	Don Joy, Cutter, Anderson Omni, McDavid Knee Stabilizer	Injuries from lateral blows: 45 in nonbraced group; 0 in braced group
Taft et al.[93]	University of North Carolina: nonbraced (1980–1982); braced (1983–1985)		No statistical difference in MCL, ACL, or meniscal injuries between nonbraced and braced periods
Teitz et al.[98]	NCAA Division I: 6307 players in 1984 (71 schools); 5,445 players in 1985 (61 schools)	Many	In 1984: 6.0% knee injury rate for nonbraced players vs. 11.0% for braced players In 1985: 6.4% knee injury rate for nonbraced players vs. 9.4% for braced players There were significantly more MCL injuries among braced players than among nonbraced players
Jackson et al.[103]	Professional football players 12 seasons (1977–1988)	McDavid, De Puy, Anderson Omni	Risk per 1,000 exposures: 25 in nonbraced group; 16 in braced group Reduced severity of MCL injuries ACL injuries unaffected

(After Montgomery and Koziris,[88] with permission.)

ble to reinjury.[75] However, because the reinjury rate is relatively low, other factors must be involved, which include the use of visual clues, status of muscle contraction, shoe and boot slippage, degree of knee flexion, the spread of impact over time and space, and the sliding or falling of the athlete.

Summary of the Rehabilitation Program

The protocol outlined above is a relatively aggressive approach, with early motion, early weight-bearing, moderate protection with a knee orthosis, rapid progression of resisted work under conditions of

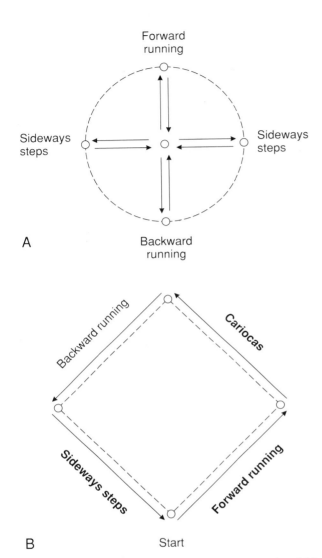

Forward
running

Sideways
steps

Sideways
steps

A

Backward
running

Backward running

Cariocas

Sideways steps

Forward running

B   Start

Fig. 15-40. Agility and strength elements should be combined into sport-specific drills using composite circuits. One could incorporate jumping activities at each corner of the circuit (not shown). The size of the circle (**A**) and the box (**B**) are adjusted to the stage of rehabilitation and requirements of the sport.

loading, and some protection from unloaded shear during the last 30 to 40 degrees of extension. There is an early emphasis on range of motion and hamstring strengthening. Later emphasis is on retraining proprioception and endurance. Final rehabilitation draws heavily on activity-specific, simulated functional training to prepare the athlete safely for rein-

tegration to full training. Education, maintenance programs, and orthoses are part of the long-term care. In some circumstances a more cautious approach is warranted. In other circumstances, particularly if graft fixation is secure and graft material is adequate or reinforced with an LAD, the program may be accelerated.

Time lines are not as essential as appreciation of the scientific and technical framework from which a logical rationale of progression may be made. The markers for safe progression and the ultimate goals must be clearly understood and appreciated by the surgeon, therapist, and patient. Within any one series of patients, some individuals require specific adjustments because of special intraoperative observations and events. The protocol need not be rigidly adhered to, and all progressions are based on muscle control and joint condition as evidenced by minimal inflammation, pain, and effusion.

In the enthusiasm for activity and progress, the pivotal role of adequate rest and recuperation must not be overlooked. The knee must be coaxed, not beaten: The "carrot is better than the stick." Long-term, progressive rehabilitation, emphasizing increased quadriceps and hamstring strength enhances the ability to successfully return to the sport. However, athletes participating in activities that involve cutting and twisting motions may be less successful in returning to preinjury levels of competition.

Knee Stiffness and the Infrapatellar Contracture Syndrome

Knee stiffness is an occasional sequel to trauma, immobilization, or infection. Payr outlined a series of changes that accompany stiffness.[77] They include adhesions of the suprapatellar pouch, quadriceps contracture, retraction of the alar folds of the patella, and then patellofemoral adhesions. Ultmately, there may be a fixed patella with progressive articular cartilage distruction secondary to invasion of fibrosclerotic pannus.[77,78] More recently, Sprague et al. classified knees with stiffness according to the arthroscopic findings: (1) those with discrete bands of adhesions traversing the suprapatellar pouch; (2) those in which there is complete obliteration of the pouch and peripatellar gutters; and (3) those with additional extracapsular bands of tissue from the proximal patella to the anterior femur.[79] The latter patients are rarely helped by simple arthroscopic débridement.

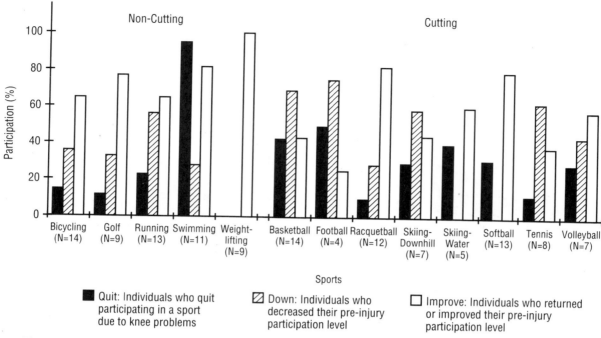

Fig. 15-41. **(A)** Percent of participants returning to noncutting and nonpivoting sports versus **(B)** those returning to highly demanding activities.

Furthermore, there is a special subgroup of patients who present with loss of range and pain, mainly secondary to entrapment and involvement of the infrapatellar structures. These patients have been classified as having the infrapatellar contracture syndrome (IPCS).[78] This syndrome may occur as primary involvement of the fat pad or secondary to prolonged immobility or nonisometric ligament repairs. Intraarticular cruciate surgery, combined with immobility due to casting, quadriceps inhibition, purposeful lack of extension exercises, an excessively anteriorly placed ACL graft or a nonisometric graft with too much tension, preventing any anterior glide of the tibia in extension, are the probable precipitating factors.[77,78]

Although as many as 5 percent of patients have an abnormal fibrosclerotic response following knee surgery, few go on to develop the full-blown IPCS. It is helpful to consider a continuum of pathology that may resolve or progress depending on the tissue response of the patient, early recognition by the physician or therapist, and adequacy of treatment. The sequence of events are outlined below.

Prodromal Stage

Nearly every patient undergoing knee surgery or sustaining a knee injury enters the prodromal stage of IPCS as a normal consequence of healing. Patients who are likely to develop IPCS should be recognized

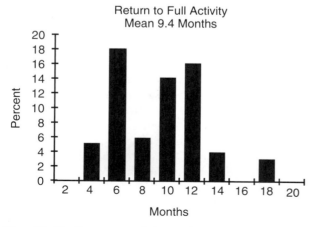

Fig. 15-42. Return to full activity is rare before 4 months; the mean in this survey was 9.4 months.

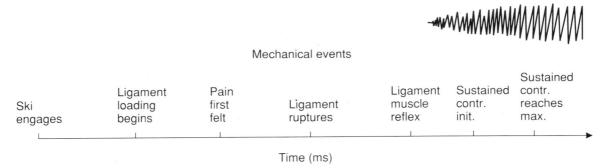

Fig. 15-43. In Pope's study, high speed application of stress causes anatomic damage before reflexes can generate enough dynamic protection. Only precontraction due to anticipation or awareness via visual clues allows full use of muscle protection against ligament injury.

at the prodromal stage, usually within 2 to 8 weeks of their surgery or injury. Periarticular inflammation and swelling combined with immobility and quadriceps weakness are common. Such patients also fail to progress during rehabilitation, are unable to gain extension, and exhibit abnormal pain and swelling.[77] Diffuse edema is present throughout the periarticular tissues, particularly in the area of the patellar tendon and fat pad. Tenderness is noted about the patellar tendon, and active motion is painful. A quadriceps lag indicates that the passive range of motion is greater than the active range. Patellar glide tests usually show decreased patellar excursion; patellar tilt is restricted, though not rigid.

Active Stage

Patients evolve to the active stage within 6 to 20 weeks of surgery. These patients may have already had manipulations or surgery that exacerbated instead of relieved their problem. Fat pad induration and patellar tendon rigidity are present. Obvious exra-articular involvement is noted. There is a severe decrease in patellar mobility in all directions, with a zero or negative patellar tilt test. A quadriceps lag is no longer present, as both active and passive knee extension and flexion are restricted.

Significant quadriceps atrophy is apparent, with patellofemoral crepitation on tracking tests. Voluntary contraction of the quadriceps fails to move the

---

Quick Facts

INFRAPATELLAR CONTRACTURE SYNDROME

Prodromal Stage

- Periarticular inflammation
- Periarticular swelling
- Quadriceps lag
- Inability to gain full extension
- Excessive pain
- Early loss of patellar motion

Active Stage

- Significantly decreased patellar mobility
- Patellar tendon rigidity
- Active and passive knee motion restricted
- Quadriceps atrophy
- Patellofemoral crepitus
- Flexion contracture gives "short leg" gait

Residual Stage

- Possibly some retained patellar mobility
- Patellofemoral crepitus
- Decreased patellofemoral joint space
- Sometimes patella infera
- Quadriceps atrophy and weakness
- Restricted flexion and extension

patella proximally. The patient demonstrates a bent knee or "short leg" gait.

Residual Stage

Patients in the residual stage generally present 8 months to several years after the onset of IPCS. Depending on the time from the onset of the syndrome, the physical findings may reveal more supple peripatellar and retinacular tissues, with some residual fat pad hypertrophy. Medial and lateral patellar glides are restricted, but not as severely as during the active stage. Significant patellofemoral arthrosis is heralded by pain and crepitus, and a decreased joint space is seen on the skyline roentgenogram. Developmental patella infera is common. Continued quadriceps atrophy and weakness are present, with restricted flexion and extension. If enough time has elapsed, many of the signs indicative of IPCS may disappear. Residual patella infera and patellofemoral arthrosis may be the only remaining symptoms.

Treatment Recommendations

Early diagnosis occasionally permits arthroscopic treatment of the syndrome. However, in advanced cases with both intra-articular and extra-articular involvement open débridement is usually necessary. Failure to recognize the extra-articular component in these cases generally necessitates repeat surgery to achieve greater motion. Early recognition and aggressive rehabilitation using early motion and muscle stimulation is, therefore, the key to prevention. Patellar mobilization techniques should be used by the therapist and taught to the patient. Anti-inflammatory medications may also prove helpful. Patients with a tendency to lateral patellar compression, patella infera, and poor pain tolerance are at risk for developing the syndrome and should be identified early and treated vigorously. Analgesics and TENS units are useful early in the recovery phases. Most patients with prodromal signs of IPCS will generally respond to this program.

If patellar mobility and knee extension are not achieved quickly, a "drop-out cast" or extension board should be considered to help achieve extension (Fig. 15-39). However, caution must be exercised when using such forceful extension measures as dropout casts, anesthetic manipulations, desubluxation hinges or traction, since precipitation and acceleration of chondral lesions may occur. Therefore, these techniques should be applied early and only

briefly (3 to 5 days) and, if unsuccessful, discontinued until *after* surgery, when they may be tried again if necessary. Quadriceps strengthening is also central to success. If extension is achieved without associated increased quadriceps strength, flexion deformity frequently recurs. Therefore it is imperative to ensure that good voluntary quadriceps contraction exists, with little or no quadriceps lag, prior to using extension drop-out casts, traction, or surgery.[79] Neuromuscular stimulators and biofeedback have proved valuable in this regard.

Approximately 5 percent of patients go on to the active stage of IPCS. Patients with stage II (active) IPCS, generally require surgery. Continued manual manipulation, forced passive motion, or traction should be avoided, as any maneuvers causing recurrent inflammation and pain only increase the severity of the disease process at this stage. The timing of surgery is critical; delays for months may be necessary to reduce inflammation and increase quadriceps strength. Patients in stage II generally have restricted extension and flexion. Attempts at mobilizing the knee usually prove futile, and it is better to work on muscle strength through the range of motion present. Also, when both flexion and extension contractures exist, it is preferable to "divide and conquer" than to attempt to correct both simultaneously. Achieving extension as soon as possible should be the priority.

Surgery for stage II IPCS usually includes both intra-articular and extra-articular débridement and release. Arthroscopy is of little help. Lateral arthroscopy should include lateral retinacular release (excluding the vastus lateralis tendon) along with débridement of hypertrophied and dysplastic fat pad tissues and the lateral patellomeniscal ligament. A limited medial arthrotomy to further débride the fat pad and exercise the medial patellomeniscal ligament is usually necessary. Attention must be paid to the fat pad attachments near the anterior horns of the medial and lateral menisci and the intercondylar extensions to the notch. If an ACL repair or reconstruction has been performed, attention must also be paid to the ligament in relation to the femur, tibia, and intercondylar notch. Nonisometric placement of the ligament necessitates removal. At the time of arthrotomy, normal patellar mobility must be restored, with passive patellar tilt exceeding 45 degrees; peripatellar tendon adhesions, as well as suprapatellar adhesions, must be released. One must also be prepared to advance the tibial tubercle proximally if patella infera is present. All incisions and portals must be meticulously closed and prophylactic antibiotics used. Nonsteroidal anti-inflammatory drugs (NSAIDs) should be given for an extended postoperative period, and if steroids are used, they should not be prescribed until all wounds have sealed (2 to 3 days). Continuous passive motion, particularly beneficial early during the postoperative recovery stages, can be combined with epidural morphine injections to aid pain control. Postoperative use of a drop-out cast, particularly at night, is usually necessary for a brief period.

Postoperatively, physical therapy is required on a daily basis. Nighttime extension splints are encouraged until active extension is demonstrated by the patient. Although it is desirable to preserve the knee flexion obtained at the time of surgery, it is far more important that knee extension be maintained; a loss of flexion can usually be rectified later with arthroscopy and manipulation. On occasion, it is necessary to include experienced psychological support because of the prolonged associated morbidity with IPCS.

Patients presenting with stage III ("burned out") IPCS have usually had multiple surgeries, yet have persistent motion loss, residual knee arthrosis, or both resulting in moderate to severe impairment. Vigorous physical therapy fails to make substantial gains in these patients because of the associated arthrosis. Likewise, corrective surgery, e.g., debridement and retinacular release, is of little benefit owing to marked articular degeneration. Surgery should be reserved for pain control and be confined to "salvage" procedures such as tibial tubercle advancement, patellectomy, Maquet osteotomy, or total knee replacement.

This important syndrome demands early recognition so preventive measures may be taken to avoid the complications of the full-blown disorder. Trauma plus immobility are central to its evolution. Hence early motion is important whenever feasible after surgery.

ROLE OF BRACING

Knee braces are considered under the headings of rehabilitative orthoses, those used for functional instability, and those used prophylactically.[80] Literature appearing during the late 1970s and early 1980s was replete with anecdotal testimonials that made it difficult to assess the efficacy of bracing in an unemotional light. It tended to polarize sports medicine

personnel into believers and nonbelievers. During the late 1980s and early 1990s, sufficient scientific documents have been published to make it clear that there are no conclusive answers regarding prophylactic braces as yet, although their role in postsurgical range control and in combating functional instability is somewhat clearer. However, it is important that studies of specific braces are not always generalized to the vast number of different makes and designs available to the athlete and clinician. Each sports medicine specialist should become familiar with the properties, fitting, and limitations of a few of these braces, so a special personal "feel" about their efficacy may be developed. The literature should be followed carefully for new developments. Degree of prominance and brace contact area, as well as comfort, fit and stability, tendency for slippage, cost, and range of motion permittted, are factors that should enter into the decision to supply a particular brace.

Rehabilitative Bracing

Rehabilitative braces are also referred to as postinjury or postsurgical motion control devices.[80–83] Interest in their area was stimulated by Anderson et al. in 1979.[81] They reported on nine athletes with mainly grade I and II medial collateral ligament injuries. They stressed the use of the brace as a rehabilitation tool and as a mechanism of returning the athlete to football within a shorter period of time. Anderson et al. followed their patients over time and documented the absence of reinjury. It is probable that the current interest in prophylactic bracing started from their work. Nevertheless, postoperative or rehabilitative braces have been largely ignored by investigators. Krackow and Vetter showed that even tightly applied casts allow significant varus-valgus motion, anteroposterior translation, and rotary motion.[51] Thus it cannot be anticipated that bracing will eliminate all motion. Hoffman confirmed this limitation with a variety of braces; although most did not create normal knee stability in patients in whom ligaments were severed, all of the braces improved anterior, valgus, and rotary stability[83] to some degree. There are several basic requirements for rehabilitative braces: They should (1) be able to limit range of motion in an adjustable fashion; (2) be comfortable and allow easy access to wound care if used postsurgically; (3) be cost-effective; (4) be adjustable to a changing contour of the limb, and (5) be able to give a measure of protection as the athlete increases stress on the re-

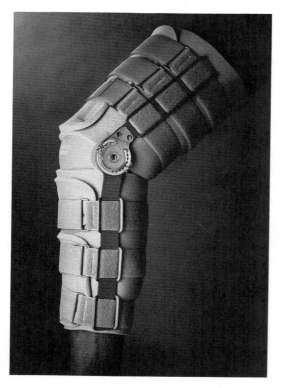

Fig. 15-44. Example of a brace suitable for postoperative support and rehabilitation (Don-Joy, Richards Co.).

covering knee during the late stages of rehabilitation (Fig. 15-44). Cawley et al. investigated several orthoses that are commonly used as rehabilitation braces.[82] Most of the braces significantly reduced both translation and rotation relative to the unbraced limb under static test conditions. These stresses, however, were well below what might be experienced during dynamic situations, particularly as rehabilitation progressed. The braces allowed 6 to 18 degrees more range than was apparently secured with pins or screws. Thus if restriction of range of motion is critical, at least 10 to 15 degrees of range should be restricted in addition to the desired endpoint.

The braces whose hinges were close to the joint prevented valgus and varus strains more effectively. The straps used with many braces were helpful in assisting the brace to function as a unit. Because many of the anterior and posterior shearing forces are internally generated, it is not reasonable to expect any brace to totally protect the individual from these forces. Education of the athlete concerning the limitations of the brace helps ensure that unreasonable risks are not taken under the assumption that the brace totally protects the knee.

Orthoses for Functional Instability

For the athlete with a functionally unstable knee, the concept of bracing may have a distinct appeal over surgical reconstruction. For the most part it means investing in a custom-made orthosis (Fig. 15-45). With few exceptions, the less expensive, off-the-shelf braces are not sufficiently effective to overcome the abnormal motion that leads to episodes of instability in the cruciate ligament-deficient knee. They may, however, help if the main problem is medial or lateral ligament attenuation without significant associated cruciate ligament damage.

Many braces protect valgus and varus stresses at low torques, but higher torques tend to overcome the brace protection.[83,84] The inability to prevent high rotary torques is a unifying theme in the literature. Nevertheless, many athletes find that their functional level increases significantly with bracing. In Colville et al.'s study of athletes with ACL-deficient knees, 22 percent returned to sport without bracing, 47 percent with bracing, 22 percent thought the brace gave some benefit, and 9 percent reported no benefit whatsoever.[85] Similarly, Coughlin et al. reported that 50 percent of their patients returned to sport, and about 75 percent of them played football or hockey or were skiers.[86] There were many complaints, including slipping down, calf cramping, pistoning, constraining, hot, heavy, and painful knees. Nevertheless, performance seems relatively little impaired when studied more objectively. Knutzen et al.'s work on running patterns using force plates and kinematic analysis revealed that there tended to be some increased force at heel strike with a decrease in knee flexion. Rotation seemed to be reduced up to 38 percent. There was also no difference in normal subjects performing agility tests such as cariocas, back-pedaling, and 10 yard sprints.[87] Testing athletes with unstable or postoperative knees during figure-of-eights, acceleration, and deceleration on slopes, stairs, and with hopping, reveals that bracing does not seem to impair function.[88] This important observation that bracing does not improve function if there is measurable muscle atrophy or weakness, re-enforces the

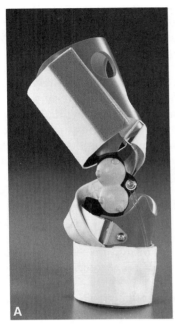 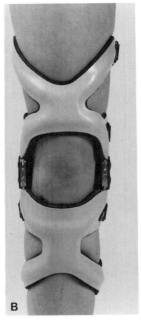 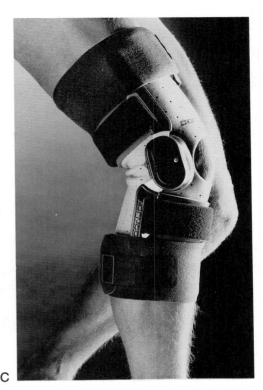

Fig. 15-45. Examples of orthoses used for functional instability. Generation II **(A)** and Double-X **(B)** are examples of polycentric, custom-made knee orthoses. **(C)** Off-the-shelf knee orthosis may be effective under specific circumstances (Don-Joy, Richards Co.).

concept that bracing is not a total treatment unless accompanied by a thorough examination and assessment and a corrective rehabilitation program for detectable muscle weakness.[88–91]

It has been postulated that some of the effectiveness of bracing is via enhanced proprioception, causing the hamstring muscles to increase their activity and perhaps contract earlier during pivoting motions, thereby enhancing stability.[89] However, further testing showed that increased hamstring activity and decreased quadriceps activity is a function of physiologic adjustment in the cruciate-deficient leg rather than attributable to bracing. The role of increased sensory feedback is probably important.

Cook et al. looked at running and cutting performance in individuals with ACL deficiency and showed that improvement may be enhanced. They cautioned, however, that the brace, in this case CTi (Innovation Sports, Irvine, CA), does not prevent abnormal anterior tibial displacement in the ACL-deficient knees and thus the long-term effect of brace wearing coupled with increased levels of physical activities are unknown, as far as the evolution of degenerative changes are concerned.[90] Bassett similarly confirmed that although bracing (Lennox Hill Derotation Brace, Orthopaedic Products, 3M Canada) consistently improved stability of the knee by a grade after manual testing, it did not eliminate abnormal motion at higher torques and hence was not a replacement for rehabilitation or, when necessary, counseling regarding activity modification.

I have had extensive clinical experience with the Double X and the Generation II orthoses (Fig. 15-45). Studies from our clinic using a straight run, figure-of-eight, slalom circuit, and the hop index have resulted in several conclusions[91]: The effectiveness of the brace was most obvious with the hop index, the figure-of-eight run, and the time taken to perform the figure-of-eight expressed as a ratio of the time for the straight run frequently independent of muscle strength and degree of instability.

Practice Point

BRACING THE UNSTABLE KNEE

- Mild to moderate ACL deficiency
- Absence of meniscal lesion
- Consider activity requirements
- Make sure quadriceps and hamstrings adequately rehabilitated
- Thigh shape and size compatible with bracing
- Comfortable and economical
- Education of patient for fit, application, and maintenance

In summarizing some of these issues with regard to clinical application, the following points should be emphasized.

1. Braces may increase static stability approximately one grade when tested by simple clinical tests.
2. Braces may improve function in sport-related tasks that require pivoting and turning.
3. Braces do not take the place of adequate rehabilitation of the hamstrings and quadriceps, and the efficacy of the brace may be enhanced by good muscle strength.
4. Because most of the subtle abnormal motions in the cruciate ligament-deficient knee are not eliminated, there is no guarantee that bracing will protect against long-term degenerative changes.
5. Sometimes counseling with regard to activity modification is a better option than bracing.
6. Little is known about the efficacy of bracing in the PCL-deficient knee, although usually there is some functional improvement with the less severe instabilities.
7. Bracing is most effective for the moderate ACL-deficient knee in the athlete with a relatively slim or muscular thigh who has a predictable instability. It is less effective in individuals with severe,

unpredictable instabilities or in athletes with short, fat thighs in whom adequate contact and control are difficult.

8. The brace is usually more effective when it is custom-made, manufactured and fitted by an experienced orthotist, and checked frequently by a knowledgeable sports physician or therapist.
9. Careful attention is given to fit, pistoning and localized pressure areas in order to prevent skin damage and difficulties with long-term wear.
10. Patient education about the fitting and application of the brace, the limitations of the device, signs of wear and tear of components, and the need for maintenance of the parts is important.
11. Bracing should be sport-specific.
    a. Some sports do not require bracing even in the face of an unstable knee, i.e., cycling and jogging.
    b. For some activities it is better to modify the activity than to wear a brace, e.g., when only specific exercises of an aerobic class produce instability.
    c. Some sports are not amenable to bracing because they hinder performance, i.e., sprinting, gymnastics. Here surgery may be a better choice.
    d. In some sports the brace may be a hazard to the individual or the opponent, e.g., wrestling, rugby, soccer. There may even be rules prohibiting the use of specific braces.
    e. There are circumstances where bracing is ideal, e.g., activities where the knee may be slightly flexed, e.g., ice hockey and skiing.
    f. In significant pivoting sports, particularly where there is good foot traction (e.g., basketball), the brace may be effective only for mild to moderate instabilities. Sometimes the effectiveness of the brace is enhanced by putting a 5 to 10 degree block to extension.
12. If a brace has been effective for a considerable period and the athlete then starts to complain of giving way, consider the following.
    a. The individual has developed poor habits of brace application, and hence a well-fitting brace becomes ineffective.
    b. The brace is broken or needs adjusting.
    c. The athlete needs a refresher rehabilitation program because of slowly decreasing muscle power, which often happens in the ACL-deficient knee despite continued activity.

d. The athlete has developed a meniscal lesion, a chondral flap, or a loose body and so requires careful evaluation and investigation.

e. The secondary restraints have stretched and the instability has progressed to sufficient severity that is not braceable.

13. Different braces allow different ranges of motion of knee flexion. With some activities this point is a major consideration.

14. The efficacy of braces is not always consistent and sometimes an athlete who has little success with one brace may do well with another. Occasionally, this difference is sport-specific, but more often it is a subtlety of fitting and anatomy.

Prophylactic Knee Bracing

Prophylactic bracing is probably the most contentious area of this general subject, and at the outset it should be stated that there are insufficient data to draw firm conclusions for or against its use. The concept has increased in popularity since 1979; and as the obvious attraction of protecting the knees from injury in sports such as football gained momentum, the chances of setting up a randomized prospective study of bracing became more difficult. Confounding features include the following.

1. Possible different effect of protecting the medial collateral ligament versus the cruciate ligament
2. Difficulty grading the severity of injury
3. Large number of braces available, all with different characteristics
4. Influence of rule changes, coaching techniques, playing surfaces, shoes and cleats, and the use of diagnostic techniques such as arthroscopy.

Studies such as that of Hansen et al., which was retrospective with no real controls, nevertheless concluded that although 11 percent of the nonbraced group and 5 percent of the braced group were injured, bracing was effective.[92] Two percent of the braced and 5 percent of the nonbraced athletes required surgery; furthermore, when they analyzed the players at greatest risk, 4 percent of the brace wearers and 25 percent of the non-brace wearers sustained ligament injury. Conversely, Taft et al., also presenting retrospective results, suggested that there were no changes in the injury rates when comparing 2 years before bracing with 5 years after bracing.[93] They did concede that bracing seemed to decrease the number of surgically treated medial collateral ligament injuries. By contrast, Rovere and Bowen retrospectively studied patients with 2 years of no bracing followed by 2 years with bracing. These investigators reported on an increased number of third degree ACL injuries, an overall increase in injuries, and specifically an increase in athletes requiring surgery.[94] Thus a selection of retrospective studies have reported a spectrum of outcomes: from bracing being efficacious, to being noncontributory, to adversely affecting the injury rate.

Jackson et al.[103] have recently recorded a decrease in risk of injury at football from 46 per 1,000 exposures to 31 through brace usage. The proportion of injuries to the MCL considered major were reduced but ACL injuries were unaffected.

Similar conflicting opinions are seen in some prospective reports. Schriner[101] reported a decrease but with no statistical significance; and Teitz et al.[98] recorded no change in severity of injury (Table 15-10).[95-98]

It appears that simple, single-hinge, off-the-shelf braces have limited ability to protect the knee. Some of the newer, off-the-shelf double-hinge knee orthoses may afford protection to certain types of impact.[99] There is a concern about prestressing the knee in some situations and throwing additional torques on proximal and distal joints (Fig. 15-46).

The ideal brace should supplement the knee ligaments, not interfere with function, not increase the risk factors, be adaptable to variations in individuals anatomy, not be harmful to others, be cost-effective, be easy to maintain, be durable, and have documented efficacy.[101,102,103] Most of the braces currently interfere with performance to some extent. Furthermore, the push to develop better and more efficacious bracing systems should not overshadow the need to be vigilant for emerging and existing dangerous techniques and the important sports medicine principle of making sport as safe as possible by removing as many harmful elements as possible. Removing and heavily penalizing blocking from behind and below the knee has done more to reduce knee ligament injuries than bracing. At the present time the decision must be left to the individual athlete, with a strong warning that all of the facts with regard to prophylactic bracing are far from clear.

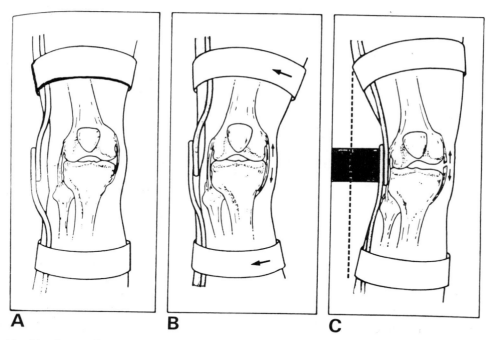

Fig. 15-46. Absolute efficacy of prophylactic knee bracing is still not established. Custom-made, well-fitting braces may protect the knee from specific stresses. There is also the danger that ill-fitting braces may prestress the knee. **(A)** Knee with normal alignment. **(B)** Varus alignment with the same brace may tend to press-stress the medial collateral ligament unless appropriately adjusted. **(C)** If the brace hinge pushes against the joint during the deformation induced by impact, a three-point bending system may be created with the hinge as a fulcrum. (From Poulos et al,[102] with permission.)

SUMMARY

There have been some exciting advances in the understanding of the biomechanics and behavior of the knee that have revolutionized the approach to surgery of the ubiquitous ACL injury and its subsequent rehabilitation. Not the least of these advances are the evolution of arthroscopically assisted techniques. Also there is the emerging appreciation of the role of proprioceptive deficits in contributing to morbidity and thus this becomes an important component of rehabilitation and bracing. There is a limited place for ligament augmentation devices and prosthetic ligaments and the future holds promise for meniscal and cruciate transplantation. The goals of knee ligament therapy are not only to improve short term function, but hopefully reduce the long term degenerative changes so prevalent in the unstable knee.

REFERENCES

1. Johnston RJ: The anterior cruciate problem. Clin Orthop 172:14, 1983
2. Robson M: Ruptured crucial ligaments and their repair by operation. Ann Surg 37:716, 1903
3. Hey-Groves EW: The crucial ligaments of the knee joint: their function rupture, and operative treatment of the same. J Bone Joint Surg 7:505, 1920
4. Smith A: The diagnosis and treatment of injuries of the crucial ligaments. Br J Surg 6:176, 1918
5. Abott LC, Saunders JB, Bost FC et al: Injuries to the ligaments of the knee joint. J Bone Joint Surg [Am] 26:503, 1944
6. Brantigan OC, Voshell AF: The mechanics of the ligaments and menisci of the knee joint. J Bone Joint Surg 23:44, 1941
7. Palmer I: On the injuries to the ligaments of the knee joint. Acta Chir Scand [Suppl] 81:53, 1938

8. Jones KG: Reconstruction of the anterior cruciate ligament: a technique using the central one-third of the patellar ligament. J Bone Joint Surg [Am] 45:925, 1963

9. Slocum DB, James SL, Larson RL et al: A clinical test for anterolateral rotary instability of the knee. Clin Orthop 118:63, 1976

10. Nicholas JA: The five-one reconstruction for anteromedial instability of the knee. J Bone Joint Surg [Am] 55:899, 1973

11. O'Donoghue D: Surgical treatment of fresh injuries to the major ligaments of the knee joint. J Bone Joint Surg [Am] 32:721, 1950

12. Galway RD, Beaupré A, MacIntosh DL: Pivot shift: a clinical sign of symptomatic anterior cruciate insufficiency. J Bone Joint Surg [Br] 54:763, 1972

13. Fetto JF, Marshall JL: Medial collateral ligament injuries of the knee: a rationale for treatment. Clin Orthop 132:296, 1978

14. Losee RE, Johnston TR, Soutwick WO: Anterior subluxation of the lateral tibial plateau. J Bone Joint Surg [Am] 60:115, 1978

15. Feagin JA (ed): The Crucial Ligament. Churchill Livingstone, New York, 1988

16. Noyes FR, Grood ES: The strength of the anterior cruciate ligament in human and rhesus monkeys. J Bone Joint Surg [Am] 58:1074, 1976

17. Czerniecki JM, Lippert F, Obrud JE: A biomechanical evaluation of tibiofemoral rotation in anterior cruciate deficient knees during walking and running. Am J Sports Med 16:327, 1988

18. Haggmark T, Eriksson E: Cylinder or mobile cast brace after knee ligament surgery. Am J Sports Med 7:48, 1979

19. Noyes FR, McGinnis GH, Grood ES: The variable functional disability of the anterior cruciate ligament deficient knee. Orthop Clin North Am 16:47, 1985

20. Magee DJ: Orthopaedic Physical Assessment. WB Saunders, Philadelphia, 1987

21. Hastings DE: The non-operative management of collateral injuries to the knee joint. Clin Orthop 147:22, 1980

22. Ellsasser JC, Reynold FC, Omohundro JR: The non-operative treatment of collateral ligament injuries of the knee in professional football players. J Bone Joint Surg [Am] 56:1185, 1974

23. Behrens F, Templeton J: Ligamentous injuries to the medial side of the knee: a one to ten-year follow up. J Bone Joint Surg [Br] 62:127, 1980

24. Holden DL, Eggert AW, Butler JE: The non-operative treatment of grade I and II medial collateral ligament injuries to the knee. Am J Sports Med 11:340, 1983

25. Frank C, Woo SLY, Amiel D et al: Medial collateral ligament healing: a multidisciplinary assessment in rabbits. Am J Sports Med 11:379, 1983

26. DeLee JC, Riley MB, Rockwood CA: Acute straight lateral instability of the knee. Am J Sports Med 11:404, 1983

27. Kannus P: Non-operative treatment of grade II and III sprains of the lateral ligament compartment of the knee. Am J Sports Med 17:83, 1989

28. Sandberg R, Balkfors B: Partial rupture of the anterior cruciate ligament: natural course. Clin Orthop 220:176, 1987

29. Noyes FR, Nooar LA, Moorman CT et al: Partial tears of the anterior cruciate ligament: progression to complete ligament deficiency. J Bone Joint Surg [Br] 71:825, 1989

30. Seto JL, Orofino AS, Morrissey MC et al: Assessment of quadriceps-hamstring strength, knee ligament stability, functional and sports activity levels five years after anterior cruciate ligament reconstruction. Am J Sports Med 16:170, 1988

31. McDaniel J, Dameron TB: Untreated ruptures of the anterior cruciate ligament: a follow up study. J Bone Joint Surg [Am] 62:696, 1980

32. Hawkins RJ, Misamore GW, Merritt TR: Follow up of acute non-operated isolated anterior cruciate ligament tears. Am J Sports Med 14:205, 1986

33. Marshall JL, Warren RF, Wickiewicz TL: Primary surgical treatment of anterior cruciate ligament lesions. Am J Sports Med 10:103, 1982

34. Gross MJ, Paterson RS, Capito CP: Acute repair of the anterior cruciate ligament with lateral capsular augmentation. Am J Sports Med 17:63, 1989

35. Jensen JE, Slocum DB, Larson RL et al: Reconstruction procedures for anterior cruciate ligament insufficiency: a computer analysis of clinical results. Am J Sports Med 11:240, 1983

36. Durkan JA, Wynne GF, Haggerty JF: Extra-articular reconstruction of the anterior cruciate ligament insufficient knee: a long term analysis of the Ellison procedure. Am J Sports Med 17:112, 1989

37. Harter RA, Osternig LR, Singer KM et al: Long-term evaluation of knee stability and function following surgical reconstruction for anterior cruciate ligament insufficiency. Am J Sports Med 16:434, 1988

38. Barton TM, Torq JS, Das M: Posterior cruciate ligament insufficiency: a review of the literature. Sports Med 1:419, 1984

39. Loos WC, Fox JM, Blazina ME e tal: Acute posterior cruciate ligament injuries. Am J Sports Med 9:86, 1981

40. Trickey EL: Injuries to the posterior cruciate ligament: diagnosis and treatment of early injuries and

reconstruction of late instability. Clin Orthop 147:76, 1980

41. Parole JM, Bergfeld JA: Long term results of non-operative treatment of isolated posterior cruciate ligament injuries in the athlete. Am J Sports Med 14:35, 1986

42. Cain TE, Schwab GH: Performance of an athlete with straight posterior knee instability. Am J Sports Med 9:203, 1981

43. Kennedy JC, Galpin RD: The use of the medial head of the gastrocnemius muscle in posterior cruciate deficient knees: indications, technique, results. Am J Sports Med 10:63, 1982

44. Fleming RE, Blatz DJ, McCarroll JR: Posterior cruciate insufficiency and posterolateral rotatory insufficiency. Am J Sports Med 9:107, 1981

45. Paulos L, Noyes FR, Grood E et al: Knee rehabilitation after anterior cruciate reconstruction and repair. Am J Sports Med 9:140, 1981

46. Eriksson E, Haggmark T: Comparison of isometric muscle training and electrical stimulation supplementary isometric muscle training in the recovery after major knee ligament surgery. Am J Sports Med 7:169, 1979

47. Eriksson E: Sports injuries of the knee ligaments: their diagnosis, treatment, rehabilitation and prevention. Med Sci Sports Exerc 8:133, 1976

48. Costill DL, Fink WJ, Habansky AJ: Muscle rehabilitation after knee surgery. Physician Sports Med 7:71, 1977

49. Solomonow M, Baratta R, D'Ambrosia R: The role of the hamstrings in the rehabilitation of the anterior cruciate ligament deficient knee in athletes. Sports Med 7:42, 1989

50. Elmqvist LG, Lorentzon R, Låström M et al: Reconstruction of the anterior cruciate ligament: long term effects of different knee angles at primary immobilization and diffferent modes of early training. Am J Sports Med 16:455, 1988

51. Krabow KA, Vetter WL: Knee motion in a long leg cast. Am J Sports Med 9:233, 1981

52. Arms SW, Pope MH, Johnson RJ et al: The biomechanics of anterior cruciate ligament rehabilitation and reconstruction. Am J Sports Med 12:8, 1984

53. Yasuda K, Sasaki T: Exercise after anterior cruciate ligament reconstruction: the force exerted on the tibia by the separate isometric contractions of the quadriceps and hamstrings. Clin Orthop 220:275, 1987

54. Morrissey MC: Reflex inhibition of thigh muscles in knee injury: causes and treatment. Sports Med 7:263, 1989

55. Arvidsson I, Eriksson E, Knutsson E et al: Reduction of pain inhibition on voluntary muscle activation by epidural analgesia. Orthopedics 9:1415, 1986

56. Young A, Stokes M, Shakespeare DT et al: The effect of intra-articular bupivacaine on quad inhibition after meniscectomy. Med Sci Sports Exerc 15:154, 1983

57. Seto JL, Brewster CE, Lombardo J et al: Rehabilitation of the knee after anterior cruciate ligament reconstruction. J Orthop Sports Phys Ther 10:8, 1989

58. Noyes FR, Mangine RE, Barber S: Early knee motion after open and arthroscopic anterior cruciate ligament reconstruction. Am J Sports Med 15:149, 1987

59. Spencer JD, Hayes KC, Alexander IJ: Knee joint effusion and quadriceps reflex inhibition in man. Arch Phys Med Rehabil 65:171, 1984

60. Renstrom R, Arms S, Stanwyck T et al: Strain within the ACL during hamstring and quadriceps activity. Am J Sports Med 14:83, 1986

61. Sherington C: Reciprocal innervation of antagonist muscles: 14th note on double reciprocal innervation. Proc R Soc Lond [Biol] 19:244, 1909

62. DeAndrade JR, Grant C, Dixon ASJ: Joint distension and reflex muscle inhibition in the knee. J Bone Joint Surg [Am] 47:313, 1965

63. Stratford P: Electromyography of the quads in subjects with normal knees and acutely effused knees. Phys Ther 62:279, 1981

64. Dvir Z, Eger G, Halperin N et al: Thigh muscle activity and anterior cruciate ligament insufficiency. Clin Biomech 4:87, 1989

65. Solomonow M, Baratta R, Zhou EE et al: The synergistic action of the anterior cruciate ligament and thigh muscles in maintaining joint stability. Am J Sports Med 15:207, 1987

66. DeLuca C: Control properties of motor units. J Exp Biol 115:125, 1985

67. Barratta R, Solomonow M, Zhou B et al: Muscular coactivation: the role of the antagonist musculature in maintaining knee stability. Am J Sports Med 16:113, 1988

68. Bilko TE, Paulos LE, Feagin JA et al: Current trends in repair and rehabilitation of complete (acute) anterior cruciate ligament injuries. Am J Sports Med 14:143, 1986

69. Yasuda K, Sasaki T: Muscle exercise after anterior cruciate ligament reconstruction: biomechanics of the simultaneous isometric contraction method of the quadriceps and hamstrings. Clin Orthop 220:266, 1987

70. Barrack RL, Skinner HB, Buckley SL: Proprioception in the anterior cruciate deficient knee. Am J Sports Med 17:1, 1989

71. Kennedy JC, Alexander IJ, Hayes KC: Nerve supply of the human knee and its functional importance. Am J Sports Med 10:329, 1982

72. Highgenboten CL, Jackson AW, Meske NB: Con-

centric and eccentric torque comparisons for knee extension and flexion in young adult males and females using the kinetic communicator. Am J Sports Med 16:234, 1988

73. Fullerton LR, Andrews JR: Mechanical block to extension following augmentation of the anterior cruciate ligament. Am J Sports Med 12:166, 1984

74. Light KE, Nuzik S, Personius W et al: Low load prolonged stretch vs. high load brief stretch in treating knee contractures. Phys Ther 64:330, 1984

75. Baugher WH, Warren RF, Marshall JL et al: Quadriceps atrophy in the anterior cruciate insufficient knee. Am J Sports Med 12:192, 1984

76. Pope MH, Johnson RJ, Brown DW et al: The role of musculature in injuries to the medial collateral ligament. J Bone Joint Surg [Am] 61:398, 1979

77. Payr E: Zür operativen Behandlung der Kniegelenksteife. Zentralbl Chir 44:809, 1917

78. Paulos LE, Rosenberg TD, Drawbert et al: Infrapatellar contraction syndrome: an unrecognized cause of knee stiffness with patellar entrapment and patella infera. Am J Sports Med 15:331, 1987

79. Sprague N, O'Conner R, Fox J: Arthroscopic treatment of post-operative knee fibroarthrosis. Clin Orthop 166:165, 1982

80. American Academy of Orthopaedic Surgeons: A Position Statement: The Use of Knee Braces. American Academy of Orthopedic Surgeons, Chicago, 1987

81. Anderson G, Zeman SC, Rosenfeld RT: The Anderson knee stabler. Physician Sports Med 7;125, 1979

82. Cawley PW, Opa RT, France EP et al: Comparison of rehabilitation knee braces: a biomechanical investigation. Am J Sports Med 17:141, 1989

83. Hofman AA, Wyatt RWB, Bourne MH et al: Knee stability in orthotic knee braces. Am J Sports Med 12:371, 1984

84. Knutzen KM, Bates BT, Hamill: Knee brace influences on tibial rotation and torque patterns of the surgical limb. J Orthop Sports Phys Ther 6:116, 1984

85. Coville MR, Lee CL, Cuillo JV: The Lennox Hill brace: an evaluation of effectiveness in treating knee instability. Am J Sports Med 14:257, 1986

86. Coughlin L, Oliver J, Beretta G: Knee bracing and anterolateral rotatory instability. Am J Sports Med 15:161, 1987

87. Knutzen KM, Bates BT, Schot P et al: A biomechanical analysis of two functional knee braces. Med Sci Sports Exerc 19:303, 1987

88. Montgomery DL, Koziris PL: The knee brace controversy. Sports Med 8:260, 1989

89. Brand TP, Hunter R, Donath M: Dynamic EMG analysis of anterior cruciate deficient legs, with and without bracing during cutting. Am J Sports Med 17:35, 1989

90. Cook FF, Tibone JE, Redfern FC: A dynamic analysis of a functional brace for anterior cruciate ligament insufficiency. Am J Sports Med 17:519, 1989

91. DaFonçeca ST: Validation of a performance test for outcome evaluation of knee function. Thesis, master of science, University of Alberta, 1989

92. Hansen BL, Ward JC, Diehl RC: The preventive use of the Anderson knee stabler in football. Physician Sports Med 13:75, 1985

93. Taft TN, Hunter S, Funderburk CH: Preventive lateral knee bracing in football. American Orthopedic Society for Sports Medicine, Nashville, 1985

94. Rovere GD, Bowen GS: The effectiveness of knee bracing for the prevention of sports injuries. Sports Med 3:309, 1986

95. Hewson GF, Mendini RA, Wang JB: Prophylactic knee bracing in college football. Am J Sports Med 14:262, 1986

96. Grace TG, Skipper BJ, Newberry JC et al: Prophylactic knee braces and injury to the lower extremity. J Bone Joint Surg [Am] 70:422, 1988

97. Garrick JG, Requa RK: Prophylactic knee bracing. Am J Sports Med 15:471, 1987

98. Teitz CC, Hermanson BK, Kronmal RA et al: Evaluation of the use of braces to prevent injury to the knee in collegiate football players. J Bone Joint Surg [Am] 69:2, 1987

99. Hansen BL, Ward JC, Diehl RC: The preventive use of the Anderson knee stabilizer in football. Physician Sports Med 13:75, 1985

100. Rovere GD, Haupt HA, Yates CS: Prophylactic knee bracing in college football. Am J Sports Med 15:111, 1987

101. Schriner JL: The effectiveness of knee bracing in preventing knee injuries in high school athletes. Med Sci Sports Exerc 17:254, 1985

102. Paulos LE, France EP, Rosenberg TD et al: The biomechanics of lateral knee bracing. Part 1. Response of the valgus restraints to loading. Am J Sports Med 15:419, 1987

103. Jackson RW, Reed SC, Dunbar F: An evaluation of knee injuries in a professional football team — Risk factors, type of injuries, and value of prophylactic knee bracing. Clin J Sports Med 1:1, 1991

Soft Tissue Injuries of the Thigh

16

Truth is the daughter of time and not authority.
—*Francis Bacon*

Muscle strains form a significant percentage of injuries in many sports, and most of these strains are into the thigh. In an Australian report of more than 1600 muscle strains, hamstring injuries were most prevalent. Different sports have different patterns; with soccer, for instance, quadriceps injuries occur with almost double the frequency of hamstring tears.[1,2] Like most statistics, however, the actual numbers represent regional considerations and methods of data collection (Table 16-1). Ice hockey in North America and soccer in Europe account for the largest percentage of adductor strains. The peak incidence for quadriceps tears is in the 16 to 20-year-old age group; hamstring tears appear most frequently in the 16 to 25-year group, and adductor tears are seen mostly in the 21 to 25-year group. By contrast, calf muscle strains tend to peak in the 35 to 50-year age group, as do Achilles tendon ruptures[2] (Fig. 16-1)

NORMAL RANGE OF MOTION

The normal ranges of motion in the knee and hip are greatly influenced by the soft tissues of the thigh, and so it is these factors that are discussed in this chapter. Although there are many devices, some sophisticated, for recording range of motion, the most available instrument is the goniometer.

Goniometer Placement for Knee Flexion and Extension

1. Axis of the goniometer is placed on the joint line where it may be palpated immediately above the head of the fibula.
2. Proximal arm lies along the lateral aspect of the thigh, pointing toward the greater trochanter.
3. Distal arm lies along the lateral aspect of the leg, pointing to the tip of the lateral malleolus.

To ensure the most accurate measurement of the range of movement of the knee, it is essential to use the type of goniometer that has long arms.

Knee Range of Motion

Knee Flexion

There are two main positions for measuring the range of movement of flexion of the knee. In the prone (face down) position, usually tightness in the rectus femoris acts as the limiting factor; the active range is about 120 degrees, whereas the forced or passive range is up to 150 degrees. In contrast, by measuring the supine (face up) position, where hip and knee flexion are combined, the limiting factor is usually apposition of soft tissue. In this case, the range is about 130 degrees of active flexion and up to 150 degrees of forced flexion.[3] Table 16-2 shows the factors involved.

Extension

As movement beyond 0 degrees is small, it is usually referred to as hyperextension. It does not mean that 0 degrees should be accepted as the normal range for all people, as particularly in women there are often a few degrees of hyperextension.[3] It is best tested with the patient lying, so the hamstrings are relaxed at their proximal attachment to the ischial tuberosity. Note that flexion is basically controlled by segments L5, S1, and S2, whereas extension is controlled by lumbar segments L2, L3, and L4 (Table 16-2).

Normally, the range of movement at the knee is recorded as degrees of flexion, but loss of range may

TABLE 16-1. Causes of 1641 Muscle Injuries

Sport	Hamstring (%)	Quadriceps (%)	Adductors (%)	Calf (%)
Rugby	53.9	44.2	43.4	18.9
Soccer	10.1	23.6	17.5	5.0
Track	14.1	15.2	10.1	14.0
Tennis	1.5	1.2	0.9	16.2
Squash	1.5	0.6	3.2	16.5
Ballet	1.8	0.6	4.6	1.5
Gymnastics	0.7	0.6	2.8	0.7
Others	13.9	11.7	15.9	26.5
Percentage of all tears	41.4	20.9	13.2	24.4
	(*n* = 680)	(*n* = 343)	(*n* = 217)	(*n* = 401)

(The data are from Australia.[2])

be referred to as degrees of limitation of extension. Here it may be pointed out that movement can be referred to as absolute (i.e., the number of degrees from a conventional zero starting point) or relative. If the term relative is used, only the direction of movement is indicated. For example, there are 0 degrees of absolute extension, but relative extension can occur from any point of flexion.

Hip Range of Motion

Hip motion is discussed more fully in Chapter 17. The average range of flexion is approximately 135 degrees with the knee flexed and having contact with the soft tissues of the thigh; the abdomen is the limiting factor. More pertinent to this chapter is the 80 to 95 degrees of hip flexion obtained with the knee in

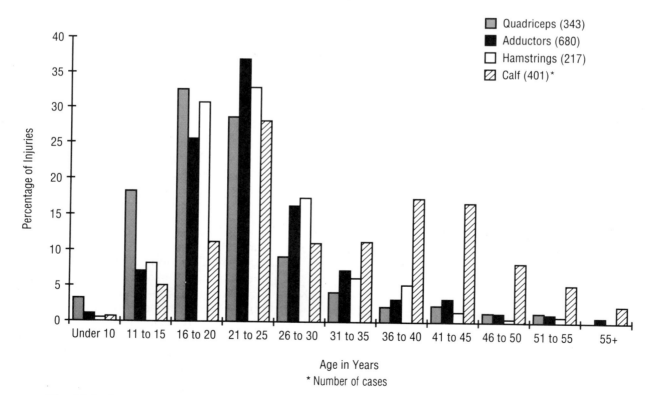

Fig. 16-1. Incidence of hamstring, quadriceps, and adductor strains peaks in the 16- to 25-year age group, whereas calf injuries are more prevalent in the 35- to 50-year range. (After Gordon,[2] with permission.)

TABLE 16-2.   Factors Affecting Motion at the Knee

Muscles Producing Motion	Nerve Supply and Segmental Control	Factors Limiting Motion
Flexion		
Biceps femoris[a]	Sciatic L5, S1, (S2)[b]	1. Contact of the leg on the thigh
Semimembranosus[a]	Sciatic L5, S1, (S2)	2. Cruciate ligaments
Semitendinosus[a]	Sciatic nerve L5, S1, (S2)	3. Tibial and fibular collateral ligaments
Sartorius	Femoral L2, 3	
Gastrocnemius	Tibial S1, 2	4. Tension in the quadriceps muscles particularly rectus femoris
Popliteus	Tibial L4, 5, (S1)	
Gracilis	Obturator L2, L3	
Extension		
Quadriceps[a]	Femoral (L2), L3, L4	1. Posterior capsule
Tensor fascia lata	Superior gluteal L5, S1, (S2)	2. Cruciate ligaments
Gluteus maximus (both above acting via iliotibial band)[c]	Inferior gluteal L5, S1, (S2)	3. Tension in hamstrings and gastrocnemius
		4. Tension in medial and lateral collateral ligaments

[a] Prime movers.
[b] Least important segment is in parentheses.
[c] May also assist flexion when iliotibial band passes posterior to the axis of motion at about 20 to 30 degrees.

> **Quick Facts**
> ### KNEE RANGE OF MOTION
>
> - *Flexion*   130 to 140 degrees
>   L3–L4 segments
> - *Extension*   5 to 10 degrees
>   L5–S1 segments

extension due to the role played by the hamstrings in limiting this motion. This range is widely discrepant in the normal population according to sex, natural joint flexibility, and sporting or recreational patterns. For instance, in the ballet dancer hamstring flexibility is such that it is frequently not the limiting factor for hip flexion. Similarly, the normally accepted 45 degrees of abduction, 55 degrees of external rotation, and 45 degrees of internal rotation are extremely variable.

STRENGTH PARAMETERS

The physiologic adaptations utilized in treatment regimens of resistance training also aid in the prevention of injury; they include increasing tendon and ligament strength as well as tendon-to-bone junction strength.[4] It has already been stressed that the strength ratios are probably as crucial as pure strength, and muscle imbalances should be actively sought.[5–10] Furthermore, assessment of total strength in all of the major lower limb muscles, particularly the proximal hip muscles, may correlate more with specific pathology than does isolated testing of any single muscle group.[11] These proximal muscles mediate force transmission from anywhere in the leg to the spine; moreover, the strength with which a segment of the body moves depends on the synergic response of proximal and distal muscles. Gleim et al. pointed out that *frequently weakness in a single muscle group is on the side contralateral to the injury*, whereas total weakness is on the ipsilateral side.[11]

With a rough correction for gravity and testing at 30 degrees per second, the hamstrings test at 50 to 60 percent of the quadriceps, whereas the hip adductors are 90 percent, the hip abductors 60 percent, and the hip flexors 55 percent (Fig. 16-2).[11] Concentric torque values and torque/body weight ratios decrease significantly at higher speeds, but the decrease is less marked with eccentric quadriceps and hamstring torques up to 180 degrees/second, as tested on a computer-controlled dynamometer (Kin Com apparatus) (Table 16-3).[12] Quadriceps torque declines more rapidly at higher speeds than does hamstring torque, and by 360 degrees/second. The hamstring/quadriceps ratio is nearer 80 percent.[13] There is usually not a significant difference between dominant

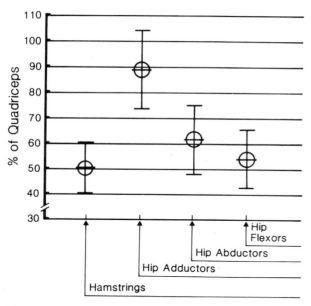

Fig. 16-2. Isokinetic testing at 30 to 60 degrees per second. With the quadriceps designated 100 percent, usually the ratios of the other thigh muscles are as shown above, with standard deviations, for the other muscle groups.

and nondominant limbs in most sports, which supports the concept of using the nondominant side as a guide to the progress of rehabilitation, bearing in mind the previous comments regarding the possibility of isolated muscle weakness in the noninjured side.[11-13]

HAMSTRING STRAINS (PULLED HAMSTRING)

The hamstring strain is caused by either a violent stretch or a rapid contraction of muscle, leading to varying degrees of tearing within the musculotendin-

ous unit. The term "hamstrings" was given to these muscles because hogs were hung up by them when slaughtered.[14] However, this apparent strength in dead animals is matched by a vulnerability in the living athlete. The hamstrings are the most frequently strained muscle in the body.[15,16] Furthermore, hamstring strains are plagued by a tendency to recur.

The injury is most commonly seen in runners, sprinters, and soccer and rugby players.[15] In Brubaker and James' series, hamstring strains accounted for 50 percent of the muscle injuries in sprinters and 20 percent of those in middle distance runners.[15] Ekstrand and Gillquist's study showed that 47 percent of the strains in soccer players involved these muscles.[17]

Anatomy

The hamstrings are composed of the semimembranosus, semitendinosus, and biceps femoris muscles (Fig. 16-3). The semimembranosus lies posteromedially on the thigh, originating from a tendon on the superolateral impression on the ischial tuberosity.[18] It receives slips from the ramus of the ischium (Fig. 16-4). This conjoint tendon interweaves with that of the semitendinosus and the long head of the biceps, eventually passing deep to them as an aponeurosis from which rises the muscle belly. The distal attachment is into the medial tibial condyle, sending important expansions to reinforce the posteromedial corner of the knee capsule.

The semitendinosus originates from the inferomedial facet of the ischial tuberosity, intimately associated, at its origin, with the biceps femoris and by its aponeurosis to semimembranosus.[18] The muscle is remarkable for the length of its tendon of insertion. It inserts by passing superior to the medial collateral ligament to attach to the tibia, posterior to the sartorius and distal to the gracilis. The latter group make up the "pes anserinus" aponeurosis, where bursae may be a source of great discomfort in runners.

TABLE 16-3. Hamstring/Quadriceps Torque Ratios with Concentric and Eccentric Contraction[a]

Contraction	Men		Women	
	30°/s	180°/s	30°/s	180°/s
Concentric	0.59 (0.07)	0.83 (0.12)	0.61 (0.09)	0.86 (0.16)
Eccentric[b]	0.67 (0.10)	0.70 (0.11)	0.65 (0.12)	0.71 (0.13)

Results are given as the mean (SD).
[a] Tested on Kin Com computerized isokinetic dynamometer.[12]
[b] Eccentric contraction affected less by speed.

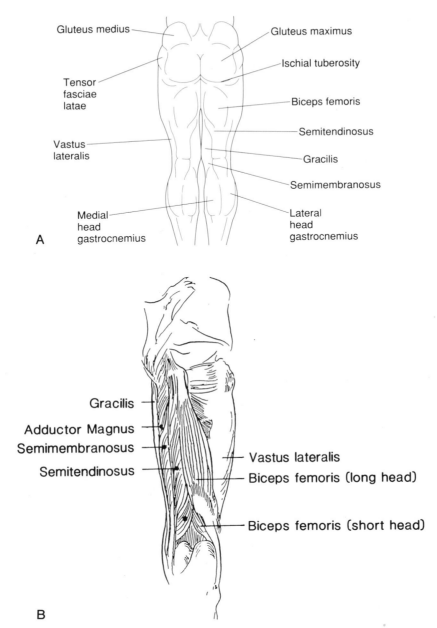

Fig. 16-3. (A) Surface markings for hamstrings. **(B)** Muscle group.

The long head of the biceps femoris, arising from the inferomedial facet of the ischial tuberosity, joins the short head when it takes origin from the lateral lip of the linear aspira on the posterior femur.[18] The conjoined muscle has a single tendon that inserts onto the head of the fibula, ensheathing the lateral collateral ligament and giving expansions to the posterolateral capsule of the knee joint.

The semimembranosus, semitendinosus, and proximal or long head of the biceps femoris are supplied by the tibial portion of the sciatic nerve, mainly from roots L5 and S1. The femoral head of the biceps femoris gains its innervation from the peroneal portion of the sciatic nerve also mainly from the L5 and S1 roots (Fig. 16-4).

The hamstring muscles have a high proportion of

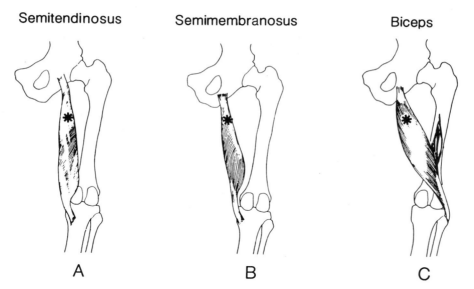

Fig. 16-4. Anatomy of hamstrings with motor points (*). **(A)** Semitendinosus. **(B)** Semimembranosus. **(C)** Biceps femoris. These are optimal points for electrical stimulation.

type II fibers;[16] which are involved with exercise of high intensity and force production (Table 16-4). This high intrinsic force production and the extrinsic stretch of the high velocity movements may be relevant to the production of tears.[16]

Function

The hamstrings help extend the hip and flex the knee by synchronizing with the other prime movers of these joints. In addition, the biceps femoris helps to rotate the flexed knee laterally, and the semimembranosis and semitendinosis rotate it medially.[19,20] There is a small component of these rotatory forces that may act at the hip. Lastly, they may assist in adduction of the abducted hip.

Because the hamstrings are two-joint muscles, they rely on external fixation (e.g., the ground), co-contraction, or fixation by other muscle groups to direct their contraction in a useful, coordinated fashion. Muscles that function over two joints have been shown to be those most commonly strained.[21,22] Much of their action is eccentric, decelerating the swinging leg when walking and running.[19,20] The faster the pace of running, the more important are the hamstrings (Fig. 16-5). To lengthen the stride, it is crucial to have adequate flexibility in these muscles. Furthermore, with the leg fixed in the stance phase, they are

TABLE 16-4.   Average Incidence of Type II Fibers

Muscle	Site	No.	% Type II
Biceps femoris long head	Proximal	10	55.2 ± 7.0
Biceps femoris long head	Distal	10	53.8 ± 4.9
Biceps femoris short head	Center	9	59.2 ± 9.3
Semitendinosus	Proximal	10	54.6 ± 4.5
Semitendinosus	Distal	10	60.4 ± 12.1
Semimembranosus	Proximal	10	51.0 ± 5.4
Semimembranosus	Distal	10	50.5 ± 6.8
Vastus lateralis	Central	10	54.5 ± 17.2
Vastus intermedius	Central	10	45.7 ± 9.7
Vastus medialis	Central	10	49.4 ± 10.8
Rectus femoris	Central	9	57.7 ± 10.7
Adductor magnus	Proximal	9	44.8 ± 8.0

(From Garrett et al.,[16] with permission.)

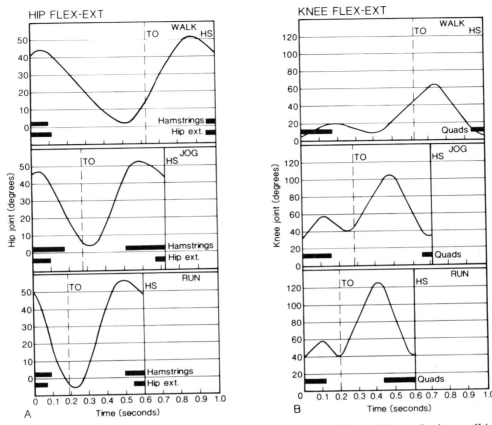

Fig. 16-5. Electromyography of the hamstrings, hip extensors, and quadriceps during walking, jogging, and running. TO = toe off, HS = head strike. (After Bateman and Trott,[19] with permission.)

important for stabilizing the knee. Through concentric contraction, the hamstrings assist in extending the hip during the support phase of running; and, finally, during take-off they assist the quadriceps in generating a vigorous push-off. At about 20 degrees from terminal extension, the mechanical efficiency of the quadriceps in extending the knee begins to decline. This motion is then enhanced by the synergic action of the gastrocnemius and hamstrings in creating an extension movement at the knee in a closed kinetic chain.

Mechanisms of Injury

Hamstring strains are mainly related to the ballistic actions common in running, specifically during the late forward swing phase and the take-off phase. There are two proposals that account for an apparent breakdown in the normal reciprocal action of the quadriceps and hamstring muscle groups. One mechanism involves excessive antagonistic force on a relaxed or lengthening hamstring muscle, which causes overstretching and injury to the hamstring. An alternative mechanism is based on a stretch being applied,

---

Quick Facts

HAMSTRING FUNCTION

- Extend hip
- Flex knee
- Biceps femoris laterally rotates flexed knee
- Semimembranosus and semitendinosus medially rotate flexed knee
- Co-contract with quadriceps to stabilize knee
- Decelerate swinging leg in gait and running

causing the hamstring to become fully elongated. The muscle responds to this stretching with rapid and excessive protective contraction, tearing the muscle fibers and intermuscular connective tissue.

Thus overstretching or rapid contraction may play a role. Contributory features include muscle tightness, muscle weakness, power imbalance, overuse, poor conditioning, improper warm-up, and inadequate healing or rehabilitation of pre-existing injuries[14,17,25,26] (Table 16-5).

The role of fatigue is difficult to assess. Fatigued muscle may relax more slowly and less completely than nonfatigued muscle, which may result in a form of physiologic contracture with a propensity to injury.[27–29] An intense workout, particularly at the end of a training session, may result in temporary loss of extensibility and range of motion at the beginning of the following day's workout.[22,26] This muscle stiffness may predispose the muscle to tearing if there has been insufficient cool down to the initial training session or warm-up for the succeeding one. This work of Ekstrand on the importance of cool down and warm-up cannot be over emphasized.[17]

The biceps femoris may be classed as a hybrid muscle innervated by two nerves. The tibial portion of the sciatic trunk supplies the long head with a proximal motor point, and the peroneal division enters the short (femoral) head more distally (Fig. 16-4). Grant suggested that the short head of the biceps evolved from the same muscular sheet as the gluteus maximus.[18] Based on this concept, the short head of the biceps should not be classed with the hamstrings, but clearly for practical purposes it cannot be considered otherwise.[31] During the running stride there are times, particularly prior to ground contact of the swinging leg, when the antagonistic groups of quadriceps and hamstrings are contracting at the same time. With the added complication of the dual innervation of the hamstrings, it is postulated that an imbalance in the contraction phase due to non-syncronous stimulation, both within the muscle group and between the antagonistic groups, may predispose to injury.[31]

Muscle Imbalance

Early reports suggested that the hamstrings should be capable of producing 60 percent of the muscle strength generated by the quadriceps muscle group. In some sports, the dominant quadriceps may have sufficient strength to alter the ratios; but usually this situation is not desirable, and every effort should be made to counteract it.[32,33]

A 10 percent or greater strength deficit between the right and left hamstring muscles is thought to predispose toward strain. These values might be angle- and speed-specific. For instance, a critical ratio of 50 percent at 90 degrees of flexion is probably equivalent to a 1 : 1 ratio at 30 degrees short of full extension. Furthermore, a 60 percent hamstring/quadriceps ratio at 45 degrees per second on isokinetic training increases to 80 percent at 300 degrees per second.[32] These ratios seem to hold true for sports as varied as middle-distance and long-distance running, as well as college football (Table 16-6).

It has already been explained that this changing ratio may not be mirrored exactly with eccentric contraction and that separate values are necessary. From the clinical point of view, it suggests that both concentric and eccentric hamstring training at high ve-

TABLE 16-5. Etiologic Factors in Hamstring Strains

Factor	Study	Year
Poor flexibility	Baker[23]	1984
Physiologic shortening due to fatigue	Ekstrand[17]	1983
Inadequate strength	Christensen[24]	1972
Inadequate endurance	Dornan[1]	1971
Contralateral hamstring imbalance	Burkett[25]	1970
Ipsilateral quadriceps/hamstring imbalance	Agre[26]	1985
Insufficient warm-up	Garrett[27]	1983
Dyssynergic contraction of the hamstrings	Grace et al.[5]	1980
Poor running style	Roy & Irvin[28]	1983
Premature return to activity	Agre[26]	1985
Inadequate rehabilitation	Coole[29]	1987
Associated with L5–S1 root irritation	Reid[4]	1985
Sudden violent stretch or contraction	Sutton[30]	1984
Action over two joints	Brewer[22]	1960

TABLE 16-6. Mean Isokinetic Values in Quadriceps and Hamstrings

Muscle	Peak Torque (ft-lb/100 lb body wt)		TRTD[a] at 60°/s (seconds)	Endurance[b]
	60°/s	180°/s		
Quadriceps	88.1	60.9	0.505	43.7
Hamstrings	56.4	44.8	0.333	32.9
Quadriceps/hamstring ratio (%)	64.0	73.6	65.9	75.3

Patient data: mixed sample (male and female); mean age 23.1 years; height 67.3 inches; weight 152.5 lb.
[a] Time to development of peak torque.
[b] Fatigue index of percent decline over 30 repetitions at 180°/s.
(From Wyatt and Edwards,[32] with permission.)

locities should be incorporated into the rehabilitation program if reinjury is to be avoided.

Practice Point
- Hamstring/quadriceps ratios change with increasing velocities.
- This change may not be mirrored exactly with eccentric work.
- High speed eccentric exercises are key to final rehabilitation.

It must be realized that these isokinetic values are a useful guide for preseason testing and postinjury rehabilitation. However, they have certain definite limitations, and not too much should be read into them. In particular:

1. Isometric, isotonic, and isokinetic strength measuring devices are inherently different in the ways in which they measure. The results derived from one device should not be generalized to any of the others.
2. Raw data from subjects of one population should be used only cautiously for another population and intrinsic normals for that particular group established at the earliest possible time.
3. The strength relations between the knee flexors and extensors are dynamic and vary as the result of physiologic and biomechanical variables, e.g., length-tension relation and speed of contraction.
4. In general, there should not be a strength deficit of more than 10 percent between the hamstrings of both sides.
5. In general, the hamstring/quadricep ratio should be more than 60 percent at isokinetic speeds of less than 90 degrees/second and more than 80 percent at speeds of 300 degrees/second.

Flexibility

Flexibility may be measured by Well's sit and reach test. Adequate flexibility is considerd when the athlete can reach the toes while the ankle is in the neutral position[25] (Fig. 16-6). The test combines back and hamstring flexibility, and it becomes slightly more specific when one leg is flexed at the hip or extended over the edge of the examining couch (Fig. 16-7).

A more appropriate test for flexibility of the hamstring group is with the patient in supine position, hip flexed to 90 and the contralateral hip extended. The knee on the test side is then extended, and the hamstring tightness is reflected in the degrees short of full extension (Fig. 16-8).

The inability to fully extend alternate knees while in the sitting position without leaning backward, the *tripod sign*, is also indication of hamstring tightness (Fig. 16-9). Care must be taken to distinguish it from radicular pain.

Although it is difficult to prove the role of flexibility in patients with hamstring tears, there have been several studies indicating that a flexibility difference between the two sides of more than 6 degrees may be a contributory factor.[17,21] However, it should be emphasized that the relation between muscle imbalance and extremity injury is obscure.[5,6] Prior to stretching exercises, local heat, either superficial or deep according to the anatomy, applied for 20 to 30 minutes facilitates the stretching exercises. Heat is effective because it increases the extensibility of collagen. Furthermore, slow passive stretching allows the collagen to "creep," utilizing its property of plasticity. These stretching exercises may be augmented by the use of physiologic reflexes, which induce relaxation or decrease the sensitivity of the muscle spindle; they include hold–relax techniques, reciprocal relaxation movements, and contract relax movements.

Ballistic movements trigger muscle spindle activity,

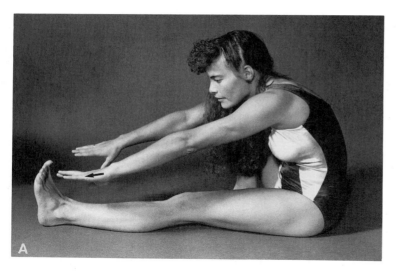

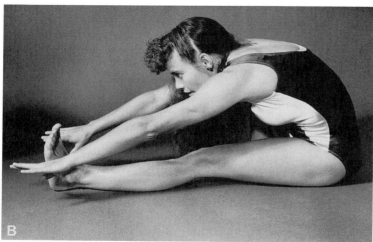

Fig. 16-6. Testing for hamstring tightness. The foot is in the neutral position. **(A)** Positive test: hamstring tight. **(B)** Negative test: flexible hamstrings or lumbar spine.

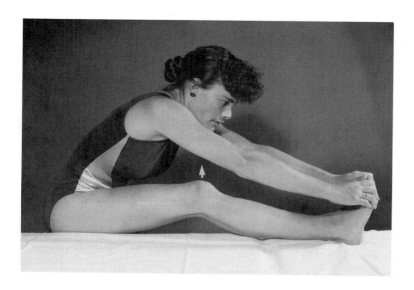

Fig. 16-7. Extension of the left leg over the examining couch locks the pelvis in extension. Hamstring contracture demonstrated by an inability to extend the knee fully while reaching to touch the toes.

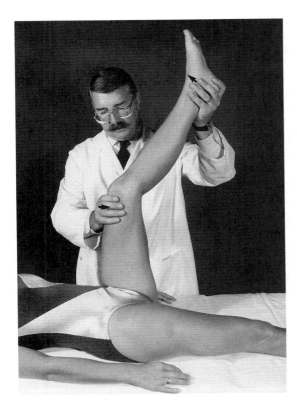

Fig. 16-8. Active or passive knee extension test with the hip flexed to 90 degrees. Hamstring tightness is illustrated by the inability to fully extend the knee.

causing protective contraction and thus preventing gain in range. However, with normal physiology, these ballistic movements can be used at the end of a stretching program and prior to commencing other activities. Furthermore, repetitive exercise within the functional range of motion, continued over a period of 15 minutes, can be equally effective in gaining range as static stretching. Highly repetitive work, e.g., cycling, also maintains range or serves as a good warm-up prior to more ballistic activity.

Site of Injury

The commonest site of hamstring tears is at the junction of the muscle with the aponeurosis. However, the muscle may tear upon the common tendon, avulse a fragment of ischium, or tear lower down in the muscle belly. The hamstring rarely pulls in the distal half of the thigh. Occasionally in the skeletally immature, the apophysis may be avulsed. The more proximal the injury, the longer the healing time;

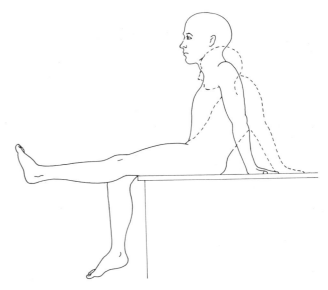

Fig. 16-9. Tripod sign. Tight hamstrings force the patient to lean backward as the knee is extended.

however, all hamstring tears are subject to healing withpainful scars and a tendency to reinjury.

Treatment

The treatment plan should evolve from consideration of the principles of healing outlined in this text (Chapter 5).

Preseason Testing

Before detailing nonoperative treatment, the value of preseason testing for muscle tightness and imbalance must be stressed as well as the institution of a prophylactic stretching program in sports associated with a high incidence of hamstring tears, e.g., football, soccer, and sprinting.[26] Any athlete with a discrepancy of more than 10 percent between the two sides or a hamstring/quadriceps ratio of 0.5 or less at slow speed isokinetic testing should be placed on a prophylactic program.[30] If isokinetic equipment is available, it would include the following at a minimum:

1. Three workouts per week.
2. Two sets of 10 repetitions each at 240, 180, 120, 60 degrees/second.
3. Complete the workout with one set at 300 degrees/second to the point of fatigue, or perform the equivalent on other exercise equipment.

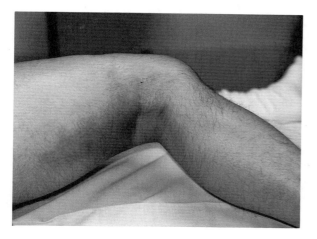

Fig. 16-10. Acute hamstring tear with tracking of hemorrhage to the knee after 2 to 3 days. However, NSAIDs are frequently very effective since inflammation and edema are usually the major component of injury and not hemorrhage in first and second degree strains. Garrett has confirmed this with CTs.[27]

Nonoperative Treatment

For those individuals with hamstring tears treated nonoperatively, the rate of progress depends on the degree of tearing and whether it is a reinjury or a chronically pulled hamstring. First degree tears may allow resumption of full training at 2 weeks, second degree tears at approximately 4 weeks, third degree injuries and reinjuries at as long as 12 weeks. Assessment of severity is based on the presence or absence of a palpable gap, the amount of pain and reflex inhibition, and the degree and ability of the swelling and bleeding to track distally (Fig. 16-10) (see Chap. 5).

The acute condition is treated in the standard mode (ice, compression, and rest) until the danger of further hemorrhage is minimized, usually 24 to 48 hours. Gentle, active range of motion is begun early, as is treatment with anti-inflammatory medication. Ambulation with crutches is used for second and third degree injuries and should not be abandoned until normal, pain-free walking is possible. Weight-

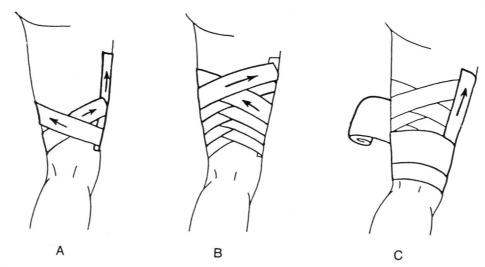

A   B   C

Fig. 16-11. Hamstring taping (method 1). The materials include skin toughener, 1.5-inch adhesive tape, a roll of 4-inch elastic tape, and a 6-inch tensor bandage. The athlete may stand or lie prone with knee slightly flexed. Tape adherent is applied. **(A)** Anchor strips are placed on either side of the thigh. They are approximately 10 inches in length and run from just above the knee to the level of the groin. **(B)** Diagonal strips are then crisscrossed upward on the posterior aspect of the thigh, starting at the distal end and working superiorly. The muscle is drawn up with it as it is pulled. **(C)** Horizontal strips may be applied from one anchor to the other, starting distally and working proximally to reinforce the crisscross pattern. Then two more anchors are placed over the original anchors. The taping is completed by a 6-inch elastic wrap around the thigh to aid in holding the crisscross tape in place. If the athlete is competing in strenuous activity, the elastic bandage should be supplemented by a 6-inch tensor bandage in the form of a hip spica to stop it from falling down.

bearing is progressed as tolerated. Supportive strapping may relieve some pain with significant tears (Figs. 16-11 and 16-12).

During the subacute period, heating modalities may be added as may active and passive stretching. These stretches are started gently and progressed as discomfort decreases (Figs. 16-13 and 16-14). Absolutely no ballistic-type activities are allowed at this point.

Practice Point

HAMSTRING TEARS (SECOND DEGREE): EARLY TREATMENT

- Ice, elevation, and compression comprise important initial treatment.
- Acute phase: do not abandon crutches until relatively normal pain-free walking is possible.
- Ensure voluntary muscle control.
- As pain subsides emphasize active range of motion.
- When 75 percent of range is reached, start resisted muscle work.

As pain decreases and range of motion is gradually restored, resisted muscle work is added and increased. Gentle isometric muscle stretching in the most pain-free range is progressed by increasing in intensity and by establishing strong isometric holds in different parts of the range of motion. Proprioceptive neuromuscular facilitation (PNF) patterns are particularly useful during these early stages, as they give the therapist good control and with correct patterning may help overcome reflex inhibition (Figs. 16-15, 16-16, and 16-17). It is essential to keep therapeutic and functional activities within the pain-free level to expedite healing and prevent reinjury. Cycling is an ideal exercise for maintenance of endurance at this time. Sometimes with significant proximal tears and avulsions the pressure of the cycle seat is uncomfortable, and thus swimming and water-running are acceptable alternatives. Ultrasound, interferential currents, and gentle cross-frictional massage may also be of benefit at the end of this stage. Further hamstring stretching is added until full range of motion is achieved. This step is critical to prevent reinjury (Figs. 16-18, 16-19 and 16-20).

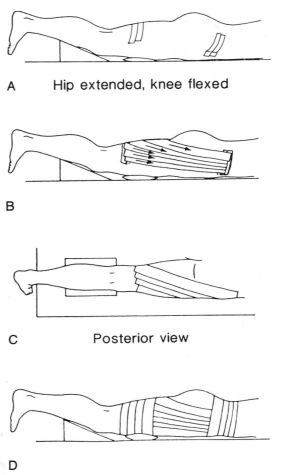

A Hip extended, knee flexed

B

C Posterior view

D

Fig. 16-12. Alternative method of hamstring taping. Materials needed are tape adherent, 1.5-inch adhesive tape, 6-inch tensor bandage, and 3- to 4-inch elastic tape. **(A)** Athlete lies prone with the knee slightly flexed and the hip minimally hyperextended; tape adherent is then applied. Using elastic tape, an anchor is placed around the distal thigh just above the knee joint. Also two adhesive tape anchors are placed along the medial iliac crest area. **(B)** Starting at the lower anchor, adhesive tape is applied from low on the thigh to the iliac crest, pulling the muscle in an upward direction. **(C)** This process is repeated using five or six strips. **(D)** Additional anchors of elastic tape around the thigh and adhesive tape around the iliac crest are applied to hold the adhesive tape in place. A hip spica using a 6-inch tensor bandage is then applied to set and secure the tape in position.

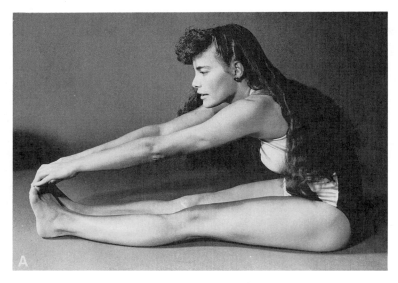

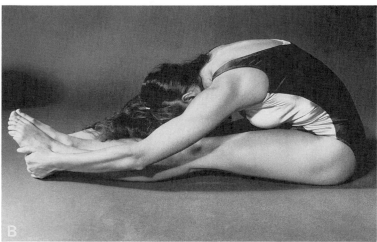

Fig. 16-13. Double hamstring stretch (sit and reach). **(A)** Grasp or touch as far down the leg as possible. **(B)** Repeat with chest to knees. Hold the stretches at least for 6 to 10 seconds.

As rehabilitation progresses, careful introduction of isokinetic work is valuable, but testing should not be considered until a strong, pain-free isometric hold is possible and range of motion is back to normal when compared to the contralateral limb (Fig. 16-21). Prior to this point, maximal isokinetic testing efforts would be dangerous. Even so, testing must be done carefully with an adequate warm-up, with the equipment set at 240/second. The test of peak torque is done at 60 degrees/second using the best of three repetitions. Results with the opposite (uninjured) leg are used as the baseline.

Jogging may be commenced when range of motion is full and peak torque at 60 degrees/second equals 70 percent of the baseline data.[8] The duration of jogging should be progressed slowly, with particular attention paid to the gradual buildup of speed. Sudden starts and stops must be avoided and adequate warm-up and gentle stretching stressed. Day-to-day monitoring is important, with the patient understanding the importance of holding back at the appearance of discomfort and informing the therapist of any reversal of a healing trend.

Taping is more useful for the chronic hamstring strain but may be used during reintroduction to activity with acute tears. It should not be used as a method of returning the athlete to activity earlier than is dictated by the functional tests and range of motion; otherwise reinjury is inevitable.

Once full range of motion has been achieved, it

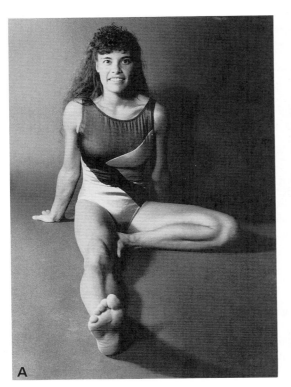

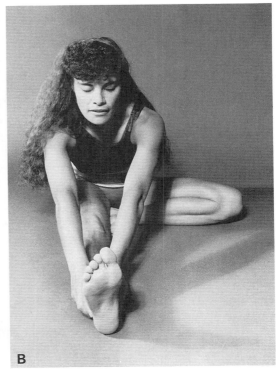

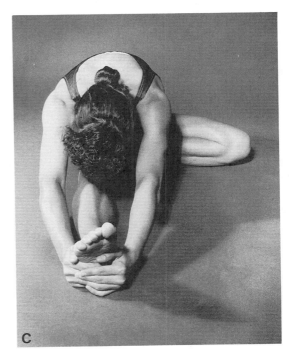

Fig. 16-14. Hurdler's stretch for hamstrings. **(A)** Starting position is sitting, one leg extended and the opposite leg abducted at the hip and flexed at the knee to allow the foot to rest on the inside of the other leg. **(B)** Hamstring is stretched by attempting to grasp as far down the leg as possible. Hold the stretch for at least 10 seconds. **(C)** When this stretch is successful or if the individual is flexible, it may be possible to reach the foot.

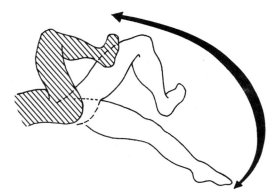

Fig. 16-15. Proprioceptive neuromuscular facilitation (PNF) patterns. Flexion–adduction–external rotation with knee extension and the antagonistic pattern of extension–abduction–internal rotation with knee flexion.

may be useful to add treatments with electrical muscle stimulation under tension to ensure maximum stretching of scar. This therapy should be applied only after heating the affected area with a suitable modality, usually ultrasound for tears near the insertion and hot packs for tears of the musculotendinous junction or the muscle belly itself.

Before return to full training, it is essential to introduce a program of controlled high velocity and high resistance eccentric work. Because the hamstrings are frequently injured and reinjured during

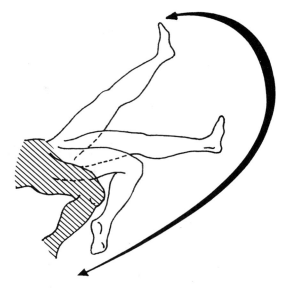

Fig. 16-17. PNF pattern (flexion–abduction–internal rotation with knee extension) and the antagonistic pattern (extension–adduction–external rotation with knee flexion).

the eccentric phase of contraction, rehabilitation must be considered incomplete if there has not been a focus on this aspect. The eccentric work must include resisted work in the outer range of muscle action.

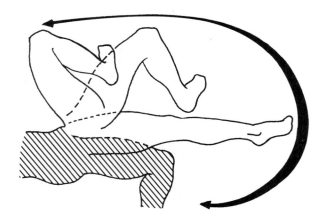

Fig. 16-16. Variation of Figure 16-17. Flexion–abduction–internal rotation with knee flexion and the antagonistic pattern of extension–abduction–external rotation with knee extension.

Practice Point

PROGRESSION OF ACTIVITIES: HAMSTRING TEARS

- Keep therapeutic and functional activities in pain-free range.
- Emphasize maintenance of cardiovascular fitness.
- Early isokinetic testing may cause reinjury.
- When full range of motion and strong resisted pain-free contraction are possible, then consider isokinetic testing.
- When patient is at 70 percent of normal, start jogging.
- Ballistic work requires at least 80 percent baseline strength.

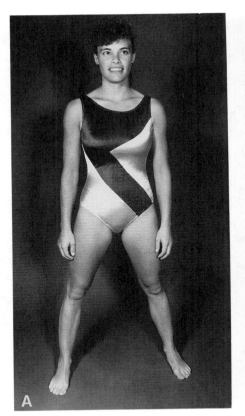
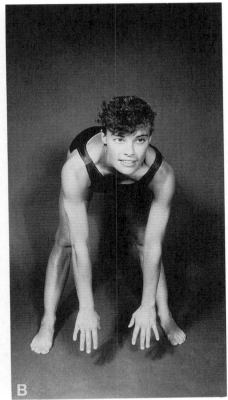
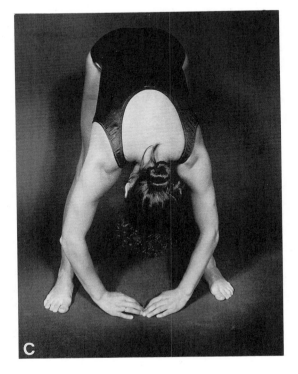

Fig. 16-18. Double hamstring straddle stretch. **(A)** Starting position is with feet about 2 feet apart. **(B)** Bend at hips, keeping knees and back straight. Hold the stretch for about 10 seconds. **(C)** Progress as range of motion increases.

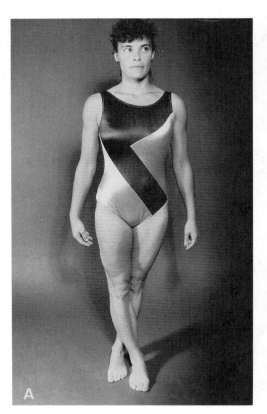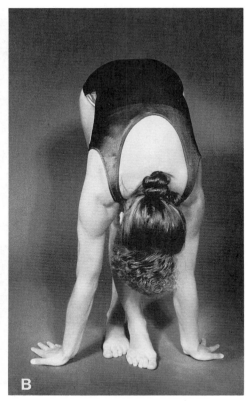

Fig. 16-19. Standing crossed hamstring stretch. **(A)** Cross the legs; the posterior leg gets the most stretch. **(B)** Bend forward and reach as low as possible; the back leg stays straight, but the front knee may bend a little. Hold stretches for at least 10 seconds.

Return to full practice in sprinting and sports requiring rapid acceleration and deceleration is allowed when good speed and agility are demonstrated, the isokinetic strength test in at least 80 percent of the baseline, and the hamstring/quadriceps ratio is 0.55 percent or more at 60 degrees/second (Fig. 16-5). In the absence of objective testing equipment, a carefully monitored progression of speed of running, sprinting, and deceleration is designed. The ability to do all maneuvers absolutely pain-free, coupled with normal strength and range of motion, is the prerequisite for returning to full training and sprinting. Once recovered, a specific warm-up and stretching program is taught to the athlete, and the importance of warm-up as a precursor to all ballistic activities for at least a year subsequent to the injury is stressed.

In general, surgery is reserved for widely separated apophyseal avulsion, ischial tuberosity separations, or large third-degree tears with considerable separa-

tion. These injuries may cause subsequent problems because of either a painful mass in the gluteal area or considerable late muscle weakness. For the most part, all other hamstring injuries may be treated nonoperatively. The decision to operate is made more readily in the elite athlete.

Chronic Hamstring Injuries

The two major contributing causes of reinjury are insufficient rehabilitation and insufficient control of the timing for progression of activities.[17,26] Many individuals sustain a reinjury within 2 months of returning to their sport, most of whom have returned to competition of their own accord whenever they felt ready after an injury.[17] Agre, during preseason testing of professional ice hockey players, found that many of these athletes had residual power and flexibility deficits due to inadequate rehabilitation of old injuries.[26]

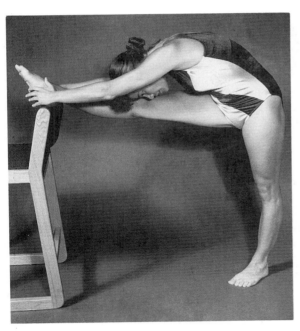

Fig. 16-20. Standing hurdler's hamstring stretch. The tension may be increased by raising the height of support.

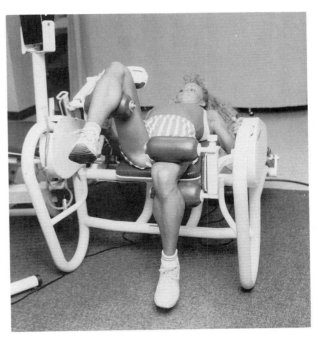

Fig. 16-21. Increasing resistance and velocity may be accomplished using this type of polykinetic apparatus. In this case it reciprocally works the hamstrings and hip extensors alternately with the hip flexors.

Differential Diagnosis

In the acute situation, hamstring strains must be differentiated from muscle cramps and delayed muscle soreness. The former is distinguished by the magnitude of the spasm, the absence of local tenderness, and the response to reciprocal relaxation PNF techniques, gentle stretching and rest. The latter is characterized by its appearance at 12 to 24 hours after exercise, the generalized nature of the tenderness, and the absence of local swelling and bruising.

Sciatica from the L5 and S1 roots may radiate mainly into the hamstrings and mimic a tear. Furthermore, radicular pathology may leave the hamstring susceptible to injury, and the association of lumbosacral root pain and hamstring tears is not uncommon. Limited straight-leg raising due to hamstring tightness, hamstring pain, or nerve root tension must be distinguished from each other. Increased pain with pressure over the nerve in the popliteal fossa with dorsiflexion of the ankle or with lifting of the head (Kernig-Lasegue's sign) during a maximal straight-leg raise point to a neural etiology. The presence of crossed sciatic pain (the well-leg-raising test), associated lumbar pain, and any distal radiation past the

knee are also indicators of radicular irritation. Obviously, distal sensory, motor, and reflex changes make the distinction easy, but the point here is to *raise the awareness of the possibility of nerve root irritation that mimics a hamstring tear* as well as the possibility of the coexistence of the tear with radicular irritation.

The association of low back pathology and its implication in the treatment of hamstring strains must be stressed.[29] Cibulka et al. demonstrated an increase in peak torque of the hamstrings in a pretest/post-test experimental design following sacroiliac joint mobilization therapy.[13] Furthermore, Muckle suggested that lower lumbar hypomobility may be a factor in recurrent hamstring strains.[33] Clinicians skilled in manipulative therapy may find it beneficial to include mobilizations of this area if they detect this association.

In 1982, Raether and Lutter described the chronic compartment syndrome of the posterior thigh that occurs in endurance athletes. It presents as an aching muscular pain, a subjective feeling of tightness not supported by findings on examination.[34] Runners often report the exact distance needed to produce the muscular aching, which was consistent in relation to duration or intensity of work. The muscle aching tends to worsen as the competitive season progresses and the muscles hypertrophy. Sometimes bilateral symptoms are present. The symptoms may be minimized by reducing exercise intensity; and, in any event, they usually disappear rapidly upon cessation of activity unless a particularly hard workout is undertaken. In this case some aching may persist into the following day.

Occasionally, fascial defects are found, but there are no pathognomonic physical signs. An index of suspicion is required as is the ability to rule out other causes of hamstring pain. The diagnosis must be established by demonstrating elevated compartment pressures by direct measurement. The treatment is prolonged abandonment of the symptom-causing activity or fasciotomy.

Summary

The importance of the hamstring muscles in high velocity eccentric motion of the lower limb has been emphasized. The complexity of the anatomy of these two joint muscles probably means that the etiology of tears is multifactorial, and analysis of those factors is important for establishing treatment protocols. The propensity to reinjury indicates the care that must be taken in progression of activities and return to sport. Lastly, with recurrent strains, a diligent search should be made for lumbosacral pathology.

QUADRICEPS INJURY

Avulsion of the Iliac Spines

Avulsion of the anterosuperior iliac spine by sartorius contraction and stretching or the anteroinferior iliac spine by the pull of the rectus femoris is unusual. If the separation is not great and the avulsed fragment is small, surgical repair is not indicated. Most of these injuries heal without significant strength deficit. Attention to gaining adequate range of motion is an important part of the rehabilitation if chronic pain is to be avoided.

Quadriceps Strains

Whereas contusion to the quadriceps is a frequent occurrence in contact sports, quadriceps strains are less common (Fig. 16-1). They are most frequently seen with soccer, weight lifting, football, rugby, and sprinting. When they do occur, it is usually the rectus femoris that tears.

Anatomy

The huge quadriceps femoris muscle group, which form the anterior aspect of the thigh, has been the center of much controversy, though some general observations may be made (Fig. 16-22). The rectus femoris, which is a two-joint muscle that may exert a force over the hip or knee, is in this group. Currier and Kumar demonstrated that it may be possible to increase the torque generated by the rectus femoris component by exercising with the hip at 60 degrees (rather than 90 degrees) of flexion.[35] The quadriceps are powerful extensors of the knee when the leg is non-weight-bearing; and, with the glutei and hamstrings, they supply the thrusts for walking, running, and jumping. The quadriceps work equally well with either the proximal or distal part fixed; and when walking, there is a phasic pattern of activity between the rectus femoris and the vastus muscles. They are quiescent during relaxed standing and show increased postural activity when the normal relations of the knee and ankle are disturbed, e.g., when wearing high-heeled shoes, or in the presence of muscle shortening or adaptive soft tissue contractures. Their role in stabilizing the knee is discussed in Chapter 15.

There are so many variables in the development of normal values that each clinic should make every effort to evolve its own standards. The values in Table 16-6 were derived from a mixed male and female population who were fit but not participating in a high level of physical activity, which is reflected in the slightly lower than anticipated peak torque values. In most serious athletes the quadriceps peak torque at speeds of 60 degrees/second and slower, expressed in foot-pounds, usually approaches the body weight in pounds, which is a reasonable rehabilitation goal.[36-38] Quadriceps strength parameters for young active females are outlined in Table 16-7.

Mechanism

Muscle belly tears are usually caused by the muscle being overstretched while contracting, as when reaching for a ball. Sudden deceleration also causes tearing, as when a hurdler catches a toe or a soccer player mistimes a kick, missing the ball and kicking the ground or the opponent. Rapid deceleration from a sprint is another common cause. The contributing factors are tight quadriceps muscles and muscle imbalance between the two legs, inadequate cool down

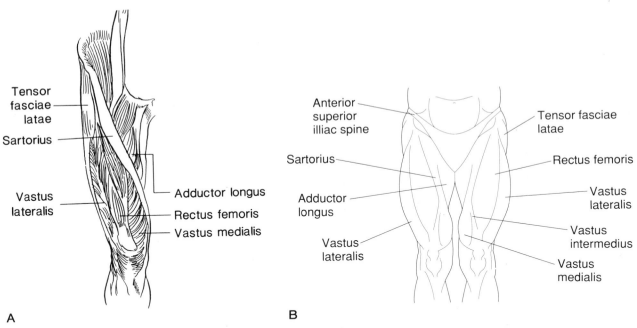

Fig. 16-22. Schematic **(A)** and surface **(B)** anatomy of the anterior thigh.

after intense exercise sessions and insufficient warm-up during the following session.[17,36]

Location

The rectus femoris muscle usually ruptures in its midsubstance, and the more rarely injured vastus lateralis and vastus intermedius rupture in their mid to upper third, through the thickest parts of their bellies (Fig. 16-23). Isolated vastus medialis tears are unusual, although with major traumatic injuries, with or

TABLE 16-7. Quadriceps Strength Scores in Women[a]

Test	Absolute Value (nm)	Relative to Body Weight (nm/kg)
Isokinetic 300°/s	48.7 ± 1.6	0.84 ± 0.03
Isokinetic 180°/s	71.5 ± 1.8	1.23 ± 0.04
Isokinetic 30°/s	125.8 ± 3.5	2.14 ± 0.06
Isometric	120.8 ± 3.8	2.06 ± 0.07
Isotonic	214.5 ± 6.9	3.65 ± 0.11

[a] Age 21.8 years (± 3.0); height 166.2 cm (± 7.0); weight 59.3 kg (± 8.9).
(Data from Hackney et al.[37])

without associated collateral ligament rupture, large tears may occur across the suprapatellar tendon and aponeurosis of the whole quadriceps. In this case the tear usually commences on the medial side and commonly goes through the entire vastus lateralis.

Quadriceps tendon rupture from the superior pole of the patella and disruption of the infrapatellar common tendon, the ligamentous patella, is either associated with previous hydrocortisone injections or ingestion, or is due to anabolic steroid abuse.[39,40] Occasionally, chronic inflammation or systemic collagen disease is the contributing factor. Disruption of the extensor apparatus around the knee is discussed in Chapter 13.

In the skeletally immature athlete there is a tendency for the tibial apophysis to be avulsed rather than traumatic disruption of the ligamentous patella.

Signs and Symptoms

First and second degree tears of the quadriceps are painful out of proportion to the damage. With a first degree injury it is usually possible to run but not sprint, jump effectively, or kick a ball. A second degree tear is not usually compatible with continuing activity. These injuries are usually caused by over-

MUSCLE STRAINS

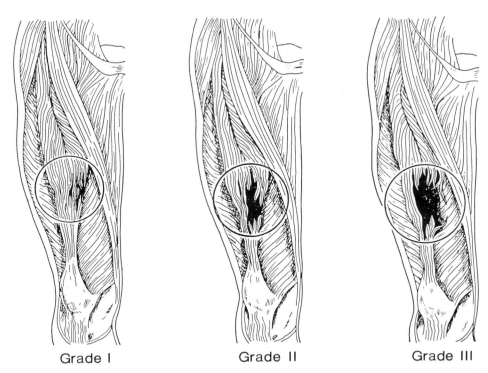

Grade I   Grade II   Grade III

Fig. 16-23. Increasingly severe tears of the rectus femoris muscle. **(A)** Grade I — minimal disruption. **(B)** Grade II — tearing with significant hemorrhage. **(C)** Grade III — complete loss of continuity and function.

stretching the contracting muscle; the same mechanism causes reinjury unless adequate range of motion is gained during the treatment. The bleeding associated with these tears tracks readily to the knee and down to the calf under the influence of motion and gravity; therefore local hemorrhage is not always a feature.

Complete tears should be easy to diagnose but in fact are frequently overlooked. In the series of simultaneous bilateral ruptures of the quadriceps tendons reported by McEachern and Plewes, three of the five cases had a delayed diagnosis despite the cardinal features of diffuse swelling around the knee, a visible or palpable defect, and an inability to do a straight-leg raise despite a functioning quadriceps muscle.[40] The defect may be filled rapidly with hemorrhage and be tense to palpation. Furthermore, the pain may prohibit adequate testing of quadriceps function. Nevertheless, careful inspection, palpation, and functional testing of muscle contraction reveal the true extent of the injury (Fig. 16-24).

Complete tears of the rectus femoris are usually more obvious because of the way in which the torn ends widely separate.

Practice Point

COMPLETE QUADRICEPS TENDON RUPTURE

- Despite its catastrophic nature, it may be misdiagnosed.
- The quadriceps may still be able to produce some extensor power through the medial and lateral retinacular bands.

Treatment

Treatment is discussed more fully under the section on muscle contusion because the concepts are similar, even though the time course may be differ-

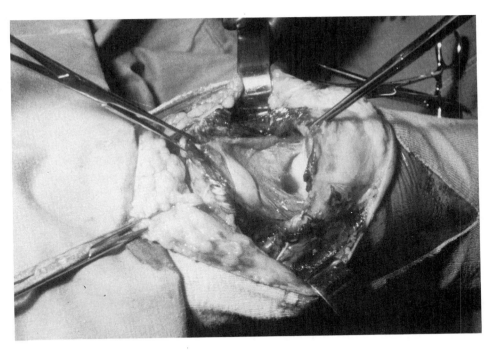

Fig. 16-24. A complete tear of the quadriceps tendon just proximal to the patella. Often some knee extension is possible through the quadriceps expansion, and the defect may be filled with hemorrhage. Thus, these severe injuries may be initially diagnosed as ligament sprains.

ent. Complete tears of the rectus femoris are usually treated nonoperatively, with excellent results (Fig. 16-25). Tears of the suprapatellar quadriceps aponeurosis and the infrapatellar tendon usually require surgical repair for adequate function, particularly in the superior athlete. Methods of repair have been described using augmentation with synthetic materials, which enables rehabilitation in the form of quadriceps contraction to begin on the first postoperative day, with full weight-bearing and active straight-leg raising at 2 weeks.[41] Almost full range of motion may be restored by 12 weeks after surgery. In view of the significant disability, the prolonged rehabilitation times with traditional methods of repair, and cast immobilization, the surgical techniques offer some distinct advantages to the athlete.

Differential Diagnosis

Muscle pain may be referred from nerve entrapment, either in the lumbar spine at the root secondary to disc disease or as a peripheral irritation. The most common peripheral entrapment that produces thigh

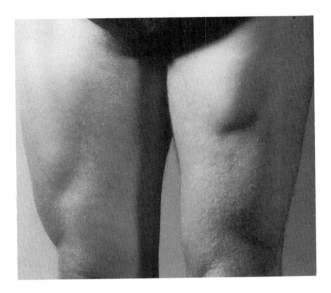

Fig. 16-25. Complete tear of the left rectus femoris. Following comprehensive rehabilitation, this injury is often compatible with excellent function.

pain is pressure on the lateral femoral cutaneous nerve in the proximal thigh.

Muscle herniation through the surrounding fascia may produce a bulging, painful mass that is made worse with activity. This situation is uncommon in the thigh, except following surgery.

Bone lesions occasionally appear first as thigh pain. Because the distal femur is a common site of both benign and malignant tumors in the young, this possibility should always be borne in mind when atypical pain is present or the pain is not responding to therapy.

Quadriceps Strains (Charlie Horse, Cork Injury)

Occasionally the huge muscle mass of the anterior thigh absorbs large impacts without apparent damage; frequently, however, locally focused blows delivered by an accelerating knee, a helmet, or the edge of a misplaced thigh pad produce a disabling injury (Fig. 16-26).[42] It is most often seen in the sports of football, rugby, soccer, basketball, and hockey. There is a suggestion that the more relaxed the muscle at the time of impact, the more severe is the injury.[43]

Quadriceps strains represent a spectrum of injury ranging from mild bruising to severe tearing of the

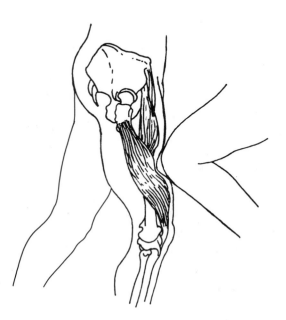

Fig. 16-26. Large anterolateral muscle mass of the thigh is exposed to direct trauma, leading to contusion.

muscle with significant localized hematoma. The contusion merges imperceptibly into the muscle strain, and the two elements usually coexist. Some degree of hematoma is probably present with any muscle contusion, although the bleeding is usually diffuse infiltration rather than an area of pooled blood.[42] The severity of the quadriceps contusion is nearly always underestimated and is frequently undertreated. Even minor injuries may cause problems, as athletes are anxious to return rapidly to their sport. However, judicious use of rest and cautious return to activity usually pay dividends, with a return to full function associated with few complications.[43]

Practice Point

QUADRICEPS CONTUSION: SEVERITY

- Severity of the injury is nearly always underestimated.
- Palpation of a solid mass that does not readily diffuse during the first few days indicates a poor prognosis.

The commonest site of injury is the anterior and lateral thigh, and the disability depends on the severity of bleeding, the amount of muscle crushed, and the experience of the physician and therapist treating the injury (Fig. 16-27).

Signs and Symptoms

Immediately after the blow the athlete experiences varying degrees of pain and, if severe, an inability to bear weight. After the initial pain, if the athlete continues to participate, the thigh becomes increasingly stiff and the quadriceps muscles become progressively unresponsive. The first aid includes ice, elevation, and compression (Fig. 16-28).

On examination there is localized pain and loss of ability to flex the knee through a full range of motion. Flexion, particularly past 90 degrees may be particularly painful, whereas active extension against firm resistance may cause rather less discomfort.[44] Indeed the severity of the contusion is often reflected in the degree of loss of range of motion. Depending on the severity, there may be a palpable, firm mass due to the hematoma and complete inability to generate a good quadriceps contraction or straight-leg raise.

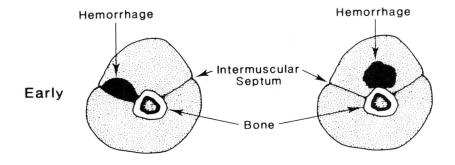

Intermuscular   **Intramuscular**

Hemorrhage   Hemorrhage

Early   Intermuscular
                                     Septum

                                     Bone

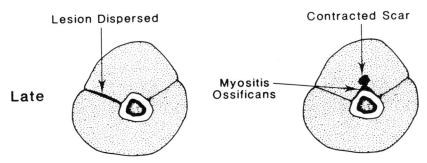

Lesion Dispersed   Contracted Scar

Late   Myositis
                                     Ossificans

Fig. 16-27. If the location of the contusion is adjacent to the intermuscular septum, tracking of the hemorrhage allows more rapid resolution and decrease in pain. The intramuscular location is associated with more protracted symptoms, greater tearing, and a tendency toward more morbidity. (After Bass AL: Rehabilitation after soft tissue trauma. Proc Royal Soc Med 59:653, 1966.)

Frequently with moderately severe hematomas, there is a sympathetic effusion which develops over a 24-hour period. Initially there is very little or no evidence of bruising, and often it never appears. If present, superficial discoloration may be seen over the lower thigh which tracks gradually past the knee, changing color with the passage of time through the various hues of hemosiderin decomposition from red to blue, light scarlet, brown and eventually, a dirty yellow.

Treatment

Phase I (Acute)

The earlier the treatment, the better the results. By the competition site, the knee should be gently flexed to the maximum allowed, and a tensor bandage and ice pack applied to encircle the leg and thigh (Table 16-8). This will produce sufficient compression to minimize bleeding. Furthermore, it allows maintenance of some of the range[44] (Fig. 16-28). After a few hours of icing the thigh with the knee held in flexion (the ice should be applied for 20 to 30 minutes at a time, and then taken off for 20 minutes), reassess the

---

Practice Point

QUADRICEPS CONTUSION: RANGE OF MOTION

- Mild   >90 degrees preserved
- Moderate   45 degrees to 90 degrees
- Severe   <45 degrees at 24 hours

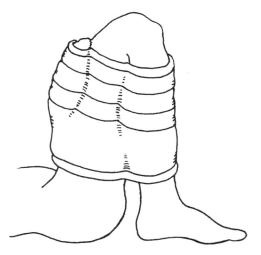

Fig. 16-28. Postcontusion adoption of the flexed position produces elevation of the thigh, internal compression by tightened fascia, external compression via the bandage, and cooling via an ice pack. Allowing the limb to rest in the flexed position is usually more conducive to maintenance of range of motion.

Practice Point

QUADRICEPS CONTUSION: COMPLICATIONS

- Development of a compartment syndrome is an unusual but severe complication.
- Deterioration of range and increasing pain should raise suspicion of developing myositis ossificans.

---

injury. If there appears to be significant damage, the ice regime is continued and the knee-flexed position adopted as frequently as possible for at least another 12 to 24 hours. If damage is mild, the athlete repeats the icing with the leg in a flexed position two or three times during the night and the following day, each time keeping the ice in place for about 20 minutes. If the leg continues to swell in spite of these measures, consideration should be given to the possibility of a developing compartment syndrome or continued

TABLE 16-8. Management of Quadriceps Contusions

Phase	Progression
Phase I: first 24–48 hours (acute)[a]	Ice: up to 20 minutes each hour Compression dressing Bed rest if severe Crutches, non- or light partial weight-bearing Gentle, active range of motion (pain-free range)
Phase II: 2–5 days (subacute)[b]	Eliminate quadriceps lag Gentle resisted exercises (no pain) Active range of motion PNF reciprocal relaxation patterns Swimming Light partial weight-bearing until 90° flexion Ultrasound or hot packs Consider NSAIDs
Phase III: (full weight-bearing)[c]	Discontinue crutches Work on active range of motion Increase resisted quadriceps work Cycling, progress to jogging High voltage galvanic stimulation Roentgenogram at 3 weeks to rule out myositis ossificans
Phase IV: (final rehabilitation)	Range of motion within 10° of normal Commence jumping, starts and stops, sprinting If progress slow, consider bone scan Test functionally to assess return to sport Consider adjustments to equipment

[a] If severe, consider aspiration or surgical drainage.
[b] If severe, consider 40 mg prednisone daily × 5 days.
[c] Critical stage for myositis ossificans. Hold if increasing pain and decreasing range.

hemorrhage. Exploring the hematoma and aspirating the blood may be a necessary option.

O'Donoghue recommended considering the possibility of aspirating large hematomas followed by local injection of the dispersal enzyme hyaluronidase.[42] In fact, he recommended it for the more severe contusions, where recovery time is a factor. The regimen includes initial injection of 1 ml of hyaluronidase repeated daily for 1 to 3 days followed by oral dispersive enzymes. However, proof of the effectiveness of this regimen is difficult to find, and the risks may be significant in terms of infection and sensitivity reactions.

In view of the possibility of sensitivity reactions, an intradermal test dose of 0.02 ml of solution should be given. A positive test is the appearance of an expanding wheal with with pseudopodia-like projections within 5 minutes and persisting for 30 minutes. There may also be local pruritus and transient vasodilation. In the presence of a history of allergies, particular care should be taken, even in the absence of a positive test. When local anesthetic is added to the hyaluronidase, the likelihood of a toxic local anesthetic reaction is increased.

If the hemorrhagic component is significant and the thigh rapidly becomes tense, hot and swollen, the possibility of a compartment syndrome should be entertained and early surgical aspiration carried out, followed by a supporting splint, a pressure dressing, and suction drainage for 24 hours.[45] Before embarking on a surgical exploration, measurements of the compartment pressures would be appropriate.[45] In addition the location and magnitude of any loculated hematoma should be assessed by MRI. The dressing is then reduced and gentle continuous passive motion on a CPM machine from 20 to 40 degrees of flexion is commenced. This is combined with attempts at getting voluntary quadriceps control.

Nearly all injuries will be treated non-operatively and, for the next 24 to 48 hours, ice packs can be applied every two to four hours for 20 minute periods. A compression bandage or supportive strapping is left in place and walking should be done non-weight-bearing, using crutches. (Fig. 16-34)

Phase II (Subacute)

The injury is reassessed at 24 hours and if full range of motion is not possible, the non-weight-bearing with crutches is continued for 2 to 5 days. After 24 hours, there should be adequate hemostasis and non-steroidal anti-inflammatory medications may be given. It is unlikely that the platelet inhibitory function would cause more bleeding if given immediately after trauma, but it may be wiser to wait.

When available, the modalities of pulsed ultrasound, and high voltage galvanic stimulation (HVGS) through direct electrode contact should be used. With HVGS, the polarity may be negative or positive, and it should be applied continuously at 80 to 120 pulses per second. The intensity should be set at the patient's sensory perception for approximately 20 to 30 minutes. At this intensity, it is possible to reduce edema without aggravating the condition.[43] As the pain lessens and range of motion starts to return, the intensity of the HVGS may be increased to produce a gentle, comfortable muscle contraction. At this time usually continuous ultrasound, appropriately adjusted for depth, is indicated. Also, quadriceps-set-

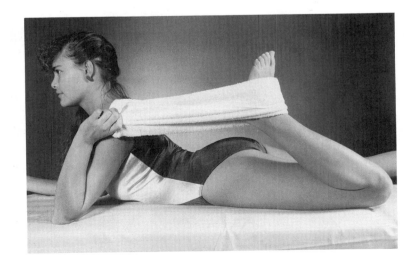

Fig. 16-29. Early treatment of a quadriceps contusion includes autoassisted gentle stretching, initially with an ice pack in place. The athlete can also be taught hold–relax techniques to obtain reciprocal relaxation and to gain range. The athlete tries to extend the knee against autoresistence for 10 seconds and then relaxes, at the same time passively pulling the leg into flexion.

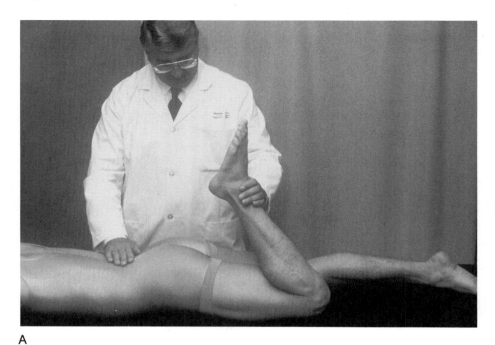

A

B

Fig. 16-30. As soon as there is sufficient range, the range of motion should be measured with the patient prone. **(A)** Normal. **(B)** A tight quadriceps causes the buttock to raise through hip flexion caused by tension in the rectus femoris (modified Ely test). Alternatively, range of motion may be measured just before hip flexion is started.

ting exercises with no resistance are commenced. The emphasis is on isometric, strongly resisted hamstring work and achieving reciprocal relaxation of the quadriceps. After each series of strong hamstring contractions the leg is taken gently, passively or actively, through a range of motion (Fig. 16-29). Anti-inflammatory medication is begun.

Initially, the range of motion is tested with the athlete lying down, with emphasis on the motion at the knee with the hip flexed. However, as soon as the patient is sufficiently comfortable, testing should be done in the prone position with the hip extended. (Fig. 16-30) This test is highly reliable as the landmarks for the goniometer are easily palpated and the endpoints of motion readily observed.[46] However, strict immobilization of the pelvis is necessary, and a strap secured across the buttocks may help in the reproducibility of testing.[47] Another option is the Ely test[48] (Fig. 16-31).

The excellent control and feedback offered by hands-on resistance applied by the therapist makes PNF techniques ideal at this stage.[49] The basic pat-

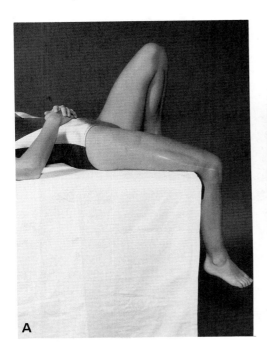

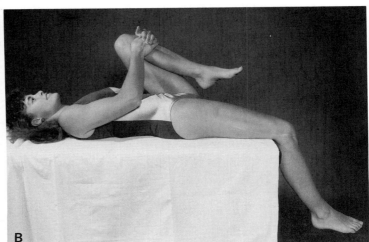

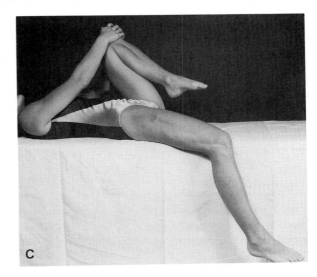

Fig. 16-31. Ely test is specific for rectus femoris tightness. Significant tightness of the whole quadriceps prevents the affected leg from dangling vertically. **(A)** Normal. **(B)** Positive test. As the contralateral hip is flexed, the tight rectus femoris produces some extension of the knee. Slight associated abduction at the hip may indicate tightness in the iliotibial band. **(C)** Alternative position with leg flexed over the side instead of over the end of the bed. The latter position enables the examiner to assess more fully the rectus femoris tightness by the tension felt with passive knee flexion.

terns have been illustrated previously and may be used to strengthen, relax, or gain range of motion in cases where there is an element of spasm or reflex inhibition (Fig. 16-15, 16-16, 16-17). Mobilization may be achieved by including knee flexion and extension in the patterns.[50] Some basic patterns are mentioned here; however, for a comprehensive repertoire of PNF exercises, consult the text by Voss et al.[49] To isolate and emphasize the knee component, it is often best to have the patient in high sitting position, and only the ankle and knee portion of the patterns are executed. The patterns shown in Figures 16-32 and 16-33 include hip motion with emphasis on the knee component.

Two specialized techniques that have particular application in the knee region are touched on briefly here. When attempting to relax tight muscle groups, try to select a reflex-inhibiting posture in order to decrease the tone as much as possible in the tight muscle group. Superimpose on it a "hold–relax" technique at the limitation of the range allowed by the tight group.

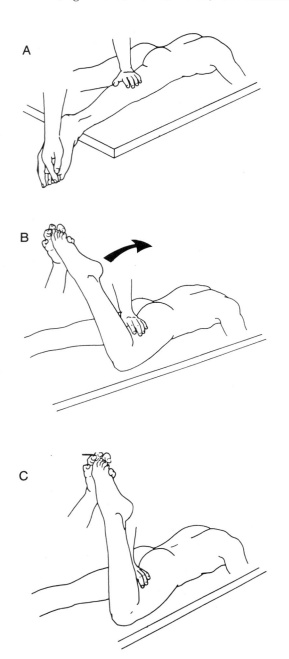

Fig. 16-32. Knee flexion pattern. **(A)** Starting position, with the tibia externally rotated. **(B)** Midposition. **(C)** End position, with the tibia internally rotated.

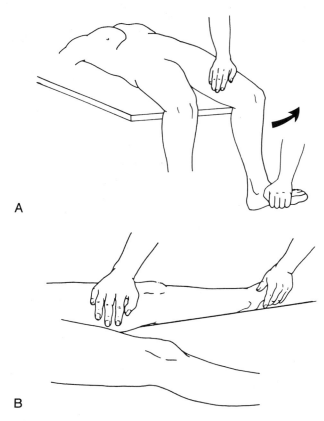

Fig. 16-33. Extensor patterns. **(A)** Extensor thrust: from flexion and internal rotation of the hip and knee to extension of the knee in external rotation. **(B)** Knee extension: from flexion and external rotation to extension with medial rotation.

Phase III (Full Weight-Bearing)

As soon as the athlete gains sufficient range to flex within 10 degrees of the opposite limb, the intensity of the exercises can be increased—both range of motion and resisted quadriceps work. If the tear is mainly in the rectus femoris, the athlete should carry out exercises with the hip at 60 degrees of flexion, achieved by leaning back. The work of Currier and Kumar has shown that this maneuver brings the rectus femoris into full contraction.[35] Jogging can be started, as can figure-of-eight circuits. The athlete frequently feels more confident with a tensor wrap or taping. With first degree tears, where early motion and non-ballistic activities are allowed, strapping may also be effective (Fig. 16-34). Exactly how this works is not fully understood.

During the early stages, there must be absolutely no forced stretching. Quadriceps-assisted stretching has a definite place, but the instructions to the patient must be clear. The patients must be supervised to ensure that they have understood the concept of gentle stretching within the range of comfort. These

stretches are designed to *maintain* a range rather than to gain it (Figs. 16-35, 16-36, and 16-37).

There is no place for massage in the early treatment of muscle contusions. "Rubbing" or "working it out"

Practice Point

EARLY TREATMENT OF CONTUSIONS

- Prompt removal from field of play
- Ice packs and pressure dressing
- Non or light partial weight-bearing
- After 24 hours, anti-inflammatory medication

Do Not

- Heat
- Forcefully stretch
- Massage
- Inject steroid

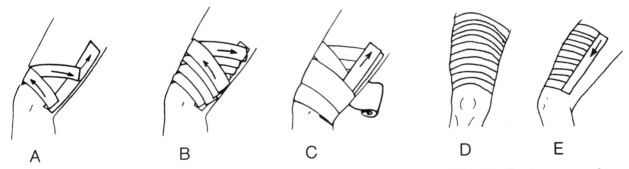

A   B   C   D   E

Fig. 16-34. Quadriceps taping. The materials needed are skin toughener, 1.5-inch adhesive tape, and a 6-inch tensor bandage. **(A)** Athlete stands with knee slightly bent. Tape adherent is applied. Two anchor strips are placed along the medial and lateral aspects of the thigh midway between the anterior and posterior aspects. These strips are about 10 inches long. **(B)** Strips of tape are then applied to the thigh using a crisscross pattern that begins 2 to 3 inches above the patella. The tapes are carried upward overlapping each other and extending from one anchor piece to the other. As the tape is applied, it is pulled up against gravity. The process is continued until the quadriceps is completely covered. **(C)** Anchors may then be placed over the original anchors, after which a 6-inch tensor bandage is applied to support and set the tape. **(D)** For further reinforcement prior to application of the bandage, tape may be applied in a horizontal fashion from one anchor to the other. Starting at the lower end, these strips are added sequentially, working up to the top. **(E)** New strips are then placed over the original anchor strips to hold the tape in place, thereby ensuring stability of the tape. The entire thigh may then be encircled with a 6-inch tensor bandage. If the athlete is going to take part in competition, the elastic bandage should also be placed around the waist in the form of a hip spica to stop it from falling down. Alternatively, an elastic thigh sleeve may be used.

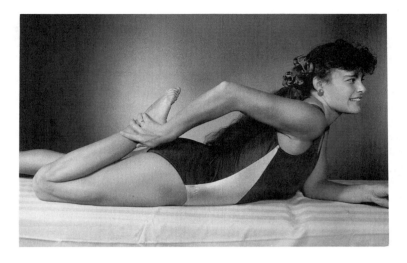

Fig. 16-35. Quadriceps stretch. Hold the top of the right foot with the right hand between the toes and ankle joint. Gently pull the right heel toward the right buttock to stretch the ankle and quadriceps. Hold an easy stretch for 10 seconds. Never stretch the knee to the point of pain. Always be in control. The stretch may be increased by contracting the right gluteal muscles while simultaneously pushing the right foot into the hand. This maneuver should stretch the rectus femoris muscle more. Hold an easy stretch for 10 or more seconds.

only increases the trauma and hemorrhage. Gentle massage may be of assistance after 10 to 14 days of healing but should not cause discomfort. Electrical stimulation-based programs may be used at this point; but unless there is an element of reflex inhibition, they are probably no more effective than voluntary isotonic and isokinetic programs.[51]

If the athlete still experiences a feeling of tightness in the muscle during the last parts of the full range of flexion, a course of electrical muscle stimulation under tension after 20 minutes of hot pack therapy often helps to mobilize and lengthen adhesions within the muscle. Progression cannot be allowed without adequate range. At this point in the program it is well to devise a stretching program the athlete may con-

tinue for the rest of the season once fully rehabilitated. (Figs. 16-36 and 16-37).

Phase IV (Final Rehabilitation)

An intensive strenghtening and conditioning program is necessary at this stage, before progressing to the fast starts and stops to acceleration, and then to full sprinting and jumping (Figs. 16-38 and 16-39). Sprinting and fast starts and stops are not allowed until the athlete can achieve full, pain-free flexion of the knee. This ability is best tested by having patients kneel and sit back with both buttocks supported on their heels (Figs. 16-40 and 16-41). Return to game fitness requires a strength difference of no more than

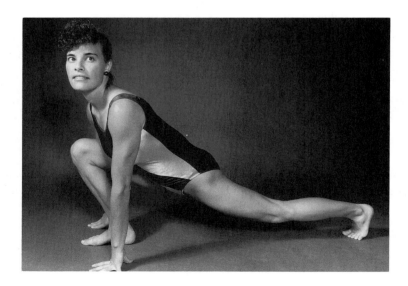

Fig. 16-36. To stretch the hip flexors and anterior thigh, move one leg forward until the knee of the forward leg is directly over the ankle, as illustrated. The thigh to be stretched is extended, and the knee should be resting on the floor. Now, without changing the position of the knee on the floor or the forward foot, lower the front of the hip downward to create an easy stretch. Hold for 30 seconds. The stretch may be felt in the front of the hip.

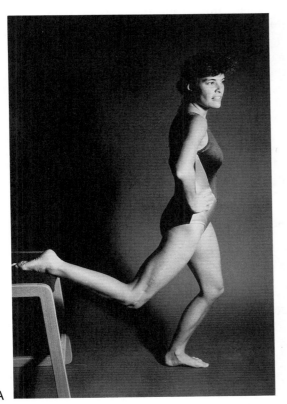 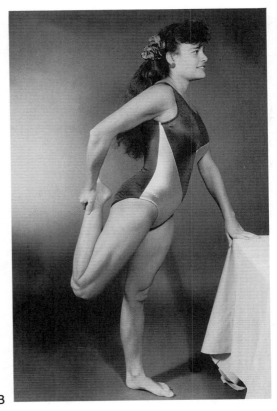

A B

Fig. 16-37. (A) Depending on the strength and balance, a supported or unsupported single leg stance is adopted with the thigh to be stretched—extended and resting on the top of a table, fence, or bar at a comfortable height as shown. Think of pulling the affected leg through (moving the leg forward) from the front of the hip to create a stretch for the iliopsoas and quadriceps. Keep the supporting knee slightly flexed and the upper body vertical. The foot on the ground should be pointed straight ahead. Alignment is important. The stretch may be progressed by increasing the flexion of the knee of the supporting leg. Hold an easy stretch for 20 seconds. Learning to feel balanced and comfortable in this stretch comes with practice. **(B)** Progression of the above stretch.

10 percent between the two sides and a hamstring/quadriceps ratio of more than 60 percent, which ensures adequate power and muscle balance. In addition, full range of motion of all parts of the quadriceps should be demonstrated by the ability to sit with the buttocks resting on the heels and then lean back to put the rectus femoris on a stretch across the hip (Figs. 16-41 and 16-42).

Protective Shells

If the athlete is to return to a contact sport, it might be advisable to fashion a protective shell of orthopast, Plastazote, or Fiberglas.[52] A second contusion soon after recovery usually produces severe signs and an

increased risk of myositis ossificans. Furthermore, those athletes who receive repeated injuries of established ectopic ossification may require some form of padding on a regular basis. If the regular protective equipment is not sufficient, a pad is custom-made. The difficulty of keeping these pads in position can sometimes be solved by stitching a pocket in a pair of cyclist's shorts that are elasticized and form-fitting.

Myositis Ossificans

Myositis ossificans is the development of ossification within the connective tissue of muscle (Fig. 16-42). It may develop to varying degrees in as many as

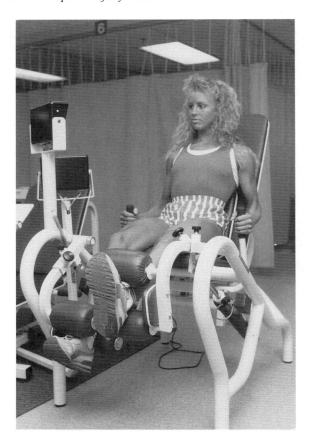

Fig. 16-38. Polykinetic quadriceps and hamstring reciprocal work at low and high speed prepares for progression to ballistic activities.

15 percent of patients with severe quadriceps contusions.[53-55]

Rothwell, in a classic article, described a typical athlete at risk.[53] A rugby player, in late teens or early twenties, is tackled while running, with the opponent's knee hitting the anterolateral aspect of his thigh.[46] He experiences intense pain and a transient feeling of paralysis of the limb as he falls to the ground, then hobbles gamely to the side of the field. After massage and ice, he tries once more to play but is usually unable to keep up with the game and so once more quits. His thigh feels much better after 10 minutes in the hot shower, but while standing around waiting for his teammates he again feels tightening of his mucles. By the next day he is barely able to bend the leg. The thigh is painful and the knee stiff, and he seeks medical help.

Examination at this time reveals a tense, swollen thigh, some 2 to 4 cm larger than that on the opposite side, maximal at 20 cm from the proximal pole of the patella. There are usually no external marks on the thigh. Active quadriceps contractions and straight-leg raising are difficult or impossible. Passive range of motion may be limited to as little as 20 to 30 degrees, and a small knee effusion may be present.

It is possible that with good treatment, careful progression, and graduated return to full activity on establishment of full range of motion and normal strength, this athlete can have an uneventful recovery. However, there are several risk factors.

1. Severity of the contusion
2. Continuing to play after injury
3. Massaging the injured area
4. Early application of heat

To these factors may be added other predisposing points.

1. Passive, forceful stretching
2. Too rapid progression of rehabilitation
3. Premature return to sport
4. Reinjury of the same area
5. Innate predisposition to ectopic bone formation

The last point is poorly understood, but it appears that some individuals show a propensity to form myositis ossificans despite a moderately small initial injury and careful progression of therapy. Attempts at correlating creatine kinase as a marker of severity of muscle damage have been unhelpful.[55,56]

Detection of Impending Ossificans

Any increase in pain or decrease in range over more than one or two treatment sessions and the persistence or return of undue warmth to palpation should signal the danger of the possibility of myositis ossificans after a quadriceps contusion. In addition to pain, the increasing hardness of the hematoma can often be palpated (Fig. 16-42).

The first roentgenographic signs on a plain film of the thigh, penetrated for soft tissue, may be present at 3 to 6 weeks (Fig. 16-43). Technetium polyphosphate scanning may reveal concentration in the soft tissues at least 1 week prior to the plain films.[57,58] Ultrasonographic scanning may also be appropriate for early localization of osteoid calcification.

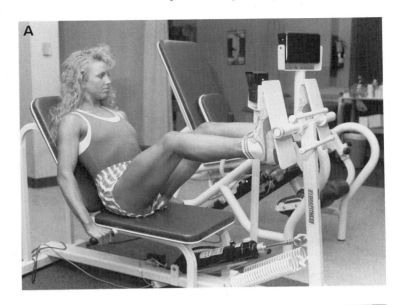

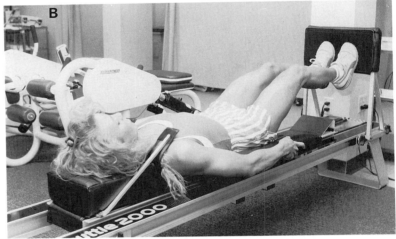

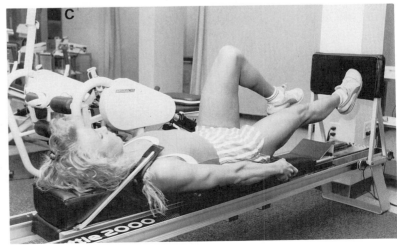

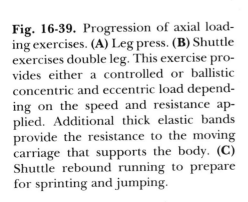

Fig. 16-39. Progression of axial loading exercises. **(A)** Leg press. **(B)** Shuttle exercises double leg. This exercise provides either a controlled or ballistic concentric and eccentric load depending on the speed and resistance applied. Additional thick elastic bands provide the resistance to the moving carriage that supports the body. **(C)** Shuttle rebound running to prepare for sprinting and jumping.

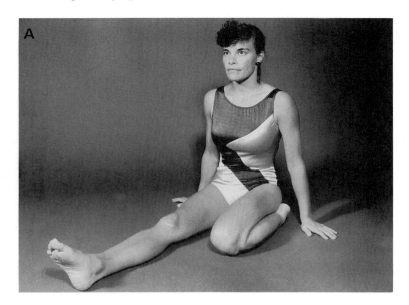

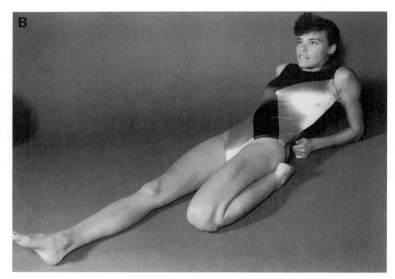

Fig. 16-40. Sitting stretch for the quadriceps. Adequate range is needed to attempt this stretch. **(A)** First sit with the leg to be stretched flexed, with the heel just to the outside of the hip. The opposite leg is extended straight out in front. **(B)** Now, slowly lean straight back until an easy stretch is felt in the quadriceps. Use hands for balance and support. Hold this easy stretch for 30 seconds. Do not let the knee lift off the floor or mat. If the knee comes up, or there is overstretching by leaning back too far, ease up on the stretch. This stretch ensures that both the quadriceps as a whole, and the rectus femoris specifically, are stretched.

Treatment

At the first sign of this complication, all resisted strengthening work and range of motion exercises should cease, and the individual should refrain from training. Anti-inflammatory agents are given and activities reduced to a minimum. After 10 days the athlete is reassessed; if the condition has not progressed, gentle range of motion and straight-leg raising exercises are begun. Progress is usually slow.

If there is no improvement, either a 7- to 10-day course of 40 mg of prednisone daily is given or a course of diphosphonates. Didronel (Etidronate disodium), which inhibits bone turnover may be tried in high risk cases. Activity is progressed when the bone mass starts to show signs of either resolving or maturing. In some instances there is a permanent loss of range. In cases where full range of motion is not possible, the normal criteria for return to sport may have to be modified. Fortunately, even large ossific masses are compatible with a full range of motion (Fig. 16-43).

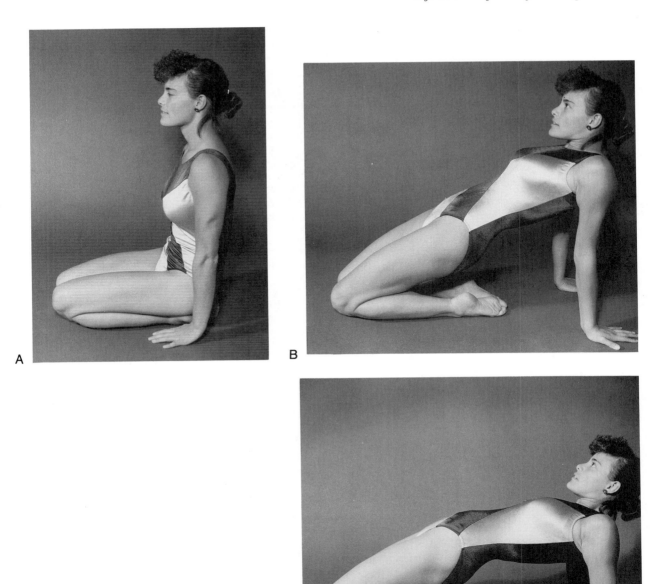

Fig. 16-41. **(A)** Starting position for the quadriceps stretch variation, which allows comparison of subtle differences between the two sides. Begin kneeling, legs together. Rest buttocks on heels. A discrepancy in range is easily seen by observing the buttock–heel difference. **(B)** From the starting position, lean backward using the arms for support and keeping the torso in a straight line with the thighs. This stretch is particularly felt in the front of the thighs. Hold the stretch for at least 10 seconds. Relax and repeat. **(C)** To maximize the stretch, if possible, continue to lean farther backward and rest on the elbows. Again, a stretch should be felt in the front of the thighs. Hold the stretch for about 10 seconds. Relax and repeat.

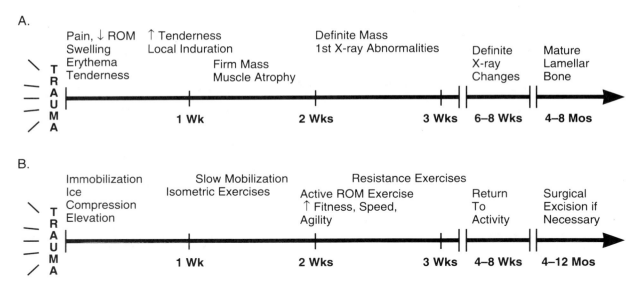

Fig. 16-42. **(A)** Clinical and radiographic events in the evolution of myositis ossificans. **(B)** Progression and conservative management of the same lesion. NSAIDs may be helpful in the early stages.

Clinical Point

CRITERIA FOR RETURN TO SPORT AFTER QUADRICEPS CONTUSION

- Normal quadriceps flexibility
- Normal quadriceps strength
- Normal muscle power balance
  -Between opposite limbs
  -Between antagonist ipsilateral leg
- Normal hip abductor/adductor ratios
- Normal hip flexor/extensor ratios
- Where applicable, fabrication of special protective padding
- No pain

Surgery

Surgical excision of a large or clinically significant mass that is limiting motion should not be undertaken unless the bone scan shows a marked quiescence of activity, which usually occurs at a minimum of 6 to 12 months. Early surgery usually results in recurrence. O'Donoghue pointed out that an adequate incision must be made to view the whole mass.[42] A computed tomographic scan helps when planning the approach that best suits the lesion (which may not be one of the traditional lateral approaches to the thigh). The mass is not covered in periosteum, and sharp dissection is necessary. Care is taken not to strip periosteum from the adjacent bone if it is attached, as it usually is. Hemostasis is important, and suction drainage is usually necessary for 24 hours.[42] It is better to discourage active range of motion for about 3 weeks, although some early, gentle, limited range on a continuous passive motion machine is advantageous. If it is necessary to remove myositic bone prior to maturation for any logistic reason, postoperative irradiation is beneficial. In any event nonsteroidal anti-inflammatory drugs (NSAIDs) are usually given for approximately 12 weeks. The use of diphosphonates may also be considered at any stage if significant risk of myositis is expected, but there is controversy as to whether they are better than simply using NSAIDs.[57,58]

Differential Diagnosis

The main dilemma with myositis ossificans is that it occurs in the same age group and site as osteogenic sarcoma. Although usually radiologically distinguishable and clinically often separable, there are distinct gross and histologic similarities. When in doubt, referral to a more experienced physician is not only appropriate but may be limb-sparing on the one hand and life-saving on the other.

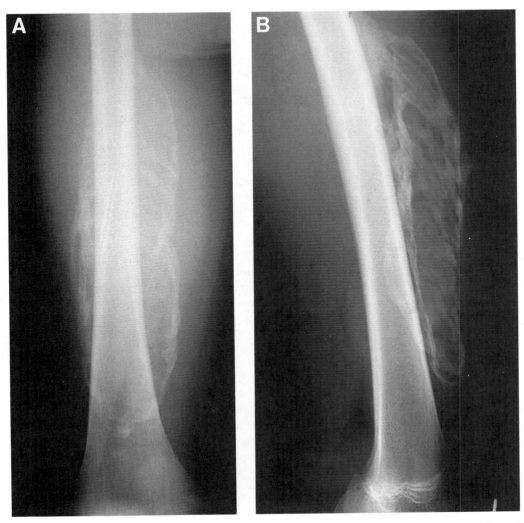

Fig. 16-43. Anteroposterior **(A)** and lateral **(B)** roentgenograms of a significant myositis ossificans lesion. Because of the deep location and attachment to bone, this individual had excellent function once range of motion was restored. However, there is a considerable predisposition to reinjury.

Summary

Prevention of quadriceps myositis ossificans begins with education. Athletes at risk, coaches, and therapists must recognize that:

1. Blunt injuries to the thigh are potentially serious.
2. Injured players should not be encouraged to continue playing.
3. Immediate first-aid measures, e.g., ice, elevation, and compression, minimize the hematoma.
4. Protected weight-bearing and avoidance of early heat, massage, and stretching reduce the tendency to form ectopic bone.
5. Judicious use of rest and slow progression during the early stages pay dividends in terms of time saved later.

ADDUCTOR STRAINS

Adductor muscle strains are frequent in ice hockey, soccer, high jump, water-skiing, and football. They usually occur at the myofascial junction and, most

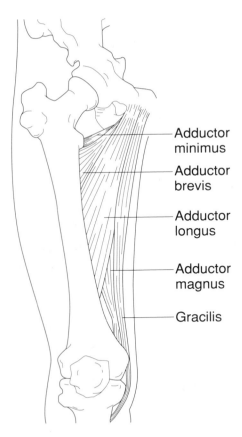

Fig. 16-44. Adductor muscles.

frequently, in adductor longus (Fig. 16-44). The usual mechanism is a sudden over-extension or stretching in the inadequately warmed up individual (Fig. 16-45).

Rarely some of the inferior pubic ramus may be avulsed, and this is discussed under the section on osteitis pubis. As with hamstring injuries, they are particularly prone to re-injury if activities are resumed prematurely. Because it is possible to continue activity in the presence of low-grade, localized groin pain, many athletes present late with chronic inflammatory lesions that take a minimum of twelve weeks to completely resolve. Occasionally, equestrian-event athletes will have a chronic but intermittent condition, which eventually is visible on roentgenogram as a spur of bone or dystrophic calcification growing into the adductor magnus or brevis origin (Fig. 16-46). Acute third-degree tears are extremely rare, and can usually be treated non-operatively. Very occasionally considerable hemorrhage results which may lead to a calcified hematoma if not adequately dispersed (Fig. 16-46).

Muscle tears are associated with inadequate range of motion and strength mismatch between the adductors of both sides.[60] Pre-season testing should seek to identify this and remedy it. Treatment consists of local therapy in the form of ice and compression at the time of injury as well as gentle range of motion after the first 12 to 24 hours, depending on the severity of injury (Fig. 16-47).

Gradually, resumption of activity commences with gentle stretching and resisted exercises, stair climbing, and cycling. The stair climbing exercise will generate good general leg strength and is an excellent precurser to running and specific adductor work (Figs. 16-48, 16-49). The cycling allows maintenance of aerobic power, and only minimally stresses the adductors. Swimming in the form of free-style, backstroke or board work can be resumed early. Controlled stretches will gradually achieve a painfree type of motion (Figs. 16-49, 16-50). Breast stroke and whip kick are not commenced until late in rehabilitation. When range of motion is within 10 degrees of the uninjured side, jogging can be commenced, but hill work and sudden starts and stops should be avoided. When jogging is comfortable, skipping is added. A continually progressive stretching program is needed to avoid re-injury (Fig. 16-51). Early isometric exercises are graduated to more rapid and vigorous resisted work (Figs. 16-52, 16-53).

When pain is absent on manual testing of muscle strength, isokinetic testing can be done. After warming up at 240 degrees/second, a test is done at 60 degrees/second. The best value of three single efforts is recorded for both sides. When the isokinetic strength deficit is less than 20 percent, compared to the good side, figure-of-eight work and wind sprints are begun. Hockey players may skate but only carrying the stick across their waist, which limits the length of stride. No sudden starts and stops are used, only figure-of-eights. Soccer players may kick the ball with the dorsum of the foot and gentle side kicking with the instep, but no full out-kicking.

When the isokinetic strength deficit is less than 10 percent and the range of motion is equal on the two sides, full activity is allowed. Treatment is continued until it is established that the overall range of motion and strength of both sides is acceptable. Usually the adductors should be 80 to 100 percent of the quadriceps power of the same leg.

The image is labeled:
Adductor minimus
Adductor brevis
Adductor longus
Adductor magnus
Gracilis

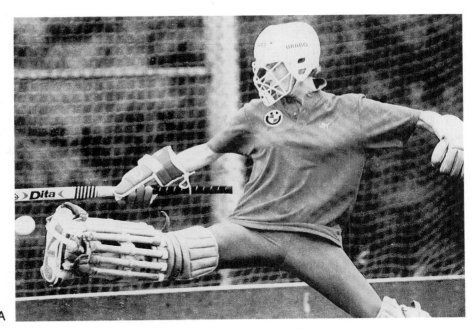

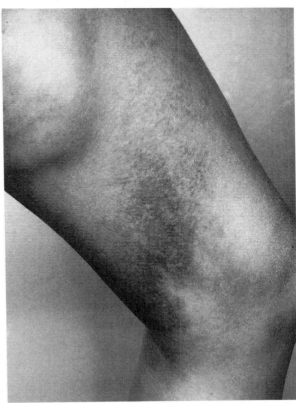

Fig. 16-45. (A) Sudden violent stretching, particularly if the athlete is inadequately warmed up, may generate an adductor tear. **(B)** Tracking of hemorrhage subsequent to a myotendinous tear.

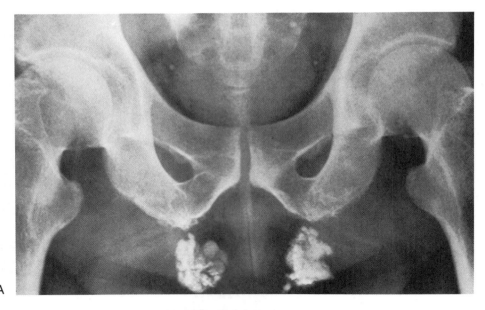

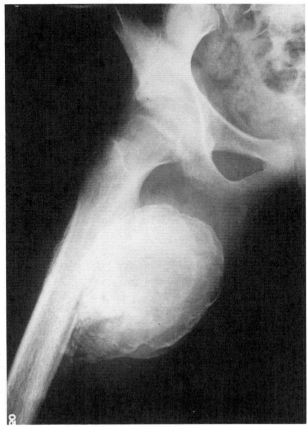

Fig. 16-46. (A) Dystrophic calcification at the origin of adductor longus in an individual who has spent many years riding horses. **(B)** Large calcified hematoma in the adductor magnus.

Internal rotation wrap

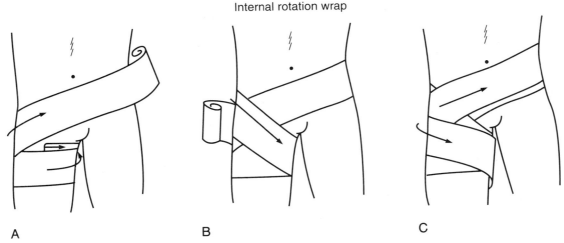

A   B   C

Fig. 16-47. Hipspica for groin strain. The materials include skin toughener, 4-inch elastic tape or a 4- to 6-inch tensor, and 1.5-inch adhesive tape. **(A)** Athlete stands with knee slightly flexed and in slight internal rotation for adductor muscle strains. **(B)** Tensor or elastic tape is applied as shown (two tensors sewed end to end are commonly used to give enough length). **(C)** At completion, 1.5-inch adhesive tape may be used to reinforce the tensor and hold it in place. If additional pressure is required, a pad may be applied over the muscle prior to application of the wrap or elastic tape.

CRAMPS

Extreme fatigue with accumulation of metabolites, undue unaccustomed exercise, strong sustained contractions, inadequate blood supply, or metabolic insufficiencies including electrolyte and mineral imbalance may precipitate cramps. Some individuals are more susceptible to cramping than others, and some muscle groups, particularly the hamstrings and gastrocnemius, are affected more frequently.

Heat cramps may occur in individuals who sweat profusely, and they are more frequent at the beginning of the warm season before acclimatization. These cramps may be more generalized and involve not only the legs but the abdominal muscles and arms. They serve as a warning to the more serious impending heat exhaustion and heat stroke.

Treatment of these cramps involves adequate hydration. In general, people suffering from cramps should ensure adequate fluid intake, minerals in the form of iron and calcium, and electrolytes such as potassium. Rarely is sodium depleted in individuals with a normal diet, except in situations of prolonged sweating in a hot climate. In these cases, the addition of more salt to the diet is all that is required. Exercise habits should be screened to see if adequate warm-up and progression of activity is being considered.

An isolated muscle cramp may be treated as follows.

1. Initially obtain a strong, resisted contraction of the antagonist. This maneuver ensures reciprocal relaxation of the agonist in this case the contracting, cramped muscle. For example, with hamstring spasm and cramp, give strong, resisted isometric work to the quadriceps. For a gastrocnemius cramp, a strong, resisted isometric contraction of the dorsiflexors suffices. The contraction should be held for several seconds after relief of the cramp.
2. This step is followed by gentle massage to the cramped muscle.
3. The cramped muscle is then gently stretched to its outer range.
4. If the cramp was particularly severe, the athlete may have to be removed from competition and hot packs applied with further massage.
5. There may be delayed muscle soreness at 24 to 48 hours after severe cramping, requiring exercise in a hot whirlpool.

In summary, the role of fitness and gradual in-

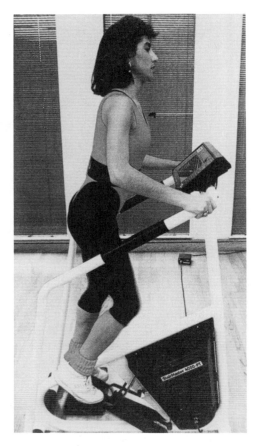

Fig. 16-48. Exercises on the step machine can be used to maintain cardiovascular fitness and general lower limb strength as soon as pain is reduced.

crease in activity level is important for the prevention of isolated cramps. In individuals with frequent cramps, consider dietary habits; and in individuals exercising in hot climates, consider electrolyte and fluid replacement.

TUMORS

The femur is one of the commonest sites for tumor in the young individual. It may be related to the large growth in length of this bone and hence the rapid cell turnover at the upper, and particularly the lower, femoral epiphyses.

Benign tumors such as bone cysts (unicameral), giant cell tumors, aneurysmal bone cysts, fibrous dysplasia, and fibrous cortical defects may produce pain if sufficiently large to cause structural change and pathologic fractures. Furthermore, osteochondroma may produce bursitis or tenderness due to friction at certain locations or may even impinge on nerves near the popliteal fossa.

In the teenager and young adult the possibility of osteosarcoma should always be borne in mind. The lower end of the femur is the commonest site. Unremitting pain, deep in nature, should always be investigated by roentgenography. Failure of the condition to respond to normal therapy for several months should raise the question of whether a second film is needed, and if further investigation is necessary in the form of scans and hematologic tests.

SUMMARY

Muscle tears and contusions are common in contact sports and activities characterized by sudden acceleration and deceleration. They present two main challenges. The first is establishing clinically the degree of injury. The second is reducing the propensity to reinjury. Early aggressive treatment aimed at dispersing the hematoma and restoring active range of motion is the key to returning the athlete to activity within the minimal time for any specific injury. Careful documentation of return of strength and strict adherence to nonballistic work until adequate rehabilitation of side-to-side deficits is necessary to prevent reinjury. The major complications of significant muscle trauma are elevated compartment pressures during the early post-trauma period and myositis ossificans later. Awareness of the potential for these problems allow early detection, which avoids a catastrophic injury in the first instance and a protracted problem in the second.

Usually the therapist is the first to detect the onset of myositis ossificans because of the decreasing range and increasing pain. Such diagnosis allows adequate adjustment of therapy and the institution of appropriate drug therapy. Tumors of the thigh musculature are rare, but the distal femur is the commonest site of osteosarcoma. Trauma does not induce malignancy, but incidental injury may bring to the physician's attention an underlying asymptomatic neoplasm, which may then be dealt with appropriately. Constant alertness to the wide differential diagnosis of all recreationally induced pain is the key.

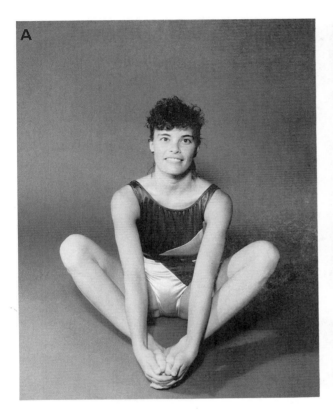 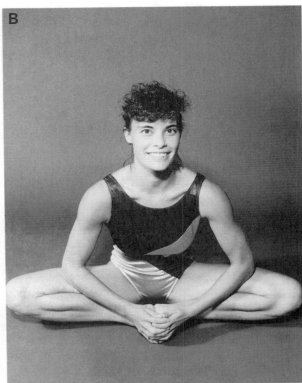

Fig. 16-49. **(A)** Starting position for the groin stretch. Sit on the floor and place the soles of the feet together. Grasp the ankles with the hands and rest the elbows on knees. **(B)** Groin stretch. Press down on the knees with the elbows until a stretch is felt in the groin. Hold this position for at least 10 seconds. Relax and repeat.

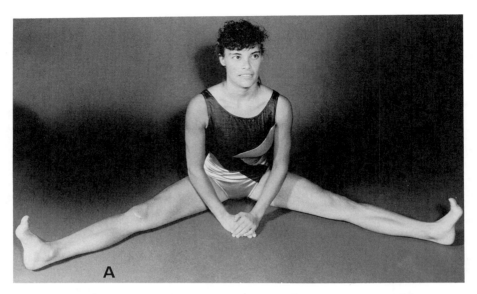

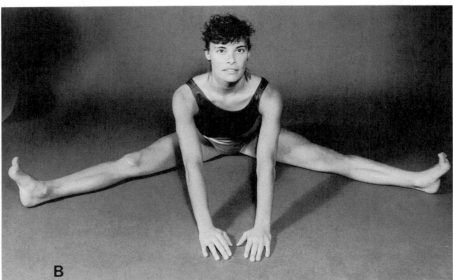

Fig. 16-50. **(A)** Starting position for the straddle stretch. Sit on the floor with the legs straddled. Keep the back and legs straight. **(B)** Straddle stretch. Lean forward to the center until a stretch is felt. Try to keep the back straight. Hold the stretch for at least 10 seconds, relax, repeat. If possible, continue leaning forward from this position and try to touch the chest to the floor.

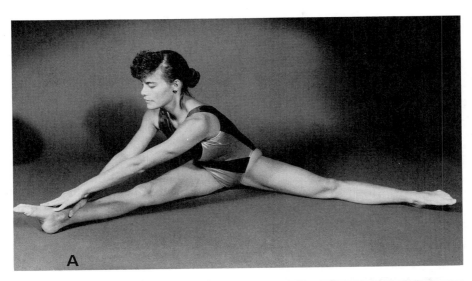

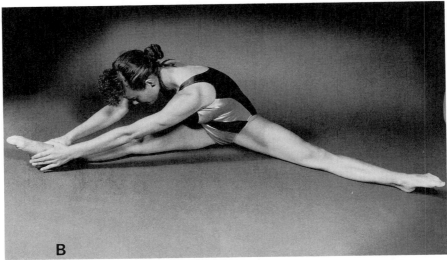

Fig. 16-51. **(A)** Straddle stretch to the right side. Sit on the floor and straddle the legs, as in Figure 16-51A. With the toes pointing toward the ceiling and the legs straight, grasp one leg with both hands and lean forward until a stretch is felt. Try to keep the back straight and concentrate on trying to touch the chest to the knee. Hold this position for about 10 seconds, relax, repeat. Repeat this stretch leaning to the opposite side. **(B)** Straddle stretch to the right with the chest to the knee.

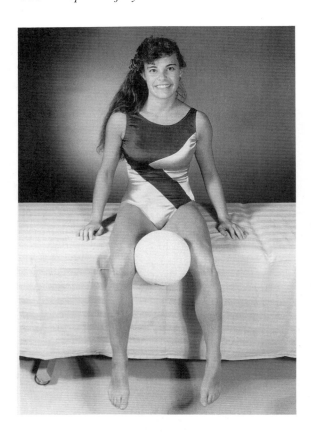

Fig. 16-52. Leg adduction. Sit on a table or chair and place a ball between the knees; squeeze for at least 6 seconds, relax, and repeat.

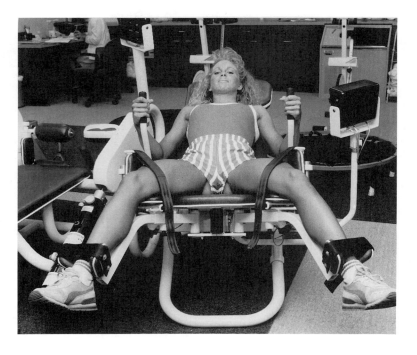

Fig. 16-53. Adduction strengthening using a polykinetic abductor and adductor exerciser. If there is a pre-existing knee problem, the thigh straps ensure that resistance is applied mainly above the knee.

REFERENCES

1. Dornan P: A report on 140 hamstring injuries. Aust J Sports Med 4:30, 1971
2. Gordon HM: Physiotherapy of muscle strains of the lower limb. Physiotherapy. J Chartered Soc Physiother 61(4):102, 1975
3. Reid DC: Functional Anatomy and Joint Mobilization. University of Alberta Press, Edmonton
4. Reid DC: Assessment and Treatment of the Injured Athlete. Teaching manual, University of Alberta, Edmonton, 1984
5. Grace TG: Muscle imbalance in extremity injury: a perplexing relationship. Sports Med 2:77, 1985
6. Grace TG, Sweetzer ER, Nelson MA et al: Isokinetic muscle imbalance and knee joint injuries. J Bone Joint Surg [Am] 66:734, 1984
7. Campbell DE, Glenn W: Foot pounds of torque of the normal knee and rehabilitation of the postmeniscectomy knee. Phys Ther 59:418, 1979
8. Heiser TM, Weber J, Sullivan G et al: Prophylaxis and management of hamstring muscle injuries in intercollegiate football players. Am J Sports Med 12:368, 1984
9. Cahill BR, Griffiths EH: Effect of pre-season conditioning on the incidence and severity of high school football knee injuries. Am J Sports Med 6:180, 1978
10. Knight JL: Strength imbalances and knee injury. Physician Sports Med 8:140, 1980
11. Gleim GW, Nicholas JA, Weldo JN: Isokinetic evaluation following leg injuries. Physician Sports Med 6:75, 1978
12. Hagerman PA, Gillespie DM, Hill ID: Effects of speed ND limb dominance on eccentric and concentric testing of the knee. J Orthop Sports Phys Ther 10:59, 1988
13. Cibulka M, Rose SJ, Delitto A et al: A comparison of two treatments for hamstring strains. Phys Ther 64:750, 1984
14. Morris AF: Sports Medicine: Prevention of Athletic Injuries. William C. Brown Publications, Iowa, 1984
15. Brubaker CE, James SL: Injuries to runners. J Sports Med 2:189, 1984
16. Garrett WE, Califf JC, Bassett FH: Histochemical correlates of hamstring injuries. Am J Sports Med 12:98, 1984
17. Ekstrand J, Gillquist J: Soccer injuries and their mechanisms: a prospective study. Med Sci Sports Exerc 15:267, 1983
18. Grant JC, Basmajian JV: Grant's Method of Anatomy. Williams & Wilkins, Baltimore, 1965
19. Bateman J, Trott A: The Foot and Ankle. Thieme-Stratton, New York, 1980
20. Mann RA, Hagy J: Biomechanics of walking, running and sprinting. Am J Sports Med 8:345, 1980
21. Agre JC, Baxter TL: Strength and flexibility characteristics of collegiate soccer players. Arch Phys Med Rehabil 62:539, 1981
22. Brewer BJ: Athletic injuries: musculotendinous unit. Clin Orthop 23:30, 1962
23. Baker BE: Current concepts in the diagnosis and treatment of musculotendinous injuries. Med Sci Sports Exerc 16:323, 1984
24. Christensen CS: Strength, the common variable in hamstring strain. Athletic Trainer 7:36, 1972
25. Burkett LN: Causative factors in hamstring strain. Med Sci Sports Exerc 2:39, 1970
26. Agre JC: Hamstring injuries: proposed etiologic factors, prevention and treatment. Sports Med 2:21, 1985
27. Garrett WE, Rich FR, Nikolaou PK et al: Computed tomography of hamstring muscle strains. Med Sci Sports Exerc 21:506, 1989
28. Roy S, Irvin R: Sports Medicine: Prevention Evaluation, Management and Rehabilitation. Prentice Hall, Englewood Cliffs, NJ, 1983
29. Coole WG: The analysis of hamstring strains and their rehabilitation. J Orthop Sports Med 4:30, 1971
30. Sutton G: Hamstring by hamstring strains: a review of the literature. J Orthop Sports Phys Ther 5:184, 1984
31. Burkett LN: Investigation into hamstring strains: the case of the hybrid muscle. J Sports Med 3:228, 1976
32. Wyatt MP, Edwards AM: Comparison of quadriceps and hamstring torque values during isokinetic exercise. J Orthop Sports Phys Ther 3:48, 1981
33. Muckle DS: Associated factors in recurrent groin and hamstring injuries. Br J Sports Med 16:37, 1982
34. Raether PM, Lutter LD: Recurrent compartment syndrome in the posterior thigh: a report of a case. Am J Sports Med 10:40, 1982
35. Currier DP, Kumar S: Knee force during isometric contraction at different hip angles. Physiother Can 34:198, 1982
36. Nicholas JA, Hershman EB: The Lower Extremity and Spine in Sports Medicine. Vol. 2. CV Mosby, St. Louis, 1986
37. Hackney AC, Deutsch DT, Gilliam TB: Assessment of maximum isometric, isotonic and isokinetic leg extensor strength in young adult females. National Strength Coaches Association Journal Aug/Sept: 28, 1984
38. Hald RD, Bottjen EJ: Effects of visual feedback on maximal and submaximal isokinetic test measurements of normal quadriceps and hamstrings. J Orthop Sports Phys Ther 9:86, 1987
39. Kennedy JC, Willis RB: The effect of local steroid injections on tendons: a biomechanical and microscopic correlative study. Am J Sports Med 4:11, 1976

40. MacEachern AG, Plewes JL: Bilateral simultaneous spontaneous rupture of the quadriceps tendons. J Bone Joint Surg [Br] 66:81, 1984

41. Levy M, Goldstein J, Rosner M: A method of repair for quadriceps tendon and patellar ligament (tendon) ruptures without cast immobilization. Clin Orthop 218:297, 1987

42. O'Donoghue DH: Treatment of Injuries to Athletes. 3rd Ed. WB Saunders, Philadelphia, 1976

43. Kalund DN: The Injured Athlete. JB Lippincott, Philadelphia, 1982

44. Reid DC, Kelly R: Selected problems of the thigh and knee to illustrate some basic techniques of rehabilitation. In Taylor AW (ed): The Scientific Aspects of Sports Training. Charles C Thomas, Springfield, IL, 1975

45. Mubarak SJ, Owen CA, Hargens AR et al: Acute compartment syndromes: diagnosis and treatment with the aid of a wick catheter. J Bone Joint Surg [Am] 60:1091, 1978

46. Torg JS, Vegso JJ, Torg E: Rehabilitation of Athletic Injuries: An Atlas of Therapeutic Exercises. Year Book Medical Publishers, Chicago, 1987

47. Magee DJ: Orthopaedic Physical Assessment. WB Saunders, Philadelphia, 1987

48. Gajdosik R: Rectus femoris muscle tightness: intratester reliability of an active knee flexion test. J Orthop Sports Phys Ther 6:289, 1985

49. Voss DE, Ionfa MK, Myers BJ: Proprioceptive Neuromuscular Facilitation. Harper & Row, New York, 1986

50. Engle RP, Canner GG: Proprioceptive neuromuscular facilitation (PNF) and modified procedures for anterior cruciate ligament instability. J Orthop Sports Phys Ther 11:230, 1989

51. Kramer JF, Semple JE: Comparison of selected strengthening techniques of normal quadriceps. Phys Can 35:300, 1983

52. Steele BE: Protective pads for athletes. Phys Sports Med 13:179, 1985

53. Rothwell A: Quadriceps hematoma: a prospective clinical study. Clin Orthop 171:97, 1982

54. Jackson DW, Feagin JA: Quadriceps contusions in young athletes. J Bone Joint Surg [Am] 55:95, 1973

55. Millar AP: Acute muscle injuries of the leg. Med J Aust 1:264, 1973

56. Thorndike A: Myositis ossificans traumatica. J Bone Joint Surg 22:315, 1940

57. Russell RGG, Smith R: Diphosphonates: experimental and clinical aspects. J Bone Joint Surg [Br] 55:66, 1973

58. Siegal BA, Engel WK, Derrer EC: Localization of technetium 99m diphosphonate in acutely injured muscle. Neurology 27:23, 1977

59. Ryan AJ: Quadriceps strain, rupture and charlie horse. Med Sci Sports 1:106, 1969

60. Merrifield HH, Cowan FJ: Groin strain injuries in ice hockey. J Sports Med 1:41, 1973

Problems of the Hip, Pelvis, and Sacroiliac Joint

17

Sydenham was called "a man of many doubts" and therein lay the secret of his great strength.
—William Osler, 1905

At first glance injuries to the pelvis and hip do not seem to have a prominent place in sports medicine. Nevertheless, contusions to the bony prominences around the pelvis are common, and the many apophyses are susceptible to inflammation and avulsion during the growth period. Furthermore, the more dramatic injuries of dislocated hip and pelvic fracture require immediate expert attention and indeed in some circumstances may even be life-threatening.

In a survey by Lloyd-Smith, at the University of British Columia Sports Medicine Clinic, which has a patient population with a bias toward running sports, approximately 5 percent of the injuries were to the hip and pelvis.[1,2] This low incidence belies their importance, as they are often difficult to diagnose and have a tendency to recur and become chronic. Many of the problems are disabling. The three most common bone problems were sacroiliitis, pelvic and femoral neck stress fractures, and osteitis pubis (Fig. 17-1). Gluteus medius strain or tendinitis, trochanteric bursitis, and hamstring strain made up most of the soft tissue injuries (Fig. 17-2).

There is always a dilemma as to how to divide (1) the trunk from the spine and (2) the pelvis from its visceral contents and the hip joint. This chapter focuses on problems of the bony pelvis, the hip joint, and conditions affecting the sacroiliac joint, but not injuries to the pelvic floor, viscera or reproductive system.

ANATOMY

The bony pelvis transmits the weight of the body through the acetabulum to the lower limbs, and, conversely, the thrusting propulsive movements of the legs are transmitted to the body. The hindlimbs extend and medially rotate from the fetal position of flexion, so the extensor muscles of the thigh in the adult lie anteriorly, on the same aspect as the flexor muscles of the hip. The broadening, flaring, and forward rotation of the iliac portion of the pelvis has evolved to allow efficient bipedalism (Fig. 17-3). Of course during evolutionary development some muscles in humans have gained in importance and significance. Other groups, which are key muscles in some of the other primates, play a surprisingly unimportant role in man's ability to stand, walk, and run.[3,4] Which of these adaptations came first is of interest only to anthropologists.

Hip Joint

The hip joint is structurally strong, with the hemispherical head of the femur fitting snugly in the acetabulum (Fig. 17-4). It is classed as a multiaxial ball and socket joint and thus has three degrees of freedom.[5] The articular surfaces are made more congruent by the triangular fibrocartilage in the acetab-

601

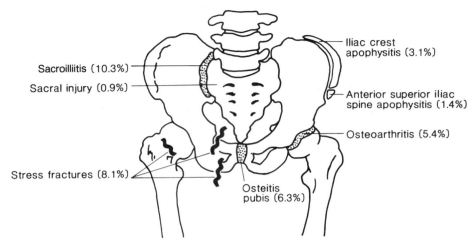

Fig. 17-1. Incidence of bony overuse injuries to the hip and pelvis. (After Lloyd-Smith et al.,[2] with permission.)

ulum. The capsule, strong and dense, is attached to the margins of the acetabulum, and it thickens around the neck of the femur by encircling fibers that form a collar, the zona orbicularis (Fig. 17-5).

The capsule is further reinforced by the iliofemoral, ischiofemoral, and pubofemoral intrinsic ligaments. These ligaments are spiral in nature, probably owing to the rotation of the lower limbs during development; they play a part in limiting the range of mo-

tion, possibly at the hip and joint. Use of the iliofemoral ligament in particular helps to stabilize the hip during gait and the weight-bearing phases of extension. It contributes significantly to the close-packed position.

The neck–shaft angle is approximately 120 to 130 degrees in the adult, and there is an average of 14 degrees of anteversion (Fig. 17-6). Because of this special arrangement of the neck of the femur in re-

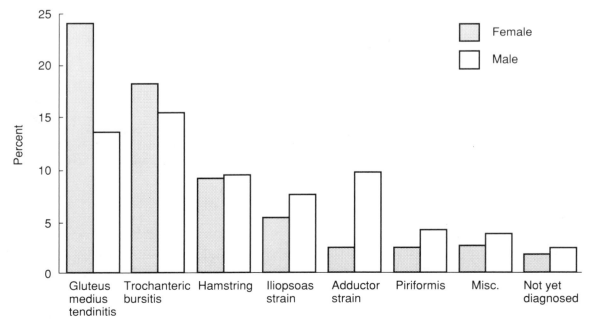

Fig. 17-2. Soft tissue overuse injuries to the hip and pelvis. They occur mainly in the running population. (Data from Lloyd-Smith et al.[2])

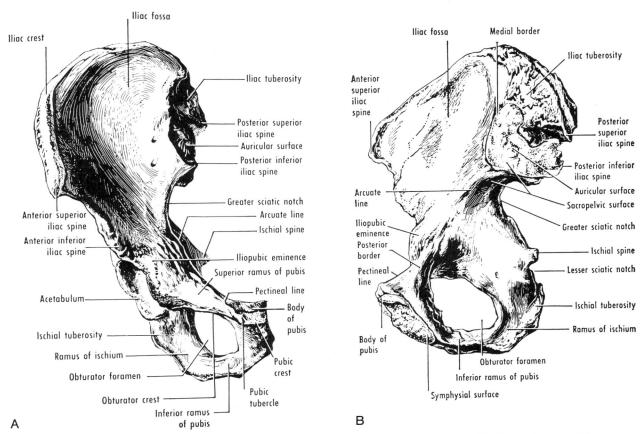

Fig. 17-3. Major bony landmarks of the pelvis. **(A)** Anteroposterior view. **(B)** Lateral view. (From Gardner et al.,[13] with permission.)

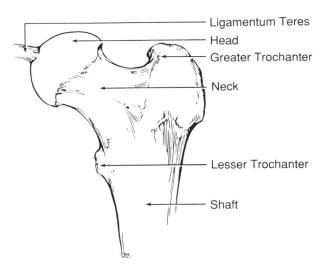

Fig. 17-4. Proximal femur with bony landmarks.

spect to the shaft, the angular movements of the thigh convert to rotatory movements in the joint. The joint is structurally secure enough to prevent significant accessory movements. (Fig. 17-7).

The resting position of the hip is at approximately 30 degrees of flexion and 30 degrees of abduction, which provides maximum capsular laxity. The capsular pattern of restriction is usually flexion lost more than abduction followed by decreased internal rotation. However, frequently internal rotation and extention are primarily affected with synovitis and thus there is neither a constant pattern of movement or degree of involvement. The close-packed position is full extension with internal rotation and abduction.

Under low loads the joint surfaces may be slightly incongruous, but under heavy loading there is excellent surface contact. Peak focal pressures during walking may be up to 1,000 pounds per square inch

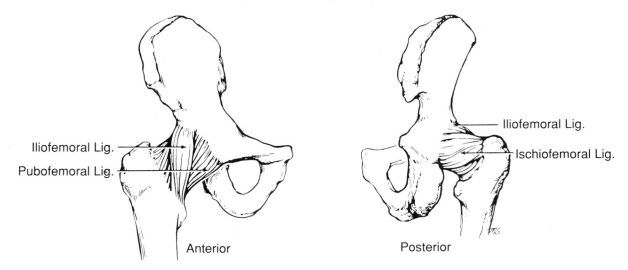

Fig. 17-5. Anterior and posterior capsular structures of the hip.

and standing from a sitting position 3,000 pounds per square inch.[6] These forces represent overall pressures of 1.3 to 5.8 times body weight when walking.

Considering the structural stability, it is amazing that a large range of motion is still possible at the hip joint. It may be accounted for in part by the fact that the neck of the femur is much smaller in circumference than the articular head.

Hip Motion

Movement of the hip is controlled by lumbar segments 2, 3, 4, and 5; and although a simplification, in general the following plan is an indication of the in-nervation of the muscle's movement of the joint. Lumbar segments 2 and 3 flex, adduct, and rotate internally, whereas lumbar segments 4 and 5 extend, abduct, and rotate externally.

Flexion

Flexion takes place through a large range of motion, approximately 140 degrees, and is usually limited by apposition of the soft tissues of the thigh on the abdomen. However, if the knee is maintained in the extended position, tension in the hamstring muscles usually drops its flexion toward 90 degrees in the untrained individual, although with adequate

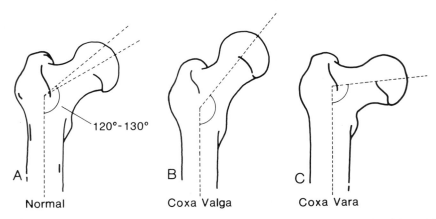

Fig. 17-6. (A) Normal neck–shaft angle (angle of inclination), approximately 120 to 130 degrees in adults. **(B)** Increased angle—coxa valga. **(C)** Decreased angle—coxa vara.

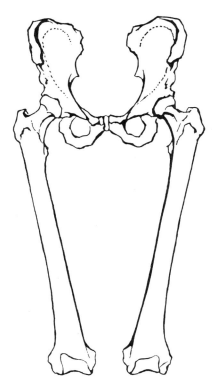

Fig. 17-7. Neck–shaft angle and the offset of the knee joints allows efficient weight transmission in the erect position. The mechanical axis is from the middle of the femoral head to the middle of the knee joint.

stretching flexion is possible way past 120 degrees, as is obvious in many ballet dancers.[7] Maximum force generated by the hip flexors is in the range of 30 to 35 degrees (Table 17-1).

Quick Facts

HIP RANGE OF MOTION[7,8]

Motion	ROM (degrees)	Range (degrees)
Flexion	150	130–150[a]
Extension	5	0–15
Abduction	45	40–50[b]
Adduction	25	20–35
External rotation	65	50–80
Internal rotation	56	45–65

[a] With knee flexion.
[b] No associated lateral rotation.

Quick Facts

HIP AGONIST/ANTAGONIST RATIOS (PERCENT)[9]

Motion	At 60 Degrees/Second		At 180 Degrees/Second	
	Male	Female	Male	Female
Flexion*-extension	75	70	70	65
Abduction*-adduction	80	75	65	60
Internal*-external	90	95	90	90

*Denotes weaker muscle.

Iliopsoas

The iliopsoas muscles have been discussed extensively by many investigators. Usually the action of the iliacus and psoas muscles are discussed separately, as the psoas muscle obviously has some direct influence on the lumbar spine. During dissection of the cadaver, the iliacus is shown to be a powerful muscle, and the psoas major is dense enough to show up as a definite shadow on roentgenograms of the lumbar region. These two muscles unite to form a tendon that is separated from the anterior capsule of the hip joint by the iliopectineal or psoas bursa (Fig. 17-8).

In normal resting posture with the weight of the body balanced over the legs, the activity in the iliopsoas is minimal. The iliofemoral ligament in this instance plays an important part in supporting the pelvis and lower limbs. However, any tilting of the pelvis or deviation of the trunk in the midline brings the iliposoas group strongly into play to maintain upright posture.

When the role of the iliopsoas is discussed in relation to internal and external rotation of the femur, many contradictions in the literature become apparent. Basmajian brought out the main point when he stressed that the iliopsoas muscle is primarily a hip flexor, and any aid that it may give to rotation is incidental and purely academic.[8] It is probable that this muscle is capable of both medial and lateral rotation according to the position of the femoral shaft in relation to the midline of the body. Iliopsoas may develop a tensile pull of about 1,000 pounds (450 kg) in the average adult; despite this fact, it is interesting

TABLE 17-1. Muscles and Segmental Supply of Hip Motion

Motion	Muscle	Nerve	Segmental Level
Flexion	*Iliacus*	Femoral	L2,L3
	Psoas	Segmentally from plexus	L2,3,4
	Rectus femoris	Femoral	L2,L3
	Sartorius	Femoral	L2,L3
	Adductor brevis[a]	Obturator	L2,L3
	Adductor magnus[a] (oblique fibers)	Obturator	L2,L3
	Pectineus	Femoral (acc. obturator)	L2,L3
	Tensor fascia lata	Superior gluteal	L4,L5,S1
Extension	*Gluteus maximus*	Inferior gluteal	L5,S1,S2
	Biceps femoris (long head)	Sciatic (tibial portion)	L5,S1,S2
	Semimembranosus	Sciatic (tibial portion)	L5,S1
	Semitendinosus	Sciatic (tibial portion)	L5,S1
	Gluteus medius	Superior gluteal	L4,L5,S1
	Adductor magnus (vertical fibers)	Sciatic	L4,L5
Abduction	*Gluteus medius*	Superior gluteal	L4,L5,S1
	Gluteus minimus	Superior gluteal	L4,L5,S1
	Tensor fascia lata	Superior gluteal	L4,L5,S1
	Sartorius	Femoral	L2,L3
	Gluteus maximus (upper fibers)	Inferior gluteal	L5,S1,2
Adduction	*Adductor brevis*	Obturator	L3,L4
	Adductor magnus	Obturator and sciatic	L3,4,5
	Adductor longus	Obturator	L3,L4
	Pectineus	Femoral (access, obturator)	L3,L4
	Gracilis	Obturator	L3,L4

Prime movers are in italics.

[a] More contribution with hip in extended position.

to note that when it is transplanted to compensate for weak or deficient abductors, flexion of the thighs is accomplished adequately by the remaining muscles.[9] If both iliopsoas muscles are paralyzed, there is some difficulty raising the body from the supine to the sitting position. With normal gait, the iliopsoas probably works to help to initiate the forward motion of the thigh during the early phase, and this action becomes progressively more important as the speed of progression increases into the sprinting posture.

The action of these muscles on the spine is normally thought of in relation to maintenance of the pelvic tilt and lumbar lordosis. Bilateral action produces flexion of the trunk, and unilateral action produces lateral flexion of the spine of the same side but rotation of the vertebra to the opposite side.[3] The following clinical points should be noted.

1. The psoas bursa may be inflamed and edematous due to a variety of conditions, which causes limitation of movement due to pain in a typical psoatic gait, i.e., leg externally rotated and adducted with the knee in slight flexion, if the pain is severe enough. This process seems to relieve the tension of the muscle and hence relieve the inflamed structures.

2. Conditions of the central nervous system (CNS) that produce flexor spasms are particularly manifested by strong contraction of the psoas muscle.

3. In addition to the above, conditions that cause chronic postural flexion of the hip, e.g., prolonged bed rest or certain running or jogging styles, may lead to adaptive shortening of the iliopsoas muscle along with the anterior capsular structures of the hip joint. It can be particularly noticeable with degenerative changes of the hip joint, and when severe, attempts to normalize the gait produce forward flexion of the trunk or excessive lordosis of the lumbar spine. This posture is not only inefficient and fatiguing, it may cause pain and secondary pathologic changes in the spine.

4. Some studies have shown that the iliopsoas works minimally up to 30 degrees of hip flexion, after which electromyographic activity from the muscle increases. When only mechanical factors such as line of pull are considered, it is obvious that the inner range for this muscle is by far the strongest.

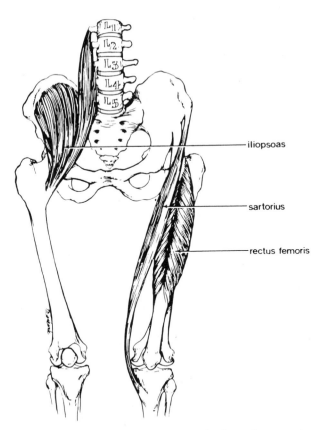

Fig. 17-8. Hip flexors. Iliopsoas is the prime mover. (After Henry,[5] with permission.)

Extension

Much has been written about the existence of true extension from the midline without associated movement of the pelvis. At best, there is probably only 10 to 20 degrees of true extension available owing to the tension in the anteriorly placed iliofemoral and ischiofemoral ligaments as well as the iliopsoas muscle.[3] Pelvic tilting and rotation appear to increase this range in the living subject; and this movement, along with lordosis of the lumbar spine, may go unnoticed unless particular attention is paid to them. Thus with re-education of hip movement, and in goniometry of this region, the pelvis must be deliberately and carefully stabilized. The prime movers are the gluteus maximus, biceps femoris, and the semimembranosus and semitendinosus (Table 17-1). These muscles generate their greatest force at about 40 to 45 degrees short of the midline. Leaning forward with the trunk alters the origin of these muscles and allows greater extensive power further into the range of extension.[9]

Gluteus Maximus

The large bulk of the gluteus maximus is associated with development of the human posture (Fig. 17-9). Anthropologically, evidence points to the fact that the gluteus medius and gluteus minimus evolved into abductors to help stabilize the pelvis during walking and running; the insignificant gluteus maximus of most primates has become progressively hypertrophied to take over the function of extension of the hip in humans.

It is, in fact, capable of producing extension and lateral rotation of the femur. During normal walking and standing there is little or no activity in the gluteus maximus, and extension is usually produced by the hamstrings. Gluteus maximus may work only to check the forward momentum of the swing leg during the normal gait cycle. In prone position, extension of the hip produces little activity in the gluteus maximus until 30 degrees is reached.[10] The main function of the gluteus maximus seems to be the following.

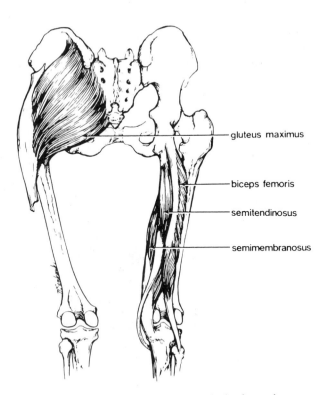

Fig. 17-9. Gluteus maximus muscle is the prime extensor of the hip but is assisted significantly by the hamstrings (biceps femoris, semitendinosus, and semimembranosus). These muscles also flex the knee. (After Henry,[5] with permission.)

1. Adding power to the extension thrust in activities such as running, jumping, and climbing stairs.
2. Working concentrically when rising from the seated position to standing and eccentrically when adopting a squatting or sitting position.
3. Controlling movements of flexion of the trunk, where they work (a) eccentrically with origin and insertion reversed to lower the trunk against gravity and (b) concentrically to return the trunk to the upright position. They exert their influence via the pelvis.

The gluteus maximus is one of the most powerful muscles in the body, and its importance in all of the propulsive movements in sport cannot be overlooked. Power to accelerate from the standing position, jumping, and pivoting require extreme control from the gluteal group.

The axis of flexion and extension is on the line connecting the centers of two femoral heads. The axis has clinical significance for the placement of hinges on an orthosis. On the surface of the body it may be located by palpating the tip of the greater trochanter, which is approximately in line, and on the level, with this axis. Thus the hinges, which are usually placed slightly anterior to the tip of the greater trochanter, also cause the least impedance to the swing of the leg in gait and flexion of the hip joint when sitting.

Abduction

The movement of abduction is limited by tightness of the adductor muscles to about 50 degrees. As the limits of this motion are approached there is a great tendency to tilt the pelvis, which prevents impingement of the greater trochanter.[11] Structurally the joint itself permits up to 90 degrees of movement if the leg is rotated laterally. In the dancer and gymnast this range is greatly exceeded. The axis of movement is horizontal, through the head of the femur. In addition to muscular tightness, range of motion is limited by the pubofemoral ligament and the medial limb of the iliofemoral ligament. Prime movers are the gluteus medius and gluteus minimus, and there is some assistance from the tensor fasciae latae (Table 17-1). The maximum power is generated by these muscles in the neutral position and decreases as the limb moves into the range of abduction.

Gluteus Medius and Gluteus Minimus

The gluteus medius and gluteus minimus muscles are abductors of the thigh and stabilizers of the pelvis (Fig. 17-10). The line of pull of the gluteus medius is a straight line from the top of the greater trochanter to the center of the hip joint. The muscle pulls almost at right angles, giving it a considerable mechanical advantage and hence the ability to exert a strong force. The anterior fibers of the group are in a position to produce medial rotation of the thigh. Muscles are electrically silent during relaxed standing. Gluteus medius and gluteus minimus contract strongly at the start of the swing phase of walking. This movement is enhanced by jogging, running, and jumping. Their contraction is a stabilizing factor that prevents the pelvis from falling on the contralateral or unsupported side. Even during normal locomotion the

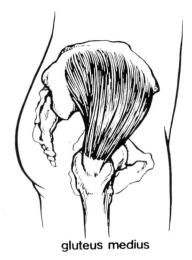
gluteus medius

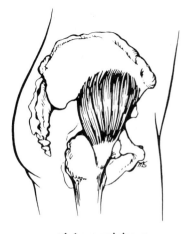
gluteus minimus

Fig. 17-10. Gluteus medius and slightly deeper gluteus minimus attaching to the greater trochanter are the prime abductors. (After Henry,[5] with permission.)

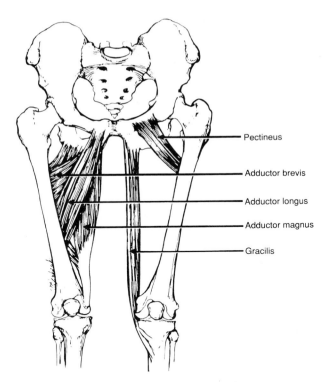

Fig. 17-11. Adductors of the hip. Adductor magnus is the most powerful; adductor longus is the most susceptible to muscle strain; and gracilis, with its distal tendon working across the knee, is frequently sacrificed for autogenous graft material for anterior cruciate ligament (ACL) reconstruction. (After Henry,[5] with permission.)

pelvis usually rises and falls on the unsupported side, a movement referred to as the Trendelenburg sign. When the movement becomes excessive, the pattern of walking is called the Trendelenburg gait. It is pathologic. These muscles, when used as prime movers for abduction, exert their most power within their ranges of motion.

> **Quick Facts**
>
> **ABDUCTION**
>
> - Usually limited by tight adductors
> - Gluteus medius and minimus prime movers
> - Weakness gives Trendelenburg lurch
> - Important muscles for balance and stabilizing pelvis

Adduction

Pure adduction is obviously limited by apposition with the opposite leg. However, if the contralateral limb is flexed, about 40 degrees of adduction is possible. The limiting factor in this instance is the lateral band of the iliofemoral (Ligamentum teres) ligament and the ligament of the head of the femur. The prime movers are the adductor magnus, adductor brevis, and adductor longus (Table 17-1; Fig. 17-11).

Hip Rotation

There are approximately 45 degrees of both internal and external rotation with the leg in either flexion or extension (Table 17-2). Internal rotation is limited by the tightness in the ischiofemoral ligament and the external rotators. Conversely, external rotation is restricted by the lateral band of the iliofemoral ligament, the pubofemoral ligament, and the tension in the internal rotators. The degree of anteversion at the femoral neck also has some bearing on the available range as does the angulation and orientation of the acetabulum to a minor degree. The major muscles producing rotation are outlined in Table 17-3 (Fig. 17-12). The external rotators are marginally stronger

TABLE 17-2. Normal Hip Rotation Related to Age and Gender

| | Normal Hip Rotation (degrees) | | | | | |
Rotation	4 Years	6 Years	8 Years	11 Years	15 Years	Adult[a]
Internal						
Women	60 (10.2)	58 (8.5)	57 (8.2)	50 (8.9)	48 (8.7)	52 (9.2)
Men	51 (7.6)	51 (9.0)	51 (9.5)	46 (7.2)	41 (7.7)	38 (7.6)
External						
Women	44 (9.6)	44 (7.6)	43 (7.9)	42 (7.4)	42 (7.0)	41 (7.7)
Men	48 (7.8)	47 (9.1)	42 (9.9)	42 (7.9)	43 (7.1)	43 (7.3)

Results are expressed as the mean (SD).
[a] Varies considerably according to population.
(From Svenningsen et al.,[18] with permission.)

The labels in the figure read: Pectineus, Adductor brevis, Adductor longus, Adductor magnus, Gracilis.

TABLE 17-3. Hip Rotation and Segmental Supply

Motion	Muscle	Nerve	Sequential Level
Internal rotation	*Gluteus medius* (ant. fibers)	Superior gluteal	L4,L5,S1
	Gluteus minimus	Superior gluteal	L4,L5,S1
	Tensor fascia lata	Superior gluteal	L4,L5,S1
External rotation	*Obturator externus*	Obturator (post br.)	L3,L4
	Obturator internus	Nerve to obturator int.	L3,L4
	Superior gemellus	Nerve to obturator int.	S1,S2
	Inferior gemellus	Nerve to quadratus fem.	L4,L5,S1
	Quadratus femoris	Nerve to quadratus fem.	L4,L5,S1
	Piriformis	Segmental from plexus	S1,S2
	Gluteus maximus	Inferior gluteal	L5,S1,S2
	Gluteus medius (post fibers)	Superior gluteal	L4,L5,S1
	Pectineus	Femoral (access. obturator)	L2,L3
	Adductor brevis[a]	Obturator	L2,L3
	Adductor longus[a]	Obturator	L2,L3
	Adductor magnus (oblique)[a]	Obutrator	L2,L3
	Sartorius	Femoral	L2,L3

Prime movers are in italics.
[a] More contribution with hip in extended position.

than the internal rotators (Table 17-4). Loss of rotational range and pain with rotation are *considered the major indicators of hip disease*.[9]

Bony Architecture

Because the pelvis is the linking system between the trunk and lower limbs, it is obvious that there is a reflection of this function in the trabecular pattern

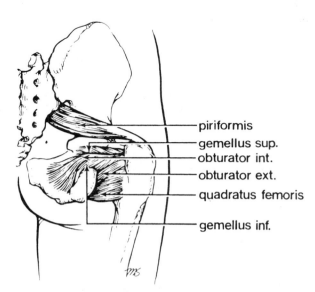

piriformis
gemellus sup.
obturator int.
obturator ext.
quadratus femoris
gemellus inf.

Fig. 17-12. Short external rotators of the hip closely approximate the hip joint capsule.

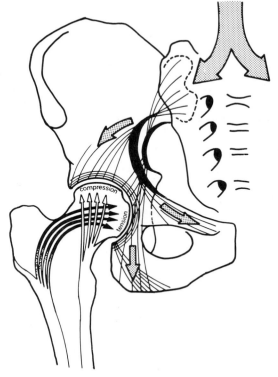

Fig. 17-13. Primary compression and tension trabeculae of the femoral neck and head carry on through the pelvis, iliac crest, and lumbar spine. (Adapted from Kapandji,[12] with permission.)

TABLE 17-4. Isokinetic Values for Hip External-Internal Rotation[a]

Rotation	Peak Torque		Normalized Peak Torque[b]		Peak Torque Ratios	
	Men	Women	Men	Women	Men	Women
Internal	27.5 (4.4)	19.1 (5.5)	34.0 (5.3)	32.8 (8.1)	1.1 (0.2)	1.2 (0.2)
External	29.5 (6.0)	21.3 (6.8)	36.3 (5.8)	36.5 (10.2)		

Results are expressed as the mean (SD).
[a] Thirty degrees per second. Torque in Newton meters.
[b] Normalized for body weight. Newson meters per Kg bwt.
(Data from Hunt et al.[19]).

of the pelvis and femur (Fig. 17-13). Its trabecular system is divided into a main and an accessory system.[12–14]

The main series consists in two sets of trabeculae, which fan out into the head and neck.

1. The first set arises from the cortical layers of the lateral aspect of the femoral shaft and terminates on the inferior aspect of the cortical layer of the femoral head. It is the "arcuate bundle of Gallois and Bosquette."
2. The second set, arising from the cortex of the internal aspect of the shaft and inferior neck, fans out vertically in an upward direction. It terminates on the cortical bone of the superior aspect of the head. This set is considered the supporting bundle for compressive forces.

The accessory system consists of two further bundles that fan out into the greater trochanter. The first bundle arises from the inner aspect of the shaft (trochanteric bundle), and the second less important vertical fibers run parallel to the greater trochanter.

The system of trabeculae rests on a strong support, i.e., the thick cortical layer of the inferior and distal aspect of the neck, known as the inferior spur of the neck or the vault of the pillar of Adams. Between the arches of the trochanter and the nucleus of the head is a zone of weakness that is intensified by osteoporosis. It is frequently referred to as Ward's triangle on the inferior neck and Babcock's triangle on the superior neck. It is a site of stress fractures.

Blood Supply

The blood supply may be considered under the headings extracapsular and intracapsular. The extracapsular blood supply is via the profunda femoris artery and is linked by encircling terminal branches: the lateral circumflex and the medial circumflex arteries (Fig. 17-14). The lateral circumflex artery supplies mainly the trochanter, the anterior femoral neck, and the metaphysis. Its contribution decreases with growth and expansion of the capital femoral circulation. The medial circumflex artery crosses with the iliopsoas muscle to the posteromedial femur and mainly traverses the intratrochanteric notch, giving off its intracapsular vessels. It anastomoses with the lateral femoral circumflex, and this basal anastomosis is mainly posterior and pericapsular. Essentially this supply remains the same throughout growth.[15]

The intracapsular supply is usually via several vessels. The first of these vessels is the medial circumflex femoral artery described above, which gives off superior and inferior retinacular vessels. The superior retinacular vessels supply the superior metaphyseal and lateral epiphyseal areas and two-thirds of the epiphyseal region. The inferior retinacular vessels provide a blood supply to the inferior metaphysis. The third set of vessels is from the obturator artery, which comes via the artery of the ligamentum teres to the medial part of the epiphysis.[16] Loss of these vessels through trauma or disease may result in avascular necrosis (Table 17-5).

Quick Facts

HIP DEVELOPMENT

Site	First Appearance (years)	Closure (years)
Femoral head	4 months	16–18
Greater trochanter	3	16–17
Lesser trochanter	11–12	16–17
Acetabulum	10–13*	16–17

*Primary centers gradually move in from birth. Secondary centers shown here.

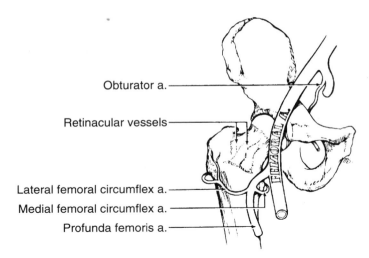

Obturator a.

Retinacular vessels

Lateral femoral circumflex a.

Medial femoral circumflex a.

Profunda femoris a.

Fig. 17-14. Major blood supply to the femoral neck and head is through an arcade formed by the lateral and medial circumflex arteries inferiorly, which gives rise to its retinacular vessels which supply the neck. It is also supplied by the obturator artery through its branch that runs with the ligamentum teres into the head of the femur. (After Henry,[5] with permission.)

TABLE 17-5. Etiology of Avascular Necrosis of the Hip

Traumatic causes
    Fractured neck of femur
    Dislocated hip
    Damage to vessels, no dislocation or fracture
    Burns
    Surgical damage to hip capsular circulation

Environment
    Caisson's disease — decompression phenomena
    High altitude

Pediatric
    Legg-Perthes disease
    Slipped epiphysis
    Congenital dislocation of hip (associated with manipulation)

Blood dyscrasia
    Sickle cell disease
    Miscellaneous hemoglobinopathies
    Hyperlipidemias
    Gaucher's disease

Miscellaneous
    Steroids
    Alcoholism[a]
    Liver disease[a]
    Renal transplant[a]
    Lupus erythematosus and other collagen disorders[a]
    Radiation

[a] Relation to avascular necrosis not clear and may be confused by the use of steroids.

Development of the Hip

The acetabulum consists of four types of cartilage during development: physeal cartilage, epiphyseal cartilage, hyaline articular cartilage, and fibrocartilage at the labrum. By age 3 years, the three components of the ilium, ischium, and pubis come together at the triradiate cartilage center in the acetabulum.[15] This triradiate cartilage allows a change in congruency of the acetabulum with the changing femoral head size during growth.

Quick Facts

CHANGING NECK–SHAFT RELATIONS

Age	Anteversion (degrees)	Neck–Shaft Angle (degrees)
Birth	40	150
3 Years	35	145
4 Years	30	140
5 Years	25	130
10–15 Years	20	125
Adult	20	120

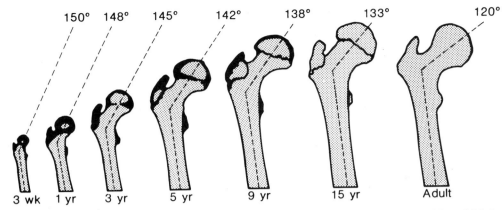

Fig. 17-15. Mean neck–shaft angle ranges from 150 degrees at birth to about 120 to 130 degrees in the adult. (Data from Von Lanz.[15])

The angle of anteversion, which is 40 degrees at birth, gradually decreases so that by about age 10 years it is reduced to 20 degrees[17–19] (Fig. 17-16). The persistance of this angle may lead to intoeing or excessive Q angle. Similarly, the neck–shaft angle, which is about 150 degrees at birth, reduces to about 120 degrees by adulthood (Fig. 17-15).[19,20]

EXAMINATION AND SPECIAL TESTS

The common problems of the hip region in sport are mainly extra-articular. However, because of the seriousness of overlooking hip disease, during examination there should be a constant awareness of the potential for these articular conditions. Some problems are seen more frequently at specific ages; thus common patterns are avascular necrosis in the child, slipped epiphysis in the adolescent, stress fractures and synovitis in the young adult, and degenerative changes in individuals over age 50.

Sometimes hip pain is easy to locate because of the association of limited range of motion and pain on rotation. However, frequent referral to the hip from back and sacroiliac pathology makes a broader examination imperative.

History

Key questions in the history concern the mode of onset, the pattern of pain distribution, the quality of the discomfort, and factors that exacerbate the pain.

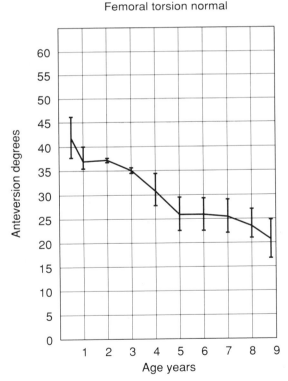

Femoral torsion normal

Fig. 17-16. Changing torsion angle anteversion of the femoral neck with the shaft. Ranging from around 40 degrees at birth, it decreases to between 15 and 25 degrees in the child. Means and standard deviations are shown. (Adapted from Crane,[17] with permission.)

Practice Point

COMMON HIP PATHOLOGY AT VARIOUS AGES

* Newborn   Congenital dislocated hip
* 2–8 Years   Avascular necrosis (Legg-Perthes)
* 10–14 Years   Slipped epiphysis
* 14–25 Years   Stress fractures, synovitis
* 20–40 Years   Avascular necrosis, synovitis, rheumatoid arthritis
* 45–60 Years   Osteoarthritis, synovitis
* 65+ Years   Stress fractures, osteoarthrosis

The relation of patients' complaints to their daily activities and occupations as well as the association with sport or recreation are particularly important, as the hip is constantly bearing weight during ambulation.

Hip pain is felt mainly in the groin and anteromedial thigh, probably through referral mechanisms linked to the obturator nerve. The pain is typically described as deep. Because of the overlapping with L4 root distribution, careful questioning regarding back pain is important. Hip pain frequently refers to the knee but rarely past it (Fig. 17-17).

Family history, trauma, and the presence of other joint symptoms may give clues to the hip problems being part of a more generalized process in the adult. Pain generated by activity, frequently associated with stiffness, and reaching a peak the morning after an exercise bout is usually synovitis in the middle-aged and elderly athlete. If frank osteoarthrosis is not already present, it may be the first sign of its impending development.

Observation

The presence of a limp, the position of the limb during gait, and the ability to sit and remove footwear give an idea of the magnitude of the pain and its probable location in the back, hip, or knee. The general body habitus in the adolescent may give an index of suspicion for slipped epiphysis. For instance, the large, overweight, sexually immature frame of the "Fröhlich" type build and the "tall for age" lean individual are associated with this condition. The general trunk, pelvis, and lower limb alignment when standing, as viewed from the rear and side, are helpful for the diagnosis and when looking for potentially correctable factors with therapy.

Examination

The key to successful examination of the hip is to be careful, systematic, and efficient. The patient's position should be changed a limited number of times (Table 17-6). The more painful the condition, the more important is this point. Attention to key points in the history and subtleties of the hip examination indicate the degree of emphasis and thoroughness that must be applied to the back and knee area.

Standing

Positive alignment and wasting of muscle are best viewed from behind, where the slope of the trapezius, scapula, spinous processes, natal cleft, and bulk of the

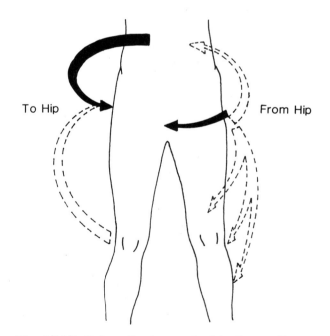

Fig. 17-17. Pain referring to the hip from adjacent structures and primary hip pain referring to both proximal and distal regions. The primary referral area for hip pain is the groin area. Solid lines are primary referral patterns from the lumbar spine and from hip to groin.

TABLE 17-6. Suggested Sequence for a Screening Hip Region Examination[a]

Standing

Observation

Posture, alignment, muscle wasting

Pelvic obliquity

Examination

Trendelenburg test

Forward flexion to touch toes

Ability to squat and duck-waddle

Specific palpation of hernia sites

Sitting

Examination

Tripod sign

Ability to cross leg over opposite thigh

Hip flexor and knee extensor strength

Reflexes if indicated

Supine

Examination

Active ROM

Flexion

Abduction and adduction

Hip flexor and knee extensor strength

Reflexes if indicated

Passive ROM

Internal and external rotation

Other passive movement as indicated

Isometric resisted

Hip flexion

Abduction and adduction

Internal and external rotation

Special tests

Joint play and quadrant tests

Thomas test for hip flexors

Rectus femoris stretch

Faber (Patrick) sacroiliac stress test

Leg length measurements

Reflexes and sensory testing if indicated[b]

Specific palpation of structures

Prone

Examination

Active, passive, and resisted hip extension

Passive medial and lateral hip rotation

Special tests

Ely test of rectus femoris tightness

Palpation

Specific areas as indicated

Side lying

Examination

Active and resisted abduction and adduction

Ober test of iliotibial band tightness

Sensory testing if indicated

[a] This sequence limits unnecessary changes in patient positioning.

[b] Some tests are repeated in different positions as indicated.

glutei can be well observed. This examination is supplemented by viewing from the side, where lumbar lordosis, hip flexion, knee flexion, and the inability to place both feet firmly on the floor without inducing flexion in one limb are noted. Subsequent tests can distinguish flexion contractures, pain, or leg length discrepancies as the main cause.[20] Palpation of specific hernia sites may be done at this juncture if indicated.

Trendelenburg Test

The Trendelenburg test assesses the ability of the hip abductors on one side to balance the contralateral unsupported side of the pelvis. The athlete is requested to stand on one leg. Normally the opposite side of the pelvis stays parallel or rises somewhat (Fig. 17-18). If the pelvis drops on the unsupported side, it constitutes a positive Trendelenburg sign. It indicates that the individual has weak abductors or an inability to control the abductors due to neural problems, pain inhibition, or mechanical factors such as an unstable insertion. The abductors, particularly the gluteus medius, are working origin and insertion reversed, as their distal attachment to the femur is the fixed point in this test. With a dislocated hip, the insertion slides up, hence a stable fixation for contraction is not available, giving the positive sign.[12] When walking, the repetitive dropping of the contralateral pelvis constitutes a Trendelenburg gait or gluteus medius lurch. The usual compensation is excessive side flexion to the affected (ipsilateral) side, which obviously constitutes an inefficient mode of progression. The commonest cause of a positive Trendelenburg sign in sport is contusion of the abductor mass or an impending stress fracture of the femoral neck, with subsequent pain inhibition.

Functional Tests

The ability to forward flex to touch the toes smoothly and without discomfort helps rule out spinal pathology and gives some indication of hamstring tightness or discomfort. Squatting and duck-waddling indicates the overall range of motion, degree of discomfort, and willingness to cooperate in the young athlete.

Sitting

The athlete should sit on the examination couch so the legs can dangle, a position that allows further assessment of the possible involvement of radicular

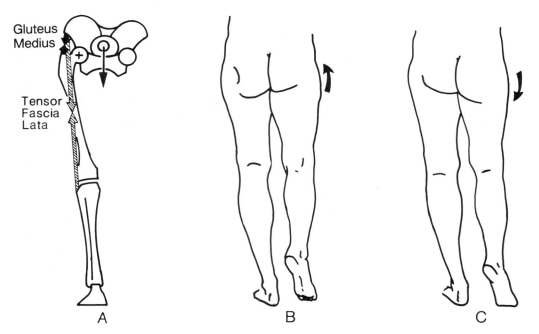

Fig. 17-18. (A) With the normal walking pattern, the unsupported side of the pelvis is controlled by the contralateral hip abductors. **(B)** Thus the pelvis remains steady or may be slightly elevated during the swing phase. **(C)** With abductor weakness on the supporting leg, the contralateral pelvis may drop, which is reflected as a positive Trendelenburg sign. (Data from Kapandji,[12] and Magee.[20])

symptoms as well as the degree of hip flexion possible. A good functional test of hip range of motion is to ask the athlete to cross one leg over the lower thigh or knee area of the contralateral leg. Note is made of any pain or difficulty. This positioning requires flexion, abduction, and external rotation. The L4 segment is judged according to the patellar tendon reflex and the quadriceps power. Furthermore, during this test the patient may lean back, the "tripod sign," which further indicates either a tight hamstring, an uncomfortable hamstring, or possibly nerve root traction of either the L5 or S1 segment. If positive, it should be supplemented by the "slump" test to rule out radicular symptoms (See Chapter 20)

Supine Position

With the patient supine (lying face up), active range of motion supplemented by passive range of motion with attention to the end feel can provide an impression of the existence of hip pathology (Figs. 17-19, 17-20). Particularly the quadrant stress tests

and overpressure on internal and external rotation help define the pathology in the hip region and even the joint itself. Furthermore, sometimes the pattern of movement is helpful. For instance, in the skeletally immature patient with slipped epiphysis, the leg tends to come up into flexion with associated external rotation, both actively and passively. Range of motion should be accurately recorded with a goniometer if the primary disease is thought to be within the hip joint.[21] Normal ranges were given earlier in the chapter.

Hip flexion is tested with the knee flexed to prevent hamstring tightness from limiting the motion. The normal range is 140 to 160 degrees (Fig. 17-21).

When testing abduction the pelvis must be fixed and the range judged from the horizontal plane. Palpation for motion of the anterosuperior iliac spine indicates when hip motion is complete. This motion is more functionally assessed with associated lateral rotation, which prevents impingement of the greater trochanter against the iliac crest, but flexion should not be permitted[11] (Fig. 17-22). Without lateral rota-

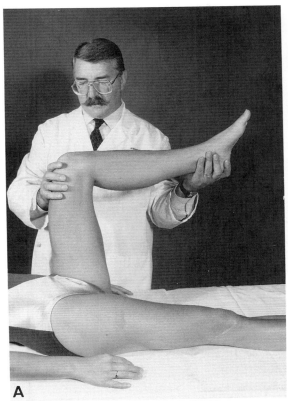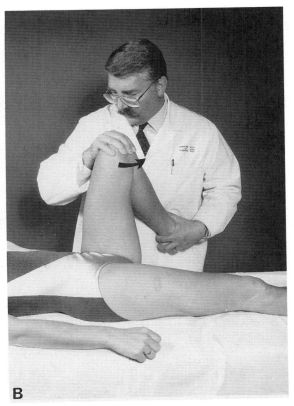

Fig. 17-19. (A) Passive internal or external rotation of the hip particularly if it is exacerbated by overpressure, **(B)** is an excellent indicator of primary hip pathology. Attention is paid to the end feel, which is the quality of the limiting factors to motion. It may be painful, soft tissue, springy or bony. This principle applies to all joints.

tion only about 30 to 50 degrees of motion is obtainable.

Hip adduction is a problem because of contact with the contralateral limb. The leg to be tested may be flexed to avoid contact; alternatively, the opposite limb may be abducted out of the way. Palpation of the ipsilateral anterosuperior iliac spine provides the most sensitive indication of when the pelvis is starting to tilt. Usually about 30 to 35 degrees is present.

Rotation with the hip and knee flexed to 90 degrees is assessed primarily to get an idea of the end feel and the proportion of internal to external rotation. In this position the joint play movement and quadrant stressing are carried out if indicated (Fig. 17-20). The patient's hip is taken into flexion and adduction. With overpressure, the hip is circled in a shallow flexion arc into abduction. The examiner tries to sense appre-

hension, pain, crepitus, or irregularities of motion, which suggest intra-articular pathology.[20,22]

Specific measurements of rotation are more accurately recorded while the patient is prone (lying face down) (Fig. 17-23). In the prone position, when the leg moves outward the hip is rotating internally; conversely, moving the leg in tests external roation. It may be appropriate to isometrically test hip flexion, the abductors and adductors, and the medial and lateral rotators at this point. Telling the patient to "hold the leg still" or "resist my pressure" or "don't let me move the leg" are instructions that they find easy to understand.

There are a series of special tests that may be performed in the supine position and are convenient to do at this juncture. They include passive straight-leg raising, the Thomas test, the rectus femoris stretch,

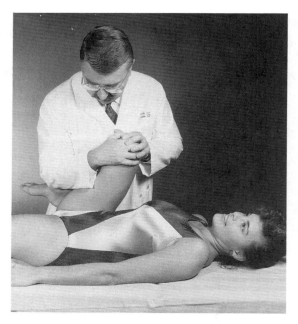

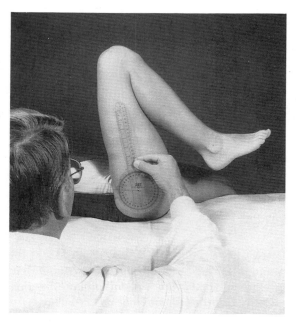

Fig. 17-20. Compression along the axis of the leg through the hip, as it is rotated through four quadrants, is also an excellent indicator of primary hip pathology and gives additional information on the end feel. These same quadrant testing techniques may be used as a therapeutic tool to facilitate regaining range.

Fig. 17-21. **(A)** Hip flexion is measured with the goniometer centered over the greater trochanter and pointing along the long axis of the thigh. The normal range is 0 degrees to 120 to 160 degrees depending on whether passive overpressure is used and on the size of the individual's thigh and abdomen.

Patrick's test, and deep tendon reflexes. These tests unmask specific muscle tightness or involvement of the spine and sacroiliac joints.

Passive Straight-Leg Raise

Passive straight-leg raise is performed by flexing the hip to 90 degrees with the knee flexed and then attempting to straighten the knee while maintaining the hip flexion. Failure to be able to fully extend the knee represents hamstring tightness, and the degree of deficiency may be recorded (Fig. 17-24). If the extended knee position is easily achieved, the leg can be continued into further flexion at the hip, and any motion past 90 degrees is recorded.

Thomas Test

The Thomas test assesses hip flexion. The examiner slides a hand into the small of the athlete's spine, after which the patient is instructed to flex the hip up until the lumbar lordosis is obliterated and the examiner feels the pressure from the athlete's back firmly

pressing down onto the hand. At this point the contralateral limb should still be resting flat on the examining couch (Fig. 17-25). In the case of an athlete, often full flexion of the hip is needed to eliminate the lordosis and flatten the back. The angle the extended leg makes with the couch indicates the degree of hip flexion contracture. It may be confirmed by pushing the flexed hip onto the table, after which either the contralateral leg, which the athlete is supporting, extends or the lumbar lordosis increases.

Rectus Femoris Stretch Test

If the Thomas test is repeated with the patient's legs dangling over the edge of the examining table, hip flexion of one limb rotates the pelvis. This rotation stretches the pelvic origin of the rectus femoris; and if this muscle is excessively tight, the contralateral limb may extend at the knee (Fig. 17-26). The examiner then attempts to flex the slightly extending knee passively to assess the degree of resistance and ascer-

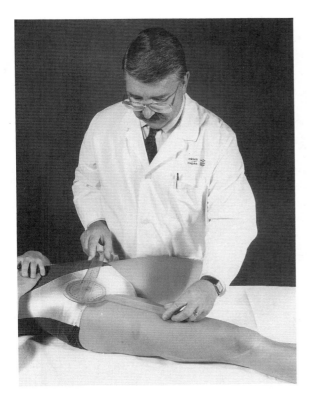

Fig. 17-22. To measure abduction and adduction, the pelvis must be stabilized. One of the more practical ways of stabilizing it is to have the patient flex the contralateral leg over the side of the examination table. One plane is between the two anterosuperior iliac spines. The other arm of the goniometer goes down along the long axis of the leg.

tain if adequate relaxation has allowed a truly positive test.

Faber (Patrick) Test

For the Faber test the examiner places the patient's test leg so that the foot and ankle rest on the contralateral knee. The flexed leg is then slowly lowered into abduction. The position at this time is flexion, abduction, and external rotation (Faber) at the hip. If the leg does not lower appropriately to an almost parallel position, there is a possible contracture at the hip joint or protective iliopsoas spasm (Fig. 17-27). Overpressure on the knee and counterpressure on the opposite pelvic brim may produce significant pain in the ipsilateral sacroiliac joint, denoting its involvement in the pathologic clinical picture.

Leg Length Measurement

Prior to measuring leg lengths the athlete is positioned appropriately by balancing the pelvis where possible. Balance indicates that the anterosuperior iliac spines (ASISs) are in the same plane, and the legs lie perpendicular to that plane approximately 20 cm apart. Although the medial or lateral malleolus may be used as the distal landmark, the lateral malleolus position is usually more reproducible and less affected by obesity or muscle wasting.

True leg length is measured from the ASISs to the lateral malleolus (Fig. 17-28). This measurement adjusts for pelvic obliquity. Differences of more than 1 cm can usually be detected reliably by this method, but lesser discrepancies are difficult to record.[23] The relation of leg length discrepancies to lower limb, sacroiliac, and back pain is not a simple one, and each case must be addressed on its own merits. Discrepancies of more than 2 cm frequently produce a noticeable limp. Once a subtle discrepancy is noted, it may be verified by using a series of increasingly thicker boards inserted under the foot until the pelvis is seen to be balanced from behind, as judged by parallel posterosuperior iliac spines (the dimples). If the discrepancy is considered significant, particularly in the growing athlete, further tests help localize the affected segment.

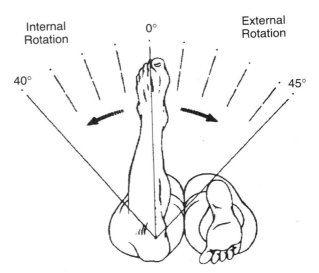

Fig. 17-23. Internal and external rotation can be specifically measured most accurately in the prone position. Approximately 45 degrees in either direction from the midline constitutes a normal range.

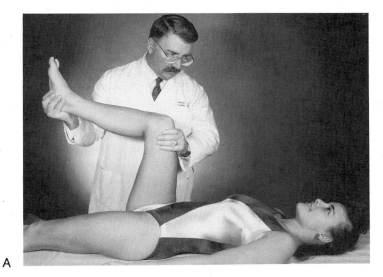

A

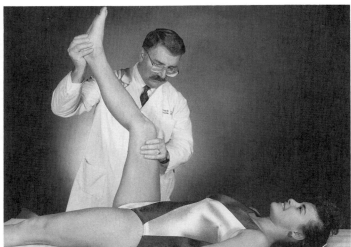

B

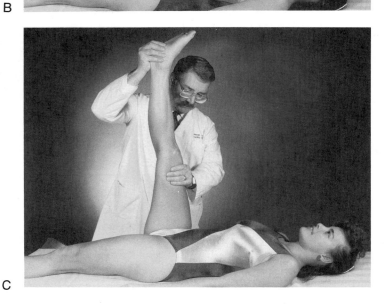

C

Fig. 17-24. **(A)** Starting position for assessing hamstring tightness is 90 degrees of flexion of the hip and knee. **(B)** As the thigh is stabilized, the leg is brought into extension; and when no further extension can be achieved, the angle short of full extension is recorded (abnormal test). **(C)** Full extension is desirable (normal test). In individuals with extremely flexible hamstrings, it is possible to take the extended knee past the neutral position. This move signifies either generalized laxity or a training phenomenon in such sports as ballet dancing and gymnastics.

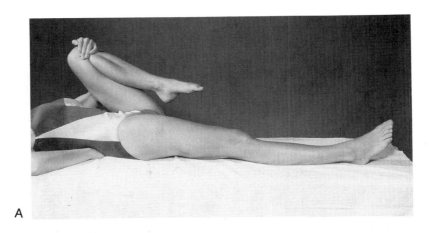

A

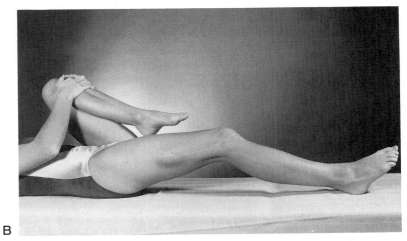

Fig. 17-25. Thomas test for hip flexor tightness. **(A)** Negative test. **(B)** Positive test as indicated by the inability to maintain a fully extended hip on the right side as the contralateral hip is brought into flexion.

B

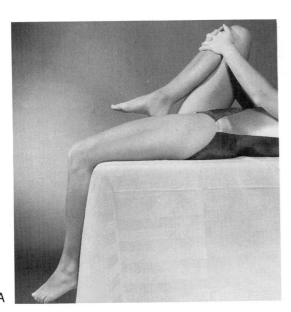

A

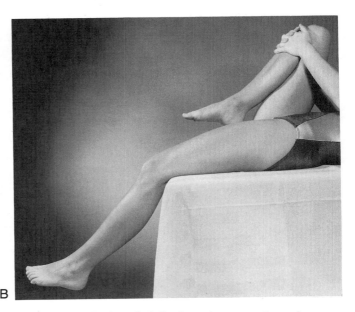

B

Fig. 17-26. Rectus femoris stretch test. **(A)** As the hip is brought into full flexion, the contralateral knee should remain at approximately 90 degrees flexed over the end of the examining couch. **(B)** Positive test is indicated by the limb extending in response to contralateral hip flexion.

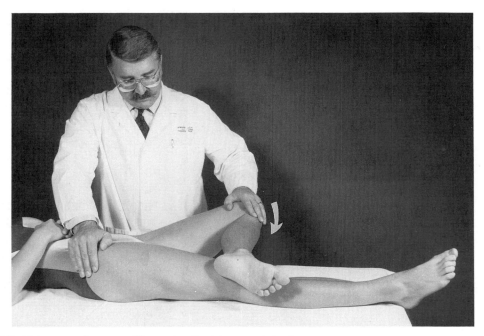

Fig. 17-27. Faber test for sacroiliac pain. Positive test is indicated by discomfort in the sacroiliac area as stress is applied. This test also unmasks limited external rotation of the hip.

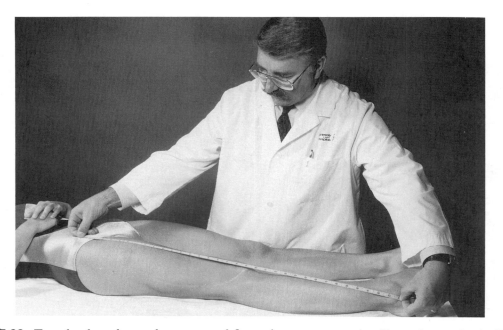

Fig. 17-28. True leg length may be measured from the anterosuperior iliac spine to the ipsilateral lateral malleolus. This measurement is possibly slightly more reproducible than measuring to the medial malleolus.

Localizing the discrepancy is important. With the legs flexed to 90 degrees at the knees, a distal segment shortening becomes apparent by viewing the height of the knees from the end of the examining couch (Fig. 17-29) Proximal segment shortening mainly involving the femur is best seen by viewing the antero-posterior relations of the two knees from the side. Discrepancies that occur secondary to hip dysplasia are suggested by Nélaton's line or Bryant's triangle, although clinical landmarks are difficult to draw accurately.

Nélaton's line is an imaginary line drawn from the ischial tuberosity to the ASIS. The greater trochanter, identified by palpation, should sit underneath this line. If it is above it, severe coxa vera or a dislocated hip is probable. The two sides should be compared (Fig. 17-29).

Bryant's triangle is best outlined on a lateral roentgenogram, although some impression can be gained from clinical measurements. Indeed the main purpose of clinical measurements is to assist in deciding the significance of the patient's symptoms and to help select appropriate films when further information is required. To outline the imaginary triangle, a perpendicular is dropped from the ASIS to the examining table; then a second line is drawn from the tip of the greater trochanter to meet the first line at a right angle (Fig. 17-29). The two sides are then compared.

Accurate recording of leg length discrepancies with exact localization to the limb segment usually requires a scanogram with an incorporated scale on the roentgenogram. Only from this information can accurate predictions be made and surgical therapy planned, when necessary, in the growing athlete.

Functional shortening, or apparent leg length discrepancy based on pelvic tilt, adductor contractures, or hip capsule tightness, may be gauged by measuring from the tip of the umbilicus or xiphisternum. Asymmetry of these landmarks affects the measurements.

Other Tests in Supine Position

Sensory testing of sequential and peripheral nerve distribution and specific palpation with the patient supine are dictated by the history and physical findings elicited up to this point in the examination (Figs. 17-30 and 17-31). Pulses should be checked and the presence of swelling, scars, and skin changes noted. The scrotum, testicles, hernia sites, and lower abdomen are palpated as indicated.

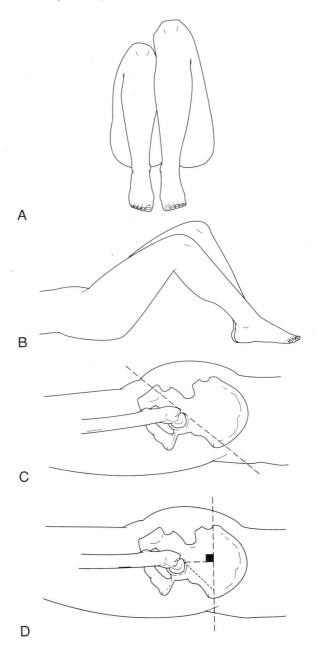

Fig. 17-29. Leg length discrepancy may be localized clinically to the tibia or the femur (if the disparity is great enough) simply by observing the patient with the knees flexed from the end (**A**) or side of the bed. (**B**) Similarly, Nélaton's line (**C**) and Bryant's triangle (**D**) give some concept of the position of the greater trochanter and hence the femoral neck. These clinical measures are indirect and are used only as a guide to direct further investigations. (Adapted from Magee.[20])

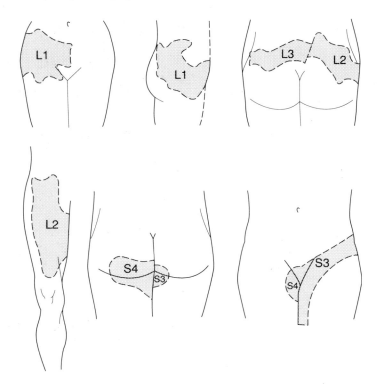

Fig. 17-30. Segmental sensory distribution (dermatomes) around the hip.

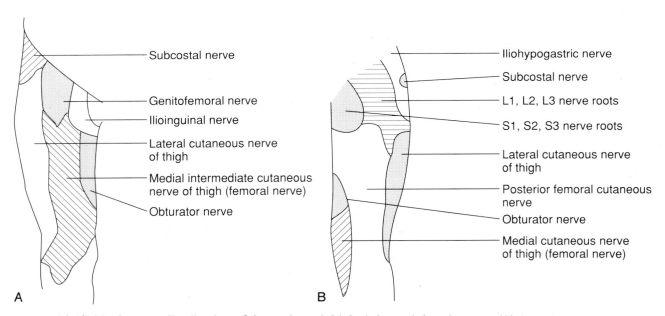

Fig. 17-31. Sensory distribution of the groin and thigh via its peripheral nerves. **(A)** Anterior view. **(B)** Posterior view. (Data from Magee.[20])

Prone Position

Active, passive, and resisted extension is checked in the prone position (lying face down). For most individuals there is limited extension at the hip, and most of the motion produced is by lumbar spine extension in the pelvic areas, particularly the lumbosacral junction. The sacroiliac joint, ischial tuberosity, and projected course of the sciatic nerve may be palpated. Two special tests are carried out in this position; the first is a femoral nerve stretch test, and the second is a test of rectus femoris tightness.

Femoral Nerve Stretch Test

The femoral nerve is put on a stretch by flexing the patient's knee to 90 degrees or more and then passively extending the hip while fixing the pelvis (Fig. 17-32). A positive test, indicated by pain along the anterior thigh in the distribution of the L2–L3 segment and the femoral nerve, is indicative of either a radicular origin of the pain or entrapment of the femoral or lateral femoral cutaneous nerve, usually at the pelvic brim adjacent to the ASIS. Occasionally, this test produces classic sciatica, in which case it suggests L5 radiculopathy.

Ely Test

The Ely test involves simple flexion of the patient's knee so the heel approximates the buttock, which is usually easily achieved. If the ipsilateral hip and buttock rise, it is probable that the rectus femoris muscle is tight (Fig. 17-33).

Side Lying Position

In the side lying position, active and resisted abduction and adduction may be tested, lateral structures may be palpated, and the Ober test for a tight iliotibial band performed.[24]

Ober Test

For the Ober test the patient flexes the lower leg at the hip and knee to stabilize the body. The lower knee may be flexed up and grasped if it appears to produce better fixation. The examiner grasps the pelvic brim to assist in the stabilization and then passively flexes, abducts, and extends the upper hip in an arc. This motion moves the iliotibial band over the trochanter. The relaxed leg is then slowly lowered by the exam-

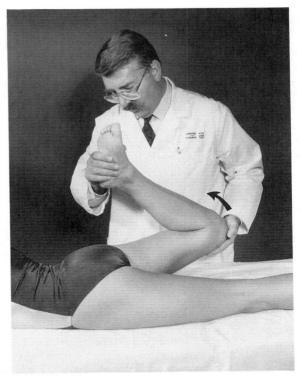

Fig. 17-32. The femoral nerve stretch test is positive if this maneuver exacerbates pain along the anterior and lateral thigh. Pain down the back of the leg in a sciatic distribution may indicated L5 root irritation; pain generated over the sacroiliac joint or lumbar sacral junction may simply indicate sacroiliac or lumbar junction pathology.

iner. With normal flexibility the upper knee reaches the level of the medial aspect of the under-leg; that is, the thigh goes past neutral.[25]

With a tight iliotibial band the thigh reaches only neutral or, more rarely, remains slightly abducted. Ober originally described performing this test with the knee flexed, which is easier for the examiner and in the neurologically involved patient population was adequate for a positive test.[24,25] However, in the young active population the test may be better performed with the knee extended, which places greater stretch on the iliotibial band and is more likely to reveal subtle tightness. (See chapter 13 for illustration.)

The sequence of the examination described may be performed in an efficient, logical manner. It may be

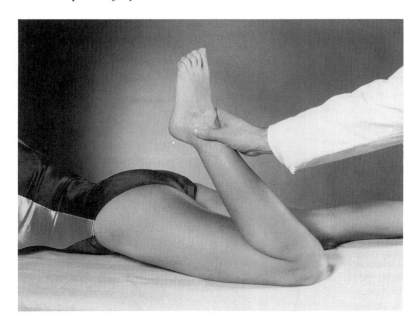

Fig. 17-33. Test for tight rectus femoris. Positive test is indicated by an inability to keep the hip extended as the knee is flexed.

adapted according to the particular inferences from the history or the dictates of positive findings during various tests.

CLICKING HIP AND BURSITIS

Snapping or Clicking Hip Sensation

The snapping or clicking hip is a frequent phenomenon among athletes and is particularly prominent in dancers.[26,27] However, fewer than one-third of individuals have associated pain. The patient frequently presents complaining of the sound or sensation of clicking, although a few patients specifically complain of the pain.[28,29] The clicking hip may be categorized as an anterior (internal, medial) clicking hip, which is distinguished from the external (lateral) type[9,30-32] (Table 17-7).

Internal Clicking Hip

There are numerous postulated causes of the internal clicking hip, including problems in the hip joint, the iliofemoral ligament, the psoas tendon, and the symphysis pubis.[33]

TABLE 17-7. Causes of Snapping (Clicking) Hips

Site and Associated Factors	Etiology	References
Medial (internal)	Iliofemoral ligament over femoral head	Howse[26]
	Iliopsoas tendon over iliopectineal eminence	Nunziata & Blumenfeld[9]
	Iliopsoas tendon over lesser trochanter	
	Subluxation of femoral head	
	Suction phenomena in joint	Quirk[27]
	Iliopsoas tendon over anteroinferior iliac spine	
Lateral (external)	Iliotibial band over greater trochanter	Binnie[28]
	Gluteus maximus tendon over trochanter	Schaberg et al.[29]
Contributing factors	Tight iliotibial band	Jones[30]
	Narrow bi-iliac width	Jacobs & Young[31]
	Imbalanced flexibility	Reid et al.[32]
	Muscle imbalance	Singleton & LeVeau[14]

Practice Point

SNAPPING OR CLICKING HIP SENSATION

- Hip joint
  -Suction phenomenon
  -Subluxation
  -Loose body
  -Osteochondromatosis
- Psoas tendon
  -Lesser trochanter
  -Iliopectineal eminence
- Symphysis pubis
  -Postpartum
  -Post-traumatic
  -Generalized ligament laxity
- Iliotibial band
  -Greater trochanter
- Biceps femoris tendon
  -Ischial tuberosity

Hip Joint

The commonest cause of a snapping hip is the suction phenomenon in the joint itself. This disorder is painless and may be present during sit-up maneuvers or with specific flexion movements of the thigh. No treatment is indicated. The more serious, rare conditions of a loose body in the joint, osteochondromatosis, and subluxation should be treated after investigation with plain films, tomograms, computed tomographic (CT) scans, or arthrograms to decide if there is evidence of impending or already present intra-articular damage. Alternatively, it has been suggested by Quirk that an individual with a large range of motion at the hip, e.g., a ballet dancer or gymnast, may have a minor subluxation of the femoral head at the extremes of range, producing a suction phenomenon within the hip.[27]

Iliofemoral Ligament and Psoas Tendon

The iliofemoral ligament may snap over the femoral head and the psoas tendon over the iliopectineal eminence or possibly the lesser trochanter (Fig. 17-34). The iliopsoas tendon may also snap over the anteroinferior iliac spine.[29]

Symphysis Pubis

After trauma, with fractures of the pelvis, or pre- or postpartum, there may be some movement at the symphysis that is symptomatic. Treatment by rest, anti-inflammatory medication, and modification of activity may be required. Rarely is surgery indicated.

External Clicking Hip

The lateral, or external, clicking hip is usually related to the gluteus maximus tendon snapping over the greater trochanter (Fig. 17-35). The contributing factors here are a tight iliotibial band, a narrow bi-iliac width, and possibly inadequate flexibility or imbalance of muscle strength.

The physical examination distinguishes the source of the click and, when present, the associated discomfort. Sometimes it is helpful to infiltrate lidocaine (xylocaine) 1 percent into the painful site to see if it relieves the symptoms. Occasionally if one is seeking to show the snapping phenomena is associated with the psoas muscle, iliopsoas bursography and cineradiography can be helpful (Fig. 17-36) for demonstrating the motion of the iliopsoas tendon over the anteroinferior iliac spine, iliopectineal eminence, or lesser trochanter. Similarly, the area around the greater trochanter may be infiltrated. Most of the discomfort due to the snapping hip phenomenon derives from the associated bursitis. In this case the internal snapping hip relates to the iliopsoas bursa, and the external snapping hip relates to the trochanteric bursa. The specific care of such bursitis is described below.

Treatment relates to identifying the contributing factors, be they muscle tightness, muscle imbalance, poor training techniques, biomechanical alignment of the lower limbs, or systemic collagen diseases. Once the contributing factors are identified, specific rehabilitation programs can be carried out along with accompanying adjustment of equipment or footwear. Occasionally, use of an orthotic is helpful. In addition anti-inflammatory medication or injections methylprednisolone (Depo-Medrol) may assist in relieving the symptoms while the activity program is modified and then subsequently progressed.

Bursitis Around the Hip

The three major sites of bursitis around the hip are the psoas bursa, the greater trochanteric bursa, and the ischial bursa (Fig. 17-37). These conditions usu-

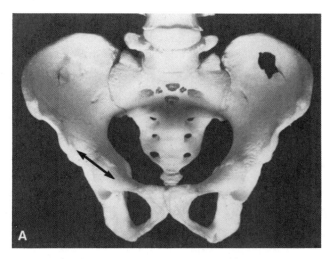

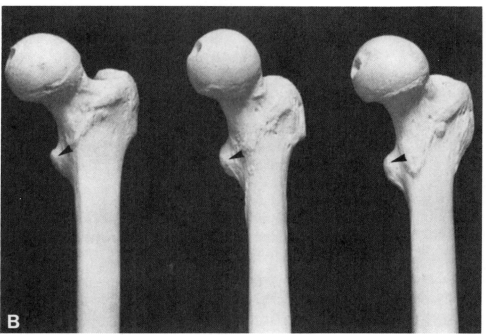

Fig. 17-34. (A) Bony pelvis. Arrows indicate the anteroinferior iliac spines laterally and the iliopectineal eminence medially with a groove between them. **(B)** Three femurs, with arrows pointing to the area of the bony prominence on the lesser trochanter over which the iliopsoas tendon may snap. (After Schaberg et al.,[29] with permission.)

ally presents with a gradual onset of pain in the anatomic region of the bursa involved that gradually progresses to become proportional to activity. Frequently when severe the pain may continue between exercise bouts, be present when first getting up in the morning, and be sufficiently uncomfortable that walking aggravates the problem. An antalgic limp is frequently present when the condition is severe.

Psoas Bursitis

The psoas bursa is usually aggravated by excessive activity. It presents with pain in the inguinal area that radiates through the femoral triangle. It may be related to the internal snapping hip syndrome. There is exquisite tenderness to palpation. Palpation of this deeply placed structure may be difficult, but with the

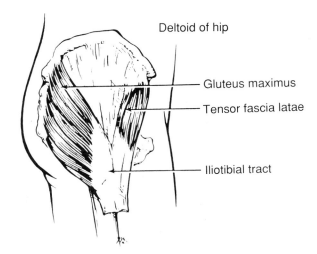

Fig. 17-35. Gluteus maximus and tensor fascia lata pulling into the iliotibial band or tract, which is separated from the trochanter by a bursa. During movements of flexion and extension of the hip, this hood of fascia slips across the trochanter and results occasionally in an external clicking hip which may or may not be associated with painful bursitis.

Deltoid of hip

Gluteus maximus

Tensor fascia latae

Iliotibial tract

hip and knee flexed to about 40 degrees, externally rotated, and supported on a pillow, sufficient muscle relaxation is achieved to facilitate placing pressure on the lesser trochanter. The extremes of rotation with the hip in flexion sometimes cause discomfort as well as resisted hip flexion if the bursitis is sufficiently acute. Otherwise, these tests are negative.

Treatment involves activity modification and nonsteroidal anti-inflammatory drugs (NSAIDs) coupled with local application of laser therapy, ultrasound, or interferential currents. If this approach is not successful, an injection of steroid may be helpful. If the athlete is not excessively lean, fluoroscopic control of the injection ensures the best chance of success. As soon as symptoms start to resolve, work should be begun on stretching the hip flexors. The psoas stretch is carried out with the athlete lying near the edge of the table on the affected side. The sound hip is flexed and held on the abdomen to fix the pelvis, and the affected leg is allowed to hang below the level of the table. The stretch is maintained for 15 seconds, and 10 repetitions should be done. Between each repetition, the leg is rested on the table. On the last repetition the leg is left in the hanging position until dis-

Fig. 17-36. Iliopsoas bursography. Contrast material in the iliopsoas bursa outlines the insertion of the tendon. Such localization may assist accurate placement of steroidal anti-inflammatory medication in recalcitrant cases of iliopsoas bursitis.

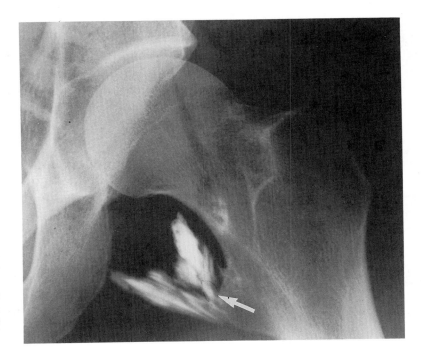

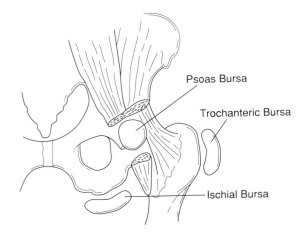

Fig. 17-37. Bursae around the hip most frequently involved in inflammatory reactions.

comfort is begun to be felt in either the groin or the back. The exercise should not be pursued beyond this point. This regimen is followed by a graduated plan for return to activity.

Trochanteric Bursitis

Trochanteric bursitis is seen frequently in runners, and it occurs sufficiently often in cross-country skiers to have the eponym "ski runner's hip." Surprisingly, ballet dancers suffer from a high incidence of trochanteric bursitis, probably related to the amount of full range, repetitive hip work and one-legged balance maneuvers. Many dancers also have imbalanced flexibility with tight iliotibial bands even in the presence of loose adductors and hamstrings.

This disorder is characterized by a burning or deep aching sensation located over or just posterior to the tip of the greater trochanter (Fig. 17-37). Unlike the iliotibial band syndrome, trochanteric bursitis may be painful with walking early during its course. The pain is made worse by activity. It is usually described as a dull ache in the hip and buttock area with a sharp pain as the hip goes from flexion to extension in the weight-bearing position. There may be referral of pain down the lateral aspect of the thigh and a sudden, sharp pain with certain movements of the hip. It is usually related to the motion of the fascia lata over the bony prominence, in which case it may be related to the external snapping hip syndrome. When the

pain is more posterior, it involves a deep component of the bursal sheath related to the gluteus medius and minimus tendons.

Trochanteric bursitis is frequently seen in runners who do a lot of road running, and then it usually occurs in the "down side" leg (related to the camber of the road). This induced functional leg length discrepancy may create extreme friction between the greater trochanter and the iliotibial tract during repetitive flexion and extension of the hip.

Although trochanteric bursitis is usually an overuse syndrome, in contact sports it may be related to direct trauma. Football, soccer, rugby, and particularly ice hockey players are susceptible to this problem. Constant trauma may produce a huge, swollen, painless or painful bursa over the area of maximum prominence of the trochanter. Occasionally "rice" bodies form within the bursa. The last group of patients have some form of generalized collagen disorders, e.g., ankylosing spondylitis, Reiter's syndrome, or even rheumatoid arthritis. These disorders do not fall within the scope of this chapter, but they stress the constant need to be aware of the coexistence of a systemic or underlying disorder in patients with activity-induced musculoskeletal problems.

The treatment is similar to that for other forms of bursitis, with the emphasis on stretching the iliotibial band should the fascia lata be tight as demonstrated by the Ober test. Interestingly, there are a group of active young individuals who develop trochanteric bursitis and who have generalized ligamentous laxity. Stretching is not required here. These patients often have a trick movement they refer to as "dislocating the hip," which in reality is the iliotibial band snapping over the trochanter.

Although rest, moist heat, and other modalities, as well as NSAIDs, usually relieve the athlete's symptoms, there are some cases that become resistant and chronically painful. When a series of local injections with local anesthetic and hydrocortisone fail, surgery may be considered. Several procedures, some complex, have been described, but the most successful is removal of an ellipse of iliotibial band along with excessive bursal tissue[34] (Fig. 17-38). It may be performed with the aid of a local anesthetic. The patient may reproduce the motion that generates pain or snapping so the most appropriate portion is excised. Postoperative weight-bearing as tolerated is permitted, with the aim of gradually returning to sport 6 to 8 weeks after surgery. There is no obvious long-term weakness.

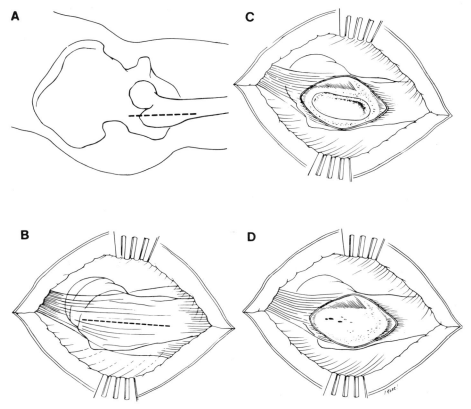

Fig. 17-38. Intractable trochanteric bursitis may be helped by excising the bursa and releasing the overlying iliotibial band. **(A)** Incision. **(B)** Exposure of the iliotibial band. **(C)** Partial excision of the band. **(D)** Excision of the trochanteric bursa.

Ischial Bursitis

Direct bruising or trauma due to the impact of a fall are the usual causes of ischial bursitis, a relatively uncommon form of bursitis. The major importance lies more in the differential diagnosis of a hamstring tear at the tendinous origin, as epiphysitis or separation in the skeletally immature patient, osteomyelitis, and several neoplasms may develop in the ischial tuberosity.[35,36] There is also a rare cause of snapping in the area as the tendinous origin of the biceps femoris muscle moves over the ischial tuberosity, the "snapping bottom." [37]

When the diagnosis of bursitis is established, treatment follows the same regimen as for the other bursa in the area. Usually the problem resolves promptly. Chronicity is unusual and the need for surgical exploration of the area rare.

Synovitis of the Hip

In the young individual, up to the age of 8 years, there is always the fear that transient synovitis of the hip may be associated with an episode of avascular necrosis. In the elderly, these episodes may precede obvious degenerative changes. In the teenage and young adult athlete, however, transient synovitis is usually related to trauma—either a fall, a direct blow, or occasionally overuse. The clinical sign is that of severe hip and groin pain aggravated by rotation. In the severe acute stage, weight-bearing may be impossible. If the synovitis does not settle rapidly with modified weight-bearing, activity and NSAIDs, concern about the diagnosis is in order. If plain roentgenograms are not revealing, a bone scan often assists in ruling out an impending stress fracture or tumor as a cause. Tomography or CT scans can reveal loose

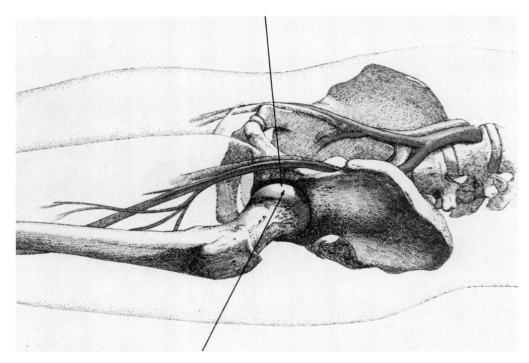

Fig. 17-39. Anatomy of the hip showing the line of the lateral approach to injection or aspiration, using the greater trochanter as a guide. An anterior approach may be selected just lateral to the femoral artery, two to three fingers' breadth below the inguinal ligament.

bodies. A blood screen should point to infection if it is the cause. Persistent sterile synovitis may be settled with an injection of cortisone (Fig. 17-39).

In-Toeing

In-toeing is a common orthopaedic disorder in children. Controversy exists regarding the evaluation and management. In-toeing can be related to increased femoral anteversion, internal tibial torsion, adduction of the forefoot, or a combination of these factors. The most common factor is said to be increased femoral anteversion. Anteversion is the angle the femoral neck makes with the femoral condyles (Fig. 17-40). The angle decreases with age. At birth it is about 40 degrees and in the adult 8 to 15 degrees (Fig. 17-40). In children older than 3 years, there is a positive correlation between internal rotation of the hip and femoral anteversion. Hip rotation is, however, dependent not only on the degree of femoral anteversion but also on the spatial orientation of the acetabulum, hip capsule, and muscles surrounding the hip. Although femoral anteversion is greatest in

children younger than 2 years of age, external hip rotation exceeds internal rotation at this age. About 16 percent of children have an in-toeing gait. The frequency decreases from 30 percent in the 4-year-old to about 4 percent in adults. Usually subjects with an in-toeing gait have a significant increase in internal rotation and decrease in external rotation. There have been attempts to correlate this alignment with knee pain in cases of squinting patella, shin pain, and other problems with in-toeing, but there are remarkably few hard scientific data to support these contentions. *Unless excessive, there is rarely any effect of these alignments on the ability to perform sport at any level of competition.*

A common clinical manifestation of increased anteversion is excessive medial rotation at the hip. The Craig test gives some approximation of the degree of anteversion (Fig. 17-40). Here the athlete lies prone with the knee flexed to 90 degrees. The greater trochanter is palpated and the hip passively rotated until the tip of the trochanter appears parallel to the examining, usually the most prominant position. The degree of anteversion is estimated by the angle the lower

Fig. 17-40. **(A)** Axial view of the right femur showing the normal ranges of anteversion and associated torsion or deformities outside that range. (From Staheli,[38] with permission.) **(B)** Rough estimation of the degree of anteversion can sometimes be obtained by passively rotating the hip until the trochanter appears by palpation to be parallel to the examining table. **(C)** Anteversion is also roughly represented by the amount of internal rotation from the neutral position (Craig test).

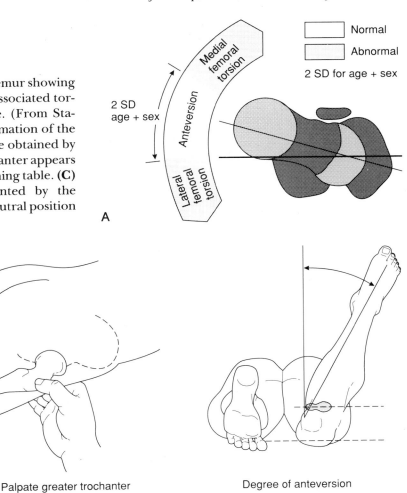

Palpate greater trochanter parallel to table

Degree of anteversion

leg makes with the vertical.[20] The Craig test, or Ryder method as it is sometimes called, is obviously more accurate in the lean individual and, at best, should only be considered an indication of the neck–shaft relation.

OSTEITIS PUBIS (TRAUMATIC ASEPTIC OSTEITIS PUBIS)

Osteitis pubis is an inflammatory lesion of the bone adjacent to the symphysis pubis. It is most commonly seen in elderly men after prostate surgery or in women after bladder neck and urethral surgery. This postprostatic syndrome was well described in 1924 by Beer.[39] Beach referred to osteitis pubis as "an ortho-

pedic disease sponsored by urologic surgery."[40,41] Osteitis pubis is also seen in postpartum women, sometimes in association with some widening and instability of the symphysis pubis. However, from the sports medicine perspective, osteitis pubis is an inflammatory lesion arising at or adjacent to the symphysis pubis as the result of repetitive minor trauma (Fig. 17-41).

There are numerous synonyms for this disorder, including rectus-adductor syndrome, traumatic inguino-leg syndrome, anterior pelvic joint syndrome, Pierson syndrome, chondritis pubis, post-traumatic osteonecrosis of the pubis, and the gracilis syndrome.[42,43] These terms seem to cover several etiologic possibilities as well as subtly different sites of maximum pain within the confines of the symphysis.

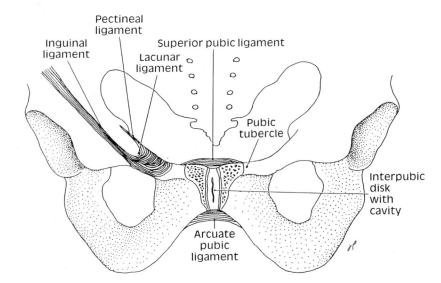

Fig. 17-41. Cross section of the symphysis pubis. (From Nicholas and Hershman,[51] with permission.)

The association of the disorder with activity was first emphasized by Pierson in 1929, when he reported groin pain in a 25-year-old man following repeated lifting of heavy boxes. Spinelli in 1932 described the syndrome in athletes, in this case mainly fencers.[43–45] The term "traumatic aseptic osteitis pubis," as coined by Shaker, is preferable in sport to indicate its traumatic and aseptic nature.[42]

The most common etiologic factor is sprinting, particularly in association with kicking or sudden direction changes. Hence the lesion is most commonly seen in soccer, ice hockey, indoor track, and basketball.[3,43] Sometimes the excessive side-to-side motion that is exaggerated by swinging the arms across the trunk while running or race walking may contribute to either the production or the perpetuation of the signs.[2] It may also be aggravated by a decreased range of rotation at the hip, which may generate increased stress on the symphysis and the sacroiliac joint in one-legged pivoting motions, including kicking. The latter has not been substantiated, however.

Signs and Symptoms

The clinical picture is fairly constant and consists in pubic symphysis tenderness and groin pain radiating to the perineal and inguinal region or along the adductor region of the thigh. It may be precipitated by adductor muscles or abdominal muscle contraction. The exact etiology of the traumatic syndrome is unsure, but it includes the following possibilities.

1. Inflammation of the symphysis pubis secondary to repetitive minor trauma
2. Aseptic necrosis of bone secondary to trauma or thrombosis of end-arteries
3. Avascular necrosis of part of the pubic bone
4. Fatigue (stress) fracture of the bone just adjacent to the symphysis
5. Minor subluxation or diastasis with or without instability or post-traumatic arthritis
6. Muscle strain with degenerative changes of the bony origin of the rectus abdominis or adductor longus

---

Practice Point

TRAUMATIC ASEPTIC OSTEITIS PUBIS
Activity-acquired osteitis pubis

- Aseptic
- Secondary to repetitive minor trauma
- May involve some damage to end-arteries
- May involve inflammatory reaction
- Maximal tenderness over symphysis
- Pain may radiate to groin or lower abdomen
- If severe gives hot bone scan
- When prolonged, association with radiologic changes

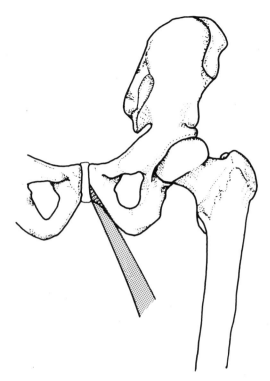

Fig. 17-42. Gracilis muscle attached to the inferior margin of the symphysis may be involved in inflammation of the symphysis complex. In this case "gracilis syndrome" is an appropriate term.

7. Gracilis tendinitis where the gracilis attaches to the inferior margin of the symphysis (Fig. 17-42)
8. Avulsion fracture (either stress or acute) involving the gracilis tendon of origin

It is probably best to reserve the term osteitis pubis for classic post-traumatic inflammation of the symphysis. When the local symptoms are more restricted to the upper surface and the rectus abdominis, it should be dealt with as rectus abdominis tendinopathy. When the symptoms are related primarily to the adductor and gracilis tendon, the term gracilis syndrome should be used. Classic osteitis pubis has some well defined radiologic changes (Table 17-8).

Radiologic Changes

Bony changes may be absent early during the symptom complex. Furthermore, variations in the appearance of the symphysis pubis are common, particularly in the adolescent (Fig. 17-43), which has led

to the assumption by some individuals that these radiologic findings are not helpful. However, in moderately severe osteitis pubis the bone scan is nearly always hot; and if athletes are followed long enough, radiologic changes always occur in the presence of protracted symptoms. Such changes include loss of definition of bone, widening of the symphysis, erosions, sclerosis, a mixed pattern of bone destruction and sclerosis, periosteal reaction, and hypertrophic changes with asymmetry[43] (Fig. 17-44).

Differential Diagnosis

Probably all of the suggested etiologies are valid and for the most part produce a similar clinical picture. However, it is necessary to consider the differential diagnosis and rule out other treatable entities (Fig. 17-45).[46]

Inguinal hernia should be ruled out if there is a dull inguinal pain after exercise and pain with coughing. The groin is examined with the patient in the supine and standing positions, looking for a visible abdominal mass that is exaggerated by increasing the intra-abdominal pressure. Palpable impact on the examining finger while pressing on the external inguinal orifice may demonstrate an incipient inguinal hernia (Table 17-8). Herniography has proved to be an ex-

---

Practice Point

TRAUMATIC OSTEITIS PUBIS: DIFFERENTIAL DIAGNOSIS

- Gracilis syndrome
- Stress fractures
- Inguinal hernia
- Ilio-inguinal ligament defects
- Orchitis or prostatitis
- Urolithiasis
- Muscle strain rectus abdominis or adductors
- Avulsion bony fragments
- Ilio-inguinal neuralgia
- Ankylosing spondylitis
- Reiter's syndrome
- Hyperparathyroidism
- Infection
- Primary and secondary tumors

TABLE 17-8.   Post-traumatic Aseptic Osteitis Pubis

Signs and Symptoms	Radiology	Treatment

Mild degree
  <6 Weeks' duration
  Pain after vigorous activity
  Settles with rest
  Tenderness over symphysis
  Resisted adduction painful
  Normal blood screen (CBC, ESR)
  Normal urinalysis
  Usually more one side than the
    other
	Plain roentgenograms, often negative
	May be hot bone scan
		Rest for 6 weeks. Only activities that
		  do not precipitate any discomfort
		NSAIDs

Moderate degree
  >6 Weeks' duration
  Pain with all vigorous activities
  Tender over symphysis
  Resisted adduction painful
  Resisted abdominal contraction
    painful
  Normal blood screen (CBC, ESR,
    HLA_{B27})
  Normal urinalysis
	Plain films may show
	  Osteolysis
	  Irregularity
	  ±Widening
	  ±Mild sclerosis
		Rest 6–12 weeks
		NSAIDs
		Consider injection if local tenderness

Severe degree
  >12 Weeks' duration
  Pain with ADL
  Pain even at rest
  Tender over symphysis
  Referred groin pains
  Passive adductor stretch painful
  Resisted adduction painful
  Resisted abdominal contraction
    painful
  Normal blood screen (CBC, ESR,
    HLA_{B27}, alkaline phosphatase)
  Normal urinalysis
	Plain films should show changes
	  Erosions
	  Irregularity
	  Fragmentation
	  Sclerosis
	  ±Widening
		Rest 3–6 months
		NSAIDs
		Consider local injection
		Oral steroids

Recurrent (intractable)
  >6 Months' duration or recur-
    rent episodes
  Local tenderness
  Varying pain severity
  Negative blood screen
  Negative urinalysis
	Hot bone scan or classic
	  plain film findings
		Consider alternate diagnosis
		Steroids (oral)
		Inject steroids
		Protracted rest
		Change recreation
		Consider surgery
		  Tenotomy
		  Fusion

cellent and sensitive diagnostic test that is capable of demonstrating a hernia in the groin, even when the physical examination has revealed nothing. Herniography is performed with an intraperitoneal injection of contrast medium through a left lower quadrant puncture.[45] (See Chapter 18.)

A diagnosis of ilioinguinal neuralgia is suspected where there has been previous abdominal surgery, e.g., appendectomy or hernia repair, or if there is a history of paresthesia.[44] Disturbed superficial sensitivity to sharp and blunt touch medially in the groin or augmented pain with the hip hyperextended are suggestive, and the diagnosis may be confirmed by blockade of the nerve with local anesthetic.[46]

Prostatitis, if present, should be confirmed by the evidence of inflammatory cells or a positive culture of prostatic secretion or urine. Rectal examination usually reveals a soft, irregular, tender prostate gland (Table 17-9).

A history of night pain or pain not related to activity should lead to a consideration of tumor, including chondroma, chondrosarcoma, chondroblastoma,

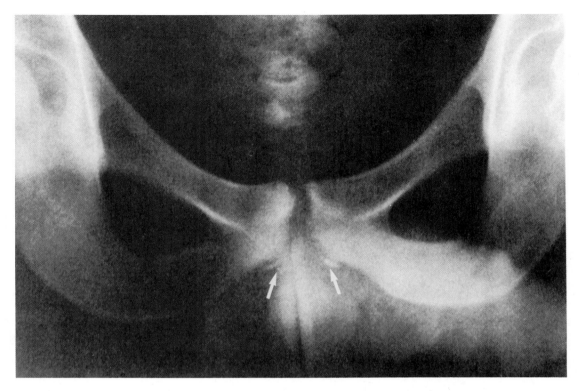

Fig. 17-43. There is considerable anatomic variation of the apophyseal center of the pubis in adolescents. It can mistakenly be identified as avulsion of the adductor longus tendon.

and Ewing sarcoma. Circulatory abnormalities of the femoral head with avascular necrosis, stress fractures, arthritis of the hip joint, and lymphadenopathy of the groin nodes enter the differential diagnosis. Finally, the history of a rapid onset of sharp pain with a sudden forceful movement should lead to consideration of an avulsion injury. Discomfort along the tendon and not on its origin from the pelvis is compatible with tendinitis. Many of these optional diagnoses for inguinal and groin pain may be delineated by plain roentgenograms and, when necessary, a bone scan.

Treatment

Treatment of osteitis pubis is based on some form of modified rest. In particular, ballistic adduction movements, rapid full range flexion and extension movements, and rapid resisted work for the rectus abdominis should be avoided. An initial trial of NSAIDs or even an injection of steroid may be tried. This injection may be directed into the symphysis; and in cases where the main symptoms are related to the adductors, the injection may be at the insertion of either the gracilis or the adductor longus. Bearing in

mind the possibility of an infective etiology, such injections should always be preceded by a complete blood count and an erythrocyte sedimentation rate (ESR). In appropriate cases, antibiotics may be necessary.

Fitness is maintained by cycling, swimming, and water-running when these motions are possible and pain-free. Return to activity must be slow. There should be no pain with activity, and a careful warm-up and stretching routine should be taught. Flexibility training is essential to prevent recurrence. Protection

---

Practice Point

PREVENTION OF OSTEITIS PUBIS RECURRENCE

- Adequate rest until all symptoms resolve
- Slow reintegration into sport
- Emphasis on full flexibility of abduction
- Education on need for careful warm-up before participation and cool down after

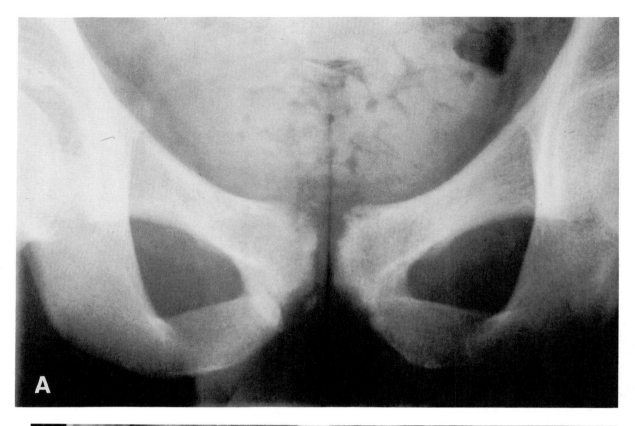

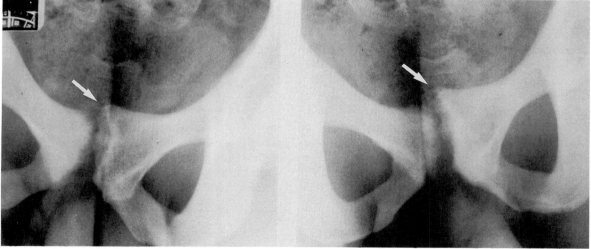

Fig. 17-44. Radiographs of traumatic aseptic osteitis pubis of the pelvis. **(A)** Subarticular erosions are observed. Note the fragmentation of the superior and inferior pubis. Other changes may include increased sclerosis on both sides of the symphysis, and osteolytic changes of the pubic rami at the origin of the gracilis muscle. **(B)** Mild instability is illustrated by having the athlete stand on the right and then the left leg (Flamingo views).

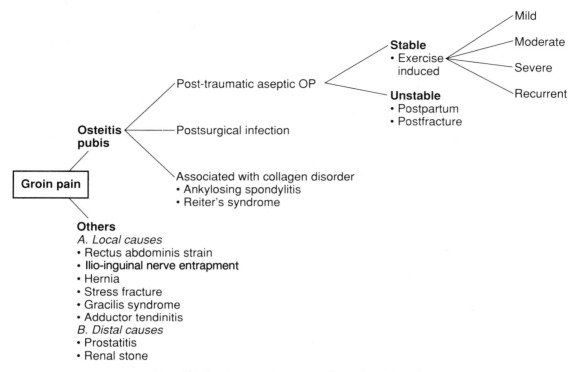

Fig. 17-45. Approach to symphyseal-groin pain.

from forceful side-foot kicking, sprinting, and sudden decelerating and turning motions is maintained until absolutely pain-free high velocity resisted adduction motion is possible on a 3 times per week basis for 2 to 3 weeks. This tolerance is best tested on hydraulic isokinetic or omnikinetic apparatus.

When conservative treatment fails, and the patient is not willing to change or abandon the sporting activity, adductor tenotomy and/or rectus abdominis tenotomy may be considered.[47] Rarely, arthrodesis (fusion) of the pubic symphysis or excision of the bony fragment, when present, is warranted in long-standing cases that have not responded to nonoperative therapy. A trial of corticosteroids in a tapered dosage regimen over 10 days to 2 weeks should be used as a final attempt to clear up the condition before surgery is carried out.

This condition is characterized by chronicity and recurrence. Therefore every effort should be made to establish an early diagnosis and to treat the initial episode aggressively in regard to medication and modalities and with adequate rest and protection in terms of the activity component.

FRACTURES AND DISLOCATIONS

Introduction

Pelvic Fractures

Pelvic fractures are classified as minor and major. Minor fractures involve avulsions and simple bone disruptions (Fig. 17-46). Major fractures involve more than one break in the ring and include displaced

---

Quick Facts

MINOR PELVIC FRACTURES

- Single pubic rami
- Wing of ilium
- Ischial ramus or body
- Avulsion fractures
- Undisplaced sacral fractures
- Coccygeal disruption

TABLE 17-9. Differential Diagnosis of Groin Pain

Diagnosis	Pain: Area of Tenderness	Referred Pain	Roentgen Changes	Bone Scan	CBC	ESR	Urinalysis	Special Tests
Osteitis pubis (traumatic aseptic)	Whole symphysis increased with resisted adduction	Groin and adductor region	Osteolysis, irregularity, sclerosis, widening, fragmentation	Positive	N	N	N	Flamingo views helpful if instability, especially postpartum
Osteitis pubis (assoc. with Reiter's syndrome or ankylosing spondylitis)	Same	Same	Same	May show other areas of involvement	Usually N	May be ↑	May have positive culture in Reiter's syndrome	May respond to antibiotics or NSAIDs HLA$_{B27}$ sometimes positive.
Osteitis pubis (after infection)	Same	Same	Same	Positive	May be ↑ WBC	May be ↑	May culture organisms	Respond to antibiotic
Gracilis syndrome	Inferior symphysis gracilis attachment Painful resisted adduction	Groin and adductor region	Occasionally inferior osteolysis or fragmentation	Negative	N	N	N	None
Adductor longus tendinitis	Proximal tendon and adductor region Usually one side	Groin and adductor region	None	Negative	N	N	N	None
Hernia	Inguinal area and symphysis Usually one side	Scrotum, groin	None	Negative	N	N	N	Palpable mass with Valsalva Positive herniography
Ilio-inguinal nerve entrapment	Inguinal area	Groin, scrotum	None	Negative	N	N	N	Usually previous abdominal surgery
Rectus abdominis strain or inguinal ligament defect	Superior pubis Rectus abdominis insertion	Lower abdomen and symphysis	None	Negative	N	N	N	Resisted abdominal contraction painful Occasionally positive herniography

N = normal; ↑ = increased.

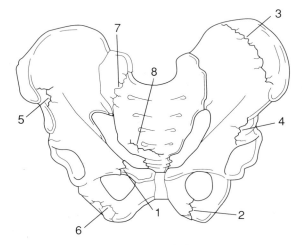

Fig. 17-46. Minor pelvic fractures include fracture of a single pubic ramus (1 and 2), fracture of the wing of the ilium (3), fracture of the ischium (4), avulsion fracture of the pelvic brim (5 and 6), and undisplaced fracture of the sacrum or coccyx (7 and 8). (Adapted from Rockwood and Green.[48])

Practice Point

MAJOR PELVIC FRACTURES

- Pelvic instability
- Significant hemorrhage
- Associated bladder and urethral injuries
- Neurologic injury with displaced sacral fractures
- May need surgical stabilization or open reduction
- All constitute an emergency

---

sacral injuries.[48] "Major" signifies potential pelvic instability or serious associated complications (Fig. 17-47). Acetabular fractures are distinguished and dealt with independently. Major pelvic fractures are rare outside of high-speed motor sports, skiing, cycling, and occasional equestrian events.

There are three patterns of major pelvic fractures. The first, the straddle type injury, involves the superior and inferior pubic or ischial rami bilaterally or in combination with a symphysis pubis disruption. The second type is the double vertical fracture, which involves one set of rami or pubis and either disruption of the sacroiliac joint or adjacent ilium. These injuries have a high associated complication rate and potential mortality. The straddle type injuries are linked to pelvic floor, urethral, and bladder damage. The double breaks in the ring are associated with nerve injury, bowel and bladder damage, and significant blood loss (Table 17-10). Major fractures comprising the third group involve the acetabular side of the hip joint. Full radiologic investigation delineates the appropriate treatment, which is frequently surgical reduction and fixation in an attempt to slow the rate of onset of post-traumatic arthritis and allow early resumption of motion. Treatment of these fractures includes first aid, treatment of shock, and transfer to a hospital as rapidly as possible.[48]

Acetabular Fractures

Acetabular fractures may occur in isolation, usually when the femoral head is driven directly into the floor of the joint, which may result in protrusion of the femoral head into the pelvis. Usually acetabular injuries are seen in association with dislocations or other pelvic fractures. Because of the intra-articular nature, careful evaluation using special views and CT scanning is necessary. Frequently open reduction is indicated.

Fractures of the Sacrum

Usually enormous forces are required to fracture the sacrum, and this injury is rarely seen in most sports. However, equestrian events, cycling, parachuting, and on occasion contact sports produce this injury. Usually the fragments are undisplaced, and the injury heals uneventfully. Complications, which include hemorrhage and trauma to the sacral nerve roots, are dramatic when they occur. Careful radiologic evaluation including CT scanning may be required to establish the need for operative intervention. The usual therapy is bed rest with slow, careful progression of weight-bearing and activity as pain subsides. However, before this treatment is pursued, a single fracture or sacroiliac injury must be distinguished from the serious, potentially fatal double fracture of the pelvic ring.

Fractures of the Coccyx

Fractures of the coccyx are produced by falling when in the sitting position and landing on the buttock. Usually separation occurs at the sacrococcygeal

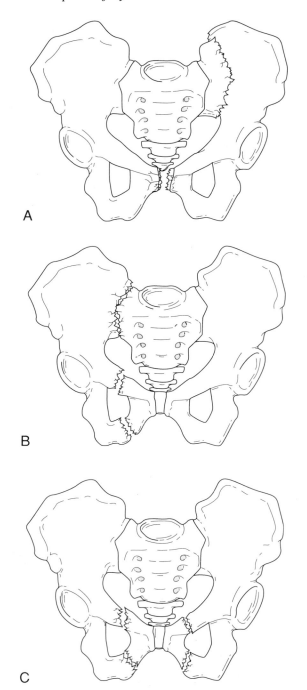

A

B

C

Fig. 17-47. Major pelvic fractures always involve two breaks in the pelvic ring. They may be any combination of the sacroiliac joint or adjacent sacrum and ischium and the pubic symphysis **(A)** or the adjacent superior and inferior pubic rami **(B)**. **(C)** The straddle fracture involves all four pubic rami. Major pelvic fracture implies instability and potentially serious associated complications of the pelvic viscera.

junction where the four coccygeal segments are united to the sacrum via a fibrocartilaginous disc.

There may be exquisite pain at the time of injury that is exacerbated by walking, running, or twisting movements as stress is placed on the ligamentous connections with the coccyx. Tenderness is seen to be present on either direct pressure over the coccyx or by moving the tip of the coccyx during a rectal examination. The lateral roentgenogram may be equivocal because of the large range of normal positions and the frequent absence of displacement. The morbidity of this injury is almost entirely related to the associated discomfort.

Treatment is directed at the symptoms. NSAIDs are helpful. Using a pillow or sitting on a thick book such as a telephone book on a firm chair allow the individual to sit forward on the ischial tuberosities and relieve pressure from the coccyx. Tight clothing may further aggravate a tender coccyx. Activity is progressed at whatever rate the resolving symptoms allow. If the coccyx remains chronically painful, injection with a steroid, with or without mobilization, may be helpful. Although excision of the coccyx is possible for an intractably painful situation, it is rarely indicated and not recommended without careful consideration.

Hip Dislocation

The hip is a structurally strong joint from both bony and ligamentous aspects, and so dislocation requires large external forces. High speed sports (e.g., skiing) and situations where heavy contact is made on the flexed adducted hip (e.g., football pile-ups) sometimes result in dislocation, and frequently there is an associated acetabular lip fracture. Approximately 90 percent of hip dislocations in sport are posterior.

Immediately after trauma the athlete is in severe pain, and the leg is usually slightly flexed, adducted, and internally rotated. Occasionally, the massive neurogenic stimulation produces "shock" irrespective of associated blood loss, which is promptly relieved with reduction. Thus blood pressure may be low or high secondary to pain stimulation. Reduction is rarely possible without some anesthesia. Treatment is splinting and rapid transfer to an institution where the diagnosis can be confirmed and reduction achieved. Severe transient or even permanent sciatic nerve damage is not uncommon with this injury.

Anterior hip dislocation, when it does occur, is associated with a blow to the extended externally rotated leg. Rarely this injury occurs when twisting away

TABLE 17-10. Blood Loss as a Complication of Pelvic Fractures

Type	Description	% Patients Transfused	Units of Whole Blood per Transfused Patient
I	Fractures without a break in the pelvic ring Wing of ilium Single pubis or ischial ramus Avulsions of anterosuperior iliac spine Avulsions of ischial tuberosity Fractures of sacrum or coccyx	28	5.5
II	Fractures with single break in the pelvic ring Both rami of one side Separation of symphysis Separation of sacroiliac joint	30	3.5
III	Double breaks in the pelvic ring Double vertical fractures Severe multiple fractures	67	11.2
IV	Fractures of the acetabulum Displaced and undisplaced With or without associated hip dislocation	24	4.0

(Data from Rockwood and Green[48] and Hauser and Perry.[49])

from a fixed hyperextended hip. The dislocation occurs with the head forcing its way out through the iliofemoral ligament and adjacent capsule. The immediate post-dislocation posture is a flexed, abducted, externally rotated position (Fig. 17-48). Management is the same as for posterior hip dislocations.

Practice Point

HIP DISLOCATION

Site	Posterior Dislocation	Anterior Dislocation
Hip	Flexed Adducted Internally rotated Trochanter & buttock prominent	Slightly Flexed Abducted Externally rotated Femoral head may be prominent
Thigh	Rests on contralateral leg	Lateral border rests on bed
Length	Appears short	Appears short
Foot	Points toward opposite leg	Points away from opposite leg

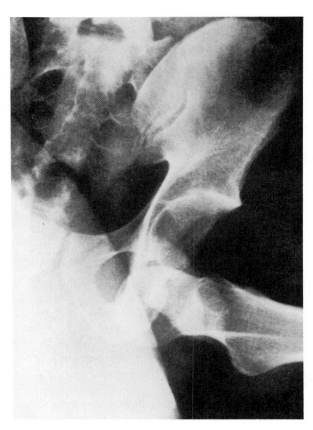

Fig. 17-48. Anterior hip dislocation. Roentgenogram shows an empty acetabulum. Clinically the athlete's leg would be flexed abducted.

Slipped Capital Femoral Epiphysis (Adolescent Coxa Vera)

A progressive or sudden slip posteroinferior of the femoral head through the epiphysis may occur in young individuals. It is important to be aware of the potential for this injury if serious short- and long-term complications are to be avoided. Although it usually presents as hip pain, particularly with rotation, the pain may be referred down the medial thigh to the knee. Occasionally, the condition is initially manifested only by knee pain. It should always be considered when a young athlete between the ages of 8 to 12 years presents with knee discomfort and no effusion. There is a 20 to 25 percent incidence of bilateral involvement.

The separation occurs through the mechanically weak zone of the epiphysis, between the hypertrophying and calcifying cells. Contributing factors include increasing shear forces as the epiphyseal plate becomes more vertical and the muscle forces and external pressures increase. The slip may occur in a slow chronic fashion, as an acute on chronic slip, or as an acute sudden separation. A disproportionate sex hormone/growth hormone ratio has been postulated but has never been substantiated.[50] The condition is frequently seen with two distinct body habitus. The first is the tall individual with a history of rapid verti-

cal growth and possibly a history of trauma, when excessive growth hormone effect could potentially widen the epiphysis. The second is the slightly obese adolescent (Fröhlich type) in whom a decrease in sex hormone response is possible[51] (Fig. 17-49).

As has been stressed, the *young athlete may present with either hip or knee pain or both*, and the subsequent symptoms depend on whether the source is the mechanical effect of a slip or the associated synovitis. The synovitis produces a painful limitation of motion with associated psoas spasm. The hip tends to be held in flexion, and there is often an antalgic or gluteal limp and an apparent leg length discrepancy if severe. The mechanical signs are due to the anterosuperior movement of the femoral neck and the apparent posteroinferior position of the head. When the patient's leg is taken passively into flexion, it tends to move into external rotation and slight abduction instead of staying in the midline (Fig. 17-49). There may be limita-

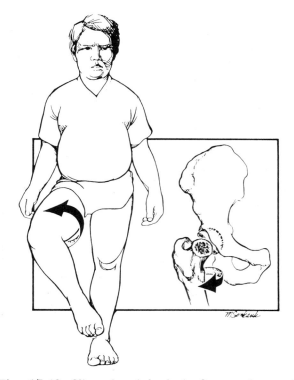

Fig. 17-49. Slipped epiphysis is frequently manifested clinically by obligatory external rotation accompanying attempts at passive flexion of the hip. **(insert)** Complete displacement, with the femoral neck rotating anteriorly and externally giving a relative posterior and inferior position to the head. (After Nicholas and Hershman,[51] with permission.)

Quick Facts

RADIOLOGIC STAGING OF SLIPPED EPIPHYSIS

- Preslip
  - No measurable displacement
  - Epiphyseal widening
  - Soft tissue swelling due to synovitis
- Minimal slip
  - Less than 1 cm of displacement
- Moderate slip
  - More than 1 cm
  - Less than two-thirds of diameter of the neck
- Severe slip
  - Displacement more than two-thirds of neck
- Complete slip
  - Loss of contact of head with neck

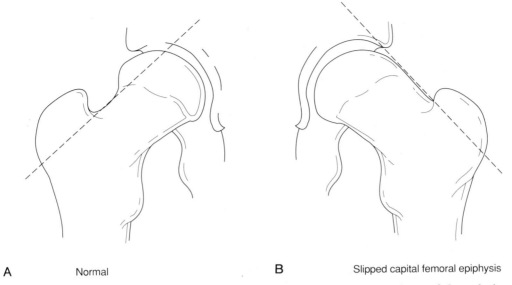

A   Normal   B   Slipped capital femoral epiphysis

Fig. 17-50. Radiologic signs of the slip may be detected by minor alterations of the relation of the head to the neck. **(A)** line drawn along the superior neck should transect some of the femoral head due to the "S" shaped silhouette. **(B)** Top of neck and head flatter, the line does not transect head.

tion of internal rotation, abduction, and flexion. There may also be a positive Trendelenburg sign and gait if severe, as well as a small but measurable true leg length discrepancy.

Radiologic evaluation may show widening of the epiphyseal line and the degree of slip. The superior line of the femoral neck fails to transect the overhanging ossified epiphysis with a minor slip (Fig. 17-50). When the slip is chronic, new bone formation may fill in the gap superiorly and inferiorly, producing the so-called coxa magna.

Treatment is aimed at reducing synovitis and preventing further slip in the early stages. When a minimal slip occurs, the head is usually pinned in situ (Fig. 17-51). There are specific limited indications for manipulation of an acute or chronic slip because of the danger of inducing avascular necrosis. When a severe chronic slip seriously affects functional range of motion, some form of osteotomy is considered. For the young active child or competitive individual, activity is resumed soon after pinning and is progressed mainly as pain allows. Full activity may be gradually undertaken by 6 weeks after operation.

Stress Fracture

Stress fracture has become a frequent diagnosis in this era of increased recreational activity, particularly among the segment of individuals who jog or participate in aerobic dance activities.[52] Although a better understanding of biomechanics and improved shoe design have modified the trend for an increase in these injuries, stress fractures of the hip and pelvis still form a small but significant injury that needs to be diagnosed early and treated effectively to avoid serious complications. Indeed, since the classic articles of Ernst,[53] Devas,[54] and Blickenstaff and Morris,[55] much emphasis has been placed on stress fractures occurring within the pelvis and femoral neck.

Femoral Neck Stress Fracture

Seen in military recruits and enthusiastic joggers, femoral neck stress fractures occur starting primarily on the tension (superior) side or the compression (inferior) side of the femoral neck (Figs. 17-52 and 17-53). Untreated they can go on to become complete and displaced fractures. (Fig. 17-54).

Diagnosis

The earliest and most frequent symptom is inguinal or anterior groin pain, which occurs in up to 87 percent of patients.[52] Occasionally, the initial complaints suggest trochanteric bursitis. Night pain occurs in a good proportion of subjects if the diagnosis is not made and the fracture progresses. Frequently, the initial symptoms start after a long run or a particularly intensive exercise bout.

On examination the most constant finding is discomfort at the extremes of hip rotation. Tenderness

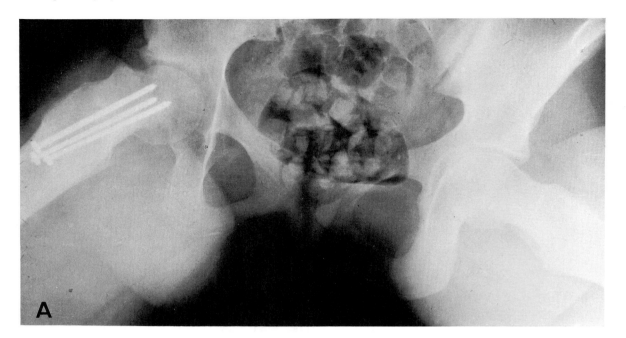

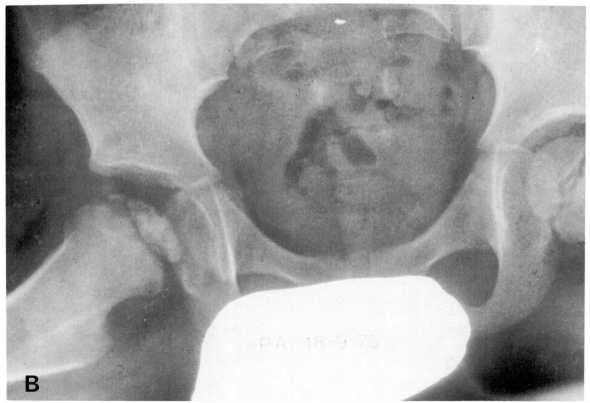

Fig. 17-51. (A) Displaced femoral capital epiphysis that has been pinned in situ. **(B)** In the young individual, avascular necrosis must always be included in the differential diagnosis of hip pain. The collapsed head is shown here.

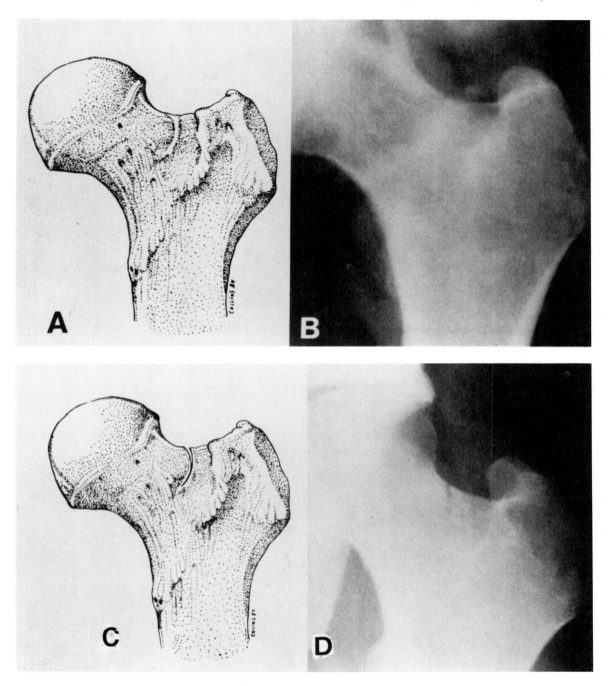

Fig. 17-52. **(A)** Stress fractures are frequently located on the superior neck, which is the tension side. **(B)** Roentgenogram of the early tension side stress reaction shows sclerosis on the superior neck. **(C)** Progression to a visible crack on superior neck. **(D)** Roentgenogram shows the tension side of the fracture. (From Fullerton and Snowdy,[52] with permission.)

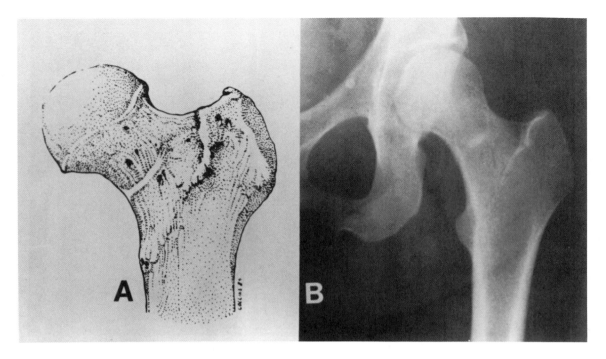

Fig. 17-53. **(A)** Location of the compression side of a femoral neck fracture. **(B)** Early cancellous reaction manifested by sclerosis on the inferior neck.

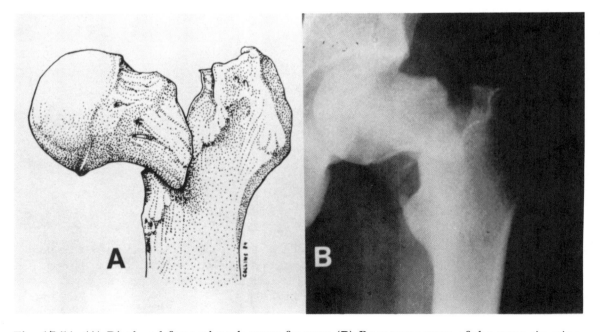

Fig. 17-54. **(A)** Displaced femoral neck stress fracture.**(B)** Roentgenogram of the same situation. (From Fullerton and Snowdy,[52] with permission.)

in the inguinal area over the hip joint is apparent in up to two-thirds of athletes. Heel percussion rarely gives a positive test. As the symptoms progress, the athlete walks with an antalgic gait. Laboratory studies, including alkaline phosphatase, calcium, phosphorus, and ESR, are rarely helpful.

Radiography

By the time the initial roentgenogram is obtained the impending fracture is usually visible, at least in retrospect. Tension side fractures frequently exhibit either endosteal or periosteal callus or an overt tension side fracture line without displacement. Eventually this fracture line widens on the tension side (superior neck) without loss of medial cortex continuity. Complete displacement will occur if activity is not modified and treatment instituted. Compression side stress fractures most commonly exhibit sclerosis on the initial roentgenograms followed by a compression (inferior neck) side cortical break. As with the superior neck fractures, this injury potentially progresses to a complete separation and displacement.

In all cases, bone scintigraphy is positive prior to the appearance of plain film studies. *Bone scintigraphy is indicated in the presence of undiagnosed, progressive, or nonresponding hip pain after a negative plain film.* The importance of the bone scan is that it gives assistance in making a more definitive diagnosis in an area where complex anatomy and a deeply placed joint make clinical evaluation difficult.

Treatment

The aims of treatment are to promote early healing, prevent development of a complete and displaced fracture, and guide a safe return to normal activity (Fig. 17-55).

Positive Bone Scan Only or Sclerosis and No Crack. Once the diagnosis is established, the initial treatment is proportional to the severity of symptoms and may range from modified bed rest to non-weight-bearing with crutches until symptoms subside. Once pain-free, weight-bearing is progressed. When significant partial weight-bearing is possible without pain, cardiovascular and general conditioning workouts are permitted with cycling or swimming. Serial roentgenograms are obtained at weekly intervals until the athlete can walk with full weight-bearing and no pain. Water-running and water-walking are progressed; and if the athlete remains pain-free, running is commenced. The initial run should be no farther than one-fourth mile, with the distance being increased by one-fourth mile every second session provided no pain or limp is experienced. If pain returns, a 2-day rest is taken and the milage reduced by one-fourth mile and then progressed again according to symptoms. If symptoms persist or distance is added so the athlete is able to run 1 mile pain-free, the hip is roentgenographed again. If healing is progressing, slow sequential resumption of former levels of activity is permitted.

Overt Fracture Line with No Displacement. Provided only one cortex is involved and there is no displacement, an initial period of bed rest or complete non-weight-bearing with crutches is necessary. It may be possible that tension side fractures are biomechanically more prone to rapid progression. In any event, caution is the key, and roentgenograms every 2 to 3 days during the first week is necessary to detect any extension or widening of the fracture line.

If healing occurs and symptoms resolve, the athlete advances through the program outlined above. If the pain does not subside or if there is evidence of fracture line extension, internal fixation with some form of hip pin is indicated, followed by return to the activity program outlined above. Some investigators believe that full activity should be restricted until pin removal at 6 months.[52] If the pin is removed, activities are restricted for about 3 months. During this interval running is resumed, but no contact sports are allowed. No activities in which athletes cannot control their own environment should be pursued, e.g., skiing, parachuting, or intensive training or competition.

Overt Fracture with Opening. Any opening or displacement, particularly on the tension side, is significant, and surgical treatment is indicated. Usually more substantial fixation is required than simple pinning, and frequently some form of hip screw and plate is used. Postoperatively the patient rests until pain subsides and then progresses to full activity as outlined and as healing occurs. The fixative device is probably better removed in an aggressively active young person; and for a displaced fracture with a hip screw with plate, a time interval of about a year is accepted, though there are no firm rules. This method obviously requires a further period of progressive rehabilitation.

Displaced Femoral Neck Fractures. Displaced femoral neck fractures must be treated as an orthopaedic emergency. Early accurate open reduction and internal fixation are necessary. The same protocol is used

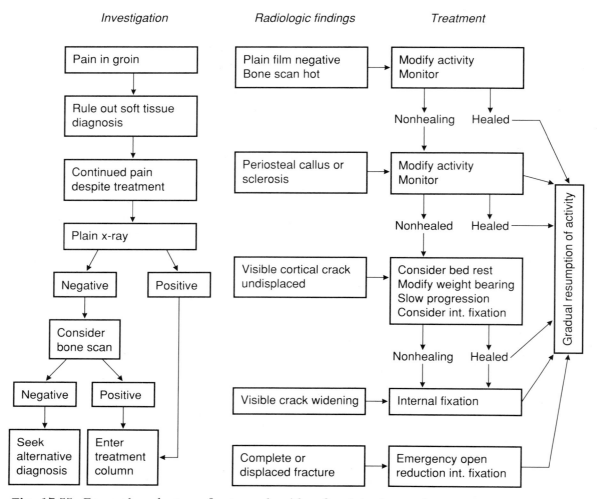

Fig. 17-55. Femoral neck stress fracture algorithm for detection and treatment

postoperatively, as outlined above. However, with displaced fractures there is a real concern about the complication of avascular necrosis of the femoral neck. If there is early evidence of avascular necrosis, a totally different protocol is required to protect the revascularizing femoral head. The ultimate prognosis for return to high level sport is poor in this situation.

Pelvic Stress Fracture

The frequent sites of pelvic stress fractures are the ischial and superior pubic rami, and the inferior ramus, the latter site being most common. Groin pain aggravated by activity is usually the presenting complaint, and single-leg standing and hopping generate or exacerbate the discomfort. Deep palpation over the pubic rami may produce severe local pain. Initial roentgenograms are falsely negative in up to 60 to 70 percent of cases. These fractures are more common in young female distance runners or postmenopausal women who have recently taken up jogging. If there is a history of amenorrhea in a young female athlete who develops stress fractures, further investigation is warranted. A dietary history is important. Occasionally, bone densitometry is part of the diagnostic work-up (Fig. 17-56).

Because stress fractures represent single breaks in the pelvic ring, treatment is largely symptomatic. Weight-bearing is graduated according to pain. A detailed activity history is obtained and analyzed for training errors in order to devise a treatment plan for

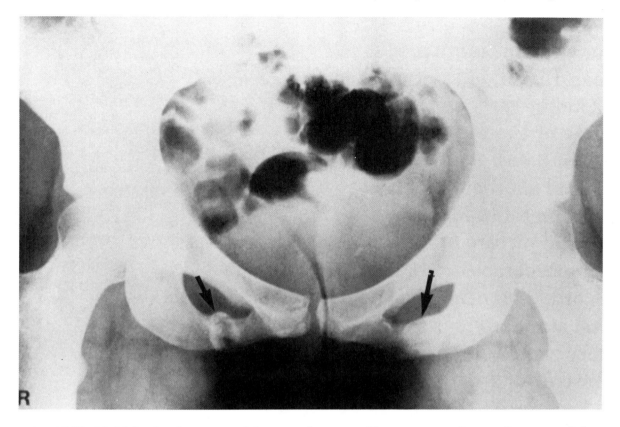

Fig. 17-56. Multiple simultaneous pelvic stress fractures. The presence of stress fractures of the pelvis in young women or multiple stress fractures in postmenopausal women should automatically generate a discussion of diet, previous pregnancies, and possibly an investigation for osteoporosis.

progressive return to activity. Unfortunately, these fractures may take as long as 2 to 6 months to heal and become asymptomatic to the degree that intensive activity can be resumed.

Practice Point

RETURN TO RUNNING WITH LOWER LIMB STRESS FRACTURES

Bone	Duration (Weeks)
Metatarsals	2–4
Fibula	3–4
Tibial shaft	4–6
Upper tibia	8–10
Femoral shaft	12–16
Femoral neck	12–20
Pelvic fracture	12–20

CONTUSIONS, MUSCLE STRAINS, AVULSIONS, AND APOPHYSEAL INJURIES

Hip Pointer (Contusion)

Hip pointer is usually a nonspecific term, and the injury is often related to a blow on the inadequately protected iliac crest. The injury may be caused by violent contact with an opponent's helmet in football, when checking in hockey, and in noncontact sports such as baseball where the player has used poor sliding technique. In volleyball, diving for the ball on hard surfaces may produce significant bruising. Because the term hip pointer is nonspecific, it sometimes includes contusions to the greater trochanter, tearing of the external oblique aponeurosis on the iliac crest, periostitis of the iliac crest, and hematomas secondary to damage to the external obliques along the iliac crest periosteum. Sometimes the term can be used to encompass even avulsion fractures of the iliac apophyses (traction epiphysitis).

There are a large number of muscles that insert onto the iliac crest, which when contracting may contribute to discomfort and pain. These muscles include the gluteus maximus and medius, tensor facia lata, sartorius, iliacus, quadratus lumborum, latissimus dorsi, external abdominal oblique, iliocostalis lumborum, and transversus abdominis. Any motion that causes rotation of the trunk or flexion to the leg may require strong contractions of these muscles, thereby causing pain.

Treatment of the classic hip contusion includes ice and compression initially. The athlete may need crutches to assist him in walking if the injury is severe. Anti-inflammatory medications are particularly helpful. Subsequently ice is coupled or replaced by ultrasound, heat, and transcutaneous electrical nerve stimulation (TENS). Padding taped over the area may serve as some protection from direct blows in contact sports. The activities are progressed as pain decreases, and the speed of progression is often modified by the presence or absence of muscle tearing or avulsion. When dealing with simple contusion, pain is the absolute guide to progression. When one of these other injuries is superimposed, activity may be delayed to allow adequate healing before progression starts.

Muscle Strains and Insertional Avulsions

Muscles usually tear at their junction with tendon, probably related to the mismatch of tensile strength. Muscle tensile strength is approximately 77 psi, whereas that of tendon is between 8,000 and 18,000 psi.[51] Similarly, the tendinous insertion into bone via the periosteal Sharpey's fibers is usually strong, and significant stress occasionally results in avulsion if the musculotendinous junction does not fail. In the skel-

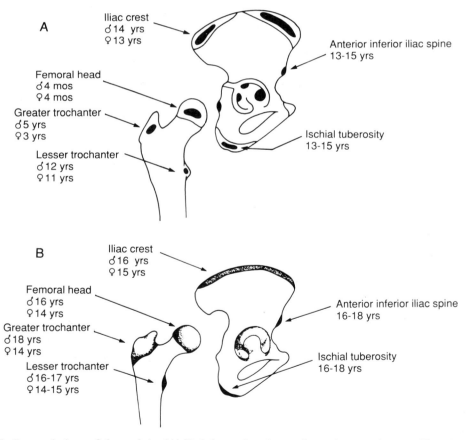

Fig. 17-57. Lateral view of the pelvis. **(A)** Epiphyseal and apophyseal secondary ossification centers. **(B)** Approximate time of fusion of the secondary centers. (Adapted from Tachdjian,[50] with permission.)

etally immature athlete the zone of hypertrophied cartilage cells is a mechanically weak link within the apophysis (traction epiphysis) and is the site of avulsion with large sudden forces[50] (Fig. 17-57). With the huge muscle masses around the pelvis, the long lever arms, and late closure of the epiphysis, the pelvis is one of the most frequent sites of avulsion in sport. Although somewhat sport-specific, the commonest sites are the ischial tuberosity, iliac crest, and antero-superior iliac spine. Less frequent are the anteroinferior iliac spine, lesser trochanter, symphysis pubis, and greater trochanter. This section deals with these areas around the pelvis where the tendon insertions form a site of potential mechanical weakness, the "locus minoris resistentia" [47] (Fig. 17-58).

Iliac Crest (External Obliques)

Either a blow to the iliac crest or abduction of the trunk on a fixed pelvis may damage the iliac crest, the apophysis, or the aponeurotic tendon of insertion of the external abdominal oblique[56] (Fig. 17-59). Athletes may even report that they felt something snap. Swelling, hemorrhage, and pain are proportional to the degree of injury, and even moderate damage usually causes a "gluteus medius" lurch when walking.

As for apophyseal injuries, a roentgenogram comparing the two sides is frequently needed to confirm the damage. It is sometimes difficult to distinguish

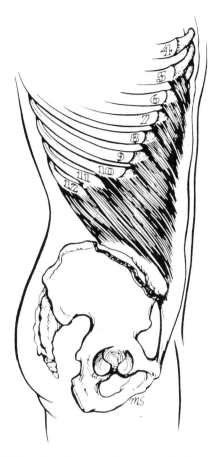

Fig. 17-59. Broad attachment of the external obliques may result in avulsion of the anterior part of the iliac crest in the young athlete.

apophyseal injury from the naturally occurring fragmentation of the iliac crest during "capping," which occurs sequentially from anterior to posterior followed by fusion from posterior to anterior in the normal adolescent (Fig. 17-60). These clinical signs are important. Furthermore, displacement of an avulsed fragment is limited by the other various soft tissue attachments. Proximal migration of the iliac crest is limited by the expansions from gluteus medius, iliacus, and tensor fascia lata.[35]

Initially, ice and compression minimize hemorrhage and edema. The degree of duration of rest is proportional to the severity of the injury. Avulsion fractures or apophyseal injuries need time to heal, as do third degree or severe second degree muscle injuries. Crutches with weight-bearing as tolerated, supportive strapping, and NSAIDs may relieve early symptoms (Table 17-11).

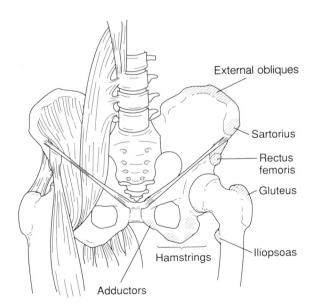

Fig. 17-58. Common sites of avulsion injuries in sports.

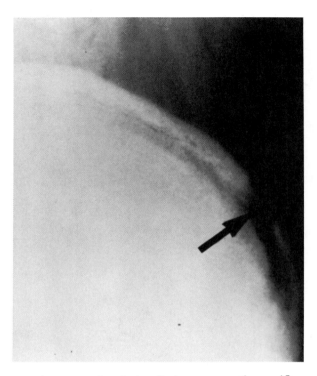

Fig. 17-60. In the skeletally immature, the ossification process (capping) of the iliac apophysis is variable. It is difficult to distinguish fractures from normal variations unless there is a broad separation accompanying the appropriate local clinical symptoms.

Ballistic activities such as jumping, twisting, and sprinting usually require complete relief of pain at rest before activities are slowly progressed. Participation in contact sports may also be delayed until tenderness is reduced. With mild injuries an early return to sports may be possible, in some cases almost immediately (Table 17-12). More severe injuries take up to 4 weeks and complete avulsions or muscle tears frequently 6 to 12 weeks. Inadequate initial therapy prolongs the duration of symptoms. Ultimately, healing occurs with little or no functional loss.

Anterosuperior Iliac Spine (Sartorius)

The anterosuperior iliac spine may be avulsed by strong contraction of the sartorius muscle (Fig. 17-61). Usually there is immediate and severe pain that radiates from the anterior iliac crest down the anterior thigh. The athlete is unable to continue participation. Examination reveals swelling and bruising over the anterior iliac crest that gradually may track

down the thigh. There is exquisite local tenderness, and flexion of the hip and knee produces pain, made worse by resistance.

Occasionally, the onset is more insidious, with increasing pain around the tendon of insertion of the muscle. Because of the limited additional soft tissue attachment, the displacement may be significant, but even in severe cases separation is rarely more than a few millimeters (up to about 2 to 3 cm) (Fig. 17-61). Comparison roentgenograms help one to appreciate the degree of displacement.

Treatment is proportional to pain but frequently requires a period of modified weight-bearing using crutches; 3 to 6 weeks are required for a bony or fibrous union. Function is usually fully restored, and surgical reattachment is rarely necessary.

Anteroinferior Iliac Spine (Rectus Femoris)

Uncontrolled contraction of the quadriceps may occur, particularly as the lower limb is being forced into extension at the hip, and flexion at the knee may cause tearing or avulsion of the rectus femoris or the anteroinferior iliac spine (Fig. 17-62). Sudden pain in the groin while hurdling, jumping, sprinting, or kicking, usually in the adolescent athlete, should lead to suspicion of this injury.

Tenderness over the muscle insertion is more difficult to isolate because of the depth of the lesion. Resistance or active contraction of the quadriceps generates pain, and combined passive flexion of the knee and extension of the hip place tension on the lesion. Migration of the anteroinferior iliac spine is not usual because of the fixation of the rectus femoris to the capsule by its reflected head. Rarely, both heads tear, and significant separation occurs. In this case, reattachment may be considered if it is thought that the healing bone will cause a mechanical block to full flexion, although it is most unusual. Late excision is also an option if symptoms persist. Generally, nonoperative treatment produces excellent functional results, however, and is similar to that outlined for the anterosuperior iliac spine injury in Table 17-12. The duration of disability is 3 to 6 weeks.

Ischial Tuberosity (Hamstrings)

Ischial tuberosity avulsion by the hamstrings, a sprinter's or gymnast's injury, is associated with sudden deceleration or stretching of the hamstrings[51]

TABLE 17-11. Treatment Principles for Muscle, Apophyseal, or Bony Avulsions

Mechanism	Overcontraction of muscle
	Frequently with eccentric loading
	Occasionally associated with direct blow
Symptoms	Sudden acute local pain at site
	Radiation down muscle
	Occasionally insidious onset
Signs	Local swelling
	Bruising proportional to injury
	Gradual tracking of bruising
	Pain with palpation at insertion site
	Pain with appropriate muscle contraction
	Rarely palpable gap
	Discomfort with muscle put on stretch
	Bilateral roentgenograms may confirm displacement
Treatment	Modified activity
	Protected weight-bearing
	Local ice and pressure as first aid
	Protective pad or strapping
	Modalities to painful area
	NSAIDs
	Restoration of range of motion
	Progressive muscle strengthening
	Gradual return to activity
	Surgery rarely indicated

All signs, symptoms, and treatment measures are proportional to the severity of the local injury and to some degree to the magnitude of the displacement and muscle involved.

(Fig. 17-63). Dancers occasionally suffer inflammation and pain in the ischial apophysis due to chronic stretching and repetitive jumping.

With avulsion, sudden pain is felt in the buttock, and usually continuation of activity is impossible. With lesser degrees of injury, activity is inhibited by the inability to generate a forceful hamstring contraction or put the hip on a stretch.

Palpation over the tuberosity is painful. There may be some swelling in the buttock area. Straight-leg raising and forceful resisted knee flexion produce pain. Roentgenograms confirm the displacement.

Treatment depends on the amount of displacement and the level of competition anticipated by the athlete (Fig. 17-64). Minimally displaced fractures are best managed by protected weight-bearing or modified activity for 2 to 4 months. Even a widely separated fragment is compatible with activity, although a large amount of callus or significant displacement may make the pressure of sitting uncomfortable, so consideration of reattachment is worthwhile even in recreational athletes. Further-

more, if the tuberosity is displaced more than 3 cm, there may be measurable loss of hamstring strength.[57] If reattachment is chosen as the treatment of choice, it is better done within the first 2 weeks.

Postoperative protection is necessary for 4 to 6 weeks. It may range from non-weight-bearing walking with crutches if good fixation is achieved to the consideration of a hip spica if the fixation is tenuous.

Superior Pubic Tubercle Avulsion and Rectus Abdominis Tendinopathy

Abdominal muscle strains usually occur within the lower rectus sheath, but occasionally the superior pubic tubercle is avulsed. The important feature here is to distinguish it from the numerous other causes of pain around the symphysis pubis or osteitis pubis.[43] Typically, an abdominal overload lesion causes pain in the lower central abdominal region when sprinting or with sudden movements such as changing direction. Abdominal exercises such as trunk curls or leg

TABLE 17-12.   Treatment Phases for Avulsion Injuries of the Hip and Pelvis

Phase	Duration (days)	Subjective Pain	Tenderness to Palpation	Range of Motion	Muscle Strength	Level of Activity	Radiographic Appearance
I: Establish diagnosis; rest and protection	0–7	Moderate to severe	Severe	Limited	Poor, pain inhibition	None to protected gait; proportional to pain and displacement	Osseous separation
II: Encourage gentle ROM	7–(14–20)	Moderate to minimal	Moderate	Improving with gentle activity and assisted exercise	Fair	Protected gait; emphasis on ROM	Osseous separation
III: Strengthening phase	14–(20–30)	Minimal with muscle contraction	Moderate	Improving; add gentle stretches	Good	Progressive ROM and strengthening	Early callus
IV: Progressive return to activity	30–(45–60)	None with strong contractions	Minimal	Full ROM	Within 15–20% of normal	Guided progressive increase in functional exercises and athletic activity	Maturing callus
V: Return to sports	45–60+	None with strong ballistic contractions	None	Normal	With 5–10% normal	Return to full training until return to competition	Maturing callus

(Data adapted from Howse.[26])

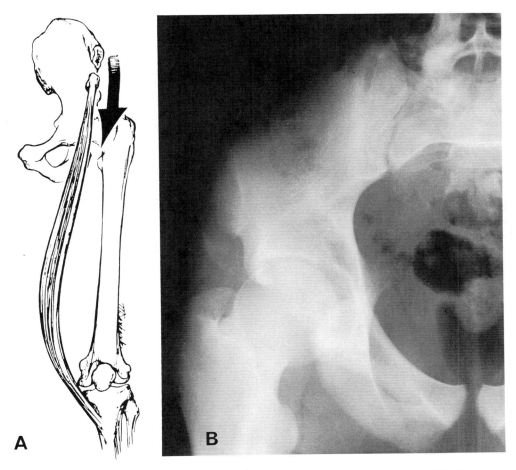

Fig. 17-61. (A) Avulsion of the anterosuperior iliac spine by the sartorius muscle. This injury is seen in sprinting, jumping, and kicking sports. (B) The separated fragment is seen on this roentgenogram.

raises are uncomfortable. There may be aching in the region after cessation of activity.

Local tenderness is usually located primarily at the insertion on the superior pubic ramus. Palpation is particularly sore just after the completion of sports activity.[57] Discomfort is aggravated by double straight-leg raising. Inguinal hernias should be ruled out by palpating all potential hernial orifices.

Conservative treatment consists in rest or modified activity, physiotherapy modalities, NSAIDs, and occasionally steroid injections. When successful, a careful progressive return to activity is mandatory. In about 40 percent of the cases of significant avulsion, particularly if initially treated inadequately, chronic pain prevents return to competitive sport. In this situation, some consideration may be given to operative intervention.

With a painful, unhealed avulsion or chronic symp-

tomatic abdominal tendinopathy, release is performed through a 10 cm transverse incision just above the symphysis pubis. The inguinal rings are left intact, and a flap of deep fascia is turned down to cover the gap created by the muscle release.[47] Postoperative care aims at allowing resumption of running at 5 weeks, depending on pain, and a return to unrestrained sports activity at 10 to 12 weeks. In a series of more than 30 patients treated in this manner by Martens et al., 70 percent had excellent and 20 percent good results; 6 percent required reoperation. At late follow-up there was no detectable muscle weakness compared to a control group. These authors stressed, however, that more intensive treatment of the acute lesion is a better option, and surgery is reserved for those who have failed conservative therapy and are unwilling to modify or give up their sport.[47]

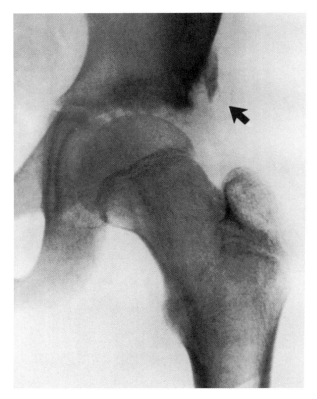

Fig. 17-62. Avulsion fractures of the anteroinferior iliac spine at the insertion of the rectus femoris.

Inferior Pubic Rami Avulsion, Gracilis Syndrome, Adductor Tendinitis

Acute traumatic avulsion of the inferior pubic ramus is rare, although a fatigue fracture involving the bony origin of the gracilis muscle at the pubic symphysis, the "gracilis syndrome," is well recognized[40] (Fig. 17-42). This injury is one of the entities that makes up the constellation of conditions broadly referred to as osteitis pubis but that should perhaps be described separately.

The gracilis muscle arises by a tendon from the inferior part of the anterior edge of the pubic symphysis and for a short distance along the border of the inferior pubic rami. Repetitive stress produces tendinitis or a stress reaction to the point of insertion causing the clinical syndrome of groin and inner thigh pain with local tenderness. Resisted adduction precipitates a sharp pain in the perineal region, often followed by a dull ache.

If the condition is simply tendinitis, the roentgeno-

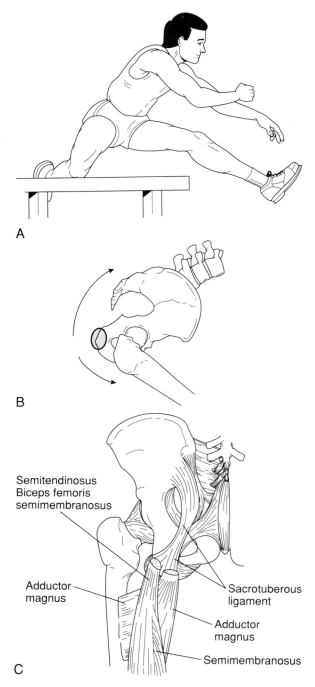

Fig. 17-63. Ischial apophyseal avulsion. **(A)** Mechanism is well demonstrated by a hurdler stumbling over a hurdle. **(B)** Counterforces generated across the ischium. **(C)** They involve the momentum of the body and contraction of the hamstrings and perhaps the adductor magnus. The sacrotuberous ligament serves to provide proximal stability. Pressure over this ligament may cause pain after an avulsion injury.

gram is negative; but if a stress fracture has occurred, the separated fragment may be visualized. However, the radiologic variations in the adolescent make interpretation difficult. Inferior rami epiphyseal centers are a normal finding.

If the usual management with modified activity, other modalities, NSAIDs, and even steroid injection is unsuccessful, surgery may be considered. If an avulsed fragment is considered the problem, it may be excised. However, if chronic adductor tendinopathy is the cause of pain, percutaneous release of the insertion of the gracilis and a small part of the adductor brevis is performed. Care must be taken to leave the adductor longus tendon intact.[40] Martens et al. reported 53 percent excellent and 25 percent good results with this procedure. A compression bandage is used postoperatively for 24 hours; running is begun at 6 weeks and full activity at 12 weeks. Attention to warm-up and stretching techniques is an important part of the follow-up.

Greater Trochanter (Gluteus Medius and Minimus)

Avulsion of the greater trochanter by the gluteus medius and minimus tendon is rare. The epiphysis appears during the fourth year of life and fuses late at about the seventeenth to nineteenth year.[50] When this injury does occur, it has serious implications for the athlete because of the importance of the abductors in stabilizing the pelvis (Fig. 17-65). Thus with other than minor degrees of separation, open reduction and internal fixation must be considered. When relatively undisplaced, the decision must be made as to the need for either protected ambulation with crutches or a hip spica. The younger the athlete, the more likely it is that spica fixation will be required.

Lesser Trochanter (Iliopsoas)

Rapid, uncontrolled rotation of the trunk on a fixed externally rotated femur may allow avulsion of a piece of the lesser trochanter in the older athlete, or the apophysis in the younger person, by the enormously strong iliopsoas muscle (Fig. 17-66). A sudden severe pain in the groin followed by an inability to bear weight comfortably comprise the usual presenting complaint. On examination, there may be minimal local swelling or visible bruising because of the depth of the involved structures. Local tenderness in the femoral triangle and decreased ability to flex the hip while in a sitting position, Ludloff's sign, are present.

Roentgenograms confirm the diagnosis, although displacement is rarely large because there are soft tissue connections from the hip joint that prevent undue retraction. Comparison with the other side helps clarify the diagnosis in the skeletally immature athlete.

In severe cases complete rest may be required for 24 to 48 hours with the hip supported in flexion. However, early gentle motion with light partial weight-bearing is the treatment of choice. Treatment involves restoring range of motion, gradual strengthening, and progressive return to activity. Surgical reattachment is rarely indicated. Occasionally, a large mass of callus forms that interferes with motion and may require surgical excision.

Gluteus Medius Strain and Tendinitis

Gluteus medius strain and tendinitis was the most common soft tissue problem in a series of 200 hip and pelvic injuries reported by Lloyd-Smith et al., comprising 18 percent of the total.[2] The report noted pain at the origin, midsubstance, and insertion. However, differentiating between gluteus medius insertion tendinitis and trochanteric bursitis can be difficult because of their proximity at the greater trochanter. The criteria given for differentiating these two entities was that inflammation of the gluteus medius tendon causes maximum tenderness just proximal to the greater trochanter and pain on resisted abduction. If the pain was located over the lateral aspect of the trochanter and there was no pain with resisted hip abduction, the entity was labeled trochanteric bursitis. In reality, it is not easy to distinguish these entities with a great degree of certainty, and the statement of Lloyd-Smith et al. that the two conditions coexisted in about 10 percent of individuals with peritrochanteric pain probably reflects this difficulty.

The mechanism of injury is unclear, but it is probably related to the seesaw tilt action of the pelvis when running (Fig. 17-67). It may lead to fatigue with overtraining, a positive functional Trendelenburg sign, and further strain on the gluteus medius of the supporting limb.[2] It is difficult to isolate specific alignment factors that predispose to this injury, but a significant leg length discrepancy would tend to increase the stresses involved in pelvic control.

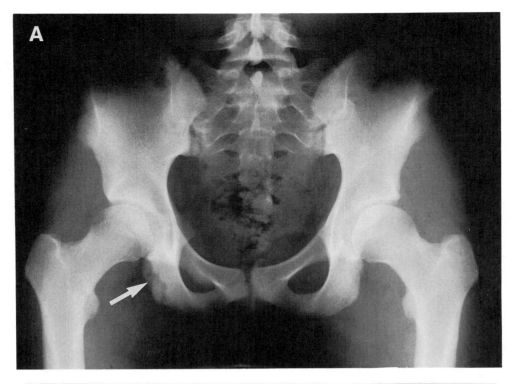

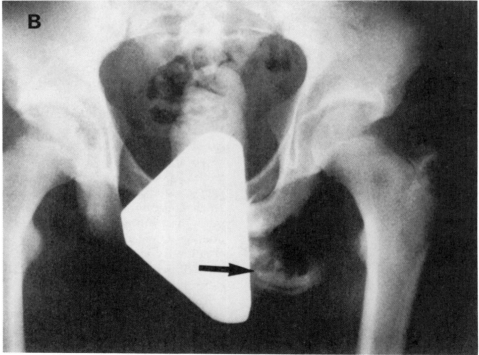

Fig. 17-64. (A) Roentgenogram of a minimally displaced avulsion fracture of a 16-year-old female figure skater. **(B)** Roetgenogram of a 14-year-old boy with a significantly displaced avulsion fracture of the ischium. *(Figure continues.)*

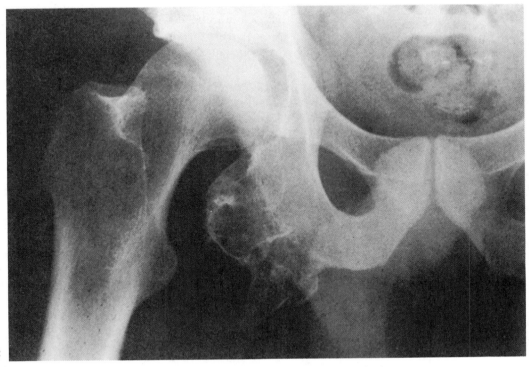

Fig. 17-64 *(Continued).* **(C)** Symptomatic excessive bone formation over the ischial tuberosity secondary to a widely displaced fragment. (After Metzmaker and Pappas,[35] with permission.)

Tensor Fascia Lata Strain

Isolated strain of the tensor fascia lata muscle is rare and may occur acutely, mostly in the muscle belly, or chronically, particularly at its insertion onto the pelvic brim.

Tensor fascia lata arises from the anterior portion of the external lip of the iliac crest and outer surface of the anterosuperior iliac spine. It lies just anterior to the gluteus medius; and because of its action of abduction and internal rotation, it is frequently classed with the gluteal group. However, it also inserts into and helps form the anterior part of the iliotibial tract, which helps flex the hip; and it indirectly stabilizes the extended knee as its femoral nerve supply suggests. With the leg fixed, the tensor fascia lata helps with pelvic support.

Strain of this muscle is not always associated with a tight iliotibial band, and often the Ober test is negative.[58] The diagnosis is made on the basis of pain over the muscle belly or origin on palpation and discomfort with resisted activity of the muscle (Fig. 17-68). Treatment follows the usual pattern for muscle strains, with protected motion and local palliative therapy, followed by progressive stretching, strengthening, and endurance work as the symptoms subside.

SACROILIAC AND ASSOCIATED SYNDROMES

This section brings together a miscellaneous group of conditions related to the sacroiliac and buttock area. The most common, sacroilliitis, involves a joint whose treatment is thwarted by controversy in the orthopaedic, physiotherapy, and sports medicine literature. Some of the subtleties relating to movement and postural changes within the sacroiliac joint are not addressed here, but generation of pain from the sacroiliac area in young active people cannot be denied and the ability to assess and treat this joint requires special skills that are holistic and multidisciplinary in nature.

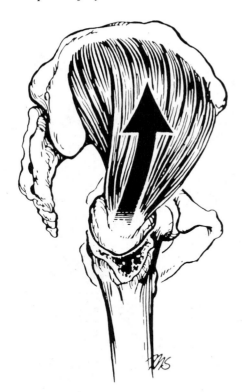

Fig. 17-65. Avulsion of the greater trochanter by the gluteus medius and minimus. This injury is rare in athletes. (After Henry,[5] with permission.)

Sacroiliac Sprains and Sacroilliitis

Sacroilliitis may be manifestation of a systemic collagen disorder such as ankylosing spondylitis or Reiter's syndrome, or it may result from single or repeated injuries. Hormone-induced laxity of the sacroiliac ligaments during pregnancy may lead to excessive painful motion that is not relieved during the postpartum period with resumption of exercise. Although much of the impact of running is dissipated through the lower limbs, the torque and shearing forces may repetitively stress the sacroiliac joint. The ilium rotates posteriorly at foot contact and remains rotated posteriorly until midstance, when it rotates anteriorly until toe-off.

Possibly excessive side-to-side or up-and-down motion when running and jogging causes repetitive stress on the joint (Fig. 17-67). Forced extension motion of the hip in ballet and gymnastics rapidly uses up available femoral head range in the acetabulum.[11] Continued extension of the hip is achieved at the expense of anteroposterior shearing and hyperextension of the lumbar spine and torque due to rotary stresses across the sacroiliac joint. In the older individual decreased rotation at the hip may also throw additional stress on the sacroiliac joint.

Contributing factors include uneven terrain resulting in an altered heel strike pattern, running on a severely cambered road, and slipping and stumbling which may cause a sudden strain. Sacroiliac pain may also be precipitated by wearing new shoes or by the use of an orthosis for some other problem.

The athlete may experience increasing discomfort in the low back and buttock region, proportional to activity. Rapid, forceful movements may produce sharp one-sided pain in the area of the sacrum followed by aching in the buttock and posterior thigh that does not usually reach the knee. Frequently there is rest pain, in the form of a dull aching in the low back after prolonged sitting. Specific stress tests via pressure and distraction on the iliac crests and the Faber's flexion abduction external rotation leverage stress test using the ipsilateral thigh may be helpful. Palpation along the joint line is often uncomfortable.

Diagnosis may be confirmed by the presence of sclerosis, osteophytes, or joint narrowing on plain films, but these signs are usually present only in longstanding cases. A bone scan may be helpful, but a hot scan should always raise the possibility of systemic disease. Blood work such as an ESR, complete blood count, and HLA$_{B27}$ antibody test help narrow the differential diagnosis. When in doubt, an injection of lidocaine into the joint under fluoroscopic control helps confirm the diagnosis of sacroilliitis if it completely removes the symptoms.

Treatment involves analysis of contributing factors such as alignment, leg length, tight or unbalanced muscles, position, and movement, and activity patterns. Anti-inflammatory medication, ice, ultrasound, TENS, and interferential current therapy are helpful. Mobilization of the joint should be considered. Re-education of the abductor power and control is important. Sometimes a sacroiliac belt permits sufficient destressing and support of the joint that all symptoms resolve, particularly in individuals with evidence of hypermobility during the postpartum period.

When symptoms are not alleviated, consideration may be given to injecting the joint with corticoste-

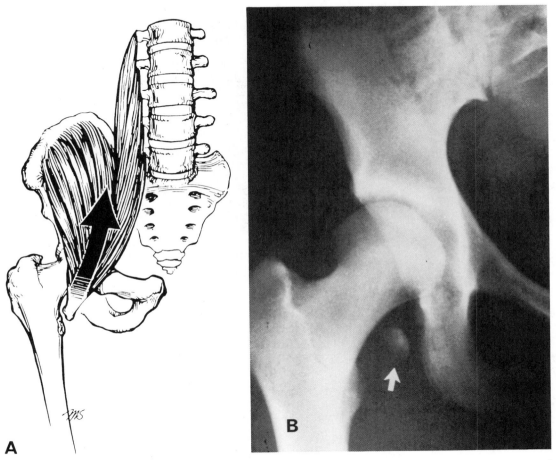

Fig. 17-66. **(A)** Lesser trochanter of the femur being avulsed. **(B)** Roentgenographic picture of a separated lesser trochanter.

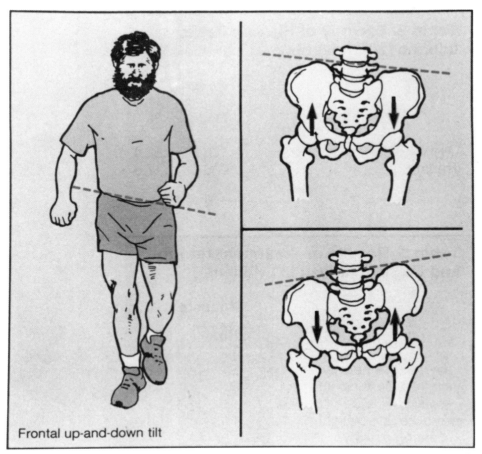

Frontal up-and-down tilt

Fig. 17-67. It is possible that some running styles that are characterized by excessive up and down motion may generate undue stress across the pelvis, contributing to trochanteric bursitis, gluteus maximus tendinitis, or sacroiliac pain. (After Lloyd-Smith et al,[2] with permission.)

roid. This difficult technique may be done through the superior aspect of the joint (Fig. 17-69). If it is unsuccessful, injection lower in the joint may be tried under fluoroscopic control. In intractable cases it has been suggested that sclerosis of the ligaments with glucose and phenol injection may be effective, but I have no experience with this technique.

Exercise-Related Stress Reaction

Stress reaction of the sacroiliac region is a rare sports-related injury. It usually presents as gradually increasing low back pain with activity. As the syndrome evolves there is pain present with prolonged standing, running, and sitting. On examination, pain with extension of the spine is one of the consistent findings, as is tenderness to palpation along the joint.

Detection of sacroiliac fractures on plain roentgenograms is difficult.[59] Bone scintigraphy is usually the best diagnostic method, so the term "stress reaction," rather than "stress fracture" is used. The sacroiliac joint is a synchrondrosis, and it is possible that the cartilaginous plates and subchondral bone are the elements damaged by stress, resulting in the positive scan. Treatment is symptomatic, and the importance of this syndrome is its role in the differential diagnosis of low back and sacroiliac pain.

Piriformis Syndrome

The sciatic nerve usually passes through the sciatic notch below the piriformis muscle and superior to the gemelli (Fig. 17-70). In about 15 percent of the pop-

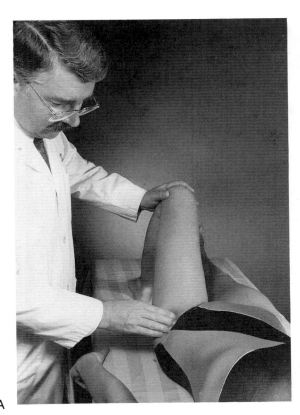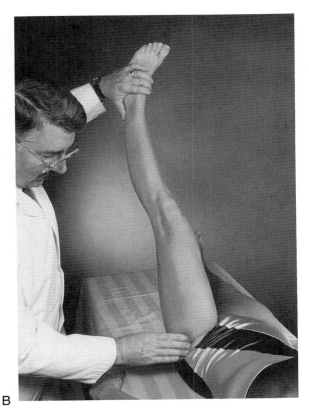

Fig. 17-68. Strain of tensor fascia lata. **(A)** Palpation of the muscle belly and origin. **(B)** Manual muscle test. The patient attempts to abduct and internally rotate the hip in the flexed position.

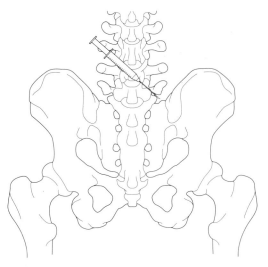

Fig. 17-69. Technique of injecting the superior part of the sacroiliac joint and the iliolumbar ligaments. The spinous process of L5 is the landmark.

ulation the nerve passes through or above the piriformis in the interval between it and gluteus minimus.[60] It is possible that trauma, hemorrhage, or spasm of the piriformis muscle can generate pressure on the sciatic nerve.

The usual complaint is numbness or tingling in the buttock and posterior thigh, sometimes with more distal referral. Low back pain is not usual. There is tenderness in the sciatic notch and over the muscle to palpation. Active or resisted external rotation may exacerbate the pain. Forced passive internal rotation may also produce symptoms and may lead to the athlete preferring to stand with the leg in slight external rotation. Straight-leg raising may be limited, and there may be a positive Faber's test.

Treatment includes relieving the acute symptoms with anti-inflammatory agents and activity modification. Attention is then turned to stretching the piriformis by adopting internal rotation positions with the adducted and flexed hip (Fig. 17-71). Muscle en-

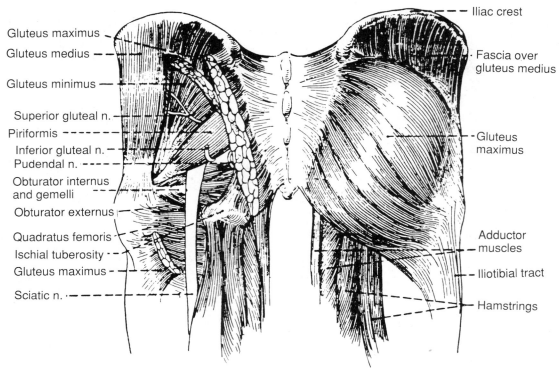

Fig. 17-70. Emergence of the sciatic nerve is variable in its relation to the piriformis. It may come above, through, or below; or the sciatic and peroneal portions may emerge independently. It is possible that spasms or tightness of the piriformis muscle could generate some neuritic pain.

ergy and hold–relax techniques may be used. Rarely, surgical decompression is considered, but the indications are few and it must be done only after careful confirmation of the diagnosis.

Superior Gluteal Nerve Entrapment Syndrome

The superior gluteal nerve entrapment syndrome, in which the superior gluteal nerve is compressed by the edge of the piriformis muscle or the muscle itself in the greater sciatic notch, is rare. It presents as aching gluteal pain and tenderness to deep palpation just lateral to the edge of the greater sciatic notch. Internal rotation of the hip tends to stretch the piriformis against the ilium, generating pain. When severe, the athlete may adopt a position of additional lumbar lordosis. There may be some weakness in the hip abductors that is related to pain inhibition or atrophy and true neurogenic weakness. When sufficiently severe, there may be a Trendelenburg lurch. The treatment of this unusual and difficult to diagnosis syndrome is similar to that of the piriformis syndrome.

Coccydynia

Coccydynia, a painful condition of the tip of the coccyx and the sacrococcygeal joint, may be the result of a direct contusion or even fracture. It was dealt with under the section on coccygeal fracture. In recalcitrant cases, consideration of injection with corticosteroid is considered, usually with an accompanying manipulation.

Entrapment of the Lateral Femoral Cutaneous Nerve (Meralgia Paresthetica)

The lateral femoral cutaneous nerve of the thigh may be entrapped as it emerges from the depth of the pelvis adjacent to the anterosuperior iliac spine. There is a fibrous or fibro-osseous tunnel through which it emerges as a single branch or occasionally multiple branches. This condition is most frequently seen during pregnancy but may also accompany direct trauma to the region of the anterosuperior iliac spine in sport; it occasionally presents as an overuse syndrome.

The athlete may complain of either tingling or

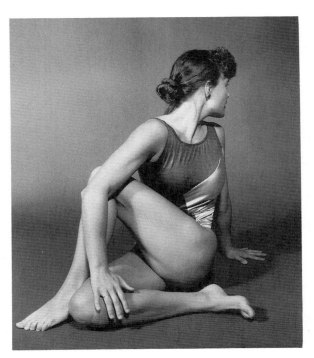

Fig. 17-71. Position adopted for stretching the piriformis.

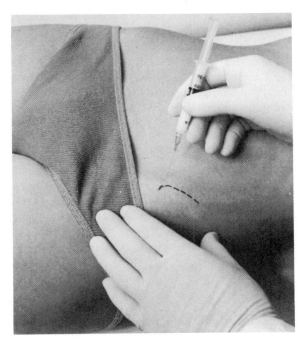

Fig. 17-73. The landmark for injecting the lateral femoral cutaneous nerve is just adjacent to the anterosuperior iliac spine. (From Béliveau,[61] with permission.)

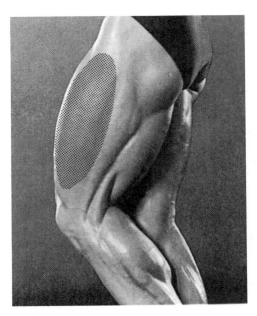

Fig. 17-72. Sensory supply of the lateral femoral cutaneous nerve of the thigh is variable. Entrapment produces tingling, pain, or numbness in the area shaded.

numbness in the distribution of the nerve that supplies the anterior and lateral aspect of the thigh (Fig. 17-72). Sensory testing may confirm it, and there may be a positive Tinel's sign to tapping at the level of the anterosuperior iliac spine and the adjacent inguinal ligament. If rest, ultrasound, laser, and NSAIDs do not relieve the problem and if the sensation is sufficiently irritating, injection of the area with methyl prednisolone (Depro-Medrol) is reasonable (Fig. 17-73).

The diagnosis should not be made without ruling out intrapelvic and spinal causes of the pathology. In situations where the diagnosis is firm, the discomfort sufficient, and the response to nonoperative treatment inadequate, surgical release of the nerve usually provides excellent relief.

SUMMARY

This chapter has focused on musculoskeletal hip and pelvic problems. Many of these conditions are difficult to diagnose either because of lack of specific symptoms or because of their depth within the body. Referral of pain to the groin should always be considered hip joint pain until this possibility is ruled out. Bone scans play an important role in isolating inflammatory conditions. The slipped epiphysis or avascular necrosis in the young, stress fracures in the distance athlete, and osteoarthritis in the older participant point to the changing spectrum of disease with age. Failure to diagnose some of these conditions has disastrous consequences should total displacement occur. Thus attention to subtle diagnostic clues is important. Some of the conditions, despite being common, are ill understood. Examples include osteitis pubis and sacroilliitis. For these entities, symptomatic treatment is the key, although some attempt has been made to outline the possible pathophysiology. It is because of the large number of clinical entities of the pelvis and hips with poor correlation to proved etiologic factors that Osler's quote is used at the beginning of the chapter. It should serve to remind us to constantly question the dogma.

REFERENCES

1. Clement DB, Taunton JE, Smart GW et al: A survey of overuse running injuries. Physician Sports Med 9:47, 1981
2. Lloyd-Smith, Clement DB, McKenzie DC et al: A survey of overuse and traumatic hip and pelvic injuries in athletes. Physician Sports Med 13:131, 1985
3. Reid DC: Functional Anatomy and Joint Mobilization. University of Alberta Press, Edmonton, 1976
4. Trotter M, Gleser GC: Estimation of stature from long bones of American whites and Negroes. Am J Phys Anthropol 10:463, 1952
5. Henry JH: The hip. In Scott WN, Nisonson B, Nicholas JA (eds): Principles of Sports Medicine. Williams & Wilkins, Baltimore, 1985
6. Hodge WA, Fijan RS, Carlson KL et al: Contact pressures in the human hip joint measured in vivo. Proc Natl Acad Sci USA 83:2879, 1986
7. Henricson AS. Fredriksson K, Persson I et al: The effect of heat and stretching on the range of hip motion. J Orthop Sports Phys Ther 6:110, 1984
8. Basmajian JV: Muscles alive. In: Their Function Revealed by Electromyography. 2nd Ed. Williams & Wilkins, Baltimore, 1967
9. Kushner S, Reid DC, Saboe L, Penrose T: Isokinetic torque values of the hip in professional ballet dancers. Submitted Clin J Sports Med, 1991
10. Inman VT, Eberhart HD, Saunders JB: The major determinants in normal and pathological gait. J Bone Joint Surg [Am] 33:543, 1953
11. Kushner S, Saboe L, Reid DC et al: Relationship of turnout to hip abduction in professional ballet dancers. Am J Sports Med 18:286, 1990
12. Kapandji IA: The Physiology of the Joint. Vol. 2. In: The Lower Limb. Churchill Livingstone, Edinburgh, 1920
13. Gardner E, Gray DJ, O'Rahilly R: Anatomy: A Regional Study of Human Structure. WB Saunders, Philadelphia, 1966
14. Singleton MC, LeVeau BF: The hip joint: structural stability and stress; a review. Phys Ther 55:145, 1959
15. Von Lanz T, Wachsmuth W: Praktische Anatomie. Julius Springer, Berlin, 1938
16. Hollingshead WH: Textbook of Anatomy. 2nd Ed. Harper & Row, New York, 1967
17. Crane L: Femoral torsion and its relation to toeing-in and toeing-out. J Bone Joint Surg [Am] 41:421, 1959
18. Svenningsen S, Terjersen T, Anflem M et al: Hip rotation and in-toeing gait. Clin Orthop 251:177, 1990
19. Hunt GC, Fromherz WA, Danoff J et al: Femoral transverse torque: an assessment method. J Orthop Sports Phys Ther 7:319, 1986
20. Magee DJ: Orthopaedic Physical Assessment. WB Saunders, Philadelphia, 1987
21. Beetham WP, Polley HF, Slocumb CH, et al: Physical Examination of the Joint. WB Saunders, Philadelphia, 1965
22. Maitland GD: The Peripheral Joints. Examination and Recording Guide. Virgo Press, Adelaide, 1973
23. Reid DC, Smith B: Leg length inequality: a review of etiology and management. Physiother Can 36:177, 1984
24. Ober FB: The role of the iliotibial and fascia lata as a factor in the causation of low-back disabilities and sciatica. J Bone Joint Surg 18:105, 1936
25. Backus R, Reid DC: Evaluating the health status of the athlete. In MacDougal JD, Wenger HA, Green HJ (eds): Physiological Testing of the Elite Athlete. 2nd Ed. Mutual Press, Ottawa, 1990
26. Howse AJG: Orthopedists aid ballet. Clin Orthop 89:52, 1972
27. Quirk R: Ballet injuries: the Australian experience. Clin Sports Med 2:507, 1983
28. Binnie JF: The snapping hip. Ann Surg 58:59, 1913
29. Schaberg JE, Harper MC, Allen WC: The snapping hip syndrome. Am J Sports Med 12:361, 1984
30. Jones FW: The anatomy of snapping hip. J Orthop Surg 2:1, 1920
31. Jacobs M, Young R: Snapping hip phenomena among dancers. Am Correct Ther J 32:92, 1978
32. Reid DC, Burnham RS, Saboe LA et al: Lower extremity flexibility patterns in classical ballet dancers and its correlation to lateral hip and knee injuries. Am J Sports Med 15:347, 1987

33. Reid DC: Prevention of hip and knee injuries in ballet dancers. Sports Med 6:295, 1988

34. Zoltan DJ, Clancy WG, Keene JS: A new operative approach to snapping hip and refractory trochanteric bursitis in athletes. Am J Sports Med 14:201, 1986

35. Metzmaker JN, Pappas AM: Avulsion fractures of the pelvis. Am J Sports Med 13:349, 1985

36. Kelly J: Ischial epiphysitis. J Bone Joint Surg [Am] 45:435, 1963

37. Rask MR: Snapping bottom: subluxation of the tendon of the biceps femoris muscle. Muscle Nerve 3:250, 1980

38. Staheli LT: Medial femoral torsion. Orthop Clin North Am 11:39, 1980

39. Beer E: Periostitis of symphysis and descending rami of the pubes following suprapubic operations. Int J Med Surg 37:224, 1924

40. Wiley JJ: Traumatic osteitis pubis: the gracilis syndrome. Am J Sports Med 11:360, 1983

41. Beach EW, Osteitis pubis: a urologic and roentgenographic study. Urol Cutan Rev 53:577, 1949

42. Shaker AM, Shaheen MA, O'Neal PJ: Traumatic aseptic osteitis pubis. Annals of Saudi Med 11:205, 1991

43. Pierson EL: Osteochondritis of the symphysis pubis. Surg Gynecol Obstet 49:834, 1929

44. Kopell HP, Thompson WAL, Postel A: Entrapment neuropathy of the iloinguinal nerve. N Engl J Med 266:16, 1962

45. Smedberg SG, Broome AE, Gullmo A et al: Herniography in athletes with groin pain. Am J Surg 149:378, 1985; Motore 4:111, 1932

46. Ekberg O, Persson NH, Abrahamsson PA et al: Longstanding groin pain in athletes: a multidisciplinary approach. Sports Med 6:56, 1988

47. Martens MA, Hansen L, Mulier JC: Adductor tendinitis and musculus rectus abdominis tendopathy. Am J Sports Med 15:353, 1987

48. Rockwood CA, Green DP (eds): Fractures in Adults. Lippincott, Philadelphia, 1984

49. Hauser CW, Perry JF: Massive haemorrhage from pelvic fractures. Minn Med 49:285, 1966

50. Tachdjian MO: Paediatric Orthopaedics. WB Saunders, Philadelphia, 1972

51. Nicholas JA, Hershman EB: The Lower Extremity and Spine in Sports Medicine. CV Mosby, St. Louis, 1986

52. Fullerton LR, Snowdy HA: Femoral neck stress fractures. Am J Sports Med 16:365, 1988

53. Ernst J: Stress fractures of the neck of the femur. J Trauma 4:71, 1964

54. Devas MB: Stress fractures of the femoral neck. J Bone Joint Surg [Br] 47:728, 1965

55. Blickenstaff LD, Morris JM: Fatigue fractures of the femoral neck. J Bone Joint Surg [Am] 48:1031, 1966

56. Godshall RW, Hansen CA: Incomplete avulsion of a portion of the iliac crest epiphysis: an injury of young athletes. J Bone Joint Surg [Am] 55:1301, 1973

57. Schlonsky J, Olix ML: Functional disability following avulsion fracture of the ischial epiphysis: a report of two cases. J Bone Joint Surg [Am] 54:641, 1972

58. Cooperman JM: Case studies: isolated strain of the tensor fasciae latae. J Orthop Sports Phys Ther 5:201, 1984

59. Marymont JV, Lynch MA, Henning CE: Exercise-related stress reaction of the sacroiliac joint: an unusual cause of low back pain in athletes. Am J Sports Med 14:320, 1986

60. Anderson BJ: An atlas of Human Anatomy. 2nd Ed. WB Saunders, Philadelphia, 1963

61. Béliveau P: Infiltrations, When? How? 40 Techniques. Editions, Science and Culture Inc. Montreal, 1990.

Injuries to the Thorax, Abdominopelvic Viscera, and Genitourinary System

18

Don't think there aren't any crocodiles because the water is calm.
—*Sam Wyche, 1990*

Torso injuries can occur in many sports, particularly those involving sudden deceleration and impact. These thoracic and abdominal injuries are easily recognized when superficial, but underlying visceral damage may be more obscure, even if significant.[1] Impacts delivered by the helmet in football and contact with the boards in hockey, falls in equestrian events and skateboarding, and high speed collisions when skiing, cycling, and car racing may result in damage to the apparently sturdy thoracic cage. Furthermore, injuries involving the respiratory and cardiac system may be immediately life-threatening and require instant expert attention for effective resuscitation.

In many contact sports there is surprisingly little protection of the lower ribs, flanks, and abdominal wall. Fortunately, the lower ribs are strong and mobile; and the abdominal and back muscles, when sufficiently tensed, protect the vulnerable viscera from significant impact.[2] The abdominal muscles are not contracted at all times, and so the deep structures are sometimes vulnerable. However, even in the lean individual there is a certain amount of abdominal and retroperitoneal fat that cushions some of the impact.

Blunt trauma to the abdomen and lower back is frequently difficult to assess, but it is mandatory to carefully estimate the degree of injury. Even small lacerations or contusions to the abdominal viscera can result in considerable bleeding and incipient shock or sepsis. Thus a high index of suspicion coupled with meticulous repeated examinations helps to ensure early diagnosis and appropriate treatment.

This chapter focuses on injuries to the thorax and abdominopelvic contents as well as the genitourinary system. The emphasis is on the signs and symptoms that denote a significant injury. The idea in all sports is to prevent rather than treat problems, which is usually achieved by utilizing appropriate, well conceived, well constructed protective equipment and

---

Quick Facts

THORACOABDOMINAL TRAUMA IN SPORT

- Reduced by adequate protective equipment
- Damaged viscera difficult to assess
- High index of suspicion necessary
- Repeated examination more efficient than single examination
- Undetected may lead to uncontrolled bleeding, shock, and sepsis

---

671

promoting good physical conditioning. Furthermore, proper medical supervision to ensure preseason fitness for participation, appropriate rest and timing of return to play after injury, and an intelligent approach to the game and to the interpretation of the rules by the coach promote safety. Unfortunately, although these guidelines are excellent for protecting the athlete from many musculoskeletal injuries, they are often less than adequate for the abdominal viscera. Many vulnerable scenarios readily spring to mind, such as the quarterback with his arm up, raised and poised for passing, or the receiver leaping with his outstretched arms to catch a pass. Furthermore, the helmet in football and the hockey stick, which can be used as a vicious weapon for spearing, can easily inflict severe trauma. Notwithstanding the above statements, it is surprising how few major visceral injuries occur in contact sports.

Prior thoracic and abdominal injuries are not usually a contraindication to participation, although there are some exceptions. Splenectomy does not usually increase the likelihood of further injury, but liver laceration and trauma of any significance probably does; and it may be well to advise the athlete to refrain from collision activities. Loss of one of the paired visceral organs is a controversial matter; but from an empiric standpoint, loss or congenital absence of a testicle or a kidney should at least warrant the advice to consider the use of protective measures for, or withdrawal from, heavy contact activities.

STABILIZING THE INJURED ATHLETE

The fundamentals of diagnosing and treating thoracic and abdominal injuries in athletes are the same as for the multiply injured or critically injured individuals who have been involved in an automobile accident. Violent sports-related contact, as well as acceleration, deceleration, and rotation maneuvers have some of the same potential for major injury. For this reason, all therapists, coaches, and medical team personnel should be skilled in the basic life support measures. As with other methods of injury, assessment must be orderly, thoughtful, and thorough in order to identify the most serious injuries.[3]

Over the years, emergency physicians and trauma surgeons have developed a systemic approach to stabilizing and managing patients that is as applicable on as it is off the playing field. This protocol includes rapid assessment followed by stabilization of the patient's condition through immediate resuscitation, followed by prevention of further injuries. After stabilization, the treatment of some injuries clearly takes precedence over that of others.[4]

Practice Point

ABCs ASSESSMENT OF MAJOR INJURIES

- **A**irway: any obstruction or inability to breath
- **B**leeding and blood pressure
- **C**onsciousness and cervical spine
- **D**igestive system and damage to abdominal wall
- **E**xcretory system and external genitalia
- **F**ractures: four limbs, deformity and motion

Checking and Clearing Airway

Clearing and maintaining an adequate airway is clearly a priority. The airway may be obstructed by the tongue falling back on the roof of the mouth and blocking air intake, a problem that is easily managed by minor repositioning of the head or insertion of an

---

Quick Facts

ABNORMAL BREATHING PATTERNS WITH TRAUMA

Pattern	Observation	Cause
Normal rate	12–20/min	
Paradoxical	Chest moves in with inspiration	Flail chest
Tachypnea	>20/min	Shallow—pain Deeper—air hunger
Periodic	Cheyne-Stokes Apneic intervals	Neurologic injury
Biot's resp.	Irregular periods of apnea Alternate work 4–5 identical depth breaks	Increased intercranial pressure

oral airway. Aspirated gum, tobacco, dentures, or tooth guards are the commonest foreign materials that block the airway. Injuries to the neck, larynx, or trachea by a direct blow from a ball, puck, kick, or stick may be sufficiently severe that only intubation or cricothyreotomy (making a direct passageway into the trachea) allow the airway to become patent. Occasionally, excessive bleeding from the back of the nose or an unstable facial fracture impedes the airway. Whatever the cause, airway management must always proceed in such a way that there is maximal protection of the cervical spine from potential injury.

Apart from the question of upper airway obstruction, it is essential to make sure the athlete can indeed carry out the mechanics of breathing. A quick check is made to confirm that the chest wall moves appropriately with the respiratory effort. When breathing is either labored or obviously inadequate, the question of equal movement of the rib cage and air entry into both lungs must be addressed. The possibility of pneumothorax is detectable by a change of breath sounds if the lung collapse is sufficient. The association of rib fractures is considered with blunt trauma, such as occurs with a fall from a horse or during boxing, football, and rugby. A flail chest secondary to fracture of several ribs in more than one place may cause paradoxical movement of the chest cage. As the rib cage expands with inspiratory effort, the unstable segment retracts (Fig. 18-1). When appropriate, evidence of a penetrating chest injury must be sought, as it may generate significant hemorrhage and can potentially produce either a pneumothorax or a tension pneumothorax (Fig. 18-2). For instance, occasionally a sword tip enters the lung apex during fencing. Increasing respiratory efforts, with no improvement of the air hunger, may be evidence of this situation. The absence of breath sounds on the affected side supports the clinical diagnosis. Finally, with the unconscious athlete, it must be established if any breathing

---

Practice Point

RECOGNITION OF BLUNT INJURY TO THE THORAX

- Difficulty getting "breath"
- Increasing shortness of breath with time
- Absent or distant breath sounds
- Paradoxical movement of rib cage
- Deviated trachea

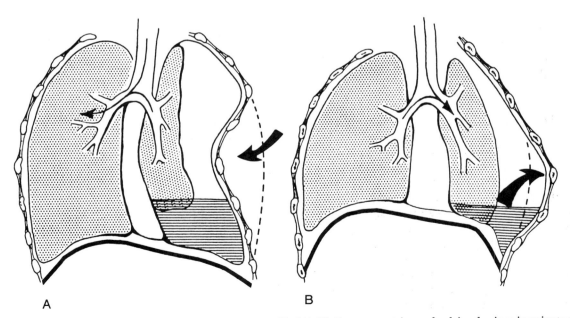

A   B

Fig. 18-1. Paradoxical motion of the chest wall. **(A)** Flail segment is sucked in during inspiratory efforts. **(B)** It is blown out during expiratory efforts. The loss of suction between the lungs and the chest wall allows the lung to collapse and cease to follow the normal respiratory excursions.

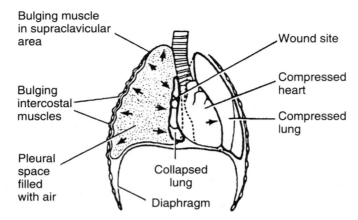

Bulging muscle in supraclavicular area

Bulging intercostal muscles

Pleural space filled with air

Wound site

Compressed heart

Compressed lung

Collapsed lung

Diaphragm

Fig. 18-2. When there is communication between the airways (or the exterior) and the interpleural space, a flap valve effect may be created. Thus with each inspiratory effort air is drawn into the pleural cavity and is trapped during the subsequent expiratory phase. Tension builds progressively in one side of the thorax, eventually resulting in pressure and shift of the mediastinal structures. This situation, referred to as a tension pneumothorax, constitutes an absolute emergency.

effort is being made. If there is respiratory arrest, resuscitation should be immediately instituted with coincidental assessment of the circulatory status.

Essentially, with the unconscious or seriously injured athlete, the airway is protected by removing any potential obstruction; and a quick search for tracheal deviation, broken ribs, and a flail chest is carried out. In the less seriously involved athlete, some idea of the effectiveness of the pulmonary system is gained by noting the depth and rate of respiration and the ability to talk without shortness of breath (dyspnea). Lack of air may generate rapid, shallow breathing, but it must also be realized that fear and panic can lead to hyperventilation and a subjective feeling of air hunger.

Management of the seriously injured athlete depends greatly on the experience and training of the individual administering the first aid. In the case of an athlete with a rapidly developing tension pneumothorax, for instance, it may range from cardiopulmonary resuscitation techniques or administration of oxygen, to insertion of an oral airway and rapid transport to hospital, to the possibility of inserting a large-bore needle or chest tube to allow breathing (Fig. 18-3). Although the latter measures may seem drastic, the seriously injured athlete with increasing dyspnea and cyanosis may require prompt life-preserving procedures to prevent a rapid demise.

When inexperience or lack of adequate equipment

Practice Point

TENSION PNEUMOTHORAX

Mechanisms

- Air leaks into pleural space with each inspiration
- Unable to be fully dispersed with expirations
- Gradual buildup of tension in the hemithorax
- Pressure pushes collapsed lung and mediastinal structure over (mediastinal shift)
- Impedes air entry to noninjured lung
- May impede venous return

Results

- Increasing air hunger
- Distension of neck veins
- Tracheal deviation
- Cyanosis

Treatment

- Rapid relief with insertion of large gauge (13 to 14) hypodermic needle
- Use second or third intercostal space in midclavicular line

Fig. 18-3. Tension pneumothorax may be rapidly relieved by inserting a 13 to 14 gauge needle into the second intercostal space, which is at the approximate level of the manubrial sternal joint in the midclavicular line. The needle is slid just over the superior aspect of the rib to avoid injury to the intercostal vessels, which run along the inferior edge. As the extrapulmonary intrathoracic air under pressure is evacuated through the needle, the tension pneumothorax is converted to a simple pneumothorax, which is better tolerated physiologically. Thus an emergent situation is converted to a semiemergent situation to allow transport and evacuation of the athlete. (Adapted from Schneider et al.,[2] with permission.)

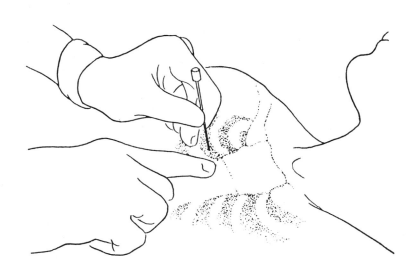

prevails, any of the warning signs of significant chest trauma (e.g., deviated trachea, flail chest, altered respiratory sounds, distended neck veins, or a rapid pulse and decreasing blood pressure) should rapidly bring the realization that prompt and urgent transfer to an area where further care can be administered may be life-saving.

Practice Point

WARNING SIGNS OF SERIOUS CHEST OR CARDIAC TRAUMA

- Neck veins distended
- Trachea deviated
- Surgical emphysema (air in tissues)
- Multiple rib fractures (flail chest)
- Chest sounds altered (tympanic or dull)
- Heart sounds faint or muffled
- Pulse rapid or irregular
- Blood pressure low

Absolute confirmation of thoracic injury usually requires a chest radiograph and sometimes more specialized tests, e.g., a computed tomography (CT) scan. Most life-threatening problems however, can be identified clinically; and in most cases, with experience, they can be treated expeditiously.

Bleeding

Visible hemorrhage can be controlled by applying direct pressure, preferably with a clean dressing, but in more dramatic circumstances with anything at hand. In the situation of a skate laceration across the neck, for instance, judicious direct pressure may be life-saving. Blind clamping within a wound by artery forceps is usually contraindicated because of the potential damage to associated nerves and other struc-

---

Practice Point

HEMORRHAGE

- Nearly all bleeding may be stemmed by appropriately placed, firm, continual pressure.
- With serious hemorrhage, often manual pressure is best.
- With major bleed, do not keep checking to see if it stopped. Apply firm manual pressure, maintain it, and transport athlete to the treatment center.

---

tures. There are few significant wounds opening on the surface that cannot be controlled with correctly applied pressure, at least until more expert help is available.

In the absence of obvious bleeding, the adequacy of circulation may be checked by feeling the peripheral arterial pulses at the radial side of the wrist, the carotid artery in the neck, and the femoral artery in the groin. One can often see, feel, or hear a precordial heartbeat. Adequate circulation and oxygenation is demonstrated by normal coloring of the face, conjunctival sacs, and fingernails. An increase in heart rate, with decreasing blood pressure, should always lead to the question of internal bleeding and incipient shock. As pressure falls, the shocky (diaphoretic) state ensues with cold, clammy extremities and frequently associated air hunger (Fig. 18-4).

Practice Point

SIX Bs

- Breath
- Brain
- Bladder
- Bleeding
- Belly
- Bones

Consciousness and Cervical Spine

The level of consciousness is established during the initial screen. If the athlete has been concussed and remains unconscious, all of the systems must be monitored to establish a baseline from which potential recovery or deterioration can be recorded. Pupil size and bilateral symmetry, pulse, blood pressure, and respiratory rate are important indicators. All unconscious patients must be treated as if they have an associated cervical spinal injury. Any complaint of neck pain from an alert patient must also be regarded as a symptom of potential serious cervical spinal injury. Screening of the limbs helps to establish if there is associated paralysis, but it is important to recall that the absence of paralysis does not necessarily rule out cervical spinal injury. During the resuscitative maneuvers and transfer, adequate immobilization of the cervical spine is mandatory. This subject is dealt with specifically in Chapter 19. Whenever head injury is

suspected or any change of peripheral motor control or sensory level is detected, it is important to minimize the use of any local anesthetics and narcotics, as it may impede assessment of the progress of central or peripheral nervous system injury.

Practice Point

All unconscious athletes must be considered to have a cervical spinal injury until proved otherwise.

General Screen

Once the stability of the athlete has been assessed, a good airway established, and obvious damage to the nervous system ruled out, a general screen ensues that initially focuses on the chest and abdomen. When there has been an obvious blow to the abdomen, tenderness or splinting with decreased respiratory movement immediately raises concern that there might be intra-abdominal bleeding. An increasing pulse, unstable blood pressure, and the absence of obvious bleeding from the limbs or the chest also raise the suspicion of an intra-abdominal bleed. Auscultation of the abdomen may sometimes already reveal decreased or absent abdominal sounds. Occasionally shoulder tip pain indicates visceral damage. In any event, any suspicion of abdominal hemorrhage indicates the need for rapid transport to a hospital.

Damage to the kidneys is difficult to detect and may present like any other intra-abdominal injury. If a

---

Practice Point

MAJOR ABDOMINAL INJURY

- Tense, tender abdomen
- Absent bowel sounds
- Decreasing blood pressure
- Increasing pulse rate
- Increasing abdominal pain and girth
- Shoulder tip pain
- Air hunger

Requires rapid transport to hospital

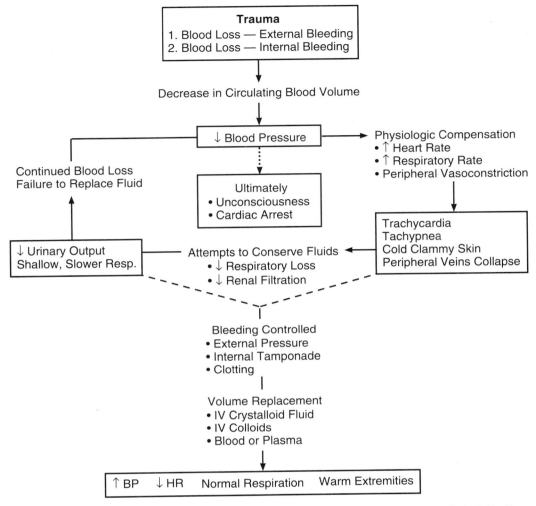

Fig. 18-4. Cardiovascular adaptations to trauma with blood loss. The resulting clinical findings are outlined in solid squares.

blow to the back has been of sufficient magnitude to prevent the individual from continuing play, he or she should be warned to observe the color of the urine over the next 24 hours to detect early signs of hematuria. Obvious wounds to the external genitalia or pelvic floor require early transport to a treatment center so a catheter can be passed and proper assessment carried out.

Fracture Care

The general screen obviously includes the extremities. Apart from monitoring the ability to move the limbs, deformity may indicate dislocation or fracture. Crepitus and excessive local pain also point to frac-

ture. If a major long bone is involved, the blood loss can rapidly amount to 1 to 2 liters or more and thus lead to shock. If the fracture is associated with an open wound, it must be assumed that there is a communication with the bone or joint, and rapid transport to the hospital becomes important. The magnitude and incidence of subsequent infections correlate directly with the time taken to get the patient to the operating room for thorough débridement of the wound. If the deformity is excessive, peripheral pulses must be checked. Circulation may nearly always be improved by gentle traction and reestablishment of the anatomic alignment of the limb. The latter should not be attempted, however, until adequate support or splints are available to maintain the limb in a good position, so movement is minimized. Dislocation of major joints may be associated with arterial damage and the potential for compartment syndromes. Thus, once more, speed of administration of first aid, resuscitative measures, and transport have a direct impact on the eventual morbidity of the injury.

Transportation

Some of the indicators of significant injury have been outlined and emphasis placed on those that require urgent transport to a treatment center. The ability to carry out this protocol in an expeditious manner depends partly on prior planning. For any sport that has a high risk of significant trauma, arrangements should have been made to have either an ambulance in attendance or a system in place whereby one can be brought to the site of injury at short notice. Provision for scoop stretchers and splints and other materials for adequate immobilization also presuppose adequate planning. One of the duties of a team physician or therapist attending any competition site is to make an initial survey of the equipment available and the arrangements that have been set up for triage. Also important is adequate stocking of the theapist's and physician's bags. Lastly, it must be mentioned that theoretic knowledge of how to transport a patient is of little use if it has not been rehearsed fairly frequently. The most experienced person should take command at the site of major injury, and field experience should take precedence over academic degrees.

Extricating and transporting a patient from a jumping pit, an ice surface, water, or a football field has nuances that require special attention and techniques. Individuals monitoring sports medically on a regular basis should make sure they are fully conversant with these special procedures.

MUSCULOSKELETAL CHEST WALL PAIN

Pain in the chest is a common symptom due to diverse causes. It may have its origin in the thoracic wall, intrathoracic structures, neck, or even areas below the diaphragm.[5] Musculoskeletal abnormalities are often the unsuspected cause of chest pain; and although the exact prevalence is unknown, it may occur in as many as 10 percent of patients who present with chest discomfort.[6] Naturally, there is

always a concern that the pain may be of cardiac origin. Knowledge of the various disorders and the pertinent clinical assessment techniques may spare the sport physician and the therapist needless anxiety and unnecessary investigations when confronted with chest pain from a noncardiac, nonpulmonary source.

Anatomy

The thorax is made up of the rib cage, which articulates posteriorly with the vertebrae and anteriorly with the sternum (Fig. 18-5). This large cavity is enclosed below by the diaphragm and above through the arch of the first rib. There is continuity with the structures of the chest and the upper limbs.[7] The obvious function of the rib cage and diaphragm is to generate respiratory efforts.

Contained within the thorax are the mediastinum and pleural cavities. The mediastinum, which divides the chest into halves, consists of the pericardium (a

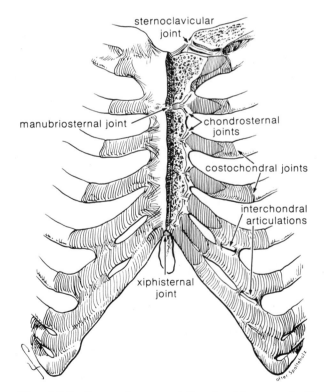

Fig. 18-5. Bony thorax outlined with a typically shaped first rib, classic second to fifth ribs, conjoined seventh to tenth ribs, and the floating eleventh and twelfth ribs. The costal articulations are shown anteriorly.

tough membrane around the heart) and the great vessels leading from the heart (Fig. 18-6). The latter include the aorta and the superior and inferior venae cavae, the roots of the pulmonary vessels. Additionally present are the trachea, the esophagus, and the many nodes that serve to filter the lymphatic drainage from the chest and to some degree the abdomen. The pleural cavities contain the lungs (Fig. 18-7). Lungs and thorax are lined with visceral and parietal pleurae, respectively, which are held together by negative pressure and form a potential space. The branches of the trachea and pulmonary vessels are centered through these cavities as they divide within the substance of the lungs.[7,8]

The ribs articulate posteriorly with the bodies and transverse processes of the thoracic vertebrae at the costovertebral and costotransverse joints (Fig. 18-8), which are true diarthrodial synovium-lined joints. The second to tenth ribs articulate by two hemifacets with two adjacent vertebrae and the intervertebral disc between them. The first, eleventh, and twelfth ribs are much more mobile than the other ribs, and each articulates with a single facet located in the body of its own vertebra.

Laterally, the ribs are joined to the costal cartilages by costochondral articulations that are synchondroses. The first seven ribs are true ribs, or vertebral sternal in nature. Their costal cartilages articulate at the sternocostal (chondrosternal) joints. The remaining five pairs are false ribs. Of the latter, cartilages of the eighth, ninth, and tenth ribs articulate with the cartilages immediatly above and below them and so form a subgroup of vertebral chrondral ribs (Fig. 18-5). The eleventh and twelfth ribs are the so-called floating ribs and are free at their cartilaginous ends.

The costal cartilage of the first rib articulates with the manubrium sterni by a synchondrosis.[7,8] The other six pairs of chondrosternal articulations are

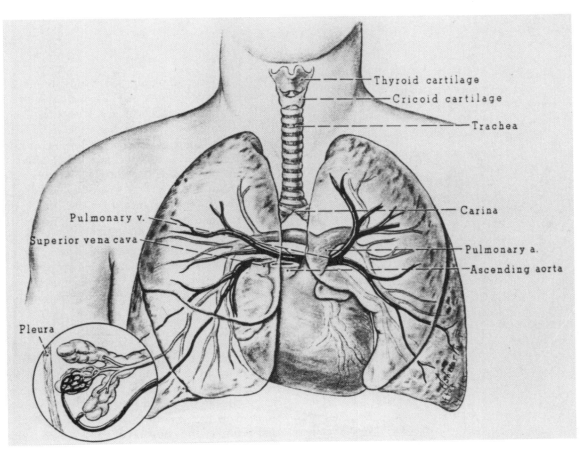

Fig. 18-6. Main structures of the mediastinum and associated lungs. (From Jacob SW, Francone CA: Structure and Function in Man, p. 381. WB Saunders, Philadelphia, 1970, with permission.)

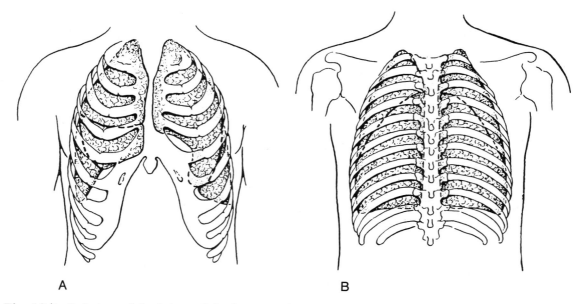

Fig. 18-7. Relation of the lobes of the lungs to the overlying thoracic cage. **(A)** Anterior view. **(B)** Posterior view.

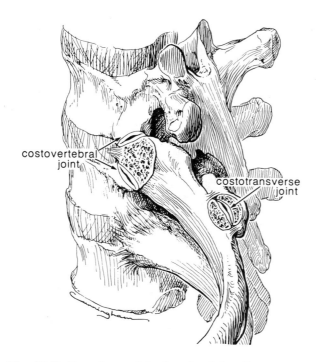

Fig. 18-8. Junctions of the heads of the ribs with the vertebral body at the controvertebral joint and with the transverse processes at the costotransverse joint.

lined with synovial membrane. Synovium-lined interchondral articulations may also occur between the fifth and ninth costal cartilages. With advancing years much of this costal cartilage is capable of becoming ossified, and some of the articulations may be obliterated. Thus the rib cage becomes less flexible.

The medial end of the clavicle articulates with the manubrium sterni and the first costal cartilage at the sternoclavicular joint. Inferiorly, the xiphoid process joins the main body of the sternum. The junction of the manubrium with the body of the sternum is a synchondrosis with a fibrocartilaginous disc uniting the two sides. Absorption of the central portion of the disc and formation of the synovium-lined cavity may occur in up to one-third of adults, and in about 10 percent of individuals the disc and joint eventually ossify.

The chest wall is largely supplied by intercostal nerves running segmentally around the chest. However, much of the shoulder girdle muscles originally developed in the lower cervical region and migrated across the chest wall, pulling their nerve supply with them. This fact accounts for pain of cervical origin that refers to the chest area, particularly in the pectoral-scapular region. The intrathoracic viscera and central diaphragm also developed in the cervical region and similarly gain their nerve supply from the cervical and thoracic segments, which offers further potential for referred pain from these viscera.

The precise diagnosis of skeletal chest wall pain syndromes rests on elucidation of a detailed history followed by a meticulous physical examination. A few carefully selected diagnostic tests are required. In view of the diverse origin of chest wall pain, the examination must extend beyond the chest to include the neck and shoulder and frequently the abdomen (Table 18-1).

Musculoskeletal chest wall pain is often well localized and nagging in nature, although it may extend well beyond its area of origin. The pain is typically made worse by movements involving the affected part—side flexion, rotation, or taking a deep breath, depending on the site of the pain. The most dominant feature of most thoracic skeletal disorders is the presence of local tenderness. Demonstration and duplication of local tenderness, which is made worse by certain movements and completed relieved by lido-

TABLE 18-1. Classification of Musculoskeletal Chest Wall Syndromes

Chest wall pain: local origin
    Arising from ribs
        Rib trauma
        Stress fracture ribs
        Slipping rib syndrome
        Tietze's syndrome
        Costovertebral arthritis
    Arising from sternum
        Sternoclavicular arthritis
        Manubrium sternal arthritis
        Painful xiphoid syndrome
    Arising from myofascial structures
        Traumatic muscle pain
        Precordial catch syndrome
        Epidemic myalgia (Bornholm's disease)
    Arising from thoracic spine
        Thoracic disc disease
        Ankylosing spondylitis
        Costovertebral arthritis
        Thoracic herpes zoster
        Fracture of thoracic vertebrae
        Osteoporosis
        Spinal tumors
Chest wall pain: remote origin
    Referred pain from cervical spine
    Referred pain from thoracic outlet
    Referred pain from shoulders
    Fibrositis syndrome
    Psychogenic regional pain syndrome

(Adapted from Fam and Smythe,[5] with permission.)

caine (Xylocaine) infiltration, is strong evidence for a musculoskeletal origin of the pain.[6] Occasionally, however, tenderness is due to underlying pleural irritation of pericarditis.

Practice Point

FEATURES OF MUSCULOSKELETAL CHEST WALL PAIN

- Onset
  - History of repetitive minor trauma or unaccustomed physical activity
- Quality
  - Often sharp, nagging, and localized to the affected side
- Posture
  - Positional component to pain
  - Exacerbated by twisting, deep breathing, or arm movements
- Signs
  - Frequently localized chest wall tenderness
  - Often relieved by local infiltration of lidocaine

The location of a specific chest wall site of discomfort should not rule out the possibility of coexistence of a second, more sinister cause of pain. Particularly in the older individual, the presence of two sources of pain in the same patient is not uncommon. Thus certain caution should be exercised when designating a benign skeletal etiology for left-sided chest pain.

Pain arising from the musculoskeltal structures of the shoulders, cervical spine, or thoracic spine may be referred to areas on the posterior or anterior chest wall. This referred pain is usually within the segmental distribution of the source, but occasionally it has a regional distribution and is deep in location. This pain has been described as being sclerotomal rather than dermatomal. The areas to which the pain is referred may have secondary reflex changes, including deep, or "myofascial," tenderness, cutaneous hyperalgesia, or circulatory disturbances.[6] A small number of tender points of asymmetric distribution grouped in a single region suggest a referred pain syndrome. A large number of tender sites spread widely and symmetrically, associated with diffuse aching and stiffness and nonrestorative sleep, suggest the fibrositis syndrome.

The initial investigations of athletes presenting with chest wall pain includes hematologic and chemical screening tests, plain chest film, and electrocardiography. Additional studies include special views of the ribs, cervical spine, or thoracic spine, sometimes supplemented by tomography or CT scanning. When inflammatory lesions are suspected, a bone scan is helpful.

Chest Injuries

This section highlights chest injuries that are related to either multiple repetitive trauma or a single major traumatic event. They include injuries to the breast, the major muscle of the chest (the pectoralis major), and the ribs.

Breast Pain

Breast Trauma

Breast injuries are observed with increasing frequency, as more women are participating in sports and recreational activities. The incidence of serious breast trauma, however, is low. Repetitive stress to the fascial attachments of the breast to the underlying pectoralis major and pectoral fascia can cause discomfort. These supporting ligaments, particularly Cooper's ligaments, hold and support the breast on the chest wall. These ligaments are not strong, being only strands of connective tissue separating the lobules of the breast. There is a tendency for a woman's breast to bounce when she runs; and depending on the size of the breast tissue, soreness or contusion may occur.[9] In the absence of a supporting brassiere, repetitive impacts of as much as 70 to 80 lb of force may occur. This effect is magnified with large-breasted women and may be a particular problem during pregnancy and in women with fibrocystic breast disease. Even individuals with small breasts may complain of extra sensitivity just before the menstrual period.

Support of the chest with a sports brassiere may help prevent premature ptosis (sagging) of the breast by reducing the stress on Cooper's suspensory ligaments. Nevertheless, because chafing is the most frequent complaint, it is important that any undergarment be carefully designed.[10] Adequate support by the brassiere should prevent a certain amount of motion of the breast relative to the chest wall and should contain at least 55 percent cotton or other suitable material for absorbance.[10] The elasticity should be minimal, with just enough to allow easy breathing. Wide nonelastic straps tend not to slide and thus are more secure on the shoulders, but they should not constitute the entire support of the brassiere. The chest strap should be designed to provide some support from below, and hooks and seams should be kept to a minimum and be well covered to preclude irritation. In large-breasted women or those with particularly sensitive breasts, further significant support can be achieved by wrapping a 4 or 6 inch elastic wrap over the brassiere. This binding can provide additional support for the chest, reducing breast motion by as much as 50 percent.[9]

Contusions do occur in contact sports, sometimes with associated hemorrhage. Application of ice, analgesia, and support allow more rapid and comfortable resolution. There is no evidence that breast injuries induce breast cancer. However, adiponecrosis or traumatic fat necrosis secondary to a direct blow can cause some concern when one is trying to differentiate a firm mass from tumor. Occasionally, this traumatic scarring causes skin retraction and a suspicious image on mammography, compounding the diagnostic dilemma.[11] Sometimes post-traumatic thrombophlebitis of the superficial veins of the chest causes acute pain with a tender cord-like swelling or skin groove. This condition, called Mondor's disease, is self-limiting and usually requires no treatment. Again, it must be differentiated from carcinoma.

Breast tenderness may be associated with specific phases of the menstrual cycle. The tenderness may be aggravated by luteal insufficiency and anovulatory cycles, which are relatively common in female endurance athletes. In addition to a supporting brassiere, it may be helpful to prescribe a natural progestogen or an antiestrogenic progestogen for the second half of the cycle.[11] When prescribing hormonal medications there should be an awareness of the potential for a positive drug test if it produces a high concentration of androgenic metabolites.

Any young woman may develop inflammation of the breast due to fibrocystic disease that is occasionally complicated by abscess. Treatment of a breast abscess consists in aspiration or formal incision and drainage. Erythromycin appears to be an effective antibiotic in most situations. Participation is continued provided there is minimal or no discomfort.

Gynecomastia

Gynecomastia is defined as excessive development of the male mammary gland. It may occur in the male adolescent and is often unilateral. The nipple can be sore and tender to pressure and may be irritated by the shirt rubbing against it during physical activity. It is rarely necessary to investigate this problem, and for the most part reassurance of the limited nature of the condition is the mainstay of treatment. Nevertheless, if the magnitude of the gynecomastia is outside the normal experience of the physician assessing the patient, adrenal, pituitary, and testicular pathology must be ruled out. Occasionally, because of psychosocial pressures, surgery may be considered for significant bilateral breast enlargement in the male.

Unfortunately, an increasing cause of gynecomastia is anabolic steroid abuse (Fig. 18-9). This condition is common in body builders and power athletes and is often associated with considerable sensitivity and discomfort. Although for the most part the breast and nipple enlargement is cyclic, after steroid intake there is a certain amount of permanence of some of the breast changes. Athletes should be warned about this possibility and every attempt made to dissuade them from continuing drug abuse.

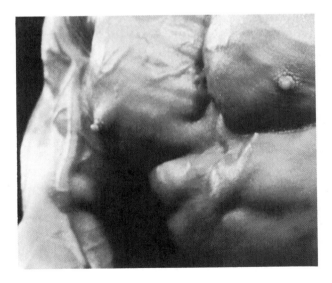

Fig. 18-9. Gynecomastia secondary to anabolic steroid abuse. Note the elevated and enlarged nipple.

Nipple Irritation (Runner's Nipple, Cyclist's Nipple, Skier's Nipple)

In association with gynecomastia, but also even with the normal chest, there may be frictional irritation of the nipple during running activities, sometimes of sufficient magnitude to cause abrasion and bleeding. Cyclists's nipple refers to a variation of this syndrome due to perspiration over the chest evaporating, which causes cooling aggravated by the wind chill, resulting in cold, painful nipples. The symptoms may last several days. Skier's nipples refer to the irritation of trouser suspenders over the chest. These symptoms occur with equal frequency in men and women and may be sufficiently uncomfortable to require some form of prophylactic treatment. For the most part, changing the type of clothing can be sufficient, but if this adjustment is inadequate the application of petroleum jelly, tape, or even special padding placed over the nipples helps avoid the irritation.[10]

Ruptured Pectoralis Major

The diagnosis and treatment of ruptured pectoralis major is dealt with more extensively in Chapter 21. The usual site of rupture is at the musculotendinous junction or near the insertion on the humerus (Fig. 18-10). Occasionally, disruption of this huge muscle occurs on the chest wall itself, and the hemorrhage and swelling can be significant (Fig. 18-11). When the major tearing occurs within the muscle, usually the sternal or the clavicular head is involved independently. Total rupture may occur during power lifting, particularly while bench-pressing. It also occurs during waterskiing, wrestling, or sudden violent deceleration maneuvers such as blocking with an outstretched arm in football or punching in boxing.[12] Unfortunately, this injury seems to be gaining prevalence in association with anabolic steroid abuse. It is likely that the muscle hypertrophy and increase in power secondary to rapid strength gain is not accompanied by a concomitant increase in tendon size.

The pain of muscle disruption is commonly accompanied by a snapping or popping sensation. Even after resolution of the hemorrhage and swelling, the muscle may be seen bunched up on the chest (Fig. 18-12).

Like all muscle injuries, the magnitude of the damage can be graded. Complete disruption is classified as grade III. Grade II involves partial disruption of

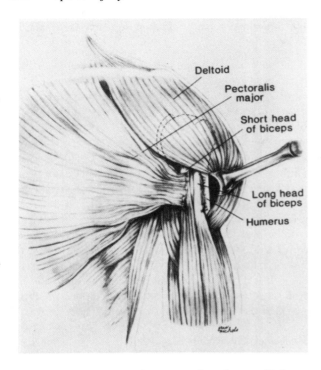

Fig. 18-10. Anatomy of the anterior chest wall showing the powerful pectoralis major and its usual site of rupture at the musculotendinous junction near the insertion. (From Kretzler and Richardson,[12] with permission.)

the muscle fibers, usually with some hemorrhage and swelling, accompanied by pain inhibition and occasionally a palpable defect. Grade I injury is a microscopic disruption with little or no hemorrhage, although there is significant discomfort and localized tenderness.

Rupture at the tendinous origin is usually complete. It is surprisingly easy to be misled by the relatively small deformity of the muscle on the chest wall in some patients, particularly if not seen acutely.[12] Occasionally, odd strands of tissue give the impression of an incomplete rupture. A webbed appearance of the anterior axilla at 90 degrees of abduction and deformity of the chest wall with resisted adduction indicate complete rupture (Fig. 18-12).

After assessing the severity of the injury, athletes with grade I and II injuries are reintegrated into activities as pain permits. In the progression from early protected range of motion and gentle strengthening to more ballistic and violent activities, there is always a risk of reinjury, and this phase of the rehabilitation

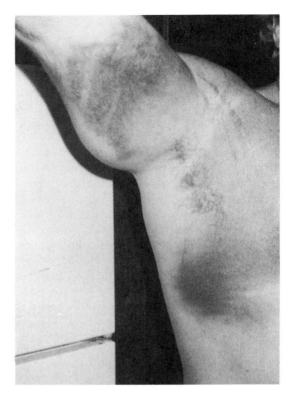

Fig. 18-11. Hemorrhage into the arm and across the chest associated with rupture of the pectoralis major.

must be supervised carefully. Re-establishment of a full range of motion is essential to prevent further injuries; once gained, the emphasis switches to restoration of full strength (Fig. 18-13).

Third degree (grade III) disruption is better treated by surgical repair in the competitive athlete involved in power sports.[13] Even late repair is compatible with significant improvement in strength.[12] However, if a nonoperative treatment is chosen, with the knowledge that there may be some minor detectable weakness during adduction and flexion maneuvers, a functional outcome is possible. Although the nonoperative tratment may leave a cosmetically unacceptable defect, the surgical treatment also leaves a scar.

Rib Fractures

With equestrian accidents and in sports that involve vehicles, multiple rib fractures are common secondary to falls and collisions. In the other contact sports, e.g., football and boxing, direct blows may

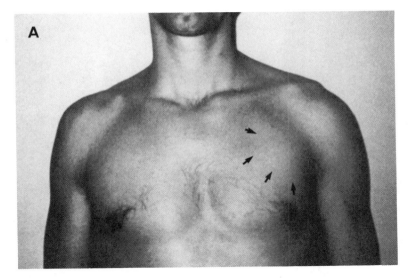

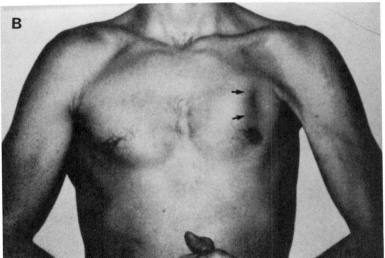

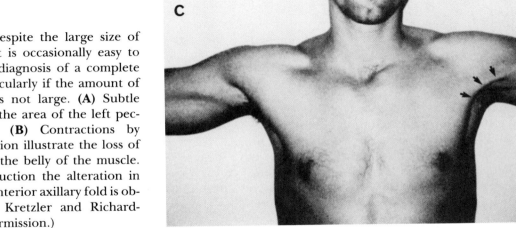

Fig. 18-12. Despite the large size of this muscle, it is occasionally easy to overlook the diagnosis of a complete rupture, particularly if the amount of hemorrhage is not large. **(A)** Subtle swelling over the area of the left pectoral region. **(B)** Contractions by forced adduction illustrate the loss of contour over the belly of the muscle. **(C)** With abduction the alteration in shape of the anterior axillary fold is obvious. (From Kretzler and Richardson,[12] with permission.)

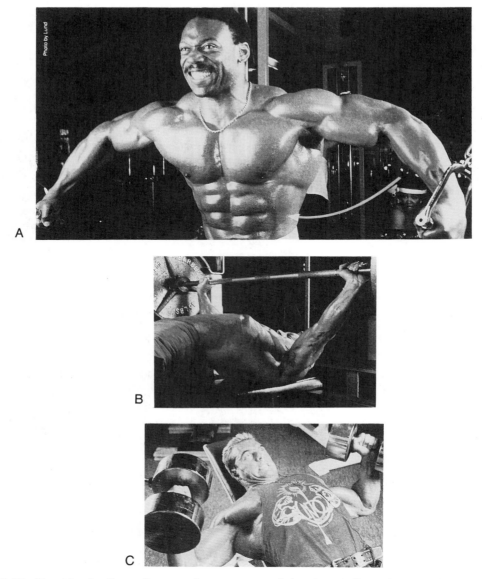

Fig. 18-13. Even in the face of a complete rupture of the pectoralis major, good strength can be achieved with sufficient exercise. **(A)** Leaning, flying exercise or resisted adduction. **(B)** Traditional bench press. **(C)** Dumbbell bench press can be done at an incline or a declining position as well as flat.

produce cracks and fractures that are usually restricted to one segment of the rib; rarely are more than one or two ribs involved. Blows to the chest by balls, e.g., a baseball or cricket ball, jabs from a hockey stick by spearing, or blows with a lacrosse stick may cause similar fractures. Occasionally, indirect forces such as violent swinging maneuvers when golfing or pitching fracture a single rib.

Clinical Picture

Rib fractures are painful and debilitating; and for the most part they are diagnosed clinically. With severe fractures, one must also entertain the existence of associated intrathoracic injury. The player usually complains of intense local pain aggravated by increased respiratory effort and by twisting or side flexing, which places tension on the involved rib. There is excruciating local tenderness; and usually rib springing in both anteroposterior and lateral directions generates discomfort at the level of the fracture. Depending on the site of the fracture, the presence or absence of displacement, the number of ribs involved, and the type of sport, this injury may eliminate the individual from competition. When possible,

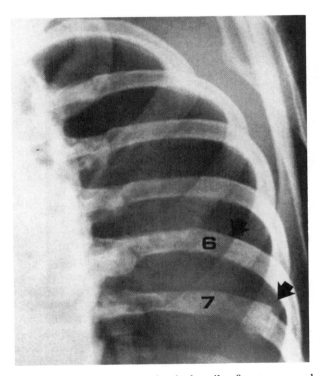

Fig. 18-14. Undisplaced sixth rib fracture and slightly displaced posterolateral fracture of the seventh rib. Frequently, special rib views or a bone scan are necessary to show rib trauma.

the diagnosis is confirmed by radiographic studies with special views of the ribs (Fig. 18-14).

Treatment

Treatment goals revolve around supplying appropriate analgesia for both comfort and to allow a full inspiratory effort. Restricted chest movement may result in atelectasis (collapse) of segments of lung parenchyma. Strapping or tight taping is neither effective or recommended since it may aggravate this tendency. Occasionally, as the discomfort subsides and the athlete is able to return to the sport, protection with a canvas rib belt or a flack jacket can be helpful. When there is excruciating, unremitting initial local pain, consideration of an intercostal block with lidocaine may be considered. The block should include the two ribs above and below the fracture site (Fig. 18-15). This measure provides temporary relief, but the technique should not be used to return the player prematurely to competition. Essentially, with rib fractures, return to competitive sports should be allowed when tenderness to palpation is minimal, no analgesics are required, and a full range of motion of the thoracic cage is possible. Sprinting and twisting abilities should also be possible without generating significant discomfort. It is not necessary to wait until there is visualization of callus on roentgenography, as it may take a considerable time and is often a late indicator of healing. Nevertheless, in the presence of an incompletely healed rib fracture, the athlete should be warned of the potential for displacement and the possible catastrophic nature of a piercing injury by a fractured rib end.

Normally, if the rib fracture was undisplaced initially, the return to activity is fairly prompt, over a period of 2 to 3 weeks for most sports. The timing also depends on the position and level of play as well as the ability to protect the chest with some form of air-inflated or flack jacket. When the initial roentgenograms show either an oblique jagged fracture or a markedly displaced rib fracture, much more caution should be used, and the time course for return to contact sport is much longer.

Stress Fractures

Stress fractures of the lower ribs are uncommon in athletes, although they have been reported in rowers, gymnasts, golfers, and tennis players. They are frequently associated with sudden increased intensity of

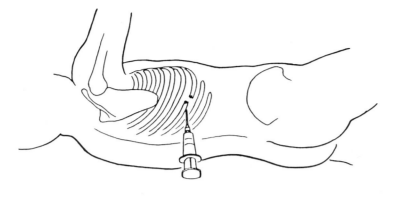

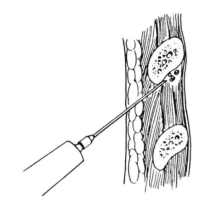

Fig. 18-15. Technique of intercostal nerve block. Local anaesthetic is infiltrated just inferior to the lower border of the rib, which brings the needle in approximation to the intercostal vessels and nerve. Usually the level of the fracture along with two ribs above and two below are infiltrated with 3 to 5 ml of 1.0 percent lidocaine (Xylocaine) or 0.25 percent bupivacaine (Marcaine). (After Schneider et al.,[2] with permission.)

training in a poorly conditioned athlete. They are difficult to see on plain chest or rib films unless callus is forming or they are displaced.[14] Hence the diagnosis is frequently made by bone scan.

Treatment is usually modification of activities. The problem resolves fairly rapidly over a period of weeks, and resumption of activities is tailored to resolution of the symptoms.

Injuries to the first rib in sport are rare because the area is not subjected to direct blows, being protected by the shoulder girdle muscles and bones. Nevertheless, indirect forces can produce stress-related fractures, usually at the subclavian sulcus. It is here that the opposing pulls of the scalene muscles in one direction and the upper digitations of serratus anterior in another generate the most torque. Frequently, the individual involved is a middle-aged athlete who is suddenly enthusiastic about a sport such as tennis and has spent the whole weekend practicing and competing. This exercise generates unaccustomed forces around the shoulder girdle. Moreover, with sudden throwing maneuvers or strong overhead movements

as in weight lifting, particularly if repetitive in nature, a stress reaction or crack may occur in the first rib. If the fracture becomes suddenly unstable, the athlete may report an acute, knife-like, excruciating pain. More often there is a gradual, insidious onset of increasing discomfort in the subclavicular area and at the base of the neck as the fracture evolves and slowly progresses. Special roentgenograms are needed to image these cracks; usually a bone scan makes the area involved obvious. The main concern with this injury is the differential diagnosis of other types of pathology to the apex of the lung and the first rib. Particularly in the older age group, the possibility of metastatic lesions from the lungs or the chest must be considered.

Major Rib Injuries

In those instances where there has been massive injury to the chest with disruption of several ribs in more than one place, a clinical examination should seek to rule out a flail segment, collapse of the lung, or bleeding into the chest cage. Furthermore, with lower rib injuries, penetration of the intra-abdominal organs, e.g., the liver, spleen, and kidneys, must also be considered. Although the thoracic cage in young athletes is elastic, a player should be carefully evaluated for visceral injury if there is any complaint of significant shortnesss of breath or, more particularly, if athletes claim they "cannot breathe at all." The following points are important for ruling out intrathoracic injury. The patient should be sufficiently undressed so the area of trauma can be directly observed for deformity, edema, and echymosis. The ribs should be palpated for abnormal movement and crepitus, as well as the reaction to anteroposterior and transverse pressure. Palpation over the area of tenderness may demonstrate crackling, which is pathognomonic of subcutaneous air or emphysema and is a sign of significant bronchial or pleural injury in the absence of an open wound to the chest.

Location of the affected ribs should focus concern for the appropriate underlying viscera, e.g., the lungs in the upper area, the liver and spleen lower down, and the kidneys adjacent to the floating ribs. Decrease in vocal fremitus may be elicited on the side of the pneumothorax or hemothorax and may be confirmed by a decrease in breath sounds on auscultation of that side. The trachea should be observed and palpated for any shift. These signs should quickly resolve if it is just a matter of a direct blow to the chest or solar plexus making initial respiratory effort difficult. If there is increasing difficulty with respiration and increasing cyanosis, consideration of some emergency procedure should be contemplated. Potential pneumothorax should be ruled out prior to transporting the patient, as it is possible that minimal attention may be given during the trip to a hospital. Insertion of a needle on the side of a tension pneumothorax can be life-saving (Fig. 18-3). Usually, if there is significant interthoracic bleeding, shock rapidly ensues.

Sternal Fractures

If an athlete's sternum is fractured, one must bear in mind the close relation to the underlying myocardium and major vessels. In the absence of obvious cardiac contusion, the clinical signs may include local tenderness to pressure and increasing pain with large inspiratory efforts. If a defect is palpable, suggesting displacement, reduction is occasionally possible by getting the athlete to lift both arms above the head and hyperextending the dorsal spine.

Contusion of the heart or hemopericardium is rare during sport; but with sternal injury, careful observation and examination of the athlete are required. If any suspicion is entertained of underlying visceral damage, a baseline electrocardiogram should be obtained for comparison with any potential subsequent changes. If the athlete shows signs of shock, pallor, diaphoresis, increasing heart rate, and decreasing blood pressure, rapid transport to hospital is necessary; a chest film is also essential to monitor and record any mediastinal widening.

Summary

Most rib injuries to athletes are contusions and minor undisplaced fractures, with little potential for significant injury. Nevertheless, the odd catastrophic situation may occur. Therefore in events where there are significant risks, qualified and experienced personnel should be in attendance who have adequate equipment available to manage these injuries. If this arrangement is not possible, some prior plans must have been made for swift and efficient transportation to a medical center.

Spontaneous Pneumothorax

Pneumothorax is the presence of air within the chest cavity, in the pleural space, leading to varying degrees of collapse of the lung. Apart from the more obvious traumatic pneumothorax, a condition of spontaneous pneumothorax is occasionally precipitated by strenuous physical activities. Rarely it occurs at rest. The incidence of idiopathic spontaneous pneumothorax has been reported to be as high as 1 in 3,000 in men between the ages of 20 and 29.[15] Defects in the periphery of the lung (usually the apex), known as bullae, may spontaneously break, with air being released into the pleural cavity. This situation in turn removes the negative pressure, which forces the lung to follow the movements of the thoracic cage. Released from this suction effect, the elastic lung collapses. The degree of the collapse is proportional to the leak.

The symptoms are similarly proportional to the magnitude of the collapse and the speed with which it occurs. The onset of the symptoms may be insidious, with gradually increasing shortness of breath and vague chest discomfort. On the other hand, the subject may have an acute and intense episode of pain and dyspnea. Pain may be referred to the shoulder tip. If large, there may be cyanosis. The diagnosis is made by percussing the chest and noting the rather tympanic note and by listening for distant or absent breath sounds. The diagnosis is confirmed by roentgenography. The film is characterized by the contrast between the absence of lung markings in the periphery and the increased density generated by the collapsed portion of the lung (Fig. 18-16). This finding can be subtle with small amounts of collapse, and it may be more easily visualized on expiration films. Diagnosis is frequently delayed 1 to 2 days. On the other hand, with a large collapse, there may be a mediastinal shift (Fig. 18-16).

Practice Point

SPONTANEOUS PNEUMOTHORAX

Suspect lung collapse if the following pertain.
- Sudden unrelieved shortnesss of breath after intense exertion
- Shoulder tip pain
- Associated vague or sharp chest discomfort

In the athlete with a small pneumothorax the only treatment required is to avoid unnecessary physical activity and to carefully monitor clinical findings and serial chest films. Usually the lung re-expands as the free air is absorbed. However, if the collapse takes up more than 30 percent of the lung, it is usual to admit the athlete to a treatment facility, with possible insertion of an intercostal chest tube (Fig. 18-17). This maneuver allows re-expansion, and the leak usually seals spontaneously within 24 hours. With a significant spontaneous pneumothorax, after discharge from hospital vigorous activities should be restricted for 2 to 3 weeks to allow thorough healing. Slow return to activity is advised after that time. It is essential to warn the athlete that other defects may coexist and that another episode may occur. Indeed recurrent episodes have been reported in up to 50 percent of cases.[15] On occasion, with a large defect or multiple recurrences, it is necessary to resect the damaged section of the lung.

Costochondral Trauma

A blow to the anterolateral part of the chest may occur during boarding in ice hockey or a pile-on in football, and it may lead to costochondral injury.

Similarly, a severe twisting injury, such as that seen in wrestling or a rugby scrum, may also lead to separation of the costal cartilage as it attaches to the sternum. The athlete may even describe feeling or hearing a "pop." After the initial sharp discomfort, a severe pain may last several days, slowly decreasing in intensity. This discomfort usually resolves over 3 to 4 weeks, although sometimes with sports that require a lot of twisting and stressing of the thorax the discomfort can persist for more than 6 weeks. The athlete may complain of a feeling of the ribs slipping out or a sensation of popping and crepitation. Usually stability is gained over the ensuing few weeks, but in some cases instability seems to persist long after the discomfort disappears.

With the lower ribs, the costochondral separation may occur at the junction of the cartilage and the bony rib. Usually this injury responds to anti-inflammatory medication and increased padding in contact sport athletes, but sometimes the problem fails to resolve, in which case careful steroid injection at the site of the separation may be considered. Only rarely is surgical resection of a chronically affected costochondral junction necessary.

Practice Point

RIB PAIN

All cases of localized rib discomfort, not resolving with appropriate rest and therapy should be investigated to rule out neoplasia.

It is important to entertain all of the appropriate differential diagnoses with this lesion, including tumor, even though there may be an obvious and apparent cause for its onset. Any case of chronic rib pain that is not relieved with the usual treatment within a short period of time requires further investigation.

Miscellaneous Conditions

Tietze's Syndrome and Costochondritis

Tietze described a benign condition of the anterior chest wall characterized by painful, nonsuppurative swelling of the cartilage at its articulations.[16] True Tietze's syndrome is rare. Frequently it is confused with another clinical syndrome, costochondritis,

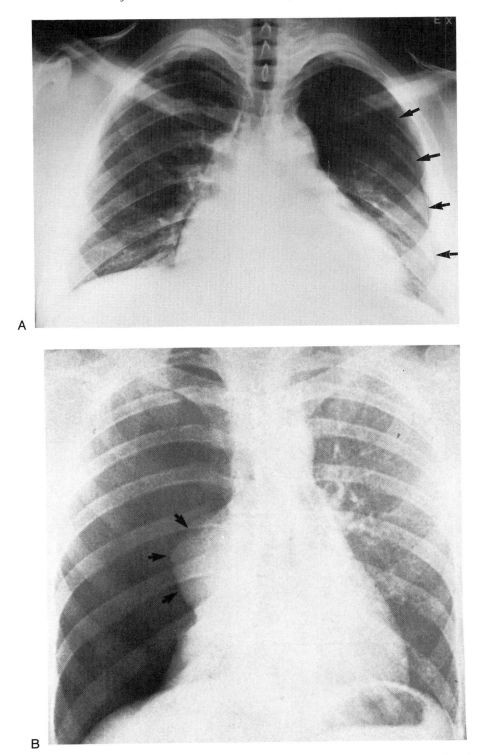

Fig. 18-16. Spontaneous pneumothorax. **(A)** Small left lung collapse is seen on an inspiration film. **(B)** Obvious complete collapse of the right lung following spontaneous pneumothorax. Expiration films will frequently make a more subtle collapse more obvious.

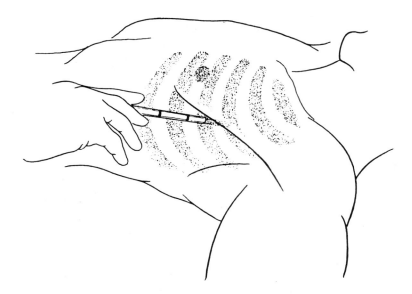

Fig. 18-17. Insertion of a chest tube. The preferred site for an apical chest tube is usually around the third intercostal space in the anterior axillary line, which is just behind the fold of the pectoralis major muscle and inferior to the axillary hairline. (After Schneider et al.,[2] with permission.)

which is also characterized by pain and tenderness of the costochondral junctions but without the swelling (Table 18-2).

Tietze's Syndrome

Tietze's Syndrome affects young people of either sex.[5,16,17] A traumatic pathogenesis has been suggested, but the cause is really unknown. In its full-blow form, there may be swelling and inflammatory changes at the perichondrium of the costal cartilages, where it has a predilection for the upper ribs, particularly the second and third costochondral junctions. The chondrosternal, manubrial sternal, sternoclavicular, and xiphisternal articulations are less commonly affected. Usually the lesion involves a single cartilage, and it is usually unilateral. Although the pain may radiate, it is usually located over the involved syn-

chondrosis. Coughing, deep breathing, and pressure over the area increases the discomfort. There are usually no systemic disturbances, and routine investigation fails to show any abnormalities. There are no characteristic radiographic findings. There is a possibility that there may be increased uptake at the involved costochondral joint on bone scanning. Essentially the diagnosis of Tietze's syndrome is made on clinical grounds after excluding other conditions that affect the costal cartilages, including trauma, rheumatoid arthritis, and tumors.

The disorder inevitably runs a self-limiting course with remissions and exacerbations. It may last only a few weeks but sometimes persists several months. The treatment consists in reassurance, local application of heat, and the use of nonsteroidal anti-inflammatory drugs (NAIDs); in cases of a particularly severe area of involvement, infiltration with steroid and lidocaine

TABLE 18-2.   Tietze's Syndrome and Costochondritis

Clinical Features	Costochondritis	Tietze's Syndrome
Frequency	Relatively common	Rare
Age group	Traumatic all ages	< 40 years
	Atraumatic > 40 years	
No. of sites affected	More than one in > 90%	One in 70%
Costochondral junction most frequently involved	Second to sixth	Second and third
Local swelling	Absent	Present
Associated conditions	Traumatic sprain	Respiratory tract infection
	Fibrositis syndrome	

(Data from Fam and Smyth.[5])

may be used. Rarely, an intercostal nerve block is needed. This syndrome has been outlined here simply to contrast it with the more frequent problem seen in young active people, costochrondritis.

Costochondritis (Costosternal Syndrome)

Costochondritis is characterized by pain and tenderness at the costochondral or costosternal articulations, without notable swelling. It has been recognized under a variety of labels, including the chest wall syndrome, anterior chest wall syndrome, and costosternal chondrodynia.[18,19] Costochondritis is in fact a relatively frequent cause of anterior chest pain, both as a primary condition and in association with the more severe problem of coronary heart disease. In the young athletic population, a certain element of trauma is involved, and the condition is usually self-limiting.

The pain involves the costochondral and costosternal regions, and frequently multiple sites of tenderness are present that usually involve the second to sixth costal cartilages. The pain in the upper costal cartilages is often mistaken for cardiac disease, whereas that of the lower costal cartilages may mimic intra-abdominal disorders. Thus it is important to distinguish this syndrome from the more dramatic underlying diseases and simultaneously rule out the coexistence of cardiac problems.

Essentially diffuse tenderness over the involved costal cartilages without swelling is a principal physical sign. It is usually exacerbated by certain movements of the chest, particularly the "crowing rooster" maneuver. This test involves extension of the cervical and thoracic spine accompanied by full extension of the arms. Other than the obvious cases of trauma, little is known about the pathogenesis of costochondritis in the absence of injury. Although the nontraumatic variety runs a self-limiting course, there are frequently more recurrences than with the traumatic type. Once again, treatment consists in reassurance and the use of analgesics or NSAIDS.

As with all cases of chronic rib pain, other causes must be ruled out, including Paget's disease, rheumatoid arthritis, and tumors. Metastatic lesions from the lung, breast, thigh, kidney, or prostate are the most frequent tumors, although occasionally primary neoplasms arise, such as osteochondroma, multiple exostosis, chondrosarcoma, multiple myeloma, and eosinophilic granuloma. Rarely, the ribs are the sites of pyogenic infections.

Slipping Rib Syndrome (Clicking Ribs, Rib Tip Syndrome)

The slipping rib syndrome is a less well known cause of mechanical rib pain. It is characterized by pain in the lower costal margins associated with increased mobility of the anterior end of the costal cartilage.[20]

Loosening of the fibrous attachments binding the lower costal cartilages to one another may allow a rib tip to curl upward and over the inner aspect of the rib above, thus putting pressure on the intercostal nerve lying between. It is probable that this syndrome has a traumatic origin. Indeed, most young athletes recall some injury to the ribs on the affected side. This relation is not always established or elicited in the history, as the onset is frequently insidious, occurring long after the initial injury as resolved.

There is usually a complaint of intermittent unilateral pain in the anterior ends of the lower costal cartilages. Occasionally, severe sharp pains are felt with certain bending maneuvers, and often a painful click is experienced over the tip of the involved costal cartilage. The involved cartilage is often tender and moves more freely on palpation. The pain may be duplicated by hooking the fingers under the anterior costal margin and pulling the rib cage anteriorly. This "hooking" maneuver may also produce a palpable click of the cartilage as it slips over the adjacent one.

Treatment includes recognizing the condition and reassuring the athlete concerned that there is no major injury. When it is not practical to teach avoidance of movement, the symptoms may be relieved with NSAIDs or occasionally injection of a steroid into the affected area. If the discomfort becomes intractable and significantly interferes with the athlete's desired activities, resection of the affected rib is considered.

Pain Due To Sternal Articulations

This section deals with pain radiating from the sternoclavicular joint, manubrial sternal joint, xiphoid cartilage, and xiphisternal joint.

Sternoclavicular Articulations

Trauma to the sternoclavicular articulation can result in degenerative changes that are usually easy to identify and localize because of their association with movements of the shoulder girdle and local crepitus in the joint. Nevertheless, these post-traumatic changes or inflammatory conditions of the joint (including rheumatoid arthritis and ankylosing spondylitis) may produce significant pain radiating to the thorax. Such pain may be confused with pain of cardiac or pulmonary origin.

There are two other obscure conditions of the sternal end of the clavicle, i.e., sternal costoclavicular hyperostosis and condensing osteitis of the clavicle.[21,22] Sternal costoclavicular hyperostosis is manifested by bilateral chronic painful swelling of the clavicles, sternum, and first ribs.[21] Radiologic changes include hyperostosis, widening and increased bone density of the clavicle and sternum, ossification of the first costal cartilage, and sternoclavicular synostosis. Increased uptake may be evident on bone scans. Blood tests are normal with the exception of an occasionally increased erythrocyte sedimentation rate (ESR) and hypergammaglobulinemia. Normal serum alkaline phosphatase and urinary hydroxyproline levels distinguish this condition from Paget's disease. The cause is unknown, but it may be related to psoriasis. Knowledge of this condition is important only in respect to the differential diagnosis of upper chest pain and the occasional associated complication of subclavian vein occlusion or thoracic outlet syndrome. The course is typically relapsing, and the symptoms often respond to NSAIDs.

The second condition, condensing osteitis of the clavicle, is characterized by unilateral or bilateral painful sclerosis and expansion of the medial end of the clavicle.[22] Skeletal scintigraphy shows increased uptake. The syndrome may be triggered by overuse or stress to the shoulder girdle, but the etiology is obscure. The clinical features include pain on abduction with occasional radiation to the ipsilateral shoulder or subscapular region. The histologic picture is one of ossifying periostitis with increasing thickness of the cancellous bone.[22] Treatment is symptomatic.

Manubriosternal Joint

Inflammation of the manubriosternal joint is an uncommon cause of upper sternal pain, although it may occur in association with ankylosing spondylitis. Because the pain may radiate to the upper chest and be aggravated by activity, it may mimic angina. Local pain and tenderness help to distinguish the condition.

Xiphoid Pain (Xiphoid Cartilage Syndrome)

Xiphoid cartilage syndrome, a rare entity, produces low substernal or epigastric pain that may radiate to the precordium or the abdomen, simulating,

respectively, cardiac or abdominal disease.[23] The xiphoid is tender to pressure, and stressing it duplicates the pain. The syndrome does not seem to be related to trauma and may be a variant of the Tietze's syndrome. NSAIDs or local injection of steroid may help severely symptomatic cases. Surgical excision of the xiphoid is reserved for painful and intractable cases.

Summary

The preceding syndromes are uncommon, but when they occur in the active individual they may be debilitating. Furthermore, their isolation and distinction from other disorders is a challenge.

Pain Due To Myofascial Structures

Stitch

A "stitch in the side" refers to a sharp pain or spasm usually in the vicinity of the right lower ribs experienced by individuals during exertion. They are either not well trained or are returning from a layoff. The possible cause of a stitch is diaphragmatic spasm, or relative local anoxia of the diaphragm and lower intercostal muscles. The high metabolic demand of the respiratory muscles during exercise may not be met immediately by an appropriate shift in circulation from the gastrointestinal tract. Thus there may be temporary relative ischemia. Training improves the efficiency of the respiratory muscles as it does for other skeletal muscles. It is possible that exercising too soon after eating aggravates this phenomena. The combination of incomplete digestion, a liver full of blood, and the circulatory demand of the rest of the upper gastrointestinal tract may make blood shunting

---

Practice Point

RELIEF OF STITCH

- Lean over to affected side.
- Press fingers into the site of pain.
- Expire through pursed lips.
- Run with arm on affected side stretched above head.
- If the above fail, lay down with knees bent and both arms raised above head.
- For repeated stitch, build up exercise tolerance more slowly.

to the respiratory muscles inefficient. Additionally, the deep breathing may stretch the distended liver capsule.[24] Although gastric distress due to intestinal gas or constipation has also been postulated, it is likely that the type of abdominal pain experienced is different from that of stitch.

Most individuals can run through the stitch by either breathing out forcibly through pursed lips or by breathing deeply and regularly, leaning slightly to the side of the stitch. If the pain is persistent or particularly uncomfortable, the athlete can usually relieve the symptom simply by lying on the back with the arms raised above the head. Once the initial stitch pain is relieved, the individual usually is able to continue training uninterrupted. Usually the stitches become less frequent as the individual becomes more fit.

Precordial Catch Syndrome (Chest Wall Twinge Syndrome)

The precordial catch syndrome is an uncommon, benign, self-limiting disorder of unknown origin characterized by episodes of brief, sharp precordial pain.[25] This variation of the "stitch," or "catch," is usually felt in the anterior chest usually to the left of the parasternal area or near the cardiac apex. The pains usually last 30 seconds to 3 minutes. They are generally aggravated by deep breathing and are usually relieved by shallow respiration, moderate activity, or assuming a more upright posture. There is no local tenderness. Little is known about the cause of this condition, and intercostal muscle spasms have been postulated, as has pain from the parietal pleura. The main concern is obviously that the pain may be from a cardiac origin. An appropriate history and examination of the patient should indicate if there is a need to investigate.

Epidemic Myalgia (Bornholm's Disease, Epidemic Pleurodynia, Devil's Grip)

Epidemic myalgia commonly affects the intercostal and upper abdominal wall muscles and more rarely the pleura. It is a sequel to an infection, most commonly with a group B Coxsackie virus.[5] After a prodrome of about 1 to 10 days, the athlete is seized with a sharp, severe pain on the lateral chest wall and occasionally the upper abdomen. This pain is intensified by respiratory effort, coughing, and other movements of the thorax. Paroxysms of fairly intense pain are often separated by relatively symptom-free intervals. The involved intercostal muscles are usually ten-

der to touch. There is associated transient pleurisy with a friction rub in a small percentage of cases. A specific diagnosis may be made by isolating the virus from the throat early in the disease or by demonstrating a rising titer of type-specific neutralizing antibodies. This self-limiting condition usually requires only symptomatic treatment.

Fibrositis Syndrome (Fibromyalgia, Myofascial Syndrome)

The myofascial syndrome is characterized by diffuse musculotendinous pain and multiple discrete tender points. The chest wall is a common site for fibrositic pain. Usually the individual is in the third and fourth decade of life.[26,27]

The term fibromyalgia, or fibrositis, should be reserved for a specific clinical entity characterized by diffuse, widespread musculoskeletal aching, pain, and stiffness, undue fatigue, and a large number of specific tender trigger areas. There is also often an association with sleep disturbance. The periscapular region, base of the neck, and chest wall are the areas most commonly involved. Fluctuation of pain from day to day is common. These symptoms are accentuated by cold, mental stress, and fatigue. Inactivity or indeed the contrary excessive exercise may also exacerbate the symptoms. Relief may be obtained by local application of heat, massage, moderate activity, and planned rest periods. There are sometimes associated nonrheumatic complaints, including tiredness, anxiety, tension headaches, numbness, and irritable bowel syndrome (Table 18-3).

The trigger points are the hallmark of this condition, and local pressure on these tender points may cause pain to radiate to distal areas, although sometimes the discomfort is local. In order of frequency, the tender points (trigger points) are found in the supraspinous fossa along the medial border of the scapula particularly near the bellies of the rhomboids, levator scapulae, and the infraspinatus, and over the anterior part of the upper chest, particularly at the costochondral junctions. This condition may be seen in association with other systemic problems, e.g., osteoarthritis, cervical lumbar disc disease, rheumatoid arthritis, and endocrine and malignant problems.

Management of diffuse fibrositis requires a great deal of understanding and patience on the part of the physician, therapist, and athlete. Treatment for the most part consists in reassurance, patient education,

TABLE 18-3.   Diagnostic Features of the Myofascial (Fibrositis) Syndrome

Pain
    Widespread musculoskeletal discomfort
    Aching in nature
    Associated with stiffness
    Typically in the neck, shoulders, and upper back
    Affected by activity, fatigue, weather, and moods
Tenderness
    Multiple discrete areas of localized tenderness
    Classic trigger point sites
General symptoms
    Disturbed, nonrestful sleep
    Frequent stiffness on awakening
    Associated tension headaches
    Often irritable bowel syndrome
    Associated labile moods or psychiatric disturbance
Investigations
    Normal screening laboratory tests
    Radiographic studies normal

supportive psychotherapy, and measures to relieve pain. If there are particularly uncomfortable trigger areas, therapeutic tools include the use of ethyl chloride sprays, transcutaneous electrical nerve stimulation (TENS), acupuncture, biofeedback, and relaxation techniques. In addition, the trigger areas may be injected with lidocaine with or without cortisone. The use of tricyclic medications, e.g., amitriptyline 10 to 50 mg, in the evenings is also convenient; but the accompanying drowsiness prohibits its use in active individuals other than as a nighttime dose.

Pain Due To Thoracic Spine Injuries

Problems of the thoracic spine, spinal cord, and spinal nerves—including traumatic lesions, disc disease, juvenile kyphosis (Scheuermann's disease), ankylosing spondylitis, and in the older age group osteoporosis involving the thoracic vertebra—may generate pain around the thoracic spine and the accompanying ribs.[28,29] These entities are dealt with in Chapter 19.

Hyperventilation

Hyperventilation may occur during periods of intense excitement, anxiety, or injury. With repetitive deep breathing at a rapid rate, carbon dioxide is removed at an increased rate, causing a pH change in the blood. Clinical signs include dizziness and tingling in the fingers and toes and the perioral area, particularly the lips. Occasionally, there are associated muscle cramps, although usually the symptoms are limited to simple lightheadedness. Nevertheless, the athlete often misinterprets the symptoms, becomes more anxious and comprehensive, breathes faster, and becomes panicky, which increases the developing symptoms.

The first line of treatment is reassurance, explanation when possible, and advice to breathe slowly and hold the breath intermittently. If these measures are not immediately effective, breathing in and out of a paper bag allows rebreathing of carbon dioxide (CO_2), increasing the CO_2 level in the lungs. This technique slows CO_2 exchange at the capillary alveolar membrane and allows gradual resumption of normal pH, thus circumventing the symptoms. The technique of rebreathing expired air is ceased when the athlete is calm and breathing in a normal fashion.

Effort Thrombosis and Pulmonary Embolus (Paget-von Schroetter Syndrome)

The first report of effort thrombosis of the subclavian vein was made by Paget in 1875.[30] The most extensive collection was that of Hughes, who reported on 320 cases from the literature[31] and suggested that the term Paget-von Schroetter syndrome be adopted.

The pathophysiology of this syndrome remains controversial. Trauma is often involved, but in many cases the condition develops spontaneously. Damage to the vein walls secondary to compression at various points with subsequent thrombosis has been suggested as the most likely sequence of events. It is intriguing that in many cases in which complete obstruction of the subclavian vein was demonstrated on venogram there was no evidence of thrombi at surgery. In these cases the term "effort thrombosis," which was to become synonymous with Paget-von Schroetter syndrome, is a misnomer.[32]

The syndrome is most commonly found on the right side of active young men. Many patients report previous bouts of strenuous activity. When the syndrome occurs in a full-blown fashion, there is often an acute onset of diffuse swelling of the arm with distension of the superficial veins (Fig. 18-18) accompanied by a variable degree of cyanosis. This bluish discoloration of the extremity is pathognomonic of the syndrome. The patient may complain of heaviness of the affected arm, and physical examination reveals an increase in the size of the extremity involved.

Although signs of arterial or plexus compression

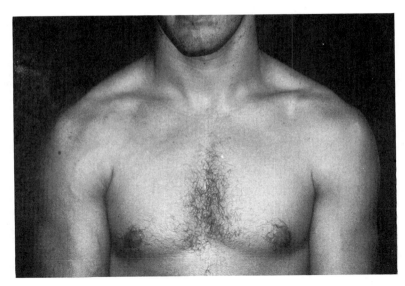

Fig. 18-18. Paget-von Schroetter syndrome. Note the swelling of the right arm with obvious venous distension extending over the shoulder and pectoral region.

may be present, usually the venous pathology is seen in isolation. In less acute forms, the athlete may simply complain of heaviness and fatigue in the upper limb. If effort thrombosis is suspected, a diligent search should be made for upper limb edema, including measuring the girth of various parts of the extremity. Upper extremity strength should be assessed because when the syndrome is long-standing some weakness results. Venous occlusion is often confirmed with an exercise test. The individual is asked to perform a workout in a fashion that usually produces the maximum symptoms and is examined immediately after this exercise bout. Occasionally, the symptoms can be exacerbated by bringing the arms into hyperabduction or into the exaggerated military position with the shoulders pulled back and depressed.

Investigations should include evaluation of the bony structures by chest roentgenogram and an anteroposterior view of the cervical spine. The venogram is the diagnostic "gold standard" technique, although CT, magnetic resonance imaging (MRI), or other diagnositc techniques such as Doppler ultrasonography may be used as indicated[33] (Fig. 18-19).

The differential diagnosis should include drug abuse, sarcoidosis, infection, hypercoagulable states including oral contraceptive use, metastatic tumor (particularly of the lung, breast, or pancreas), or medical causes of poor circulation including heart disease, polycythemia, dehydration, or the nephrotic syndrome. It is important to differentiate between

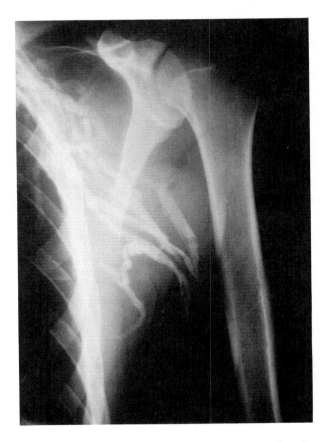

Fig. 18-19. Effort thrombosis. Venogram showing venous occlusion in the left axillary region with extensive collateral dilatation.

venous and arterial occlusion. Patients with venous thrombosis usually have the symptoms that have been described, i.e., superficial venous distension, increased arm size, and diffuse aching in the limb aggravated by activity. Classic arterial occlusion is accompanied by more dramatic presentation of a cold, pale, pulseless extremity. There may be a feeling of decreased strength, and there may be tingling and sensory changes in the hand.

Upper extremity thrombosis is rare, occurring in approximately 1 to 2 percent of all patients with deep vein thrombosis. By contrast, it is associated with effort thrombosis in about 20 to 30 percent of cases. In this situation the acute pain and swelling are more dramatic in the affected extremity. When the diagnosis is confirmed by venogram, because of the danger of pulmonary embolus the patient should be anticoagulated using heparin (with careful monitoring, followed by warfarin (Coumadin). The duration of oral anticoagulation therapy is empirically placed at about 3 months. All activities should be curtailed initially, after which, depending on the resolution of symptoms, reintroduction to activity is allowed.

The literature reports the risk of pulmonary embolus as high, probably because most cases in series involve a large number of people with underlying medical conditions. In the young, fit athlete, the risk of pulmonary embolus is probably relatively low. Nevertheless, because of the potential risk of a fatal pulmonary embolus, aggressive medical therapy is indicated. Some investigators recommend that treatment include resection of the first rib, although it is not usually necessary.

ASSOCIATED CARDIAC PROBLEMS

This book features mainly orthopaedic and musculoskeletal problems. When dealing with the torso, however, it is necessary to consider some of the associated cardiac problems. This section is limited to conditions that preclude participation, the detection of risk for sudden death in sport, myocardial contusion, emergency protocols, and brief consideration of exercise prescription, and recognition of risk factors.[34,35]

Conditions Precluding Participation

Extrasystoles without a detectable underlying organic problem and physiologic heart murmurs are the commonest cardiac signs detected at preseason test-

ing. The decision to dismiss these findings and allow full sports participation requires experience and judgment. When in doubt, an electrocardiogram (ECG) and possibly a cardiac consultation are appropriate. Essentially there are four questions that must be addressed: (1) What is the cardiac lesion? (2) What risk for morbidity or mortality does the lesion pose? (3) In what activity does the athlete participate? (4) What is the extent of the athlete's participation?[36]

Practice Point

EXTRASYSTOLES OR MURMURS

- Is there a cardiac lesion?
- What risk does the lesion pose?
- What is the activity of the athlete?
- What is the intensity of participation?

Athlete's Heart

The variations under the eponym of "athlete's heart" require some consideration. It is suggested that athletes who engage in isotonic-type activities — distance running and swimming, for example — tend to develop large left ventricular chambers. Athletes involved in relatively isometric exertion, e.g., weight lifting, accommodate with thick left ventricular walls.[37] Methods of measuring cardiac chamber and wall size, however, have shown that these adaptations are by no means universal, and cardiomegaly is not as prevalent as previously thought.[38]

The significance of the constellation of changes (sinus bradycardia, chamber dilatation, and muscle hypertrophy) is variable depending on the clinical context. In a tertiary care setting, an individual with a systolic heart murmur, increased voltage on the ECG, a ventricular free wall ratio of greater than 1 to 3, merits consideration of the diagnosis of cardiomyopathy. In a primary care context, with an active young person, the athletic heart syndrome is an equally valid consideration.

Note that the conditioned athletic heart usually has a normal or enlarged left end diastolic diameter and symmetrical myocardial thickening. With the cardiomyopathic individual, there is usually enzymatic septal hypertrophy, and the ventricular cavity is encroached upon.[35]

The ECG variations associated with the athlete's heart are (1) changes in impulse formation and conduction and (2) waveform changes. With respect to the former, slowing of the resting heartbeat (bradycardia) is a well known association with progressive fitness. What is less well appreciated is that, in the setting of this sinus bradycardia, junctional escape rhythms may occur at rest.[38,39] First degree atrioventricular (AV) block is common. Unusual waveforms include tall and peaked T waves in the precordial leads; occasionally, T wave inversion and ST segment elevation are seen.[38] Thus, when confronted with these ECG abnormalities it is important to rule out organic heart disease, particularly hypertrophic cardiomyopathy. Help is obtained from the family history, and normalization of the ECG changes with adequate exertion, sympathomimetic or vagolytic drugs.[35] Treadmill testing, Holter monitoring, gallium scanning, and/or an angiogram are further diagnostic aids.

Quick Facts

ATHLETE'S HEART

The ability to generate efficient increased cardiac output with activity
- Frequently, left ventricular enlargement
- May have thick left ventricular walls
- Sinus bradycardia (slower resting pulse)
- Associated ECG changes

Mitral Valve Prolapse

Mitral valve prolapse (MVP) is the most common cause of mitral insufficiency in the athlete. It occurs predominantly in the female athlete at an incidence estimated to be about 7 percent.[38] MVP classically is associated with a murmur or a click on auscultation. Because these findings are inconsistent, sometimes being present on one examination and absent on another, it may be the athlete's complaint of chest pain or the discovery of ectopic beats that triggers the diagnosis. Suspicion of MVP warrants a cardiology consultation and probably an echocardiogram in a competitive athlete. MVP has been associated with sudden death in sport, probably secondary to major ventricular rhythm disturbances, e.g., premature ventricular contractions, runs of tachycardia, or both. It is also seen in association with Marfan syn-

drome. However, it is probably permissible to allow young athletes to compete if they have no cardiomegaly, a normal resting ECG, or only minor repolarization abnormalities. They must not have any significant ventricular irritability with exercise.[38]

Practice Point

MITRAL VALVE PROLAPSE

- Systolic murmur
- Midsystolic click
- Irregular heart rate
- Premature ventricular contraction
- Dizziness or fainting
- Chest pain with exertion
- Echocardiogram positive

Full work-up required before return to participation

Hypertension

Accurate recording of blood pressure is a prerequisite for any clinical decisions and advice. Note that an appropriate size cuff must be used (Fig. 18-20).

In adults systolic pressure is indicated by the first appearance of Korotkoff's sounds, and the diastolic value is recorded when they disappear. These points are the so-called phase I and phase V sounds.[40] In children the phase IV sound, when there is distinct muffling, is utilized, as it is occasionally in some adults in whom faint sounds continue down to very low readings.

Quick Facts

RECOMMENDED BLOOD PRESSURE CUFF SIZE

Patient	Arm Circumference (cm)	Cuff Bladder Width (cm)	Cuff Length (cm)
Infant	75–13	5	8
Child	13–20	8	13
Small adult	17–26	11	17
Adult	24–32	13	24
Large adult	32–42	17	32

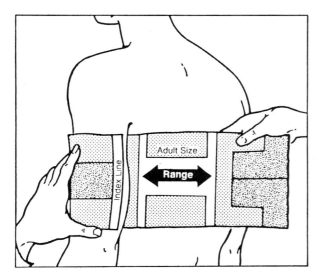

Fig. 18-20. For maximum reducibility of blood pressure recordings, the appropriate size cuff is necessary. Index line should fall within the range indicated. Many athletes have arms that are far too large for the standard adult cuff.

In athletes 18 years and older, a diastolic pressure of more than 90 mmHg is abnormal. A high reading should be observed on at least three occasions in the most relaxed atmosphere for confirmation. Elevated systolic readings should be followed with care, as they may be a predictor of evolving hypertension. It is difficult to assess the immediate risks and dangers of hypertension to the young athlete, and it seems reasonable to permit most athletes with mild to moderate hypertension to participate in organized sport.[40] Mild hypertension may be managed by body weight control, sodium restriction, and relaxation techniques.[41] Unresponsive moderate hypertension and markedly elevated blood pressures usually require medication. It is beyond the scope of this text to discuss these subjects further. Adequate investigation of renal functional and cardiac status are mandatory before initiating drug therapy, and in all cases of hypertension in the young age group long-term follow-up is important.

Other Common Problems

Hypertrophic obstructive cardiomyopathy is the most frequent totally unsuspected cause of mortality in athletes. Mitral and aortic stenosis, cyanotic heart disease, pulmonary hypertension, and active myoper-

icarditis are absolute contraindications for collision and contact sports and are relative contraindications for noncontact sports. The presence of a well investigated, diagnosed cardiac problem allows some established guidelines to be utilized with the discretion of a cardiologist (Table 18-4). However, it is the more subtle or new problems that are particularly worrisome. Currently we are unable to screen for every potential lethal condition. Essentially, *a history of fainting with exertion, chest pain, a constellation of significant known risk factors, and the presence of a murmur are indicators of the need to examine the individual more carefully* and when necessary refer for a thorough workup. The latter includes a cardiology consult, electrocardiography, echocardiography, and stress testing when appropriate[42,43] (Table 18-5).

Emergency Evaluation of Chest Pain

Ischemic heart disease with myocardial infarction, dissecting aortic aneurysm, and pulmonary embolus are among the potentially catastrophic causes of chest pain.[44] However, relatively minor conditions such as muscle strain, esophagitis, and many of the costochondral syndromes described in the previous section may mimic the more serious conditions. Nevertheless, when initially attending a person with chest pain, the possibility of the more significant causes, particularly unstable angina or myocardial infarction, must remain uppermost in one's mind. Particularly in any individual who is dyspneic, diaphoretic, or who has severe chest discomfort, there must be provisions made for stabilization and resuscitation along with the assessment. When suspicion is high, administration of oxygen and, if available, cardiac monitoring and establishment of an intravenous line are appropriate. The latter is important because if the individual's condition deteriorates, intravenous access becomes difficult owing to hypotension and collapsing veins. Thus at a time when rapid administration of medication is required, access is most difficult.

In the presence of stable vital signs, the history is obtained with special reference to the nature of the chest pain and its onset. The terms "heaviness," "tightness," and "squeezing pain" in the left upper chest typically describe angina or myocardial infarction. The pain may be located in the substernal or epigastric area, but on occasion it is felt only in the jaw or the arms. Chest pain occasionally radiates to both arms. Pain radiating to the jaw or the lower teeth is highly suggestive of myocardial infarction. Chest pain

TABLE 18-4. Heart Problems and Activity

Defect	Recreational Restriction	Examples of Allowable Recreation	Peak Load Allowed (cal/min)	Examples of Work Allowed[a]
Aortic Insufficiency				
Mild, with normal ECG and heart	None	All recreational activity allowed	2.6–4.9	Lifting objects 20 lb max.
Moderate, with cardiac enlargement	Mild	All but those requiring violent, prolonged exertion	2.6–4.9	Lifting objects 20 lb max.
Severe, without signs of QRS-T angle abnormality on ECG	Moderate	Baseball, volleyball, noncompetitive activities	≤2.5	Mostly sitting, some walking, lifting 10 lb max.
Severe, with signs of QRS-T angle	Severe	Golf with cart, bowling, walking and swimming at own pace	≤2.5	Mostly sitting, some walking, lifting 10 lb max.
Aortic Stenosis[b]				
Mild, with or without surgery	None	All recreational activity allowed	2.6–4.9	Lifting objects 20 lb max.
Moderate, with or without surgery	Mild	All but those requiring violent, prolonged exertion	2.6–4.9	Lifting objects 20 lb max.
Severe, with or without surgery[c]	Moderate	Baseball, volleyball, noncompetitive activities	≤2.5	Mostly sitting, some walking, lifting 10 lb max.
Atrial Septal Defect				
Unoperated or successfully operated with normal pulmonary artery pressure[d]	None	All recreational activity allowed	≥7.6	Lifting objects ≥100 lb
Unoperated or successfully operated, with pulmonary artery pressure <0.50 systemic	None	All recreational activity allowed	5.0–7.5	Lifting objects 50 lb max.
With severe pulmonary vascular disease[e]	Moderate	Baseball, volleyball, noncompetitive activities	2.6–4.9	Lifting objects 20 lb max.
Chronic Congestive Heart Failure	Severe	Golf with cart, bowling, walking and swimming at own pace	≤2.5	Mostly sitting, some walking, lifting 10 lb max.
Coarctation of the Aorta				
Unoperated, without severe systemic hypertension and no significant aortic valve disease	None	All recreational activity allowed	5.0–7.5	Lifting objects 50 lb max.
Postoperative, with normal pressure and no significant valve disease	None	All recreational activity allowed	5.0–7.5	Lifting objects 50 lb max.
Mitral Insufficiency				
With little or no cardiac enlargement	None	All recreational activity allowed	5.0–7.5	Lifting object 50 lb max.
With moderate to marked cardiac enlargement	Moderate	Baseball, volleyball, noncompetitive activities	2.6–4.9	Lifting objects 20 lb max.
Myocarditis, Active	Severe	Golf with cart, bowling, walking at own pace		
Patent Ductus Arteriosus				
Unoperated or operated, with normal pulmonary artery pressure	None	All recreational activity allowed	≥7.6	Lifting objects 100 lb or more
Unoperated or operated, with pulmonary hypertension (pulmonary artery pressure <0.05 systemic)[e]	None	All recreational activity allowed	5.0–7.5	Lifting objects 50 lb max.

(Continued)

TABLE 18-4 *(continued).* **Heart Problems and Activity**

Defect	Recreational Restriction	Examples of Allowable Recreation	Peak Load Allowed (cal/min)	Examples of Work Allowed[a]
noperated or operated, with severe pulmonary vascular disease[e]	Moderate	Baseball, volleyball, non-competitive activities	2.6–4.9	Lifting objects 20 lb max.
Prosthetic valve replacement	Moderate	Baseball, volleyball, non-competitive activities	2.6–4.9	Lifting objects 20 lb max.
Pulmonary stenosis				
Mild to moderate (peak systolic gradient <50 mmHg) with or without surgery	None	All recreational activity allowed	≥7.6	Lifting objects ≥100 lb
Severe (peak systolic gradient 80 mmHg)	Moderate	Baseball, volleyball, non-competitive activities	≥7.6	Lifting objects ≥100 lb
Tetralogy of Fallot				
Postoperative, right ventricle pulmonary artery gradient <50 mmHg without overflow patch	None	All recreational activity allowed	5.0–7.5	Lifting objects 50 lb max.
Postoperative, right ventricle pulmonary artery gradient <50 mmHg with outflow patch and pulmonary insufficient	Mild	All activities but those requiring violent, prolonged exertion	2.6–4.9	Lifting objects 20 lb max.
Ventricular septal defect				
Unoperated or operated, with normal pulmonary pressure[d]	None	All recreational activity allowed	≥7.6	Lifting objects ≥100 lb
Unoperated or operated, with pulmonary hypertension (pulmonary artery pressure <0.50 systolic)[e]	None	All recreational activity allowed	5.0–7.5	Lifting objects 50 lb max.
Unoperated or operated, with severe pulmonary vascular disease[e]	Moderate	Baseball, volleyball, non-competitive activities	2.6–4.9	Lifting objects 20 lb max.
*Other mild forms of heart disease—*not requiring surgery and without natural history of progressive disability	None	All recreational activity allowed	≥7.6	Lifting objects ≥100 lb
*Other severe defects—*not operated or amenable to surgery	Severe	Golf with cart, bowling, walking, swimming	≤2.5	Mostly sitting, some walking, lifting 10 lb max.

a As classified in the *Dictionary of Occupational Titles.*
b Definition of severity by gradient not included because of individual patient variability.
c Patients with severe aortic stenosis may or may not have ECG abnormalities.
d Assuming surgery performed during childhood with abolishment of gradient.
e Restricted to low altitude, except airplane travel.
(Adapted from a position statement, American Heart Association. Activity guidelines for young patients with heart disease.)

described by patients as the worst they have ever experienced, particularly when not relieved by changes in position or rest, suggests infarction.

Cardiac syncope, a transient loss of consciousness related to an arrythmia, is occasionally associated with chest pain as well as with palpitations. Shortness of breath, generalized weakness, dizziness, nausea, and vomiting are suggestive of infarction. A history of myocardial infarction in the older age group helps confirm a suspicion of coronary artery disease. Particularly if the individual says the pain is identical to that experienced during a previous episode of infarction, the diagnosis must be assumed accurate.

The presence of risk factors for chest pain and coronary artery disease include cigarette smoking, hypertension, elevated cholesterol levels, diabetes, and a positive family history[45] (Table 18-5). The use of cocaine in sport is an established risk factor for myo-

TABLE 18-5.   Coronary Risk Factors and Physical Activity

Risk Factor	Effect of Physical Activity
Age	Risk enhanced in 40- to 49-year age group commencing an activity program.
Family history	May be enhanced risk if relatives also died while active.
Physical inactivity	Increases risk at given power output, but inactive subject not prone to overexertion.
Sudden unaccustomed activity	Insufficient time for development of normal cardiovascular adaptations.
Excess body mass, obesity	Increases risk of given power output, but inactive subject not prone to overexertion.
Type A personality	Risk due to excessive competitiveness, overachieving, and failure to follow exercise prescription.
Smoking habits	Reduces benefits of vigorous physical activity, probably through disturbances of cardiac rhythm.
Hypertension	Increases chance that cardiac work rate will exceed ischemic threshold.
Fainting with exertion	May signal undetected hypertrophic obstructive cardiomyopathy, mitral valve disease, or arrhythmias with exertion, all of which are risks of sudden death.
Cocaine abuse	Associated with cardiomyopathy and ischemia.
Abnormal exercise ECG	Deep horizontal or downward sloping ST segmental depression and angina pain increase the risk of exercise.
Other factors	Exercise has no acute adverse interaction with an abnormal lipid profile or glucose tolerance curve. Women seem relatively immune to exercise-induced cardiac death.

cardial ischemia and infarction. With a history of recent cocaine use, even patients in their teens and twenties may have coronary ischemic attacks and infarction.

Quick Facts

POSSIBLE RISK FACTORS FOR CORONARY ARTERY DISEASE[a]

- Total cholesterol
  >5.2 mmol/l at 30+ years
  >4.6 mmol/l at 18–29 years
- Low density lipoprotein cholesterol
  >3.4 mmol/l at 30+ years
  >3.0 mmol/l at 18–19 years
- High density lipoprotein cholesterol
  <0.9 mmol/l or triglycerides 2.3 mmol/l

  [a] TC/HDL ratio >5/1

Without elaborate equipment the physical examination is often less sensitive than the history for detecting potential coronary ischemia. The appearance of pallor, perspiration, and coolness of the skin, particularly in the extremities, suggest hypotension. Distension of the neck veins with the patient in the upright or semiupright position suggests that the right ventricle is failing to pump effectively; and if the systolic pressure is high, the entire heart may not be pumping adequately. Wheezing is suggestive of pulmonary edema. Murmurs may be difficult to hear in emergency situations, but the presence of a loud systolic murmur may be indicative of a papillary muscle rupture, which signifies a potentially lethal complication. An aortic diastolic murmur associated with sharp chest pain radiating to the back may indicate dissecting thoracic aneurysm. Stabilization, establishment of a tentative diagnosis, and provision for resuscitation should be rapidly followed by transport to the nearest treatment facility.

Sudden Death in Sport

Sudden death in sport can occur at any age and without any history of illness. It may be due to hypertrophic cardiomyopathy, coronary artery anomalies, coronary atherosclerosis, myocarditis, arrhythmias, rupture of the myocardium or aorta, aneurysm, aortic stenosis, or mitral valve prolapse.

Atherosclerotic coronary artery disease is the usual cause of sudden death in individuals over 40 years of age, whereas congenital conditions, specifically hypertrophic cardiomyopathy, is the most common cause in young, conditioned athletes. It is possible that this condition is largely genetic, so screening of

---

Quick Facts

CAUSES OF SUDDEN DEATH IN ATHLETES

- Myocardial ischemia
  - Atherosclerotic coronary artery disease
  - Coronary artery spasm
  - Coronary artery thrombosis
- Structural abnormalities
  - Hypertrophic cardiomyopathy
  - Mitral valve prolapse
  - Valvular heart disease
  - Marfan's syndrome
- Arrhythmias
- Miscellaneous causes
  - Subarachnoid hemorrhage
  - Gastrointestinal hemorrhage
  - Myocarditis

---

trophic cardiomyopathy. Its presence should raise suspicion for the disorder. The typical systolic ejection type cardiac murmur is generally transmitted widely and can mimic combined lesions of mitral regurgitation and aortic stenosis. This murmur often increases with standing owing to the reduction in left ventricular volume. It also tends to increase during the phases of the Valsalva's maneuver when the heart accelerates. Thus this simple bedside technique should be used as a screening device during auscultation of all athletes who have systolic heart murmurs. The absence of this sign does not exclude the diagnosis, however. It has been suggested that one should consider hypertrophic cardiomyopathy in athletes with prominent freckles[45] because the skin lesions of lentiginosis mimic freckles. However, those of lentiginosis differ from typical freckles in that they appear at or soon after birth, increase in number until puberty, and do not darken or increase when exposed to the sun.

individuals with a family is indicated once the syndrome has been identified. It is considered an absolute contraindication for competitive strenuous activity.

Cardiomyopathy of unknown cause is subclassified into dilated, restrictive, and hypertrophic types. Theories about the underlying cause of hypertrophic cardiomyopathy with its usually associated subaortic obstruction (idiopathic hypertrophic subaortic stenosis) range from congenital variations of the ventricular septum to abnormal development of the sympathetic nervous system with inappropriate or abnormal stimulation of the myocardium. There are strong autosomal dominant features in most of the proved cases of hypertrophic obstructive cardiomyopathy.

In a large percentage of athletes symptoms are conspicuously absent. When present, they may include chest pain, near-syncopal or syncopal episodes, inappropriate dyspnea, and palpitations. The chest pain may not be typical of angina pectoris, and it is frequently described in unusual terms, e.g., a pressure sensation on the chest. It is possible that the syncopal episodes are related to underlying cardiac rhythm disorders or to the obstructive hemodynamic features of the disease.

Auscultation may reveal a fourth heart sound (S_4 gallop), as it is nearly always present with hyper-

---

Practice Point

HYPERTROPHIC CARDIOMYOPATHY

- May be no symptoms
- Clinical symptoms
  - Near syncopal or syncopal episodes
  - Chest pain
  - Palpitations
  - Shortness of breath
- Auscultation findings
  - Fourth heart sound
  - Systolic ejection murmur
  - Increased with Valsalva's maneuver
- ECG findings
  - Deep septal Q waves
  - Left ventricular hypertrophy
  - Repolarization changes
- Occasional association with "freckles" of lentiginosis variety

---

The ECG of hypertrophic cardiomyopathy sometimes shows a deep septal Q wave that may be mistaken for an old myocardial infarction. Such Q waves are seen in about one-third of cases. The most common ECG abnormalities are those of left ventricular hypertrophy and repolarization changes. The clinical suspicion, along with any ECG abnormality, should trigger the need for further investigation. Echocardiography and cardiac catheterization help confirm the diagnosis in most athletes. Once the diagnosis of hypertrophic cardiomyopathy has been established, these athletes should be restricted from vigorous exercise; and it may be necessary to treat them with β-blockers and antiarrhythmic agents.

Cardiac Arrest

Cardiac arrest occurs only rarely in young athletes with no evidence of coronary artery pathology. However, conditions that deprive the heart of oxygen or blood, e.g., respiratory distress associated with severe exercise-induced asthma, or trauma with hemorrhage or some form of toxic episode such as carbon monoxide poisoning, occasionally occur. Usually clinical recognition of the cardiac arrest is fairly straightforward, as the individual is in either extreme distress or unconscious, with an absent pulse and severely altered or absent respiration.[46] This section deals with the three most common scenarios of cardiac arrest, i.e., ventricular tachycardia, ventricular fibrillation, and asystole.

Cardiopulmonary Resuscitation Techniques

The aim of cardiopulmonary resuscitation (CPR) is to maintain cerebral and myocardial viability while the underlying cause of the cardiac arrest is determined and corrected. These basic life support techniques are continued until adequate equipment and a competent cardiac life support team arrives, often in the form of paramedical personnel in a vehicle equipped with life-support systems.

Cardiopulmonary resuscitation is most effective when instituted immediately at the scene and preferably when accompanying defibrillation, if indicated, can be administered within 5 to 10 minutes. The three major components of CPR include opening and maintaining an airway, ventilation, and closed chest cardiac massage.

Establishing an Airway

A check for airway obstruction by foreign objects (e.g., a mouthguard, broken teeth, chewing gum, tobacco) is essential. An airway may be established by several methods including the mandibular and chin lift and the head-tilt method (Fig. 18-21). The object of these maneuvers is to allow the tongue to fall away from the back of the throat, thereby establishing a patent airway. This airway is then reinforced if possible by introducing an oral or oropharyngeal airway. In a trauma victim, with suspected neck injury, the initial step for opening the airway is the chin lift or jaw thrust without head tilt.

Practice Point

ESTABLISHING AN AIRWAY

- Don't head tilt if there is any possibility of a neck injury
- Use chin lift or jaw thrust

Ventilation

If spontaneous breathing is not present, mouth-to-mouth or mouth-to-nose ventilation is attempted; or in a well equipped facility a bag-valve, mask, and oxygen are used (Fig. 18-21). After two initial ventilations the carotid pulse is checked.

Cardiac Massage

If no pulse is evident by either carotid artery palpation or peripheral pulse, closed chest cardiac massage should be instituted. Chest compression is performed

---

Practice Point

PRINCIPLES OF ONE- VERSUS TWO-RESCUER CPR

- One rescuer
  - Four groups of 15 chest compressions per minute at rate of 80 per minute (to achieve actual rate of 60 per minute)
  - Two quick lung inflations between chest compression sequences (15 : 2[a])
- Two rescuers
  - Five chest compressions at rate of 60 per minute without pauses
  - One lung inflation interposed between each set of five compressions (5 : 1[a])

[a] Compression/ventilation ratios for easy memorization.

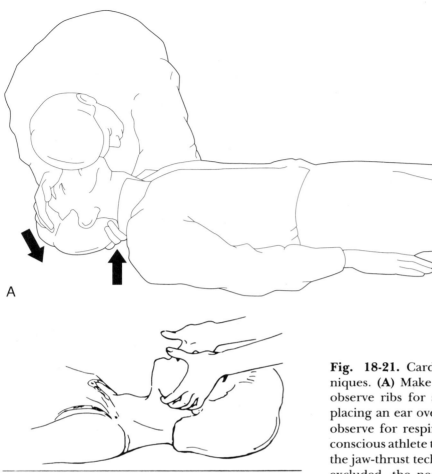

A

B

Fig. 18-21. Cardiopulmonary resuscitation techniques. **(A)** Make sure the airway is clear and then observe ribs for spontaneous respiratory effort by placing an ear over the mouth and at the same time observe for respiratory movements. **(B)** In the unconscious athlete the airway can be improved by using the jaw-thrust technique. If cervical injury cannot be excluded, the neck should not be hyperextended. *(Figure continues.)*

by locating the midpoint of the sternum, palpating the xiphoid sternal junction, and identifying a point two fingers' breadth cranially from that (Fig. 18-22). The heel of the hand is placed over this point; and, using one hand to reinforce the other with the fingers interlocked, thrusting maneuvers are carried out that depress the sternum approximately 1.5 to 2.0 inches in the adult.

Whenever possible individuals administering the massage should try to position themselves so they effectively use their body weight, ensuring that fatigue does not rapidly ensue. If only one person is present, two initial ventilations over 2 to 3 seconds are followed by 15 chest compressions and then two more ventilations. This pattern is continued. With two people available, five chest compressions to one ventilation is usually an efficient system that is kept up until

spontaneous circulation is restored or a qualified individual has decided that resuscitation should be discontinued (Fig. 18-23). Hopefully, within a short period of time, both personnel and equipment arrive to provide more advanced life support techniques, such as intubation, defibrillation, and drug therapy.

Although CPR techniques are undoubtedly efficient for 5 to 10 minutes, their ability to sustain adequate oxygenation to vital neural structures gradually deteriorates with time. Thus equipment for defibrillation, intubation, and intravenous access, along with a definitive diagnosis to distinguish primary cardiac from other secondary causes of cardiac arrest, are urgently required.

In summary, although cardiac arrest is not a common phenomenon in the recreational and sporting environment, prompt management using CPR tech-

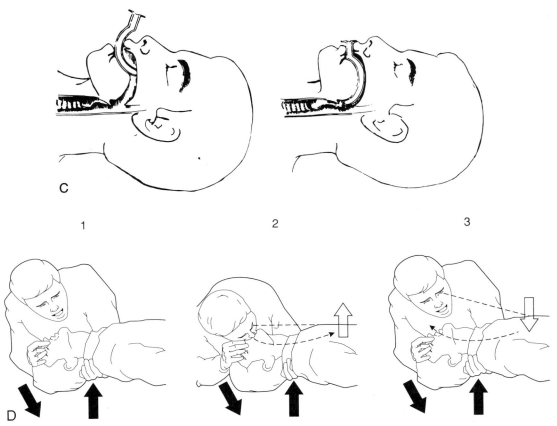

Fig. 18-21 *(Continued)*. **(C)** Oral airway facilitates patency of the upper airway and is inserted by pushing it over the tongue and then rotating it 180 degrees as it is gently introduced so it sits back over the tongue. **(D)** If no spontaneous respiratory efforts are occurring, mouth-to-mouth resuscitation can be performed by pinching off the nose and blowing air into the athlete's lungs. If a good seal is achieved either directly or via an adapted airway, it is important to make sure the rib cage moves adequately. If it does not, the airway should be rechecked.

niques can provide sufficient time to allow assessment and, when possible, institution of more advanced cardiac support techniques. It is obvious that knowledgeable equipping of the physician's or therapist's bag and carefully planned furnishing of the sport's venue, along with provisions for emergency access, are the hallmarks of an experienced and professional sports medicine individual and organization.

Specific Common Problems

Ventricular Tachycardia

Ventricular tachycardia results in inefficient ejection of blood from the left ventricle and hence circulatory collapse. A drop in blood pressure results in weakness, palpitations, occasionally chest pain, and eventually loss of pulse and consciousness. Patients may then recover spontaneously or respond to resuscitation. Alternatively, ventricular fibrillation or asystole may ensue. Ventricular tachycardia may be confirmed by typical ECG tracings (Fig. 18-24).

Initial treatment consists in a precordial thump, which is a sharp blow delivered to the mediastinum from approximately 8 to 12 inches with a closed fist. This sharp sudden movement of the rib cage is capable of generating an electrical current within the myocardium of approximately 30 to 40 joules, which may be sufficient to convert the dysrhythmia. If the ventricular tachycardia persists in a deteriorating patient who is pulseless and unconscious, immediate

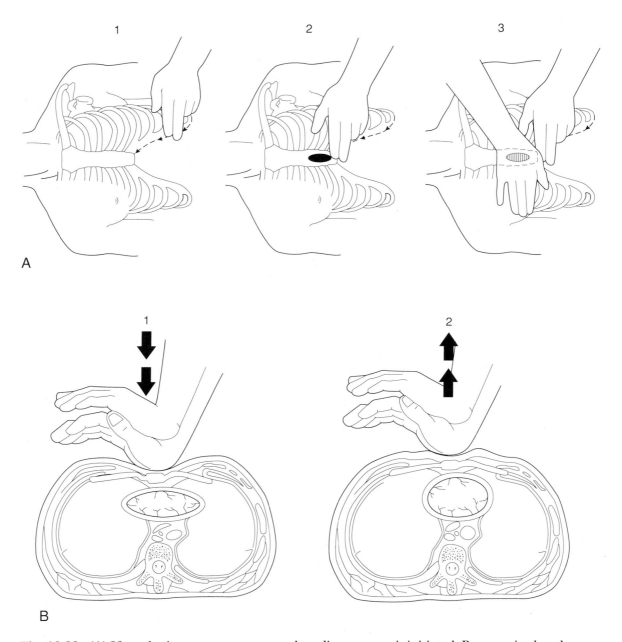

Fig. 18-22. (A) If a pulse is not present, external cardiac massage is initiated. Pressure is placed over the lower half of the sternum with the heel of the hand. The correct place is located by palpating the tip of the xiphoid and pushing through the sternum in the midline one to two fingers' breadth above it. **(B)** Downward thrust compresses the heart between the sternum and the vertebral body, exerting a pumping action. *(Figure continues.)*

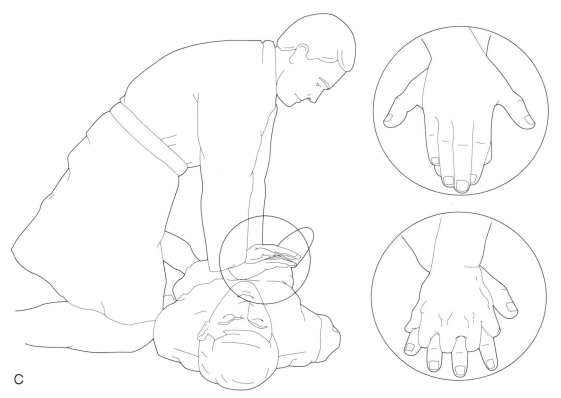

C

Fig. 18-22 *(Continued).* **(C)** By keeping the elbows relatively straight, the body weight can be used with an appropriate pressure to prevent fatigue. The fingers may be locked or kept separately to facilitate efficient use of the hands.

cardioversion with a defibrillator is appropriate. If cardioversion is achieved but the heart rate is unstable, a lidocaine bolus of 1 mg/kg is infused followed by an infusion of 2 to 4 mg/minute with a further attempt at cardioversion using the previously successful technique.

Ventricular Fibrillation

Ventricular fibrillation is the most common cause of cardiac arrest in the emergency setting. Its ECG pattern is classic, with a variable-amplitude, irregular zigzag waveform (Fig. 18-25). Once recognized, the patient should be defibrillated if equipment is available; otherwise, support and cardiac massage are carried out until arrival at an adequate facility. When cardioversion equipment is available and if defibrillation is successful and a reasonable cardiac output pulse is established, all that is necessary are monitoring and correction of the acid-base status as needed while transfer is arranged.

A dose of 200 to 300 joules in an unsynchronized mode is necessary to convert ventricular fibrillation. If fibrillation persists, this dose is repeated immediately. If the response is inadequate, a third defibrillation effort using 360 joules is carried out (Fig. 18-25).

Basic airway management with administration of oxygen and external cardiac massage should proceed in an efficient manner between defibrillatory efforts.

Probably the most efficient method of defibrillation is to position one paddle over the apex of the heart and the second paddle anteriorly over the second intercostal space, just to the right of the sternum. Firm pressure of about 25 lb is used on each paddle, with adequate coupling gel or paste. A slight change of positions is required with each defibrillatory effort to help balance the lowering of the transthoracic resistance, and prevent the current delivered to the patient's heart from increasing with each resuscitation effort.

If ventricular fibrillation persists despite defibrillation, epinephrine in doses ranging from 0.5 to 1.0 mg

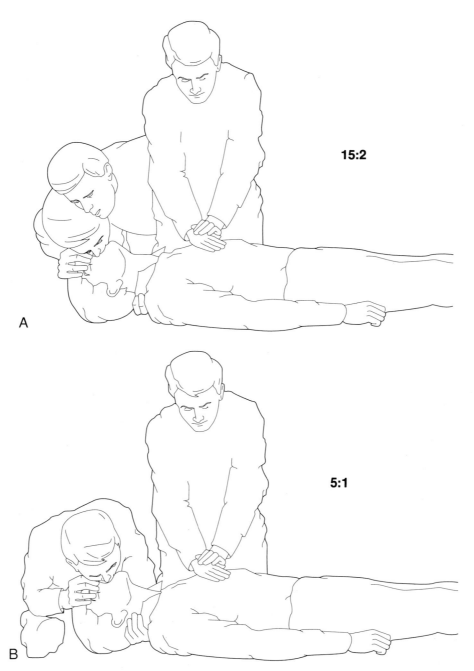

15:2

5:1

A

B

Fig. 18-23. (A) With only one resuscitator present, 15 cardiac compressions are followed by two breaths. **(B)** If there are two individuals available, the ratio should be five to one. Timing is important to ensure there is no delay in cardiac resuscitation and no drop in blood pressure during the respiratory efforts.

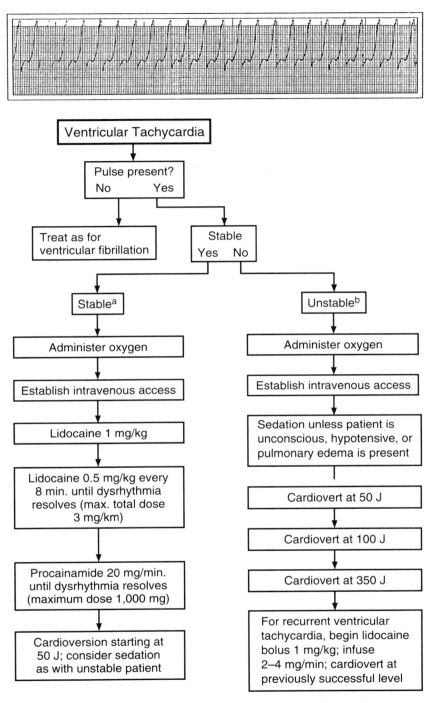

a If patient becomes unstable at any time move to "Unstable" arm of algorithm
b Unstable indicates chest pain, dyspnea, hypotension (BP<90 mmHg), or pulmonary edema.

Fig. 18-24. The symptomatic individual with ventricular tachycardia requires emergency treatment. Typical tracings and a proposed approach for resuscitation.

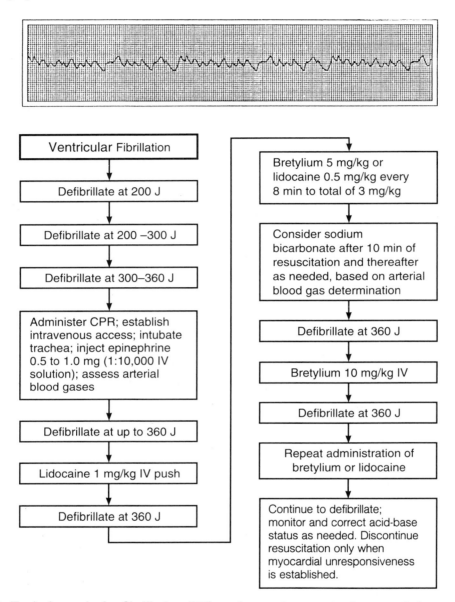

Fig. 18-25. Typical ventricular fibrillation (VF) tracings and a proposed approach for resuscitation. Survival from VF demands rapid, early electrical countershock.

improves coronary and cerebral blood flow. For endotracheal instillation, epinephrine should be diluted with 10 ml of normal saline or sterile water before administration. After epinephrine administration a further attempt at defibrillation with 360 joules should be attempted.

Ventricular fibrillation requires addition of an antidysrhythmia drug. Lidocaine is the most widely recommended first-line medication, as it tends to raise the fibrillatory threshold of the myocardial tissue. The recommended loading dose is 1 mg/kg body weight intravenously, followed by a constant infusion of 1 to 4 mg/minute. One-half the loading dose is repeated in 10 minutes and ensures adequate serum levels. Usually the total of the two loading doses should not exceed 3 mg/kg. Further defibrillation attempts at 360 joules follow the antidysrhythmia therapy.[46]

Sodium bicarbonate may be required for maintenance of the appropriate acid-base level to prevent acidosis. There is some controversy regarding its administration, but an initial dose in the absence of arterial blood gases is approximately 1 mg/kg intravenously about 10 minutes after resuscitation is begun. Furthermore, sodium bicarbonate should be administered only when ventilation has been adequately controlled either by endotracheal intubation with a good bag-and-valve ventilation technique or a controlled-volume cycle ventilator. The sodium bicarbonate combines with water to form carbon dioxide, which must be eliminated by adequate ventilation; otherwise the acidosis persists. Further therapy should be dictated by arterial blood gas levels. After each administration of sodium bicarbonate, the line should be flushed because the bicarbonate solution precipitates calcium chloride and partially inactivates any subsequently administered epinephrine.

Practice Point
SODIUM BICARBONATE

- Sodium bicarbonate should be used only after application of more definitive interventions such as prompt defibrillation, effective chest compression, establishment of an airway at hyperventilation with 100 percent oxygen and such drugs as epinephrine
- Coordinate use with clinical circumstances suggesting metabolic acidosis

---

Asystole

Asystole is the absence of any discernible cardiac rhythm. A slightly wavy or flat line is the typical ECG tracing. Asystole may be the outcome of defibrillation of a ventricular fibrillation or tachycardia, or it may follow unsuccessful attempts at resuscitation. Asystole is treated by vigorous CPR techniques while intravenous access is established and, whenever possible, intubation and the administration of 100 percent oxygen (Fig. 18-26).

Empirically, atropine 1 mg followed by another 1 mg dose in a few minutes may block vagal impulses. Although the role of vagal stimulation is not clear in asystole, this preconditioning may be helpful. It is also necessary to stabilize the acid-base level; and so sodium bicarbonate may be given at appropriate intervals. The use of a defibrillator may also stimulate the heart into a contraction pattern if good acid-base balance is preserved.

Electromechanical disassociation and idioventricular rhythms are two other conditions that lead to an ineffective cardiac contraction and thus insufficient cardiac output. Electromechanical dissociation appears on the ECG as a narrow QRS rhythm (<0.12 ms) in the absence of a pulse. Pulseless idioventricular rhythm is similar to electromechanical dissociation, except that the QRS complex is more than 0.12 ms. Therapy for both these dysrhythmias includes administration of epinephrine and sodium bicarbonate in the same manner as has been described for asystole.

Cardiac Contusion, Tamponade, and Major Vessel Damage

Blunt trauma to the chest may result in contusion of the myocardium or hemorrhage into the pericardial sac.

Cardiac Contusion

The signs of cardiac contusion vary with the degree of myocardial damage. At one extreme minor chest pain is experienced, and at the other sudden cardiac arrest is the result. Gradations of injury between these two extremes may produce tachycardia, arrhythmias, ECG changes, and a decrease in cardiac output. Any suspicion of cardiac contusion requires hospitalization and careful monitoring until the severity and prognosis are established.

Cardiac Tamponade

Blunt trauma may result in bleeding or an accumulation of edematous exudation into the pericardial sac. The volume and rate of accumulation determine the symptoms; but even relatively small volumes of fluid, accumulating rapidly, can result in cardiac tamponade. Tension within the pericardial sac limits venous inflow and thus diastolic filling of the heart, and the cardiac output rapidly declines. Tachycardia and elevation of the venous pressure appear as compensatory mechanisms. Shock and death rapidly evolve if the tamponade is not relieved. This condition obviously is an emergent one, and the major chance of survival rests with recognition and rapid transport to an appropriate facility.

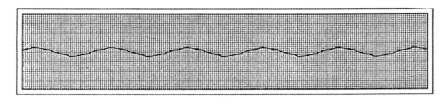

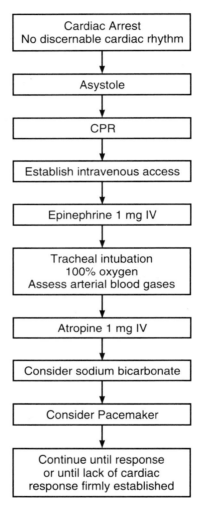

Cardiac Arrest
No discernable cardiac rhythm

Asystole

CPR

Establish intravenous access

Epinephrine 1 mg IV

Tracheal intubation
100% oxygen
Assess arterial blood gases

Atropine 1 mg IV

Consider sodium bicarbonate

Consider Pacemaker

Continue until response
or until lack of cardiac
response firmly established

Fig. 18-26. Emergency protocol for the patient with flat or slight wavy tracings of a cardiac arrest and no discernible cardiac rhythm. Intubation is preferable, however, cardiopulmonary resuscitation and the use of epinephrine are more important initially if the patient can be ventilated without intubation. (Endotracheal epinephrine may be used.)

Major Vessel Damage

Sudden deceleration, as seen in falls at speed from a horse, toboggan, or bobsled or with skiing or vehicular accidents, may result in tremendous torques at the junction of fixed and mobile portions of the great vessels. The heart and aortic arch may swing forward, lacerating or transecting the fixed descending aorta or its associated vessels. Rapid exsanguination is a frequent outcome; but recognition of major blood loss and impending shock, with immediate transport of the athlete, may be life-saving. When possible, establishing an intravenous route for infusion of fluids is important. The diagnosis is usually established by detecting widening of the mediastinum on an anteroposterior chest roetgenogram and is confirmed by arteriography when necessary.

ABDOMEN

This section deals primarily with the effects of trauma to the abdominal wall and its contents. The abdomen is left surprisingly vulnerable in many contact sports; and yet the efficiency of the ribs, pelvis, and abdominal musculature in preventing serious injury is borne out by the low incidence of serious visceral trauma in most published series. With both trauma and disease, local pain and discomfort may be complicated by remote referral (Fig. 18-27).

It is customary to divide the abdomen into either quadrants or nine regions for descriptive purposes and to correlate these regions with underlying visceral pain (Fig. 18-28). A combination of local tenderness and common referral pattern of pain helps identify the source of the discomfort. (Table 18-6).

Abdominal Wall

The strength of the abdominal wall resides in both the power of the muscles to contract and their ability to be flexible and absorb blows (Fig. 18-29). In sports where direct contact is expected from missiles, e.g., pucks, hard balls, sticks, and bats, the protective padding is generally well conceived and designed. It is probably easiest to consider injuries to the abdominal wall according to the level of injury, i.e., skin, subcutaneous tissue, and muscle. In addition, there are obviously separate categories for blunt versus penetrating trauma.

After abdominal surgery there is always concern regarding the strength of the healing wounds. Usually a period of 2 weeks is required to allow adequate collagen strength to develop, followed by slow resumption of sport depending on the size and location of the wound, the absence of complications, and the type of activity anticipated (Table 18-7).

Skin

Most injuries to the skin are abrasions or friction burns due to contact with the ground during sliding, although occasionally the skin is chafed by ill-fitting equipment. Essentially, skin wounds are best handled by carefully cleansing the surface to remove any contamination. If the wound is moist or bleeding it should be covered with a light, occlusive, nonstick dressing. Petrolatum-impregnated fine mesh gauzes are inexpensive and effective. The surface of the protective dressing should be firmly adherent around the

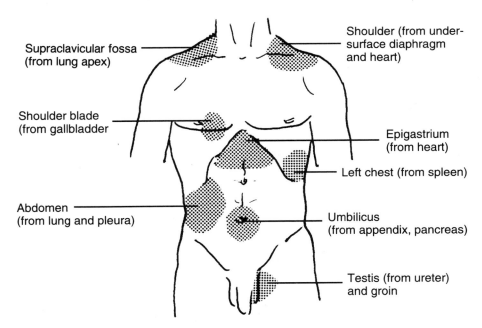

Fig. 18-27. Referred pain from thoracic and visceral structures.

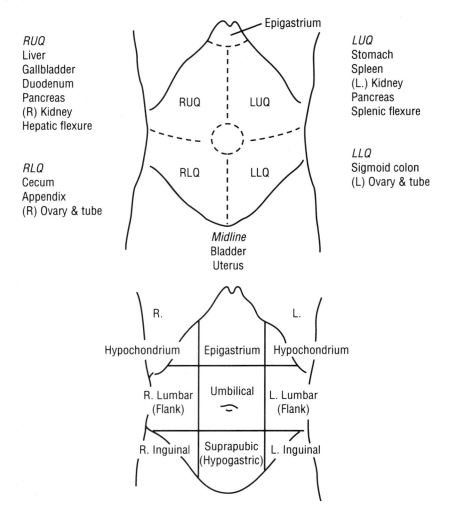

RUQ
Liver
Gallbladder
Duodenum
Pancreas
(R) Kidney
Hepatic flexure

LUQ
Stomach
Spleen
(L.) Kidney
Pancreas
Splenic flexure

RLQ
Cecum
Appendix
(R) Ovary & tube

LLQ
Sigmoid colon
(L) Ovary & tube

Epigastrium

Midline
Bladder
Uterus

R.   L.
Hypochondrium   Epigastrium   Hypochondrium
R. Lumbar   Umbilical   L. Lumbar
(Flank)   (Flank)
R. Inguinal   Suprapubic   L. Inguinal
(Hypogastric)

Fig. 18-28. **(A)** Four quadrants of the abdomen with associated underlying viscera. **(B)** More refined nine major areas.

abrasion so friction is generated over the dressing and not over the damaged area itself.

With abdominal wall lacerations the main concern is depth. Any question that the laceration involves the abdominal wall muscles or deeper is an indication for immediate hospital referral. These deep wounds should not be contaminated further by the application of ointments or creams; rather, they should be given first aid in the form if irrigation with sterile water, providone-iodine (Betadine), or an alcohol based solution (Savlon) and then covered with a hemostatic type dressing suitable for transferring the patient.

The trunk and abdomen are occasionally the sites

of dermatitis generated by foreign material in the protective equipment. The fiberglass of hockey stick blades, for instance, may easily get onto the surface of undergarments or pads and then be rubbed into the skin, causing an irritation rash. Treatment for this type of injury is application of steroid-base cream followed by counseling to prevent recurrence.

Subcutaneous Tissue

Bleeding into the subcutaneous fat and connective tissue may appear traumatic but is rarely significant. Early application of ice and compression limits its extent. Occasionally, subcutaneous hematomas are

TABLE 18-6. Correlates of the Nine Regions of the Abdomen

Right hypochondrium
 Right lobe of liver
 Gallbladder
 Portion of duodenum
 Hepatic flexure of colon
 Portion of right kidney
 Right suprarenal gland

Right lumbar (flank) region
 Ascending colon
 Lower half of right kidney
 Portion of duodenum and jejunum

Right inguinal region
 Cecum
 Appendix
 Lower end of ileum
 Right ureter
 Right spermatic cord
 Right ovary and fallopian tube

Epigastrium
 Pyloric end of stomach
 Duodenum
 Pancreas
 Portion of liver

Umbilical region
 Omentum
 Mesentery
 Lower part of duodenum
 Jejunum and ileum

Hypogastric (suprapublic) region
 Ileum
 Bladder
 Uterus (during pregnancy)

Left hypochondrium
 Stomach
 Spleen
 Tail of pancreas
 Splenic flexure of colon
 Upper pole of left kidney
 Suprarenal gland

Left lumbar (flank) region
 Descending colon
 Lower half of left kidney
 Portions of jejunum and ileum

Left inguinal region
 Sigmoid colon
 Left ureter
 Left spermatic cord
 Left ovary and fallopian tube

sufficiently large that they require a pressure dressing or even aspiration if a fluctuant collection is present.

A few precautions should be taken with regard to sterile technique. Any decision to openly drain an area should be carried out by an experienced physician under ideal circumstances. Finally, subcutaneous hematomas, particularly if not associated with significant trauma, should trigger the suspicion of an underlying blood dyscrasia. The more common abnormalities encountered in young athletes are leukemia and idiopathic thrombocytopenic purpura. These conditions can be screened for by a complete blood count and a platelet count.

Muscle

The major muscle groups of the abdominal wall are the two rectus muscles running parallel from the costal margins to the pubis, the external and internal obliques, and the transversus muscles (Figs. 18-29 and 18-30). Posteriorly, the sheaths of these muscles enclose the large paravertebral masses of the erector spinae and quadratus lumborum. These muscles may be injured in the same way as other large muscle groups, i.e., by direct contusion or strains. Injury to the back extensors is discussed in Chapter 19, and the common contusions and avulsions of the oblique muscles are dealt with in Chapter 17. This section therefore deals with strains and hematomas of the rectus abdominis.

Rupture of the rectus abdominis muscle with damage to either the epigastric artery or intramuscular vessels may result in a hematoma that, if large, usually soon tamponades within the sheath. Eighty percent of rectus abdominis hematomas occur below the umbilicus.[47] Occasionally, with violent stretching movements, the inferior epigastric artery ruptures and hemorrhages into the sheath without accompanying muscle damage.

Frequently the diagnosis of torn abdominal muscle is delayed, and usually the initial diagnosis is that of an intra-abdominal problem. Sudden abdominal pain, with or without local swelling, is the first sign. A mass is more common above the line of Douglas (arcuate line), where the tough posterior sheath makes it more obvious. There may be the bluish discoloration of bruising over the abdomen 3 to 4 days after injury.[48] Bluish discoloration around the periumbilical area is known as Cullen's sign. These signs aid diagnosis. First, the abdominal mass, when present, is palpable

TABLE 18-7.   Recommended Time Before Returning to Activity After Abdominal Operations

| | Weeks of Delay | | | |
Operation	Return to Classes	Supervised Progressive Exercise and Conditioning	Noncontact Sports	All Activities Including Contact Sports
Indirect hernia repair (children)	1	2	3	4
Small indirect hernia repair	1	3	4	6
Appendectomy	1	3	4	6
Other uncomplicated abdominal operations	2	4	8	12

(After Schneider et al.,[2] with permission.)

with the athlete both sitting and lying. Second, it is not movable because of the restriction imposed on it by the rectus sheath. Third, the swelling is usually limited to the rectus abdominis muscle and does not pass the midline or the lateral borders of the muscle.[49] These signs are more obvious in the lean individual.

Resisted trunk or hip flexion is painful. Early there may be increasing pain and tenderness with guarding, and it is this finding that raises the concern of intra-abdominal pathology. Rectal examination is normal. Hyperextension of the spine places tension on the muscle and sheath, which are likewise tender. The athlete is usually more comfortable lying in the supported flexed position.[48] If confirmation is required, CT scanning or MRI usually delineates the swelling and hematoma.

Treatment consists in application of ice, modified activity, and early use of NSAIDs. Activities that require sudden stretching, twisting, or flexion of the trunk are progressed cautiously, depending on the size of the hematoma and the degree of associated muscle tearing. Similarly, exercises and progress are modified if the obliques are the main muscles involved. On occasion, because of continued hemorrhage or because of a tense, painful hematoma, surgical exploration and evacuation of clot are necessary. Rarely, continued hemorrhage from the epigastric vessels has culminated in death.[50] By contrast, small tears and hematomas may clear rapidly with initial ice application followed by hot packs and cautious return to sport. After any injury to the trunk or after any abdominal surgery, a special effort must be made to restore both strength and endurance to the abdominal musculature (Figs. 18-31 through 18-34).

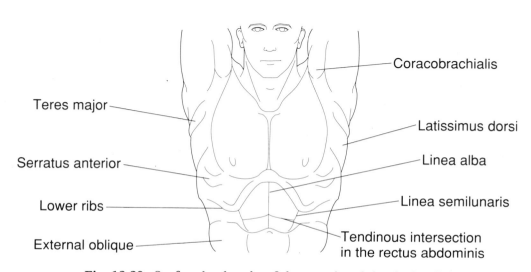

Fig. 18-29. Surface landmarks of the anterior abdominal wall.

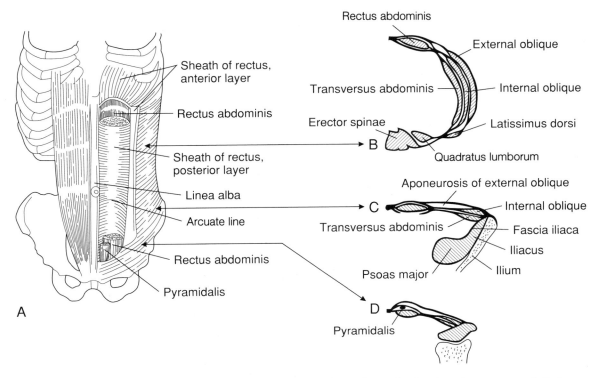

Fig. 18-30. (A) Rectus sheath. **(B–D)** Transverse sections through the sheath at sequentially lower levels showing the anatomic relations of the rectus abdominis and the oblique muscles.

Blows to the Solar Plexus

An unguarded blow to the abdomen when the abdominal muscles are relaxed results in the athlete being winded. There is inability to breathe freely; and if severe, athletes feel as if they are suffocating, or indeed, even in danger of dying. The cause of the respiratory difficulty is unknown, but diaphragmatic spasm and transient contusion to the sympathetic celiac plexus have been postulated. The physician or therapist arriving on the scene should first make sure there is no block to the upper airway by the mouthpiece, tongue, or foreign object and then loosen the equipment or belt around the abdomen. The knees should be allowed to flex, and the athlete should lean forward over the flexed knees. After the first few difficult breaths, normal respiration is usually rapidly restored.

The main point about this common occurrence is that to be winded in this manner does represent an unguarded, unprotected blow to the abdomen; hence there is some danger of intra-abdominal injury. Careful observation of the athlete during the rest of the game or practice is in order, with a careful repeated examination at the end of the session to make sure significant rib or visceral injury has not been overlooked.

Practice Point

WINDED ATHLETE

- Check airway.
- Encourage relaxation.
- Prevent fear and hysteria.
- Loosen restrictive belt.
- Flex up knees.
- Encourage athlete to sit up and lean forward.
- Ensure there is no significant rib, lung, or intra-abdominal injury.

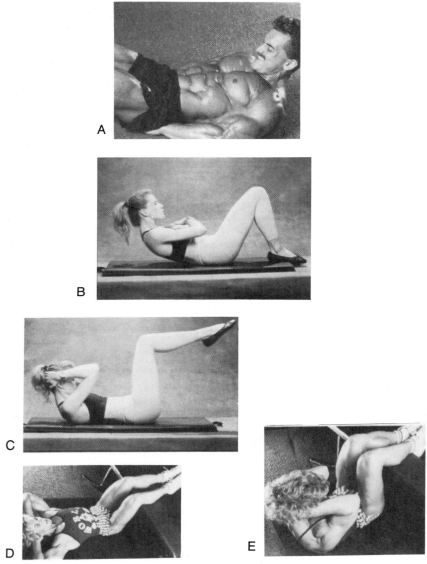

Fig. 18-31. Initial sequence of exercises for the rectus abdominis. **(A)** Abdominal crunch with arms at the sides. **(B)** Roll up with the arms across the chest. **(C)** Roll up with the arms by the head. It is important for individuals who have any propensity for cervical discomfort not to pull on the neck. Legs are held in the flexed position. Alternatively, the abdominal roll-up may be performed with the legs supported on a bench. **(D)** Start position. **(E)** Finish.

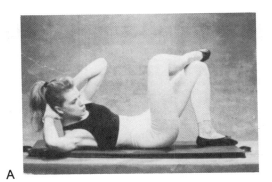

A

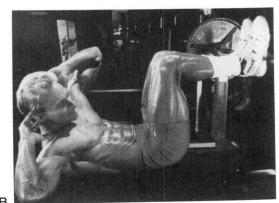

B

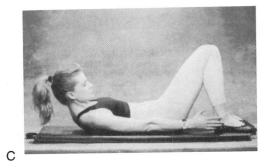

C

Fig. 18-32. Sequence of exercises for the obliques. **(A)** Diagonal curl-up. This exercise should be done in a smooth, twisting maneuver; and like most abdominal exercises, it requires many repetitions for maximum benefit. **(B)** Twisting crunches. This exercise is an effective, safe way to tone the midsection. The athlete should be cautioned about pulling on the back of the head, particularly older individuals, as it may aggravate cervical pathology. **(C)** Heel-touch starting in the lying position with the knees flexed. The head and shoulders are just slightly elevated while simultaneously reaching down with the hand to touch the heel. This maneuver is continued with alternating sides.

Intra-abdominal Trauma

Adequate examination of the abdomen is an essential skill. The athlete must be in a relaxed position so abdominal movement with respiration can be observed. The absence of splinting (keeping the abdominal muscles tight) and the differentiation of guarding from normal muscle tone is confirmed. Gentle but deep palpation for tenderness and elicitation of rebound pain with release of the deep pressure are important.

The clues to injury, in addition to rigidity of the abdomen, are the absence of bowel sounds to auscultation and the presence of blood from the rectum or genitourinary system. Initial careful and sequential monitoring of blood pressure are important steps for

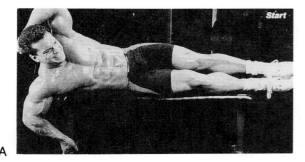

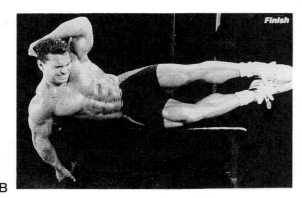

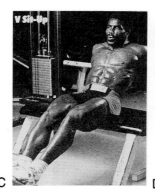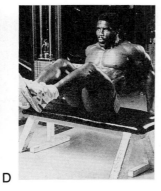

Fig. 18-33. Advanced exercises for abdominal musculature. **(A)** Starting position for the side crunch. **(B)** Finishing position. **(C)** V sit-up for the rectus abdominis; starting position. **(D)** Finishing position.

establishing baselines if significant bleeding is suspected. The normal patterns of referred pain to the shoulders, back, or groin also need consideration (Fig. 18-27).

There must be an awareness that some blunt trauma is associated with a delayed onset of hemorrhage. Thus athletes who sustain significant injury

---

> **Quick Facts**
>
> **ABDOMINAL CONTENTS**
>
> - Solid organs
>   - Liver
>   - Pancreas
>   - Spleen
>   - Kidneys
>   - Adrenal glands
> - Hollow viscera
>   - Stomach
>   - Small bowel
>   - Large bowel
>   - Ureters
>   - Major blood vessels

should be given adequate advice regarding this potential. Appropriate follow-up is also necessary. The nature of the sport and the chances of reinjury are important factors when deciding whether an individual can return to play either immediately or during subsequent days after abdominal trauma.

> **Practice Point**
>
> **INDICATORS OF BLUNT ABDOMINAL INJURY**
>
> *Encourage the athlete to relax.*
> - Absence of normal respiratory motion of abdomen
> - Guarding on palpation (splinting)
> - Localized tenderness on palpation
> - Rebound pain with release of deep pressure
> - Absence of normal bowel sounds
> - Referred pain to shoulder tip or back
> - Falling blood pressure, increasing pulse rate

Splenic Injury and Infectious Mononucleosis

The spleen is located on the posterior wall of the abdomen along the ninth, tenth, and eleventh ribs (Figs. 18-35 and 18-40). The normal spleen is rarely

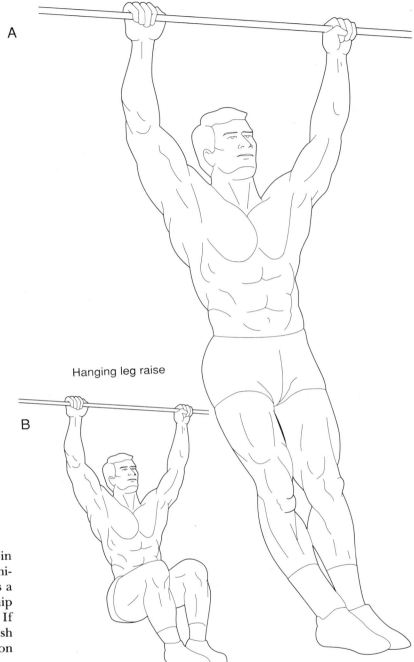

Hanging leg raise

Fig. 18-34. For any athlete involved in sports that require extensive abdominal strength, the hanging-leg raise is a powerful exercise. It also works the hip flexors. **(A)** Start position. **(B)** Finish. If a good curl-up is achieved at the finish position, there is a strong influence on the abdominals.

damaged even in sports with significant contact. After certain systemic disorders, however, it may be enlarged and more vulnerable. The most common of these conditions is infectious mononucleosis. In this situation the spleen is large and weak owing to white pulp hyperplasia and extensive lymphocytic infiltration. A blow to the left upper abdominal quadrant may easily damage a spleen in this condition. The capsular and trabecular changes are evident after about 14 to 28 days of the disorder, and thus the

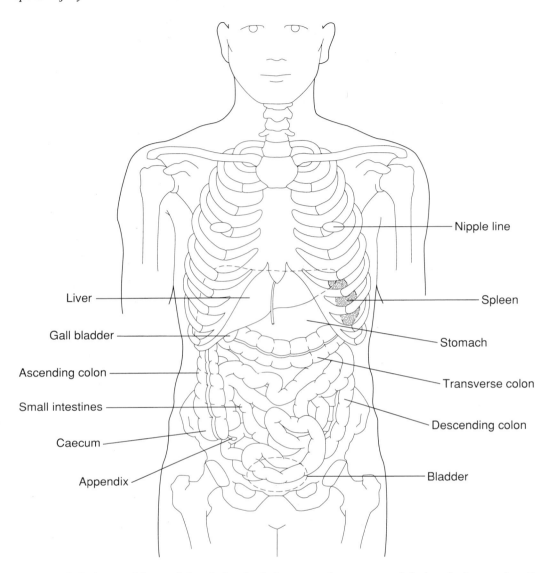

Fig. 18-35. Relative positions of the abdominal viscera and organs, and their relation to the rib cage and pelvis.

spleen is more vulnerable after the initial 2 weeks of the condition. For this reason, once mononucleosis has been diagnosed, athletes should be advised to restrict themselves from contact activities until the splenic enlargement recedes.

Infectious mononucleosis is a common condition among young athletes. The presenting signs are a sore throat, fever, fatigue, and lassitude. Careful examination usually reveals lymphadenopathy in either the neck region, the axillae, the groin, or the abdomen. The spleen should be palpated gently and carefully.

Individuals should be advised to rest for the duration of the fever, after which they can resume ordinary activities. Before returning to competitive situations, however, they should feel generally well and have regained normal stength; moreover, the spleen and liver sizes should be established as having returned to normal. Liver enzymes (e.g., serum glutamic oxalo-acetic transaminase, serum glutamic-pyruvic transaminase, and bilirubin), complete blood count, (CBC), ESR, and urinalysis should be normal.[51] For most individuals, the return to contact sport is usually possible at about 3 months. In some situations of high contact activities where there has been significant risk of splenic rupture, return may be delayed for up to 6 months.

Although some physicians believe the risk of ruptured spleen is low, it is still the most frequent cause of death due to abdominal injury in sport. In 17 of 22 splenic ruptures occurring in football, eight of the athletes had had a prior diagnosis of infectious mononucleosis. Because delayed rupture has been reported, even at some months after the initial infection when the splenic size appeared to have returned to normal, the athlete should be cautioned to report any onset of acute abdominal discomfort immediately.

Practice Point

INFECTIOUS MONONUCLEOSIS

- Rest for duration of fever
- spleen vulnerable to trauma after 14 days
- Return to training after lymphadenopathy resolved and energy levels raised
- Contact sports when spleen returned to normal, liver enzymes, CBC, and urinalysis normal
- Any acute abdominal discomfort after return to sport report immediately

---

Even a normal spleen can be ruptured with or without an accompanying lower rib fracture. Once the initial sharp pain has subsided, the presenting features are the continuation of a dull, left-sided flank pain. In some instances where there is a slow leak of blood, the patient may experience a symptom-free period followed by the development of left shoulder tip pain, referred to as Kehr's sign. It is thought to represent free intraperitoneal blood irritating the diaphragm and causing reflex discomfort. It is possible that this free blood may irritate the right hemidiaphragm, in which case the pain would be referred to the right shoulder tip.[52]

Delayed rupture can follow injuries that cause subcapsular hematomas. Essentially, the diagnosis of subcapsular hematoma depends on a high index of suspicion confirmed by repeated abdominal examinations and, when necessary, CT scanning.

With minor and moderate splenic injuries, where blood loss is within reasonable limits and systemic signs are stable, the main treatment is rest and observation. Rapid significant blood loss and extensive splenic injury require splenectomy. After splenectomy, usually about a 3-month period is needed for healing of the abdominal musculature and regaining adequate strength before return to vigorous activity. Most authorities recommend a 6-month interval before returning to contact sport.

Liver Damage

Right upper quadrant contusions may damage the liver and produce subcapsular hemorrhage, which generally results in significant pain and tenderness to palpation. Lacerations of the liver are rare in contact sports; and if an index of suspicion is maintained after severe right upper abdominal blows, ultrasonography or CT scanning can help with a definitive diagnosis.

Pancreatic Injury

The pancreas is seated well at the back of the abdominal wall, nestled in the duodenum, and is rarely damaged by sporting injuries. The pancreas rests on the vertebral column, however, and is thus at risk during deceleration injuries, such as would occur in motor vehicle sports. Pancreatic injury may be suspected if the pain is epigastric, radiating to the back, after blunt trauma. There may be some tenderness in the midline over the vertebral column. Usually reflex ileus is present with loss of normal bowel sounds and gradually progressing abdominal distension. As with many intra-abdominal conditions, the temperature may eventually be elevated. Diagnosis is confirmed by the elevation of serum amylase, serum lipase, and the amylase/creatine ratio. Ultrasonography and CT scanning are most useful.

Diaphragm

Most traumatic ruptures of the diaphragm are due to massive blunt abdominal injury. They usually occur on the left because there is a certain amount of protection from the liver on the right. Occasionally, the traumatic opening is large, permitting interthoracic displacement of the abdominal viscera, which causes significant respiratory distress and collapse of the left lung. Although it is possible to diagnose this problem based on the change in breath sounds, the condition is usually detected on a plain film of the abdomen and chest. Immediate transfer to hospital is obviously required with operative management.

Rupture of Hollow Viscera

Although such injuries rarely occur, kicks and blows to the abdomen, landing awkwardly against an uneven parallel bar, pile-ons in football, and spearing in hockey are capable of rupturing the hollow viscera of the abdomen.[52] In addition, visceral injuries may result from rodeo and equestrian accidents; therefore after a fall riders should be checked carefully for internal injuries. Ruptured hollow viscera usually produce pain, guarding, tenderness, loss of bowel-sounds, abdominal rigidity, and possibly signs of shock such as clammy, sweaty skin and a falling blood pressure. Free blood in the abdomen may irritate the diaphragm and cause shoulder tip pain. Occasionally, bleeding of the viscus wall and its accompanying blood vessels causes free blood to pool in the abdomen. This problem may be confirmed, in the appropriate setting, by an abdominal tap.

An abdominal tap or peritoneal lavage is preceded by sterile preparation of the abdomen and after making sure the bladder is empty with a catheter if necessary. Approximately 1 liter of fluid is then instilled into the abdomen and siphoned back into a glass tube. If the examiner is unable to read newsprint through the fluid-filled tube, the tap is considered positive. This degree of haziness is considered significant because it indicates that there are at least 20,000 to 30,000 cells per milliliter of fluid. Despite this dra-matic method of detecting intra-abdominal injury, serial examination is often the most efficient. With a small visceral injury, the signs may take several hours and sometimes even several days for pain and guarding and shock to develop. Plain roentgenography, with both upright and right-sided decubitus abdominal films, may illustrate free air from the viscus under the diaphragm or along the abdominal wall. For the film to have maximal value, the athlete should remain sitting upright or in the decubitus position for approximately 3 minutes so the air can percolate to the uppermost position.[53]

Intermucosal hemorrhage may leak into the content of the bowel. Therefore the athlete should be warned to check the stool after a significant injury to rule out this other, more overt source of hemorrhage.

Stomach

Blunt injury to the stomach in sport is unusual, but direct spearing of the epigastrium may indeed damage the gastric wall. Blood is found in a nasogastric aspirate if this injury is suspected, and there is early peritoneal irritation because of the acidity of the stomach content. Free air is also usually evident on plain roentgenograms. Obviously the treatment is prompt abdominal exploration and repair of the injury.

Duodenum, Jejunum, Ileum

Blunt injury to the abdomen may result in isolated retroperitoneal rupture of the duodenum. Sometimes a fall, landing heavily on the back, has also caused this injury. It is thought that at the time of the blow the air within the duodenum may be trapped between the closed pylorus and the sharply angulated duodenojejunal junction. This has almost the effect of a blast from within the lumen, causing rupture or laceration. This injury can be easily overlooked because it is retroperitoneal and the intra-abdominal signs may be minimal initially. There may be coincidental injury to the ribs, spine, or other solid organs such as the liver and spleen. Most of the small intestinal disruptions occur distal to the duodenum in the proximal half of the jejunum or the distal ileum. A history of persistent abdominal pain with a progression of abdominal signs should lead to a suspicion of these injuries. The severity of signs and symptoms may vary considerably, but frequently onset of a

---

Practice Point

INTERPRETATION OF PERITONEAL LAVAGE

Lavage Result	Incidence of Significant Injury (%)	Therapeutic Plan
Strongly positive (>20 ml blood)	95	Surgery Required
Weakly positive (<20 ml blood)	25	In-patient observation
Negative (and stable)	<1	Re-evaluate at 24 hours

chemical peritonitis makes the diagnosis of visceral damage more likely. The diagnostic studies include lavage and the presence of free air seen on roentgenogram; occasionally, minor injuries are detected through a gastrografin swallow. Treatment is surgical.

Large Bowel Injury

Blunt injury with rupture of the large intestine is associated with massive peritoneal contamination and frequently injury to other abdominal organs. It is surprising, however, that the onset of significant abdominal signs may not occur promptly if there is an isolated small rupture, until there is significant bacterial escape into the peritoneal cavity and infection becomes established. At this point, severe peritonitis may ensue. Prompt treatment is necessary and may involve colonic resection with or without colostomy.

Hernias

It may seem obvious that the enormous forces and increased intra-abdominal pressure generated by heavy lifting activities may contribute to the formation of hernias in athletes. It is probably true, however, that nearly all hernias develop on the basis of some congenital weakness in the arrangement of the abdominal muscles and fascia (Fig. 18-36). The three most common hernias in adults are the indirect and direct inguinal hernias and the femoral hernia.

Indirect hernias account for approximately 50 to 70 percent of all hernias. Occurring primarily in men under the age of 30,[52] they develop as the result of a weakness in the processus vaginalis. A diverticulum of the perineal membrane is usually obliterated in women, thus decreasing their susceptibility. This sac extends through the processus into the inguinal canal and occasionally extends into the scrotum (Fig. 18-37). Large indirect hernias may reduce spontane-

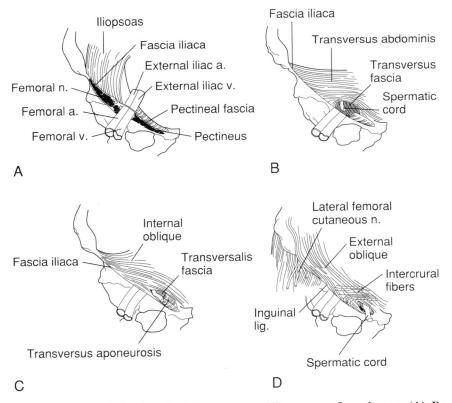

Fig. 18-36. Arrangement of the inguinal ligament and its areas of weakness. **(A)** Passage of the femoral artery and vein. **(B)** Transversus muscles with the transversalis fascia forming the inner part of the inguinal ring. **(C)** Internal oblique muscle forming the major part of the canal. **(D)** External oblique with the intercrural fibers comprising the external inguinal ring.

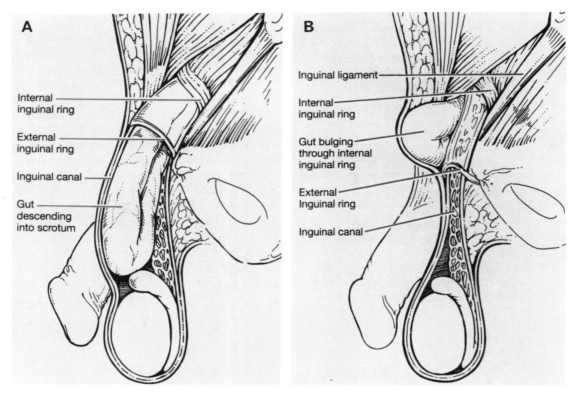

Fig. 18-37. **(A)** Indirect hernia with the gut extending through the inguinal canal down into the scrotum. **(B)** Direct hernia bulging through the weakened fascia just adjacent to the inguinal ligament and the epigastric vessels.

ously because they do not easily extend into the inguinal canal.

Direct hernias are the result of a weakness in the area of fascia known as Hesselbach's triangle. This area is bordered by the rectus abdominis muscle, the inguinal ligament, and the epigastric vessels (Fig. 18-37). Direct hernias occur more frequently in men over the age of 40. Scrotal swelling is rare with direct hernias because the sac does not extend into the inguinal canal.

Femoral hernias occur much less frequently. The fascial weakness for this type of hernia is similar to that of the direct inguinal hernia except that the sac extends posterior to the inguinal ligament. It emerges below the ligament and medial to the femoral artery and vein. Femoral hernias affect primarily women.

Symptoms of all these hernias vary, and often the first complaints are an aching sensation in the groin frequently accompanied by tender swelling. Indirect hernias are palpable by invaginating the scrotum with a finger and palpating the soft mass that bulges fur-

ther with coughing (Fig. 18-38). Frequently, small hernias are asymptomatic and detected only incidentally. They are usually more prominent when the athlete stands. Incarcerated hernias, i.e., irreducible hernias, may bring on symptoms of bowel obstruction or, in more significant cases, toxicity. Occasionally, these hernias twist on themselves and produce a strangulating hernia in which there is a considerable danger of the hernial sac becoming gangrenous.

If the hernias are sufficiently large or symptomatic, surgical repair is warranted. After surgery a period of healing is required, depending on the size of the defect. Walking, mild upper extremity exercises, and cycling are usually allowed by the sixth week after surgery for individuals with indirect hernias; return to noncontact sports is permitted at 7 to 8 weeks and to contact sports at 8 to 10 weeks.

Repairs of direct inguinal and femoral hernias are generally more extensive and thus require a longer recovery. It is usual to prohibit all strenuous activities for 3 weeks after surgery; return to noncontact sports

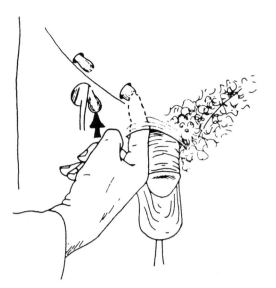

Fig. 18-38. Inguinal hernias in men may be palpated by invaginating the scrotum and feeling the mass or pressure of the lesion, particularly with coughing. Arrow represents the site of the more uncommon femoral hernia.

is allowed by about 8 weeks and contact sports by about 12 weeks. Activities that stretch or pull the abdominal muscles are usually avoided during the first interval following hernia repair.

Another common site for hernias is the anterior abdominal wall. These hernias may be classified as incisional, umbilical, diastasis recti, or linea alba defects (Fig. 18-39). Their size dictates the amount of bulge, which increases as the intra-abdominal pressure rises. The athlete may simply complain of aching in the region of the defect during activities that stretch or stress the abdominals. Sometimes there are no symptoms. Treatment depends on the size of the defect, the discomfort experienced, and the potential for incarceration or strangulation.[52]

GENITOURINARY SYSTEM

Renal Trauma

The kidneys are vital for controlling the acid-base balance of the body, disposing of toxic by-products in the urine, controlling salt and water balance, and influencing blood pressure and hematocrit via the release of angiotensin and erythropoietin. Thus any renal injury is potentially significant.

The kidney is vulnerable to blunt trauma in collision sports such as football, rugby, or ice hockey. Despite being somewhat protected by the eleventh and twelfth ribs and an excellent surrounding perirenal fat pad and psoas muscles, contusions to the renal system are well documented in the literature[54,55] (Fig. 18-40). Rupture or damage to the ureters, however, is rare in sport. An index of suspicion must be maintained when a collision results in severe or protracted flank pain. Pain may refer posteriorly to the costovertebral angle and anteriorly to the lower abdomen. In many instances the decision to investigate further depends more on the appearance of gross blood in the urine than the evolution of retroperitoneal or abdominal signs. However, not all patients with hematuria require further imaging studies. Essentially, these tests are recommended with (1) blunt trauma

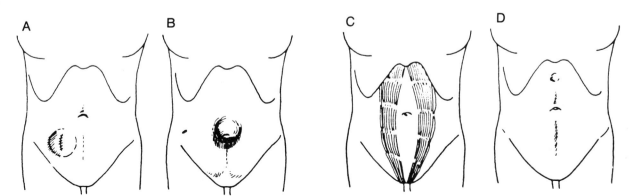

Fig. 18-39. Potential sites of herniation. **(A)** Stretching or dehiscing of an incision. **(B)** Periumbilical hernia. **(C)** Diastasis of the rectal sheath and weakened linear alba. **(D)** Rectal sheath defect.

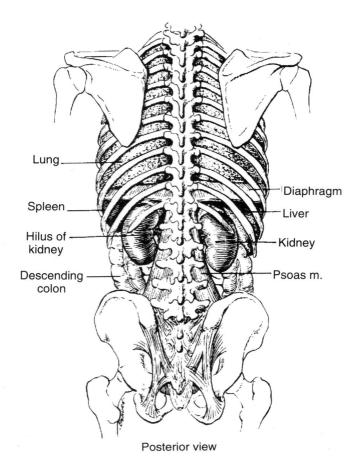

Posterior view

Fig. 18-40. Relations of the ribs and the posterior musculature to the kidneys, liver, and spleen.

and gross hematuria, (2) blunt trauma with microscopic hematuria and a systolic blood pressure (BP) less than 90 mmHg, and (3) obviously penetrating abdominal flank trauma with hematuria.[56]

The presence of microscopic or even a minimal amount of obvious bleeding in the first voided urine specimen after a traumatic incident obviously may indicate urinary tract injury. However, the amount of blood does not necessarily correspond with the magnitude of the trauma.[57]

Renal injury may be graded as renal contusion (grade I), cortical lacerations without extravasation (grade II), deep cortical and calix lacerations (grade III), or vascular pedicle injury (grade IV). The abdominal and flank examination should help assess the degree of injury and the presence of palpable mass. If there are signs of shock, hemorrhage must be assumed, and all investigation and treatment must be expedited. Proper clinical staging of the renal trauma awaits intravenous pyelography (IVP) or CT evaluation (Fig. 18-41). The greater the degree of renal injury, the more likely it is that the CT scan can determine the nature and extent of the injury better than the IVP. If the kidney is not visualized on an IVP, one of the following conditions should be considered: (1)

Practice Point

INDICATION FOR INTRAVENOUS PYELOGRAM WITH SUSPECTED RENAL TRAUMA

- Blunt trauma and gross hematuria
- Blunt trauma, microscopic hematuria, BP <90 mmHg
- Penetrating flank wounds and hematuria

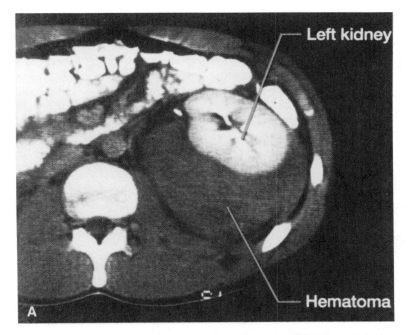

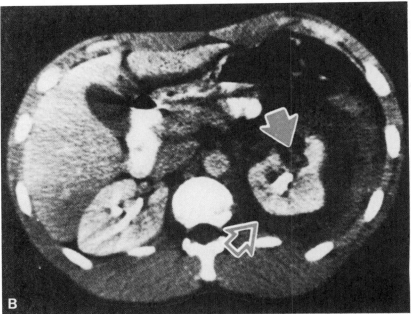

Fig. 18-41. (A) CT scan showing the left kidney almost surrounded by a large hematoma. **(B)** CT slice showing left upper pole cortical laceration with a significant perirenal hematoma. (After Freitas,[55] with permission.)

total vascular pedicle avulsion; (2) arterial thrombosis; (3) vascular spasm; (4) congenital absence; or (5) previous surgical excision of the kidney. Such a finding on the IVP indicates that renal arteriography or contrast-enhanced CT scanning is necessary.

After initiation of emergency care to treat shock and associated injuries, early management of blunt renal trauma depends on complete definition of the extent of the injury. Surgical intervention is indicated only in those few athletes who have persistent retroperitoneal bleeding, urinary extravasation, nonviable renal tissue, or renal vascular pedicle injury. Most athletes with blunt renal trauma can be managed nonoperatively, and spontaneous healing and return of good renal function are to be expected.

Careful follow-up with measurements of blood

pressure and perhaps an IVP at 3 to 6 months is recommended for individuals with a grade II or greater renal injury. This protocol detects late complications, e.g., renal vascular hypertension and hydronephrosis, early so that more permanent injuries can be avoided.

Hematuria, Hemoglobinuria, Myoglobinuria, Proteinuria

Direct damage to the bladder usually is associated only with massive pelvic injury. However, gross hematuria is sometimes seen after strenuous activity, particularly long distance running, and has earned the name "runner's bladder."[58,59] Routine urinalysis show that microhematuria is present in up to 20 percent of marathoners and in 50 to 70 percent of ultramarathoners after a race, but it normally resolves within 1 to 2 days. Blacklock described "kissing lesions," which consisted of a brim of contused bladder tissue encircling a central area of normal urothelium mostly over the posterior bladder wall, bladder neck, and trigone. It was postulated that repeated trauma to the posterior bladder wall from the impact of running generated these lesions. They appeared to be self-limited, resolving within about a week. Patients prone to this abnormality are cautioned not to run with a totally empty bladder, as it seems to worsen the situation. Blood seen at the beginning of urination may indicate a urethral source, whereas blood seen at the end may be from the bladder or higher; this finding is by no means diagnostic, however. Patients who present with gross hematuria should be carefully evaluated with urography and cystoscopy to rule out potentially more serious causes. In addition, the urine should be examined for casts and protein, which may indicate primary parenchymal disease of the kidney coexisting with the repetitive trauma-induced hematuria.

Some athletes present with smoke or tea-colored urine after their athletic endeavors, a condition called "athletic pseudonephritis." It may be due to a combination of hematuria, proteinuria, hemoglobinuria, and myoglobinuria. These conditions are the consequences of the breakdown of red blood cells and microscopic muscle trauma due to excessive physical activity. Like microscopic hematuria, the proteinuria usually clears in 1 to 2 days. Frequently however, if associated with red blood cell casts, it is possible that blunt trauma, particularly in contact sports, is implicated, rather than just excessive exercise. Evidently these findings are common during race-walking events. It is postulated that continuous minor renal trauma, increases in renal vein pressure, dehydration, and perhaps even transient renal ischemia are causes. Nearly always these repetitive exercise-related problems resolve within about 24 to 48 hours. If so, they do not require further evaluation.[51] It should be recalled that sometimes running or exercise unmasks early stage bladder cancer. Initial screening includes a CBC, serum chemistries, urine cultures, or even protein electrophoresis. Renal ultrasonography or intravenous pyelography should then precede cystoscopy, CT, or MRI, depending on the patient's history.

Urinalysis

Normal urine is sterile. A red blood cell (RBC) count of three RBCs per high power field from centrifuged urine sediment is also considered normal for men and four to five RBCs for women. Alternatively, 1000 RBCs per milliliter of urine is acceptable. Any value exceeding these figures indicates the need for a repeat specimen for further evaluation and perhaps calls for other tests of the genitourinary system.

A careful history should be obtained to document any use of analgesics, NSAIDs, or anticoagulants, all of which may produce bleeding. Furthermore, a history of previous oropharyngeal infections that may give rise to poststreptococcal glomerulonephritis,

---

Practice Point

HAMATURIA-PROTEINURIA

- If it occurs after exercise, rest athlete and repeat test in 2 days.
- If hematuria persists or is gross, consider investigation.

Sources

- Terminal hematuria—possibly bladder neck or prostate
- Initial hematuria—urethra
- Total hematuria—bladder, ureter, or kidney
- Clots—nonglomerular bleeding
- Large, thick clots—possibly bladder
- Small specks or thick stringy clots—upper urinary tract

Practice Point

SIGNIFICANT HISTORY ASSOCIATED WITH HEMATURIA

- Colicky flank pain radiating to groin—renal stone
- Perineal pain, dysuria, terminal hematuria—prostatitis
- Penile discharge, microscopic hematuria—urethritis
- Dysuria, urgency, frequency—cystitis
- Easy bruising, easy bleeding, gross hematuria—blood dyscrasia
- Blunt trauma to flank—renal contusion

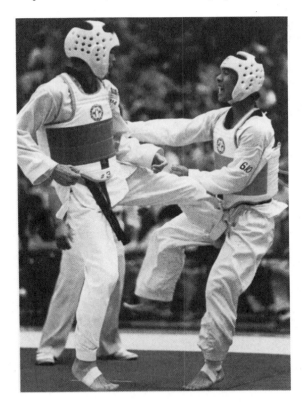

Fig. 18-42. A direct blow to the groin can cause injury to the external genitalia, particularly the scrotal contents with men.

blood dyscrasia in the family, or recent trauma must be elicited. Note is made of urinary tract infections, along with abnormal voiding patterns such as painful urination (dysuria). If there is protein in the urine, serum creatinine should be evaluated or even consideration given to a creatinine clearance test. If the possibility of a streptococcal infection exists, an antistreptolysin O titer, complement levels, and an ESR should be obtained. In athletes of black, southern European, or Mediterranean ancestry, a test for sickle cell anemia is appropriate. It should also be remembered that certain drugs (e.g., nitrofurantoin and quinine) and some foods (e.g., excessive intake of beet juice or V-8 juice) may discolor the urine.

Male Genitalia

The male genitalia, although not anatomically as protected as the kidneys and bladder, are seldom injured during athletic activities. Nevertheless, in contact sports where inadequate protective devices are worn, significant injury may occur (Fig. 18-42). Furthermore, continuous pressure over the perineal region may produce transient paresthesias. Sexually transmitted diseases, e.g., nongonococcal urethritis, condyloma acuminatum, and herpes progenitalis, are common urologic problems in both sexes.

The male genitalia are potentially exposed to direct trauma. The testes usually sit in the scrotum, which is the optimal environment for sperm production. The prepubertal testicle is approximately the size of a peanut, and the adult testes are more the size of a walnut and smooth. An empty scrotum may signify testicular retraction via the cremasteric reflex but should raise the suspicion of absence or failure to descend. This situation should always be reviewed by a urologist for consideration of operative treatment because of the potential long-term problem of infertility and testicular carcinoma.[60,61]

Penis

Direct injuries to the penis in sport is rare with the exception of a few direct blows leading to vascular damage and bleeding and straddle-type injuries with direct blows to the pubis. Trauma may result from direct blows by football helmets or sticks. These same mechanisms may also lead to damage to the urethra; usually in sport these injuries resolve without specific treatment. However, if they are of sufficient magnitude, a retrograde urethrogram can be obtained, which can indicate if surgical treatment is necessary.

Perineum (Pudendal Nerve Neuropraxia and Urethral Injury)

Transient paresthesia, or numbness, in the perineum and penis or in the female external genitalia due to pressure on the pudendal nerve, usually after cycling, has been well reported. The "bicyclist's penis" is usually neuropraxic, but the problem resolves spontaneously with no apparent sequelae. There have also been reports of transient urinary retention following long episodes of cycling. Both of these considerations are usually resolved by adjusting saddle height and tilt and the duration of exercise bouts. Intermittently raising up on the pedals, transiently relieving pressure, is helpful.

Scrotum and Contents

Direct contusion of the scrotum may result in a severe testiclular injury. The tunica albuginea, which covers the vascular and tubercle components of the testes, may rupture with forceful impact. (Fig. 18-43). It is sometimes difficult to distinguish a contusion from a more severe injury because of the scrotal swelling. The ruptured testicle requires emergency surgery, so it is important to make an accurate diagnosis.

Furthermore, blunt trauma to the inguinal region may result in rupture of the pampiniform plexus of veins that constitute part of the spermatic cord.[61] Engorgement of these veins constitutes a varicocele. Patients with a varicocele are at increased risk of injury to the pampiniform plexus.[60] If the plexus is ruptured by a groin impact or a high scrotal impact, rapid accumulation of blood in the scrotum (a hematocele) occurs (Fig. 18-44). If the bleeding is massive and tense, it may be indistinguishable from bleeding caused by rupture of the testicles.[62] The degree of pain is not a reliable indicator of which structure is involved. Usually the less severe traumatic injuries of scrotum or testicular contusions are seen. If there is no significant scrotal swelling and the testicles can be examined completely to ensure they are intact, only symptomatic treatment is required. If the scrotal swelling precludes a good examination, occasionally transillumination is helpful. A hematocele does not transilluminate well. If the testicular shadow can be seen by good transillumination, the swelling is probably a hydrocele (Fig. 18-44). In any event, significant scrotal hemorrhage or swelling is an indication for referral to a urologist. Aspiration of the scrotum is rarely indicated for diagnositc reasons, and the risk of

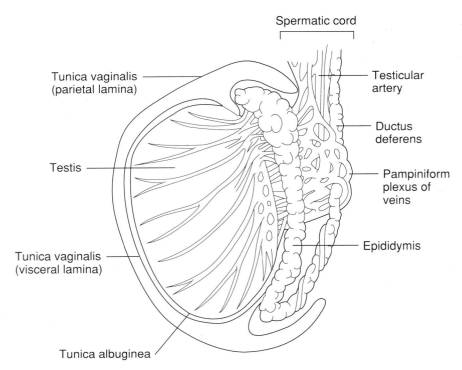

Fig. 18-43. Anatomy of the normal testicle.

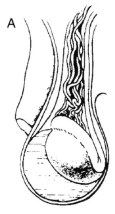 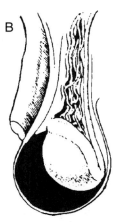

Hydrocele   Hematocele

Fig. 18-44. (A) Irritation of the tunica of the testicle may generate swelling or hydrocele formation. It usually transilluminates well. **(B)** Blood within a hydrocele following trauma produces a hematocele. Tense swelling of the scrotum should be assessed carefully by someone with experience because of the implications regarding permanent testicular damage.

introducing infection overrides any therapeutic gain in most cases. In the case of a reactive hydrocele, the fluid usually absorbs without specific treatment. In the case of a hematocele, the blood collection frequently recurs unless the underlying problem is resolved.[62,63]

If the condition is a simple scrotal or testicular contusion, support of the scrotum (occasionally with the use of cold packs) is helpful. NSAIDs may reduce the swelling and edema, thereby reducing the discomfort. Ambulatory activities are progressed as the pain and swelling subside. In more severe cases, bed rest may be required for 12 to 24 hours. If the testicle is not palpable or the scrotum does not transilluminate, testicular rupture cannot be ruled out, and prompt referral to a urologist is indicated.[61] A report by Nolten et al. suggested that some individuals demonstrating infertility in their thirties had had significant testicular trauma during their teens, which points to the need for adequate protective equipment and careful evaluation of the initial trauma.[64]

Torsion of the testicle may occur by rotational twisting of the vascular pedicle and spermatic cord, producing varying degrees of venous and arterial insufficiency (Fig. 18-45). There is probably an element

of congenital variation in the testicular suspension that makes certain individuals more susceptible. This condition constitutes an emergency, because if corrected within 6 to 8 hours recovery is close to 100 percent.

It is usually seen at about the time of puberty, and the individual presents with acute testicular pain, sometimes with associated nausea and vomiting. The testicle is painful and frequently firmer than normal to palpation. Elevation does not relieve the pain. There may be considerable heat due to the inflammation. The cremasteric reflex is absent. Early recognition and referral are important because usually surgical correction is warranted.

Female Genitalia

Direct blows to the perineum occasionally lead to vulvar hematomas, which may be treated by application of ice packs and NSAIDs. Occasionally, with an inexperienced water-skiier, water enters the vulva and vagina under high pressure, resulting in contusion or tearing of the vaginal wall. In addition, inflammation of the fallopian tube (salpingitis) has been described after such injuries. Salpingitis usually presents with upper quadrant iliac fossa pain about 3 days after the forced vaginal douche. Usually these injuries are easily preventable by wearing a nylon-reinforced suit or a wetsuit.

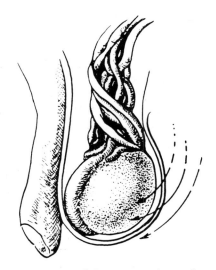

Fig. 18-45. Torsion of the spermatic cord around the tunica vaginalis.

Perineal Rashes (Tinea Cruris, Jock Itch)

Jock itch (tinea cruris) is a common fungal infection affecting the crural or perineal folds and adjacent skin of the proximal thighs. It derives its name from its common association with the use of athletic supports (jock straps).[65]

Itching in the genital area may be marked and distressing. The rash begins as small patches of erythema and scaling and less commonly as vesicles and crusting. Commencing in the crural folds and inner thigh, it may spread to the perineal area, buttocks, and less commonly the abdomen.[65] The skin changes may be chronic and subtle, with redness and scaling at the leading margin and the central clearing that is so characteristic of other ringworm (mycotic, fungal) infections. Some lesions are acutely inflamed, particularly if there is an element of mechanical irritation or excoriations due to scratching the irritation. In some cases only diffuse thickening and darkening (lichenification) are present.

Most cases of jock itch are caused by *Trichophyton rubrum*, which has an affinity for the stratum corneum (superficial layers of the epidermis). A warm, moist environment enhances fungal growth. Diagnosis is based on the classic appearance and, if necessary, visualization of branching fungal filaments (hyphae) under low power microscopy after staining scrapings from the lesion with a 10 to 20 percent solution of potassium hydroxide.

Treatment involves education, hygiene, and antifungal medication. Keeping the perineal area dry by the use of powder, looser-fitting underwear, and frequent changes and washing of the jock strap or training undergarments go a long way to clearing up the condition and preventing recurrence. Careful drying after showering and the use of absorbent powders after thoroughly rinsing off all of the soap is important. Early lesions frequently respond to a sulfa-based shampoo such as Selsun. More resistant cases may require antifungal compounds such as naftifine (Naftin), ciclopirox (Loprox), or one of the many other imidazole agents. Cream preparations are preferable to ointments and should be applied sparingly twice daily. Acute, weeping lesions may respond to Burow's Solution (5 percent aluminum diacetate; Domeboro) applied two or three times daily.[65] If stored in the refrigerator, the coolness of the medication provides extra relief on application. Occasionally, the combination of an antifungal agent and a topical corticosteroid is required, or even systemic agents. If this stage is reached, it may be well to consult a dermatologist.

The differential diagnosis includes candidiasis, seborrheic dermatitis, psoriasis, erythrasma, and lichen simplex chronicus.[66] Candidiasis (a yeast infection) is usually more moist, red, and tender and may affect the scrotum and penis or the external labial folds in women. Seborrheic dermatitis and psoriasis typically affect areas in addition to the groin. Erythrasma is related to a gram-positive bacterial infection and is characteristically an asymptomatic, reddish brown rash with no central clearing. Any source of inflammation in the groin area, particularly irritation due to soap, may precipitate itching and chronic scratching. This situation sets up a cycle of further itching (pruritis) and scratching that may ultimately lead to lichenification.

In summary, prevention is the main thrust of treatment for tinea cruris and centers around not presenting an ideal environment of warm, moist, dead cells and repeated reinoculation. Attention to thoroughly rinsing off the soap after washing, drying meticulously, and wearing more loosely fitting undergarments is central to effective prevention and treatment. This condition is presented here because of its frequency. Failure to respond to therapy should raise a consideration of other lesions or an unusual infecting organism.

Other Lesions

A discussion of other perineal and genital lesions —venereal warts, syphilitic lesions, herpetic infections, and penile and urethral discharges due to venereal disease—is beyond the scope of this book.

SUMMARY

This chapter has dealt with injuries to the chest and the abdominopelvic viscera. It has departed from the usual emphasis of the book, the musculoskeletal system. Many of the true emergencies in sports medicine relate to abdominopelvic injuries, and hence protocols have been outlined for significant chest contusion, pneumothorax, tension pneumothorax, cardiac arrest, and blunt abdominal trauma with hemorrhage. Recognition of these major catastrophic injuries frequently makes the difference between survival of athletes or their demise. Although the injuries are traumatic and massive, often the first aid procedures are simple and require only rudimentary knowledge.

Some of the skills require practice, and sensible sports medicine therapists and physicians maintain these skills with periodic practice. Injuries to the genitourinary system, which may present a diagnostic challenge, range from the rather insidious microhematuria experienced in the distance athlete, to the occult renal trauma experienced in contact sports, to the emergent situation of testicular torsion. Gross hematuria must never be shrugged off as an innocent finding. Guidelines were presented about the appropriateness of initial investigations. Recognition of significant testicular damage or torsion may save a testicle and prevent long-term problems that can arise concerning altered fertility.

Three major concerns emerge from this chapter: (1) the existence of the intent to injure seen in some sports; (2) the lack of adequate protective equipment in others; and finally (3) the refusal to wear appropriately adjusted equipment that is available. These three factors combine to produce worrisome, unnecessary statistics that indicate the potential for catastrophe with sports medicine injuries.

REFERENCES

1. Eichelberger MR: Torso injuries in athletes. Physician Sports Med 9:87, 1981
2. Schneider RC, Kennedy JC, Plant ML: Sports Injuries. Mechanisms, Prevention and Treatment. Williams & Wilkins, Baltimore, 1985
3. Moncure AC, Wilkins EW: Injuries involving the abdomen, viscera, and genitourinary system. In Kulund DN (ed): The Injured Athlete. 2nd Ed. JB Lippincott, London, 1988
4. Rund DA: Managing multiple trauma: how to stabilize the injured athlete. Physician Sports Med 18:20, 1990
5. Fam AG, Smythe HA: Musculoskeletal chest wall pain. Can Med Assoc J 133:379, 1985
6. Smythe HA: Fibrositis and other diffuse musculoskeletal syndromes. In Kelley WN, Harris ED, Ruddy S et al (eds): Textbook of Rheumatology. 1st Ed. WB Saunders, Philadelphia, 1981
7. Grant JCB: Grant's Atlas of Anatomy. 5th Ed. Williams & Wilkins, Baltimore, 1962
8. Williams PL, Warwick R (eds): Gray's Anatomy. 36th Ed. Churchill Livingstone, Edinburgh, 1980
9. Gehlsen G, Albohm M: Evaluation of sports bras. Physician Sports Med 8:89, 1980
10. Hunter LY, Torgan C: The bra controversy: are sport bras a necessity? Physician Sports Med 10:75, 1982
11. Baeyens L: Breast problems in athletes. Physician Sports Med 15:25, 1987
12. Kretzler HH, Richardson AB: Rupture of the pectoralis major muscle. Am J Sports Med 17:453, 1989
13. McEntire JE, Hess WE, Coleman SS: Rupture of pectoralis major muscle: a report of eleven injuries and a review of fifty-six cases. J Bone Joint Surg [Am] 54:1040, 1972
14. Holden DL, Jackson DW: Stress fractures of the ribs in female rowers. Am J Sports Med 13:342, 1985
15. Pfeiffer RP, Young TR: Case reports: spontaneous pneumothorax in a jogger. Physician Sports Med 8:65, 1980
16. Tietze A: Über eine eigenartige Häufung von Fällen dystrophie der Rippenknorpel. Berl Klin Wochenschr 58:829, 1921
17. Dunlop RF: Tietze revisited. Clin Orthop 62:223, 1969
18. Wolfe E. Stern S: Costosternal syndrome: its frequency and importance in differential diagnosis of coronary heart disease. Arch Intern Med 136:189, 1976
19. Talucci RC, Webb WR: Costal chrondritis: the costal arch. Ann Thorac Surg 35:318, 1983
20. Heinz GL, Zavala DC: Slipping rib syndrome: diagnosis using the "hooking maneuver." JAMA 237:794, 1977
21. Resnick D. Sternocostoclavicular hyperostosis. J Bone Joint Surg [Am] 63:1329, 1981
22. Cone RO, Resnick D. Goergen TG et al: Condensing osteitis of the clavicle. AJR 141:387, 1983
23. Oren BG: Pain at the xiphisternal joint. N Engl J Med 274:1035, 1966
24. Stamford B: A "stitch" in the side. Physician Sports Med 13:187, 1985
25. Sparrow MJ, Bird EL: "Precordial catch": a benign syndrome of chest pain in young persons. NZ Med J 88:325, 1978
26. Bennett RM: Fibrositis: does it exist and can it be treated. J Musculoskeletal Med 1:57, 1984
27. Wolfe F, Cathey MA: Prevalence of primary and secondary fibrositis. J Rheumatol 10:965, 1983
28. Rodnan G, McEwan C, Wallace SL (eds): Primer on the Rheumatic Disease. 7th Ed. Prepared by The Committee of the American Rheumatism Association Section of the Arthritis Foundation. The Arthritis Society, Toronto, 1973
29. Rothman RH, Simeone FA (eds): The Spine. Vols. I & II. WB Saunders, Philadelphia, 1975
30. Paget J: Clinical Lectures and Essays. Longmans, Green, London, 1875
31. Hughes ESR: Venous obstruction in the upper extremity (Paget-Schroetter's syndrome). Int Abstr Surg 88:89, 1949
32. Huber EC, Storey HD: Effort thrombosis in a runner. Physician Sports Med 18:76, 1990
33. Wright RS, Lipscomb B: Acute occlusion of the subclavian vein in an athlete: diagnosis, etiology and surgical management. J Sports Med 2:343, 1975
34. American Heart Association: Position statement: ac-

tivity guidelines for young patients with heart disease. Physician Sports Med 4:47, 1976

35. Hara JH, Puffer JC: The pre-participation physical exam. In Mellion MB (ed): Office Management of Sports Injuries and Athletic Problems. CV Mosby, St. Louis, 1988
36. Rose KD: Relationship of cardiac problems to athletic participation. JAMA 208:2319, 1969
37. Morganworth J, Maun BJ, Henry WL et al: Comparative left ventricular dimensions in trained athletes. Ann Intern Med 82:521, 1975
38. Grossman M, Baker BE: Current cardiology problems in sports medicine. Am J Sports Med 12:262, 1984
39. Lichtman J, O'Rourke RA, Klein A et al: Electrocardiograms in the athlete. Arch Intern Med 132:763, 1973
40. Walther RJ, Tifft CP: High blood pressure in the competitive athlete: guidelines and recommendations. Physician Sports Med 13:93, 1985
41. Goodman DS: Report of the National Cholesterol Education Program export panel on detection, evaluation, and treatment of high blood cholesterol in adults. Arch Intern Med 148:36, 1988
42. Grossman M, Baker BE: Current cardiology problems in sports medicine. Am J Sports Med 13:262, 1984
43. Cantwell JD: Hypertrophic cardiomyopathy and the athlete. Physician Sports Med 12:111, 1984
44. Rund DA: Emergency evaluation of chest pain. Physician Sports Med 18:69, 1990
45. Maron BJ, Roberts WC, McAllister HA et al: Sudden death in young athletes. Circulation 62:218, 1980
46. Rund DA: Cardiac arrest. Physician Sports Med 18:97, 1990
47. DeShazo WF: Haematoma of the rectus abdominis in football. Physician Sports Med 12:73, 1984
48. Michel R, Oxorn H: Hematoma of the rectus abdominis muscle. Can Med Assoc J 105:72, 1971
49. Manier JW: Rectus sheath hematomas. Am J Gastroenterol 57:443, 1972

50. Ducatman BS, Ludwig J, Hurt RD: Fatal rectus sheath hematoma. JAMA 249:924, 1983
51. Eichner ER: Hematuria—a diagnostic challenge. Physician Sports Med 18:53, 1990
52. Danneker DA, Mandetta DF, Rockower R: Case report: intra-abdominal injury in a gymnast. Physician Sports Med 7:119, 1979
53. Williams RD, Patton R: Athletic injuries to the abdomen and thorax. Am J Surg 98:447, 1959
54. Reilly BM: Practical Strategies in Outpatient Medicine. WB Saunders, Toronto, 1984
55. Freitas JE: Renal imaging following blunt trauma. Physician Sports Med 17:59, 1989
56. Mee SL, McAninch JW: Indications for radiographic assessment in suspected renal trauma. Urol Clin North Am 16:187, 1989
57. Bright TC, White K, Peters PC: Significance of hematuria after trauma. J Urol 120:455, 1978
58. York JP: Sports and the male genitourinary system: kidneys and bladder. Physician Sports Med 18:9, 1990
59. Blacklock NJ: Bladder trauma in the long distance runner: "10,000 metres haematuria." Br J Urol 49:129, 1977
60. York JP: Sports and the male genitourinary system. Physician Sports Med 18:92, 1990
61. Hooves DL: How I manage testicular injury. Physician Sports Med 14:127, 1986
62. McMaster JH (ed): The ABC's of Sports Medicine. Robert E. Kriegar, Malabar, FL, 1982
63. Noujaim SE, Nagle CE: Acute scrotal injuries in athletes: evaluation by diagnostic imaging. Physician Sports Med 17:125, 1989
64. Nolten WE, Lorenman SG, Viosca SP et al: Remote testicular trauma as a cause of infertility. Clin Res 38:147, 1990
65. Ramsey ML: How I manage jock itch. Physician Sports Med 18:63, 1990
66. Lamberg SI: Dermatology in Primary Care: A Problem Oriented Guide. WB Saunders, Philadelphia, 1986

Injuries and Conditions of the Neck and Spine 19

Many authors use statistics the way a drunk uses a lamp-post: For support rather than illumination.
— Anonymous

Spinal injuries and conditions related to the nerves and paravertebral structures do not form a large block of injuries, although their potential seriousness, difficulty in diagnosis, and possibility of protracted symptoms with significant loss of practice and game time brings them into prominence. In some sports these problems have a distressingly high incidence, whereas in others the spine seems almost immune from involvement. This chapter focuses on the potentially catastrophic injuries of spinal fractures as well as traction of compression injuries to the brachial plexus and the common conditions of the thoracic and lumbar spine. The emphasis is on: (1) detection, particularly of those conditions in danger of being overlooked; (2) diagnosis, with special reference to severity and prognosis; and (3) guidelines for return to activity.

INJURIES TO THE NECK

During one review of 1,500 high school football injuries documented over one season, 5 percent were concussions and 4 percent neck injuries. Similarly, of the 2,400 football injuries reported during a survey at the University of California, 6 percent of the injuries were to the head and 5 percent were neck injuries.[1] These potentially serious injuries account for a large proportion of the medical problems in a collision sport such as football. Indeed, they are outnumbered only by trauma to the ankles, knees, and thighs.

Anatomic Considerations

The cervical vertebrae are small and delicate and in the human species have evolved to accommodate a large range of motion so the head can be placed in a position to see through a wide arc, greatly increasing the visual fields Fig. 19–1. In some animals the neck has evolved so that the head can move in the range suitable for obtaining food at a distance without the use of forelimbs. The giraffe is an excellent example, but this function is hardly a consideration in the human. In other animals, the head often supports a large rack of horns, e.g., the elk. To deal with such enormous weight the anatomy of the neck has evolved in such a way that a large amount of elastic recoil can be obtained from the ligaments, in particular the ligamentum nuchae and flavum. Once more, it is not a consideration in the human. However, in some sports, the neck has to become weight-bearing, such as with the movement of bridging in wrestling, or it must be able to absorb impact, as is seen when a linebacker tackles a runningback and the helmets collide. Furthermore, the neck may indeed be required to sustain tremendous torque loads such as occurs with a rugby tackle. It is obvious, then, that the otherwise frail anatomy of the cervical spine must be gradually and sequentially adapted by exercise and range of motion work to accept these stresses. Nevertheless, even the most muscular individual cannot protect the cervical spine under all circumstances in these sports.

Musculature

Just below the occiput several massive muscles support and control the head; they are separated from their fellow of the opposite side by the midline tough yet flexible ligamentum nuchae. These muscles include the trapezius, splenius, and semispinalis capitis (Fig. 19-2). They arise from the lower cervical and upper thoracic vertebral arches and insert on the skull.[2] They are influenced by shoulder, upper tho-

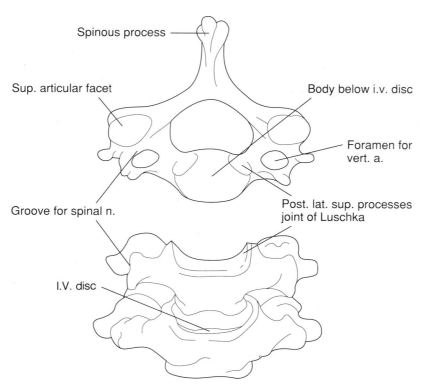

Spinous process

Sup. articular facet

Body below i.v. disc

Foramen for vert. a.

Groove for spinal n.

Post. lat. sup. processes joint of Luschka

I.V. disc

Fig. 19-1. Typical cervical vertebra is characterized by a relatively large spinal canal, a foramen for the vertebral artery, and a small body. There are also the associated joints of Luschka, which help provide lateral stability, although their importance lies in their relation to adjacent nerves and vessels.

racic, and particularly lower cervical postures and pathology, which may result in associated spasm, dyssynergy, and weakness of these muscles. This spasm may be linked to the tension headaches seen with neck and shoulder girdle problems.

Deeper in the suboccipital region are the intrinsic muscles, which control the motions between the occiput C1 and C2 and to some degree the vertebrae below. Despite their obvious function, derived from observations of their attachments, the subtle interplay during activity can only be surmised (Fig. 19-32).

These muscles form the suboccipital triangle, which is important for its main content, the vertebral artery, on its way from the foramen transversarium of the atlas, where it pierces the dura mater and enters the foramen magnum.[3,4] Anteriorly, the rectus capitis anterior and lateralis, longus capitis, longus colli (cervicis), and sternomastoid generate flexion, side flexion, and work synergically with rotation. Although the movements of these small muscles are impossible to isolate, their sequential innervation (myotomes) may be assessed grossly with key motion of the neck, along with the upper limb segmental screen.

Range of Motion

Most movement in the cervical spine occurs at the atlanto-occipital and atlantoaxial joints. In fact, this movement accounts for approximately 50 percent of cervical spine motion. There is no consensus in the literature as to the amount of motion possible at each level, so the principles themselves are important and only approximate ranges are presented.[5-7]

Atlanto-occipital Joints

The atlanto-occipital joint articulation is characterized mainly by flexion and extension with a total range of 15 to 30 degrees, although there is a wide discrepancy of ranges reported in the literature. Similarly, there is disagreement about side flexion, which averages about 5 to 10 degrees. There is no or little rotation.

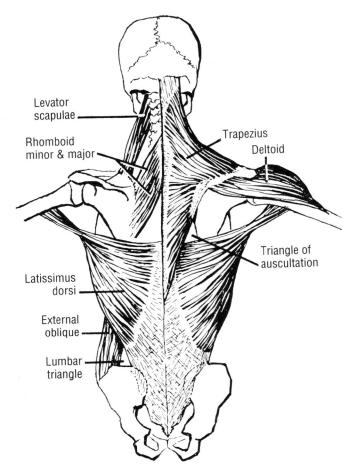

Fig. 19-2. Right trapezius and latissimus dorsi cover most of the back and connect the upper limb to the axial skeleton right down to the pelvis. (After Gardner et al.[7])

Atlantoaxial Articulation (C1 – C2)

There is an even greater variation of reported ranges at C1 – C2. Rotation is the prime motion (30 to 90 degrees) depending on the laxity of the capsule and the alar and transverse ligaments. This motion is a complex one that involves some vertical approximation as the inferior facets of the atlas slide off the summits of the convex superior facets of the axis. Additionally, there are about 10 degrees of flexion, 5 degrees of extension, and 5 degrees of side flexion at the C1 – C2 articulation.

C3 – C7

Lower down the spine there is significant flexion centering around C5 – C6 and extension of C6 – C7. During all of these movements there is usually a grad-

ual intersegmental flow. Motion between C1 and C2 may occur relatively independently, but below C2 normal movement is always a combined motion at all levels. As the articular processes move over each other, the disc deforms to permit the range (Fig. 19-3). The total range varies between 30 and 50 degrees of flexion and 35 and 60 degrees of extension. Rotation is always accompanied by side flexion.

Although neck movement is considerable, there are definite endpoints to cervical spinal range of motion. Forward flexion is stopped by the apposition of the chin on the chest. Side flexion is, to some degree, limited by the apposition of the ear on the elevated shoulder, although often this is beyond the normal range of motion. In rotation, which is limited by capsular and ligament restraints and extension where apposition of the spinous processes are important,

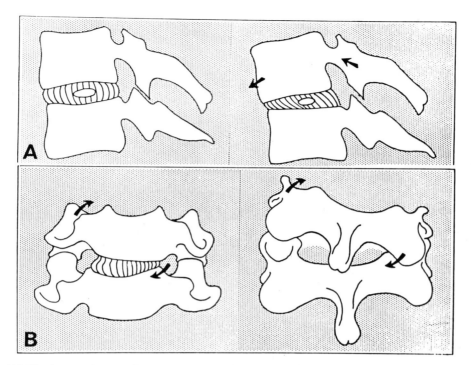

Fig. 19-3. **(A)** Flexion and extension requires considerable deformity of the disc in the cervical spine. **(B)** Rotation and side flexion movements are linked because of the shape of the articular facets.

the lack of soft tissue apposition may allow unguarded motion to damage these structures.

Definitely with extension, the apposition of the occiput on the back is way beyond the normal range of motion of the cervical spine. For these reasons, in situations where the head and neck are forced beyond

their normal range the ligamentous muscular, and nervous systems can be stretched, torn, and damaged. In particular, we must realize that the brachial plexus, which is fixed at the neural foramina and the arm, has only limited tolerance to being stretched. Indeed the neck may be particularly vulnerable, as the mechanisms of injury are diverse, making prophylaxis difficult.

Quick Facts

CERVICAL SPINE MOTION

- Atlanto-occipital motion
  - Flexion 15 degrees
  - Extension 15 degrees
- Atlantoaxial motion
  - Rotation 45 degrees
  - Flexion 10 to 15 degrees
  - Extension 10 to 15 degrees
  - Lateral gliding
  - Vertical approximation
- C2–C7 motion
  - Flexion-extension 55 degrees
  - Rotation
  - Lateral flexion

Quick Facts

MECHANISMS OF INJURY

- Forced excessive range of motion
- Direct compression injury to head
- Fall with superimposed opponent's body weight
- Equipment failure or design directly responsible due to features or illegal use
- Illegal procedures
- Attempting maneuvers beyond skill level
- Evolving dangerous techniques
- Fall from height
- Violence as the object of the sport

Von Luschka Joints

The bony lips (uncinate processes) extending upward from the lateral margins of the upper surfaces of the bodies of C3 to C7 are Luschka joints (uncovertebral).[2] Considered by some as synovial articulations, their importance lies in their intimate relation to the vertebral arteries, cervical nerves, sympathetic rami, and discs (Fig. 19-1). With degenerative and hypertrophic changes, each of these structures may be affected by its contiguous Luschka articulations.

Plexus Concept

The typical spinal nerve, formed by the union of dorsal and ventral roots, divides outside the intervertebral foramen into a dorsal and a ventral ramus.[4,8] In general, the dorsal rami of spinal nerves supply the skin of the medial two-thirds of the back from the top of the head to the coccyx, the deep (intrinsic) muscles of the back, and the zygoapophyseal vertebral joints. Each dorsal ramus supplies the strip of skin and muscle and the zygoapophyseal joint located at the level of its origin. The ventral rami of spinal nerves supply the rest of the spinally innervated muscles, skin, and joints of the neck, trunk, and extremities.[3] The ventral rami, except those from T2 to T11, form plexuses; i.e., they join with higher or lower ventral rami (or both) to form networks from which peripheral nerves may arise containing nerve fibers derived from more than one spinal cord segment, in contrast to the dorsal rami, which generally do not form plexuses and are therefore themselves unisegmental peripheral nerves (Fig. 19-4).

The brachial plexus is usually formed from the ventral rami of C5–T1 spinal nerves. The ventral rami of C5 and C6 fuse to form the superior trunk; the ventral ramus of C7 continues on as the middle trunk, and the ventral rami of C8 and T1 form the lower trunk. Thus injuries may occur at four general levels: (1) above the plexus, involving the spinal cord and manifesting signs of an upper motor neuron lesion (in sport usually the result of a spinal fracture or disloca-

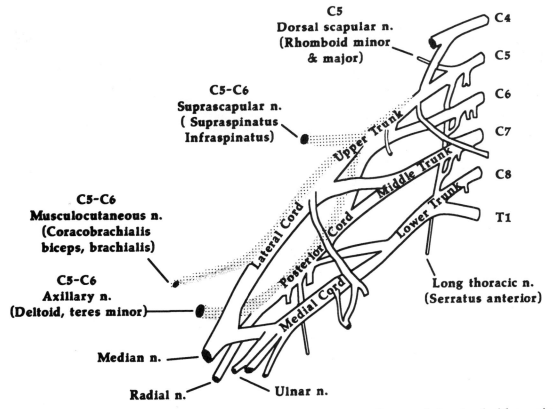

Fig. 19-4. Brachial plexus. The shaded portions are the nerves most frequently involved with traction injuries in sport, as well as dislocations of the shoulder. (Adapted from Speer and Bassett,[8] with permission.)

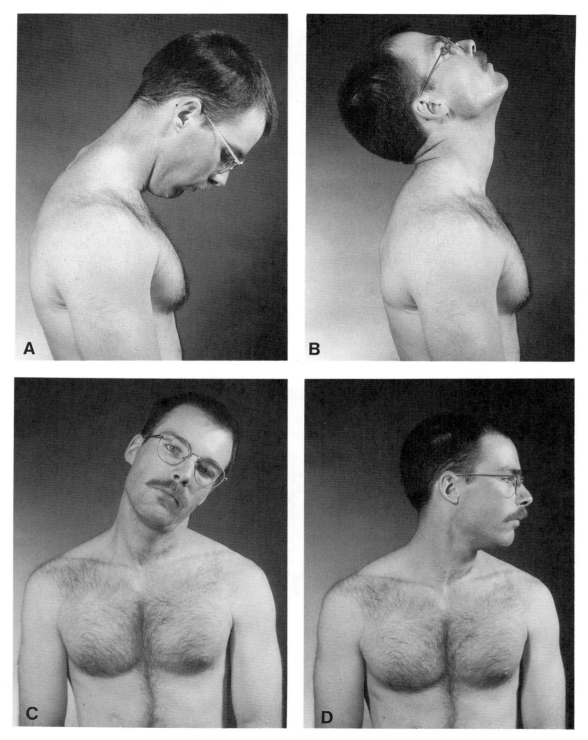

Fig. 19-5. Active range of motion of the cervical spine. **(A)** Flexion. **(B)** Extension. **(C)** Side flexion. **(D)** Rotation.

tion): (2) at the level of the roots, producing definite segmental signs (dermatomes and myotomes) and symptoms (in sports, commonly secondary to either a traction injury or disc protrusion); (3) within the plexus (trunks and cords), requiring careful application of anatomic knowledge to localize (usually arising secondary to traction injuries), and (4) within the peripheral nerve, producing a distinct pattern of sensory and motor disturbance (in sport frequently secondary to direct blows, dislocations at the shoulder, or pressure or repetitive traction injuries).

Examination of the Cervical Spine

Examination of the neck involves a screen of the whole upper limb. Details of the history indicate where the emphasis should be.

History

The two major points in the history include firmly establishing the chief complaint. If there is pain or numbness, the exact distribution and associated features such as headaches, disturbed vision, or hearing disturbances are significant. A second important factor is the nature of the onset—whether traumatic and acute or slow and insidious in nature.

The association of pain with positions of the head and with coughing or sneezing may give some indication of a radicular origin. An attempt should be made to distinguish primary shoulder and periscapular postural problems referring into the neck from that due to primary neck pathology radiating into the shoulder and down the upper limb.

Physical Examination

The physical examination begins with a careful inspection of posture, assessing rotational deformity such as wryneck, postural deformities such as poking chin, and the presence or absence of obvious wasting or deformity. An unusually low posterior hairline may indicate associated congenital malformations of the spine. Symmetry of the scapula is also important.

Active range of motion is shown in Fig. 19-5. Side flexion of the neck combined with rotation into flexion or extension while depressing the opposite shoulder approximates the neuroforamina on the ipsilateral side. It also puts traction on the contralateral side. If pain is increased, particularly in a root distribution, it may indicate (1) irritation of the nerve root,

(2) foraminal encroachment, (3) adhesions around the dural sleeve, or (4) changes in the facet joint and capsule.

This maneuver is followed by overpressure and distraction to see if it reproduces, exacerbates, or generates pain in the shoulder and upper limb (Fig. 19-6).

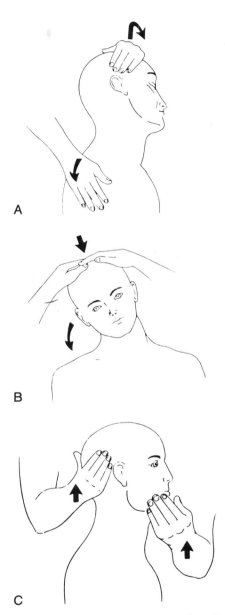

Fig. 19-6. Stress test of the cervical spine for eliciting radicular pain. **(A)** Cervical quadrant test for the lower cervical spine on the left. **(B)** Foraminal compression test. **(C)** Cervical distraction. (From Magee,[9] with permission.)

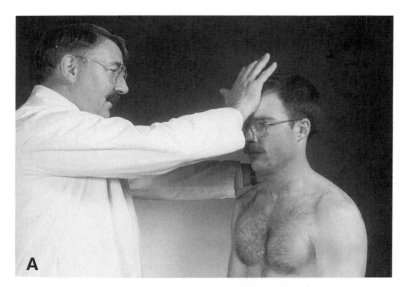

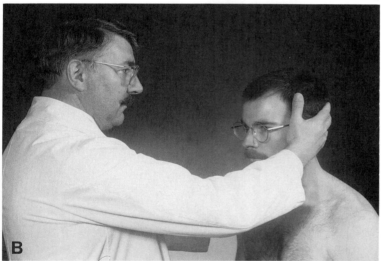

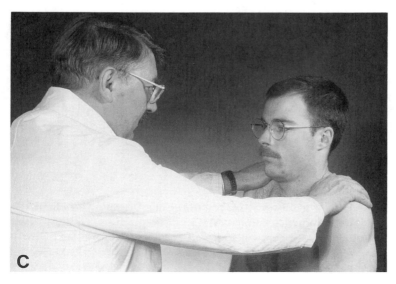

Fig. 19-7. Screen of muscle strength of the upper limb organized according to myotomes. **(A)** Neck flexion (C1–C2). **(B)** Neck side flexion (C3). **(C)** Shoulder shugging (C4). *(Figure continues.)*

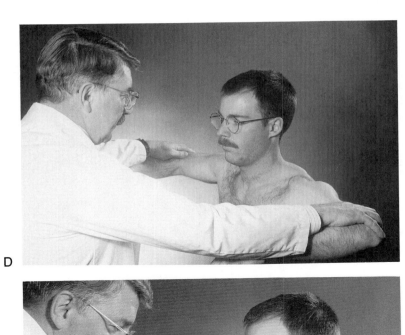

D

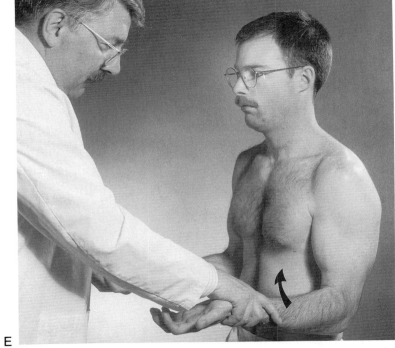

E

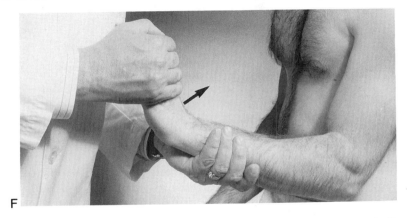

F

Fig. 19-7 *(Continued).* **(D)** Shoulder abduction (C5). **(E)** Elbow flexion (C5–6). **(F)** Wrist extensions (C6–7). *(Figure continues.)*

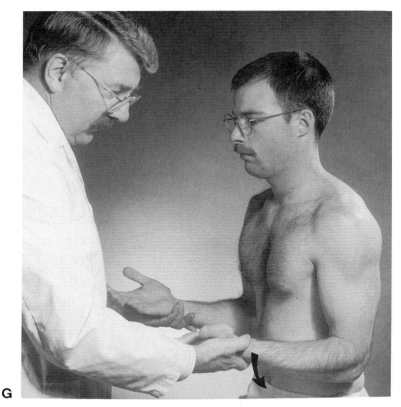

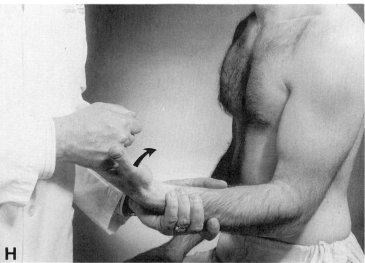

Fig. 19-7 *(Continued).* **(G)** Elbow extension (C7). **(H)** Wrist flexion (C7–8). *(Figure continues.)*

This test should be done with care and modified according to details found in the history. It is difficult to record cervical spinal motion accurately, and frequently some estimate of the percent of normal motion by comparing the two sides for rotation and side flexion is adequate. A quick screen of upper limb motion by asking the athlete to elevate fully through flexion and abduction is also helpful. If appropriate resisted isometric neck motion not only confirms the willingness to exert an effort but may exacerbate pain in a certain pattern (Fig. 19-7).

Initial palpation can be done with the patient in the

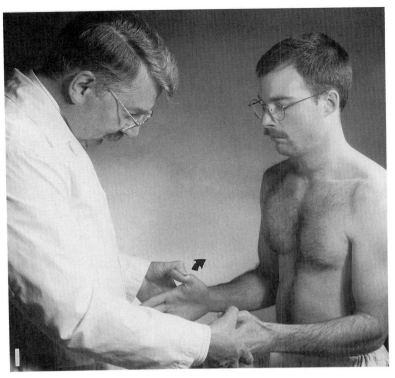

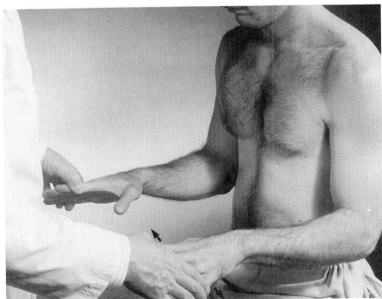

Fig. 19-7 *(Continued).* **(I)** Thumb extension (C8). **(J)** Finger abduction (T1).

sitting position and the examiner standing behind the patient. Palpation can be carried out along the spinous processes and the paraspinal areas. The sternoclavicular joint, clavicle, and acromioclavicular joint are palpated as are the periscapular areas, particularly the supraspinous fossa and the medial borders of

the scapulas, which are common trigger point areas. The supraclavicular area is carefully assessed for the possible presence of abnormal nodes which may indicate infection or neoplasm. This palpation is later repeated with the patient lying down. Passive range of motion is tested as dictated by the history.

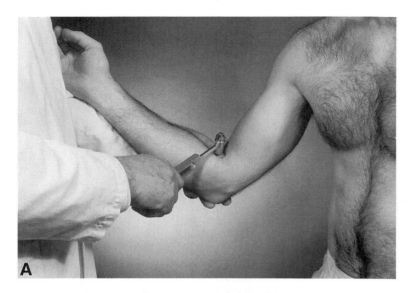

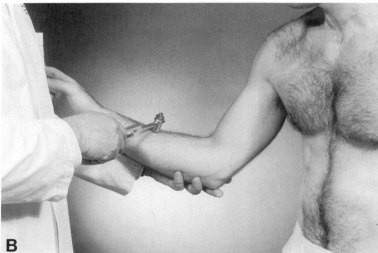

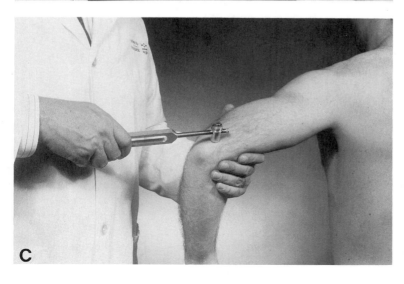

Fig. 19-8. Upper limb reflexes. **(A)** Biceps (C5–C6). **(B)** Brachioradialis (C6). **(C)** Triceps (C7).

Neurologic Screen

For efficiency a neurologic screen of the upper limb should be done at this point, initially testing strength and reflexes (Fig. 19-8). If there is specific indication in the history, cranial nerves can be tested at this point. Sensory testing is aimed at distinguishing root from peripheral nerve involvement[7-9] (Fig. 19-9). By this time the degree of neural involvement should be obvious, as should the probable level: central, segmental, or peripheral (Tables 19-1 and 19-2).

The athlete is then placed in the lying position with the head supported, and gentle palpation is carried out along the cervical spine. The patient then moves so the (supported) head extends over the end of the examining couch, and in this position passive motion can be tested. This examination is supplemented by rotational overpressure traction and, when necessary, attempts to localize motion and pain to the various segments of the cervical spine.

Special Diagnostic Maneuvers

Specific diagnostic maneuvers are added when the history or previous screen suggests clinical relevance.

Vertebral Artery Competence

When traction or cervical manipulation is selected as appropriate treatment, the possibility of a vascular pathology must be considered in the older age group. The vertebral artery test is then essential.[9] With the patient sitting or lying, the head is passively moved to

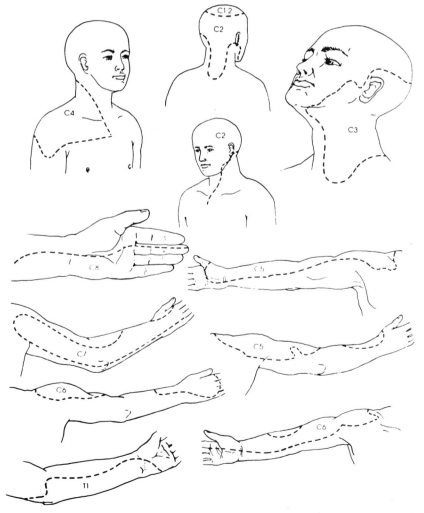

Fig. 19-9. Dermatomes of the cervical spine. (After Magee,[9] with permission.)

TABLE 19-1. Tests for Segmental Innervation of Upper Limb

Disc	Root	Reflex	Muscles	Test Movement	Sensory Area and Nerve
C4–C5	C5	Biceps reflex	Deltoid (biceps)	Shoulder abduction	Lateral arm tip of deltoid (Upper lateral cutaneous N of forearm)
C5–C6	C6	Brachioradialis reflex (biceps reflex)	Biceps (wrist extension)	Elbow flexion	Lateral forearm (Lateral cutaneous N of forearm)
C6–C7	C7	Triceps reflex	Triceps (extensor digitorum, flexor carpis ulnaris, and radialis)	Elbow extension	Middle finger (Median N)
C7–T1	C8	—	Flexor digitorum superficialis (hand intrinsics)	Cutaneous nerve	Ring and little finger (Ulner N)
T1–T2	T1	—	Hand intrinsics	Abduction and adduction fingers	Medial forearm (Medial cutaneous N of forearm)

take the neck into extension and side flexion. From this position the neck is rotated to the same side and held for approximately 30 seconds (Fig. 19-10). Dizziness or nystagmus indicates inadequate vertebral artery flow. Alternatively, if the test produces dyssesthesias in the arm, nerve root pressure in the lower cervical region is suggested. Greater tension on the upper cervical area is achieved by starting the maneuver with an anterior glide of the head, effectively poking the chin followed by extension, side flexion, and rotation. When used for root traction, these maneuvers are referred to as quadrant tests.

Brachial Plexus Tension (Traction) Test

The brachial plexus tension test, popularized by Elvey, was designed to place tension on nerve roots and nerve sheaths, particularly C5, to elucidate the cervical component of shoulder pain.[10] It is critical that neither the shoulder joints nor the cervical spine is stressed during the maneuvers. The stages of the test are as follows (Fig. 19-11).

1. Patient lies with the arm abducted slightly behind the coronal plane, just to the point of painful limitation.

TABLE 19-2. Testing for Major Upper Limb Peripheral Nerve Injuries

Nerve	Motor Test	Sensation Test
Axillary nerve	Shoulder abduction	Lateral arm—deltoid area on upper arm
Musculocutaneous nerve	Elbow flexion	Lateral forearm
Radial nerve	Extensor carpi radialis—wrist extension	Dorsal web space between thumb and index finger
Posterior interosseous branch of radial	Extensor pollicis longus—thumb extension Abductor digiti minimi—abduction little finger Abductor pollicis brevis Opponens pollicis	
Ulnar nerve	Abduction—little finger	Distal ulnar aspect of forearm—little finger
Median nerve	Thumb pinch Opposition of thumb Abduction of thumb	Distal radial aspect of forearm—index finger
Anterior interosseous branch of median	Flexor pollicis longus—thumb pinch to 2nd finger Deltoid—shoulder abduction Biceps—elbow flexion	

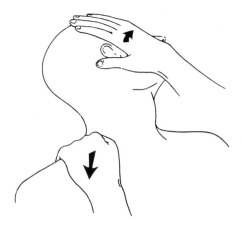

Fig. 19-10. Several maneuvers that apply traction to the cervical spine by a combination of side flexion and rotation are designed to test the irritability of the nerve roots and the patency of the vertebral artery. Referred pain or dysesthesia constitutes a positive test for nerve root irritation, and dizziness or vertigo suggests undue vertebral artery pressure.

2. Arm is brought back a little, just short of pain, and passively externally rotated at the shoulder (with the elbow kept in extension).
3. Once more the rotation is reduced to a position just short of pain. The forearm is then fully supinated, fixing and supporting the arm to prevent shoulder movement. The elbow is then carefully flexed.

Reproduction of symptoms implies a cervical origin of the discomfort. The symptoms may be magnified by performing the test in slight cervical flexion by having the head on a pillow or rotating the head away from the side being tested.

Other Tests

The cervical spine roentgenogram assists in establishing normal alignments, thereby ruling out specific pathology. The anteroposterior view is useful for visualizing the relations of the spinous processes and the presence or absence of cervical ribs.

The lateral view is usually the most helpful and can be used to visualize the position of the odontoid process, the width of the soft tissue shadows,[11,12] and the space available in the spinal canal; it can also be used to gain a preliminary impression of the facet joints and to detect the presence or absence of cervical spondylosis, as indicated by disc narrowing and osteophytes (Figs. 19-12 and 19-13). Flexion-extension lateral views also give good indications of the segmental flow of motion. In the post-traumatic situation, angulation and wedging are also apparent in the lateral view. Subluxation and dislocation are usually discernible on the lateral view. Bilateral facet subluxation allows more than 3.5 mm forward motion of one vertebra on another (Fig. 19-14). However, unilateral facet subluxation or dislocation is much more subtle and is frequently missed.[12] These are best seen by examining the facet joint relation in the oblique film. Another indicator of the abnormal anatomic relation is an angle of more than 11 degrees between vertebral bodies, usually associated with spreading of the spinous processes (Fig. 19-14).

Should the C1–C2 relation come into question, through-the-mouth anteroposterior views clearly outline the odontoid process, its anatomic variations, and the presence or absence of post-traumatic changes.[14] The odontoid-atlas space is normally no more than 3 mm in healthy adults or 5 mm in children less than 8 years of age (Fig. 19-15). Larger dimensions may denote damage to the transverse ligament. Fractures of the lateral masses of C1 with displacement are usually detected by carefully evaluating the space between the odontoid and the lateral masses and comparing the two sides. Fracture versus rotational subluxation versus anatomic variations are confirmed by viewing soft tissue shadows and, when appropriate, repeating the views with rotation of the head to both sides. (See Fig. 19-19.)

Views of the facet joints and the intervertebral foramina are best outlined with oblique roentgenograms. These views clearly show abnormal facet relations as well as osteophytic impingement and changes in the neuroforamina.

Clinical Points

SCREENING FOR CERVICAL TRAUMA

- Three-view cervical screen is adequate.
  -Lateral view
  -Anteroposterior view
  Open-mouth odontoid view
- CT may be used if the above is technically inadequate.

Supplementary examination includes computed tomography (CT) and magnetic resonance imaging (MRI), which provide more details of the soft tissues.

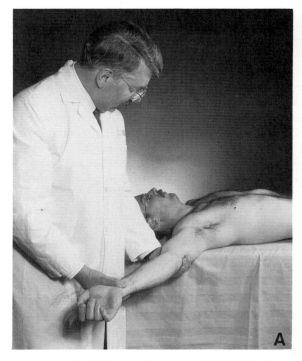
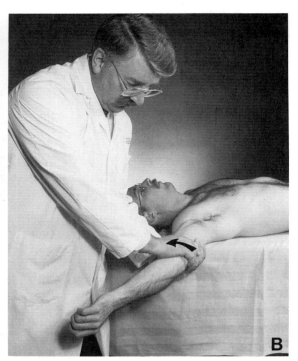
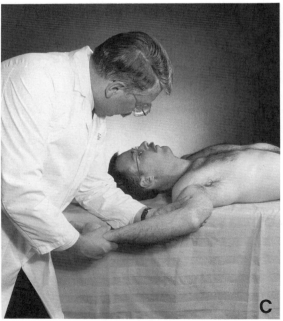

Fig. 19-11. Elvey's brachial plexus traction test. **(A)** Shoulder abduction is maintained just short of the point of pain onset. **(B)** External rotation is maintained just short of the point of pain onset. **(C)** Forearm supination is maintained while the elbow is flexed. A positive test generates pain with each maneuver and is indicative primarily of midcervical root irritation.

Some caution is necessary at this point, however, as many of the normal variations are still being defined. For example, in a significant percentage of the population, MRI scans reveal disc protrusions. Many of these individuals are asymptomatic, emphasizing the point that radiographic abnormalities should be considered only in the light of the accompanying history and physical examination. Bone scans are occasionally helpful for ruling out post-traumatic changes when roentgenographic findings are equivocal.

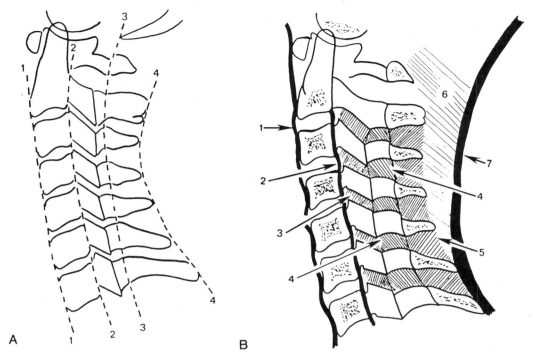

Fig. 19-12. Four main bony contour lines are seen on the normal lateral cervical spinal roentgenogram. **(A)** 1 = Anterior vertebral margins; 2 and 3 = extent of the vertebral canal; 4 = tips of the spinous processes. **(B)** Lines 1 to 4 are used to infer integrity of the anterior and middle supporting columns. Lines 5 to 7 are designated poster column. (1) anterior longitudinal ligament, (2) posterior longitudinal ligament, (3) ligamentum flavum, (4) facet joint capsules, (5) interspinous ligament, (6) ligamentum nuchae, and (7) supraspinous ligament.

Classification of Nerve Injury

Nerve injuries may be classified into three grades of severity. These grades, however, are not absolute, and there is a spectrum of clinical severity found within each grade[15-19] (Table 19-3).

Grade I

Grade I nerve injury is the neuropraxia of Sedden and the grade I nerve injury of Sunderland.[17,19] There is interruption of physiologic function without significant anatomic damage. There should be no degeneration within the nerve. Classically there is a transitory loss or alteration of motor or sensory function lasting seconds to minutes. The physical examination rapidly returns to normal. There is debate as to whether persistent symptoms lasting 10 to 12 hours or longer may still fall into this category, provided there is no eventual electrophysiologic evidence of denervation. In an attempt to resolve this question, the subclassifica-

tions of mild, moderate, and severe are possible (though not necessarily accurate).

A mild grade I injury involves transient weakness, numbness, or paresthesia. If the symptoms persist more than a few minutes, the injury is considered moderate; and if they remain at 10 to 12 hours, they are classified as severe. This classification presupposes that electromyography (EMG) will not detect denervation at 18 to 21 days. Thus it is a fine clinical judgment. The prognosis for all grade I injuries should be 100 percent recovery.

Grade II

Grade II injury is the axonotmesis of Sedden and grade II and III injuries of Sunderland.[17,19] This level of injury assumes some reaction of degeneration within an intact neurolemmal sheath. There is a persisting motor or sensory loss that lasts longer than 2 weeks. At 18 to 21 days, the EMG is abnormal, and

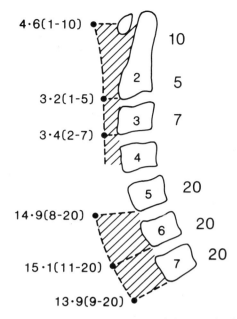

Fig. 19-13. Soft tissue swelling of the cervical spine. The normal widths (and ranges), in millimeters, are given along with the upper limits of normal (figures at right). Upper cervical pathology is usually judged in front of the body of C2, and lower cervical pathology is usually judged by the width anteriorly to C6.

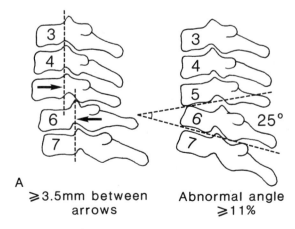

Fig. 19-14. Abnormal cervical spine relations. **(A)** Forward displacement of more than 3.5 mm is indicative of at least facet subluxation and **(B)** abnormal angulation of more than 11 degrees between the cervical vertebrae indicates disruption of the supraspinus and interspinous ligaments as well as, potentially, the anterior stabilizing elements. In this example, the angulation is 25 degrees.

there may be some persisting abnormality up to 1 year. The clinical recovery is often 100 percent; but according to the site and severity of the initial injury, there is an anticipated 60 to 80 percent electrophysiologic recovery for the more serious injuries, provided the existing factors are removed or in cases of constant pressure the duration of the pathologic compression has not been long.

Grade III

Grade III injury is the neurotmesis of Sedden and grade IV and V injuries of Sunderland.[17-19] There has been disruption of the neurolemmal sheaths of all or part of the nerve; usually more than 60 percent. The reaction of degeneration is complete; and depending on the treatment, site, severity of injury, and makeup of the nerve involved, recovery ranges from 0 to 30 percent, and rarely more. Fortunately, there is a certain amount of "sprouting" of motor units, so remaining nerve fibers innervate a greater number of muscle fibers. Clinical improvement may be more dramatic than electrophysiologic recovery, as other muscles take over the function and existing recovered muscle may be hypertrophied.

Other specific tests, e.g., nerve conduction studies and EMG, have a definite role in sorting out the magnitude and location of peripheral nerve involvement. Occasionally, when there is combined neck and shoulder pathology, studies of the shoulder may include arthrograms to differentiate the magnitude and extent of the shoulder disease.

Traumatic Radiculopathy (Burners, Stingers, Pinched Nerve Syndrome)

Sport/recreation is the second leading cause of spinal cord injury. The catastrophic consequences of these injuries have led to enlightened preseason training programs, better protective equipment, and rule changes.[14,20] Such measures have dramatically reduced the severity of head and neck injuries associated with many sports.[21-24] Nevertheless, there are some neurogenic symptom complexes that occur frequently in contact sport, particularly football, that are treated with less respect than they deserve.[24-30] In a 1983 survey of more than 3,000 secondary school and varsity football teams, 25 percent reported a history of neck injury. Of these, significant numbers reported neck pain, numbness, tingling, or burning of the upper extremities and upper limb weakness.[30-34] These episodes, clumped together under

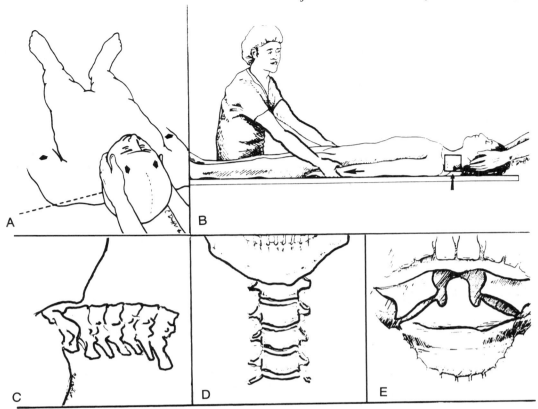

Fig. 19-15. Roentgenographic evaluation of cervical spine. **(A)** Stabilize head and neck. **(B)** Consider traction on upper limbs to depress shoulder to get better view of C7. When clinically and logistically possible, the initial series of roentgenograms after trauma should include a **(C)** lateral, **(D)** anteroposterior, and **(E)** through-the-mouth odontoid view. If there are technical difficulties, the most information can be gained from a simple lateral view. Any suspicion or failure to adequately visualize the cervical spine including C6, C7, and the odontoid process should constitute an indication for further examination by CT scan if the clinical indications warrant it.

TABLE 19-3.   Classification of Nerve Injury

Severity (Sedden)	Pathophysiology	Grade (Sunderland)[a]		Symptoms[a]	Recovery Potential (%)[a]
Neuropraxia (grade I)	Physiologic interruption of function	I	Mild	Transient dysesthesia and weakness	100
			Moderate	Symptoms persist more than a few minutes	
			Severe	Symptoms remain 10–12 hours	
Axonotmesis (grade II)	Some reaction of degeneration within an intact neurolemmal sheath	II		Persisting motor or sensory loss beyond 10–12 hours	100
		III		Persisting motor or sensory loss beyond 2 weeks; electrophysiologic abnormalities	60–80
Neurotmesis (grade III)	Reaction of degeneration of separated axons	IV		Disruption of neurolemmal sheath; may have part of nerve intact	30–60
		V		Complete separation of whole nerve	0–30

[a] Not always clear division of grades, symptoms, and neurologic recovery.

the heading of "burners" or "stingers" are frequently treated with an inappropriate nonchalance. These episodes were often related to the continued use of illegal blocking and tackling techniques involving primary contact with the head; and for many, these symptoms were recurrent. Indeed, 40 percent of cervical spinal injuries in football occur during tackling, most frequently to a defensive back.[35,36]

Torg classified cervical spinal injury into: (1) fractures and dislocations of the cervical spine with quadriplegia; (2) fractures and dislocations of the cervical spine without neurologic involvement; and (3) degenerative changes and occult fractures resulting from repetitive noncatastrophic injuries and brachial plexus (stretch-pinch) syndromes.[37] The latter being synonemous with the terms "bursars" or "stingers."

Clinical Presentation of Burners or Stingers

Classically, the athlete experiences transient upper extremity dysesthesia, pain, and weakness. This episode usually follows an ipsilateral or, less commonly, a contralateral shoulder blow that may be associated with cervical spinal extension, lateral flexion, or both.[25,27,29,31,34] Alternatively, direct cervical compression with slight flexion, as epitomized by the illegal spearing technique of football, may produce the symptoms.[37]

Symptoms range from brief "knife-like" shooting pains confined to the shoulder area to transient numbness and paralysis of the whole arm. Occasionally, the dysesthesia is bilateral. Persistent neurologic dysfunction has been reported.[38,39,50] Unfortunately, there is confusion in the literature as to the mechanism, pathology, and severity of these injuries. The lesion is variously reported to be located in the spinal cord, nerve root, brachial plexus, or peripheral nerve.[34,39-42]

The frequent occurrence and lack of evidence for location or permanence of the neurologic injury contributes to a diversity of treatment formats. Options vary from uninterrupted continuation of play to complete cessation of sport. Treatment typically consists in a brief on-the-field assessment followed by return to play. Athletes may receive bolstering of the cervical spine or shoulder and instruction about altering tackling techniques. Only rarely is there rigid immobilization until fracture or dislocation has been ruled out. Most often the episode is ignored, with expectation of an immediate full recovery. It is common for athletes to admit to sustaining burners as

TABLE 19-4.   Duration of Symptoms Due to Burners

Symptom Duration	Frequency (%)
Initial dysesthetic pain	
≤1 minute	57
≥5 minutes	35
Unknown	18
Continued subjective weakness	
None	34
8 hours	12
24 hours	12
≥2–3 weeks	42

frequently as one per game for an entire season without undergoing a detailed neurologic assessment or any specific therapy. This casual approach to neurologic symptoms is perhaps more pronounced in the management of burners than any other sport injury. It is incompatible with the usual regard given to neuropathology in other situations.

Much of the discussion in this section is based on the work of Bergfield and his colleagues as well as our own study using standard clinical history and physical examination procedures, full cervical spinal radiographs, electrophysiologic studies, and isokinetic muscle testing.[30,39] In our study, a significant number of athletes tested had persistent neurologic signs or symptoms 3 weeks after their latest burner episode (Table 19-4). The common site of occurrence of burners has perhaps de-emphasized them as a significant neurologic injury. Nevertheless, persistent neurologic deficits demonstrated by these athletes highlight the need for careful clinical evaluation following a burner. The immediate mandatory examination must include evaluation of sensory and motor func-

---

Clinical Point

EVALUATION OF THE "BURNER" SYNDROME: MINIMUM ASSESSMENT

- Cervical spine palpation for midline tenderness
- Range of motion, including quadrant stressing
- Sensory testing of upper limb, including shoulder
- Strength testing for bilateral symmetry

tion, pain, swelling, tenderness, and range of motion. The examiner must recognize that *the term burner describes a symptom complex and does not imply a specific diagnosis, severity, nerve injury, or prognosis.*

Criteria for Return to Play

An athlete experiencing a first-time burner with arm symptoms only should be withheld from competition until residual symptoms and signs have fully resolved. Specifically, there should be no cervical tenderness, a full range of cervical motion with no pain on slight overpressure (quadrant stressing), and no reproduction of signs with compression. McKeag and Cantu suggested that the single most useful clinical test for eliciting radicular symptoms is to tilt the head toward the side of the burner, extend it, and then apply axial compression.[43] An effective assessment requires diligent serial clinical examinations and full cooperation from the athlete.

For athletes experiencing recurrent burners, contact sports should be discontinued until further investigations have been completed. Such investigations should include a radiologic examination of the cervical spine and, where available, isokinetic testing. However, in the absence of objective quantification of muscle strength, careful clinical assessment may indicate the need for EMG studies. When initially evaluating the athlete on the field, any detection of significant cervical tenderness, restricted range of cervical motion, or palpable deformity should indicate the need to move the athlete using full spinal precautions until a radiographic evaluation has been completed.

Radiographic Evaluation

Radiographic abnormalities are frequently found in athletes with severe or recurrent burners. Cervical spine, anteroposterior, oblique, lateral flexion and extension, and odontoid views should be obtained on athletes with recurrent burners and those with residual neurologic signs and symptoms. If an acute traumatic spinal injury is suspected, flexion and extension views should be omitted until screening lateral views are done (Fig. 19-16).

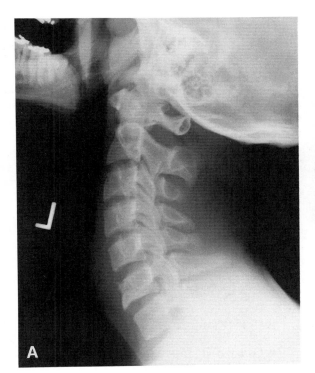
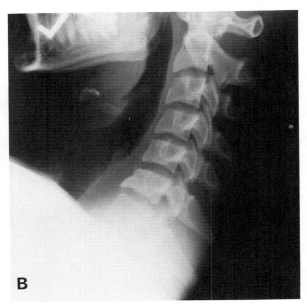

Fig. 19-16. (A) This football player presented with repeated episodes of burners. Radiographs show evidence of an old C6 anterior crush. Evaluation of **(A)** and **(B)** flexion films show no evidence of instability.

Twelve percent of the athletes in our series had relative spinal stenosis. Torg et al. focused attention on the potential risk associated with congenital spinal stenosis.[42] They suggested measuring spinal stenosis on the lateral roentgenogram using a ratio method to eliminate radiographic magnification error. In their study of 32 players with the syndrome of transient quadriplegia, which they attributed to neuropraxia of the spinal cord, 24 were found to have vertebral canal/vertebral body ratios of less than 0.80[41,42] (Fig. 19-17). This figure was compared to a ratio of 0.98 or more in the control group.

Brief episodes of bilateral arm pain or transient quadriplegia constitute one of a constellation of clinical pictures that have been previously lumped together under the heading "burners." Torg et al. suggested that it is a different entity and that there is no evidence that neuropraxia of the spinal cord predisposes an individual to permanent neurologic injury.

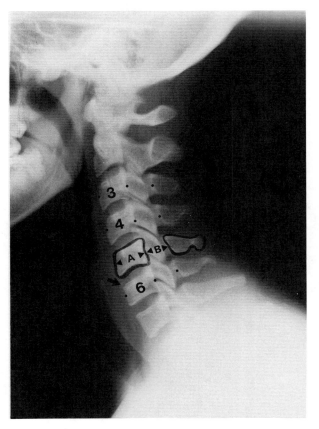

Fig. 19-17. Relative spinal stenosis in an individual according to the Torg index (vertebral canal/vertebral body ratio of less than 0.80).

However, patients who have this syndrome in association with instability of the cervical or chronic degenerative changes should be precluded from further participation in contact sports.[41] Those who have congenital spinal stenosis in association with congenital abnormality should be treated on an individual basis. By contrast, in the same journal issue as that of Torg et al.'s report, Ladd and Scranton suggested that an episode of transient quadriplegia calls for a full neurologic work-up including either a CT scan or a myelogram.[50] They further suggested that individuals with spinal senosis of the cervical spine should be advised to discontinue participation in contact sports. This area obviously is still controversial.

A more recent study by Oder et al., using the Torg ratio in 224 football players, noted that 32 percent of the 124 professionals and 34 percent of the 100 rookies had a ratio of less than 0.80 at one or more levels from C3 to C6.[44] The question then arises as to what to do with a player who has transient neurologic signs and relative spinal stenosis on the lateral roentgenogram. In view of the fact that approximately one-third of football players apparent have ratios of less than 0.80, it is not immediately apparent that this parameter predisposes the athlete to either transient or permanent neurologic sequelae. Thus any decision for return to play or advice regarding vulnerability should include other factors, e.g., results of a thorough neurologic assessment, the severity and frequency of the symptoms, and the duration of the signs. In situations where the clinical picture raises concern, further evaluation, including MRI with flexion and extension sagittal images, CT scans, or myelography may give some indication of the absolute canal size, as well as any potential lesions, such as disc protrusions, that may contribute to cord or nerve root encroachment.[44,45] Only then should a defini-

---

Clinical Point

SIGNIFICANCE OF RELATIVE SPINAL STENOSIS

Depends on:

- Canal/body ratio less than 0.80
- Magnitude of symptoms
- Frequency of "burner" episodes
- Duration of symptoms

tive conclusion be drawn on the implications of the stenosis.

Ligamentous instability contraindicates further contact sport participation (Fig. 19-18). It is impossible to know the relation between the spinal canal and neural tissue at the moment of injury. A subluxation may spontaneously reduce, and displacement would not be evident on plain lateral views. Hence a lack of displacement does not rule out significant pathology, and clinical findings and the history must take precedence over plain roentgenograms. Concurrent bilateral burners may indicate spinal instability; and *any athlete with bilateral symptoms, no matter how transient, should be removed from play until instability has been ruled out.* Specific radiologic studies must include at

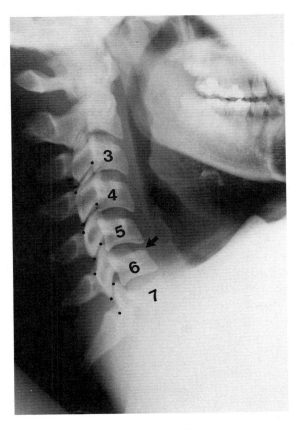

Fig. 19-18. Widening of the interspinous space, small chip of bone from the superior body of C6 (arrow), and localized increased facet excursion in flexion-extension views: C5–C6 gives an indication of potential segmental instability in this athlete suffering from recurrent burners.

least lateral flexion and extension views (Fig. 19-16). Furthermore, when symptoms are suggestive of more proximal pathology, particularly high cervical tenderness, a careful evaluation of C1–C2 is in order (Fig. 19-19).[12,45,46]

Individuals with degenerative spondylosis must be considered on an individual basis. The rigors of contact sports, particularly football, wrestling, and soccer, may result in increased radiologic evidence of facet joint changes, including sclerosis, joint space narrowing, and osteophyte formation. Although there is no direct relation between radiographic changes and symptomatology, significant degenerative changes combined with chronic nerve root irritation are known to affect activities of daily living. Because this symptom complex has the potential to progress, athletes should be alerted to this possibility and decide whether to continue a sport. Athletes with degenerative change and frequent or protracted burners should be encouraged to give up the provocative activities. Because of the diversity of signs, symptoms, radiographic change, and level of play, individuals with degenerative spondylosis must be counseled on an individual basis.

A large cervical rib or associated anomalies may also predispose an individual to burners and stingers. The cervical rib develops during intrauterine life more often with a prefixed than a postfixed brachial plexus. One hypothesis suggests that the bony anomalies are due to the variations in the manner in which the spinal nerves combine to form the brachial plexus.[19,45] Thus resistance encountered by the small first thoracic nerve root in a prefixed plexus during development allows formation of the cervical rib. Cervical ribs are found in approximately 0.5 to 1.0 percent of the population, and approximately one-half of the cases are unilateral, with the left side being more commonly affected than the right. The presence of a cervical rib modifies the anatomy of the region; the scalene muscles are often displaced medially, and the insertion of the scalene medius is extended to the accessory rib. The cervical rib is usually attached to the first rib by a fibrous band. The presence of the accessory rib leads to narrowing of the interscalene triangle and abnormal angulation of the subclavian artery and the lower trunk of the brachial plexus. A cervical rib more than about 5.5 cm in length may put unnecessary stretch on the seventh cervical nerve root, particularly during circumduction movements of the arm or forced side flexion of the neck with depression of the shoulder.

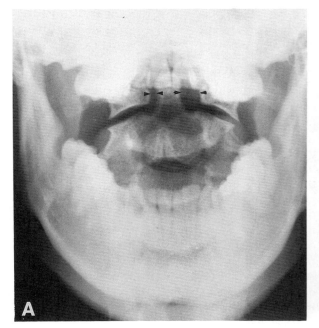

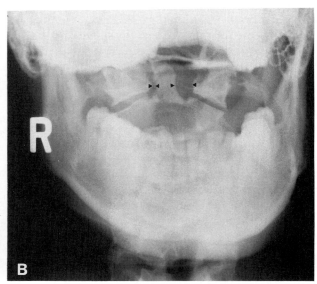

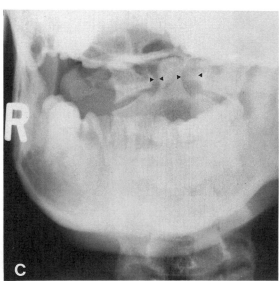

Fig. 19-19. Young hockey player complained of recurrent episodes of stingers. **(A)** Note the disproportionate gap between the odontoid and the C1 articular process on the left. **(B)** With right rotation this space (arrowheads) is maintained. **(C)** With left rotation the gap (arrowheads) is similarly maintained. This fixed position with rotation distinguishes a rotatory subluxation from an anatomic variance.

Electrodiagnostic Investigation

Electrodiagnostic investigation is of limited help in documenting the presence or prognosis of neurologic injuries. Needle EMG evidence of denervation is only present when trauma is severe enough to cause death of the motor axons (axonotmesis or neurotmesis). Nerve trauma and burners represent a spectrum of injury severity. To document the milder but more

common neuropraxic lesion electrophysiologically, nerve conduction stimulation must be done proximal to the lesion. Lesions located at the distal portion of the nerve root or at the proximal brachial plexus level can be identified by needle nerve root stimulation techniques.[47-53] This procedure is poorly tolerated by most patients.

Evidence of muscular weakness on clinical testing that persists at 72 hours after injury is most likely to

TABLE 19-5. Clinical and EMG Abnormalities Following "Burner" Syndrome

Muscle	Initial Motor Weakness (No.)	Weakness at Follow-Up (No.)	EMG Abnormalities No.	EMG Abnormalities %	Lesion Site[a] Location	Lesion Site[a] No.
Supraspinatus	7	1	4	20	Upper trunk	11
Infraspinatus	7	0	6	30	Root	
Rhomboids	—	—	2	10	C5	2
Deltoid	18	5	14	70	C6	1
Biceps	8	0	7	35	C7	1
Triceps	1	1	1	5	Axillary n.	4
Brachioradialis	1	0	5	25	Suprascap. n.	1
Pronator teres	1	0	—	—		—
Wrist extensors	1	0	—	—	Total	21

[a] Lesion site is not intended to correlate with other columns but to emphasize diversity of lesion location.
(Data from et al.,[39] with permission.)

correlate best with electrodiagnostic studies[8] (Table 19-5). Prognostically, if denervation is present, reinnervation occurs by collateral sprouting of adjacent motor axons and axonal regeneration. This process progresses at the rate of approximately 1 mm a day, which may mean many months for nerve recovery. Moreover, the extent of nerve recovery tends to be less complete as the site of injury becomes more proximal. Because EMG evidence of previous nerve injury (especially findings of reinnervation) persists for a long time, it should not be used as a criterion for return to sport. This fact was emphasized by Bergfeld et al.,[39] who found that 80 percent of athletes tested 1 to 7 years after a burner still had abnormal EMG findings consistent with reinnervation.

For athletes with predominantly sensory complaints, EMG studies may not provide helpful information. Nerve root lesions often occur proximal to the dorsal root ganglion, and intact cell bodies keep distal portions of the sensory nerves alive and conducting normally.

Muscle Strength Testing

Athletes generally have strong muscles. Even physically powerful and skilled examiners can miss significant weakness using manual muscle testing techniques. Although we had experienced examiners for our series, many of the athletes who were classed as having normal manual muscle testing proved to have significant defects on isokinetic testing. Thus when available, the use of isokinetic testing to ensure an objective measure of strength prior to return to play is an excellent tool.

Clinical Point

MUSCLE WEAKNESS AND THE BURNER SYNDROME

Isokinetic strength evaluation demonstrates many relative strength deficits that are difficult to discern or not apparent on manual muscle testing.

Cervical Neck Rolls and Collars

To prevent further episodes in athletes who sustain repetitive burners or stingers, neck rolls or cervical collars are frequently used, although the exact mechanism of action by which they are successful is ill understood. Gibbs reported on their efficacy over a 10-year period in football players at Harvard University feeling that cervical collars could assist in protecting players with a history of burners.[33]

Summary

The C5–C6 area is the most common level of involvement identified radiographically and with EMG studies. However, the lack of concurrence between clinical (symptoms and signs), radiographic, EMG, and isokinetic results suggests that each test is providing slightly different information. The large variety of pathologies and diagnoses has reinforced the need to recognize burner as a symptom complex. Furthermore, it reinforces the potentially serious nature of some injuries and the need for more aggressive investigation prior to resuming activity.

The location and severity of a neurologic injury following forced cervical lateral flexion and shoulder compression are variable, and the diagnosis of a "burner" or "stinger" does not imply specific nerve injury or indicate a prognosis. Medical staff dealing with burners must not assume full recovery with no permanent neurologic dysfunction based simply on clinical examination. Individuals sustaining recurrent burners should be investigated, the findings reviewed, and athletes advised regarding their risks. Burners should be recognized as a potential threat to neurologic function.

1. A significant number of athletes have persistent neurologic symptoms and signs after a burner. When clinical findings suggest acute bone or ligamentous injury, or if there have been recurrent burners, full cervical spinal radiography should be done. Although evidence of acute spinal trauma is rare, abnormalities that preclude continuation of contact sport may be evident.
2. Simultaneous bilateral burners or the presence of midline cervical tenderness should be treated as a potential traumatic instability until ruled out by appropriate radiographic studies and clinical examination.
3. Spinal stenosis, as judged by the Torg ratio, is prevalent in football players. Hence decisions regarding risk should be based on supplementary clinical data and more definitive tests when associated with multiple burner episodes or residual symptoms. Other congenital variations, including cervical ribs, blocked (unsegmented) vertebrae, and minor spinal dysrhaphism, must be considered on an individual basis.
4. When degenerative changes are present, continuation of participation is permissible so long as the burner episodes are transient. If the symptoms start to become protracted or interfere with activities of daily living, discontinuing participation at that sport is recommended.
5. Electrodiagnostic testing provides useful information about location and severity of nerve injury. Nevertheless, EMG cannot be used as an indicator of readiness to participate in contact sport.
6. Isokinetic strength testing provides an objective measure of muscle power. In athletes who are strong, manual muscle strength testing fails to reflect subtle changes in torque. By itself, isokinetic testing is a poor guideline of when it is safe to

return to sport, but it does serve as a useful adjunct to other clinical and radiologic information.

The diversity of pathologies and diagnoses emphasizes the burner as a symptom complex. Medical personnel dealing with athletes must be aware that the site and severity of neurologic injury is variable. Appropriate precautions must be taken to prevent damage to the neural system. If the person responsible for medical care has doubt about the extent of the injury, the athlete should be removed from play and properly immobilized until a definitive diagnosis is made.[48-53]

To distinguish a mild transient injury from those that may lead to permanent paralysis if inadequately managed, the following rules are helpful.

1. If in doubt, do not make final decisions on the field or sidelines where things are difficult at the best of times. Take the player to the dressing room and reassess the injury carefully.
2. Do it immediately, not at the end of the game. There is a tendency for athletes to "sneak" back onto the field of play.
3. Adequately undress the player to visualize and inspect the area properly. It may require careful removal of equipment.
4. Make a decision that errs on the side of safety.
5. When in doubt, send the athlete for roentgenography.

Specifically, the following points may indicate a severe injury.

1. Significant tenderness over the trapezius and sternomastoid
2. Restricted range of voluntary motion
3. Obvious midline deformity to palpation, specifically a step or gap between spinous processes
4. Extreme tenderness in the midline over the ligamentum nuchae and spinous processes
5. Weakness or paresthesias in more than one extremity, particularly if it involves the lower limbs with cervical spinal injury

It is apparent that during preseason medical examinations individuals with a history of multiple burner or stinger episodes and those who are in vulnerable positions, e.g., linebackers or fullbacks, should have a careful neurologic examination and perhaps appropriate roentgenograms. For these individuals reduction of risks includes a neck strengthening program and minimizing contact time in practice. The physical

---

Practice Point

BURNERS AND STINGERS

- Risk factors
  - History of stinger episodes
  - Position—linebacker, fullback
  - Cervical spinal anatomic variations
- Reduction of risk
  - Preseason medical examinations
  - Neck strengthening program
  - Minimizing contact time during practice
  - Teaching blocking and tackling techniques that minimize the use of the head as a major weapon
  - Change position of injury-prone players

---

barrier provided by neck rolls or cervical collars is difficult to quantify. Nevertheless, frequently the addition of one of these devices to the shoulder pads or neck seems to reduce the incidence of burners. Emphasis should be on teaching correct techniques of blocking and tackling that minimize the use of the head as a major weapon; and if these efforts are unsuccessful, consider changing the position of the injury-prone player so he is less at risk.

Changing tackling techniques must be done with care if the desired end result of reducing all neck injuries is to be achieved. Torg et al. estimated that the compressive load limits for cervical vertebral bodies are between 750 and 1000 lb. If this load is reached in an axial compressive mode with the head slightly flexed, a compressive fracture of the vertebral body may occur.[13] Extending the neck to keep the face up may create uneven forces around the cervical vertebrae and is equally difficult to protect by simple muscle contraction. In an attempt to reduce catastrophic injuries, coaches are being encouraged to teach tackling with the head rotated and laterally flexed to prevent using it as a weapon.[13,21] This commonly used hitting position may not be as safe as it seems, though, as the athlete is unable to generate maximum muscle power in this side-flexed rotated position. The impact thus forces the neck beyond its physiologic limit, generating a traction injury, i.e., a "stinger." Emphasis must be placed on contracting the large neck muscles, hunching the shoulders, and

using the arms for initial contact when blocking and tackling in order to reduce the risk of injury.

Burning Hand Syndrome and Neuropraxia of the Cervical Cord

The burning hand syndrome is a transient neurologic deficit first described by Maroon in 1977 and subsequently refined by Wilberger. The syndrome is now recognized as a variant of the central cord syndrome.[38,40] The characteristic complaint is burning paresthesias and dysesthesias in both arms or hands and occasionally in the legs; weakness does not occur. This syndrome differs from the "pinched nerve" or "stinger," which occurs at least once during the career of more than 50 percent of athletes.[45] A stinger or burner is a minor nerve root or brachial plexus stretch injury rather than a spinal cord injury.

Burning hands syndrome is associated with a bony or ligamentous spinal abnormality in approximately 50 percent of affected individuals. Thus any athlete with this syndrome should be treated as having a significant spinal cord injury until proved otherwise. If a spinal injury has been ruled out, somatosensory-evoked potentials may be useful for documenting physiologic cord dysfunction. In some instances MRI can document an anatomic cord abnormality such as swelling or a hyperintense intramedullary lesion.

In 1986 Torg et al.[41] reported on a condition they termed neuropraxis of the cervical cord with associated transient quadriplegia. Torg et al. thought that the cervical spinal films of these individuals showed abnormalities. Of the 32 cases, 17 had developmental cervical canal stenosis: 4 of the 32 athletes showed evidence of ligamentous instability, 6 had acute or chronic intervertebral disk disease, and 5 had congenital cervical anomalies. The quadriplegia lasted 1 minute to 48 hours, and in all cases it resolved completely. MRI was done on only one patient, and no intrinsic cord abnormalities were demonstrated. Based on their findings (Table 19-6) Torg et al. concluded, "The young patient who has had an episode of neuropraxia of the cervical spinal cord, with or without transient quadriplegia, is not predisposed to permanent neurologic injury because of it."[41]

To determine the relative risk of future neurologic consequences to athletes, Ladd and Scranton conducted a retrospective analysis on 117 quadriplegic athletes listed in the National Football Head and Neck Registry.[30] None reported episodes of transient

TABLE 19-6.   Outcome in Athletes with (Neuropraxia) Transient Quadriplegia of the Cord (n = 35)

Of the 17 athletes with developmental cervical spinal stenosis (follow-up 3–5 years)
    9 Stopped all sports after first episode of TQ
    3 Continued sports but stopped after second episode of TQ
    1 Continued sports despite two more episodes of TQ
    3 Continued sports with no subsequent TQ
    1 Underwent laminectomy and returned to sports with no subsequent TQ
Of the 5 athletes with congenital cervical anomaly (follow-up 1–5 years)
    4 Stopped all sports
    1 Returned to sports with no subsequent TQ
Of the 6 athletes with degenerative disc disease (follow-up 1–5 years)
    3 Stopped all sports
    2 Underwent anterior cervical discectomy but did not return to sports
    1 Continued sports with no subsequent TQ
Of the 4 athletes with ligamentous instability (follow-up 1–5 years)
    2 Stopped all sports after first episode of TQ
    1 Stopped all sports after three more episodes of TQ
    1 Continued sports with no subsequent TQ

TQ = transient quadriplegia.
(Adapted from Torg et al.,[41] with permission.)

motor weakness prior to their permanent cord injury; only one reported prior transient sensory symptoms.[50]

When faced with an athlete who has suffered a transient neurologic deficit, a thorough work-up is necessary to rule out bony or ligamentous injury to the spine. Plain cervical spinal films with flexion and extension views are essential. A CT scan, or polytomography, or both may be necessary to evaluate subtle bony injuries. If no bony or ligamentous abnormalities are identified in a patient with transient neurologic deficit, the physician must rule out ongoing extrinsic cord or nerve root compression or intrinsic cord abnormalities. It is most readily accomplished by MRI. Somatosensory-evoked potentials may also help to document physiologic cord dysfunction. Special concerns should be raised if any intrinsic abnormalities are seen on MRI or are documented by somatosensory-evoked potentials, as these results provide direct evidence of an overt, though mild, spinal cord injury and preclude a return to sports. If no evidence of spinal cord injury is found and no bony or ligamentous problems are identified, return to com-

petition is probably safe. A second episode of transient neurologic deficit should initiate another complete work-up. If all the studies remain normal, a return to competition is possible but concern should be raised about the recurrent nature of the problem and consideration given to limiting further athletic activities.

Brachial Plexus Neuritis

Acute brachial neuropathy is an uncommon entity characterized by shoulder pain and disability. Characteristically, the pain is intense and may continue for several hours to 2 to 3 weeks despite rest and analgesics. There is usually no history of trauma, although sometimes the pain follows a bout of intense strenuous activity. The literature also recalls some association with antecedent illness, immunization, exposure to toxic substances, and viral infections. Bergfield et al. reported a series that included athletes in both contact and noncontact sports, all of whom had had an insidious onset of shoulder pain during the sport. None of these athletes, however, could relate it to a specific traumatic episode.[39]

The condition has been described in the literature under a variety of names, including multiple neuritis, localized neuritis of the shoulder girdle, acute brachial radiculitis, Parsonage-Turner syndrome, brachial plexus neuropathy, and paralytic brachial neuritis.[54–58] Weakness either appears with pain or, more often, develops as the pain recedes. The athlete often notices the weakness during activity. A distribution of muscle involvement is variable but usually includes muscles of the shoulder girdle or proximal arm.

Because most of the affected muscles receive their

Clinical Point

ACUTE BRACHIAL NEURITIS

- Onset with contact and noncontact sports
- Rather acute onset of pain
- Not obviously related to trauma
- Severe pain may continue despite rest
- Patches of brachial plexus or peripheral nerve involvement
- Usually dominant arm

innervation via the brachial plexus, particularly the upper trunk, this entity is frequently classified as a brachial plexopathy. However, Bergfield et al. pointed out that the patterns of involvement encountered on EMG examination are not always consistent with such localization. Their series included (1) involvement of muscles that are not innervated by the plexus, e.g., the serratus anterior and trapezius; (2) severe denervation limited to muscles innervated by a single peripheral nerve or two peripheral nerves, e.g., the suprascapular nerve, axillary nerve, or anterior interosseous nerve; (3) severe denervation restricted to a single muscle, with sparing of muscles innervated by the same portion of the plexus or even the same nerve trunk; (4) significant involvement of the motor component of the nerve with sparing of the sensory axons. Occasionally, an individual has more than one attack. Usually laboratory studies are not helpful.

Treatment of the acute brachial neuropathy is divided into two phases. The initial phase includes the time from the onset of symptoms until the resolution of pain. During this phase the extremity is rested, particularly if activity is associated with increased symptoms. Analgesics are given for pain control, and if necessary a sling is used to support and rest the limb. As the pain diminishes, the patient enters a second phase of treatment, which is rehabilitation. Rehabilitation is directed toward increasing the strength and endurance of the muscles that have been involved. Return to sport is usually allowed when the athlete has regained sufficient control of the limb. Intensive training and activity are probably not advisable even though there is rapid recovery; rather, one should wait for the recovery curve to plateau. Although most individuals return to their sport, many report a subjective feeling of residual weakness, and a few retain significant denervation patterns, as indicated by persistent winging of the scapula or poor control of the shoulder girdle.

Levator Scapula Syndrome

The levator scapula syndrome, first described by Moseley in 1945 as the superior scapula syndrome, and a similar disorder, the scapula costal syndrome, reported in 1969 by Shull, may in fact be variations of the previously described brachial neuropathy.[59–61] The levator scapula syndrome is a form of tendinitis in patients with neck, shoulder, and upper back pain. It may be likened in some ways to lateral epicondylitis (tennis elbow) in its etiology and treatment principles. With both conditions, acute or chronic overload mechanisms are present. It is postulated that the inflammation occurs in or near the insertion of the levator scapula tendons.

The levator scapula muscles elevate the scapula while rotating the glenoid cavity downward. It also helps in neck rotation. When both levator scapulae contract together and the origin insertion is reversed, they serve as a rein to neck flexion. The muscle, originating at the transverse processes of the cervical vertebrae C1 – C4, has a broad insertion onto the supermedial border of the scapula. It is innervated by the third and fourth cervical nerve roots and gains its circulation via the transverse and descending cervical arteries (Fig. 19-20).

The syndrome presents as local or generalized pain in the area of the levator scapulae, sometimes precipitated by a direct blow and frequently related to occupations that require carrying heavy objects. Many of the individuals in Estwanik's series had their discomfort aggravated by swimming, wrestling, gymnastics, boxing, karate, weight lifting, sailing, or golf.[59] The pain may appear only during the activity or may be made worse by postural positions or even be present during sleeping.

Physical Examination

Because the levator scapula muscle is deep, the patient is usually unable to pinpoint the site of the pain. If the patient is placed in the prone position with the elbows adducted to support weight on the elbow and forearm, both scapulae protrude, exposing the superomedial border for examination (Fig. 19-21). It should be stressed that the superomedial border of the scapula is normally somewhat tender, so the two sides should be compared before judging the value of the local tenderness. Symmetrically increased tenderness suggests fibromyalgia. Generally, there is a specific point of tenderness at the levator scapula insertion and pressure may precipitate the patient's symptoms. There may be associated areas of trigger point tenderness along the trapezius, but such tenderness is probably related to the chronicity of the symptoms.

The levator scapula syndrome can be clinically confused with many disorders that generate discomfort around the neck and shoulders and the upper back. Thus cervical radiculopathies, cervical spondylosis, fibromyalgia, myofascial syndrome, and referral of

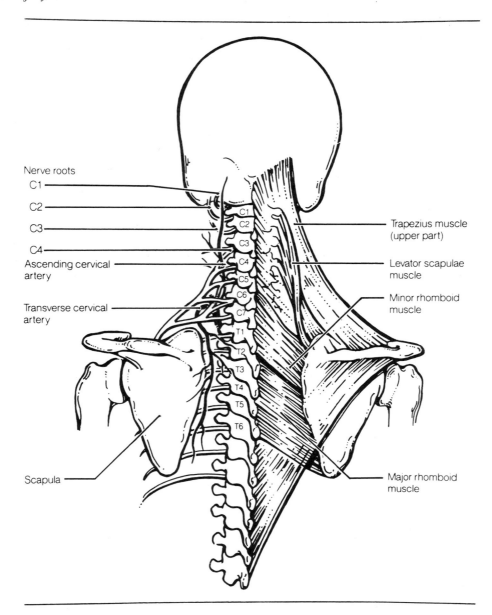

Fig. 19-20. Levator scapula muscles, which originate from the transverse processes of C1–C4. Insertions are at the superomedial border of the scapula, and they are innervated by the third and fourth cervical roots. (Adapted from Estwanik,[59] with permission.)

discomfort due to shoulder pathology must be included in the differential diagnosis.

Treatment

Treatment consists in aggressive stretching and strengthening exercises after initial relief of the most severe symptoms. Such symptoms can be initially re-

duced by nonsteroidal anti-inflammatory drugs (NSAIDs) and physiotherapy in the form of "spray and stretch" (ethyl chloride, ice massage) and phonophoresis. Occasionally, transverse friction to the trigger points is helpful. It must be stressed that the key is stretching of the tight muscles as well as postural correction and ultimately strengthening.

If the patient does not improve rapidly, the most

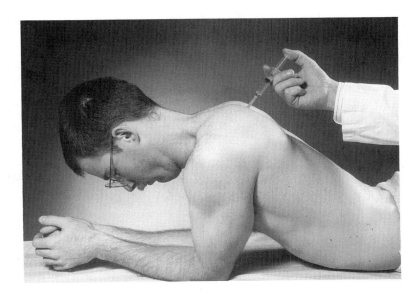

Fig. 19-21. To facilitate examination for the levator scapula syndrome as well as establish a safe position for an injection, the patient assumes a prone position with the elbows adducted so they touch the examination table approximately at shoulder level. This position allows prominence of and access to the medial border of the scapula bilaterally.

tender area can be injected using 1 ml of 1 percent lidocaine (Xylocaine) or 1 ml of 0.25 percent bupivacaine (Marcaine) along with 1 ml of corticosteroid. The position adopted for palpating the tendon can similarly be adopted for the injection techniques (Fig. 19-21). It is important to adopt the position described for the injection, as it reduces the risk of causing a pneumothorax.

In the past this syndrome has been underdiagnosed because it was not well recognized. By the same token it is just as inefficient to overdiagnose it and use it as a catch-all term for all periscapular pain. Finally, pain in this area is occasionally referred from the chest via a lung tumor and from the abdomen secondary to gallbladder disease.

Serratus Anterior Palsy

Serratus anterior palsy is one of the most common exercise- and traction-induced palsies in sport. Classically, the athlete reports a history of feeling weakness of the shoulder girdle specifically with inability to abduct fully. The history may include an activity that is compatible with excessive pressure across the trapezius at the base of the neck, and in this situation it is usually called backpack palsy. Prolonged stretching and pressure over Erb's point may generate paralysis of the muscle and is frequently seen with individuals carrying heavy packs that are poorly loaded. Occasionally, it occurs after a sudden exertion and is accompanied by a feeling of weakness. Thus in weight lifters it is possible that the injury is generated either by a sudden jerking and pulling movement rather than by direct pressure. The serratus anterior nerve is also involved after direct trauma or viral infections. As with many exercise-induced or traction-induced nerve palsies, pain in the area of the neck or shoulder is frequently the presenting complaint.

The physical test that confirms the diagnosis is weakness with protraction of the shoulder. This sign is clearly demonstrated by asking the individual to push with both hands against the wall while leaning forward. The medial border of the scapula immediately becomes prominent.[54] (See Chapter 21.)

Treatment involves de-stressing the muscle while the nerve recovers, which means that the athlete's "workouts" or exercises must be analyzed and undue fatigue and stress to the serratus anterior eliminated. The shoulder should be taken passively through a full range several times a day to maintain capsular dimensions. Attention to posture is important as these individuals tend to develop a small scoliosis secondary to the muscle imbalance. Recovery is usually slow, and a 6 to 12-month period (at least) is usually required to allow the nerve to regenerate. Full recovery is not necessary for excellent or even normal function. Most individuals show permanent evidence of some persisting denervation. Exercises specifically for the serratus anterior are begun when resisted protraction of the shoulder starts to produce a less obvious scapular or chest wall deformity. By this time, reinnervation is usually sufficient to allow benefit from direct exercise.

Acute Torticollis (Cervical Lock Syndrome, Wryneck)

The acute torticollis syndrome is a sudden onset of neck pain resulting in the athlete adopting a "cock robin" attitude of the head with side flexion and rotation. Frequently the athletes are awakened from sleep by the pain or when they wake up in the morning they find that they have an acute, stiff, sore neck. Associated neurologic findings are rare. The etiology is usually unknown; and although there may be a preceding episode of intense activity, sitting in an awkward posture for a period of time, or indeed a minor muscle strain, usually there are no outstanding features in the history. Occasionally, a sore throat or infection of the pharynx is the precipitating cause.

Attempts to move the patient's neck seem to generate more pain and spasm. The manipulative therapy theory suggests that it is primarily the facet joints opposite the side to which the head is flexed that are involved. "Unlocking" these joints is attempted by gentle, oscillatory mobilization of the joint and judiciously applied traction. Treatment is enhanced by muscle relaxants, analgesics, and local application of heat. Worsening of the patient's pain by gentle mobilization constitutes a contraindication for this type of treatment. Failure of this condition to resolve rapidly should generate a search for underlying malignant, inflammatory, or infectious pathology.

Anterior Neck Trauma

Any blow to the anterior neck can cause serious airway compromise due to crushing of the trachea, larynx, and hyoid bone against the unyielding spine with a hammer and anvil "effect." [62,63] Trauma to the larynx and trachea occur most frequently in hockey. Injury may also arise from a hit or blow during soccer, wrestling, or the martial arts (Fig. 19-22). Apart from crushing the anterior structures, late injuries may result from edema, hemorrhage, or laryngospasm. Sharp skate blades used for figure skating or hockey may lacerate the structures of the anterior neck.

Vascular Injury

Although uncommon, there have been several catastrophic injuries caused by a skate blade lacerating the anterior neck. This injury is dramatic, as all of the structures in front of the neck bleed profusely. Should the laceration be sufficiently deep, there is hemorrhage from the jugular vein and even the ca-

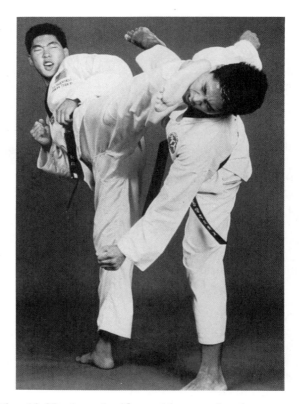

Fig. 19-22. Any significant blow to the throat can cause a subtle but potentially fatal injury, as the airway may be compromised either immediately or over the ensuing hours owing to evolving edema. Voice change, dysphagia, or sudden onset of a cough should raise suspicion. (Photo Jimmy Kim, All Sport 1989, with permission.)

Quick Facts

SPORTS ASSOCIATED WITH LARYNGEAL INJURY (50 Cases)[a]

- Hockey   40
- Football   4
- Softball   3
- Soccer   1
- Wrestling   1
- Lacrosse   1
- Gymnastics   1

([a] Data from McCutcheon and Anderson.[62])

rotid system. The incidence of this injury could be reduced by wearing a throat protector wrapped around the neck or by a more rigid system that requires a face mask and helmet.

If this injury should occur, prompt attention can be life-saving. The major concern is to stem the rapid flow of blood and exsanguination, which is usually achievable simply by direct pressure followed promptly by an assessment of the status of the airway. If the airway is involved, it may be necessary to carry out an emergency cricothyreotomy (insertion of a large-gauge needle). Once pressure over the bleeding area has been applied, it should not be released, and the first-aider and victim should remain together during rapid transport to hospital before the wound is reinspected. In cases of lesser bleeding, experienced therapists or medical personnel may elect to explore the wound rapidly and reposition the pressure more effectively. Preferably, sterile material is applied to the wound followed by direct manual pressure. Unless good visualization is achieved and the helping individual has surgical experience, it is often dangerous to clamp a bleeding neck wound blindly. Only a cool head and rapid action can save an individual bleeding profusely from a deep neck wound.

Practice Point

MASSIVE BLEEDING FROM THE NECK

- Firm, accurate pressure that is maintained until transport to a medical facility may be life-saving.

Laryngeal and Tracheal Injury

Anatomy

The larynx and trachea are bounded anteriorly by the strap muscles and skin, laterally by the sternomastoid muscles, and posteriorly by the esophagus and cervical vertebrae.[64] The larynx consists of a framework of cartilage that supports and protects the upper airway and vocal cords (Fig. 19-23). Although the hyoid bone is not an anatomic division of the larynx, it is an important supporting structure for the upper airway, as are the cartilages of the trachea. Specialized respiratory mucous membrane forms the inner lining of the pharynx, larynx, and trachea.

Several anatomic spaces lie between this membranous lining and the underlying muscles, nerves, blood vessels, cartilages, and ligaments. After trauma, these spaces are prone to edema and hemorrhage, which may obstruct the airway or interfere with the vocal cords and thus the voice.

Mechanism of Injuries

Blunt impact to the anterior larynx may crush it and cause fractures of the cartilaginous structures. This injury occurs more easily when the neck is in a hyperextended position. Because it is the most prominent structure, the thyroid cartilage (Adam's apple) is the most commonly injured cartilage. The symptoms may be obvious immediately and may range from mild changes in voice or respiration to life-threatening obstruction. On the other hand, the symptoms may be delayed, caused by accumulating edema. This situation often presents as the dangerous scenario of a young athlete leaving the field of play to return home, only to get into increasing respiratory difficulty en route. As the swelling starts to impede respiration, panic and agitation cause an increase in respiratory rate, compounding the problem and producing an increasingly severe emergency situation. Edema is usually maximal within 6 hours, but it may occur as long as 24 to 48 hours after the injury. Thus late airway obstruction as the result of edema or a developing and expanding hematoma must always be considered and the individual warned appropriately.

Practice Point

INJURIES TO THE TRACHEA OR LARYNX

- Symptoms may be delayed as edema or hemorrhage accumulate.
- Laryngeal spasm may effectively close the larynx.
- Breathing may be obstructed.
- There may be a life-threatening situation.

If the athlete does not have significant obvious signs of fracture or discontinuity of the airway, the most important initial measure is reassurance. The head should be placed in a chin-up position to straighten the airway. If there has been a sufficient

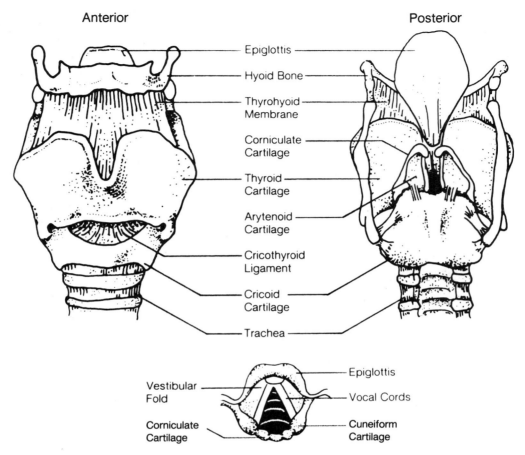

Fig. 19-23. Anatomy of the laryngeal area. (After McCutcheon and Anderson,[62] with permission.)

contusion, application of an ice pack may be appropriate.

Sudden inability to breathe produces immediate panic, and the athlete becomes agitated. Reassurance therefore is a major part of the treatment. If the athlete has any effective respiration, administration of oxygen is helpful. If the degree of obstruction is sufficient to make respiration ineffective or if there is increasing subcutaneous emphysema, confirming the discontinuity of the airway, it is necessary to establish an artificial airway immediately. Airway obstruction for more than 4 minutes may cause brain damage. Because the obstruction is usually below the oral cavity, an oral airway is ineffective. An inexperienced person should not try to intubate an agitated player lying on the ice or playing field, as it is a difficult maneuver and may stimulate further laryngeal obstruction and spasm. Moreover, the tube often is inserted in the esophagus, compounding the problem.

Tracheostomy, usually lower than the second tracheal ring, is desirable. It establishes an airway below the level of obstruction and avoids disruption of the injured area. However, this procedure may require half an hour and is best done in the surgical environment by an experienced individual. Hence the physician or therapist at the scene of the accident may need to carry out a cricothyreotomy.[62,64]

Laryngospasm

Laryngospasm may occur reflexively after traumatic stimulation of visceral nerve endings in the abdomen or thorax or secondary to a direct blow to the front of the neck. Spasm of the adductor muscles of the true vocal cords pulls them tightly together in a shutter-like fashion.[64] At the same time, the pre-epiglottic muscles become rounded and pressed against the upper surface of the false vocal cords in

Practice Point

SIGNS AND SYMPTOMS OF TRACHEAL OR LARYNGEAL INJURY

- Shortness of breath (dyspnea)
- Loss of voice (aphonia) or hoarseness
- Hemorrhage with blood-tinged sputum
- Local pain and tenderness
- Cough
- Loss of contour of the Adam's apple (thyroid cartilage)
- Subcutaneous emphysema
- If obstruction
  -Dyspnea (shortness of breath)
  -Stridor (difficult respiration)
  -Cyanosis (blue lips and forehead)
  -Loss of consciousness

the manner of a ball and valve, causing complete obstruction.[65]

Clinically, the athlete is agitated, may thrash around, and with persistent spasm becomes cyanotic and may even lose consciousness. These individuals are aphonic and may even be unable to cough. If only the shutter mechanism is occurring, the athlete may have stridorous respiration. First aid includes forcing

Practice Point

IMMEDIATE TREATMENT OF ANTERIOR NECK TRAUMA OR SPASM

- Ensure airway.
- If obvious deformity, manually straighten airway.
- Pull chin forward by tilting angle of jaw to relieve laryngospasm.
- Pull tongue forward to stretch hyoepiglottic ligament.
- If life-threatening airway obstruction is not relieved by above, perform emergency cricothyreotomy: Insert 14–18 gauge needle through cricothyroid ligament.

the chin forward by strong pressure behind the angle of the jaw. This forward movement is transmitted to the hyoid bone and hyo-epiglottic ligament, pulling it away from the false cords and opening the laryngeal passage. Another neck maneuver, advocated by some anesthesiologists, is to grasp the base of the tongue, pulling it forward and thereby stretching the hyo-epiglottic ligament and breaking the ball- and-valve effect. As the spasm starts to relax, usually within a minute, a loud inspiratory, crowing sound is heard.[62] Delivering 100 percent oxygen by mask helps the patient recover more rapidly. No attempts should be made to suction the oropharynx, as the catheter may trigger another laryngeal spasm. Once the athlete has recovered from this emergency situation, rapid transit to hospital is important.

Cricothyreotomy

Cricothyreotomy is used for the emergency treatment of laryngeal injuries where the airway is obstructed. The patient's head is placed in the chin-up position with a rolled towel under the neck. The thyroid cartilage prominence is identified with the forefinger of the nondominant hand, and the fingers slide down the midline to the lower margin of the thyroid cartilage.

The site of incision is the midpoint of the membrane that runs from this point to the upper margin of the cricoid cartilage caudally (Fig. 19-24). If materials are immediately available, the area is swabbed with povidone-iodine (Betadine). If the individual is alert and conscious, the area is injected with local anesthetic subcutaneously or sprayed with ethyl chloride. With the thumb and middle finger of the nondominant hand on either side of the airway to stabilize the cricothyroid membrane, a vertical incision is made in the midline 1 to 2 cm through the skin and then an incision through the cricothyroid membrane itself. As the blade pops through the cricothyroid membrane, it is turned 90 degrees to spread the incision. A small clamp or surgical scissors can be put into the wound to enlarge the incision. Great care is taken to avoid damaging the posterior wall of the larynx. At this point, a number 5 or 6 (7 to 9 mm) tracheotomy tube can be inserted (Fig. 19-24). The tracheostomy tube stylet is removed, and the tube is secured with ties to avoid external dislodgement. Free side-to-side movement of the tracheostomy tube and audible movement of air through the tube indicate a good position.

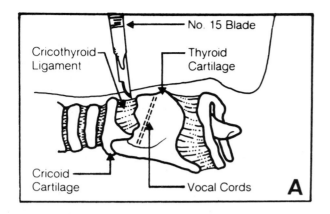

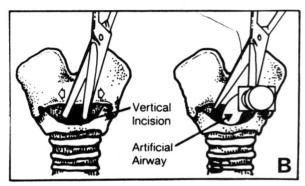

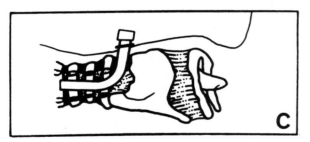

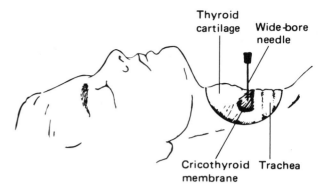

Fig. 19-25. If it is not possible to remove the upper airway obstruction, consideration is given to insertion of a wide-bore needle through the cricothyroid membrane into the trachea.

An emergency cricothyreotomy cannula is available that needs no equipment and can be inserted within minutes. It consists of a 7-gauge curved trocar with a tip sharp enough to be pushed through the cricothyroid membrane. The sharp tip is retracted to avoid mucosal laceration after incision of the trocar to a specific mark (approximately 0.5 inch up the barrel of the tube). The tube is then gently inserted in a manner similar to that for inserting the tracheostomy tube.[62] It should be remembered that a large (18 gauge or larger) needle inserted just above the sternal notch by any person on the scene can be lifesaving, and it is a relatively simple procedure (Fig. 19-25).

Obstructed Airway

Should an athlete inhale gum, tobacco, tooth shield, or any other foreign material, the Heimlich maneuver may be appropriate. The resuscitator assumes a position behind the individual, supporting the patient's body as it leans forward (Fig. 19-26). Place the fist, thumbside in against the soft area above the navel and below the rib cage. Cover the fist with the other hand and push quickly inward and upward to expel air from the lungs. If this maneuver is not effective, a needle tracheostomy can be carried out as described in the previous section.

SPINAL FRACTURES

Epidemiology

Sports and recreationally induced spinal fractures have received relatively little attention in view of the potentially serious impact they may have on the life of

Fig. 19-24. Procedure for inserting a cricothyroid airway. **(A)** Cricothyroid ligament incised. **(B)** Airway inserted. **(C)** Airway in place with stylet removed. (After McCutcheon and Anderson,[62] with permission.)

Cricothyreotomy is better than an emergency "tracheotomy," as the landmarks are easily identified even in the heavily muscled or obese neck. Moreover, bleeding is less because there are no major vital vessels in the midline. The thyroid gland is avoided as well. The procedure also requires less experience and if performed efficiently can be completed in 1 to 2 minutes. The disadvantage is that with some subepiglottic injuries the artificial airway is not below the level of obstruction.

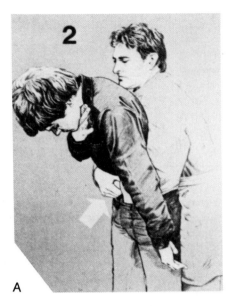

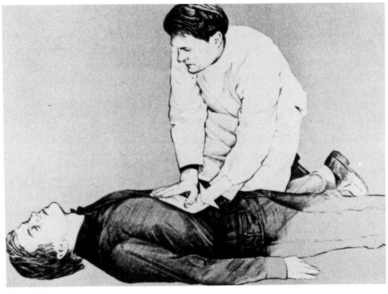

Fig. 19-26. Emergency procedures for assisting clearance of an obstructed airway. Heimlich maneuver. **(A)** Place a fist in the soft area above the navel. Cover with other hand. Give one or several sharp thrusts inwards and upwards to expel object. **(B)** The same maneuver done with the athlete lying.

the individual.[66-70] Some of these injuries result directly from equipment or permissible techniques within the sport and therefore allow for modification of rules and equipment should statistics prove a definite causal relation.[66-72] Furthermore, there has been a suggestion that the incidence of spinal fractures is perhaps increasing, and therefore the epidemiology and pathomechanics of these injuries become in-

creasingly important so preventive measures may be instituted.[73-77]

In our series of 1,081 spinal fractures, 134 (12 percent) were sport or recreationally induced[20] (Table 19-7). Of the population surveyed, 262 patients had neurologic deficits. Indeed although sports and recreation comprised the fourth most common cause of spinal fractures, it was the second common-

TABLE 19-7. Cause of Spinal Injury

Cause	Absolute No.	Percent of All Causes	Associated Neural Deficit		
			Absolute No.	Percent of Cause with Defect	Percent of All Defects
MVA	579	53	146	25	56
Occupational	171	16	43	25	16
Domestic	159	15	9	6	3
Sport/recreational	134	12	53	40	21
Others	38	4	11	29	4
Total	1,081	100	262		

MVA = motor vehicle accident.

est cause of patients becoming paralyzed, temporarily or permanently[20] (Fig. 19-27). Tator and Palm reported that 34 percent of neurologically associated spinal fractures were due to motor vehicle accidents, 29 percent were work-related injuries, and 15 percent were due to sports and recreation.[78]

Specific Sports

Diving

Diving is the sport with the highest incidence of spinal fractures. Alarmingly, many of these fractures have been associated with neurologic deficiencies (Table 19-8). In our series, considering only those with neurologic problems, we have a corrected figure of 45 percent of all sports-related injuries being due to diving; and they comprise 9.2 percent of spinal cord injuries from all causes. This figure compares to

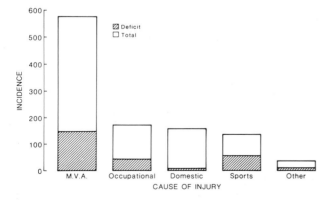

Fig. 19-27. Although sports- and recreation-induced spinal fractures rank only fourth in frequency, they are the second most frequent cause of injury with associated neurologic deficit. M.V.A. = motor vehicle accident.

the 10.4 percent reported by Tator in Eastern Canada, 14 percent by Sutton, and 8.3 percent by Cheshire from Australia.[79-80] In areas of the world with less sunshine and fewer private pools for water sports, accidents on lakes and rivers tend to occur at a lower frequency[56-59] (Table 19-9).

The average diving injury is a cervical fracture, usually between C4 and C6, with an associated complete motor and sensory lesion and a poor prognosis for functionally useful recovery. It is this last fact that makes it such a disastrous statistic (Table 19-8). Diving off a beach, a pier, or into a private pool is the commonest cause of this injury. The mechanism is

---

Practice Point

GUIDELINES FOR REDUCING DIVING INJURIES

- Do not dive into water shallower than twice your height.
- Do not dive into unfamiliar water.
- Check out first what is underneath the surface.
- Do not assume the water is deep enough.
- Remember the influence of tides on water depth.
- Do not dive near dredging or construction work, as water levels change and dangerous objects may be underneath the surface.
- Do not dive until area is clear of other swimmers.
- Do not drink and dive.
- Limit horseplay to safe areas, not as part of diving.

TABLE 19-8. Sport/Recreation Activity as a Cause of Spine Trauma

Sport/Recreation	Absolute Frequency (No.)	%	% With Neurologic Deficit for Particular Sport	
			Absolute Frequency (No.)	%
Diving	34	25	24	71
Snowmobile	16	12	7	44
Equestrian	16	12	4	25
Parachute/ skydiving[a]	14	10	3	21
All-terrain vehicles[b]	12	9	4	33
Toboggan	11	8	1	10
Bicycle	4	4	1	25
Rugby	4	4	1	25
Ice hockey	3	2	1	33
Downhill skiing	3	2	1	33
Surfing	3	2	1	33
Football	2	1	0	0
Mountaineering	2	1	1	50
Other[c]	10	8	4	40
Total	134	100	53	

[a] Includes hang-gliding and ultralight plane.
[b] Includes motocross racing, dirt-biking and all-terrain (three-wheel) vehicular sports; each with four cases.
[c] Includes only one case of trampoline injury.

usually striking the bottom, invariably secondary to there being insufficient depth of water. Alcohol abuse often contributes to poor judgment. The fact that the increasing incidence of diving injuries is mostly due to accidents in private pools, often with the complicating feature of alcohol ingestion, points to the potential preventability of these injuries with adequate supervision and responsibility.

Indeed the dangers of private pools have not been emphasized enough when we add the statistics of infant mortality to those associated with neck injury. For instance, in Arizona, a landlocked desert, drowning is the number one cause of death for children under the age of 4 years.[79] It is obvious that most of these injuries are preventable, and public education programs could play an important role, particularly as there are indications that these injuries are increasing and are typically severe if not death-causing. Indeed, a group of Florida neurosurgeons have embarked on an aggressive educational campaign aimed mainly at teenagers using a "Feet First—First Time" slogan. They claimed to have reduced the incidence of spinal cord injury by 40 percent in the Florida area. Even though expensive, this type of campaign will ultimately be cost-effective if it is successful. Furthermore, perhaps some considerations should be given to different pool designs and construction. Any diver can hit the bottom from a high dive, irrespective of

TABLE 19-9. Diving as Cause of Traumatic Spinal Cord Injury[a]

Site	Study (First Author)	Total Cases (All Causes)	Percent Due To	
			Sport	Diving
USA	Key[80]	318	5.0	2.2
Norway	Zrubecky 1974[a]	725	8.2	4.4
England	Krause[81]	619	6.9	5.3
Austria	Gione 1974[a]	112	10.7	8.0
Australia (Victoria)	Cheshire 1967	325	12.6	8.3
Alberta	Reid 1991[1]	262	21.0	9.2
Ontario	Tator[78]	358	15.4	10.6
Australia (Brisbane)	Sutton 1973[a]	207	17.9	14.0

[a] Other areas taken from papers by Krutzke[82] and Tator and Palm.[78]

depth. There is thus a need to teach "avoidance maneuvers" to be practiced immediately upon hitting the water. The ability to use these moves with high dives comes with training and experience.

Snowmobile Accidents

Snowmobile accidents account for about 12 percent of spinal fractures, and 44 percent of these individuals have associated spinal cord injuries.[70,84,85] These statistics are important because along with head injuries spinal cord injuries are the major cause of morbidity. Wenzel and Peters reported that cervical fracture was implicated in 20 percent of the fatal injuries.[83] Other contributing factors to significant injury are alcohol abuse, inadequate lighting, young drivers, and driving in illegal areas. In one study, 21 percent of the fractures were in people who had been drinking. In Wenzel and Peters' report alcohol was involved in 61 percent of the fatalities. It is of particular concern that many of these injuries are occurring in young individuals[83] (Table 19-10).

Equestrian Injuries

It is estimated that more than 80 million people in North America ride a horse at least once annually and about two million of these riders are under the age of

20 years.[87] Furthermore, about 25 percent of these injuries are associated with spinal cord and cauda equina damage, with one-third involving the cervical spine and two-thirds the thoracolumbar junction (Table 19-11). A particularly large number of horses are available around farming communities, where, additionally, rodeo riding is a popular sport. Special note should be made, however, that show jumping and recreational horse riding account for a significant percentage of the injuries, despite the apparent risk that at first glance seems to be associated with the rodeo. Perhaps these experienced riders developed techniques of falling that help protect the spine. It is important that head or facial trauma accounts for more than half the injuries, and 80 percent of these individuals sustain a closed head injury. If an effective, properly secured helmet, which is readily available, were worn, most of these severe head injuries could be prevented.[87]

All-Terrain Vehicles

The emergence of the all-terrain vehicle as an important factor in spinal fractures is worrying. Motocross racing and dirt-bikes also contribute to the statistic. With the all-terrain vehicles the main mechanism of injury is falling over backward, supporting the concept that the all-terrain vehicle is an inherently unstable machine. Furthermore, because parents seem to consider these vehicles almost as toys, unless more safety standards are introduced and the hazards of these machines are fully outlined the general public is likely to continue to believe in the exaggerated situations depicted in the advertisements of these motor vehicles, and the incidence of associated spinal trauma in young people will continue to rise.

Football

The low frequency of football-related spinal fractures reflects a steady improvement.[66,67,79,84,85] When spinal fractures do occur, the mechanism is usually axial loading with the cervical spine slightly flexed (Fig. 19-28). Axial loading occurs when the head is stopped, the trunk is still moving, and the spine is crushed between the two. From 1976 to 1987, about 49 percent of nonquadriplegic cervical spinal injuries and 52 percent of the quadriplegic injuries were attributed to this mechanism. In the past, the fractures were often produced by the fulcrum supplied by a single-bar face mask giving the hyperflexion injury of

TABLE 19-10. Spinal Cord Injury by Age

Sport	Mean (Yrs)	SD	Range
Diving	22.00	5.85	12–39
Equestrian	35.81	11.69	17–52
Snowmobile	26.93	7.71	12–39
Parachute/skydiving	26.00	5.72	19–41
All-terrain vehicle	27.33	9.35	16–46
Toboggan	20.82	9.29	8–35
Bicycle	42.00	26.91	12–64
Rugby	26.75	2.50	24–30
Downhill skiing	18.33	6.81	13–26
Ice hockey	19.33	4.51	15–24
Surfing	40.00	17.06	26–59
Mountaineering	24.00	5.66	20–28
Football	17.00	1.41	16–18
Soccer	24.00[a]		
Water skiing	28.00[a]		
Frisbee	27.00[a]		
Dancing	14.00[a]		
Badminton	72.00[a]		
Caber throw	50.00[a]		
Trampoline	5.00[a]		
Wrestling	20.00[a]		
Rope swing	21.00[a]		

[a] One subject only.

TABLE 19-11. Sport/Recreation by Spinal Level

Sport	Absolute Frequency		Thoraco/lumbar
	C1–C3	C4–C7	
Diving	2	30	2
Equestrian	1	5	10
Snowmobile	0	3	13
Parachute/skydiving	0	0	14
All-terrain vehicle	0	4	8
Toboggan	1	2	8
Bicycle	1	1	2
Rugby	0	3	1
Ice hockey	0	2	1
Downhill skiing	0	0	3
Surfing	1	2	0
Football	0	1	1
Mountaineering	0	0	2
Other	0	5	5
Total	6	58	70

Schneider as well as a hyperextension mechanism where the back of the football helmet forms a guillotine. These injuries have gradually been eliminated owing to changes in equipment manufacturing and fitting. Most importantly, the rules eliminating spearing, head butting, and face tackling have also had a significant impact on decreasing the frequency of serious neurologic injuries.[27,74] It is believed that axial compression is responsible for similar injuries occurring in other collision sports. The success of the preventive measures in football based on an understanding of how the injury occurs should serve as a model for similar studies in other risky sports.

In our series alone, the incidence of permanent quadriplegia decreased from 34 cases in 1976 to a low of 5 cases in 1984, illustrating the potential efficacy of preventive programs involving rule and equipment changes.[85] In addition, the importance of cervical musculature strength has been repeatedly emphasized and incorporated more frequently into the preseason training programs as well as the ongoing conditioning exercises during the season. These rule changes and training techniques are particularly important for those in the younger age group. Although it is conceivable that neck rolls may play a minor role in protecting against spinal root traction injuries, they offer little protection against cord damage secondary to fracture and fracture-dislocation.

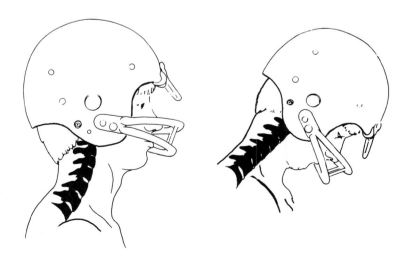

Fig. 19-28. When the neck is in the normal upright anatomic position, the cervical spine is slightly extended because of the natural cervical lordosis. When the neck is flexed to approximately 30 degrees, the cervical spine is straight and thus converted to a segmented column. In this position, loading tends to produce a burst-type injury. (Adapted from Torg et al.,[68] with permission.)

Rugby

Rugby spinal trauma has been widely researched and its high frequency reported.[67,75,86,88] In North America these figures are still relatively low, but in Britain, New Zealand, and Australia, where rugby is one of the sports played most frequently at all levels of school and community, the incidence is higher.[69,75,77] These injuries are often of sufficient severity to cause either death or complete quadriplegia. Unfortunately, there is a suggestion that the incidence is increasing.

The most vulnerable age for the rugby player is between 15 and 21, and the injury is often related to aggressive and dangerous play, particularly in the scrums. The front row of players are most vulnerable, particularly when the scrum collapses and the players are unable to extricate themselves. The arms are trapped above shoulder level, and the neck is frequently forced into hyperflexion. For this reason, new rules have been introduced for the under-nine-teens to "de-power" the scrums, rucks, and mauls. These rules have been adopted for international competition as well. The rule changes include keeping the head and shoulders above the level of the hips in the scrum, no charging, and penalties assessed for collapsing, popping, and wheeling. The importance of these rule changes cannot be overemphasized when it is appreciated that worldwide rugby along with diving is the number one cause of sport and recreational spinal fractures.

Neck strengthening needs to be emphasized far more in rugby, as frequently injuries occur at slower velocities than with other sports and are more amenable to prevention. The neck can be significantly strengthened: A gain in circumference of 3 cm in 6 weeks is possible.[40,42]

Ice Hockey

Tator, in a national survey of spinal cord injuries in hockey players, concluded that the incidence is possibly rising.[96] He estimated that, on a per capita basis, hockey in Canada now causes approximately twice as many cases of quadriplegia annually as does football in the United States. There has been much speculation about the reason for the sudden surge of hockey-related spinal trauma including larger, stronger players, changes in attitudes of the coaches and referees, and improved helmets and face masks leading to a false sense of security.[73,89] Although the hockey helmet does protect the skull, it does not appreciably alter the dynamics of the neck during a collision.[90] Inevitably, the mechanism of injury is an axial load during flexion as the individual collides with the boards. Ice hockey has implemented a new rule forbidding checking from behind into boards as well as stricter enforcement of boarding, cross-checking, and other stick penalties. There has also been a serious effort to educate people involved in hockey — players, coaches, and referees — as to the seriousness of the problem.

Trampolining and Gymnastics

At one point it appeared that trampolining would produce an ever increasing number of spinal injuries.[53] A virtual ban of trampolines in the school system and better ways of spotting, improved techniques, and more safety rules have led to a decreasing incidence. Inasmuch as trampolines are often used by gymnasts and divers to practice difficult moves, an ongoing appreciation of the safety precautions must be present.

Skydiving

Spinal injuries with skydiving are mainly thoracolumbar fractures. Parachuters usually land feet first, with the feet together to absorb the shock of the fall. This landing technique involves slight flexion of the hips and spine and sudden rotation to the side while rolling to the ground. Thus the mechanism of injury theoretically usually involves flexion and rotation, producing either a wedge compression or a burst-type fracture. Many recreational skydivers have relatively little training prior to their first dives; and despite advertisements to the contrary, many are ill-equipped to carry out this type of recreational activity without additional training.[91]

Recognizing Spinal Injury

With the excitement and tension of sporting competition, it is easy to overlook a serious vertebral fracture[12,38] (Fig. 19-29). It is important to recognize that all fractures may not be associated with neurologic injury. In fact, a surprising degree of displacement of the spine may be present without an initial neurologic deficit (Fig. 19-30).

Careful palpation for pain in the midline over the spinous processes, undue spasm and discomfort, or any palpable defect must be treated as a spinal fracture until proved otherwise. Bilateral pain, pins and

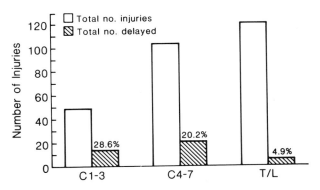

Fig. 19-29. Despite good clinical signs and frequently evidence on roentgenographic films, the incidence of missed diagnosis of cervical spinal injuries is unacceptably high by the person initially assessing the patient.

Clinical Point

SPINE FRACTURES

Even significantly displaced spinal fractures may not be associated with paralysis.

needles, or numbness in the hands is usually indicative of a more severe injury and should not be treated merely as a "pinched nerve" syndrome. Furthermore, bilateral or unilateral leg or foot dysesthesia after cervical injury should be considered evidence of spinal cord damage until proved otherwise, as should persistent unilateral tingling or numbness. Any player who has received a cervical spine injury should

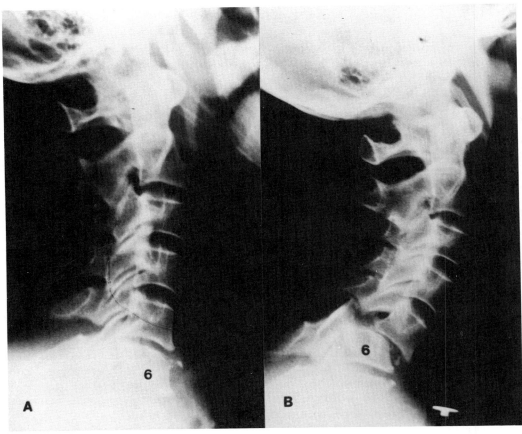

Fig. 19-30. Fracture was initially overlooked in this patient. **(A)** There was loss of the C5 disc space and a small fragment anteriorly. **(B)** Two weeks later this man presented with increasing pain and weakness in his arms. Bilateral facet dislocation is evident. Had he returned to his sport of horse polo, the result might have been catastrophic.

not be moved on the field until a complete interrogation or assessment has been carried out on the spot and the examiner is convinced a major injury does not exist. If one adheres to these rules, the risk of getting into the unpleasant and disastrous situation of being party to furthering neurologic injury in an already injured athlete should be minimized. Great caution is urged with the initial movement after injury. It is tragic that a missed diagnosis may endanger a neurologically intact individual to secondary neurologic deterioration.

Conclusion

In North America, there are approximately 30 cases of acute spinal cord injury due to sports-related trauma annually for every one million people. Because approximately half of these injuries result in complete quadriplegia, the economic burden to society approaches a phenomenal figure, which of course does not take into account the human suffering.[78,82,92-95]

A significant percentage of spinal trauma occurs as a result of recreational activity in sports. Although diving features among the most frequent etiologic factor of the high association of spinal cord injury, rugby, equestrian activities, hockey, and to some degree football share the load. Public education is obviously essential. The incidence of snowmobile and all-terrain vehicular injuries is rising continually, and there is a worrisome statistic of associated alcohol abuse and young, inexperienced drivers. Rule changes in football have proved successful, and there is hope that the changes in rugby and hockey will achieve the same results. The catastrophic nature of spinal trauma with spinal cord injury cannot be overemphasized, and an awareness of the frequency can alert the medical staff attending sporting events of the ever present need to be careful when assessing injured athletes before moving them, thereby avoiding the risk of compounding an already serious situation.

Principles of Moving a Spine-Injured Athlete

Proper organization of emergency treatment and turning of the spinal injured athlete requires experience and practice. The method depends on whether the athlete is conscious or unconscious and the environment in which the accident has taken place. There are special problems related to accidents in the swimming pool or water, on the ice surface in hockey, and

on the spongy landing surfaces of a jumping pit; the pads and helmets of football and hockey players and the triage of skiers on the ski slopes also require special attention.

Quick Facts

PREPARATION FOR HANDLING EMERGENCIES

- Ensure that appropriate equipment on site — or its accessibility.
- Ensure that plan for evacuation is in place.
  - Phone numbers
  - Access plan
  - Communication links
- Make sure personnel are properly trained for nuances of environment, sport, and equipment.

Essentially, the first thing that must be done is to establish that there is a patent airway and the level of consciousness by direct questioning and examination. Then reassure the individual while at the same time asking about sensation and ability to move the limbs. The most experienced person present should take command. The head and neck is stabilized while a primary screen is carried out to assess the extent of the injury. If necessary, turning is then organized. This step must be done with adequate personnel and preferably with a spinal board or stretcher and equipment to stabilize the head and neck once the athlete is transferred to the board.

Practice Point

EMERGENCY MANAGEMENT OF SPINAL INJURIES

- Establish airway patency.
- Most experienced person takes command.
- Stabilize head.
- Carry out primary screen.
- Send for ambulance.
- Organize turning.
- Carry out secondary screen.
- Check if adequately stabilized.

Someone should have already been sent to arrange for evacuation. Prior arrangement should have been made regarding the necessary details of location and access to an ambulance. When turning and transferring are completed and the individual is stabilized on the spinal board or stretcher, a secondary screen is carried out to ensure that other significant injuries have not been overlooked. Certainly with many high speed sports there is a close association of spinal fracture with peripheral injuries.

Rescue Techniques in the Water

As soon as it is established that somebody is seriously hurt in the water, the lifeguard or person in charge should ask all other individuals to carefully and slowly clear the pool, making as little disturbance and as few waves as possible. Frequently, spine-injured or unconscious persons are lying head down, so the first task is to turn them in order to make them float face up as quickly as possible to prevent drowning. At the same time, the head and neck must be aligned to prevent further damage. The maintenance of alignment can make all the difference between an individual being neurologically intact or seriously paralyzed after sustaining a spinal cord injury. There is a vast difference in recovery potential between incomplete and complete neurologic situations.

There are two basic techniques used to stabilize the head. The newest method is called the head splint technique. The rescuer brings the victim's arms forward along the head (Fig. 19-31). The victim's upper arms should be *pressed* against the head to create a splint. While moving the victim forward in the water, the victim's torso should be rotated toward the rescuer bringing the head to rest in the crooked arm until help arrives or until the spinal board can be slid into the water. With the assistance of several others, the injured athlete can then be transferred onto the board.

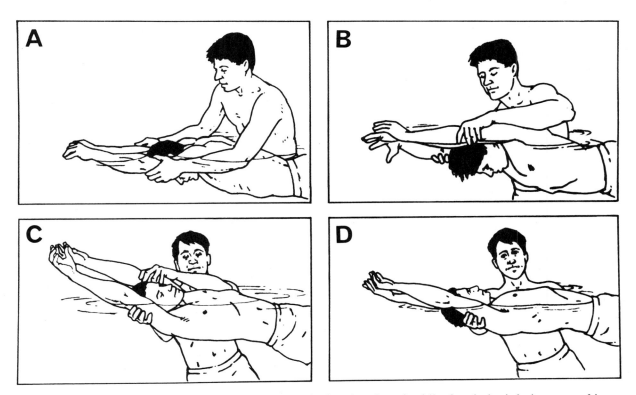

Fig. 19-31. Head splint technique immobilizes the head and neck while the victim is being turned in the water. **(A)** Rescuer extends the victim's arms forward alongside the head. **(B)** Victim's arms are pressed against the head to create a splint. **(C)** Victim is moved forward while rotating his torso. **(D)** Victim's head is brought to rest in the crook of the rescuer's arms. As the turning process proceeds, the rescuer lowers himself into the water to help maintain the splinting action and to facilitate a smooth turn. (From Samples,[95] with permission.)

The second technique, the head and chin support, has been used for some time. It requires a little more practice. The rescuer places one forearm under the victim and along the sternum with the hands supporting the chin. The rescuer's other forearm is placed along the victim's spine with the hands supporting the back of the head. Thus the front and back of the victim's torso and the front and back of the head are held in the vice supplied by the rescuer's forearms and hands. Careful turning is then carried out.

Spinal boards and cervical collars should be standard equipment at any pool. Unfortunately, many of these injuries occur away from public swimming facilities, in private pools where appropriate equipment is not available. The emergency personnel should be ready to perform artificial respiration; and because there are frequent respiratory problems, the rescuer might be tempted to hyperextend the victim's neck to open the airway and perform the appropriate respiration. The neck should be kept immobile; and preferably, instead of hyperextending it the rescuer should place his or her fingers behind the angle of the mandible and pull up on both sides of the jaw to open the airway (jaw thrust).[92]

Football

The large shoulder pads of football prevent adequate use of a simple cervical collar. Furthermore, they wedge the shoulders high, so removal of a helmet allows the head to flop back into hyperextension. For this reason it is probably better not to remove the helmet unless there is difficulty of ventilation or an open head injury is suspected. The face mask is removed rapidly, the individual reassured, and after careful placement on a spinal board the helmet is left in place and used as part of the securing mechanism of the head. It can be removed when the individual arrives at the emergency department of the hospital.

Ice Hockey

The ice surface presents a surprisingly difficult challenge for individuals who have never practiced turning a hockey player on the slippery surface. Once again, it is difficult to apply most of the cervical collars available because of the back of shoulder pads. For this reason, it is probably better not to remove the helmet unless it is necessary to do so because of some other indication such as respiration or head injury.

The hockey helmet is not as large as the football helmet, and it may be necessary to put some padding underneath to prevent the head from falling back.

The small child, although not often sustaining a spinal cord injury, has a disproportionately large head, which has the same effect as a helmet worn without shoulder pads: It therefore thrusts the head forward into flexion. Thus in a young individual, it might be necessary to put padding under the shoulders and torso to keep the head in the neutral position as far as flexion and extension are concerned.

THORACOLUMBAR SPINE

The extremes of spinal motion are commonplace in many sporting activities, sometimes under heavy loading and sometimes at great velocities. It is little wonder, then, that back pain is a frequent complaint among athletes. Unfortunately, it can be a significant disabling problem.

In many athletes low back pain resolves within 1 to 2 weeks without seeking medical care. Those who do seek evaluation usually have had a significant problem for many weeks or months. Often they have tried to continue in their sport until they are no longer capable of performing. When this approach fails they turn to the therapist or physician for help with what is now often a chronic and difficult problem. At this point, a thorough understanding of the differential diagnosis, careful history and physical examination, correct diagnostic procedures, and a functional rehabilitation program frequently lead to an earlier return of the athlete to their sport.

The healthy spine is capable of withstanding enormous stress, seemingly without ill effects. By contrast, once the spine has undergone some adverse structural, postural, or degenerative changes, it becomes a temperamental unit that may respond unpredictably, even to the most minor stress. Thus a reasonable question is: "What makes a spine healthy?" There is no simple answer, but good muscle strength on all of

---

Quick Facts

WHAT MAKES A SPINE HEALTHY

- Genetics
- Muscle strength and muscle balance
- Flexibility
- Posture
- Body weight
- Adaptation to stresses

the trunk musculature, adequate flexibility, a mechanically sound posture, and reasonable body weight are important factors. Gradual adaptation to specific tasks and demands is also crucial. Above all, however, is the genetically dictated makeup of the spine, with all of the immeasurable subtleties of biochemical, physiologic, and anatomic structure.

When trying to read and evaluate the literature on back problems, one is confused by the inaccurate use of terminology and by the introduction of nonmedical jargon by various paramedical groups. Terminology is important. It must be accurate so there is a minimum of ambiguity when trying to communicate.

Anatomy

Muscles of the Back

The superficial layer of the back is made up of the huge trapezius muscle above (which controls the head, neck, and shoulder girdle) and the latissimus dorsi muscle below (which links arm motion to that of the spine and pelvis) (Fig. 19-2). If these muscles are removed, the underlying intrinsic muscles are seen occupying a pair of broad gutters on each side of the spinous process. This muscle is the erector spinae, attached below to the iliac crest. It passes the length of the spine as a deep and superficial layer, limited laterally by the line of the costal angles, the transverse processes of the cervical vertebrae, and on up to the occiput and mastoid processes.

The deepest part of the erector spinae is made up of bundles that control and run from one vertebral segment to the next. Collectively they are called the rotatores, the multifidus, and the semispinalis (Fig. 19-32). Covering these muscles is the more superficial part of the erector spinae, passing as three bundles, each extending over several segments. The lateral column (iliocostalis) inserts onto the ribs, the middle column (longissimus) inserts onto the thoracic and cervical transverse processes and the mastoid

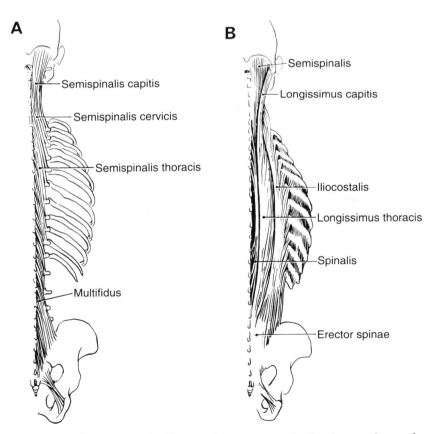

Fig. 19-32. **(A)** Multifidus and semispinalis, or "oblique group." The deepest layer, the rotatores, are not exposed. **(B)** Superficial layer of erector spinae, which splits into three basic columns; spinalis, longissimus, and iliocostalis.

TABLE 19-12. Muscles of the Lumbar Spine: Their Action and Innervation

Muscles Involved	Innervation
Forward flexion	
Psoas major	L1–L3
Rectus abdominis	T6–T12
External abdominal oblique	T7–T12
Internal abdominal oblique	T7–T12, L1
Transversus abdominis	T7–T12, L1
Extension	
Latissimus dorsi	Thoracodorsal (C6–C8)
Erector spinae	L1–L3
Transversospinalis	L1–L5
Interspinales	L1–L5
Quadratus lumborum	T12, L1–L4
Side flexion	
Latissimus dorsi	Thoracodorsal (C6–C8)
Erector spinae	L1–L3
Transversospinalis	L1–L5
Intertransversarii	L1–L5
Quadratus lumborum	T12, L1–L4
Psoas major	L1–L3
External abdominal oblique	T7–T12
Rotation[a]	—

[a] Little rotation occurs in the lumbar spine because of the shape of the facet joints.

process, and the most medial column (spinalis) is confined to the thoracic area from spine to spine as the name implies (Fig. 19-32). The more superficial the fibers, the larger is the number of segments traversed, so that some fibers cover three to six segments.[3]

These muscles work in a complex fashion in conjunction with the support offered by the lumbosacral fascia and spinal ligaments. Thus their activity is often peculiar to an individual, and postural advice should be given with this point in mind. They react strongly with positive spasm in conditions of the spine, often contributing significantly to the pain. This is most noticeable in lumbar disc disease. As prime movers, they work eccentrically, lowering the trunk in a forward flexed position, as well concentrically when assuming an erect stance (Table 19-12). In the fully leaning position they may show amazingly little activity, even electrical silence, as the stresses are transferred to ligaments. Thus unguarded movements may leave the ligaments, and perhaps the disc, vulnerable.[49]

Spinal Motion

In the thoracic spine the articular facet direction for T1 through T10 lie almost in the coronal plane and angle posteriorly at about 60 degrees. The transitional facet articulation between T11 and T12 is closer to the sagittal plane. Approximately 5 degrees of flexion and extension takes place at each vertebral level; motion being limited by the direction of the facets and narrowness of the discs. Lateral flexion is similarly limited to 5 degrees on each side for each vertebral level, the ribs preventing further motion. In addition, the contact of the lower facet with the upper root of the transverse process of the vertebra below means that a certain amount of rotation usually accompanies the side flexion. There are approximately 3 to 5 degrees of rotation each side for the first nine thoracic vertebrae and slightly less for the last three. This motion again is limited by the ribs.

The normal range of motion in the lumbar spine is considerable. Motion is greatest between the fourth and fifth vertebrae, amounting to some 24 degrees. The overall motion from full flexion to full extension in the lumbar spine is in the range of 80 degrees (Fig. 19-33). This motion may seem adequate, but without supplementary flexion from the hips it is unimpressive. Most flexion during athletic activities is achieved at the hips, and it can be increased by systematic and gradual stretching of the hamstrings. The term hyperflexion of the spine is used; but there is no adequate definition or method of measuring it, and so the term is not truly applicable.

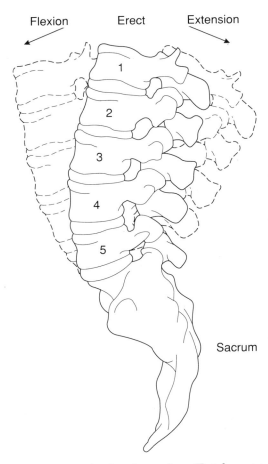

Degrees Of Movement		
Segmental		Total
L1-2	11	83
L2-3	12	72
L3-4	18	60
L4-5	24	42
L5-S1	18	18

Flexion   Erect   Extension

1

2

3

4

5

Sacrum

Fig. 19-33. Segmental flexion and extension motion in the lumbar spine. Total range of motion approximates 80 to 90 degrees.

Extension is the close, packed position of the spine and thus is the position at which the facet joints lock. Movement past this point may be achieved only at the expense of the vertebral disc unit. For this reason, it is frequently associated with pathology. Because there is little or no actual extension of the hip joint, increasing the range of extension is difficult. Thus activities in which extreme extension maneuvers are used frequently stress the spinal elements. Efforts at further extension must be accompanied by rotation of the pelvis, stressing the sacroiliac joints. The term hyperextension has often been used to signify a hypermobile condition of the lumbar spine due to generalized ligamentous laxity or stretching of the ligament disc material. However, once again there is no adequate definition and certainly no point at which extension becomes hyperextension; therefore the term is probably not useful and is indeed somewhat confusing.

Spinal Posture

There is no uniform agreement within the literature as to the normal line of gravity through the spine. It is generally accepted as falling slightly posterior to the coronal suture, through the external auditory meatus, the vertebral body at the cervical thoracic junction, through S2, posterior to the hip joint, anterior to the knee joint, and through the line of the lateral malleolus. There is obviously considerable variation. General body morphology and relaxed versus imposed posture alter these dimensions slightly. Distinct from active range of motion, one must consider the static posture of the spine and hence the terms lordosis, hyperlordosis, and kyphosis. The main point is that any alterations of the line of gravity through one curve automatically requires adjustment through another.

The normal thoracic curve is kyphotic, usually 15 to

30 degrees. *Kyphosis* in the lumbar spine is seen only under abnormal circumstances such as with fractures, congenital abnormalities, and disturbances of collagen production. Thus the term kyphosis should never be used to describe the physiologic extremes of normal posture in the lumbar spine.

By contrast, *lordosis* is the normal position of the lumbar spine. The angle between the fifth vertebra and the top of the sacrum contributes most of the lordotic curve. There is usually a steady curve of the other vertebrae above the sacrum. The normal lumbosacral angle is in the region of 120 to 130 degrees. Excessive lordosis at the lumbosacral angle is in the region of 95 to 100 degrees. Once again it is tempting to use the term hyperlordosis, but clinically it is impossible to define this term and so it is better to avoid it. Much of the smooth lordotic curve is made up of the shape of the discs, with only wedging of the L4 vertebral body being significant.

Decreased lordosis may be a significant cause of ligamentous back pain in the nonathletic population, with the exception of obese individuals and pregnant women. However, increased lordosis is the bane of the athlete. Resolution of forces show that excessive lordosis may throw considerable stress on the posterior elements of the spine as well as the anterior longitudinal ligament. This situation is particularly prominent when extrinsic forces are added to the body weight, as occurs during a collision of interior football linemen as they come off a three-point stance and make contact with their opponents.

Intervertebral Disc

The intervertebral disc comprises approximately 25 percent of the total length of the spinal column.[96] The height of the disc in relation to the vertebral bodies varies in each area, being 22 to 33 percent in the cervical region, 16 to 20 percent in the thoracic area, and approximately 33 percent in the lumbar region. The functions of the discs include binding the vertebrae together, allowing motion, absorbing shock, and serving as the primary load distributor between vertebral segments. Indeed the disc is a self-contained fluid-elastic system that absorbs shock during vertebral loading and permits transient compression.[97] With the various movements of the spine, it distributes the pressure more equally so there is no concentration of compressive forces around the edges of the vertebral body. The nucleus pulposus in the young individual is approximately 80 percent

water and therefore is largely incompressible, but it can be deformed. The ability of the nucleus to change shape accounts for the compressibility of the disc as a whole. The annulus fibrosus, a strong structure made up of interlacing cross-fibers of collagen, contains the nucleus. Fibers of each layer run obliquely, adjacent layers crossing each other to reinforce, strengthen, and permit better resistance to torsion and motion. The outer fibers of the annulus are attached to the vertebrae through Sharpey's fibers. The annulus, which tends to be thicker anteriorly than posteriorly, may be stretched and therefore provides some inherent elasticity to the spine. Additional reinforcement anteriorly and posteriorly is provided by the longitudinal ligaments.

Quick Facts

FUNCTION OF THE INTERVERTEBRAL DISC

- Binds vertebrae together
- Allows motion
- Absorbs shock
- Distributes load between segments
- Contributes to lordosis

In the cervical region the disc is large in comparison to the vertebral body, thicker anteriorly, and contributes significantly to the normal cervical curve. In the thoracic region the heights of the discs are approximately equal anteriorly and posteriorly, and therefore much of the thoracic curve is related to the shape of the vertebral bodies. In the lumbar region, the discs are thicker anteriorly than posteriorly and hence contribute significantly to the lumbar curve.

Not much is known about the innervation of the disc, but the sinuvertebral nerve (meningeal recurrent), which innervates the posterior longitudinal ligament, probably innervates the posterior part of the annulus but not the nucleus. Nachemson has noted that during some static positions in motion the disc pressure increases significantly.[97] In a 70 kg subject the load on the L3 disc is approximately 140 kg when sitting and 100 kg when standing; when tilting forward from a standing position and lifting a 50 kg weight, this load increases to 300 kg. Because theoretically these forces are greater than a disc can tolerate, there must be other mechanisms to help disburse the force (Table 19-13). It is possible that intraabdominal pressure is one of these factors.

Because both the annulus and the reinforcing ligaments are thinner posteriorly, particularly at the lateral limits of the posterior longitudinal ligaments, most disc protrusions occur posterolaterally. It is also in this area of the disc that eccentric loading tends to put additional stress. The posterior longitudinal ligament is a richly innervated structure, and it is possible that much of the back pain due to disc protrusion arises in this structure.

During the course of a day, the water content and shape of the disc change sufficiently for an adult man to lose as much as 2 cm of height. This height is usually regained during sleeping when the pressure on the disc is decreased and the water content increases. The ability of the disc to transmit pressure may relate directly to the water content of the nucleus, and this ability changes with age. The nucleus is approximately 88 percent water in the newborn, reducing to 70 to 75 percent water by age 70, representing an approximately 20 percent reduction. During aging the gel of the nucleus is replaced to some degree by collagen, and there is sometimes degenerative calcifi-

cation. This factor has an influence not only on the weight-relieving properties of the disc but also on the propensity for nuclear material to extrude.

Assessment

The healthy spine, like most joints of the body, is an incredibly efficient and versatile structure. Most of the day-to-day forces do not reach even 20 percent of its ultimate failure point. By contrast, the diseased back, even with only moderate changes, is a brittle, sensitive, much less accommodating structure, and even day-to-day activities may stress it to 80 percent of its ultimate tolerance. Therefore the key to a pain-free spine, particularly with the superimposed stresses of sport and recreation, is a healthy spine.

TABLE 19-13. Approximate Load on L3 Disc in 70-kg Individual in Various Positions, Movements, Maneuvers, and Exercises

Activity	Load (kg)
Supine in traction (30 kg)	10
Supine lying	30
Standing	70
Walking	85
Twisting	90
Bending sideways	95
Upright sitting, no support	100
Coughing	110
Jumping	110
Isometric abdominal muscle exercise	110
Bilateral straight-leg raising, supine	120
Straining	120
Laughing	120
Bending forward 20°	120
Active back hyperextension, prone	150
Sit-up exercise with knees extended	175
Sit-up exercise with knees bent	180
Bending forward 20° with 10 kg in each hand	185
Lifting of 20 kg, back straight, knees bent	210
Lifting of 20 kg, back bent, knees straight	340

(After Nachemson and Effström,[74] with permission.)

> **Practice Point**
>
> **AGE-RELATED SPINAL PATHOLOGY**
>
> - Young child
>   - Genetic disturbances of formation and growth, e.g., unsegmented vertebrae
> - Adolescent
>   - Affected by growth spurt and increasing stress, e.g., scoliosis, Scheuermann's kyphosis, spondylolysis
> - Young adult
>   - Risk-taking activities, e.g., spinal fractures, muscle and ligament sprain
> - Middle age
>   - Disc becomes vulnerable, e.g., disc protrusion
> - Elderly
>   - Degenerative changes and neoplasia, e.g., osteoarthrosis and secondary tumor

What makes the spine healthy? Muscle strength, flexibility, and posture contribute; but genetic influences are probably the prime reason some people are susceptible to spinal pathology and others appear to absorb stress comfortably. Nevertheless, each spine is susceptible, in different ways, at different points of our lives. In children we see problems related to genetic disturbances of growth and anatomic variation. In adolescents there are problems related to the growth spurts, e.g., scoliosis. In the teenager the bone is starting to mature, but stresses and torques are rising exponentially, and there are problems associated with the stress, e.g., spondylolysis and Scheuermann's disease. In the young adult postural back pain predominates, with chronic ligamentous strains and trauma related to risk-taking activities. During middle age the disc becomes vulnerable, as it changes its histologic structure. Finally, in the elderly as the disc narrows and the facet joints are exposed to more pressure, degenerative changes occur. In addition, secondary neoplastic changes are more common.

In sport and recreation, the spine is stressed in many ways, including the high loading of weight lifting, speed and torque as seen in the figure skater with sudden impacts in the extended position, the thrusting and pushing with the spine in the extremes of motion by football linemen, the high repetitive loading of gymnasts, the rotation stresses in discus and javelin throwers, the torques during wind-up and delivery of the baseball pitcher, and finally the prolonged postural stresses seen in cyclists. It is with this background in mind that the athlete's history is obtained and the examination focused for individuals with athletically acquired back pain.

History

The chief complaint must be clearly established. In particular, it is important to know whether the complaint is of back pain, leg pain, or both. Isolated back pain is usually not discogenic in young individuals unless there is a central protrusion. Furthermore, if leg discomfort is present, it is important to know whether it is pain, dysesthesia, or numbness. Mild radicular irritation produces pain or dysesthesia, whereas significant protrusions produce numbness. Bilaterality of the symptoms suggests either a central protrusion or some other cause of pain. The nature of the onset and the association with trauma may point

toward contusion, muscle tear, ligament strain, or acute discogenic disease.

There are some key points that differentiate the more benign common problems from those that constitute potentially serious back pain. Significant back pain in individuals under the age of 10 should raise the question of tumor or discitis. Spinal tumors in individuals of this age group have, on the average, up to a 2-year delay in diagnosis. Similarly, back pain for the first time in anyone over the age of 60, with no history of aching or discomfort, should also introduce the possibility of tumor.

Unexplained weight loss, altered bowel habits (particularly in men), intermenstrual bleeding, chronic cough, and the presence of night pain should similarly raise the question of neoplasia. Altered bladder function is important to note because it signifies a significant problem that is potentially irreversible if not treated promptly. Altered balance, visual disturbance, and associated upper limb dysfunction raise the question of generalized neuro-

---

> **Practice Point**
>
> **SCREENING QUESTION FOR MORE SINISTER CAUSES OF BACK PAIN**
>
> - Pain in individual less than 10 years of age
> - First time back pain in individual more than 60 years of age
> - Unexplained weight loss
> - Chronic cough
> - Night pain
> - Intermenstrual bleeding
> - Altered bowel function (rectal bleeding)
> - Altered bladder control
> - Associated visual disturbance, balance problems, or upper limb dysesthesias

---

> **Practice Point**
>
> **ONE-QUESTION TEST: RADICULAR PAIN**
>
> Between the knee and the ankle, is the pain at the front, side, or back of the leg?
>
> Front = L4
> Side = L5
> Back = S1

logic disease and thus also require further investigation. Essentially these questions screen for more sinister causes of back discomfort; if the responses to these possibilities are negative, one can focus on expanding the history of the evolution of the presenting complaint (Table 19-14).

It is specifically important to note the level of activity, the goals of the individual, and the degree to which pain is either aggravated by or interferes with training and competition. In this regard, a detailed

TABLE 19-14.   Segmental Innervation of Viscera and Referred Pain

Structures	Segmental Innervation	Possible Areas of Pain Referral
Cardiopulmonary system		
Heart	T1–T5	Cervical anterior upper thorax
		Left upper extremity
Lungs and bronchi	T5–T6	Ipsilateral thoracic spine
		Cervical (diaphragm involved)
Digestive system		
Esophagus	T4–T6	Substernal and upper abdominal
Stomach	T6–T10	Upper abdominal
		Middle and lower thoracic spine
Small intestine	T7–T10	Middle thoracic spine
Pancreas	T6–T10	Upper abdominal
		Lower thoracic spine
		Upper lumbar spine
Gallbladder	T7–T9	Right upper abdominal
		Right middle and lower thoracic spine, including caudal aspect of scapula
Liver	T7–T9	Right middle and lower thoracic spine
		Right cervical spine
Common bile duct	T6–T10	Upper abdominal
		Middle thoracic spine
Large intestine	T11–L1	Lower abdominal
		Middle lumbar spine
Sigmoid colon	T11–T12	Upper sacral
		Suprapubic
		Left lower quadrant of abdomen
Genital system		
Uterus including uterine ligaments	T10–L1, S2–S4	Lumbosacral junction
		Sacral
		Thoracolumbar
Ovaries	T10–T11	Lower abdominal
		Sacral
Testes	T10–T11	Lower abdominal
		Sacral
Urinary system		
Kidney	T10–L1	Lumbar spine (ipsilateral)
		Lower abdominal
		Upper abdominal
Ureter	T11–L2, S2–S4	Groin
		Upper abdominal
		Suprapubic
		Medial, proximal thigh
		Thoracolumbar
Urinary bladder	T11–L2, S2–S4	Sacral apex
		Suprapubic
		Thoracolumbar
Prostate gland	T11–L1, S2–S4	Sacral
		Testes
		Thoracolumbar

history is required to pinpoint the level of discomfort during each of the activities, as well as the duration and intensity of the pain after the activity has stopped. It is these questions that will guide the rate and progression of treatment.

Examination

For an efficient examination of the back, it is important to be organized and to place the patient in as few positions as possible.

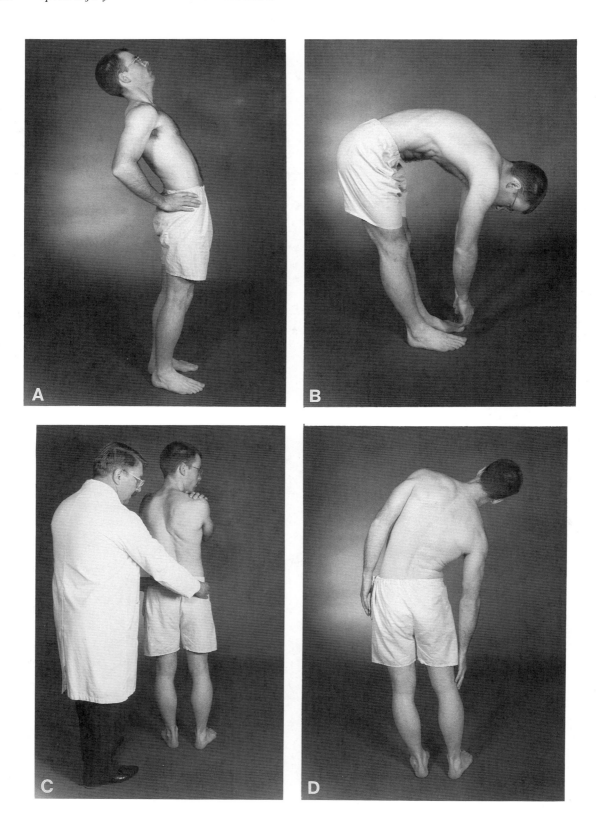

Standing

With the patient sufficiently undressed the posture can be observed with particular reference to shoulder height, scoliosis, iliac crests, and obvious leg length differences. Apparent spasm of the paravertebral muscle mass can be confirmed by gentle palpation. The important landmarks on the back are the vertebra prominens (which may be C7 or T1), the top of the scapula (which is T2), base of the spine of the scapula (T4), inferior angle of the scapula (T7), the lowest rib (T12), the tops of the iliac crest (approximately at the bottom of L4), and the posterosuperior iliac spine (marked by dimples lying at about the S1–S2 junction).

Practice Point

SURFACE LANDMARKS ON BACK

• Vertebra prominens	C7 or T1
• Top of scapula	T2
• Base of spine of scapula	T4
• Inferior angle of scapula	T7
• Lowest rib insertion	T12
• Top of iliac crest	L4
• Dimples marking the posterosuperior iliac spines	S1–S2

The individual is asked to bend forward, and the amount of motion and the ease at which this movement is achieved is observed. Special reference is made to the way the person straightens, noting if there is splinting of the back instead of uncurling and if most of the motion comes from the hip. If there has been a complaint of sciatica, forward flexion may trigger sciatic scoliosis or increased pain down the leg. If scoliosis is present, leaning forward reveals prominence of the rib hump in the thoracic region and the paravertebral muscles over the spinous process in the lower back (2-minute scoliosis screening test) (Fig. 19-34).

The Schober test can be used to assess the range of motion during forward flexion (Fig. 19-35). The vertebra prominens is marked, and a 30 cm segment from this point incorporates most of the thoracic spine. With flexion this distance should increase 3 cm. Lumbar spinal motion is tested by marking a 10 cm segment up from the dimples. With full forward flexion this distance should increase 5 cm. If there is restricted thoracic motion, this test should be supplemented by measuring the inspiratory excursion of the chest to make sure there is adequate rib motion. This point is particularly important if ankylosing spondylitis is suspected in the young athlete.

The patient is asked to lean backward in an extension motion. This maneuver gives the overall impression of "extension pattern" pain, which is often largely mechanical, versus "flexion pattern" pain, which is frequently discogenic. If there is considerably increased point tenderness with extension and spondylolysis is suspected, this test is supplemented by asking the individual to lean back, standing first on one leg and then the other, to see if it localizes the low back discomfort.

Rotation is checked by fixing the pelvis and asking the patient to look over the shoulders; lateral flexion is achieved by asking the individual to slide the arms down either side of the leg, reaching as low as possible. The most reproducible measurement of lateral flexion is recorded from the starting position of the fingertips to the ending position of the fingertips as they slide down the side of the leg.[98] This measurement may also be used as an index of the severity of back pain and to record its progress (Fig. 19-35).

The athlete is then asked to walk on the heels and toes, which gives some indication of muscle control. A series of heel raises with either leg assesses gastrocnemius strength and S1 root function; this parameter is difficult to test manually. While the heel raise is being performed, the examiner can also look for evidence of a Trendelenburg sign, which may indicate hip disease and pain or gluteus medius weakness. The ability to squat also provides some functional information. The patient is asked to squat as far as possible, bouncing two or three times before returning to the stand-

---

Fig. 19-34. Assessment of spine motion in standing. (**A**) extension (**B**) flexion. These motions will divide the problem into two broad patterns. In addition the rib hump, or unilateral prominence of the erector spinae, in a true structural scoliosis is well visualized in forward flexion (the 2-minute screening test). (**C**) Rotation requires fixation of the pelvis (alternately done in sitting). (**D**) Side flexion.

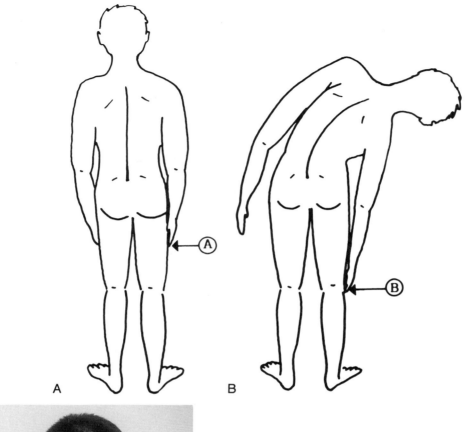

A   B

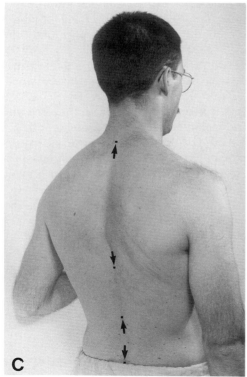

C

Fig. 19-35. Lateral bending recorded by **(A)** measurements of the distance between the starting and **(B)** finishing positions of the fingertips. **(C)** The Schober's test can be used to document adequate thoracic and lumbar spine motion. The 30 cm segment distal to the vertebra prominens representing the thoracic spine should increase by 3 cm during flexion. The 10 cm segment proximal to the dimples (S1–2) represents the lumbar spine and should increase by 5 cm during full flexion. In addition, pelvic asymmetry may give a clue to leg-length discrepancy.

ing position. If the patient can do this maneuver readily, it serves as a "quick" screen for lower limb joint disease. Caution is observed when asking older individuals or patients with known significant arthrosis to perform this test (Fig. 19-36).

Sitting Position

In the sitting position, the patients are asked to extend first one leg and then the other. If they have to lean back (tripod sign), it is a sign of undue tension on either the sciatic nerve or the hamstrings (Fig. 19-37). A slump test may then be performed that prestresses the dura by neck and thoracic spinal flexion. This movement is a sensitive test of radicular irritation (Fig. 19-38).

While sitting, the strength of the hip flexors, the quadriceps, the dorsiflexors, and the toe extensors are easily tested. Similarly, Achilles and quadriceps

jerks can be elicited in this position and retested when the patient assumes the lying position. The examinator may prefer to perform these tests when the patient is in the lying position.

Lying Position

The patient is then asked to assume a lying position, and the gastrocnemius (S1) and quadriceps (L4) reflexes are easily retested. The medial hamstring reflex for L5 can be added (Table 19-15) (Fig. 19-39). Where indicated the superficial reflexes (cremasteric T12-L1) and the abdominal (thoracic segments) may be added, as well as the test for long tract cord involvement using the Babinski's extensor plantar reflex (Fig. 19-40). It must be emphasized that an equivocal Achilles tendon jerk is not accepted as abnormal unless retested with the patient kneeling with the feet over the end of a stool.

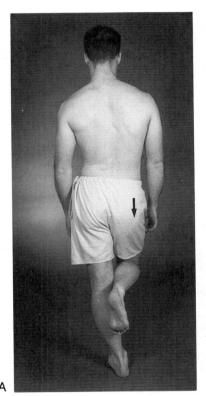 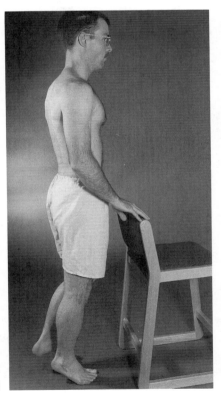 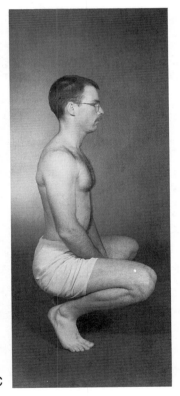

A   B   C

Fig. 19-36. Initial screening and standing is supplemented by **(A)** one legged stance to eliminate abductor weakness or pain inhibition from the hip or the supporting side (Trendelenburg test). The test is demonstrated here as mildly positive with the right hip dropping. **(B)** Heel raises to evaluate the S1 root and gastrocnemius strength, and **(C)** the so-called "quick test" in which a squat is performed supplemented by two or three bouncing maneuvers. The latter test helps to eliminate the dilemma of hip or knee arthrosis as a cause of the patient's symptoms.

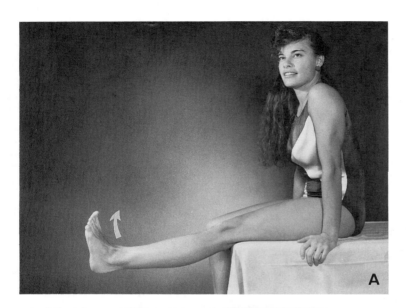

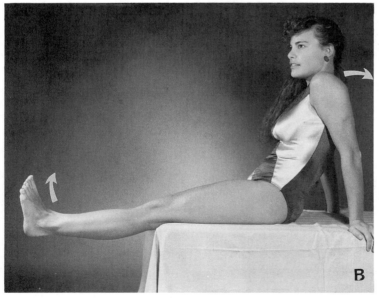

Fig. 19-37. Tripod test. In the sitting position, the patient is asked to extend the leg. **(A)** Normal test. **(B)** Positive tripod sign, which is the position adapted by the patient either because of tight hamstrings or to relieve stress on the sciatic nerve.

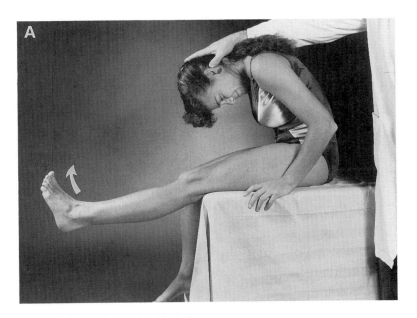

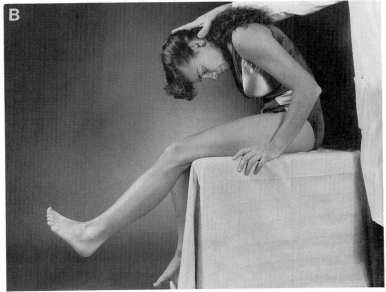

Fig. 19-38. Slump test. By flexing the patient's neck and thorax prior to leg extension, the dura and nerve roots are prestressed, increasing the sensitivity of the test. This is equivalent to a Kernig-Lasègue test for nerve root and dural irritation which is done in the lying position.

TABLE 19-15. Reflex Arcs and Clinical Significance[a]

Reflex	Site of Stimulus	Normal Response	Segment
Deep tendons			
Biceps	Biceps tendon	Flexion of elbow	C5–C6
Brachioradialis	Styloid process of radius	Flexion and pronation of elbow	C6
Triceps	Tendon just above olecranon	Extension of elbow	C7–C8
Patellar	Patellar tendon	Extension of knee	L3–L4
Medial hamstring	Semitendinosus at knee	Muscle belly contraction	L5
Achilles	Achilles tendon	Plantar flexion	S1, S2
Superficial			
Upper abdominal	Stroke upper abdomen	Umbilicus moves up and toward the side being stroked	T7–T9
Lower abdominal	Stroke lower abdomen	Umbilicus moves down	T11–T12
Cremasteric	Stroke upper inner thigh	Scrotum elevates	T12–L1
Plantar	Stroke sole of foot	Flexion of toes	S1–S2
Pathologic			
Babinski	Stroke lateral aspect of the sole of the foot	Extension of big toe; fanning of the other toes[b]	Sign of pyramidal tract disease

[a] Reflexes judged by comparing with opposite side and normal expected response. Recorded as hyperactive (+++), brisk (++), normal (+), decrease (−) or absent (0).

[b] Normal response in flexion of toe, extension is a pathologic reaction.

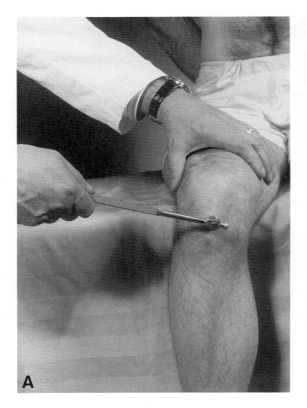
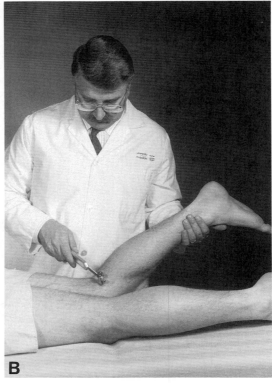

Fig. 19-39. Screening the deep tendon reflexes. **(A)** The quadriceps patella tendon reflex tap (L3–L4). **(B)** Medial hamstring reflex. *(Figure continues.)*

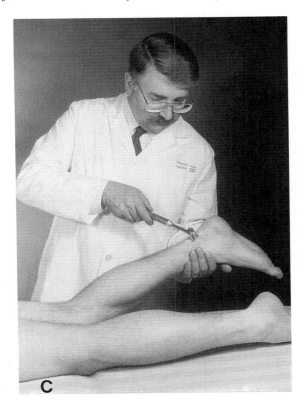

Fig. 19-39 *(Continued).* **(C)** Achilles tendon reflex. If for any reason the results of these tests are equivocal, the hamstring reflex is retested in the prone position and the Achilles reflex with the patient kneeling. All reflexes may be augmented by having the patient ''clench'' their teeth and locking the fingers and tensing the upper limb muscles.

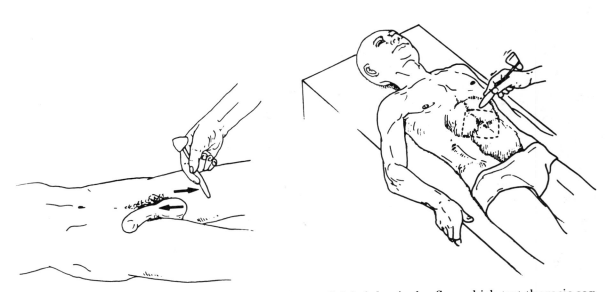

Fig. 19-40. Cremasteric reflex (T12–L1) and superficial abdominal reflex, which test thoracic segments. (Superior to umbilicus, T7–T9, below umbilicus T11–12.)

In the lying position the hips may be taken up into flexion and rotated, which helps rule out primary hip disease as a cause of back pain or, conversely, the back as a cause of hip discomfort. Painful hip rotation is the *sine qua non* of hip disease.

Muscle tightness can be tested using the Thomas test for hip flexors, the Ely test for quadriceps, and the straight-leg raising test for hamstrings. The gastrocnemius and soleus can be tested by flexing the leg over the edge of the examination couch. Muscle strength of the abductors and adductors may be tested in this position and, depending on preference,

several other muscle groups instead of in the sitting position (Fig. 19-41). A correlation with appropriate myotomes is performed (Table 19-16). The principles of muscle testing include (1) placing the test joints in a neutral, pain-free resting position; (2) applying isometric pressure with a simple command such as "don't let me move you," or "hold it there"; (3) holding the contraction for at least 5 seconds, as fatigue unmasks subtle weakness; (4) whenever possible testing the two sides simultaneously or consecutively for comparison with normal; and (5) when pain or joint disease is a factor, attempting to minimize position

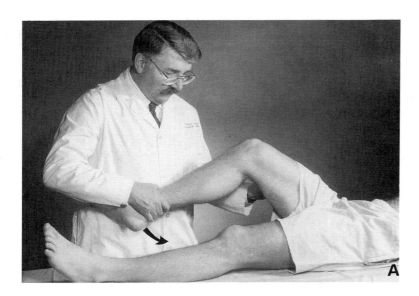

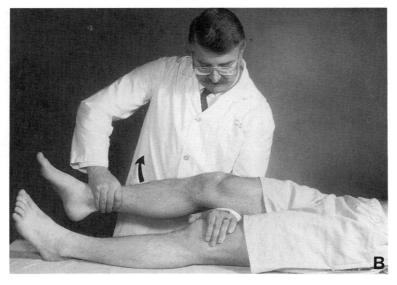

Fig. 19-41. Positioning and testing of segmental levels and myotomes.* **(A)** Hip flexion (L2–L3) **(B)**, knee extension (L3–L4). *(Figure continues.)*

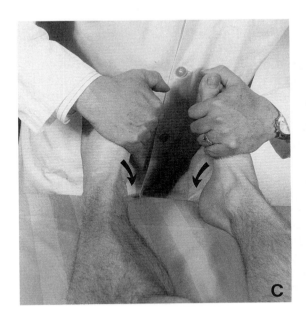

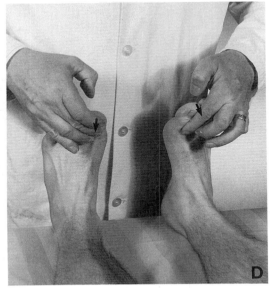

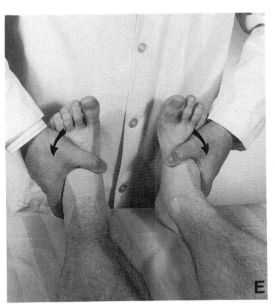

Fig. 19-41 *(Continued).* **(C)** Foot dorsi-flexion with inversion (L4–5), **(D)** extension of the great toe (L5), **(E)** eversion of ankle (S1).

(Figure continues.)

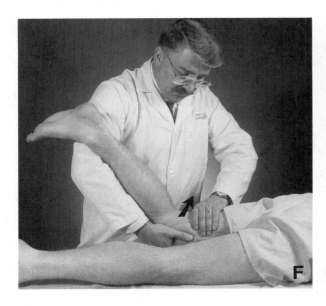

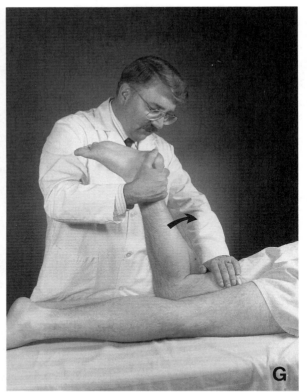

Fig. 19-41 *(Continued).* **(F)** Hip extension (L5-S1), and **(G)** knee flexion (L5-S1).

* Although significant variations exist in various texts, these levels are the ones most commonly used to screen for radicular problems.

changes for the patient, leaving the most uncomfortable test until last and avoiding direct pressure over painful joints.

The screen for altered sensation completes the sensory examination (Figs. 19-42 and 19-43). Leg length should be measured, and the pulses are confirmed by palpation, which helps rule out any periph-

eral vascular involvement. Particularly in the elderly athlete, it is necessary sometimes to distinguish neural from vascular claudication. The abdomen can be palpated if no obvious cause of pathology has been found to this point. In the older individual, abdominal palpation is an important routine part of the screen.

TABLE 19-16.   Myotomes of the Lower Limb[a]

Nerve Root	Test Action	Muscles
L1–L2	Hip flexion	Psoas, iliacus, sartorius, gracilis, pectineus, adductor longus, adductor brevis
L3	Knee extension	Quadriceps, adductor longus, magnus, and brevis
L4	Ankle dorsiflexion	Tibialis anterior, quadriceps, tensor fascia lata, adductor magnus, obturator externus, tibialis posterior
L5	Toe extension Ankle inversion Knee flexion	Extensor hallucis longus, extensor digitorum longus, gluteus medius and minimus, obturator internus, semimembranosus, semitendinosus
S1	Ankle plantar flexion Ankle eversion Hip extension	Gastrocnemius, soleus, gluteus maximus, obturator internus, piriformis, biceps femoris, semitendinosus, popliteus, eroneus longus and brevis, extensor digitorum brevis
S2		Piriformis, soleus, gastrocnemius, flexor digitorum longus, flexor hallucis longus, intrinsic foot muscles

[a] There may be small segmental contributions from other levels.

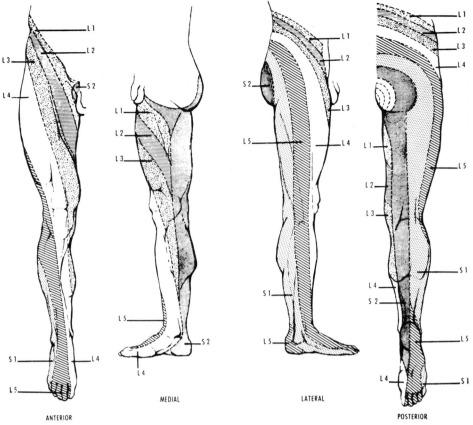

Fig. 19-42. Segmental sensory levels.

Side Lying Position

The sacroiliac joint may be stressed by the flexion, abduction, external rotation (FABER test) prior to turning the individual on the side (Fig. 19-44). If the FABER test is positive, further confirmation of sacroiliac pathology can be obtained by compressing the sides of the pelvis to further stress the sacroiliac joints. The Ober test may be done for abductor tightness. If necessary, a rectal examination is performed, which should be a compulsory part of the examination for men over age 40 and any athlete who has altered bowel habits.

Prone Lying Position

The athlete can now turn to the prone lying position, which facilitates testing hip extensor power. Asking the athlete to squeeze the buttocks together allows palpation of the gluteal tone, which is often significantly altered with an S1 disc lesion. Knee flexion strength is best tested in this position.

Practice Point

CORRELATION OF PLAIN FILMS WITH SYMPTOMS

- Poor correlation
  - Spondylosis
  - Scoliosis
  - Spondylolysis
  - Degenerative disc changes
- Better correlation
  - Spondylolisthesis
  - Scheuermann's kyphosis
  - Ankylosing spondylitis
  - Osteopenia

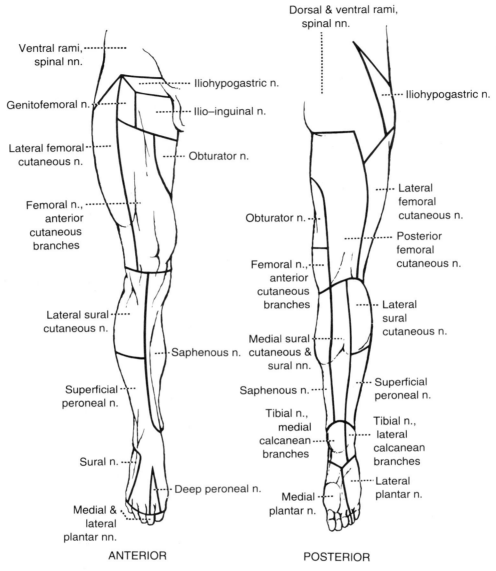

Ventral rami, spinal nn.

Genitofemoral n.

Iliohypogastric n.

Ilio–inguinal n.

Lateral femoral cutaneous n.

Obturator n.

Femoral n., anterior cutaneous branches

Lateral sural cutaneous n.

Saphenous n.

Superficial peroneal n.

Sural n.

Deep peroneal n.

Medial & lateral plantar nn.

ANTERIOR

Dorsal & ventral rami, spinal nn.

Iliohypogastric n.

Lateral femoral cutaneous n.

Obturator n.

Posterior femoral cutaneous n.

Femoral n., anterior cutaneous branches

Lateral sural cutaneous n.

Medial sural cutaneous & sural nn.

Saphenous n.

Superficial peroneal n.

Tibial n., medial calcanean branches

Tibial n., lateral calcanean branches

Medial plantar n.

Lateral plantar n.

POSTERIOR

Fig. 19-43. Sensory areas supplied by specific sensory nerves.

The femoral nerve stretch test may yield several important pieces of information (Fig. 19-45). If forced hip extension with knee flexion produces pain down the anterolateral thigh, it indicates tension on the femoral nerve or the L3 or L4 root. If the maneuver triggers classic sciatic pain, it is pathognomonic of L5 root irritation. If there is little or no peripheral pain but discomfort in the low back area, associated palpation may reveal the source as being either sacroiliac or low lumbar, probably nondiscogenic.

The paravertebral muscle, spinous processes, and sacroiliac area are carefully palpated. Sometimes pain can be localized by stressing the area over each spinous process, seeking painful mobile segments.

Based on these findings, laboratory tests and appropriate radiologic investigations may be ordered. Routine roentgenograms should probably include only anteroposterior and lateral views of the lumbar spine. About 90 percent of the information is obtainable from the lateral view. Oblique views usually offer

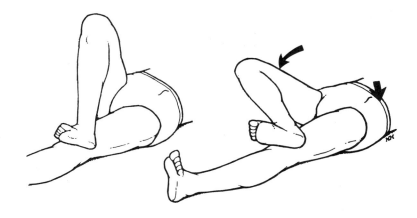

Fig. 19-44. Patrick, or FABER, test (flexion, abduction, and external rotation) is performed by pushing down over the flexed knee and the contralateral anterosuperior iliac spine. A positive test is pain felt in the area of the sacroiliac joint on the side of the anterosuperior iliac spine being stressed.

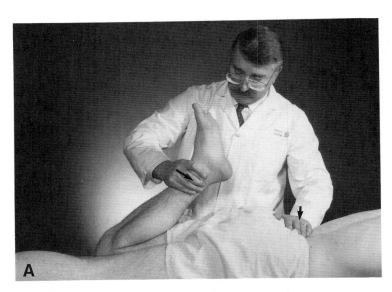

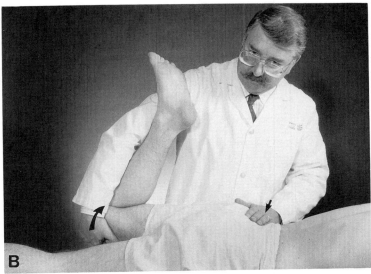

Fig. 19-45. Femoral nerve stretch test. **(A)** Knee flexion may give lateral thigh pain (possibly indicative of lateral femoral cutaneous nerve irritation) or anterior thigh pain (L4 root traction). **(B)** These signs are exacerbated by associated hip tension. Posterior leg pain may be indicative of L5 root irritation. Back or sacroiliac pain may be produced by the stress across the lumbosacral junction.

little additional information except in cases of suspected spondylolysis. They simply add expense and expose the patient to considerably more radiation.

Plain films assist in the detection of traumatic disruption of the bony elements, tumor, infection, degenerative changes, and spondylolysis. However, there is often a poor correlation between radiologic changes and disease. Further investigation is usually based on the magnitude of symptoms, suspicious history, or failure to respond to therapy. It includes bone scanning, CT, and MRI.

Back Pain

For a complete and safe approach to the diagnosis of back pain and sciatica, it is necessary to consider extrinsic and intrinsic causes (Fig. 19-46). The extrinsic causes include abdominal, vascular, pelvic, and hip pathology. The likelihood of each depends on the age of the individual, family history, and the type of trauma precipitating the back discomfort. Intrinsic causes include tumor; and, particularly in the middle-aged female athlete, one should think of secondary tumor from the breast. In the older male athlete, consider metastasis from prostatic cancer.

Infection is a possibility, as is discitis in the very young. In individuals from areas where tuberculosis is still a problem, this infection must be part of the differential diagnosis. Metabolic disturbances include Paget's disease and rare conditions such as

ochronosis. Inflammatory problems of the spine lead to a consideration of ankylosising spondylitis in young men and rheumatoid arthritis in women. Under the heading of congenital causes one would include predisposing structural defects. Despite all these possible etiologies, in the young athlete the commonest single cause of back pain is trauma, either a repetitive minor injury or a single episode that produces muscle tears, ligament sprains, endplate

---

Quick Facts

MECHANISMS OF BACK INJURY IN SPORT

- Chronic stressful position: field hockey, jogging
- Repetitive loading: rowing
- Hard repetitive contact: football, hockey
- Lifting human bodies: ballet, figure skating
- Hyperextended lumbar spine: gymnastics, football
- Stressing an immature spine: weight training, gymnastics
- Sudden violent muscle contraction: throwing sports

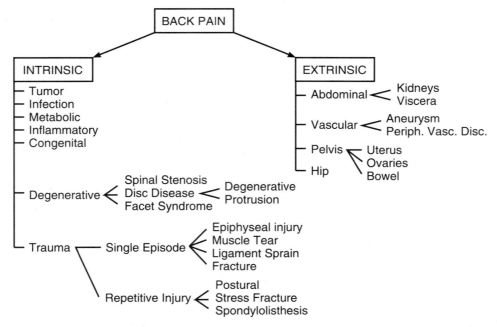

Fig. 19-46. Back pain etiology with intrinsic and extrinsic causes.

(growth) injury, or fractures. Repetitive minor trauma may be in the form of the habitual postures of some sports or the repetitive movements in others, e.g., rowers.

In the older athlete degenerative conditions predominate, leading to disc disease, facet syndrome, and spinal stenosis. Only those secondary conditions that are common in the athlete are discussed in any detail.

Muscle Contusion, Strain, Avulsion

Muscle contusions are common in many of the collision sports; and for the most part, disability is short-lived and can be treated symptomatically. The immediate application of ice minimizes bleeding as for any other acute soft tissue injury. If there is still significant discomfort after 24 hours, heat is sometimes helpful, as are NSAIDs. The area can be protected from further contusion, and the athlete returns to activity as allowed by pain and discomfort. If the contusion is significant, awareness of a potential underlying visceral injury is mandatory, particularly of the spleen and kidneys. (See Chapter 18.)

Muscle strains occur with torsional and twisting activities, e.g., javelin throwing, gymnastics, and hockey. These strains are usually first or second degree in nature. They produce acute pain and spasm but resolve rapidly if treated by modified activity and rest. Occasionally, these muscle injuries are more significant and may be associated with avulsion of the transverse processes by the quadratus lumborum or iliopsoas, or the iliac crest by the external obliques. In this situation up to 3 months may be required before the individual can resume full contact activities, although return to fairly vigorous training is possible before this time. The pain may be significant during the first 2 to 3 weeks, requiring a thoracolumbar orthosis to help with mobility. As the acute spasm settles, activity is progressed within the tolerance of pain, with care to avoid ballistic type movements for 6 weeks. A 12-week period is usually required before full return to activity in sports that require rapid movements through a full range or sudden deceleration and twisting.

A related but less common condition is the quadratus lumborum syndrome. It is characterized by posterior iliac crest pain and tenderness, with occasional pain referred into the groin and thigh. There is tenderness along the posterior iliac crest just adjacent to the iliolumbar ligaments that is aggravated by resisted side flexion and extension with rotation. This chronic inflammatory response of the tendinous insertion of the quadratus lumborum muscle usually resolves with a local injection of 3 to 4 ml of local anesthetic used to dilute 1 ml of corticosteroid.

Ligament Sprain

Ligament sprains fall into two basic categories, i.e., chronic postural sprain and acute traumatic strain. The acute traumatic sprain presents similarly to muscle injury; only the site of maximal tenderness with palpation and the relatively less discomfort on resisted isometric contraction of the muscle help differentiate the conditions. The treatment is essentially the same as for muscle injury, with local heat and NSAIDs being the mainstays. Activity is modified according to symptoms, with gradual progression back to full participation.

The location of a chronic ligamentous sprain depends on the activity of the athlete as well as the predisposition according to body build, musculature, and posture. There are three major sites of these sprains. The first is in the cervical area, referring pain into the trapezius. The second is located in the interscapular region, and the third is the lumbosacral area. Often the chronic ligamentous sprain is brought on by repetitive activities associated with certain sports, e.g., judo and karate, and is aggravated by the activities of daily living, e.g., chronically poor posture at a desk or while driving. Hence this problem requires careful investigation into the individual's day-to-day activities as well as the sporting component. Therapy relates to correcting posture and analyzing the kinematics of the movements that are contributing to the problem in addition to treating the local discomfort. Mobilization of stiff segments and attention to adequate muscle strength and endurance are vital elements of treatment. Occasionally, if there is an inflammatory component to the problem, NSAIDs help, but more frequently the inflammatory element is minimal.

In athletes who lift heavy objects while rotating and bending their backs, as well as individuals who have an occupation that requires repetitive activities such as lifting boxes off a truck, the pathology is frequently a chronic sprain of the iliolumbar ligament. This ligament connects the transverse processes of the fifth lumbar vertebrae and the iliac crest. There may be local discomfort, pain in the gluteal area, and even referred pain down the back of the thigh. The pain is exacerbated by extension and lateral bending away from the involved side. There is local tenderness on the posterior portion of one or both iliac crests just adjacent to the transverse processes.

If the condition does not resolve with NSAIDs, local application of ultrasound or laser, and modified activities, it can often be relieved by an injection of corticosteroid.[100]

Sacroiliac Pain

Sacroiliac disorders are discussed in Chapter 17. Nevertheless, it is important to mention here the sacroiliac problems in the differential diagnosis of lumbosacral discomfort, buttock pain, and referred pain down the posterior thigh. Usually it is possible to isolate the sacroiliac joint as being the source of the discomfort when (1) there is local pain to palpation over the joint line itself; (2) the back pain is frequently unilateral and low; and (3) the stress test to the sacroiliac joint is positive (Figs. 19-44 and 19-47). There may also be unilateral pain when hopping. Abnormal motion of the joint may be present that is either excessive or (more frequently) decreased, a condition referred to as sacroiliac fixation (Fig. 19-48). If fixation is present it is an indication of the potential benefits of mobilizing the joint. The diagnosis can be confirmed by injecting lidocaine (Xylocaine) into the

sacroiliac joint itself, which should obliterate the discomfort.

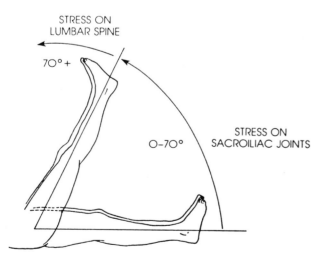

Fig. 19-47. Bilateral straight-leg raising test. The examiner supports and lifts both legs simultaneously. Usually the stress is mainly in the sacroiliac joint in the first 70 degrees; subsequently, movement is concentrated on the lumbosacral junction. The patient is asked to locate exactly the area of unpleasant sensation or pain. (After Magee,[9] with permission.)

Practice Point

CONSIDER SACROILIAC PAIN

- Pain over sacroiliac joint and buttock
- Back pain unilateral and low
- Pain on stressing S1 joint
- Unilateral pain on hopping
- Pain resolves with lidocaine injection into S1 joint

Spondylolysis and Spondylolisthesis

Spondylolysis is a defect in the neural arch, usually in the pars interarticularis. Spondylolisthesis is a slipping of one vertebra forward on another (Fig. 19-49). These terms were coined in 1853 by Kilian.[101] From a practical standpoint, spondylolisthesis may be divided into degenerative and isthmic (pars defect) varieties, and it is the latter that is discussed here.

Although congenital defects that occur during formation of the neural arches of the vertebrae may result in spina bifida, spondylolysis has never been found in the newborn. The youngest reported case was a 3.5-month-old infant recorded in 1971. The occurrence of spondylolysis increases markedly between the ages of 5.5 and 6.5 years; and by the age of 7.0 years it is present in about 5 percent of the popu-

---

Practice Point

SPONDYLOLYSIS AND SPONDYLOLISTHESIS: CLINICAL PRESENTATION

- Dull backache
- Aggravated by activity
- Buttock pain
- Possibly sciatica from root irritation
- Spasm of erector spinae muscles
- Hamstring spasm, limited straight-leg raise
- Occasional increased lumbar lordosis (low slip)
- Transverse crease across back (high slip)

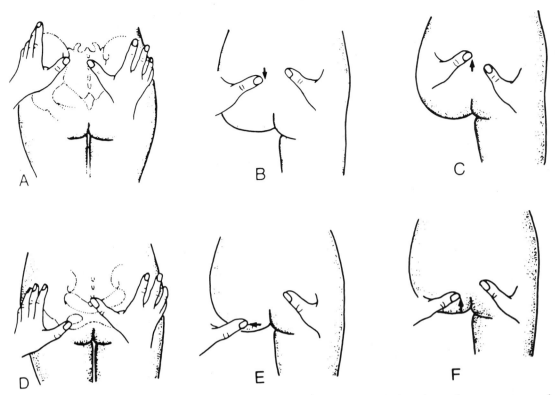

Fig. 19-48. Test for left sacroiliac fixation. **(A)** Examiner places the left thumb on the posterosuperior spine and the right thumb over the sacral spinous process. **(B)** When movement is normal, the examiner's left thumb moves downward as the patient raises the left leg. **(C)** When the joint is fixed, the examiner's left thumb moves upward as the patient raises the left leg. **(D)** Examiner's left thumb is over the ischial tuberosity, and the right thumb is over the apex of the sacrum. **(E)** With normal motion, the examiner's left thumb moves laterally as the patient raises the left leg. **(F)** When the joint is fixed, the examiner's left thumb moves slightly upward as the patient raises the leg. (From Kirkaldy-Willis,[130] with permission.)

lation. The incidence remains at this level in the white adult, although an incidence of 7 to 10 percent is seen among Japanese adults, and Eskimos north of the Yukon may have an incidence of 20 to 50 percent. In active individuals the defect may become symptomatic, or fresh stress fractures may occur during the teenage years.

Although the defect is frequently present, few actually progress to a slip. When slips do develop, it is often between the ages of 10 and 15 years; and there is rarely an increase in the slip after age 20. In summary, there is probably a congenital predisposition to spondylolysis that is precipitated by postural and environmental stress.

Approximately 90 percent of the slips occur at the L5–S1 level. The amount of slip is graded according to the percent slip of the superior vertebrae on the inferior vertebrae. A minimal slip is categorized as grade 1; and if more than 75 percent of the vertebra has slipped, it is a grade IV slip (Fig. 19-50). Between these extremes are grade II and III slips.

That vigorous activity plays some role in the etiology is beyond doubt.[88] There is an incidence of approximately 11 percent in female gymnasts, and the condition occurs frequently in high jumpers and hurdlers. Hoshini subjected the spines of 677 male high school athletes to roentgenography in 1978 and found that spondylolytic neural arches were present in more than 20 percent.[102] He noted that about 25 percent of the athletes with spondylolysis had back

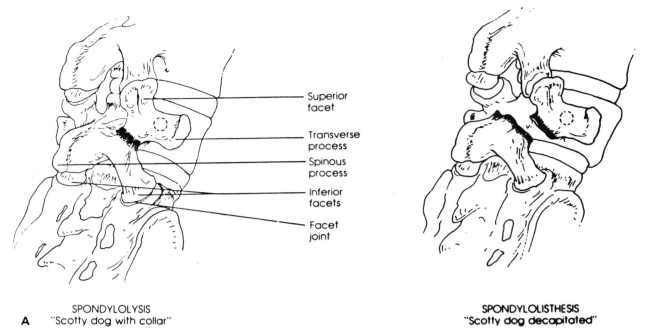

SPONDYLOLYSIS
"Scotty dog with collar"

A

SPONDYLOLISTHESIS
"Scotty dog decapitated"

Fig. 19-49. **(A)** Spondylolysis with a defect in the pars interarticularis. **(B)** Spondylolisthesis. In this instance the vertebra has slipped, and the apparent "collar on the Scotty dog" widens. This picture is seen in the oblique roentgenographic view. (After Magee,[9] with permission.)

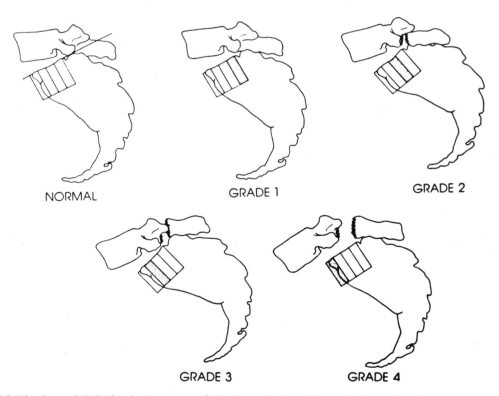

NORMAL

GRADE 1

GRADE 2

GRADE 3

GRADE 4

Fig. 19-50. Spondylolisthesis. Amount of slip is graded I to IV by dividing the adjacent vertebral body into quadrants. Should the superior vertebrae completely dislocate anteriorly it is referred to as a spondyloptosis.

pain, in contrast to only about 15 percent of those with intact neural arches. Hoshini also drew attention to the high incidence of associated anomalies, such as spina bifida and partial sacrolization of the lumbar spine. Wiltse in 1957 noted that all but one of 14 adolescents with spondylolysis were engaged in vigorous sports at the time of the onset of their back pain.[103] Spondylolysis has been reported in up to 30 percent of weight lifters between the ages of 18 and 24 who experience back pain. Finally, Fergusson in 1974 reported that half of the interior linemen on one football team complained of back pain and that of these men one-half had spondylolysis.[104] That is, one-fourth of the interior linemen on one football team suffered from back pain with spondylolysis as a cause.

Although these statistics are impressive, the presence of a radiologic defect does not automatically make it the source of low back pain. Back pain aggravated by forced extension of the spine and a hot bone scan, are strong evidence that the defect is the source of discomfort. Similarly, the presence of documented lumbar instability on lateral flexion extension views and progressive slip over time point to the defect as the source. There should be a reluctance to indict lysis as the source of low back pain in the absence of the above clinical and radiologic findings. Particular attention should be paid to the young athlete developing acute low back pain with severe paraspinal muscle spasm. Eventually, many of these individuals are shown to have roentgenographic evidence of spondylolysis. There may be an association of spina bifida of the fifth lumbar vertebrae with spondylolysis, which may indicate that the developmental defect in this vertebra causes an instability that may predispose to the development of a fracture of the neural arch. Furthermore, the greater body weight and muscle strength in those with spondylolysis suggests that these factors may also contribute to its development by allowing a greater torque to be exerted on the spine during twisting actions and hyperextension maneuvers.

Young female gymnasts are particularly predisposed to lower back troubles. The frequency of somersaulting and back arching in modern gymnastics leads to an increase in back stress. Seventy-five percent of international women gymnasts suffer from lower back pain. Excessive lordosis present in a significant proportion of these women may predispose them to problems.[105]

Unsupervised weight training or the combination of an extensive weight program emphasizing poorly performed squats, leaping exercises, and repetitive back extension with rotation, particularly when combined with repetitive back extension and twisting at high velocities in sport, leave the young athlete susceptible to this condition.[106]

Practice Point

DEFECT/PAIN (0 TO 25 PERCENT SLIP): TREATMENT

- Training modification
- Correction of techniques
- Hamstring stretching
- Anti-inflammatory medication
- Bone scan if symptoms do not resolve

It is important to detect early stress fractures so the aggravating activities can be restricted for a period of time. The presenting complaint is usually low back pain and aching aggravated by activity, particularly repetitive loaded extension maneuvers. Occasionally, there are sharp, shooting pains and sometimes aching into the buttock. Single-legged back extension or arching may aggravate and localize the symptoms to one side or the other (Fig. 19-51). The diagnosis is confirmed by oblique roentgenograms. If the symptoms are present and the history suggestive, a bone scan helps confirm the diagnosis. It is critical, in cases of a well developed defect, to document any tendency toward a progressive slip.

Treatment consists in avoiding aggravating activities and rest. The average time for returning to pain-free competition is about 7 months. If these lesions are not detected early, they can be the source of prolonged and considerable disability. In some cases it is possible for the athlete to continue training wearing a special lumbar brace.

Practice Point

CONSIDER BRACE

- Pain continues despite decreased activity.
- Athlete unable to train in key situations.
- Increasing slip is suggested.
- Bone scan confirms spondylolysis is hot.

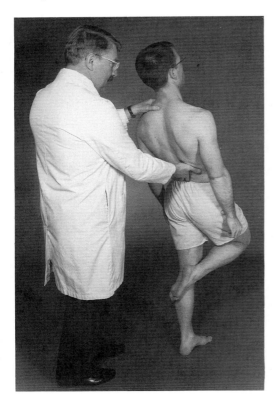

Fig. 19-51. In cases of suspected spondylolysis or spondylolisthesis, one-legged back extension may help localize the pain specifically to one or the other side of the low back. A positive test is aggravation of the symptoms with mainly a unilateral focus.

If the pain becomes unremitting, the slip progresses despite treatment, or reflex changes and muscle weakness start to develop, discontinuance of vigorous activity is necessary. Furthermore, if the slip is more than 25 percent, caution should be exercised about allowing contact sports unless the patient is absolutely asymptomatic and lack of progression has been documented.

Practice Point

SURGERY CONSIDERED

- Progression of slip despite rest
- Progression of hard neurologic signs
- Any evidence of spinal cord involvement
- Intractable pain despite treatment

In a few individuals, progression of the slip and evolution of neurologic signs make necessary the consideration of surgical intervention. Such surgery usually involves only fusion occasionally associated with decompression.

Back Pain in Runners

Chronic low back pain may affect 9 to 12 percent of distance runners.[107] Because running training forms the basis for endurance work in many sports, the importance of any running-acquired injury cannot be overemphasized. The prevalence and treatment of running-related back discomfort may be considered under the headings of anatomy, terrain, technique, equipment, and pre-existing pathology.

Practice Point

BACK PAIN IN RUNNERS

- Anatomic factors
  -Tight hip flexors
  -Tight hamstrings
  -Leg length discrepancies
  -Loss of disc height
  -Excessive body weight
- Terrain
  -Camber of roads
  -Hill work
- Technique and style
  -Forward lean versus upright stance
  -Overstriding
  -Excessive sway or pelvic tilt
  -Distance and intensity
- Equipment
  -Footwear
  -Orthosis
- Pre-existing disease
  -Degenerative disc
  -Spinal stenosis
  -Protruding disc
  -Vascular insufficiency

There is a tendency for selected muscle tightness in runners and in those involved in running sports such as soccer and field hockey.[108] In particular, tight hip flexors produce a greater tendency to forward lean and a shorter stride. Similarly, tight hamstrings may decrease stride length.[109] Perhaps overstriding in the presence of this pattern of tightness results in increased stress at the lumbosacral junction and sacroiliac joints. An excessive sway and tight abductors may also increase lumbosacral stress. A leg length discrepancy or running on the camber of the road may place undue stress on the spine.

Training techniques that include inadequate time for progression of distance, speed, and hill work may precipitate back pain. Running styles must be individualized; and if there is significant back pain, the athlete's style should be analyzed. Runners who are overweight may be particularly susceptible.

The stress induced by running is high, but fortunately usually fewer than 1 to 2 percent of impact forces reach the lumbar spine because the physiologic shock is absorbed through the lower limb joints. Nevertheless, poor or worn footwear, a rigid orthosis, or an inappropriately prescribed orthosis may generate a multitude of lower limb problems including back pain.

Some compressive loading is unavoidable when running. Compressive forces narrow the intervertebral discs when the osmotic pressure within the nucleus pulposus is exceeded.[110] Loss of disc height may be reflected in changes in stature; which thus forms an indirect measurement of the associated spinal shrinkage. Shrinkage increases with running speed, probably because of increased stress, and is always greatest during the first 15 to 30 minutes; the shrinkage ranges from 3 to 10 mm.[111,112] If there is pre-existing facet joint or disc disease, it is possible that this shrinkage adversely affects the local pathology, resulting in pain or inflammation. This point has not been satisfactorily correlated, however.

Certainly individuals with pre-existing disease may find that running adversely affects the problem, although it is not universally true. Athletes who have periodic radicular symptoms may have to limit their mileage and select flat terrain. Similarly, individuals with repeated flare-ups of facet joint inflammation may have to modify their style or consider swimming or walking as an alternative activity. Claudication symptoms may be due to vascular or neural causes. Usually if the pathology is atherosclerosis, activity must be curtailed to within the tolerance of the muscles and the ability of the circulation to support exercise. When neural claudication is the cause of leg symptoms, modification of style and terrain may provide remarkable relief. Usually a more forward lean and avoidance of steep hills is necessary. Ultimately,

with both vascular and neural causes, surgical therapy may be the answer.

Individuals with repeated episodes of backache when running should take the following precautionary measures.

1. If overweight, decrease body fat.
2. Experiment with stride length and particularly avoid overstriding.
3. Do not overstride to increase speed, as it increases leg shock.[112]
4. When appropriate, use maximum shock-absorbing shoes and orthoses. Consider heel motion control, and do not use footwear to the point that the shoes have lost all ability to assist in stress dissipation.
5. Warm up and stretch thoroughly and conscientiously, concentrating on hip flexors, hamstrings, and abductors.
6. Increase the strength of the abdominal muscles.
7. Consider alternating running with nonimpact activities such as swimming or cycling.
8. Adjust for significant leg length discrepancies.
9. Avoid training errors of sudden increases in intensity, duration, and distance. Do not increase any of these parameters more than 10 percent in 1 week and increase only one of them at a time. Progress each independently.
10. Consider running on the best terrain available. Keep off concrete when possible. Avoid excessive hill work.

Paying attention to the above suggestions may assist in decreasing the frequency of attacks of back pain and allow successful progression of activity. However, for some individuals, the establishment of more realistic goals is the most important treatment modality.

Radiculopathy (Radicular Back and Leg Pain)

Radicular pain in athletes is nearly always to the sciatic nerve and is invariably secondary to disc protrusion. This subject is discussed below along with some other common radicular complaints.

Sciatica (Disc Protrusion)

The intervertebral disc in young individuals is incredibly strong. Although there is a large amount of jelly-like nucleus in its center, disc protrusion rarely occurs because of the integrity of the surrounding annulus. Thus disc protrusion in the young is un-usual, although with the multiple stresses of some sports there is perhaps a slightly higher incidence of disc prolapse and radicular irritation in the young athlete. The treatment goal is to resolve the symptoms and to try and prevent them from becoming asso-ciated with hard neurologic findings. To do it while guiding the individual back into activity presents a difficult challenge. At birth the disc is approximately 88 percent water; and as this water content decreases with age, so does the ability of the disc to withstand stress. In the older individual the annulus is fre-quently worn and structurally weak, and the nuclear material has changed in consistency and amount. Thus radicular symptoms are not usually due to disc protrusion but, rather, to impingement on osteo-phytes in the narrowed intervertebral foramen or lat-eral recess. It is in the age group from 30 to 50 that there is the more fragile combination of accumulat-ing damage to the annulus and a large bulging nu-cleus. Hence the risk of disc protrusion is greatest, usually posterolaterally when the annulus is weakest (Table 19-17).

To better understand the consequences of a col-lapsed intervertebral disc, it is probably better to use standard terminology. The term *bulging* or *protruded disc* refers to some eccentric accumulation of the nu-cleus with slight deformity of the annulus. A *prolapsed disc* is one in which the eccentric nucleus produces a definite deformity as it works its way through the fibers of the annulus. An *extruded disc* refers to the situation in which the nuclear material comes out into the canal and runs the risk of impinging on the adja-cent nerve roots. Finally, with a *sequestrated disc,* this nuclear material has separated from the disc itself and potentially migrates (Fig. 19-52).

Understanding of the pathophysiology of disc her-niation is relatively recent. Although Domenico Co-tugno gave an excellent description of sciatica in 1764, and Von Luschka in 1858 described a soft, grayish nob of tissue on the surface of the posterior longitudinal ligament and speculated that it could eventually lead to cord compression,[113,114] it re-mained for Mixter and Barr in 1934 to publish their classic paper "on the prolapsed intervertebral disc as a cause of sciatic pain."[115] Even then, the concept was not universally accepted until the signal work of Smyth and Wright, who left nylon threads attached to the nerve root and disc at surgery and then carefully outlined the following observations.[113–116]

1. Traction on the nerve root produced a character-istic distribution of pain.
2. The pain was proportional to the pressure.
3. An inflamed nerve root produced more symptoms than a normal nerve root.
4. Pain can be referred to the back or the buttock from the dura and the longitudinal ligaments.
5. Referred pain from the L4 and L5 nerve roots may produce symptoms in the foot. Pain from the other structures rarely went past the knee.
6. Pain is relieved when the pressure is removed.

With this irrefutable evidence, it seemed that diag-nosis would soon become clear and a treatment plan standardized. However, there is still much contro-versy regarding all aspects of the management of disc disease.

Physical Findings

To localize the lesion it is necessary to record a combination of sensory alteration such as pain, dys-esthesia, or numbness, the distribution of muscle weakness and wasting, and altered segmental reflexes (Table 19-18). Of these problems, muscle weakness and wasting and loss of a reflex are considered hard neurologic signs. Any significant involvement of bowel or bladder constitutes a situation in which im-mediate relief of the pressure on the nerves or conus must be considered in order to stop the situation from becoming permanent. It requires immediate diagnosis and perhaps urgent surgical therapy.

TABLE 19-17. Incidence of Disc Disease and Protrusion with Age

Young Age	Middle Age	Old Age
Healthy disc	Slightly degenerative disc	Narrowed dystrophic disc
Tough annulus	Wear changes on peripheral annulus	Worn annulus
Large nucleus	Still relatively large nucleus	Minimal nucleus available
Disc protrusion rare: usually with significant trauma	Disc protrusion common; often with minor trauma	Disc protrusion unusual

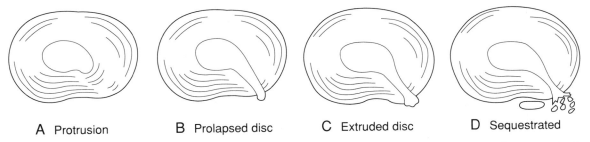

A   Protrusion   B   Prolapsed disc   C   Extruded disc   D   Sequestrated

Fig. 19-52. Classification of prolapsed (herniated) intervertebral discs. A sequence of progressively more eccentric position of the nucleus **(A)** protruded **(B)** prolapse **(C)** extrusion, which culminates in **(D)** a sequestrated disc in which the nuclear material is free in the canal. It may then move up and down, impinging on adjacent nerve roots. (From MacNab,[113] with permission.)

Because of the anatomic relation of the disc to the emerging nerve roots, there is not always a clear segmental picture. Indeed particularly at the L5–S1 disc, one would expect a more centrally protruding nucleus to press on the S1 root, but a lateral and superior protrusion easily irritates the L5 root. A similar situation occurs at the L4–L5 level in which the L5 root is usually irritated, but the L4 root can be easily involved with a superiorly migrating excursion. A large protrusion at L4–L5 may affect multiple roots. Of particular relevance is cauda equina pressure, which results in bowel and bladder symptoms[14] (Fig. 19-53).

Shiquing et al., observing a series of patients with sciatica who came to surgical exploration, noted that: (1) a small central protrusion at L4–L5 or L5–S1 usually compresses the dura and causes back pain only; (2) a massive central prolapse is in contact with both dura and bilateral nerve roots and may cause pain in the back and bilateral sciatica; (3) a lateral protrusion usually compresses the sheath of the nerve root alone, thus producing only sciatic pain; (4) an intermediate placed protrusion may be in contact with both the dura and the spinal nerve root on one side, producing back pain and unilateral sciatica; and (5) protrusion in the axillary position of the junction of the root with the cord usually causes pain in the back and sciatica, as well as limitation of straight-leg raising of the contralateral limb in most patients[114] (Fig. 19-54). This type of protrusion is aggravated by side flexion away from the side of the lesion and is released slightly by side flexion to the side of the lesion (Fig. 19-55). Sometimes this bending to one side (sciatic scoliosis) is due entirely to spasm, and so

reduction of the listing relieves symptoms. However, if the scoliosis is serving the purpose of reducing radicular pressure, attempts to straighten the spine aggravates the symptoms until the protrusion becomes

---

Practice Point

DIFFERENTIAL FEATURES OF RADICULOPATHIES

Symptom	L3–L4 (L4 Root)	L4–L5 (L5 Root)	L5–S1 (S1 Root)
Pain	Lumbar region and flank	Lumbar region, groin, sacroiliac area	Lumbar region, groin, sacroiliac area
Radiation	Anteromedial thigh	Lateral thigh, leg, dorsum of foot, hallux	Buttock, posterior, thigh, leg, lateral foot
Sensory loss	Medial shin	Hallux area	Lateral foot
Weakness	Quadriceps	Extensor hallux	Gastrocnemius
Reduced deep tendon reflex	Quadriceps	Medial hamstrings	Ankle jerk
Straight-leg raising	Normal	Reduced	Reduced

TABLE 19-18. Lumbar Root Syndromes

Root	Dermatome	Muscle Weakness	Reflexes Affected and Tension Test	Paresthesias
L1	Back; over trochanter, groin	None	None	Groin, after holding posture, which causes pain
L2	Back; front of thigh to knee	Psoas Hip adductors	None	Occasionally front of thigh
L3	Back; upper buttock; front of thigh and knee; medial lower leg	Psoas Quadriceps Thigh wasting	Knee jerk sluggish; femoral stretch test positive; pain on full SLR	Inner knee, anterior lower leg
L4	Inner buttock; outer thigh, inside of leg; dorsum of foot; big toe	Tibialis anterior Extensor hallucis	SLR limited; neck flexion increases pain; weak or absent knee jerk; side flexion limited	Medial aspect of calf and ankle
L5	Buttock; back and side of thigh; lateral aspect of leg; dorsum of foot; inner half of sole and first, second, and third toes	Extensor hallucis peroneals Gluteus medius Ankle dorsiflexors Hamstrings Calf wasting	SLR limited to one side; neck-flexion increases pain; ankle jerk decreased; crossed-leg raising sometimes painful	Lateral aspect of leg, medial three toes
S1	Buttock; back of thigh and lower leg	Calf and hamstrings Peroneals, plantar flexors Wasting of gluteals	SLR limited	Lateral two toes, lateral foot, lateral leg to knee, plantar aspect of foot
Sacral roots 2–4	Perineum; genitals; lower sacrum	Bladder, rectum		Saddle area, genitals; impotence if massive posterior protrusion

SLR = straight-leg raise.

less painful. Furthermore, to some degree mild irritation of the root is signified by pain, whereas more extensive and protracted pressure may result in numbness, muscle weakness, and reflex changes.

There are some classic presentations of radiculopathy (Table 19-18). The L4 root produces pain mainly in the lumbar region and flank radiating into the anteromedial thigh, with occasional sensory loss along the anteromedial shin. The major weakness is in the quadriceps. The patellar tendon reflex is affected. Straight-leg raising may be normal, but the femoral nerve stretch test is markedly positive, producing pain along the anteromedial thigh. An L5 root impingement results in pain radiating to the lateral thigh and the dorsum of the foot, with or without back pain. Sensory loss is mainly in the region of the big toe, on the dorsal surface. The weakness is in the extensor hallucis longus and the inverters. The medial hamstring reflex is affected. With this lesion, all of the sciatic nerve tension tests are frequently positive. In addition, the femoral nerve stretch test produces pain that radiates along the posterior thigh in the sciatic distribution, rather than anteriorly and

medially, as when the L4 root is affected. The S1 root may produce pain in the groin and the sacroiliac areas, along the buttock and posterior thigh, and down to the lateral foot. When sensory loss occurs, it is usually in the area of the lateral side of the foot. The gastrocnemius may be weak, and the gluteus maximus may lose some of its tone. The affected reflex is the ankle jerk. S1 root impingement is usually sensitive to all of the sciatic nerve tension tests.

The important nerve root stretch tests include standing with forward bending to touch the toes, sitting alternately extending one leg and then the other, sitting bent forward and extending leg and then the other (the slump test), and the straight-leg raising test (Lasègue sign) (Fig. 19-56). The Lasègue sign can be enhanced by flexing up the head (Kernig-Lasègue) or by pressing in the middle of the fossa, placing further tension on the tibial component of the sciatic nerve (Figs. 19-57 and 19-58). In each case a positive test is an increase in symptoms in the distribution of the appropriate root. Usually the more severe the radiculopathy, the more sensitive is the nerve root and the more rapidly are signs evident after starting the test.

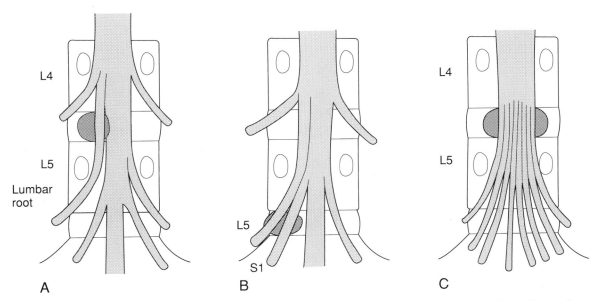

Fig. 19-53. Possible effects according to the level of disc herniation. **(A)** Herniation of the disc between L4 and L5 compresses the fifth lumbar root. **(B)** Large herniation of the L5–S1 disc may compromise not only the nerve root crossing the disc (first sacral nerve root) but also the nerve root emerging through the foramen (fifth lumbar nerve root). **(C)** Small central protrusion of the disc may compress the dura mater and usually causes pain in the back only, but massive central sequestration of the disc at the L4–L5 level may involve all the nerve roots in the cauda equina and thus may result in bowel and bladder paralysis. (From MacNab,[113] with permission.)

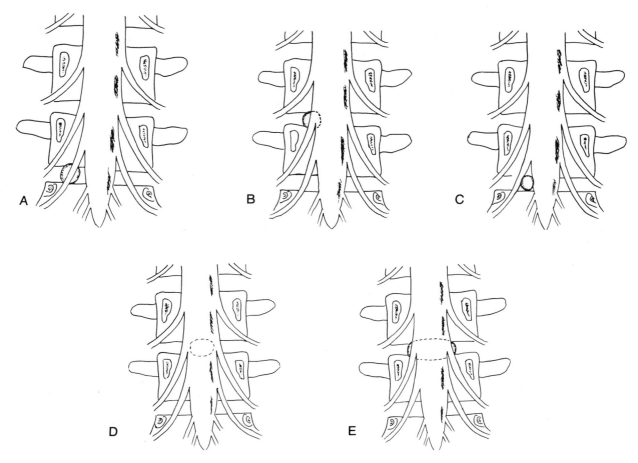

Fig. 19-54. Effects of position of the protrusion on symptoms. **(A)** Lateral protrusion that compresses the sheath of the nerve root alone usually causes only sciatic pain. **(B)** Intermediate protrusion in contact with both the dura mater and the spinal nerve usually causes pain in the back and unilateral sciatica. **(C)** Protrusion in the axilla of the root causes back pain and sciatica as well as limitation of straight-leg raising of the contralateral lower limb in most patients (well leg, straight-leg raising test positive). **(D)** Small central protrusion may produce only back pain. **(E)** Large central protrusion may produce back pain and bilateral sciatica.

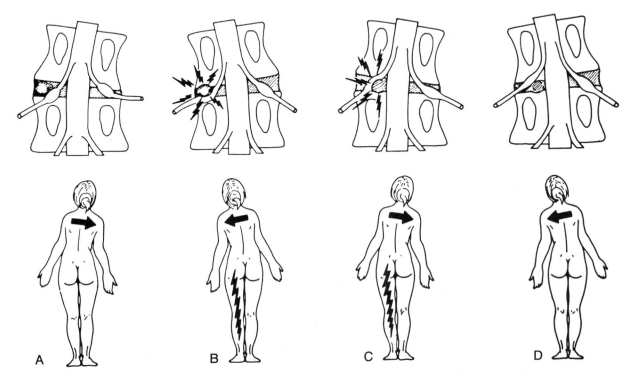

Fig. 19-55. Effect of position of the protrusion on scoliosis. Patients with herniated discs sometimes list to one side (sciatic scoliosis). This mechanism tends to alleviate nerve root irritation but may also be the result of spasm. **(A)** When the herniation is lateral to the nerve root, the list is to the side opposite the sciatica because **(B)** a list of the same side would tend to increase the pain owing to pressure on the nerve root possibly secondary to further bulging of the disc. **(C & D)** Conversely, when the herniation is medial to the nerve root (axillary position), leaning away from the side of the sciatica tends to increase the tension over the protrusion whereas a list toward the side of the sciatica provides symptomatic relief. (From White AA, Panjabi MM: Clinical Biomechanics of the Spine. p. 299. JB Lippincott, Philadelphia, 1978, with permission.)

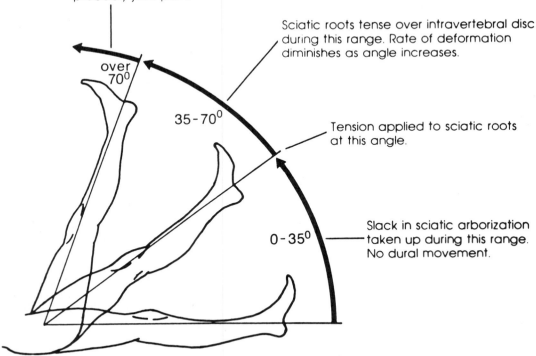

Practically no further deformation of roots occurs during further straight leg raising. Pain is probably joint pain.

Sciatic roots tense over intravertebral disc during this range. Rate of deformation diminishes as angle increases.

over 70⁰

35-70⁰

Tension applied to sciatic roots at this angle.

0-35⁰

Slack in sciatic arborization taken up during this range. No dural movement.

Fig. 19-56. Dynamics of the single straight-leg raising test. Even the most severe radicular pain usually enables approximately 30 degrees of straight-leg raising. Subsequently, there is increasing tension on the sciatic nerve roots. Caution should be used when interpreting this test if the athlete is flexible, as increased sciatic signs may not become apparent until well past the normal expected range because of the acquired increased flexibility of all structures. (Modified from Fahrni, WH: Canadian J Surg 9:44, 1966.)

The well-leg-raising (cross-sciatic reflex) test, described by Fajersztajn in 1901, is also important.[117] Fajersztajn described the foot dorsiflexion and neck flexion tests as well, which are performed with the leg raised to the point of producing sciatic pain; these additional maneuvers compound the discomfort. It has already been mentioned that the femoral nerve stretch test may produce sciatic pain when the L5 root is involved.

Probably the most unequivocal signs of disc protrusion are pain on contralateral straight-leg raising, an abnormal reflex, and measurable muscle wasting or significant weakness.[9,117,118] If there is a question as to whether the patient is cooperating with strength assessment, the Hoover test may unmask a functional component to the symptoms. Normally, significant effort to elevate one leg results in downward pressure by the contralateral limb (Fig. 19-59).

Practice Point

CAUDA EQUINA INVOLVEMENT

- Central disc
  - Asymmetric muscle weakness in legs
  - Radicular sensory loss over sacrum, perineum, and back of thigh
  - Impotence; urinary frequency or retention
- Lateral disc
  - Segmental root pain
  - Segmental weakness and wasting
  - Altered sequential reflex
  - Late development of sphincter disturbance

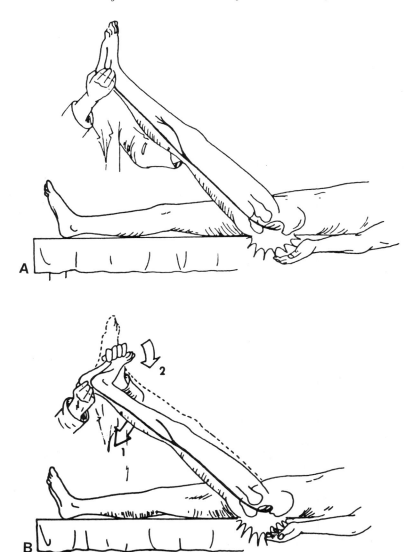

Fig. 19-57. Straight-leg raising test can be enhanced by **(A)** elevating the head (Kernig-Lasègue sign) or **(B)** passively dorsiflexing the foot. Both of these mechanisms increase dural tension and should exacerbate the sciatic symptoms. (From Reilly BM: Practical Strategies in Outpatient Medicine. p. 10. WB Saunders, Philadelphia, 1984.)

Other Diagnostic Tests

If the history is compatible with the physical findings and a diagnosis of protruded intervertebral disc is made, the radiologic and laboratory workup depends on the duration and intensity of the symptoms. In all cases plain films of the spine are warranted. However, specialized tests such as CT, CT myelogram, and MRI are reserved for: (1) confirming the diagnosis if the athlete does not respond to treatment; (2) confirming the diagnosis if the symptoms are recurrent; (3) presurgical testing to localize the site and extent of the protrusion; or (4) cases in which

an alternate cause for the radiculitis is suspected. A word of caution is necessary, however, as a significant percentage of the population have bulging discs that are asymptomatic. Therefore surgical decisions should depend on the clinical picture and radiologic findings confirming the site of pathology.

Treatment Principles

Treatment depends on the severity and chronicity of symptoms at presentation, the type of activity in which the athlete participates, and the normal daily activity and occupation (Table 19-19). Sciatica is not

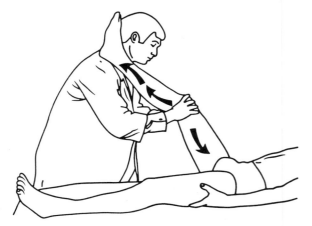

Practice Point

DISCOGENIC PAIN: TREATMENT

- Treat proportional to signs.
- Modify or discontinue activity.
- Consider short period of bed rest.
- Give some combination of NSAIDs, analgesics, muscle relaxants.
- Set up rehabilitation protocol.

Fig. 19-58. Bowstring sign. The straight-leg raise is performed until significant sciatic discomfort is felt. The knee is then flexed to slightly relieve this sensation. At this point, pressure on the popliteal nerve in the fossa should once more exacerbate the discomfort. This test is used primarily to contrast it with the response of pressure over the hamstring insertion in an attempt to delineate the true symptoms from a patient who may have a functional overlay. (After MacNab,[113] with permission.)

an automatic reason to discontinue all training and competition, but it is a symptom that must always be taken seriously, investigated adequately, and a treatment plan devised that provides maximal chance of uneventful recovery. Above all, the progression of neurologic signs is to be avoided.

If the athlete presents with sciatica, associated hard neurologic signs, and bladder involvement, a full investigation is required and perhaps immediate decompressive surgery. If there is no evidence of bladder or bowel involvement, significant restriction of activity for up to 3 weeks is appropriate. The same is true of individuals with intense sciatic pain and paravertebral muscle spasm, even without hard neurologic signs.

During these first few weeks, analgesics, NSAIDs, and perhaps antispasmodic medication are given proportional to the symptoms. Absolute bed rest is not necessary, but the therapist can discuss with the patient the various positions that most relieve stress on the disc, including lying with the legs flexed and pillows under the thighs or side lying with the knees flexed and pillows between the legs. Prolonged sitting

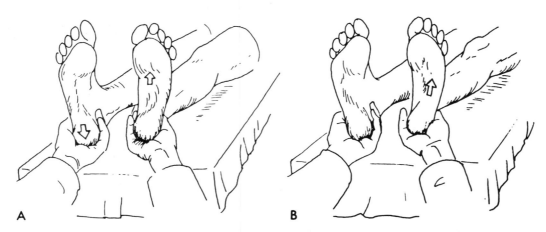

Fig. 19-59. Hoover test. **(A)** Normally a significant voluntary effort by the patient to elevate one limb results in palpable downward pressure by the heel of the contralateral limb. **(B)** Failure of the examiner to experience this involuntary downward pressure suggests that some of the weakness is possibly feigned. (From Reilly BM: Practical Strategies in Outpatient Medicine. p. 10. WB Saunders, Philadelphia, 1984, with permission.)

TABLE 19-19.   Treatment Guidelines for Athletes Presenting with Sciatica

Condition at Presentation	Investigation	Treatment
Sciatica. Reflex changes. Muscle weakness. Bladder function altered.	CT scan or MRI urgently	Consider immediate surgical decompression.
Sciatica. Reflex changes. Muscle weakness. Normal bowel and bladder function. Acute onset.	Plain roentgenograms of lumbar spine. If improves in 10–14 days, follow patient. If not, consider CT, MRI, or myelogram.	Complete withdrawal from sport. Modified bed rest for few days according to pain. NSAIDs, analgesics. If improves, progress treatment as per symptoms.
Sciatica. Reflex changes. Muscle weakness. Normal bladder function. Repeat or chronic.	Consider above investigations immediately.	Treat as above.
Sciatica, sensory changes, mild or no reflex changes. Normal muscle strength. Bladder normal.	Plain lumbar spine roentgenograms. If no improvement at 6 weeks, consider further investigation.	Take careful activity history. Elicit aggravating factors. Two weeks rest from sport. Immediate physiotherapy. NSAIDs. If no improvement, further modify activity. If improves, progress PRN.
Sciatica only. Sensory normal. Muscle normal.	Plain roentgenograms of lumbar spine. If no improvement at 6 weeks, consider further investigation.	Detailed activity history. Modify activity appropriately. Physiotherapy. NSAIDs. If improves progress.
Sciatica with atypical features such as fever, weight loss, chronic cough, abdominal pain, altered bowel habit or rectal bleeding, long tract signs or onset in very young or elderly.	Plain roentgenograms of lumbar spine. Consider complete blood screen. ESR. Acid and alkaline phosphatase. Bone scan. Where diagnosis not apparent, CT or MRI. Chest film.	Treat according to magnitude of symptoms and findings of screening tests.

and standing usually aggravate the condition, as they increase intradiscal pressure. Local heat or ice may help the spasm. A careful history is needed to decide not only the precipitating factor but the contributing factor that may have to be altered or rectified as the athlete is gradually returned to activity.

As the spasm subsides, therapy is progressed to include gentle pelvic tilting exercises and possibly grade I or II mobilization. With decreasing pain, further activity is allowed and traction considered. If

---

Practice Point

WHEN TO RETURN TO SPORT

- Sciatica with soft signs: 6 to 12 weeks
- Sciatica with hard signs: 12 to 24 weeks
- Analyze sport and back stresses.
- Plan a reintegration program.
- Progress depends on response to activity.
- Any deterioration of clinical signs requires immediate re-evaluation.

---

there are no significant signs of improvement at 2 to 3 weeks, further investigation is probably indicated.

If the athlete presents with only moderate sciatica and no other signs, or if the more seriously involved individual improves to this point, therapy is based on a detailed activity history. Lifting, repetitive bending, prolonged stressful postures, and rapid twisting activities are ruled out. Running is allowed if it does not increase the symptoms. Only about 1 to 5 percent of the stress resulting from landing on the ground when running reaches the lumbar spine, and hence the spine is relatively protected. As the athlete improves, abdominal and extensor muscle strength must be restored and improved; poor techniques or body mechanics must be analyzed and corrected before progression back to activity is allowed. In the individual with less involvement, full activity may be expected within 3 to 6 weeks. In those with more serious involvement, 3 to 6 months is more realistic.

In selected patients, e.g., a male ballet dancer or figure skater who is required to lift a partner, some adjustment of the roles and routines are possible. Nevertheless, these athletes occasionally benefit from wearing a corset or a custom-made thoracolumbar orthosis during the first few months after return to activity. A particularly large weight lifting belt helps others. Although the biomechanics of such devices is not clear, in special situations they are helpful adjuncts to reintegration into activity.

If symptoms resume, stopping the activity on a permanent basis is seriously considered, particulary for weight lifters, footballers, or people practicing the martial arts. Sometimes a complete year off from the sport allows a slow return to the activity. Alternatively, if symptoms are related to a definite nerve root and a significant disc protrusion is visualized on CT scanning that coincides with the clinical signs and symptoms, surgical decompression may allow resumption of activity by selected patients.

Whatever the severity of the initial radicular symptoms, once an athlete has been demonstrated to have discogenic pathology, it must be assumed that there is a risk and predisposition to further episodes. Thus an important part of the treatment is counseling, education, and instruction about techniques to maximally protect the back. The simple illustration that lifting a 20 kg weight using good techniques may result in stresses of 240 kg across the L4−L5 disc, whereas lifting the same weight with poor attention to detail may increase the load to 400 kg, may help press home the principle.

Quick Facts
INTRADISCAL PRESSURES

Condition	Pressure (kg)
Relaxed standing	95
Sitting	125
Lifting 20 kg — good technique	240
Lifting 20 kg — poor technique	400

Role of Traction

Lumbar traction can be an effective adjunct to treatment of a number of common muculoskeletal complaints including facet joint pain, disc degeneration, and disc protrusion. It is the skill of the therapist that frequently provides optimal efficacy. The choice of manual traction, postural traction, sustained horizontal traction, and inversion therapy should be based on the patient's presenting complaints, gentle tentative trials and slow progression, and the absence

of contraindications (Table 19-20). For patients with lumbar disc protrusion, correctly applied traction may reduce the bulging disc, but the mechanical effect is usually transient.[119] However, symptomatic relief may be much longer lasting and hence is a useful part of the athlete's therapy.

Mechanical traction should always be applied cautiously, so treatment progress may be based on the response to the previous session. To produce effective distraction of the disc, 80 to 200 lb of traction is needed to overcome the inertia of the body and the friction of the table. This statement does not mean that this amount is the starting poundage or that the maximum weight is desirable. There should be a buildup to effective, comfortable traction, and the therapist must be prepared to abandon the technique if it is not working. Initially, treatment times should be kept relatively short because most distraction is achieved fairly rapidly, with only a small amount of creep occurring after the first 5 to 10 minutes. Also, after a while the distracted disc may imbibe fluid. Thus when pressure is released there may be a relative increase in intradiscal volume and pressure relative to the pretraction values. Traction times of 10 minutes

---

TABLE 19-20. Lumbar Traction

Physiologic effects
  Separation of vertebral bodies
  Distraction and gliding of the facet joints
  Tensing of the ligamentous structures of the spinal segment
  Widening of the intervertebral foramen
  Straightening of the spinal curves
  Stretching of the spinal musculature

Indications
  Herniated discus pulposus with disc protrusion
  Degenerative disc disease (stenosis of the intervertebral foramen)
  Joint dysfunction (hypomobility)
  Facet joint symptoms

Contraindications and precautions
  Structural compromise secondary to tumor, infection, or disease
      Patients with vascular compromise
      Fractures
      Any condition where movement is contraindicated
  Acute strains, sprains, and inflammation aggravated by traction
  Intervertebral segment instability
  Pregnancy
  Osteoporosis
  Hiatus hernia

for sustained traction and 15 minutes intermittently are probably safe and maximally efficacious.

Gravity-facilitated (inversion) traction has an obvious appeal, and many such systems are available. There is little question that these systems have the ability to distract the disc spaces.[119,120]

Quick Facts

AVERAGE SEPARATION OF DISC SPACES WITH GRAVITY-ASSISTED TRACTION

- Relieve spasm prior to therapy.
- May distract facet joints
- May distract disc space
  L3–L4: 1.5 mm
  L4–L5: 1.6 mm
  L5–S1: 2.0 mm

It is important to be cognizant of the cardiovascular effects. The heart rate may drop approximately 16 beats per minute, and the systolic and diastolic pressures increase by 16 to 17 mmHg.[120,121] It is probably unwise to add an exercise routine to the inverted position. The patients may complain of headaches; blurred vision; conjunctival injection; periorbital and phalangeal petechiae; dry eyes (contact lens wearers); feelings of chest discomfort; ankle, calf, and thigh discomfort; and nasal stuffiness. There is also decreased lower limb blood flow. Thus if this technique is considered, adjustments must be made if the above

---

Practice Point

CONTRAINDICATIONS TO GRAVITY-ASSISTED TRACTION

- Hypertension
- Peripheral vascular disease
- Cataracts
- Glaucoma
- Chronic obstructive pulmonary disease
- Labile asthma
- Hemophilia
- Pregnancy

---

symptoms are experienced, and due regard must be given to any specific contraindications.

Surgical Treatment

Should the symptoms of radiculitis secondary to disc protrusion fail to resolve, a surgical option may be appropriate. Such surgery includes chemonucleolysis, percutaneous suction excision, or open discectomy.

Chemonucleolysis. Chymopapain is a proteolytic enzyme found in the latex of the pawpaw (*Carica papaya*). In 1941 Jansen and Balls isolated chymopapain, and in 1959 Hirsch first proposed its use as an enzyme to dissolve disc material.[122]

Practice Point

IDEAL CANDIDATE FOR CHYMOPAPAIN INJECTION

- Single level disc disease
- Nonsequestrated disc
- Confirmed level and diagnosis
- Short duration of symptoms
- No muscle weakness
- Minimal associated degenerative changes

It disrupts the fine chondromucoprotein structure, destroys the water-binding capacity of the nucleus, and reduces the pressure it can exert. Used for

---

Practice Point

CONTRAINDICATIONS TO CHYMOPAPAIN INJECTIONS

- Pregnancy
- Allergy to meat tenderizer
- Uncertain diagnosis
- Complete block on myelogram
- Cauda equina syndrome (poor sphincter control)
- Severe progressive paralysis
- Spinal stenosis
- Tumor
- Prior injection of chymopapain

the correct indications, successful treatment results in resolution of the sciatica, pain-free straight-leg raising, and ultimately narrowing of the disc space. For the athlete it is a technique that allows shorter interruption of training. Although the sciatica improves quickly, there may be acute intermittent backache for up to 24 hours and dull backache lasting up to a month — frequently worse in muscular individuals. Light work is allowed at 3 weeks and gradual resumption of full training starting at 6 weeks after injection.

Percutaneous Suction Excision. Percutaneous discectomy is performed by introducing an aspiration probe (nucleosome) through a hole in the annulus and into the disc space. The probe is a cutting instrument as well as a suction instrument, and aspiration occurs concurrently with the morcellation.[123,124] The instrument is introduced into the disc space, as with the chymopapain technique, by fluoroscopic or CT control. This technique may even be considered on an outpatient basis for selected patients. It may be used in large athletes, who are difficult to operate on or without a large incision using standard techniques; and it may be done with local anesthesia. Its use is appropriate for disc herniation still contained by the annulus or the posterior longitudinal ligament. It should not be used in individuals who have extruded or free fragments of disc in the spinal canal, and it is difficult to enter at the L5–S1 level.

Practice Point

PREREQUISITES FOR SUCTION DISCECTOMY

- Persistent sciatic pain
- Failure to respond to nonoperative therapy
- Neurologic signs such as reflex, sensory, and motor change deficits
- Presence of positive radicular tension signs
- Clear evidence of level of involvement and extent of protrusion

---

Except in special circumstances, resumption of activity and full training are usually possible along the same time lines as for open discectomy. There are some advantages, however, in that epidural bleeding and perineurial fibrosis are reduced and the portal is established away from the neural elements should further herniation occur. There is also preservation of spinal stability.[124]

Open Discectomy. In well selected patients direct open diskectomy provides an excellent outcome in 80 percent and improvement in another 18 percent. It is the standard against which all other procedures must be judged. Furthermore, return to activity and full training occur at approximately the same time as when the percutaneous techniques are used, i.e., ambulation the day of surgery, return to light activity at 3 weeks, and gradual resumption of full training beginning at 6 to 8 weeks depending on the preoperative condition and the type of activity.

Practice Point

OPEN DISCECTOMY INDICATIONS

- Absolute indications
  -Bladder bowel paralysis (cauda equina)
  -Marked progressive weakness of central disc
  -Progressive neurologic deficit and ineffective nonoperative therapy
  -Failure of conservative treatment in emotionally stable person
- Relative indications
  -Recurrent episodes of incapacitating sciatica
  -Pain unrelieved by complete rest from activity

Differential Diagnosis

The differential diagnosis of sciatica has already been alluded to; but apart from the usual conditions, the most frequent misdiagnosis in athletes is the confusion between sciatica and hamstring tears. Usually, distinguishing these two entities is easy once an awareness of the possibility of disc protrusion is entertained. However, in the young sprinter or running athlete, vague or even sharp posterior thigh pain is easily treated as a hamstring tear unless the injury is carefully evaluated.

Piriformis Syndrome

The piriformis syndrome is a rare condition characterized by pain and paresthesias located in the buttocks, often radiating to the posterior thigh.[125] Symptoms are frequently made worse by hip abduction and internal rotation. True neurologic deficits are uncommon. Symptoms are usually unilateral and probably related to an entrapment neuropathy caused by pressure on the sciatic nerve or adjacent inflammation from the sacroiliac joint on pelvic viscera, spasm, or trauma to the piriformis muscle. This diagnosis has been supported by an abnormal appearance of the piriformis muscle on CT scans or MRI.

In 1924 Yoemans mentioned that spasm of the piriformis muscle, in connection with degenerative changes of the sacroiliac joint, may generate sciatic pain.[126] Freiberg and Vinke proposed a clinical test using forced internal rotation of the hip with the legs extended to demonstrate the presence of pain in the piriformis.[127] Beaton and Anson reported on piriformis muscle anomalies, but it was left to Robinson in 1947 to coin the term "piriformis syndrome."[128]

Anatomically, the sciatic nerve usually passes between the piriformis muscle and the gemellus. The piriformis muscle itself arises from the pelvic surface of the sacrum, exiting from the pelvis through the greater sciatic foramen and inserting onto the upper border of the greater trochanter. In about 20 percent of the population the muscle is split, and one or both parts of the sciatic nerve pass through the muscle belly. In 10 percent of the population the tibial and peroneal portions of the sciatic nerve are not enclosed in a common sheath; and one portion, usually the peroneal division, may pierce the muscle. The piriformis muscle functions as an external rotator of the hip when the thigh is extended and an abductor of the joint when the thigh is flexed.

The clinical tests are the Freiberg sign, which is passive internal rotation of the leg generating pain, and the Pace sign, which is discomfort on resistance to abduction and external rotation of the thigh.[129] Furthermore, voluntary adduction, flexion, and internal rotation (Lasègue sign) also may generate pain.

Treatment for this condition includes stretching the piriformis muscle, ultrasound, injection of muscular trigger points with local anesthetics and corticosteroids, and in a few cases surgical section of the tendons of the piriformis.

Anterolateral Groin and Thigh Pain

The syndrome of entrapment of the lateral cutaneous nerve of the thigh has already been described (p. 666). The iliohypogastric, ilioinguinal, and genitofemoral nerve may be entrapped during their passage from the lumbar spine through the abdominal wall and onto their points of distribution. Frequently, the common denominator for the latter nerves is pain around the pubis in the inguinal area, the groin, and the scrotum.[130] The diagnosis is difficult. It should be entertained particularly if there had been previous abdominal surgery (Table 19-21). All other diagnostic possibilities should be eliminated including osteitis pubis and inguinal hernias. The classic clinical findings are presented in Table 19-21.

Thoracic Disc Disease

Symptomatic thoracic disc disease is rare. When it does occur, it usually is located in the lower thoracic segments. It most often affects men in their fifth decade, although in the active athlete it is seen occasionally secondary to trauma. If the disc does herniate, the pain radiates anteriorly and should be distinguished from cardiac pain or any of the other previously described chest conditions. Posterolateral disc protrusion may result in compression of a nerve root producing unilateral dermatomal chest wall pain. There is limited free space in the thoracic spinal canal, and even moderately sized posterior thoracic disc herniations may lead to cord compression and spinal paraparesis. Early on, the pain is exacerbated by coughing and sneezing or straining when lifting. If long tract signs are involved, there may be feeling of weakness or heaviness in the lower limbs, bowel disturbance, altered balance, and ultimately detectable weakening and sensory change. The diagnosis, once confirmed, should be treated promptly by rest. If there are hard neurologic signs, particularly long tract signs, usually prompt surgical intervention is indicated.

Degenerative Disc Disease

The repetitive stress of some activities produces ligamentous back pain. During the natural course of aging degenerative changes may occur within the disc that result in narrowing (Fig. 19-60). Such narrowing, in turn, places additional stress on the facet joints, which may develop degenerative changes, articular surface narrowing, synovitis, and osteophyte formation. Furthermore, as the disc narrows, the ligaments crossing the segment and the annular fibers may slacken sufficiently to allow increased segmental motion during flexion and extension. Ultimately, as disc narrowing progresses, large osteophytes may meet, join, and once more produce a stable segment (Fig. 19-61).

TABLE 19-21. Lumbar Cutaneous Entrapment Syndrome

Feature	Iliohypogastric Nerve	Ilioinguinal Nerve	Genitofemoral Nerve	Lateral Cutaneous of Thigh Nerve
Injury site	Above inguinal canal	Posterior to anterosuperior iliac spine; inguinal canal; femoral region	Posterior abdominal wall; inguinal region	Junction of inguinal ligament and anterosuperior spine
Pain distribution	Above pubis	Groin; scrotum; back	Groin; scrotum; upper thigh	Lateral anterior upper thigh
Point of maximum tenderness	Point of entrapment or where nerve emerges through external oblique muscle	Medial to anterosuperior iliac spine or inguinal canal	Internal inguinal ring	Anterosuperior iliac spine
Treatment	Neurolysis, consider neurectomy	Nerve block, neurolysis; consider neurectomy	Nerve block; consider excision of portion of main trunk of nerve	Nerve block; release by division of ligament

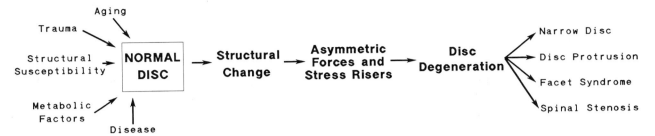

Fig. 19-60. Stresses impinging on a normal disc. These changes may evolve to either a collapsed disc or to degeneration, which may culminate in arthrosis.

Facet Joint Syndrome and Unstable Segments

Recurrent flare-ups of facet joint pain and synovitis produce what is called the facet joint syndrome (posterior facet syndrome). Pain is aggravated by extension and may be referred to the buttock and the posterior thigh (Fig. 19-62). Segmental sequential instability may cause a flare-up of pain in a similar pattern.[131] The increasing involvement in aerobic exercises and the interest of progressively older individuals in keeping fit and participating and competing in a variety of sports have produced a large population of athletes with back pain resulting from their pre-existing underlying degenerative processes.

Essentially, the hypermobile segment and facet joint syndrome are treated in a similar manner. The basis is patient education. The athlete must (1) analyze the specific component of the exercise that seems to cause a flare-up of their back pain; (2) learn to recognize the impending flare-up and treat it prophylactically; and (3) be prepared to change their activity pattern entirely.

Flare-ups of pain are best treated by taking NSAIDs as soon as the prodrome of impending symptoms appears. Therapy includes traction, mobilization, or manipulation plus exercise analysis and instruction. When the degenerative changes are associated with radiculopathy due to nerve root irritation by osteophytes, symptoms may be more recalcitrant. Although not universally accepted, occasionally facet joint injection or extradural corticosteroid injection alleviates particularly severe flare-ups.[132]

Spinal Stenosis

Encroachment of the spinal canal, usually by hypertrophic bone and frequently in the lateral recesses, produces signs of neural claudication[130,131] that may be particularly problematic in running athletes. They describe the onset of leg aching or numbness, usually at a predictable point in their run. The leg may feel heavy, and if they ignore the symptoms weakness may develop even to the point of footdrop with L4–L5 level involvement. It may occasionally produce bilateral leg symptoms. Back pain is usually a feature. The differential diagnosis includes chronic exercise-induced compartment syndrome, vascular claudication, diabetic neuropathy, and disc hernia-

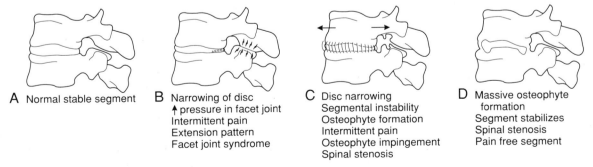

A Normal stable segment

B Narrowing of disc
↑ pressure in facet joint
Intermittent pain
Extension pattern
Facet joint syndrome

C Disc narrowing
Segmental instability
Osteophyte formation
Intermittent pain
Osteophyte impingement
Spinal stenosis

D Massive osteophyte
formation
Segment stabilizes
Spinal stenosis
Pain free segment

Fig. 19-61. Sequential evolution of disc degeneration. **(A)** Normal disk, **(B)** early changes, **(C)** significant narrowing with segmental instability evolving into **(D)** a potential stabilized segment with decreasing symptoms or alternatively spinal stenosis with radicular signs.

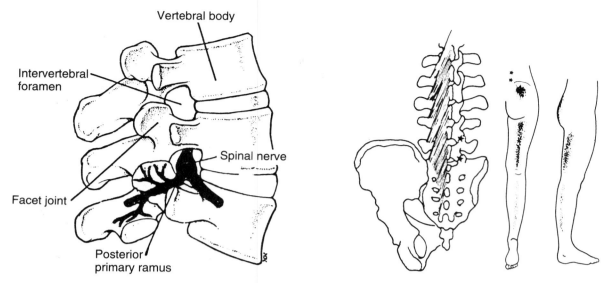

Fig. 19-62. Facet joint syndrome. Innervation of the facet joint. The synovial joint may become inflamed and produce intermittent symptoms that are frequently referred to the area of the buttock and posterior thigh. They must be differentiated from radicular irritation and sciatica.

tion. Vascular claudication is characterized by pain more than numbness, and the discomfort resolves rapidly after resting. Usually the pulses are altered, and there may be signs of dystrophic changes in the skin if the vascular disease is severe enough. Unlike neural claudication, which is frequently affected by the positional posture of the spine, vascular claudication is not. The definitive test is an arteriogram. Exercise-induced compartment syndrome is not usually associated with back pain, and the numbness is clearly in a peripheral nerve distribution rather than segmental in nature. The definitive test is resting and exercise compartment pressure measurements. Confirmation of decreased canal size is based on CT scanning, which reinforces the clinical impression of spinal stenosis.

Treatment of spinal stenosis may involve a change of running style or distance, keeping off hilly terrain, and possibly changing the activity to swimming or cycling. If the stenosis is severe, surgical decompression is warranted.

General Conditions

There are three conditions that are common enough always to be considered in the differential diagnosis of back pain in the young athlete.[133-135] Ankylosing spondylitis is an inflammatory collagen disorder; Scheuermann's disease is probably related to trauma, to a great extent in the active young individual; and Reiter's syndrome is related to an infective etiology.

Ankylosing Spondylitis (Marie-Strümpell Disease)

Ankylosing spondylitis is an inflammatory disorder that particularly affects the spine. It frequently starts in the thoracic spine, in the costovertebral and sacroiliac joints. It may present initially as a backache, chronic in nature, with morning stiffness; it is aggravated by exercise. Frequently, the onset is insidious. Eventually there may be ossification in the ligaments around these joints.

Although more usually found in young men, it is occasionally diagnosed in women. Its onset is generally during the late teens and seldom after the age of 30 years. The inflammatory process involves the synovial lining of the spinal joints, and eventually the whole spine may become stiff. The athlete may first experience a gradual onset of vague low back pain that is aggravated by sudden movements and not completely relieved by rest. There may be pain and tenderness in the sacroiliac regions. After a year or so, the disease may spread to involve much of the spine, and the patient notices that the back is not only painful but also stiff. Involvement of the costovertebral joints causes pain on deep breathing. A decrease in normal chest expansion may be an early clinical sign.

Furthermore, the Schober test with forward flexion may detect early loss of mobility (Fig. 19-35). The Schober test is performed by marking off the vertebra prominens and then measuring 30 cm from that point down the midline of the thoracic spine. In forward flexion the length of this section should increase approximately 3 cm. A refinement of this test measures 10 cm superiorly from the line drawn between the dimples marking the posterior superior iliac spine. This 10 cm section includes a large portion of the lumbar segments and in forward flexion increases approximately 5 cm in young, healthy individuals.

Practice Point

ANKYLOSING SPONDYLITIS

- Pain usually thoracolumbar area
- Frequently proportional to activity
- Complaints of spinal stiffness
- Chest expansion decreased
- Spinal motion decreased
- Hot scan at sacroiliac joint (80 percent)
- Antibodies (HLA-B$_{27}$) (80 percent)

The presence of a hot bone scan involving either the spinal segment or the costovertebral joints—specifically increased uptake in a disproportionate pattern in the area of the sacroiliac joints—helps confirm the diagnosis. Furthermore, the presence of an HLA-B$_{27}$ antigen, which is present in approximately 80 percent of people affected by this disease, is further evidence when superimposed on a good clinical history.

The treatment of ankylosing spondylitis is mainly symptomatic. It includes modification of painful activities and long-term use of intermittent courses of NSAIDs. Therapy is centered around maintaining mobility, when possible, or at least counteracting the progressive gravity-induced deformities. Postural exercises to keep the spine straight comprise the main thrust of successful treatment.

Thus when the disease is confirmed, a regular, specific exercise program must be designed. It is important to counsel the young athlete, as ankylosing spondylitis is frequently a lifelong problem. However, when the issue is approached with realism and sympathy, it does not always include total withdrawal from all physical activities. Indeed such an approach would be entirely wrong, as the disease is a spectrum and may arrest in a mild form. Every effort should be made to keep the person active within the limits of practicality.

Scheuermann's Disease

Scheuermann's osteochondritis is an ill-understood condition that affects up to 8 percent of the population and in which there may be inflammatory changes in the ring apophysis and altered growth, particularly in the thoracic spine.[136] Changes in the endplate may allow herniation of the disc into the vertebral body (Fig. 19-63). It is twice as common in girls as in boys. Scheuermann's osteochondritis in its most developed form may lead to Scheuermann's kyphosis, with a typical age of onset at 12 to 13 years.

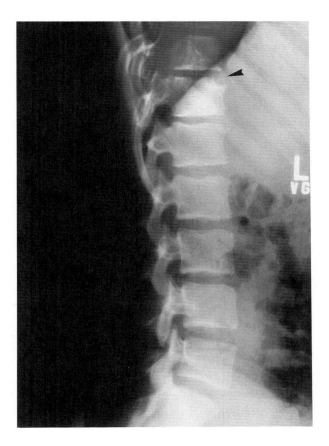

Fig. 19-63. Endplate changes are frequently seen with Scheuermann's disease, and this erosion in the anterior body may represent an anterior Schmorl's node (arrow).

Quick Facts

SCHEUERMANN'S OSTEOCHONDRITIS

- Onset typically 12 to 13 years of age
- Pain and deformity at apex of kyphosis
- Pain greater if associated lumbar involvement
- Etiology unknown
- Some cases related to sports trauma

Young athletes may complain of pain in the middle of the thoracic spine or in the upper lumbar region, aggravated by activity.[136] Ultimately, these activities, if they include repeated bending and stressing the spine, may potentially aggravate a slowly increasing kyphotic deformity. Eventually, the increased thoracic kyphosis is associated with some roundness of the shoulders and tightness of the anterior muscles of the shoulder group, including the pectoral and anterior deltoid muscles. There is often associated hamstring tightness with this condition and exaggerated lumbar lordosis.

The radiologic findings of Scheuermann's kyphosis include irregular vertebral endplates, apparent narrowing of disc spaces, progressive kyphosis, and wedging of three or more disc vertebrae. This wedging should be 5 degrees or more in at least one vertebra, and the dorsal kyphosis should be more than 35 degrees to constitute classic Scheuermann's disease. In addition, one may see bulging into the vertebral body through the endplates, the so-called Schmorl's nodes.

In the early stages, treatment of this condition requires some modification of activity proportional to

---

Quick Facts

RADIOLOGIC CRITERIA FOR SCHEUERMANN'S DISEASE

- Irregular vertebral endplates
- Apparent narrowing of disc space
- Kyphosis of more than 35 degrees
- Affects three or more adjacent vertebrae
- Five degrees or more wedging of at least one vertebra
- Schmorl's nodes

---

the pain. If there appears to be progressive kyphosis, it may be necessary to counsel the young individual about sports such as gymnastics, weight training, and heavy lifting activities. Indeed the relation to these vigorous activities is not clear, but Oseid noted that 75 percent of young female gymnasts competing in international gymnastics suffered from intermittent back discomfort, and a large number of these girls had radiologic changes consistent with those of Scheuermann's disease.[133-136]

If the curve continues to progress and reaches the upper limit of what would be considered acceptable, a custom-made thoracolumbar orthosis combined with a specific back extension and mobilizing exercise routine may help control the progression. This therapy is aimed at increasing the lumbar lordosis and extension of the thoracic spine. In exceptional circumstances there is continued progression of the curve; and some form of operative intervention, with the possibility of fusion, must be considered.

Reiter's Syndrome

Reiter's syndrome comprises urethritis, conjunctivitis, and some form of arthritis. It is a disease of young people and is thought to be a venereal type disease. It is relatively common and often presents with sacroiliac pain, back pain, and swelling of one of the peripheral joints. A bone scan reveals the joints to be hot. The erythrocyte sedimentation rate is elevated. Treatment often comprises antibiotic therapy. Restriction of activity during the active phase of this disease is also necessary.

SUMMARY

The spine, like most joints, has incredible resilience, enormous ability to absorb stress, and amazing endurance provided it is structurally sound and healthy. These abilities deteriorate rapidly with even minimal pathology.

The spine is vulnerable during the adolescent period owing to the growth plates, during early adult life owing to risk-taking activities, and during middle and old age owing to increasing stiffness and degenerative changes. Nevertheless, the overall incidence of back pain in athletes is low.

The advent of intensive weight training schedules for young athletes has resulted in back pain becoming an issue between physicians and coaches. The hyperextended, lordotic position adopted during many weight training routines and competitive sports, e.g., gymnastics and ballet, has taken its toll, with an increasing incidence of spondylolysis. The chronic repetitive stresses of jogging and aerobic dance have also produced a small but significant population with back pain, either ligamentous in nature or secondary to irritation of pre-existing degenerative spinal segments. The role of balanced muscle strength and adequate flexibility in minimizing the risks of back pain cannot be overemphasized.

Probably sacroiliac pain is seen more frequently in the athlete than other segments of the population. Recognition of this syndrome is important. The decision of when to return athletes to their sport after discogenic disease is sometimes difficult, and often prolonged modification of activity is the wisest approach.

The ultimate back problem is fracture with associated paralysis, and in this regard sport and recreation comprise the fourth commonest cause of spinal fracture and the second commonest cause of paralysis. These statistics are obviously unacceptable, and attempts to increase public awareness are essential.

In conclusion, it can be seen that there are many causes of back pain in the young athlete, and as a group they may be particularly vulnerable to back pain. There are inherent stresses in some sports that obviously predispose to back problems. Some individuals are structurally unsuited for participation in certain sports, and it may be necessary to advise them to discontinue activities entirely or to use their energies in a different sport that does not stress the back to the same degree.

The terminology to describe anatomy, kinetics, and conditions of the spine should be exact. Failure to use standard terminology results in confusion. Early diagnosis and treatment cuts down the length of time necessary to restore the athlete to full activity. It may also prevent progression of a ligamentous problem to a condition that may involve a stress fracture with its associated prolonged healing time.

1. Exercise and a healthy life style should produce a healthy spine.
2. Most recreational activities are associated with a low incidence of back pain.
3. There are exceptions due to high repetitious loading, torques, lifting, and chronic postures.
4. The spine is particularly vulnerable during adolescence.
5. Risk-taking, alcohol, and breaking rules lead to catastrophic injury.
6. Healthy genes produce healthy backs; thus individuals must learn their own inherent weaknesses and limitations.

Empirically, healthy living should not be dangerous for the spine, but unfortunately it is easy to make it so in some of the circumstances outlined in this chapter.

REFERENCES

1. Reid DC, Saboe LA: Spinal trauma in sports and recreation. Clin J Sport Med 1:75, 1991
2. Robinson RA, Southwick WO: Surgical approaches to the cervical spine. Instruc Course Lect. Am Acad Orthop Surg 17:3707, 1960
3. Basmajian JV: A fresh look at the intrinsic muscles of the back. Am Surg 42:685, 1976
4. Grant JCB: An Atlas of Anatomy. 6th Ed. Williams & Wilkins, Baltimore, 1962
5. Kent BE: Anatomy of the trunk. Phys Ther 54:850, 1974
6. Maigne R: Orthopaedic Medicine (translated and edited by Liberson WT). Charles C Thomas, Springfield, IL, 1972
7. Gardner R, Gray B, O'Rahilly R: Anatomy. 3rd Ed. WB Saunders, Philadelphia, 1969
8. Speer KP, Bassett FH: The prolonged burner syndrome. Am J Sports Med 18:591, 1990
9. Magee DJ: Orthopaedic Physical Assessment. WB Saunders, Philadelphia, 1987
10. Elvey RL: Brachial plexus tension tests and the pathoanatomical origin of arm pain. In Idczak IM (ed): Biomechanical Aspects of Manipulation Therapy. Lincoln Institute of Health Sciences, Carlton, Australia, 1981
11. Reid DC: Spinal trauma—general principles and cervical injury. In Dickson RA (ed): Spinal Surgery Science and Practice. Butterworth, London, 1990
12. Reid DC, Saboe L, Henderson R, Miller J: Evaluation of cervical fractures and rate of missed diagnosis. J Trauma 27:980, 1987
13. Torg JS, Glasgow SG: Criteria for return to contact activities following cervical spine injury. Clin J Sport Med 1:12, 1991
14. Ross SE, Schwab CW, David ET et al: Clearing the cervical spine: initial radiographic evaluation. J Trauma 27:1055, 1987
15. Clancy WG, Grand RL, Bergfeld JA: Upper trunk brachial plexus injuries in contact sports. Am J Sports Med 5:209, 1977
16. Fielding JW: Cineroentgenography of the normal cervical spine. J Bone Joint Surg [Am] 39a:1280, 1957
17. Sedden H: Surgical Disorders of the Peripheral Nerves. Churchill Livingstone, Edinburgh, 1972

18. Hohl M: Normal motion of the upper portion of the cervical spine. J Bone Joint Surg [Am] 46a:1777, 1964

19. Sunderland S: Nerves and Nerve Injuries. 2nd Ed. Churchill Livingstone, Edinburgh, 1988

20. Reid DC, Saboe LA, Allan G: Spine trauma associated with off-road vehicles. Physician Sports Med 16:143, 1988

21. Hodgson VR: Reducing serious injury in sports. Interschool Athletic Admin 7:11, 1980

22. Franco JL, Heszog A: A comparative assessment of neck muscle strength and vertebral stability. J Orthop Sports Phys Ther 9:351, 1987

23. Schneider RD: Head and Neck Injuries in Football: Mechanisms, Treatment and Prevention. p. 77. Williams & Wilkins, Baltimore, 1973

24. Albright JP, McAuley E, Martin RK et al: Head and neck injuries in college football: an eight year analysis. Am J Sports Med 13:147, 1985

25. Bateman JE: Nerve injuries about the shoulder in sports. J Bone Joint Surg [Am] 49:785, 1967

26. Gerberich SG, Preist JD, Boen JR et al: Spinal trauma and symptoms in high school football players. Physician Sports Med 11:122, 1983

27. Chrisman OD, Snook GA, Stanitis JM et al: Lateral-flexion neck injuries in athletic competition. JAMA 192:117, 1965

28. Torg JS, Quedenfeld TC, Burstein A et al: National Football Head and Neck Registry: report on cervical quadriplegia: 1971 to 1975. Am J Sports Med 7:127, 1979

29. Funk FJ, Wells RE: Injuries of the cervical spine in football. Clin Orthop; 109:50, 1975

30. Watkins RG, Dillin WH, Maxwell J: Cervical spine injuries in football players. In Hochschuler SH (ed): Spinal Injuries in Sports. Hanley and Belfus, Philadelphia, 1990

31. Maroon JC: Burning hands in football spinal cord injuries. JAMA 238:2049, 1977

32. Poindexter DP, Johnson EW: Football shoulder and neck injury: a study of the "stinger." Arch Phys Med Rehabil 65:601, 1984

33. Gibbs R: A protective collar for cervical radiculopathy. Physician Sports Med 12:139, 1984

34. Robertson WC JR, Eichman PL, Clancy WG: Upper trunk brachial plexopathy in football players. JAMA 241:1480, 1976

35. Hershman EB, Wilbourn AJ, Bergfield JA: Acute brachial neuropathy in athletes. Am J Sports Med 17:655, 1989

36. Mueller FO, Schindler RD: Annual Survey of Football Injury Research. 1931–1987. National Collegiate Athletic Association and American Football Coaches Association, Mission, KS, 1987

37. Torg JS, Vegso JJ, O'Neill MJ et al: The epidemiologic, pathologic, biomechanical and cinematographic analysis of football induced cervical spine trauma. Am J Sports Med 18:50, 1990

38. Wilberger JE, Maroon JC: Cervical spine injuries in athletes. Physician Sports Med 18:57, 1990

39. Bergfeld JA, Hershman EB, Wilbourn AJ: Brachial injuries in athletes. Orthop Trans 12:743, 1988

40. Sovio OM, Van Peteghan PK, Schweigel JF: Cervical spine injuries in rugby players. Can Med Assoc J 130:36, 1984

41. Torg JS, Pavlov H, Genuario SE et al: Neurapraxia of the cervical spinal cord with transient quadriplegia. J Bone Joint Surg [Am] 68a:1354, 1986

42. Masoon JC, Kevin T, Rehhopf P: System for preventing acute neck injury. Physician Sports Med 5:76, 1977

43. McKeag DB, Cantu RC: Neck pain in a football player: a case conference from the American College of Sports Medicine. Physician Sports Med 18:115, 1990

44. Oder JM, Watkins RG, Dillin WH et al: Incidence of cervical spinal stenosis in professional and rookie football players. Am J Sports Med 18:507, 1990

45. Feldick HG, Albright JP: Football survey reveals "missed" neck injuries. Physician Sports Med 4:77, 1976

46. Reid DC, Leung P: A study of the odontoid process. Adv Orthop 12:147, 1989

47. MacLean IC, Taylor RS: Nerve root stimulation to evaluate brachial plexus conduction. p. 47. In: Abstracts of Communication of the Fifth International Congress of Electromyography, Rochester, Minnesota, 1975

48. Basmajian JV: Muscles Alive: Their Functions Revealed by Electromyography. 3rd Ed. Williams & Wilkins, Baltimore, 1974

49. Schneider RC, Kennedy JC (eds): Sports Injuries. Mechanisms, Prevention, and Treatment. Williams & Wilkins, Baltimore, 1985

50. Ladd AL, Scranton PE: Congenital cervical spinal stenosis presenting as transient quadriplegia in athletes: report of two cases. J Bone Joint Surg [Am] 68a:1371, 1986

51. DiBenedetto M, Markey K: Electrodiagnostic localization of traumatic upper trunk brachial plexopathy. Arch Phys Med Rehabil 65:15, 1984

52. DiBenedetto M, Chardhry U, Markey K: Proximal nerve condition: brachial plexus. Muscle Nerve 5:564, 1982

53. Stanish WD, Lamb H: Isolated paralysis of the serratus anterior muscle: a weight training injury. Am J Sports Med 6:385, 1978

54. Hershman EB, Willbourn AJ, Bergfeld JA: Acute brachial neuropathy in athletes. Am J Sports Med 17:655, 1989

55. Burnard ED, Fox TG: Multiple neuritis of the

shoulder girdle: report of 9 cases occurring in second New Zealand Expeditionary Force. NZ Med J 41:243, 1942

56. Parsonage MJ, Tuner JWA: Neuralgic amyotrophy: shoulder girdle syndrome. Lancet 1:973, 1948

57. Tsairis P, Dyck PJ, Mulder DW: Natural history of brachial plexus neuropathy: report on 99 cases. Arch Neurol 27:109, 1972

58. Dixon GJ, Dick TBS: Acute brachial radiculitis: course and prognosis. Lancet 2:707, 1945

59. Estwanik JJ: Levator scapulae syndrome. Physician Sports Med 17:57, 1989

60. Moseley HF: Shoulder Lesions. Charles C Thomas, Springfield, IL, 1945

61. Shull JR: Scapulocostal syndrome: clinical aspects. South Med J 62:956, 1969

62. McCutcheon ML, Anderson JL: How I manage sports injuries to the larynx. Physician Sports Med 13:100, 1985

63. Storey MD, Schatz CF, Brown KW: Anterior neck trauma. Physician Sports Med 17:85, 1989

64. Fabian RL: Sports injury to the larynx and trachea Physician Sports Med 17:111, 1989

65. Fink B: The etiology and treatment of laryngospasm. Anesthesiology 17:569, 1956

66. Gerberich SG, Priest JD, Boen JR et al: Spinal trauma and symptoms in high school football players. Physician Sports Med 11:122, 1983

67. Schneider RC: Head and Neck Injuries in Football: Mechanisms, Treatment and Prevention. Williams & Wilkins, Baltimore, 1973

68. Torg JS, Vegso JJ, O'Neill MJ et al: The epidemiologic, pathologic, biomechanical and cinematographic analysis of football-induced cervical spine trauma. Adv Orthop Surg 13:220, 1990

69. Scher AT: Rugby injuries to the cervical spinal cord. S Afr Med J 57:37, 1980

70. Reid DC: Spine fractures in winter sports. In Torg JS (ed): Athletic Injuries to the Head, Neck and Face. 2nd Ed. Year Book Medical Publishers, Chicago, 1991

71. Hayes D: Reducing risks in hockey: analysis of equipment and injuries. Physician Sports Med 6:67, 1978

72. Kewalramani LS, Krauss JF: Cervical spine injuries resulting from collison sports. Paraplegia 19:303, 1981

73. Albright JP, McAuley E, Martin RK et al: Head and neck injuries in college football: an eight year analysis. Am J Sports Med 13:147, 1985

74. Nachemson A, Effström G: Intravital dynamic pressure measurements in lumbar disc. Scand J Rehabil Med [Suppl 1] 1970

75. Burry HC, Gowland H: Cervical injury in rugby football—a New Zealand survey. Br J Sports Med 15:56, 1981

76. Feriencik K: Trends in ice hockey injuries: 1965 to 1977. Physician Sports Med 7:81, 1979

77. McCoy GF, Piggot J, Macafee AL et al: Injuries of the cervical spine in schoolboy rugby football. J Bone Joint Surg [Br] 66b:500, 1984

78. Tator CH, Palm J: Spinal injuries in diving: incidence high and rising. Ontario Med Rev 48:628, 1981

79. Burd B: Infant swimming classes: immersed in controversy. Physician Sports Med 114:239, 1986

80. Key AG, Retief PJM: Spinal cord injuries: an analysis of 300 new lesions. Paraplegia 7:243, 1970

81. Kraus JF, Franti CE, Riggin RS et al: Incidence of traumatic spinal cord lesions. J Chronic Dis 28:471, 1975

82. Krutzke JF: Epidemiology of spinal cord injury. Exp Neurol 48:163, 1975

83. Wenzel FJ, Peters RA: A ten year survey of snowmobile accidents: injuries and fatalities in Wisconsin. Physician and Sportsmed 14:140, 1986

84. Feldick HG, Albright JP: Football survey reveals missed neck injuries. Physician Sports Med 4:77, 1976

85. Murphy P: Still too many neck injuries. Physician Sports Med 13:29, 1985

86. O'Carroll PF, Sheehan JM, Gregg TM: Cervical spine injuries in rugby football. Ir Med J 74:377, 1981

87. Barone G, Rodgers BM: Pediatric equestrian injuries: a 14-year review. J Trauma 29:245, 1989

88. Silver JR: Injuries to the spine sustained in rugby. Br Med J 288:37, 1984

89. Clarke KS, Powell JW: Football helmets and neurotrauma an epidemiological overview of three seasons. Med Sci Sports 11:138, 1979

90. Bishop PJ, Norman RW, Wells R et al: Changes in the centre of mass and movement of inertia of a headform induced by a hockey helmet and face shield. Can J Appl Sport Sci 8:19, 1983

91. Rodrigo J, Boyd R: Lumbar spine injuries in military parachute jumpers. Physician Sports Med 7:9, 1979

92. Schneider RC: Serious and fatal neurosurgical football injuries. Clin Neurosurg 12:226, 1964

93. Schneider RC, Reifel E, Crisler HO et al: Serious and fatal football injuries involving the head and spinal cord. JAMA 177:362, 1961

94. Carvell JE, Fuller DJ, Duthie RB et al: Rugby football injuries to the cervical spine. Br Med J 286:49, 1983

95. Samples P: Spinal cord injuries: the high cost of careless diving. Physician Sports Med 17:143, 1989

96. Tabor CH, Edmonds VE: Sports and recreation are a rising cause of spinal cord injury. Physician Sports Med 14:157, 1986

97. Nachemson A: The load in lumbar disc in different positions of the body. Clin Orthop 45:107, 1966

98. Mellin GP: Accuracy of measuring lateral flexion of the spine with a tape. Clin Biomech 1:85, 1986

99. Schober P: Lendenwirbelsaule und Kreuzschmerzen. Munch Med Wochenschr 84:336, 1937

100. Namey TC, An HS: Sorting out the causes of sciatica. Mod Med Can 40:672, 1985

101. Kilian H: De spondylolisthesi, gravissimae pelvangustiae causa nuper detetta, commentatia, anatomica-obstetrica. Bonni Formis Caroli Georgia 2:315, 1853

102. Hoshini H: Spondylolysis in athletes. Physician Sports Med 8:75, 1980

103. Wiltse LL: Etiology of spondylolisthesis. Clin Orthop 10:48, 1957

104. Fergusson RJ, McMaster JH, Stanitski CL: Low back pain in college football linemen. J Sports Med 2:63, 1974

105. Billings RA, Burry HC, Jones R: Low back injury in sport. Rheumatol Rehabil 16:236, 1977

106. Brady TA, Cahill BR, Bodnar LM: Weight training-related injuries in the high school athlete. Am J Sports Med 10:1, 1982

107. Devereaux MD, Lachmann SM: Athletes attending a sports injury clinic: a review. Br J Sports Med 17:137, 1980

108. Ekstrand J, Gillquist J: The frequency of muscle tightness and injuries in soccer players. Am J Sports Med 10:75, 1982

109. Bach DK, Green DS, Jensen GM et al: A comparison of muscular tightness in runners and non-runners and the relation of muscular tightness to low back pain in runners. J Orthop Sports Phys Ther 6:315, 1985

110. Hirch C: The reaction of the intervertebral disc to compression forces. J Bone Joint Surg [Am] 37a:118, 1955

111. Garbutt G, Bocock MG, Reilly T et al: Running speed and spinal shrinkage in runners with and without low back pain. Med Sci Sports Exerc 22:769, 1990

112. Clarke TE, Frederick EC, Hamill C: The effect of varied stride rate and length upon shank deceleration during ground contact in running. Med Sci Sports Exerc 170:376, 1983

113. MacNab I: Backache. Williams & Wilkins, Baltimore, 1977

114. Shiquing X, Quanzhi Z, Dehao F et al: Significance of the straight-leg raising test in the diagnosis and clinical evaluation of lower lumbar intervertebral-disc protrusion. J Bone Joint Surg [Am] 69a:517, 1987

115. Mixter WJ, Barr JS: Rupture of the intervertebral disc with involvement of the spinal canal. N Engl J Med 211:210, 1934

116. Smyth MJ, Wright V: Sciatica and the intervertebral disc: an experimental study. Clin Orthop 129:9, 1977

117. Fajersztajn J: Weber das gekreutze Ishiasphänomen. Wien Klin Wochenschr 14:41, 1901

118. Kerr RS, Cadoux-Hudson TA, Adams CB: The value of accurate clinical assessment in the surgical management of the lumbar disc protrusion. J Neurol Neurosurg Psychiatry 51:169, 1988

119. Mathews J: Dynamic discography: a study of lumbar traction. Ann Phys Med 9:275, 1968

120. Kane MD, Karl RD, Swain JH: Effects of gravity facilitated traction on intervertebral dimensions of the lumbar spine. J Orthop Sports Phys Ther 6:281, 1985

121. Goldman RM, Tarr RS, Pinchuk BG et al: The effects of oscillating inversion on systemic blood pressure, pulse, intraocular pressure, and central retinal arterial pressure. Physician Sports Med 13:93, 1985

122. Jansen EF, Balls AK: Chymopapain: a new crystalline proteinase from papaya latex. J Biochem 137:459, 1941

123. Kambin P, Sampson S: Posterolateral percutaneous suction-excision of herniated lumbar intervertebral discs: report of interim results. Clin Orthop 207:37, 1986

124. Maroon JC, Onik G, Dey A: Percutaneous automated discectomy in athletes. Physician Sports Med 16:61, 1988

125. Jankiewicz JJ, Hennrikus WL, Houkom JA: The appearance of piriformis syndrome in computed tomography and magnetic resonance imaging. Clin Orthop 262:205, 1991

126. Yoemans W: The relation of arthritis of the sacroiliac joint to sciatica. Lancet 2:1119, 1978

127. Freiberg AH, Vinke TA: Sciatica and the sacroiliac joint. J Bone Joint Surg 16:126, 1934

128. Robinson D: Piriformis syndrome in relation to sciatic pain. Am J Surg 73:355, 1947

129. Pace JB: Commonly overlooked pain syndromes responsive to simple therapy. Postgrad Med 53:107, 1975

130. Kirkaldy-Willis WH: Managing Low Back Pain. p. 94. Churchill Livingstone, New York, 1983

131. Bernard TN, Kirkaldy-Willis WH: Recognizing specific characteristics of non-specific low back pain. Clin Orthop 217:266, 1987

132. Dilke TFW, Burry HC, Grahame R: Extradural corticosteroid injection in management of lumbar nerve root compression. Br Med J 2:635, 1973

133. Stanitski CL: Low back pain in young athletes. Physician Sports Med 10:77, 1982
134. Fisk JW, Baigent ML, Hill PD: Scheuermann's disease: clinical and radiologic survey of 17 and 18 year olds. Am J Phys Med 63:18, 1984
135. Micheli LJ: Low back pain in the adolescent differential diagnosis. Am J Sports Med 7:362, 1979
136. Bradford D, Moe J, Montalvo F: Scheuermann's kyphosis and round back deformity. J Bone Joint Surg [Am] 56a:740, 1974

Injuries to the Head and Face

20

A doctor at a boxing match is like a priest at a hanging.
— *Anonymous*

Over the last few years there has been a phenomenal increase in participation in all kinds of recreational endeavors. The obvious advantage is the potential for improving the health of a nation. There are risks, however, and a plethora of injuries has been generated, lending impetus to the development of the specialty of sports medicine and therapy.[1] Whereas minor and temporary trauma are easily acceptable as part of the risk of participation, long-lasting and catastrophic injuries are not, and the risks must be reduced to an absolute minimum. Cranial and facial injuries are mostly in the latter categories, and this chapter focuses on their prevention and treatment.

Quick Facts

RISK ODDS PER YEAR OF EXPOSURE

1 : 10,000,000	Extremely low risk
1 : 1,000,000	Very low risk
1 : 100,000	Low risk
1 : 10,000	Medium risk
1 : 1,000	High risk

Risk statistics are difficult to obtain, and care must be taken with their interpretation (Table 20-1). However, if they are used to record trends in different sports, specifically to identify significant increases or changes in injury pattern, they become important triggering mechanisms for more careful scrutiny. In football, for example, rule changes and improved equipment have dramatically reduced head and neck fatalities over a 30-year period.[2] (Fig. 20-1). Similarly, the signal work of Pashby and his colleagues generated increasing public awareness of the danger of serious eye injuries, the importance of standards for protective glasses, and ultimately the reduction of risks.[3] Preventing and managing injuries to the head, neck, and face exemplify the need for a multidisciplinary approach with both medical and nonmedical personnel involved. Physical educators, sports scientists, coaches, therapists, and physicians must be constantly aware of the need for educating the public in order to keep serious and catastrophic injury statistics to a minimum. Certain sports have traditionally been regarded as having a high inherent risk of nervous system injury. Among them are boxing, wrestling, martial arts, football, rugby, vehicle racing (automobile and motorcycle), equestrian events, sky diving, hang-gliding, trampolining, hockey, and gymnastics.[4–12] Ironically, the apparently safe pastime of jogging suffers from the highest fatality rate, due to the risk of being hit by a car. Recreational cyclists are at similar risk. The magnitude of this problem is exemplified by the recorded 500,000 cycle injuries per year in the state of Indiana alone. However, when vehicle accidents are eliminated, 80 percent of serious head trauma results from the collision sports. Unfortunately, despite the frequency of some significant injuries, protocols for management are difficult to establish. Nevertheless, a cautious approach to these problems reduces long-term problems and in some cases prevents a catastrophic outcome.[13]

HEAD INJURIES

The overall incidence of head injury in sport is in the area of 5 percent. The highest risk of head injury is to racing car drivers followed closely by jockeys.

TABLE 20-1.   Risk Odds for Activities per Year of Participation[a]

Activity	Death	Major Injury
Mountain climbing (dedicated experts)	1:167	1:23
Hang gliding	1:560	1:56
Parachuting	1:570	
Motor cycling	1:1,100	
Sailplaning (gliding)	1:1,710	
Mountain climbing (all levels)	1:1,750	
Boxing (professional)	1:2,200	
Scuba diving	1:2,400	
Automobile use	1:4,000	
Snowmobiling	1:7,600	
Mountain hiking	1:15,700	1:1,570
Boating		
Canoes and kayaks	1:13,200	
Motorized boats	1:24,000	
Sailboats	1:38,000	
Football		
College	1:33,000	1:18
High school	1:81,000	
Skiing downhill		
Racing	1:40,000	
Recreational	1:1,430,000	1:30

[a] These figures are only approximates of relative risks.
(Adapted from Reif,[1] with permission.)

Although with some activities it is an incidental side effect of contact and collisions that are part of the sport, unfortunately head injuries frequently result from illegal procedures (Fig. 20-2). Indeed, in boxing, cerebral injury from a "knockout" is part of the object of the activity. The puck in hockey and the ball in cricket and baseball are frequently the cause of concussion. These missiles travel at great speeds and are quite hard. In soccer, for instance, despite its plastic coating, the ball remains a factor that may contribute to concussion. On average, it travels at 60 to 120 km/hour (37 to 74 mph) and may exert an impact of over 100 kp. Probably however, most significant injuries in soccer are caused by inadvertently clashing skulls while heading the ball.[14]

Head injuries result in concussion, contusion, laceration, or compression of the cranial contents by bleeding or swelling. They may be further considered

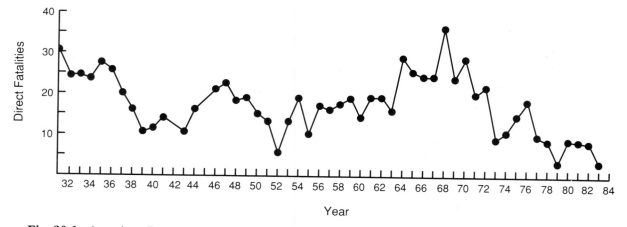

Fig. 20-1. American Football Coaches Association football fatality data from 1932 to 1983. Although the incidence has fluctuated, there has been a steady decline since approximately 1968 and influenced by the introduction of specific rules discouraging spearing in 1976. (From Torg,[2] with permission.)

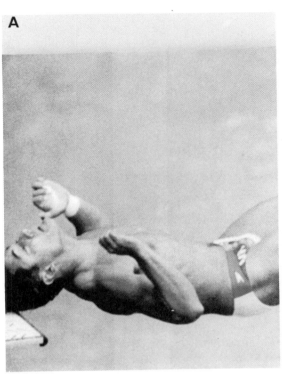

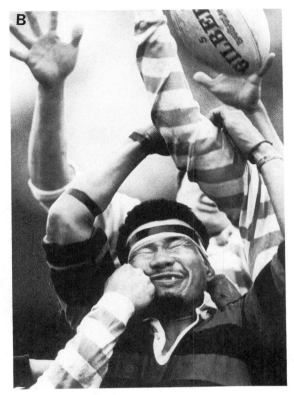

Fig. 20-2. Injuries to the head and neck may be the result of **(A)** accidental collisions and dangerous techniques or **(B)** more deliberate illegal maneuvers.

as open or closed injuries, the latter frequently presenting a worrisome diagnostic challenge to assign severity with any degree of certainty. Acute subdural hematomas are the major cause of death in sport-induced head trauma. Concussion is fortunately more common than cerebral contusion in sport. Cantu suggested that more than 250,000 concussions a year occur in football alone in the United States.[15]

The term concussion implies that there is minimal structural damage to the brain despite an interruption of its function. The definition is one of a short-lived traumatically induced disorientation or loss of consciousness that is not associated with evidence of permanent damage to the brain. However, the exact correlation of symptoms with pathology is imprecise, and there may be some neural loss, shearing injury to white matter, petechial hemorrhage, and, with cumulative insults, cerebral atrophy. Cerebral contusion suggests that there is bleeding and bruising of the brain tissue itself. The more severe degrees of concussion may be associated with cerebral contusion. Naturally, a contusion is more serious as an initial

injury and because of the subsequent scarring that may occur and residual permanent brain damage.

It is important also to realize the distinction between the direct blow versus the contrecoup injury (Fig. 20-3). The direct blow, or coup, is the injury produced by the force applied to the head. This injury can be protected against by adequate helmets and head gear. The contrecoup injury is due to acceleration of the brain within the decelerating cranium. For instance, a blow to the back of the head may cause a contrecoup injury to the frontal and temporal lobes. Unconsciousness or concussion frequently results from a rotational (angular) acceleration injury where there may be associated torsion on the vessels. It is more difficult to protect against acceleration-deceleration injuries because much of the movement is indirectly generated within the cranium.[15,16]

Concussions

Concussions, which have been defined as a physiologic interruption of brain activity, may be classified into mild (grade I), moderate (grade II), and severe

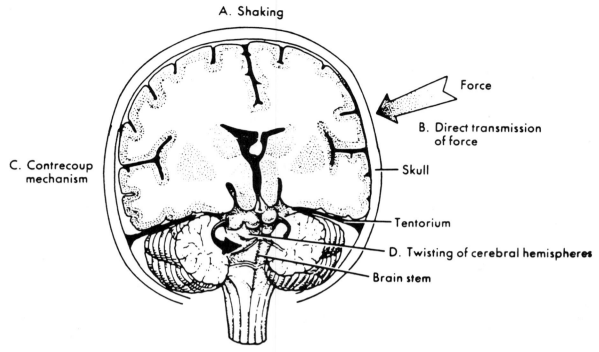

Fig. 20-3. Mechanisms of sustaining brain damage. **(A)** Shaking of the brain due to vibration. **(B)** Direct transmission of a force by a blow. **(C)** Contracoup mechanism due to rapid acceleration and deceleration and perhaps with rotational injuries. It is the most dangerous mechanism of all because of the difficulty of counteracting it with protective equipment. **(D)** Twisting or swirling of the cerebral hemisphere on the brainstem due to rotational movements of the head. (Adapted from Booker and Thibadeau,[16] with permission.)

(grade III), although there is no universal acceptance of a finite grading system (Table 20-2). In reality these are all closed head injuries.

It is important to realize that these definitions stem out of the inability of crude measuring systems to record and correlate the wide spectrum of potential damage to the brain with specific clinical pictures. Thus the grading system is only a mechanism of triggering a safe clinical approach to concussion. Naturally, these grades are overlapping, and the more severe concussion runs imperceptibly into a cerebral contusion. Fortunately, concussions in sport are mild. They are accompanied by disturbances of short-term memory and data processing. Although dramatic physiologic disturbances may occur, they are frequently not clinically apparent. The altered performance is easily overlooked, subjecting the athlete to further risk. Hence concussions are a potentially hazardous injury, particularly to the athlete who walks and talks and appears to be normal after the injury.[17]

There is a trend among sports physicians and ther-

Practice Point

CONCUSSION

- Loss of consciousness is not necessary for a potentially severe concussion or injury.
- Amnesia is the common denominator.
- After first concussion, risk of second is increased.

---

apists to take a more conservative approach than previously. This change in attitude is due to increasing awareness of: (1) the reduced ability to process information after a concussion; (2) the severity and duration of the functional impairment being greater with repeated concussions, suggesting a cumulative effect; and (3) that there is a protracted period, which may extend over weeks to months, during which subtle mental functioning is disturbed.[18,19] It is estimated that after individuals suffer one concussion, if they

TABLE 20-2. Signs and Symptoms of Concussion[a]

Mild cerebral concussion: first degree (approx. 90%)
    May be no obvious signs
    Brief period of slight mental confusion
    No loss of consciousness
    Some dizziness
    Minimal unsteadiness
    Brief loss of judgment

Moderate cerebral concussion: second degree (approx. 10%)
    Transitory unconsciousness (up to 2 minutes)
    Subsequent momentary mental confusion or disorientation
    Unsteadiness up to 10 minutes
    Minimal retrograde amnesia ($>$ 30 minutes)
    Variable period of tinnitus (ringing in the ears)
    Dizziness of moderate severity
    Transient headache

Severe cerebral concussion: third degree (less than 1%)
    Unconscious for prolonged interval ($\geq$ 2 minutes)
    Prolonged and significant retrograde amnesia ($\geq$ 24 hours)
    Marked unsteadiness (lasting over 10 minutes)
    Severe headache
    Severe tinnitus
    Severe dizziness and possible nausea
    Possible convulsions
    Serous discharge from nose or ear[a]
    Blood from ear[a]
    Cranial vault deformity[b]
    Facial asymmetry or dysesthesia[b]

One or all signs may be present.
[a] Suggestive of basal skull fracture.
[b] Suggestive of skull or facial bone fractures.

return to play, the chance of a second concussion occurring is more than four times greater than that of their nonconcussed teammates. Neuropsychological testing and post-traumatic complaints of headaches and memory loss frequently resolve together, and the athlete usually is restored to preinjury status by 5 days. The most important post-traumatic intellectual impairment appears to be a deficit in sustained attention and concentration and the rapid assimilation of new material. Cantu pointed out that if this information is not serious enough to make a physician wary, the work of Saunders and Harbough on the second impact syndrome should.[20] With this condition, fatal brain swelling follows minor head contact in players who have symptoms from a prior concussion. This syndrome is fortunately rare, but when present its consequences are catastrophic, emphasizing the need to be aware of subtle residual signs resulting from concussive impacts. The following guidelines are not absolute and each physician must use clinical judgment commensurate with their training and experience.

Practice Point

SEVERITY OF CONCUSSION

Grade	Criteria[a]
I (mild)	No LOC, PTA $<$ 30 min
II (moderate)	LOC $<$ 2 min or PTA $>$ 30 min
III (severe)	LOC $\geq$ 2 min or PTA $\geq$ 24 hr

[a] LOC = loss of consciousness; PTA = post-traumatic amnesia.

Grade I (Mild)

The mild concussion is perhaps the most difficult to recognize and grade. There may be no obvious signs. The athlete often describes it as being "dinged" or having their "bell rung." There may be a brief period of slight mental confusion, some dizziness, minimal unsteadiness, and a brief loss of judgment. There should be no loss of consciousness. The athletes themselves frequently report that the only way they know they have been hit is because they cannot remember the plays. Indeed not clearly remembering recent events and difficulty interpreting new information are the hallmarks of this level of concussion and hence should be incorporated in the testing procedure. Removal from the field of play is mandatory. The following paragraphs deal specifically with football, but the principles are easily extrapolated to other sports.

After an initial mild concussion, return to competition is deferred until all symptoms, e.g., headaches, dizziness, and impaired orientation, have resolved, and memory and concentration are restored. In the absence of overt physical signs, ability to answer questions, add or subtract figures, and remember number sequences are useful (Table 20-3). Running and agility work on the sideline without impairment or the triggering of a headache are also helpful tests.[15]

A second mild concussion during the same game or within a few days should probably mandate removal from competition and contact for about 2 weeks. All symptoms, e.g., headache, must be absent for a week during rest and exertion.[15] If symptoms persist past 24 hours or start to increase in severity, a computed tomography (CT) or magnetic resonance imaging (MRI) scan should be considered to rule out frontal and temporal lobe contusion. Furthermore, a second concussion during one game should trigger the need to review the situation carefully to see if poor skill, technique, or judgment is a contributing factor, as each is potentially remediable. Equipment should also be checked to ensure that it is adequate, properly maintained, and correctly adjusted and worn. Possibly a specific neck strengthening program may be instituted even though its value in some circumstances is questionable. There is some suggestion that three or more concussions, particularly if they are within a 6 to 8 week period, should raise the possibility of suggesting that the athlete terminate the season.

Grade II (Moderate)

The moderate cerebral concussion is characterized by a transitory unconsciousness of up to 5 minutes. Many grading systems place longer periods of unconsciousness in the moderate category, but from a pragmatic point of view, greater than 2 minutes should place the athlete into the severe category. Considerable clinical judgment is needed if the unconscious period is brief. There is some subsequent mental confusion, dizziness of moderate severity, and sometimes a transient headache. There is a period of unsteadiness on the feet and a variable period of ringing in the ears, or tinnitus (Table 20-3). There is

---

TABLE 20-3. Brief Neurologic Examination (After Concussion)

Verbal
    Quality of speech (no slurring)
    Appropriateness
    Memory (events of the day)
    Cognitive (add or repeat number sequences, use $100 - 7$ to demonstrate ability to concentrate

Visual
    Pupil equality of size and reaction
    Movement (track penlight)
    Absence of nystagmus
    Gross visual fields (arms stretched, observe finger movement)

Motor
    Coordinated movement (finger–nose test)
    Equal strength (test key muscles)
    Balance (stand on one limb, extend arms)
    Line walk
    Romberg test (standing, feet together, eyes closed): falling to one side is a positive test

Reflex
    Elbows, knees
    Plantar response if doubt

Sensory
    Touch or pinch in each limb
    Response to pain (if impaired consciousness)

Practice Point

GUIDELINES FOR RETURN TO CONTACT ACTIVITY AFTER CONCUSSION

Grade	1st Concussion	2nd Concussion	3rd Concussion
I (mild)	May return to play if asymptomatic[a]	Return to play if has been asymptomatic for 1 week	Consider terminating season; may return if asymptomatic
II (moderate)	Return to play after asymptomatic for 1 week	Minimum of 1 month; may return to play then if has been asymptomatic for 1 week; consider terminating season	Terminate season; may return to play next season if asymptomatic
III (severe)	Minimum of 1 month; may then return to play if has been asymptomatic for 1 week[a]	Terminate season; may return to play next season if asymptomatic	

[a] No headaches, dizziness, or impaired orientation, concentration, or memory during rest or activity

minimal retrograde amnesia, and perhaps the fact that this symptom persists for a significant period after the injury is more significant than the immediate postinjury loss of memory for preinjury events.

If the athlete has no neck symptoms after regaining consciousness, removal on a spine board is not usually necessary. The athlete is, however, removed from the game and must be examined by an experienced physician. Return to practice may be as soon as 1 week after all symptoms have resolved during rest and exercise. After a second moderate concussion, return to play should be deferred for at least a month.[15] Three grade II concussions suggest the need for further neurologic investigation and termination of the season. Abnormalities on a CT or MRI scan would make the latter decision irrefutable.

Grade III (Severe)

The severe cerebral concussion produces an unconscious period of more than 2 minutes. There may be prolonged and significant retrograde amnesia after this injury. Sometimes there is marked unsteadiness on the feet lasting for more than 10 minutes and a persistent headache. The ringing in the ears (tinnitus) can be prolonged. There is often severe dizziness, and there may be some nausea. Convulsions have been triggered by third degree cerebral concussion. Initial treatment should be the same as that of a suggested cervical spinal fracture. The athlete should be transferred on a spinal fracture board, with head and neck immobilized.[13] It should be added that because this injury merges into a cerebral contusion, it is mandatory that individuals in this category are taken immediately to hospital. The main concern is an intracranial bleed. For optimal diagnostic accuracy an MRI scan is capable of detecting edema and hemorrhage (Fig. 20-4). It has the disadvantage relative to CT in that it is not possible to perform rapid scanning in unstable patients who may require immediate surgery.[21] The athlete should be prohibited from competition for at least 1 month, and there should be no symptoms with rest or exercise for a week. Two severe concussions are an indication to desist for the rest of the season. It is possible for the athlete to return to play the next season if totally asymptomatic. Athletes who have required intracranial surgery or who have hydrocephalus should be strongly advised against return to contact sports.

In summary, the following may serve as a guide (Table 20-4): No players should be returned to the game until they have been thoroughly assessed, which entails at least one or two plays if the individual has been momentarily dazed, suffers from mild dizziness, has mild tinnitus, or claims they saw stars or colors. This information must be elicited by close questioning of the player, ignoring their anxiousness to get back into the game. There should be a quick neuro-

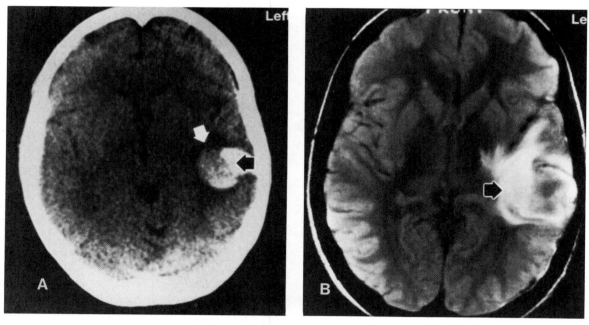

Fig. 20-4. **(A)** Axial section from a nonenhanced CT scan after head injury. Note the acute hemorrhage surrounded by edema in the left parietal area (arrows). **(B)** One week later an MRI scan shows the spreading edema (arrow) and the greater sensitivity in delineating cerebral tissue. (From Hayes and Nagle,[21] with permission.)

logic assessment, which includes determination of adequate visual fields, lack of double vision, good recall, and orientation.

The mild concussion is easy to overlook when one is busy watching as a spectator, rather than observing the players as a therapist. The main decision is whether the player should be returned to the game or be sent to hospital for observation. As stated, there is no problem with a severe concussion, but there is some problem with the less severe forms.

The player should not be returned to the game unless assessed by a medical doctor if, in addition to the above findings, there is unsteadiness, mild headache, disorientation, moderate dizziness, some amnesia, and moderate ringing in the ears.

The player needs a complete neurologic assessment and should not be returned to the game and probably should be sent to hospital if, in addition to the above signs; there are severe headaches, prolonged amnesia, amnesia for the second time in one game, one side of the body numb, one side of the body tingling, unsteadiness lasting for more than 10 minutes, muscle weakness, severe ringing in the ears, lethargy, facial asymmetry or hyperirritability (Table

---

> **Practice Point**
>
> **CONCUSSION: FACTORS TO CONSIDER**
>
> - Severity of current injury
> - Magnitude of postinjury symptoms
> - Results of tests (MRI, CT, neuropsychological)
> - History of previous concussions
> - Likelihood of reinjury (high versus low risk sport)
> - Level of competition (elite versus recreational)
> - Availability of protection

20-4). Blood from the ear canal or discharge other than blood from the nose is suggestive of a basal skull fracture. Indeed, any sign of paralysis or numbness down one side of the body, lethargy, blood from the ear canal, discharge from the nose, or muscle weakness constitutes a medical emergency. The individual should be moved cautiously and sent immediately by

TABLE 20-4. Criteria for Level of Assessment and Appropriate Action

Criteria	Do Not Return For at Least One Play.	Needs Assessment By Doctor. Remove from Game.	Needs Medical Evaluation. Return to Game is Contraindicated. Probably Send to Hospital.
Momentarily dazed[a]	X		
Mild dizziness	X		
Mild tinnitus	X		
Saw stars or colors	X		
Loss of consciousness <2 minutes			
Slight unsteadiness		X	
Mild headache		X	
Disorientation		X	
Moderate dizziness		X	
Amnesia (slight and first occasion)		X	
Moderate tinnitus		X	
Loss of consciousness ≥2 minutes			
Severe headache			X
Prolonged amnesia			X
Or amnesia with minimal trauma			X
Or amnesia for second time in 1 day			X
Unsteadiness lasting more than 10 minutes			X
Muscle weakness			X
Severe tinnitus			X
Lethargy			X
One side of body numb[b]			X
One side of body tingles[b]			X
Facial asymmetry or facial dyesthesia[b]			X
Hyperirritability			X
Discharge other than blood from nose[b]			X
Blood from the ear canal[b]			X
Bruising behind the ear (Battle's sign)[b]			X
Asymmetric pupils[b]			X

[a] More than one episode in a game requires removal from competition until full assessment. More than three concussions in a season requires removal from sport until full neurologic assessment.

[b] May indicate basal skull or sinus fracture; constitutes criteria for emergent, rapid transport to hospital.

Practice Point

CONCUSSION ASSESSMENT

- No return to activity until no neurologic symptoms at rest
- No return to contact sport unless no neurologic symptoms at a relatively intense level of activity
- Headaches with activity an important sign

Practice Point

REFER TO NEUROSURGICAL CENTER IF FEASIBLE

- Penetrating cranial injury
- Deteriorating level of consciousness
- Lateral deficit (hemiparesis)
- Prolonged unconsciousness
- Associated injuries requiring narcotic use
- Cerebrospinal fluid leak
- Post-traumatic seizures
- Preschool children with skull fracture

ambulance to a hospital. It must be recalled that there is a high association of neck fractures with severe head injuries, and for this reason the head should be stabilized and, when appropriate, a cervical collar placed around the neck.

To ensure detection of a potentially serious injury, remember that serial evaluations are more valuable than a single test. Be alert for other injuries, especially those of the neck. *Do not use ammonia ampules* (smelling salts). There is no place for them on the football field, the hockey rink, or for other contact sports where concussions are possible. If the player takes some time to recover, it is better to let nature take its course and then assess the extent of the damage. In any case, if there is an accompanying neck injury, and the player jerks his head away from the smelling salts, he may compound a cervical spinal problem. In all cases be conservative and seek medical help whenever necessary. A neural watch should be instituted by the medical person in attendance at the event followed by a simplified version by the athlete's roommate during the following night if the injury is significant (Table 20-5). Preferably, the individual should be awakened hourly during the night. The responsible person should be warned to bring the athlete back to the hospital for further evaluation if there are increasingly severe headaches, vomiting, restlessness and irritability, dizziness, or drowsiness or if the athlete is difficult to awaken or has a seizure (convulsions). The roommate should be warned not to give these athletes alcohol, not to allow them to drive, and to try to ensure that they rest quietly. Furthermore, the injured athlete should not play again without a doctor's clearance.

Practice Point

Serial evaluations are more valuable than a single examination.

There are some neurologic tests that can be carried out to assess expanding lesions. They are outlined in the following section.

Intracranial Injury

Although serious intracranial injury is rare, coverage of high risk activities by medical personnel requires anticipation of potential catastrophic injury.

TABLE 20-5. Neural Watch Chart

Test	Level	Time[a]
I. Vital signs	Blood pressure Pulse Respiration Temperature	
II. Conscious and . . .	Oriented Disoriented Restless Combative	
III. Speech	Clear Rambling Garbled None	
IV. Will awaken to	Name Shaking Light pain Strong pain	
V. Nonverbal reaction to pain	Appropriate Inappropriate "Decerebrate" None	
VI. Pupils	Size on right Size on left Reacts on right Reacts on left	
VII. Ability to move	Right arm Left arm Right leg Left leg	

[a] Record the time that each check is performed in columns on the right.
(From Schneider,[22] with permission.)

Adequate supplies and prior arrangement of evacuation and transport routes are important. The more remote the competition site, the more important it becomes. Significant impact-related brain injuries are invariably accompanied by secondary cardiopulmonary and metabolic changes, which if not corrected significantly complicate the evolution and magnitude of these injuries.[23,24] Thus the initial assessment and management of the brain-injured athlete may have as much impact on the outcome as the subsequent neurosurgical measures.[25] The principal secondary systemic insults to the brain include hypoxemia and hypotension. The net effect is additional ischemic-hypoxic brain damage superimposed on the primary insult (Table 20-6). Hypotension usually reflects associated injuries with blood loss. On-site physicians are in an ideal position to initiate the critical steps that may provide the chance of optimal recovery from the head injury.

TABLE 20-6. Cumulative Insults to the Injured Brain

Mechanism
  Concussion
  Contusion
  Laceration
  Compression

Secondary intracranial insult
  Brain edema
  Vasospasm
  Seizures
  Hemorrhage
  Infection

Secondary systemic insult
  Hypoxemia
  Hypotension
  Anemia
  Hyperthermia
  Hyponatremia

Quick Facts

ESSENTIAL SUPPORT FACILITIES AT HIGH RISK VENUES

- Supplies
  -Airways
  -Injectable sedative for seizures (pheno-barbitol)
  -Cervical collar
  -IV infusion set (normal saline, mannitol 20%)
- Information
  -Nearest hospital
  -Athlete's medical history
  -Access routes
- Facilities
  -Stretchers
  -First-aid personnel
  -First-aid station
  -Provisions for transport
- Communication
  -Two way communication; site of injury to ambulance or to hospital

Assessment of Severity

A brief history of the mechanism of the injury, duration of unconsciousness, and any known associated problems such as diabetes are rapidly obtained from the personnel at the scene of the accident. Establish that the airway is patent and carry out any steps necessary to ensure good ventilation. This point is particularly important when there is an associated facial injury. Protection of the cervical spine is mandatory if the athlete is still unconscious or confused.

A rapid scan should follow in an attempt to judge the magnitude of the cerebral injury. If alert, establishing the duration of the post-traumatic amnesia is a useful guide to severity. It is followed by a rapid screen of pupils, posture, and reflexes. Although the Glasgow Coma Scale is universally accepted and understood, it may be difficult to administer at the scene of the accident (Table 20-7). Nevertheless, some attempt must be made to establish a careful baseline of neurologic status. (Particularly if there is associated facial injury, the cranial nerves should be rapidly screened.) Only then can educated judgments regarding the most appropriate therapy be made based on subsequent subtle changes in the athlete's neurologic status.[26]

Because there is a significant association of major cranial trauma with injury to other parts of the body, the secondary screen should seek out intrathoracic

TABLE 20-7. Glasgow Coma Scale[a]

Condition	Score
Eye opening	
Spontaneous	4
To verbal command	3
To pain	2
None	1
Best motor response	
Follows commands	6
Localizes stimuli[b]	5
Withdraws	4
Flexion posturing	3
Extension posturing	2
No movement	1
Verbal response[c]	
Oriented	5
Confused	4
Inappropriate words	3
Incomprehensible sounds	2
No verbal response	1

[a] To be repeated over time to record changing neurologic status (total 3 to 15). A score of 10 or lower signifies significant intracranial injury or elevated intercranial pressure and requires immediate transport to hospital.

[b] Apply knuckles to sternum and observe arm movements.

[c] Arouse patient with painful stimulus if necessary.

Practice Point

NEUROLOGIC SCAN

- Pupils
  - -Size
  - -Equality
  - -Reactivity
- Movements
  - -Present appropriate
  - -Present inappropriate
  - -Absent
- Posture
  - -Normal
  - -Flexion
  - -Extension
  - -Flaccid
- Reflexes
  - -Corneal
  - -Deep tendon
  - -Gag
  - -Carinal
  - -Caloric

---

and intra-abdominal hemorrhage as well as axial and limb fractures.

Epidural (Extradural) Hemorrhage

Epidural hemorrhage is bleeding between the cranial vault and the dura (Fig. 20-5). It is usually related to a tear of the middle meningeal artery or one of its branches. A blow to the temporal region may particu-

larly involve this vessel. The classic clinical description involves the following.

1. Loss of consciousness at the time of trauma.
2. Regaining of consciousness followed by its loss some hours later ("the Lucid interval").
3. Appearance during the second episode of a deep coma from which the patient does not spontaneously recover.

A subdural or even intracerebral hematoma may present in an identical manner. Unrecognized and untreated, the mortality is close to 100 percent for large bleeds (Fig. 20-6). Even treated these lesions

---

Clinical Point

NEUROLOGIC TESTING FOR A SIGNIFICANT DANGEROUS OR EXPANDING LESION

Test	Abnormality
State of consciousness	Degree or impairment in words
Pupils	Inequality in size
Heart	Unusual slowing
Eye movements	Nystagmus "dancing eyes"
Outstretched arms	Drift unilaterally, down or outward
Finger-to-nose test (with eyes closed)	Asymmetry
Heel-to-knee test (with eyes closed)	Asymmetry
Romberg test (standing with eyes closed)	Falling
Tandem walk (heel to toe walking on a straight line)	Inability to perform

---

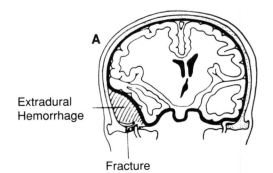
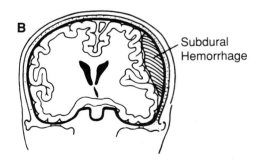

Fig. 20-5. Expanding intracranial lesions. **(A)** Extradural (epidural) hemorrhage. **(B)** Subdural hemorrhage between the arachnoid and the dura. (From Roy and Irvin,[26] with permission.)

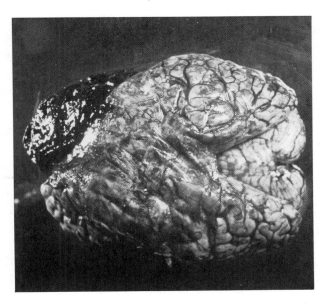

Fig. 20-6. Large subdural hematoma adjacent to the right frontal lobe.

may have a significant mortality rate unless recognized promptly. The individual in fact may not regain consciousness after the first episode. Recognition of localizing signs or the onset of lethargy or drowsiness following concussion is the key to early diagnosis. An increasingly severe headache or progressive dilatation of one pupil, on the side of the hemorrhage, followed by weakness usually on the side opposite the damage, herald impending loss of consciousness. Any suspicion of this lesion necessitates prompt removal of the individual to hospital. Simple screening tests for detection of a significant expanding lesion include assessing appropriate verbal responses, checking pupil size and visual fields, the finger–nose and heel–knee test, Romberg's test, and tandem walking. Should equipment or facilities be available, there is an emergency protocol for management of head injuries (Table 20-8).

Precautions and Contraindications for Participation

Conditions That Absolutely Contraindicate Contact Sport Competition

1. Symptomatic (neurologic or pain-producing) abnormalities about the foramen magnum
2. Congenital spinal anomaly with potential instability that would render the spinal cord vulnerable (e.g., Klippel-Feil syndrome or significant spinal fracture or dislocation)
3. Temporary quadriplegia, no matter what the etiology or degree of recovery (until thoroughly assessed)
4. Spinal cord abnormalities (e.g., syringomyelia, arteriovenous malformation)
5. Permanent central neurologic sequelae from a head injury (e.g., organic dementia, homonymous hemianopsia)
6. Spontaneous subarachnoid hemorrhage from any cause
7. Cervicomedullary-vascular injury with or without recovery

TABLE 20-8. Suggested Emergency Care of the Severely Head-Injured Patient

1. Establish reliable airway. Intubation indicated in all comatose patients and when deterioration in evidence.
2. Total body resuscitation and stabilization (multiple trauma).
3. Neurologic evaluation and documentation for later comparisons.
4. Restriction of intravenous fluids except to combat hypovolemic shock (i.e., normal saline, or Ringer's lactate at 30–50 ml/hour).
5. Hyperventilation (assisted or controlled) in an attempt to maintain PCO_2 at 25–30 torr, PO_2 at >80 torr; and pH 7.55.
6. Decadron 100 mg IV stat, then 20 mg IV q6h ("megadose" short-duration therapy).*
7. Indwelling bladder catheter to prevent distension and monitor adequate renal function and intake.
8. Mannitol 0.5–1.0 g/kg IV (20% solution rapidly or IV bolus) for any severe head injury or deteriorating neurologic condition.
9. Skull roentgenograms when appropriate and safe.
10. Cervical spinal roentgenograms: always in unconscious head-injured patients (AP and lateral views with arms pulled down on lateral view if necessary, must see C6–C7).
11. Expeditious transfer to fully equipped and staffed neurosurgical center with CT scanner, intracranial pressure monitoring, and available ICU bed.
12. If significant delays are encountered owing to clinical instability or transportation problems, additional neurosurgical phone consultation is recommended.
13. Patient should be kept in a head-elevated position (45 degrees preferred); "normo"tensive (100/70–160/90 mmHg); "normo" thermic (37°–37.8° rectal) Tylenol 1 gram q 4h for temperature $>39°C$ prn. Sedated if agitated (phenobarbital 32–65 mg IV prn), morphine sulfate (2–4 mg prn, or valium (5–10 mg prn). Keep seizure-free: treat seizures with IV dilantin, phenobarbital, or valium).

* There is considerable disagreement as to the efficacy of steroids.

Conditions That Strongly Suggest Elimination of Contact Sports

1. Recurrent concussion with repeated postconcussion syndrome
2. Repeated painful injury to the cervical spine (particularly with demonstrable radiographic changes (e.g., spondylosis)
3. Any intracranial condition requiring operative intervention (subdural or epidural hematoma)

Conditions That Require Discontinuation of Contact Sports for Remainder of Season

1. Seizure secondary to head trauma, single or multiple, focal or generalized. Particular attention must be paid to determination of the etiology to exclude any pre-existing cerebral abnormality
2. Brachial plexus injury producing significant neurologic impairment
3. Ruptured intervertebral disc, with or without surgery
4. Prolonged postconcussion syndrome

Conditions That Require Removal from Remainder of Game

1. Concussion with residual effects (retrograde amnesia, confusion, headache, unexplained behavior)
2. Brachial plexus injury (pinched nerve syndrome, burner, stinger) in which there is a question about the possibility of a cervical spinal fracture.

Head Injury in Boxing

In boxing one would anticipate a high incidence of concussion and facial injuries, and it is so, particularly in the professional ranks.[26] There is evidence that the repeated minor trauma received by boxers in a large number of fights over many years contributes to early dementia. This condition is seen often enough to be recognized by anyone associated with boxing and is affectionately referred to as "punch drunkenness." Autopsies on the brains of 12 professional fighters, two of whom were world champions, showed that compared to age-matched controls there is a definite increase in brain destruction in boxers. These men admittedly had fought in the brutal heyday of boxing before the 1940s. Most of them had as many as 700 fights in 15 years, which is approximately one competitive fight a week for their entire career. The British boxing board of control has tried to claim that

with the modern protective head gear, new rules, and good adjudication this situation does not exist today, but one would have to doubt this statement. Unfortunately, many boxers break the rules, and governing bodies turn a blind eye. Similar situations occur in kick-boxing and some of the martial arts. It has been also demonstrated that some professional soccer players, after years of heading the ball, have a syndrome akin to mild punch drunkenness.[26-30]

Quick Facts

RECOGNITION OF PUNCH DRUNK SYNDROME[a]

- Slight mental confusion
- Slowness of thought
- Personality change
- Memory impairment
- Hand tremor
- Nodding head movements
- Unsteady gait
- Dysarthria (slurring of speech)

[a] These signs may progress slowly over many years

In Jordon et al.'s 10-year review of boxing injuries at the United States Olympic Training Center[28] and Welch et al.'s report of injuries sustained by 2,100 cadets at the U.S. Military Academy, the occurrence of cerebral injury was 6.5 percent and 7.4 percent,[29] respectively, none of which resulted in obvious neurologic deficits. The low frequency among boxers in these programs represent the relatively controlled environment. However a 2-year survey of professional boxers in New York State showed that 89.7 percent of the injuries were craniocerebral, and they represented "knockouts" or "technical knockouts"; these were probably at least moderate concussions.[30] It is the latter situation that gives rise to concern (Fig. 20-7).

Death In the Ring

As many as 10,000 Americans die each year in sports-related accidents. The number sounds surprising, but drowning while participating in recreational swimming, boating, fishing, and hunting account for about 70 percent of that total. Why, then, is

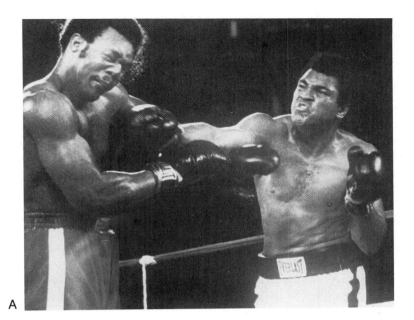

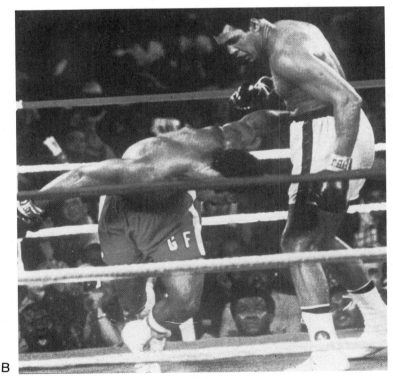

Fig. 20-7. (A) In boxing it is often the second punch delivered when the opponent is not protecting his head that produces the most cerebral damage. **(B)** Furthermore, because of the relaxed muscles of the neck the head can be twisted, causing a dangerous rotational insult to the brain.

there so much concern when someone dies in the ring?

The death of a boxer during a fight evokes feelings of individual and collective guilt because we witness the events leading up to it. Although we no longer

have "fights to the finish," most expect a fighter to disable his opponent before the bout ends.[31] The best way for a boxer to fulfill these expectations is to produce a concussion that renders the opponent temporarily unconscious or a series of concussions that leaves him on his feet but helpless. There is a suggestion that it is often the second blow that is catastrophic, following an initial blow that reduces the ability of the boxer to initiate appropriate defensive action including tensing of the neck muscles (Fig. 20-7). Fights may be won by points scored, incapacity due to severe lacerations, fractures, dislocations, or a solar plexus blow, or even through a combination of dehydration and heat exhaustion. However, the knockout is an unequivocal win. Indeed, a fighter's record is not considered strong unless it is heavily loaded with knockouts.

There is a delayed recovery of intellectual function after concussion, and the effects of successive concussions are probably cumulative. The memory cognitive system is fragile, and concussion may cause retrograde or postinjury amnesia.

It is difficult to judge accurately when the concussive effects of a knockout have worn off and it is safe to fight again. Electroencephalograms are too insensitive. CT is capable of revealing small brain hemorrhages at selected sites, and MRI is even more sensitive. The latter tests should probably be linked with some sophisticated psychological instrument of brain function to ensure the greatest protection for the boxer. Nevertheless, repeated knockouts are bound to take their toll on brain function. Defects in the septum pellucidum are well documented. Spillane found such defects using air encephalography of the brains of five former boxers aged 33 to 69.[32] All showed symptoms of chronic brain disorder, and two had cerebral atrophy. In 1963 Mawdsley and Ferguson used the same means to demonstrate dilated cerebral ventricles and cortical atrophy in former boxers.[30] Finally there are Corsellis' studies at autopsy of the brains of retired boxers who died between 57 and 96 years of age.[31] During life all had developed intellectual impairment and other symptoms such as paranoia. Half had parkinsonism, and a significant number had become hemiplegic owing to cerebrovascular hemorrhages.

Considering such severe consequences, it is not remarkable that boxing has been banned permanently in Sweden and Czechoslovakia and was not allowed from 1965 to 1969 in Connecticut. Because the sport is still regulated by individual states, broad recommendations of the American Medical Association and other interested groups have gone largely unheeded. Nothing has come of several attempts in New York to introduce the British rule of continuing knockdown counts after the bell ends the round.

What is needed at the moment is a better way to determine if a boxer is suffering progressive brain damage and should be stopped from fighting. The Paced Auditory Serial Addition Test used by Gronwall and Wrightson is one such test and could be applied after a knockout or more frequently with a fighter who accepts many bouts a year. The test has particular relevance to boxing because it deals with the ability to process information rapidly. Although this faculty is critical to any athlete, it is particularly important that the boxer protect himself from unnecessary punishment.

Certainly in the light of the evidence of considerable brain damage over a period of time, there is an added responsibility for the physician attending the fight and the trainer or therapist looking after the practice sessions to step in when necessary. Unfortunately, the point at which it happens depends on the attitude and personality of the medical person concerned.

Several points are important in regard to trying to prevent boxing injuries.

1. Adhere to the official rules regarding the amount of tape and bandage that can be placed inside a glove.
2. Use sufficiently padded gloves during practice sessions. The padding in the glove should not be manipulated. A combination of thinned padding and altered taping can produce as much as 30 percent difference in impact between the two gloves.
3. Mouth guards should be worn at all times to protect the teeth and mandible and reduce concussions. They provide an impact-absorbing surface.
4. Use head gear to protect against impact injuries. It provides absorbing material around the head.
5. Use Vaseline or lubricants liberally over the facial skin and the eyebrows to increase its plasticity and provide a more frictionless surface. It is particularly important to cover all old lacerations, as scar tissue tears easily.
6. Use good shock-absorbing ring floors. The materials should be soft and flexible enough to reduce the concussions and cerebral contusion injuries that are caused when a boxer's head contacts the floor.
7. Competent training and officiating is one of the most effective ways of avoiding serious injury. Potentially dangerous situations have to be identified before they occur. Better officials and trainers are

needed who are capable of recognizing minor injuries and potential risk situations.

Unquestionably, improvements occurred during the late 1980s, but if one looks critically throughout the ranks of boxing, at all levels, there is still a long way to go. Furthermore, because much of the cerebral damage is due to rotational and deceleration injuries to the brain, even the best equipment cannot completely eliminate cerebral damage. An analogy of this concept is one of a bartender sliding beer along a bar; it does not spill unless it tips (rotation) or is suddenly stopped (deceleration). It should be added that the brain is not the same consistency as beer, but enough alcohol eventually makes it become that way. The concept of the second blow and multiple punches when the boxer is not in a state to fully initiate protective reflexes has been stressed.

Helmets

The helmet is an integral piece of protective equipment in many sports. It usually protects well against direct blows, but it must be sport-specific.[32,33] The helmet must fit well, be lightweight and comfortable, not interfere unduly with vision and hearing, be durable, and be available at a reasonable cost. The helmet should meet the safety standards set up by the National Standards Association and should undergo frequent inspection, maintenance, and appropriate adjustments. Familiarization with the design and the fitting of specific headgear designed for individual sports is essential for involved individuals. Certain factors determine a helmet's protective abilities.

1. *Dispersion.* This factor depends on the construction and quality of the shell. To disperse an impact force, the helmet must be made of a rigid material with a uniformity of construction on the exterior. The inside of the shell must be padded with a material able to absorb energy. A one-piece molded construction or a highly integrated two-piece shell is recommended. The helmet must be able to disperse the impact force over as large an area as possible.
2. *Deflection.* The contour of the helmet should create an oblique surface that can deflect a direct blow from the head or away from the central axis, thereby decreasing the force impact. The outer shell should be smooth and round, with minimal slots and ridges.
3. *Absorption.* This factor is provided by the inner lining or padding of the helmet. The type of liner determines its ability to absorb forces. The helmet should be light and comfortable and meet the demands of the specific sport (Fig. 20-8).

Headaches

Transient headaches are common and, unless they are unduly severe or frequent, should not arouse anxiety in the young athlete. However, headaches may be a manifestation of intracranial disease or tumor. They may also result from systemic conditions, e.g., infection and hypertension, or local diseases of the ears, eyes, and mouth (Table 20-9). Thus a careful history and physical examination are important, and no athlete should be dismissed without a

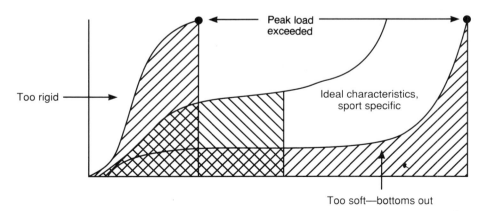

Fig. 20-8. Suspension of a helmet must be carefully designed, as too rigid mechanisms allow transmission of forces in excess of the peak load needed to produce head injury. Conversely, too much give allows the suspension to bottom out, similarly delivering forces in excessive peak load. The helmet needs to be specific for each sport.

TABLE 20-9. Common Extracranial Causes of Headaches (Referred Pain)

Type	Precipitating Cause	Symptoms	Diagnosis	Treatment
Eye	Eye strain or inflammation	Frontal or supraorbital pain	Association of eye pain	Refraction Treat inflammation
Ear	Otitis media	Temporal or aural pain; unilateral	Drum injected Fever	Antibiotics Decongestant
Sinuses	(1) Maxillary sinusitis, infective or inflammatory	Pain over cheek Associated tenderness	Pain on percussion Positive x-ray film Associated dental caries	Steam inhalation Decongestant Antibiotics Tooth care
	(2) Frontal sinusitis	Frontal headaches Directly over sinus May radiate behind eyes	Morning headache Tenderness to pressure	Steam inhalation Decongestant Antibiotics Tooth care
Oral cavity	(1) Dental caries	May be bilateral	Precipitated by cold drinks	Dental care
	(2) Temporomandibular joint disease	Associated pain in jaws	Aggravated by chewing, opening mouth wide	Orthodontic care
	(3) Ninth nerve stimulation	Swallowing cold drink or ice cream	Per history	Self-limiting

thorough consideration of the potentially serious causes of headaches.

The most common headache syndromes are outlined in Table 20-10, and a few are discussed in greater detail. There are some specific complaints which may suggest significant intracranial disease, meningitis, cerebral edema, and impending neurologic catastrophes.[34]

1. Onset of severe headache with vomiting and neck stiffness
2. Headaches accompanied by loss of consciousness, slow pulse, or increased drowsiness
3. Headaches accompanied by progressive failure of vision
4. Associated memory loss, disturbance, or a definite change in personality
5. Associated convulsions
6. Sudden change in a chronic headache pattern
7. Continually worsening headaches over several days
8. Early morning headaches sufficient to awaken the individual
9. Headaches of subacute onset that are significantly aggravated by the Valsalva's maneuver of coughing or sneezing
10. Highly localized chronic pain
11. Increasing headaches after a definite episode of intracranial trauma, e.g., concussion or cerebral contusion
12. Headaches accompanied by hypertension or increasing high blood pressure

Although the above signs and symptoms do not themselves indicate serious underlying pathology, they should at least serve to trigger further investigation.

Quick Facts

CLASSIFICATION OF COMMON HEADACHES

Type	Cause
Post-traumatic	Postconcussion or head injury
Psychogenic	Tension, anxiety
Intracranial	Exertion, hangover, subarachnoid hemorrhage, tumor, infection
Extracranial	Sinus infection, dental caries, eye strain
Migraine	Vascular spasm

Post-traumatic headaches have value in that they help decide the length of time a player should take off from contact sports following a concussion. Athletes

TABLE 20-10. Common Intracranial and General Causes of Headaches

Type	Precipitating Cause	Symptoms	Diagnosis	Treatment
Post-traumatic	Concussion or contusion	Generalized	Per history	Modifying activity Follow carefully
Hangover	Alcohol	Generalized	Per history	Self-limiting
Exertional	Running High intensity practice Coughing and bending	Generalized Frequently frontal	Concurrent with activity	Occasionally NSAIDs Activity modification
Migraine (classic)	Vasoconstriction and then vasodilation during paroxysmal attacks	Headache transient Hours to days Prodrome Associated nausea Blurred vision	Family history Unilateral throbbing Aggravated by oral contraceptives	Individualized treatment Medication Decrease precipitating factors
Migraine (common)	Tension, vasoconstriction	May be bilateral	Possibly aura	Medication
Infectious disease	Subacute infection	Vague fatigue Generalized headache Fever	Per history	Treat cause Observe Decrease activity level
Steroid and NSAIDs	Sodium and water retention	Generalized headache	Per history	Stop or change drugs
Heat injury	Metabolic heat production Hyperthermia	Generalized headache Piloerection, chills Overbreathing	Temp. elevated $39.5°-42°C$	Water Cooling Observation
Tension	Stress and anxiety	Intermittent, fronto-occipital tightness	Constant, tight, band-like	Counselling Medication Relaxation
Cluster headaches	Vasodilation and vasoconstriction Usually no visual or other associated problems	Unilateral Paroxysmal Unilateral rhinorrhea Facial flushing	May recur for days or weeks then disappear for months or years	Medication

should not train intensively or compete while this headache persists.

Cluster headaches are a highly distinctive type of vascular headaches. They usually begin when the athlete is in the late teens or twenties; and unlike migraine, predominantly males are affected.[35] They are called cluster headaches because of their temporal distribution. Sufferers may have one or several headaches per day, over several consecutive days, for several weeks or even months. Then they may be headache-free for a variable interval, sometimes up to several years. The headaches usually appear at exactly the same time of day, frequently awakening the individual from sleep. They commonly affect the eye or the area around it.

Unlike migraines, in which the pain is classically throbbing or pulsating, patients describe cluster headaches as a pain that is boring, stabbing, piercing, or knife-like (Table 20-11). They are possibly the most painful of the benign headaches. Fortunately, in contrast to migraines, they mostly last only about 30 minutes to 2 hours. Also, unlike migraines, they are not usually accompanied by nausea and vomiting. The eye on the affected side may be red and tearing, and there may be nasal congestion, rhinorrhea, miosis, ptosis, and facial flushing.[35] These symptoms may occur, but less frequently, with migraine, as both headache types have a vascular basis. There may be a strong link to smoking and alcohol. The treatment is highly individ-

TABLE 20-11. Characteristics of Cluster Versus Migraine Headaches

Cluster	Migraine
Male predominance	Female predominance
Clustered in time	Exacerbation and remission with no precise clustering in time
Pain in and around the eye Unilateral (but shifting) Pain stabbing, piercing, knife-like	Pain constant or pulsating Often bilateral
Short duration 30 minutes to 1–2 hour	Often last hours to days
No prodrome	Usually a definite prodrome
Nausea and vomiting rare	Frequently accompanied by nausea and vomiting
May wake patient from sleep	
Often agitated and hyperactive during attack	Prefer to be in quiet, dark room
Frequently has associated Horner's syndrome	Less frequent Horner's syndrome
Not usually hereditary	Often a strong family history
Attacks linked to tobacco and alcohol	Also triggered by alcohol

ual and experience is required to juggle the most effective combination of prophylactic and therapeutic medication.

There is a relatively rare type of headache called *benign exertional headache,* which may be defined as one that is triggered by and transiently interrupts complete comfort during exertional activities, e.g., running, bending, and weight lifting. It comes on rapidly, and its duration is usually brief, no longer than 4 to 6 hours.[36] Any of the prostaglandin inhibitors seems to provide temporary relief. Indomethacin has been widely discussed in the literature, however some of the better tolerated nonsteroidal anti-inflammatory drugs (NSAIDs) are effective. It may be necessary to reduce the amount of activity or, in some cases, change the nature of the sport.[35] The use of prophylactic loading doses routinely before exercise is not a sensible approach. The exertional headache must be distinguished from more ominous types of headaches associated with intracranial lesions, e.g., brain tumors, aneurysms, or vascular anomalies, as well as the more common cluster, fatigue, or migraine headaches.[36]

Pinching or entrapment of the high cervical nerve roots as well as tension due to poor posture may lead to *occipital headaches.* The therapist should be aware of these various causes and be prepared to send any athlete who exhibits more than the usual degree or frequency of headaches for neurologic evaluation.

Fainting (Syncope)

The term *syncope* evolves from Greek, meaning "a cutting short." Fainting, or syncope, occurs when there is sudden loss of consciousness, associated decreased muscle tone, and a resultant fall to the ground (unless supported in time). Usually it is a benign event in young athletes, and the only initial concern is to establish that there is an adequate airway and no secondary injury has resulted from the fall. Usually consciousness, muscle control, and alertness return within a minute. The fainting has usually resulted from a brief, abrupt fall in blood pressure and hence decreased cerebral circulation, which in turn generates either electrical or biomechanical dysfunction of both cerebral hemispheres or the reticular activating system.[37] If this classic sequence of rapid recovery is not followed or if fainting occurs frequently, a search for an underlying condition is necessary.

In many instances the cause of fainting is unknown. Classically, immobility may lead to insufficient lower limb muscular activity to assist in adequate venous return, thus decreasing cardiac output. Alternatively, suddenly ceasing vigorous activity may have the same effect, as there is widespread vasodilation demanding a vigorously reinforced, muscle-enhanced venous return. These last two mechanisms account for the fainting "guardsman" and the "collapsing" nonexhausted, normothermic runner at the end of a race. The third common mechanism is due to vasovagal tone. Increased vagal stimulation results in bradycardia, causing the cardiac output and blood pressure to fall. This situation may contribute to the hypotensive episodes of people standing in crowds but is usually in response to intense emotional stress, e.g., expecting an injection, the sight of a needle, or while awaiting competition.

Most syncopal episodes result from an abrupt decrease in cerebral perfusion. Orthostatic syncope occurs when an individual moves abruptly from the supine or crouched position to standing. In an intensely trained athlete, occasionally dehydration contributes to this loss of postural reflexes. Fainting may also be commonly related to antihypertensive drugs, diabetic neuropathy, or prolonged bed rest due to illness or surgery.

Cardiac dysrhythmias or a cardiac event such as an infarct can also cause dizziness and fainting. When associated with diaphoresis (sweating and cold, clammy skin), chest or arm pain, shortness of breath, or a positive cardiac history, one of these significant cardiac causes must be considered and appropriate therapy, transport, and follow-up for diagnosis and treatment organized.

Practice Point

FAINTING

Most syncopal episodes are benign. Concern is necessary if the following factors are present.
- Frequent episodes
- Associated with chest pain
- Associated with shortness of breath
- While on antihypertensive medication
- In the presence of strong cardiac history
- Related to exertion and presence of significant heart murmur
- Significant associated seizure activity
- Prolonged unconscious period

Pulmonary embolism may cause syncope and be difficult to detect. Typically there is chest pain, shortness of breath, and tachycardia. A history of recent surgery, prolonged immobilization of a leg, and the use of birth control pills may be contributory.

Hypovolemia due to occult blood loss presents usually as orthostatic syncope. A positive tilt test may help confirm it. A test is considered positive when there is a pulse increase of more than 30 beats per minute when moving from the lying to the standing position. This criterion has been correlated with an acute blood volume loss of 1,000 ml. Occult blood loss by rectal bleeding or in the stool from a higher gastrointestinal bleed is common, although a history of blunt trauma to the flank or abdomen in the athlete, particularly if there are local signs, should raise the suspicion of damage to the viscera.

Severe vertigo may cause the individual to fall but does not cause loss of consciousness. Seizure activity with classic fainting is uncommon, although a few clonic movements may be observed. With generalized seizures, a phase of overall stiffening (tonic phase) is followed by jerking muscular movements (clonic phase). The duration and magnitude distinguish them from simple recovery from syncope. There may also be a postictal phase (after seizure) of somnolence and confusion, which may persist 30 to 60 minutes.

If the period of unconsciousness is protracted, alcohol ingestion, hypoglycemia, hyperglycemia, diabetic ketoacidosis, heat stroke, cerebrovascular accident, hemorrhage, or closed head injury must be considered. Knowledge of the circumstances, medical history, and immediate precipitating events help diagnose the cause of what is in reality stupor or coma and not a syncopal episode.[38]

Quick Facts

CAUSES OF SYNCOPE

Cause	%
Unknown	38
Vasovagal	37
First seizure	9
Orthostatic	8
Cardiac	4
Others	4

(After Hitchcock and Bechtol,[37] with permission.)

With most isolated cases of classic syncope, no specific treatment is required. However, more frequent or atypical fainting spells should trigger appropriate investigations to rule out or elicit an underlying cause. Lastly, *fainting with exertion, particularly in association with a significant heart murmur, may be a warning sign of a cardiac anomaly that may lead to sudden death in sport.* Thus it should be appropriately investigated.

"Weight Lifter's" Blackout

Loss of consciousness during weight lifting is a phenomenon with which competitors are all too familiar. While lifting a maximum load "they become dizzy and confused or may fall suddenly to the floor.'' This type of fainting or syncope was most common during completion of the first phase of the lift called "the clean and jerk." It is possible that the loss of consciousness is associated with an increase in thoracic and abdominal pressures. However, it might be related to the overbreathing of most weight lifters during the period immediately before lifting.

Weight lifters overbreathe as one of various stratagems, e.g., posturing, shouting, and stamping, which they believe allows maximum effort. It is hoped that these maneuvers will overcome the inhibiting mechanisms that normally prevent application of full muscular power. The combination of hyperventilation, with raised intrathoracic pressure by any variation of the Valsalva's maneuver, is well recognized as a mechanism of reducing cerebral blood flow and inducing immediate syncope. It may be performed at will, as in the "mess trick," or "fainting lark."

Weight lifters susceptible to these "blackouts" should reduce hyperventilation, and the squatting phase should be as brief as possible. The weight to be lifted should be raised as quickly as practical.

ESSENTIALS OF THE NEUROLOGIC EXAMINATION

The neurologic examination is adapted to the particular circumstances. The key points for evaluating concussion and intracerebral injury have already been outlined, along with a neural watch chart and the Glasgow Coma Scale. This section briefly reviews tests for localization of neural deficits and lesions, commencing with tests for cranial nerve function followed by screening of cerebellar function. The tests of peripheral motor and sensory function are outlined in Chapter 19.

Cranial Nerves

The cranial nerves are screened in sequence except for III, IV, and VI, which are tested together because they control eye movement, and IX and X because of their influence over the tongue and phalangeal sensation and motion[39] (Table 20-12).

I: Olfactory nerve. Before testing the olfactory nerve, obstruction of the nasal passages should be

TABLE 20-12.   Screening Cranial Nerves

Cranial Nerve No.	Common Name	Function	Test
I	Olfactory	Sense of smell	Identify familiar odors: coffee, tobacco
II	Optic	Vision	Visual fields
III	Oculomotor	Eye movement Pupil constriction; elevate lid	Upward, downward and medial gaze; reaction to light; associated with upward gaze
IV	Trochlea	Superior oblique	Downward and lateral gaze
V	Trigeminal	Sensory to face; muscles of mastication	Corneal reflex; sensory face; grit teeth
VI	Abducens	Lateral rectus	Lateral gaze
VII	Facial	Facial expression Taste anterior tongue	Close eye tight; smile, whistle
VIII	Vestibulocochlear (acoustic nerve)	Hearing; balance	Hear watch tick
IX	Glossopharyngeal	Muscles of pharynx Sensory posterior tongue	Gag reflex; ability to swallow
X	Vagus	Muscles of palate; pharynx and larynx; autonomic heart, lungs, viscera	As for cranial IX
XI	Accessory	Sternomastoid and trapezius	Resisted shoulder shrug
XII	Hypoglossal	Voluntary muscles of tongue	Tongue protrusion

determined. With the eyes closed, the athlete is asked to identify familiar odors, e.g., coffee, tobacco, peppermint. Test each side separately. Disorders of the sense of smell may be caused by conditions affecting either the primary olfactory receptors in the nasal mucosa or the neurons of the olfactory bulb and tract.

II: Optic nerve. Visual acuity is tested with the Snellen charts. Corrected and uncorrected vision is recorded. To test the visual fields, the athlete covers one eye and then focuses on the examiner's nose with the open eye. The examiner brings the fingers in from a wide arc starting at each quadrant, asking the athlete to report as soon as the finger comes into view. Any persistent gross defect must be tested with more sophisticated apparatus. These screening maneuvers test the path from the retina to the optic lobe, and some localization is possible by the pattern of visual loss (Fig. 20-9).

III, IV, VI: Oculomotor, Trochlear, Abducens. These nerves are tested as a unit, as they supply all the muscles for eye movement. In addition, the oculomotor nerve supplies the muscles that constrict the pupils and elevate the lid. Eye motion is checked by the ability of the athlete to track the examiner's finger in the six cardinal positions of gaze (Fig. 20-10). The pupillary reaction is assessed by shining a light to confirm constriction. When the oculomotor nerve is affected, upward gaze and lid elevation are difficult. If the trochlear nerve is affected, the athlete cannot look downward and laterally. If the abducens is involved, the patient cannot look laterally with the affected eye.

V: Trigeminal nerve. This nerve supplies sensation

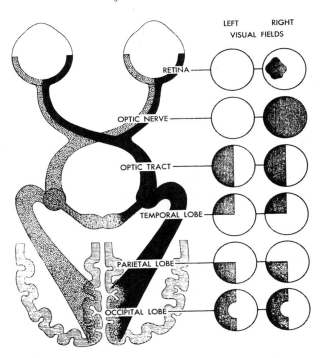

Fig. 20-9. Neural pathways for vision showing the pattern of visual field impairment with damage at the various levels of the retina, optic nerve, optic track, temporal lobe, parietal lobe, and occipital lobe.

to the face and the corneal reflex. It may be checked by testing sensation and by observing if the patient blinks in response to a light touch of a wisp of cotton on the cornea. Avoid stroking only the sclera. The last component, innervation of the muscles of mastication may be tested by asking the athlete to grit the

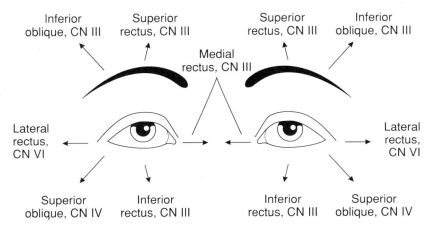

Fig. 20-10. Six cardinal fields of gaze that test cranial nerves III, IV, and VI.

teeth. A maxillary reflex may be elicited by tapping the middle of the chin with a reflex hammer while the athlete's mouth is slightly open. The nuclei for the trigeminal nerve reside in medulla and the pons.

VII: Facial nerve. The facial nerve innervates the muscles of facial expression. It is tested by asking the athlete to wrinkle the forehead, frown, smile, raise the eyebrows, and whistle. Asymmetry is noted. The nuclei are in the lower pons and upper medulla.

VIII: Acoustic nerve. Special equipment is necessary to examine the vestibular component, and hence it is not routinely tested. The external ear is examined with an otoscope to ensure that no canal obstruction is present, e.g., a buildup of wax. Hearing is tested by moving a watch away from the ear until the ticking is no longer audible.

IX, X: Glossopharyngeal and Vagus. The pharyngeal gag reflex is tested by touching each side of the pharynx with a tongue depressor. Normal function of the vagus nerve alone is revealed by the patient's ability to swallow and speak clearly without hoarseness, by symmetric movements of the vocal cords, and by symmetric movements of the soft palate when the athlete says "ah."

XI: Accessory nerve. The sternomastoid and trapezius muscles are tested by neck rotation and side flexion and shoulder shrugging, respectively. The nuclei are located in the medulla and the first five to six cervical segments.

XII. Hypoglossal nerve. The athlete is asked to protrude the tongue, and any deviation is noted. The strength is tested by asking the individual to push the tongue from side to side against the resistance of a tongue depressor. The nucleus is in the medulla.

Cerebellar Function

The tests for cerebral function essentially evaluate balance and coordination.

1. *Finger–nose test.* With the eyes open, the athlete touches a finger to the nose and then touches the examiner's finger. The examiner changes the position of his or her finger. The motion is repeated with increasing rapidity as the examiner moves his or her own finger. The test is repeated for each hand.
2. *Rapid alternating motion test.* Rapid motion is tested by getting the athlete to tap the back of the hand rapidly.
3. *Heel–toe test.* The patient is lying and carries the heel to touch alternately the toe and knee of the

opposite leg. This exercise is done with increasing speed or with eyes closed.
4. *Tandem walking.* The athlete is asked to walk in heel-toe fashion, initially with the eyes open and then with eyes closed. There should be a minimum of swaying.
5. Romberg test. The athlete stands with arms extended forward at shoulder height and eyes closed. A positive test is falling to one side.

This examination is obviously supplemented by examination of the limbs for intact sensation, reflexes, and muscle power.

INJURIES TO THE FACE

Facial injuries are common in sports where there are missiles, e.g., hockey pucks, baseballs, and cricket balls (Table 20-13). Racquets and hockey sticks are also formidable weapons. Moreover, high velocity, direct contact, as in football, hockey, rugby, and boxing, jeopardize facial structures (Fig. 20-11). The first-aid management of these injuries is emphasized here.

Quick Facts
BALL AND RACQUET SPEEDS

Missile	Speed (mph)
Racquetball	
Ball	85–110
Racquet	85–90
Squash	
Ball	130–140
Racquet	95–110
Tennis ball	90–110
Handball	60–70
Shuttlecock (initial speed)	130–135
Cricket ball	80–110
Baseball (hardball)	80–105
Puck (hockey)	80–130
Football	35–75

Laceration

There are several points that must be adhered to when cleaning, dressing, and protecting a wound from contamination. Bleeding should be stopped by simple pressure to enable assessment of the magni-

TABLE 20-13. Average Annual Rate of Facial Injuries in Collegiate Sports

Activity	Injuries Per 100 Athletes (No.)		
	Eye	Maxillofacial	Mouth/Teeth
Ice hockey	3.8	14.3	9.3
Wrestling	2.8	2.9	2.0
Basketball (men)	1.3	2.1	2.7
Field hockey (women)	1.1	1.7	2.4
Basketball (women)	1.4	1.0	2.1
Football	0.7	1.6	0.8
Soccer	0.3	1.1	1.1

(From Torg,[2] with permission.)

tude of the wound. Lacerations are nearly always less severe than they look at first (Fig. 20-12). The basic principles are as follows.

1. There is a danger of tattooing when dirt is taken deep into a wound. This material stays in the dermis and is not excreted onto the surface as is the case with a superficial wound. When there is any doubt about inadequate cleaning because of an inability to achieve anesthesia or because of fear of stimulating further bleeding, the athlete must be sent to the hospital for débridement.
2. Wounds heal best and bleeding is minimized when the edges of the wound are brought closely together. Frequently there is no need for sutures, and skin tapes are adequate. Preparation of the surrounding skin with a sticky material such as tincture of benzoin allows better adherence of the tapes.
3. If excessive sweating is anticipated or there is a possibility of further direct abrasion or contin-

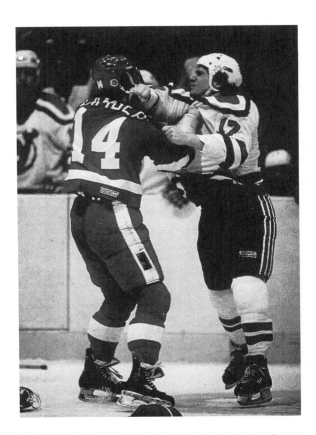

Fig. 20-11. Many of the facial injuries in hockey are due to the illegal use of a stick or fighting. Stricter adherence to the rules can decrease these injuries, and the use of protective equipment can further minimize injury from the puck.

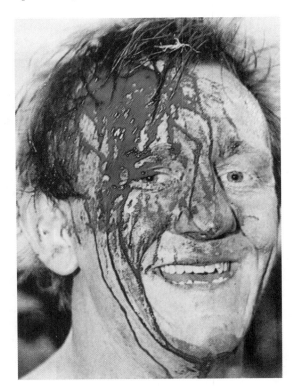

Fig. 20-12. Facial lacerations look much worse than they are because of the amount of rapid hemorrhage. Once this wound has been cleaned, its magnitude can be assessed and the appropriate decisions made as to whether skin taping or suturing is required.

ued oozing, even small wounds are better sutured.

4. Wounds that cross the border of the lips or eyebrow or enter the eyelids require expert, careful
approximation to prevent future puckering and
unsightly scarring.

5. Deep wounds of the eyelids should be seen by a
specialist to rule out eye injury and to prevent
later scar contracture and poor lid closure.

6. It is rarely necessary to suture the inside of the
mouth. If there is a deep wound or a flap that may
get caught in the teeth with chewing, suturing is
necessary. In those cases frequent gargling with
salt water and possibly antibiotics reduces the
potential for infection.

7. Most facial sutures should be removed at 5 to 7
days to minimize the eventual scar.

8. One must be cognizant of the danger of spreading infection. Local signs include increased redness, pain, or the appearance of pus. Systemic
signs include a fever, palpable nodes, and a feeling of malaise. When in doubt, a swab should be
prepared for culture and antibiotics started.

9. The tetanus organism is ubiquitous and can be a
contaminant of almost any wound. It is an obli-
gate anaerobe and thrives best where there is
devitalized tissue and lowered oxygen tensions.
Any significant cut, particularly if it is a penetrating wound with a small exit, should have adequate tetanus prophylaxis.

10. Tetanus immunization.

General principles of the *tetanus immunization* are
as follows. The attending physician must determine
for each patient with a wound, individually, what is
required for adequate prophylaxis against tetanus.[40]

1. Regardless of the active immunization status of
the patient, meticulous surgical care, including removal of all devitalized tissue and foreign bodies,
should be provided immediately for all wounds.
Such care is essential as part of the prophylaxis
against tetanus.

2. Passive immunization with tetanus immune globu-
lin-human (human TAT) must be considered individually for each patient. The characteristics of the
wound, the conditions under which it was incurred, its treatment, its age, and the previous
active immunization status of the patient must be
considered. Passive immunization is not indicated,
however, if the patient has ever received two or
more injections of toxoid.

3. A written record of the immunization provided is
given to all traumatized patients, instructing them
to carry the record at all times and if indicated to
complete active immunization. For precise tetanus prophylaxis, an accurate and immediately
available history regarding previous active immunization against tetanus is required.

4. Immunization in adults requires at least three injections of toxoid. A routine booster of absorbed
toxoid is indicated every 10 years thereafter.

Previously immunized individuals: When the attending physician has determined that the patient has
been previously fully immunized and the last dose of
toxoid was given within 10 years:

1. For tetanus-prone wounds and if more than 5
years has elapsed since the last dose, give 0.5 ml
absorbed toxoids. If excessive prior toxoid injections have been given, this booster may be omitted.

2. When the patient has had two or more prior injections of toxoid and received the last dose more
than 10 years previously, give 0.5 ml absorbed
toxoid for both tetanus-prone and non-tetanus-
prone wounds. Passive immunization is not considered necessary.

Individuals NOT adequately immunized: When the
patient has received only one or no prior injection of
toxoid or the immunization history is unknown:

1. For non-tetanus-prone wounds, give 0.5 ml absorbed toxoid.

2. For tetanus-prone wounds:
   a. Give 0.5 ml absorbed toxoid.
   b. Give 250 units (or more) of human TAT.
   c. Consider providing antibiotics, although the
   effectiveness of antibiotics for prophylaxis of
   tetanus remains unproved.
   d. Use different syringes and sites of injection.

Eye Injuries

The eye is usually well protected by the supraorbital
ridge and the cheek. Nevertheless, trauma to the eye
by a ball, racquet, puck, or any other missile may
cause traumatic cataracts (Fig. 20-13). Furthermore,
partial and total retinal detachments can result in
total blindness. All eye injuries should be treated with
absolute respect. If the individual complains of a sudden loss or change in vision, double vision, black
spots, flashing lights, or undue pain, a consultation
should be sought. Approximately 1 percent of all

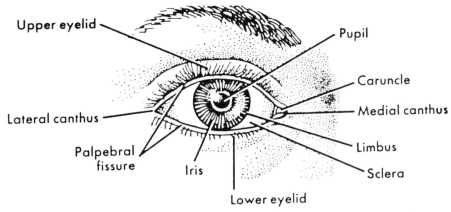

Fig. 20-13. Normal anatomy of the eye showing major landmarks. (After Booker and Thibadeau,[16] with permission.)

sporting trauma affects the eye. Pashby collated more than 3,000 injuries, of which 346 resulted in blind eyes[41] (Table 20-14).

The puck and highsticking at hockey predominated as mechanism of eye injury during the 1970s. A massive educational campaign has since resulted in compulsory eye protection at several levels of hockey and has dramatically reduced the incidence. Subsequently, racquet sports became the major problem, and the development of closed eye guards have had an impact on these injuries. A continuing campaign is necessary to further reduce these largely unnecessary statistics.

the lids open except in cases of chemical burns where irrigation is mandatory. The degree of sensitivity to light (photophobia) is noted. A careful check is made for foreign material, scratches, abrasion, and hemorrhage. The size and shape of the pupil and its normal constriction with light are established, which indicates optic nerve and retinal function. The six cardinal eye movements of lateral gaze, upward and downward gaze, and the oblique positions of up and right, down and right, up and left, down and left are checked to determine neuromuscular control (Fig. 20-10). Visual acuity may be documented with the standard chart or a near vision chart held 14 inches from the eyes. With experience and training, the opthalmoscope is used to check the retina; fluorescein is used to better visualize abrasions; and, ideally, a slit lamp examination of the cornea is performed.

Quick Facts

FORCES ON IMPACT OF SQUASH AND RACQUETBALLS

- Racquetball
  -1.4 oz ball at 128 mph   29.0 ft lb
  -1.4 oz ball at 78 mph   17.8 ft lb
- Squash
  -70+ ball (1.25 oz) at 100 mph   23.6 ft lb
  -International ball (0.846 oz) at   16.0 ft lb
    100 mph

Examination Principles

The examination principles are outlined in Table 20-15. Essentially, the eye is carefully inspected, although there should be some reservation with forcing

---

Practice Point

EQUIPMENT FOR ON-THE-SPOT EXAMINATION

- Penlight
- Vision card
- Sterile fluorescein strips
- Sterile eye pads
- Sterile irrigating saline
- Sterile swabs
- Eye shield
- Tape

TABLE 20-14. Canadian Ophthalmological Society Survey of Eye Injuries in Canadian Sports

Sport	1972–3	1974–5	1976–7	1977–8	1978–9	1979–80	1980–1	1981–2	1982–3	1983–4	1984–5	1985–6	Total
Hockey	287 (20)	258 (43)	90 (12)	52 (8)	43 (13)	85 (21)	68 (20)	119 (18)	115 (13)	124 (12)	121 (18)	123 (22)	1,485 (220)
Racquet sp.			48 (3)	12 (1)	28 (1)	58 (1)	103 (4)	100 (3)	88 (5)	115 (6)	81 (6)	83 (1)	716 (31)
Baseball			19 (2)	2	2	10	15	41 (5)	68 (3)	56 (3)	43 (2)	32 (3)	288 (18)
Ball hockey			24 (3)	8	9 (2)	27 (2)	22 (4)	10 (2)	19 (3)	25 (2)	29 (1)	28	201 (19)
Football			13 (1)	2	3	1	8	4	27 (1)	22 (1)	15 (1)	10	105 (4)
Golf			5 (1)	0	1	0	0	5 (4)	7 (2)	3 (2)	4 (1)	5 (2)	31 (12)
Skiing			1 (1)	1	3 (2)	0	0	3 (2)	0	2 (1)	4	2 (1)	16 (7)
Volleyball			3 (3)	0	0	6	3	2	3	4 (1)	0	2	23 (4)
Basketball			0	1	0	0	2	4	5	5	1	2	18
Broomball			2 (2)	0	0	2	2	3	3	2	0	1	15 (2)
Lacrosse			3	1	1	0	0	0	3	4	1	1	14
Hunting			0	0	0	0	4 (1)	0	0	1	5 (2)	1	11 (3)
Snowmobiling			2 (1)	0	1	0	0	1 (1)	0	1	1	2 (1)	8 (3)
Water polo			1	0	0	0	3	1	0	0	1	1	7
Boxing			0	0	0	0	0	0	0	0	2	1	3
War games			0	0	0	0	0	0	0	0	26 (14)	8 (2)	34 (16)
Equestrian			0	0	0	0	0	0	0	0	1 (1)	0	1 (1)
Other sports			5	0	0	7	0	5 (1)	6 (1)	9 (2)	15 (1)	5 (1)	52 (6)
Total	287 (20)	258 (43)	216 (29)	79 (9)	91 (18)	201 (24)	227 (29)	298 (36)	342 (28)	377 (30)	345 (47)	307 (33)	3,028 (346)

Numbers in parentheses indicate the blind eyes.
(From Pashby,[41] with permission.)

TABLE 20-15. First-Aid Protocol After Eye Injury

1. Inspect the lids and brows for laceration or hematoma.
2. Inspect the conjunctival sac for hemorrhage, laceration, or foreign body.
3. Evert the upper lid for a foreign body or dislocated contact lens.
4. Examine the cornea for a foreign body, abrasion, or laceration.
5. Remove contact lens if significant eye injury to prevent eye drying out.
6. To show most abrasions, use a fluorescein strip, moistened by a drop of sterile saline, and place in the inferior conjunctival fornix.
7. Assess the depth and clarity of the anterior chamber compared to its fellow eye.
8. Compare the sizes and shapes of the pupils and their reactions to light.
9. Check central vision with a reading card and compare with the fellow eye (always with correction by glasses or contact lenses). It is helpful to know any preinjury problems. If visual acuity is less than 20/40, refer to an ophthalmologist.
10. Check peripheral vision by confrontation perimetry. Have the patient fixate on the examiner's nose and identify the number of fingers held up in all fields of gaze (while occluding the other eye). The normal range is 85 degrees temporally, 65 degrees downward, 60 degrees nasally and 45 degrees upward. Comparison may be made with examiner's own visual field.
11. Assess ocular motility by asking the patient to make the six cardinal movements (looking right and left, up and down, left and up, right and up, left and down, right and down). If any diplopia (double vision), refer to an ophthalmologist.
12. Compare the eyes to see if there is any evidence of enophthalmos or proptosis.
13. Intraocular examination by a physician with an ophthalmoscope.

Conjunctivitis (Red Eye) and Subconjunctival Hemorrhages

Inflammation of the conjunctiva usually is secondary to irritation, often contact lenses. Spontaneous resolution follows removal of the irritant. Unless associated with pain, photophobia, or altered vision, it is usually treated by observation. It must be distinguished from iritis, where the inflammation is in a halo around the iris. This distinction may need examination by an expert. Subconjunctival hemorrhage may be secondary to rupture of a vessel spontaneously or traumatically and resolves spontaneously within 1 to 3 weeks.

Orbital Hemorrhage

Orbital hemorrhage is usually the result of blunt trauma. Proptosis (bulging of the eyeball) may occur with restricted extraocular motility.[41] In severe cases vascular supply to the retina and optic nerve may be compromised, causing visual loss. First aid includes immediate application of ice pack compresses to reduce edema and aid hemostasis, followed by prompt examination or referral to an expert before the swelling becomes severe.

Lacerations

Lid lacerations must be treated with care. They are usually sutured by an expert if they cross the margin of the lid. Scarring may eventually produce lid deformity (ectropion), which results in the lid not retaining fluid and hence drying of the eyes. Laceration into the corner may involve the lacrimal gland.

Minor *conjunctival lacerations* do not require repairs. Subconjunctival hemorrhage is dramatic but usually asymptomatic.

Corneal lacerations, if large, may result in extrusion of ocular contents with additional pressure. Hence an eye shield should be used over a lightly applied dressing prior to referral to hospital.

Corneal Abrasion and Foreign Particle in Eye

Corneal abrasions may be due to a scratch or to some foreign material, e.g., dirt, in the eye. The abrasions are characterized by tearing, photophobia, blepharospasm, and pain. Superficial foreign bodies can usually be brushed off the corner with a cotton swab (Q-tip) or irrigated off with sterile saline. If the foreign material is difficult to visualize, the lid may be everted (Fig. 20-14). After removal of any particulate matter in the eye, the presence and extent of the abrasion are confirmed by fluorescein staining with or without the aid of topical anesthesia (Fig. 20-15). Frequently there is some denuding of the corneal epithelium, which has the potential to recover fully.[43] Treatment usually consists in a firm sterile pad dressing, possibly with topical antibiotic and adequate analgesia, and re-examination every 24 hours until healing is established[42] (Fig. 20-16).

Hyphema

Hyphema is a collection of blood in the anterior chamber of the eye (Fig. 20-17). At first dispersed, it may settle with a visible level. It commonly comprises more than 25 percent of sports-related eye injuries.[41]

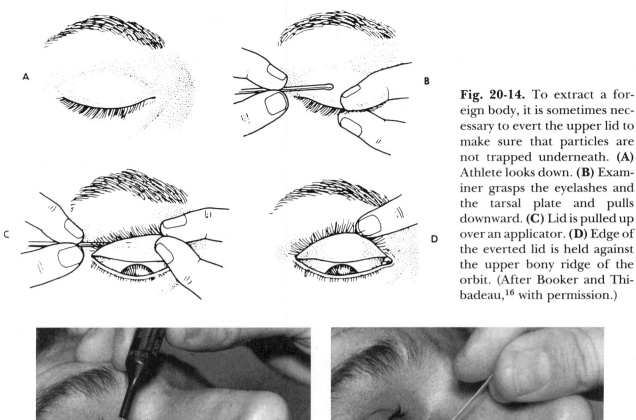

Fig. 20-14. To extract a foreign body, it is sometimes necessary to evert the upper lid to make sure that particles are not trapped underneath. **(A)** Athlete looks down. **(B)** Examiner grasps the eyelashes and the tarsal plate and pulls downward. **(C)** Lid is pulled up over an applicator. **(D)** Edge of the everted lid is held against the upper bony ridge of the orbit. (After Booker and Thibadeau,[16] with permission.)

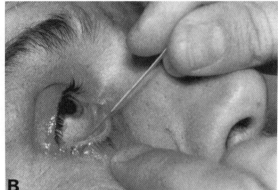

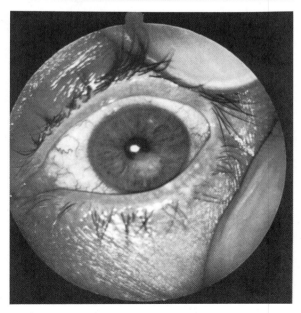

Fig. 20-15. **(A)** Examination of the eye. Sterile saline or, when necessary, local anesthetic of proparacaine hydrochloride 0.5 percent. The athlete looks directly up, and the eyelid is depressed by stretching the skin and applying pressure over the inferior orbital rim. **(B)** Sterile fluorescein-impregnated paper strips available in individual sterile packets help to stain in the eye. **(C)** This method assists in visualizing corneal abrasions. Unstained abrasions are often difficult to see. (After Bedford MA: Color atlas of ophthalmological diagnosis. Year Book Medical Publishers, Chicago, 1971, with permission.)

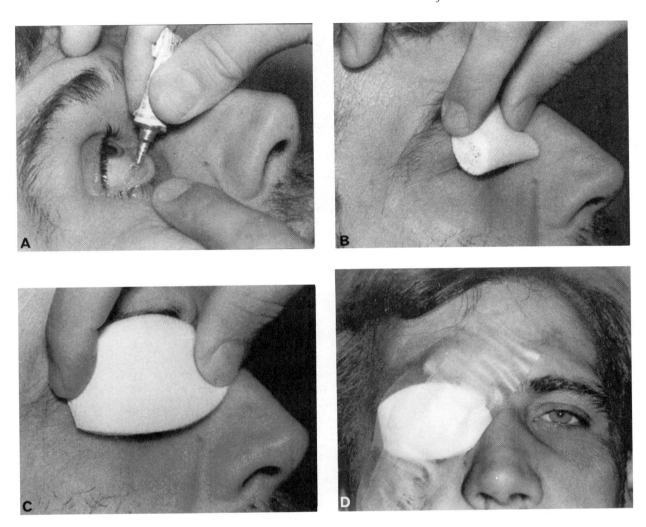

Fig. 20-16. Application of a dressing to an eye. **(A)** Consider instilling some antibiotic ointment, e.g., chloramphenicol (Chloromycetin). **(B)** Apply a fold of sterile pad lightly over the closed eye. **(C)** Place an unfolded sterile pad lightly over the closed eye. **(D)** Place several strips of tape diagonally from the forehead to cheek with enough pressure to keep the eye closed when the noninjured eye is open. Wrinkling of the skin usually denotes that the pressure is adequate. When necessary, a hard shield is placed to prevent the athlete from raising the intraocular pressure by rubbing the injured eye. (The cut-out bottom of a paper cup may be used if nothing else available.)

Minor hyphema is detectable only with slit lamp examination. The affected pupil is usually irregularly larger than the opposite one, and vision may be slightly or dramatically reduced. Most hyphema resolves within a few days, but 15 percent of individuals suffer a second bleed, usually between the second to fifth day. Treatment involves rest, with elevation of the head, for 5 days, usually in hospital. A second bleed reduces the chance of full recovery. Late com-

plications include post-traumatic glaucoma and cataract. Hence all of these injuries require ophthalmologic consultation (Fig. 20-17).

Retinal Injury

Retinal hemorrhages may follow blunt trauma. If they are in the macular area, visual loss may ensue. Retinal tears are not uncommon and may result in

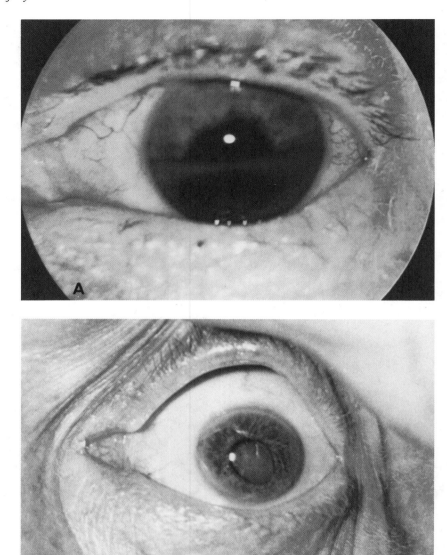

Fig. 20-17. **(A)** Collection of blood in the anterior chamber of the eye (hyphema). **(B)** Late complication of a direct blow, the post-traumatic cataract.

detachment (Fig. 20-18). They may also follow a concussive injury, occasionally delayed for several weeks. Retinal detachment is described as being like "a curtain falling in front of the eye" or as lights "flashing on and off." There may be floating black specks across the eye. The immediate treatment requires protection from further injury until a full assessment can be made and definitive treatment planned. If a proper eye shield is not available, the base of a paper cup often suffices. For severe injuries, it is best to

patch both eyes, which provides complete rest and leaves the athlete in total darkness. Hence constant reassurance is necessary.

Fracture of the Bony Orbit

Blow-out fractures of orbit may be caused by a puck or ball in the eye, boxing accidents, or collisions where a finger or racquet hits someone directly in the orbit. This impact generates forces within the orbit as

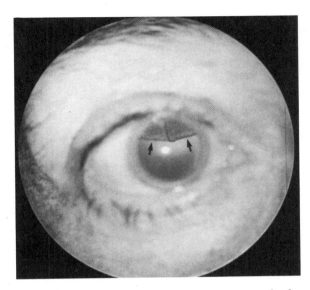

Fig. 20-18. Retinal detachment is seen as a shadow across (arrows) the pupil when attempting to view the retina. (After Bedford MA: Color Atlas of ophthalmological diagnosis. Year Book Medical Publishers, Chicago, 1971, with permission.)

the eyeball deforms and may result in excessive pressure on the orbital walls, particularly the inferior floor, which happens to be also the roof of the maxillary sinus. A variable quantity of the lower part of the orbit is incarcerated in the roof of the maxillary sinus, which may result in double vision when the patient looks upward as the entrapped inferior rectus muscle of the eye prevents concentric gaze. It can also be detected as a difference in the gap between the limbus and lower lid on the affected side with upward gazing (Fig. 20-19). After a significant blow to the bridge of the nose or the eye, athletes should be prevented from blowing their nose until normal eye movements are established. Blowing one's nose in the presence of an inferior orbital fracture may allow the contents of the maxillary sinus to track into the orbit (Fig. 20-20). Once more, prevention is the key, and high risk sport such as court games should not be played without adequate eye protection.[43]

Contact Lenses

Contact lenses must be removed from an unconscious athlete, as the decreased amount of moisture in the eye causes the lens to stick to eye surface. Hard contact lenses must be removed immediately, whereas a soft lens can usually be left in for some time without significant damage to the eye.

Removal of a Hard Contact Lens.

1. Shine a penlight on the side of the eye to cast a shadow on the surface. Hard contact lenses are 1/3 inch in diameter and often tinted.
2. Remove using a suction cup. Hold the eyelids apart with the thumb and forefinger. Place the suction cup directly onto the lens and remove it. Slide the contact lens off the suction cup and store it in a lens case.

Removal of a Soft Contact Lens.

1. Pull down the lower lid with the middle finger, and place the index finger on the lens. These lenses are large, clear, and flexible and may be difficult to locate.

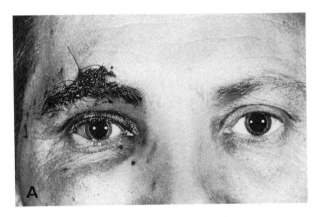

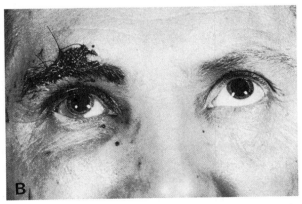

Fig. 20-19. After entrapment of the inferior rectus muscle in the floor of the orbit with a right blow-out fracture the upward gaze is not concentric. **(A)** Normal while looking directly forward. **(B)** As the patient looks up, the right eye does not move adequately, producing double vision. Note the different distance between the limbus and the lower lid of the two eyes.

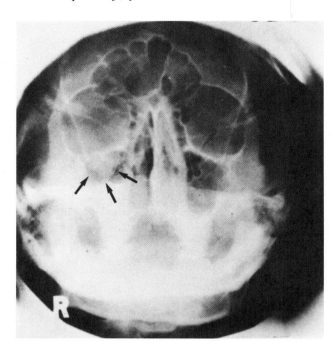

Fig. 20-20. Right inferior orbital wall fracture. Note the opacity of the right orbit (arrows) possibly secondary to hemorrhage, edema, and some infraorbital fat and muscle pushed down into the sinus.

2. Slide the lens onto the white part of the eye. Compress the lens between the thumb and finger in a pinching motion and remove the lens from the eye. Store it immediately in a lens case.

Note. Do not attempt to remove any contact lens with cotton swabs, toothpicks, or fingernails.

Protective Eye Wear

Athletes who participate in sports where there is a significant risk of being hit in the eye by a missile should wear some eye protection[43] (Fig. 20-21). The protective eye wear should meet the standards of the American Society of Testing and Materials (ASTM) or the Canadian Standards Association (CSA) in North America and of comparable bodies elsewhere. The frame should be constructed of a resilient plastic, with reinforced temples, hinges, and nosepiece. Adequate cushioning should protect the eyebrow and nasal bridge from sharp edges. The lenses should be made of polycarbonate material that is 3 mm thick. Eye guards without lenses do not provide adequate protection from compressible tennis and racquetballs hitting at high velocities. Polycarbonate is an

impact-resistant plastic that was introduced during the 1960s for bullet-proof windows. It is at least ten times stronger than industrial thickness CR39 plastic. It is also 50 percent lighter than crown glass and 10 percent lighter than CR39 plastic. It is thus ideal for protective eye wear.[41] It may be used for a wide prescription range.

One-Eyed Athlete

Anyone whose best corrected vision is 20/200 or worse in the poorer eye is effectively blind in that eye. Anyone whose best corrected vision is 20/40 or better is effectivley two-eyed. However, if the level of vision falls between 20/40 and 20/200 the definition of "one-eyed" is pragmatic and depends on the individual's sport and life style. If an athlete's status is in question, wearing an occluder over the better eye for a few days usually allows a realistic assessment of the individual's status and a more objective basis for discussion as to whether participating in an activity presents a significant risk and the need for eye protectors for all activities. One-eyed athletes have reduced visual fields and depth perception. Thus injury

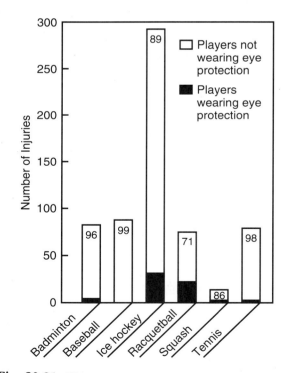

Fig. 20-21. Players injuring their eyes, showing the small number of those who wear adequate eye protection versus those who do not.

to the remaining eye would be catastrophic. Boxing is the only sport that is totally contraindicated because there is no available protective eye wear. Wrestling should be discouraged, as protective eye wear is inadequate. For virtually all other sports, preventive eye wear is available and must be worn.

Practice Point

VISUAL ACUITY

- Athletes with a best correct vision of 20/200 are effectively blind in that eye.

Nasal Injuries

Nasal injuries occur frequently in sport, and many are abrasions and contusions. In one study of English boarding school children, 20 percent of the fractures were to the nose, an injury second in frequency only to arm fractures.[44] Many nasal injuries are due to fighting in sports such as rugby and ice hockey. Collisions while heading the ball in soccer or a direct blow by a squash racquet are examples of accidental injury.

For the most part, protective equipment has reduced but not eliminated the more serious injuries.[43] It is usually worn only for high risk sports, e.g., foot-

ball; but for moderate to high risk activities such as racquet games, baseball, and hockey, facial protection is rarely used. For example, only the catcher in baseball and the net-minder in hockey usually wear a mask. When it is not mandatory, athletes decline face protection on the grounds of discomfort, difficulty breathing, and restricted vision. Peer pressure also plays a significant role in not wearing adequate protective equipment.

Nasal fractures have both functional and cosmetic significance, particularly during adolescence, when the nose is growing. Furthermore, recurrent fractures are seen in many individuals, producing cumulative functional problems.[45] Familiarity has bred contempt, and the frequent cursory examination fails to assess fully the magnitude of the injury. A thorough knowledge of both cartilaginous and bony structures is needed to decide and implement early successful treatment and avoid late complications and reoperation[46] (Fig. 20-22).

Contusions and Hematomas

Most swelling and hematomas are important only in that they may obscure underlying damage. Large hematomas, however, may eventually produce thickening and deformity; and septal hematomas occasionally result in necrosis of the septum, which if suf-

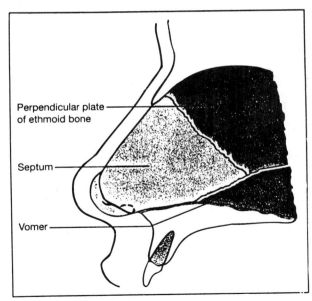
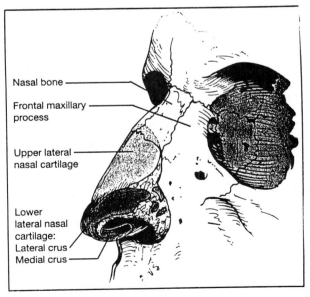

Fig. 20-22. (A) Structural support of the nose is provided by the paired nasal bones and the upper and lower lateral cartilages. **(B)** Internal support is provided by the septum, vomer, and perpendicular plate of the ethmoid bone.

ficiently widespread may lead to collapse of the nasal septum, producing a "saddle nose" deformity. Decompression should be performed early to these large hematomas followed by packing or splinting to decrease reaccumulation.

Abrasions and Lacerations

Most abrasions are treatable by simple cleaning to remove all debris that might leave a tattoo. The wound is then allowed to dry and crust, avoiding topical antibiotic ointments. Large, deep skin defects that could result in scar contracture need grafting, usually with postauricular skin for the best match.

Practice Point

NASAL CONTUSIONS AND LACERATIONS

- Septal hematomas may cause cartilage damage.
- They may need drainage.
- Careful cleaning of abrasions prevents tattooing.
- Use a brush to scrape if necessary.
- Lacerations exposing cartilage require meticulous attention.

Lacerations are dealt with according to the principles outlined earlier. Most can be cleaned and approximated with skin tapes. They heal rapidly. Lacerations extending to or through the nasal cartilage require more care. The mucosal and skin surfaces must be closed, and no cartilage should be removed or left exposed. Significant wounds need the care of an experienced practitioner or plastic surgeon.

Epistaxis (Bleeding)

Most nasal bleeding stops easily. The source of hemorrhage may be anterior or posterior. Anterior bleeding is usually from the vessels in the anterior septum (Kiesselbach's area) (Fig. 20-22). Such bleeding is controlled by pinching the nose for 2 to 5 minutes or, if unsuccessful, packing, with or without silver nitrate stick cauterization. These vessels are easily visualized. Profuse bleeding after fracture is generally from the anterior ethmoidal artery and

usually requires reduction of the displaced segment and packing.

Practice Point

EPISTAXIS (NOSEBLEEDS)

- Key to diagnosis is adequate visualization.
- Anterior bleeds usually stop with pressure.
- Posterior bleeds may need positioning and packing.
- Significant blood loss is possible, and failure to stem profuse hemorrhage should signal a need for early consultation.

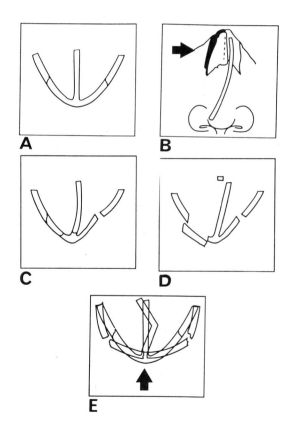

Fig. 20-23. (A) Normal nasal bones: septal pyramid. **(B)** Lateral nasal blow causing ipsilateral nasal fracturing and concomitant septal fracture. **(C)** Fracturing of the ipsilateral nasal bone without septal fracture. **(D)** Fracturing of the ipsilateral nasal bone and out-fracturing of the contralateral bone with septal fracture. **(E)** Direct blow to the front of the nose causes splaying of the nasal bone and septal fractures.

Posterior bleeding drains mostly into the throat and is generally from the posterior ethmoidal artery. Profuse hemorrhage is controlled by head elevation and nasal packs of half-ribbon gauze (Vaseline or Xeroform). For uncontrollable bleeding, a small Foley catheter may be inserted into the nostril and the balloon inflated and withdrawn until snug while consultation with a specialist is arranged.[45]

Nasal Fractures

Diagnosis of nasal fracture is based on a thorough history and examination. The history includes the nasal appearance before injury; but in view of the high incidence of refracture, this picture is not always easy to obtain accurately (Fig. 20-23). The ability to breathe through each nostril and the absence of associated facial numbness are key points during the examination. An adequate internal examination requires adequate lighting and preferably a nasal speculum. The most common signs of nasal fracture are epistaxis, swelling of the nasal dorsum, subsequent ecchymosis around the eyes, tenderness, crepitus, and obvious deformity (Fig. 20-24). Anterior, lateral, and oblique roentgenograms may give some information but are frequently falsely negative.

First aid includes stopping hemorrhage; then, if adequate examination is not possible because of edema, the patient is re-examined after the swelling resolves. Definitive treatment is best done within 4 days for children and 10 to 12 days in adults.[45] Re-

---

Practice Point

NASAL FRACTURES

- Diagnosis is essentially clinical.
- Check for associated facial bone injury.
- Reduce immediately after injury, prior to swelling, if possible.
- If not possible, wait until edema subsides.
- Septal position is the key to a good airway.

---

duction is best achieved and maintained when good visualization is possible and edema is resolving. Other than simple septal deviation, these injuries are best treated by experienced personnel. For contact sports special protective equipment should be worn until healing is well under way to prevent further injury or redisplacement. Occasionally, open reduction or late rhinoplasty is required to correct a residual deformity where the airway is impaired or the cosmetic results are unacceptable.[46]

Ears

There are three major areas regarding the ears that are of concern in sport: (1) trauma to the ear; (2) effects of water in the canal; and (3) noise-induced deafness.

The external ear consists of an auricle (Pinna) and

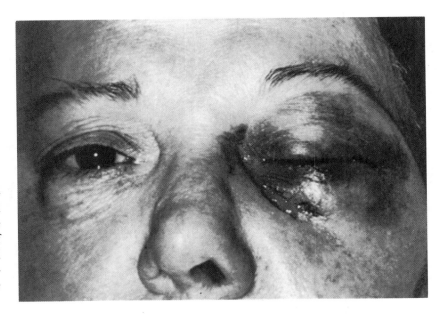

Fig. 20-24. Displaced nasal fracture and associated periorbital ecchymosis. Concern should be expressed about the condition of the eye, the possible infraorbital fractures, and the long-term effect of the displacement on the airway.

an external acoustic meatus, both of which are designed to collect sound waves and transmit them into the external auditory canal and hence the eardrum (tympanic membrane) (Fig. 20-25). The auricle has multiple eminences and depressions supported by a thin fibrocartilaginous plate connected to surrounding structures by ligaments and muscles. The lateral surface is covered by firmly adherent skin. The tympanic membrane separates the external from the middle ear, which contains the small ossicles necessary for sound transfer (Fig. 20-26). The middle ear connects with the pharynx via the eustachian tube, which allows equalization of air pressures when patent and forms a channel for the transmission of throat infection to the middle ear, particularly in children where the canal is short. The inner ear, entirely protected by bone, contains the cochlea and semicircular canals for transmission of hearing and balance sensors, respectively.

Cauliflower Ear (Scrum Ear, Hematoma Auris)

Cauliflower ear is the name given to the eventual deformity of the pinna that results from significant or

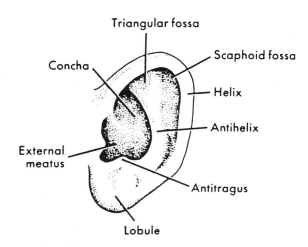

Fig. 20-25. Surface landmarks of the ear.

repetitive trauma, edema, and scarring. The cauliflower ear is seen commonly in sports such as wrestling, rugby, and boxing. Friction or blows to the ear may cause edema or hemorrhage between the skin and the cartilage (Fig. 20-27). The usual site of hematoma is between the skin and the perichondrium, but

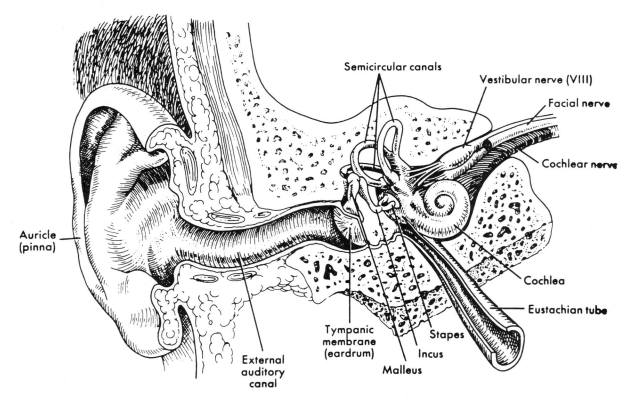

Fig. 20-26. Components of the outer, middle, and inner ear (After Booker and Thibadeau,[16] with permission.)

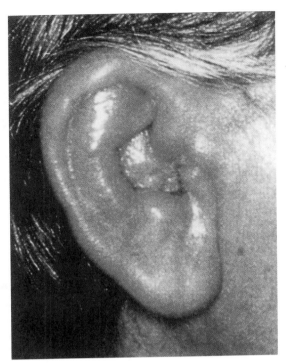

Fig. 20-27. Cauliflower ear. Hematoma or edema with fluctuant swelling obscures the normal contours of the auricle.

it may occur between the perichondrium and the auricular cartilage or within the cartilage itself.[47] Upon reabsorption a certain amount of scar is left that eventually contracts and deforms the pinna, leaving it susceptible to further injury. Although considered unsightly by most, the severe cauliflower ear is accepted as a "badge of courage" in some communities, and hence there is often reluctance to allow treatment. However, at least young wrestlers and boxers should be protected from their own folly.

Clinical Point

CAULIFLOWER (SCRUM) EAR

- Frictional injury
- Formation of edema and/or hematoma
- Development of granulation and fibrosis
- Contracture and deformity

- *Look for warning signs and protect.*
  -Aspirate significant hematoma.
  -Apply pressure dressing.

Treatment is best instituted before major injury ensues. Any signs of redness should be treated by application of Vaseline over the ears to reduce friction or protection in the form of ear guards or bandages. Ice and pressure applied at the end of practice or game, whenever there are apparent hot spots, also helps. If there is an intense inflammation of the ear, excessive edema can be prevented by forming a pressure dressing over the ear itself. Should there be a large accumulation of serum or blood, it may be best to aspirate or drain the fluid under sterile conditions. Large hematomas, if left, may cause pressure necrosis of the cartilage with early significant deformity. When it is necessary to make incisions for drainage, appropriate anesthesia is achieved by blocking anteriorly and posteriorly at the base of the pinna (Fig. 20-28). Reaccumulation is then prevented by application of a cast. Such a cast may be made from cotton batting and collodion, which solidifies the batting in the shape of the ear and external canal.[48] This internal splint collodion-impregnated batting or Webril is placed in the helix and white wool in the concha, providing a firmer mold than cotton alone. It is held in place with further pressure by an external bandage. Alternatively, plaster of paris casts or silicone molds have been used.[49] Some individuals advocate holding the dressing in place with buttons and through-and-through sutures, but this measure is rarely necessary.

If any open drainage technique is used, the wound must be checked at regular intervals, every 2 to 3 days, to ensure that the fluid has not reaccumulated and that there is absence of infection. Local or general erythema, increasing pain, warmth, fever, or pus should trigger the immediate use of antibiotics. Because the most common organisms are *Staphylococcus aureus* and frequently *Pseudomonas*, it is wise to swab for cultures and use broad-spectrum antibiotics.

Swimming Pool Ears (Otitis Externa)

Swimming ear (swimming pool ear) is a painful form of otitis externa with possible bacterial or fungal superinfection.[50] Some swimmers seem particularly prone and are constantly troubled, even to the point of totally disrupting training routines. Competitive swimmers, divers, water skiers, and scuba divers may be affected.

Presentation and Pathophysiology

Symptoms of swimmer's ear include (1) itching, (2) extreme pain, (3) discharge, and (4) even partial hear-

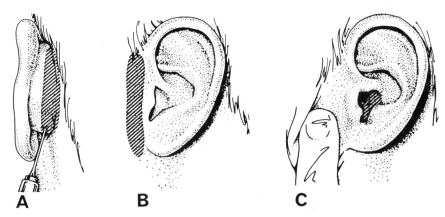

Fig. 20-28. Evacuation of a hematoma from the ear and application of a pressure dressing may require local anesthesia. **(A)** Lidocaine 1 percent is administered to the external ear in the posterior sulcus and **(B)** in the skin and subcutaneous tissue anterior to the helix, tragus and lobule. **(C)** External meatus may require additional infiltration, as may the various quadrants. After aspirating the hematoma, a pressure dressing is applied. If necessary it may be secured by two buttons loosely sewn through the auricle, one in each side, using a tie-through suture technique.

ing loss. These problems must be treated promptly at the first sign of trouble if a chronic condition is to be avoided.

Quick Facts

OTITIS EXTERNA (SWIMMING POOL EAR)

- Initial symptom: itch (may become painful)
- Hearing loss (seldom)
- Due to
  -Prolonged contact with water
  -Removal of normal wax
  -Trauma during ear cleaning
- Results in pH change in ear canal
- Secondary infection possible, bacterial usually and occasionally fungal

---

The ear canal is approximately 2.5 cm long. The outer cartilaginous portion, approximately 1.0 cm, contains hair cells and sebaceous glands. The secretions from these glands mix with sloughed epithelial elements to form an acidic waxy barrier (cerumen, ear wax). The interosseous portion has virtually no subcutaneous tissue underneath the epithelium and does not secrete cerumen. It is therefore more vulnerable.[50]

In the normal ear, nature has provided an efficient mechanism for defense. There is a natural migration of meatal skin, which, as it grows, moves from the region of the eardrum (tympanic membrane) to the meatal opening, taking to the outside world debris and dried wax (cerumen). This contaminating material then further dries, pulverizes, and disappears. The ear also has a normal flora of organisms, which also have a protective function.

Experiments have shown that even the dirtiest of water does not cause inflammation or infection when the skin of the canal is unbroken and is covered by a good layer of normal wax. The meatus, if full of water from a swim, a bath, or a shower, soon empties with movements of the head and dries by evaporation without the use of a towel. Thus the fleeting application of water can do little harm. Longer contact, as with frequent swimming or diving, especially underwater swimming (e.g., scuba diving), may be hazardous. The water macerates the ear, and the chlorine compounds the problem by destroying the protective keratin layer.

The usual flora of the ear consists predominantly of gram-positive oranisms, which may be replaced by a secondary gram-negative bacterial invasion. This situation particularly pertains when normal hygiene is poor and dangerous cleaning habits are used. Cerumen plugs may trap water in the ear (Fig. 20-29).

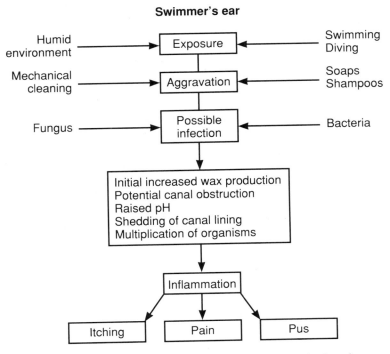

Fig. 20-29. Flow chart of the evolution of otitis externa (swimming pool ear).

Prophylaxis

Keeping the normal wax and bacterial flora in the ear probably constitutes the best protection.[51]

1. Never let shampoo or soap get into ear.
2. When showering, avoid letting water run into the ear.
3. Take time to drain ears and to dry outside of ears when leaving pool.
4. No attempt is made to dry the canal by touching, rubbing, or probing.
5. Never use sharp objects to dry ears.
6. Do not use cotton-tipped swabs in the ear.
7. A few drops of baby oil in the ears before swimming or showering can keep the skin oily and help protect them. Alternatively, the instillation of alcohol eardrops after swimming is allowed, which may help change the pH toward acidity.[51]
8. Do not use ear plugs. Ear plugs or cotton batting soaked in oil is not a good idea prophylactically, as they may break the protective lining of the ear canal and aggravate the drum directly and indirectly by preventing the equalization of pressures during sudden emersion. A tight-fitting swimming cap may be an alternative.

Treatment

1. Athlete may have to stop swimming for a variable length of time.
2. Reinforce healthy "ear" habits as described.
3. Swimmer should be educated to consult a physician whenever the problem is severe or recurrent.
4. If the problem is infection, antibiotic powders lightly insufflated or topical antibiotic eardrops, e.g., polymyxin B-neomycin-hydrocortisone (Cortisporin) otic drops or colistin sulfate (Coly-Mycin),[51] may be necessary.
5. If the ear is painful, a strong analgesic may be required initially.
6. As a rule, applications that absorb fluid from the tissues should be avoided, as are strong chemical disinfectants. However, in problem cases 5 percent acetic acid or 3 percent boric acid with 85 percent isopropyl alcohol or any other acidifying solution such as aluminate sulfate-calcium acetate (Domeboro) applied immediately after swimming may be effective. The eardrum must be intact and the canal not too inflamed.
7. Swimmers are usually able to resume water activity

in 7 to 10 days if they are able to tolerate alcohol eardrops.

Noise-Induced Deafness

A highly specific sports injury is the noise-induced tinnitus and deafness experienced by marksmen. The Walsh-Healy Act of 1969 established the 85 decibel figure for broadband industrial noise as the maximal permissible 8 hour working environment noise level.[52] Greater duration or intensity than this level may result in significant hearing loss.

In contrast to continuous environmental noises, sudden loud sounds also present a danger. Impulse noise results from sudden explosions. A high sound pressure develops rapidly, lasts only a few milliseconds, and subsides as rapidly as it develops. Hearing loss due to the acoustic trauma of repetitive impulse noise has been recognized. All shotguns, center firing, and rim firing weapons exceed the damage-risk level of 150 dB with the exception of the smaller 0.22 cartridges. To minimize the potential trauma, the following points are worth considering. First, firing on flat open terrain minimizes noise. When adjacent to solid masses, as when firing in indoor ranges, ear protectors should be worn. These ear defenders are of various descriptions and may provide 20 to 45 decibels of noise reduction. Well designed and carefully made ear protectors afford the most protection.[53]

Barotrauma

The barometric pressure outside and inside the body at sea level is 14.7 lb per square inch. For every 33 feet of descent in the sea, the pressure increases by approximately that same amount.[50] There is a constant need to equilibrate the pressures within the air-filled cavities of the head, e.g., sinuses and middle ear. It demands that the eustachian tube and the sinus ostia be patent.

"Ear squeeze" may develop during a diving descent. Pressure differentials cause swelling of the epithelium of the middle ear and vascular dilation. These changes may be adaptations to auto-regulate the pressures by decreasing the volume of the cavity.[50] Gross engorgement may further occlude the ostia and prevent equalization of pressure. There may be transudation or even vessel rupture and bleeding in the middle ear. With ear squeeze the diver notices ear pain, decreased hearing, ringing in the ears (tinnitus),

and, if the adjacent sinuses are involved or there is bleeding, blood-tinged sputum.

If the external canal is blocked by cerumen, a diving hood, or an ear plug, an artificial air-filled cavity external to the tympanic membrane is formed. The middle ear becomes overpressurized in relation to the closed artificial external cavity and the tympanic membrane distends outward, a "reverse ear squeeze." This phenomenon is similar to that experienced during the rapid descent of an aircraft.

Divers should attempt to keep the external opening of the ear patent by ensuring that there is not a wax plug buildup. They should not dive if suffering from sinusitis, allergic rhinitis, or severe upper respiratory tract infection. Antihistamines taken as a decongestant may cause a rebound phenomenon that involves mucous membrane swelling and may thus lead to barotrauma. Repeated problems should stimulate the diver to seek medical attention to rule out osteoma, large adenoids, or congenitally small openings of the eustachian tubes.

Tympanic Membrane Rupture

A blow to the unprotected ear in water polo, diving, surfing, skiing, or, more rarely, boxing and football may rupture the tympanic membrane. The rupture occurs with a pop and a suddenly decreased ability to hear. Bleeding may be apparent. If cold water enters the defect, labyrinth stimulation may cause dizziness and nausea, panicking a swimmer or diver.

The ruptured membrane should be carefully observed each day until healing to ensure that associated infection does not develop. Antibiotic drops should not contain steroid, as it may delay healing. Healing is usually rapid.

Teeth

Sport-related dental injuries, though decreasing in number, are common, particularly in sports that do not require the use of mouth protection.[54] The healing mechanisms of teeth differ markedly from other repair processes in the body, and even as long as 2 years after trauma the status of the injured tooth may be in question. To be reasonably sure the tooth has survived significant trauma, the tooth's response to temperature and pressure and an x-ray examination of the alveoli enclosed within the gum must remain normal for approximately 5 years. First aid for dental injuries is not necessarily complicated and centers on three principles: (1) determine the source of any oral bleeding; (2) assess the mobility of the teeth suspected of being injuried; and (3) prevent further problems during the healing phase (Fig. 20-30).

Castaldi[54] pointed out that most authorities on dental trauma agree on the following tenets.

1. The less traumatic the injury, the more likely it is that the tooth will return to normal.
2. The rate of recovery is closely related to adequate, prompt first aid, particularly when a tooth is completely avulsed from the gum. It is essential that the tooth is not permitted to dry out, and it should be reimplanted and splinted within an hour of the avulsed injury.[54] A dislodged tooth left out of the mouth for longer than 30 to 60 minutes has little chance of being saved.
3. Roentgenographic evaluation of all significantly injured teeth is appropriate within the 24 to 48 hour period after trauma to rule out root fractures (Fig. 20-31). These films serve as a baseline for future studies and for following the evolution of post-traumatic changes within the tooth and surrounding alveolar bone.
4. The use of a properly fitted mouth protector

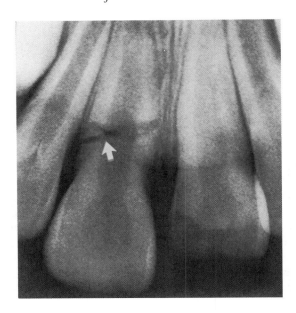

Fig. 20-31. Asymptomatic tooth fracture at the level of the root (arrow) that had occurred sometime prior to the roentgenogram. This type of fracture may heal. Conversely, the root may be resorbed or become inflamed resulting in loss of the tooth.

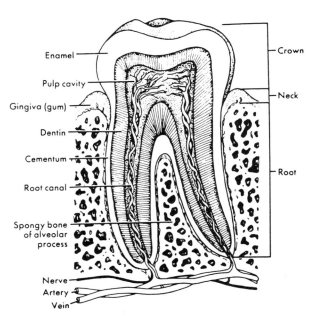

Fig. 20-30. Normal anatomy of the tooth showing the crown, neck, and root. The latter is buried in the alveolar bone of the jaw. The layers of the tooth comprise the outer enamel, the dentine, and the inner pulp along with the nerves and vessels. (After Booker and Thibadeau,[16] with permission.)

unequivocally reduces the number and severity of dental injuries.

Assessment of Dental Injury

Identifying the Source of Bleeding

A direct blow to the mouth often damages the inner surface of the lips. It is important to distinguish this injury from seepage of blood around the base of the tooth. Carefully sponging away the excessive blood and occasionally rinsing the mouth may make it possible to distinguish the exact source of bleeding.

Loose Teeth

The extent of the damage to the tooth is not always obvious immediately, because although the exposed tooth appears normal there may be a fracture of the crown or the root. Furthermore, the tooth may be loosened in the alveolar bone, which can compromise or even sever the tooth from the blood supply and thus jeopardize any chance of significant recovery.

The potentially damaged teeth should be examined by the finger pressure test. The finger is placed on the biting edge of the tooth, and mild pressure is exerted inward toward the tongue and then outward toward the lips (Fig. 20-32). Normal teeth move only slightly under such pressure. Therefore if the degree of movement is similar to that of adjacent teeth, and there is no triggering of pain or prolonged feeling of numbness, it is probable that the damage is only to the gums surrounding the tooth. If an injured tooth remains in the bone after it has been shifted, the dental artery vein or nerve may be compromised. If the tooth is slightly depressed in the bone, is loose, or feels numb or painful to pressure, the athlete should be given emergency care by a dentist. If these symptoms are absent, the athlete can resume play. It should be recalled that if an injured tooth is not quickly repositioned by firm finger pressure, it may die and become discolored. The venous blood stagnates in the tooth, and the hemoglobin seeps into the dentin, turning the tooth pink then dull yellow and finally gray.

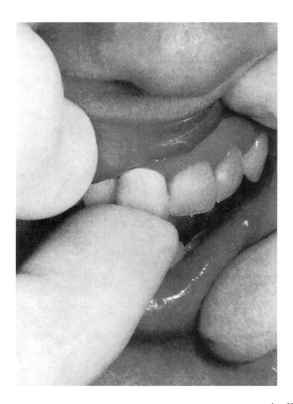

Fig. 20-32. Finger pressure test on traumatically loosened teeth. The therapist or physician exerts some mild pressure on the tooth, first inward toward the tongue then outward toward the lips.

Avulsed Teeth

An avulsed tooth should be cleaned of all dirt and debris by flushing it with sterile water if available; if sterile water is not available, tap water will suffice. The tooth should then be repositioned in its socket. It is understandable that nonexperienced personnel may hesitate to reimplant an avulsed tooth, but providing it is repositioned with its correct orientation, it constitutes the best first aid because it prevents the tooth from drying and minimizes the changes within the tooth and gum. If reimplanted within 30 minutes there is up to a 90 percent chance of the tooth being retained.

An alternative to immediate reimplantation is to wash the tooth, wrap it in a sterile gauze sponge, moisten it with tap water, and make immediate arrangements for dental consultation. It is possible that the best storage medium for a tooth is milk, but it is often impractical in a sport environment. Keeping the avulsed tooth under the tongue is also a resonable environment, but obviously it has its risk in that the athlete can accidentally swallow the tooth. The main principle is that reimplantation and splinting should be done within an hour of injury. An avulsed tooth is therefore a definite sports medicine emergency. If reimplantation is successful, it may take up to 5 years before one is certain that the dentition has indeed returned to normal.

Tooth Fractures

Small cracks in the enamel may be of little consequence but should be assessed by a dentist. Fractured teeth are classified according to the level, size, and structures involved (Fig. 20-33).

Practice Point

SMALL CORNER FRACTURE (CHIPPED TOOTH)

- Finger pressure test is negative (no pain or movement).
- Tooth is not sensitive to air on inhalation.
- Athlete may continue to play.
- Tooth should undergo roentgenography within 24 hours.

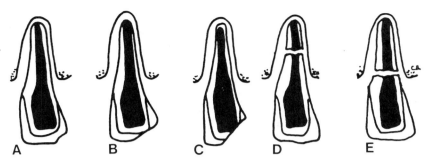

Fig. 20-33. Increasingly severe fractures of the tooth. **(A)** Small corner fracture involving only the enamel. **(B)** Some slight exposure of the dentine (large corner fracture). **(C)** Large corner fracture, with the nerve root pulp exposed. **(D)** Fracture close to the apex of the root. **(E)** Fracture at the level of the gum, which surprisingly has slightly less favorable outcome than the fracture in Fig. **D**.

Small Corner Fractures. A small chip off the corner of a tooth that is not sensitive to air when the player inhales vigorously through the mouth and is not loose is compatible with continuation of play. If the tooth has a particularly sharp edge, the tongue must be kept away from the fracture margins; if there is any suggestion of loosening, it is appropriate to make arrangements for dental roentgenography and the chip corner attended to preferably within 24 hours (Fig. 20-34).

Large Corner Fractures. If the break in the tooth exposes dentin, there is usually sensitivity to inhaled cold air, unless the tooth is so severely damaged that it is numb. By looking up into the tooth, the pulp may be visualized (Fig. 20-34). If this pulp is exposed, the athlete should receive dental treatment. If the pulp is not exposed and the tooth is sensitive only to air, the athlete may be permitted to resume play. If there is increasing sensitivity, the athlete should be removed from play. It is preferable to arrange for dental consultation within 2 to 3 hours of the injury so a full assessment is available. Pain relief with analgesics or local anesthetic may be necessary.

Major Fractures. With severe fractures, fairly extensive dental treatment is required often culminating in root canal treatment followed by implantation of a cast-metal cap over which an artificial crown is fitted (Fig. 20-35). Root canal work involves removing the

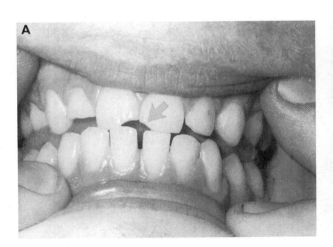
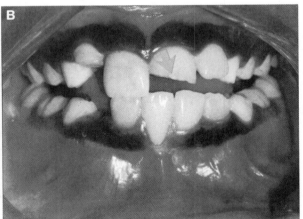

Fig. 20-34. Fractures of the teeth. **(A)** Small corner fracture (arrow). **(B)** Large corner fracture of the upper incisor (arrow). This fracture usually exposes the dentine, causing hypersensitivity to inhaled air.

Practice Point

LARGER CORNER FRACTURE (MAJOR CHIP)

- Dentine exposed
- Tooth sensitive to air on inhalation
- May be numb initially
- If pulp (nerve root) not exposed may continue to play
- Dental treatment in 2 to 3 hours arranged
- If pulp exposed, receive immediate dental care

---

pulp (nerve root) from the canal, sterilizing the canal, and then filling and sealing it.

Prevention of Dental Injury

Incidences. Universally, only football, boxing, and ice hockey currently require the use of face masks and mouth guards. Although these devices do not entirely eliminate oral and facial trauma, they do greatly reduce the risk of dental injuries. It is interesting that youth baseball (athletes under age 14), although not considered a high injury sport, has by far the highest incidence of head and facial injuries in athletes. Fortunately, excellent educational programs sponsored by the American Dental Association has induced an interest and awareness of the danger of oral injury. The use of mouth guards is increasing, and gradually

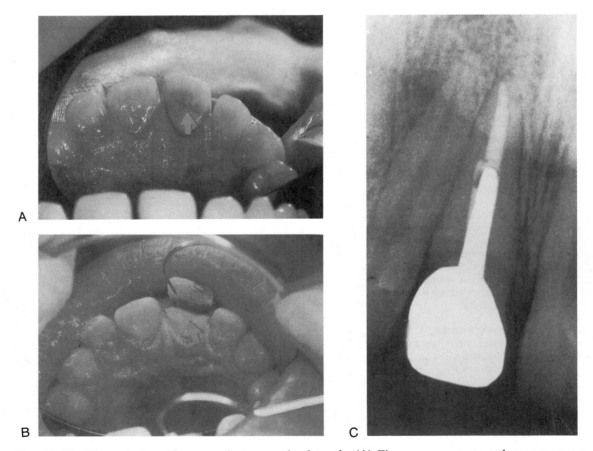

Fig. 20-35. Lingual view of a severely traumatized tooth. **(A)** Finger pressure test demonstrates a vertical fracture extending across the entire width of the crown. **(B)** It is treated by root canal treatment. **(C)** Metal posts are inserted to accomodate the crown.

they are being used more often in field hockey, lacrosse, basketball, and rugby.

Functions of Mouth Guards. The mouth guard (tooth guard, gum shield, mouth protector) should be a relatively inexpensive item that is fabricated to fit over the teeth and a certain amount of the gums. It is intended to prevent injuries to the teeth and to absorb some of the impact to the facial structures, reducing the incidence of fractures, dislocations, and concussions.[55] It should fit comfortably within the jaw and interfere minimally with respiration, particularly under exercise conditions. In some sports it should allow easy communication. Mouth guards should be able to be positioned accurately within the jaw to facilitate maximum efficiency and should be difficult to malposition. They should cover the surface of all the teeth, be light and strong, and be easy to clean. Finally, they should be resilient and not easily traumatized by external forces or by chewing.

Types of Mouth Guards. There are essentially three classes of mouth guards: (1) stock, or off the shelf (ready to wear), mouth guards; (2) mouth-formed guards (boil and bite); and (3) custom-fabricated models. Each of these mouth guards provides protection against injuries; and although they cover all of the teeth, they are usually constructed for the upper arch. In recent years, construction of one-piece mouth guards fitting over both the mandible and maxilla have been discouraged. The most effective mouth guard is the custom-made model because the size fitting is slightly better. It also overcomes the objections raised by the athlete concerning speech and breathing for the most part.

There is one more type of mouth guard, the external mouth guard, which is usually used by ice hockey players or occasionally football players. It is flexible, movable, and attached by a strap to the helmet or the face guard.

Off the Shelf Mouth Guard. Stock mouth guards are inexpensive, readily available, and usually made of rubber, polyvinylchloride, or a polyvinylacetate copolymer. They are usually slightly bulky. Their fit is such that they usually remain in place only so long as the jaws are closed. Thus they are not effective in maximizing the ability to breathe through the open mouth. They are, however, acceptable and preferable to not wearing any mouth guard.

Mouth-Formed Guards. Mouth-formed guards are of two varieties: shell-liner and thermal plastic type. The shell-liner type consists of a preformed outer shell of polyvinylchloride that fits loosely over the maxillary teeth. The liner is a plasticized acrylic gel or silicone rubber. These substances are mixed and put in a shell, placed in the mouth, and finger-fitted; they set in a few minutes.

The second type is preformed from a thermal plastic copolymer of polyvinylacetate-polyethylene. These guards are popular because they are easily purchased and manipulated and can be formed by the coach, athlete, or therapist. The mouth guard is immersed in boiling water for approximately 15 to 45 seconds and then dipped in cold water for 1 second; it is immediately transferred, while wet, into the mouth and adapted to the contour of the teeth. The athlete may mold the material by finger and tongue pressure and by biting gently. Unfortunately, the material often becomes distorted and loose, although it can be reformed by repeating the procedure. It has the disadvantage that equal thickness protection is not always achieved throughout the area of dentition. If it is not carefully molded on the periphery of the inner lip and gum, contusions, cuts, and abrasions may be generated. These thermoplastic protectors are popular because of their decreased bulk and cost; furthermore, they can be worn over fixed interoral orthodontic applicances. Unfortunately, a significant number of mouth-formed guards do not adequately cover all teeth and do not meet the NCAA requirements. A wider variety of sizes, particularly large sizes, are necessary to accommodate athletes with greater arch lengths.[55]

Custom-Made Mouth Protectors. The primary material is a thermoplastic polymer of polyvinylacetate-polyethylene. Because they are so well fitted, they are more efficient in terms of their fixation and thus allow more physiologic use of the oral airway. These guards have the disadvantage of requiring experienced personnel to fit them accurately.

Care of Mouth Guards. It is important that the athlete be educated in the care of the mouth guard. There should be an adequate denture cup or plastic container so the guard can be rinsed and kept after each use. Usually cold soapy water should be used for cleaning. The guard may be damaged or cracked as a result of excessive chewing on top of the guard and the athlete should be cautioned against this practice. Periodically, the mouth guard should be checked to see that it not only fits well but is not unduly damaged.[56]

Specific Sports. *Hockey.* In 1977 Rontal et al. presented statistics on facial injuries in hockey that were of great concern. In the 7- to 10-year age groups, 7 percent of players had facial injuries.[57] Those age 10 to 19 had an incidence of up to 66 percent; 95 percent of college players had sustained these injuries; and 93 percent of nongoalie National Hockey League (NHL) players had sustained facial injuries. Goalies were indexed separately; and although in the youngest groups the incidence was negligible because of the mandatory face mask rule, 76 percent of college goalies had injuries, as did 74 percent of goalies in the NHL. Many of these injuries involved the teeth as well as the facial bone. The loss of teeth was such that one of ten nongoalies lost a tooth at the high school level; and at the college level, six of ten nongoalies lost a tooth. In the professional group, there was an average of two teeth lost per player. The fundamental cause of these injuries was the hockey stick, which fact stimulated the effort to make mouth guards and masks obligatory.

The rule governing the use of mouth guards in hockey is ambiguous and seems to allow versions of the guard that covers only the anterior teeth. The Amateur Hockey Association of the United States has expanded this rule to try to ensure that the guard covers all of the maxillary teeth.

Field Hockey. In field hockey, mouth guards are commonly used, but they are not mandatory. The hazard presented by a fast moving stick suggests that the mouth guard is a sensible addition to the basic equipment.

Lacrosse. Lacrosse is another sport in which a stick is used as a potential weapon. The helmet that is worn protects the face to some extent, but the accessory use of a mouth guard would lower the incidence of injury even more.

Basketball. Although basketball is considered by some as a relatively noncontact sport, there is a large element of aggression with many of the maneuvers; "flying elbows" are the commonest missiles. There is no mandatory rule demanding the use of a mouth guard, but many college athletic associations encourage its use. It is easy to visualize many other situations in noncontact sports in which mouth guards do add protection to dentition and minimize facial trauma. It is also obvious that additional action is required by many sport governing bodies to ensure maximal safety of at least the younger individuals participating in the activities.

Facial Fractures and Jaw Injuries

Minor fractures of the facial bones including the nose are common in contact sports, whereas major facial smashes are relatively rare[58] (Fig. 20-36). The latter are seen only in high velocity sports such as skiing, equestrian events, and sports involving vehicles. Most of these fractures are undisplaced and require a certain index of suspicion for diagnosis (Table 20-16). On the other hand, some constitute major injuries and are associated with cranial nerve problems, cosmetic defects, and malocclusion. Thus it is essential to ensure an accurate diagnosis and, in many circumstances, referral to an experienced practitioner who can carry out the necessary treatment. With severe facial fractures there may be airway compromise, which must be assessed carefully. If the athletes are unconscious, they should not be transported on their backs as it may cause further difficulty with the airway, particularly if there is associated hemorrhage. Nevertheless, because of the potential association with cervical spinal fracture, they should be treated with spinal precautions and where possible transported in the semiprone position.

Practice Point

RECOGNITION OF FACIAL FRACTURES

- Malalignment of teeth (bite)
- Biting down hard on tongue depressor causes pain at fracture site
- Asymmetry of cheek, nose, jaw
- Black eyes
- Eye movements asymmetric, causing diplopia (double vision) or blurred vision
- Loose or missing teeth
- Altered talking or swallowing
- Altered sense of smell

Maxillary Fractures

Fractures of the maxilla are usually diagnosed by attempting to move the upper jaw while stabilizing the head with the other hand. It is usual to classify these maxillary injuries, according to the anatomic location of the fracture lines, as LeFort I, II, or III injury[58] (Fig. 20-37).

The LeFort I injury is separation of the palate from the superior portion of the maxilla. It is usually secondary to a shearing force hitting the maxilla. The fracture lines extend horizontally across the maxilla at about the level of the floor of the nose, thereby shearing off the hard palate and the upper dental alveolus. Essentially, the maxilla is separated from the

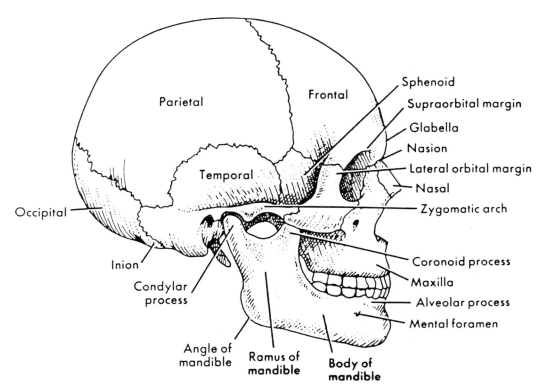

Fig. 20-36. Bony anatomy of the skull, face, and jaw. (After Booker and Thibadeau,[16] with permission.)

rest of the face, and only the tooth-bearing segment moves with pressure.

The LeFort II injury is generally the result of a blow landing on the middle of the face. The nasal bones and middle and lower portions of the maxilla separate from the zygoma and the frontal bone complex. This injury has also been referred to as a pyramidal fracture. The fracture line extends obliquely upward and medially through the body of the maxilla toward the apex of the nose on both sides. The nasal bones and

TABLE 20-16. **Symptoms and Findings of Facial Bone Injuries**

Injury	Symptoms	Examination Findings
Maxillary fracture	Pain with chewing Lip and cheek anesthesia Diplopia (double vision) Flattening face	Palpable fracture fragment Middle one-third mobility Subcutaneous emphysema (air underneath skin) Malocclusion Extraocular muscle dysfunction
Nasal bone fracture	Epistaxis Nasal obstruction Pain and swelling Decreased smell sensation	Deformity of external nose or septum Intranasal bleeding Septal hematoma
Mandibular fracture	Skin damage over fracture site Mandibular deformity Pain with mastication Lower lip anesthesia	Mobile fracture fragments Palpable irregularity at fracture site Intraoral lacerations Malocclusion
Zygoma fracture	Diplopia Cheek anesthesia Cheek flattening Epistaxis	Palpable fracture Cheek anesthesia Extraocular muscle dysfunction

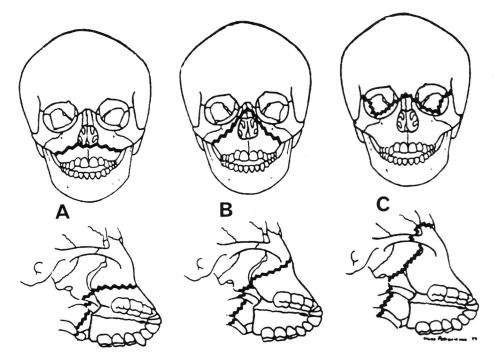

Fig. 20-37. Fractures of the facial bones. **(A)** LeFort I. **(B)** LeFort II. **(C)** LeFort III. (After Sanders,[58] with permission.)

midportion of the face as well as the maxilla are obviously involved. With overpressure there is movement of the entire midface (Fig. 20-38). With displacement there may be a step deformity along the infraorbital area extending down across the zygoma. Because of the frequent involvement of the infraorbital nerve there may be altered sensation along the cheeks. Occasionally there is cerebrospinal fluid (CSF) leak from the nose or the ear with this fracture.

LeFort III fracture involves the zygoma and maxilla, which along with the ethmoid bone are separated from the frontal bone and cranial vault. Essentially the middle third of the face separates from the upper third of the face. It is a craniofacial separation with a fracture line extending from one frontal zygomatic suture line across the cranial facial junction to the other side. When displaced it may dish in the whole front of the face, and is associated with varying degrees of disturbance of the sensory supply to the face. There is frequently CSF leak from the nose or ears.

Although the LeFort injuries have been described as classic symmetric injuries, it is obviously possible to have a combination of one level of injury on one side of the face with a different degree of injury on the

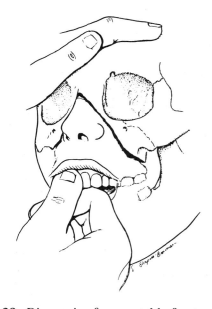

Fig. 20-38. Diagnosis of an unstable fracture by stabilizing the head and mobilizing the fracture by pressure through the tooth and palate. (After Torg,[2] with permission.)

contralateral side. All of these injuries are serious and require the attention of experienced plastic surgeons.

Mandibular Fractures

Fractures of the mandible in sport are most commonly found at the condyle and the body, followed by fractures at the angle[57,59] (Fig. 20-39). Diagnosis is based on clinical signs and symptoms and then confirmed with various roentgenographic views of the mandible including the panoramic view, which helps to eliminate superimposed shadows. Subsequent to a blow on the chin or face, the manifestations of a mandibular fracture range from isolated pain on palpation and pressure to edema, ecchymosis or gross displacement. It must be remembered that all fractures involving the dentulous alveolar bone are classified as compound or open and thus require special attention.

Examination is carried out by careful palpation along the inferior border of the mandible looking for evidence of a step defect. Placing the small finger in the external auditory meatus bilaterally and getting the athlete to open and close the mouth allows palpation of tenderness and the feeling of movement of the condyle as the mouth opens and closes. Mobility between segments is detected by firmly grasping the mandible on either side of the suspected site of fracture and gently manipulating it (Table 20-17). Inspection of dental occlusion also allows judgment of symmetry. Mandibular fractures compounded into the oral cavity are often accompanied by blood-tinged saliva with a distinctive odor as well as bruising on the floor of the mouth. Altered sensation in the distribution in the mandibular division of the trigeminal nerve may be associated with fractures of the angle or body of the mandible. The sensory area extends over the chin and lower lip.[59,60] If a panoramic roentgenogram is not available, open and closed lateral oblique films eliminate some of the superimposition of structures over the condyles, ramus, and posterior body.

The initial treatment of a patient with a mandibular fracture includes maintenance of the airway, stopping hemorrhage, and when necessary some form of immobilization of the fractured segments. With severe jaw fractures, especially in the unconscious patient, the anterior muscular support of the tongue may be lost, which tends to occlude the airway. If a head bandage is applied to temporarily immobilize the jaw, the mandible itself must be pulled upward and not backward, as the latter movement would further occlude the airway (Fig. 20-40).

Definitive therapy aims at reducing any displacement and providing good dental occlusion. Open reduction with wiring of the jaw was the classic method of treatment, but there is now some support for intraoral placement of plates, circumventing the need for jaw fixation.[59] Furthermore, rigid internal fixation of fractures with a variety of appliances, by eliminating the need for prolonged immobilization of the jaw, allows earlier return to function. These treatment options should be dealt with only by properly trained individuals.

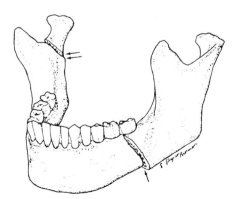

Fig. 20-39. Mandible with associated common fractures through either the condyle (two arrows) or the body (arrow). (After Torg,[2] with permission.)

Practice Point

SIGNS AND SYMPTOMS OF MANDIBULAR FRACTURES

- Deviation of the chin
- Abnormal movement
- Loss of occlusion
- Pain on movement
- Crepitus on movement
- Bleeding around the teeth
- Anesthesia of the chin secondary to mandibular nerve involvment
- Limited opening of the mouth
- Inability to move the jaw from side to side
- Open bite deformity (malocclusion)

Occasionally a blow to the jaw causes dislocation, effectively locking the jaw in one position. It is ex-

TABLE 20-17.   Signs and Symptoms of Facial Fractures

Site	Signs and Symptoms

Unilateral condyle	Affected side
	    Pain in joint, worse on moving
	    Tenderness and swelling
	    Absence (or abnormality) of movements of condyle head
	    Deviation of mandible towards this side
	Opposite side
	    Open bite
	    Limitation of lateral excursion to that side

Bilateral condyle	Pain, tenderness, and swelling over both joints Anterior open bite Restricted lateral movements Absence of movement of condyle heads
Body of the mandible	Pain on moving jaw Trismus Movement and crepitus at site of fracture Step deformity of lower border of mandible Derangement of the occlusion Dental anesthesia Hematoma in the floor of mouth and buccal mucosa
Malar area	Depression of the prominence of the cheek Step deformity in the infraorbital ridge Subconjunctival hemorrhage and diplopia Infraorbital nerve anesthesia Hematoma intraorally over the malar buttress Blood in the antrum Trismus due to the coronoid process impacting against the displaced malar or zygomatic arch Circumorbital ecchymosis
LeFort I	Floating palate Blood in the antrum Bilateral hematoma in buccal sulcus Deranged occlusion with anterior open bite
LeFort II	Gross swelling and, after edema subsides, dish-faced deformity Subconjunctival hemorrhage and diplopia Bilateral infraorbital nerve anesthesia Bilateral hematoma intraorally over malar buttresses Retroposed upper dental arch with anterior open bite
LeFort III	Gross swelling; after edema subsides, dish-faced deformity Subconjunctival hemorrhage and sometimes diplopia Retroposed upper dental arch with anterior open bite Cerebrospinal fluid leak from nose Signs of head injury

tremely painful. Reduction is usually possible with firm downward and backward pressure, without anesthesia (Fig. 20-41).

Injuries to the Zygoma (Cheek)

The zygomatic process of the maxilla is prominent and often receives the impact of punches and blows to the face. When seen immediately after impact, the face may be flattened on the affected side, but this deformity is frequently soon hidden by edema or hemorrhage (Fig. 20-42). Mandibular movement may be painful. There may be double vision (diplopia), anesthesia in the infraorbital nerve distribution over the front of the cheek, and associated epistaxis (nosebleed). Occasionally, there is injury to the eye with these fractures because of the proximity. Periorbital ecchymosis is common. These injuries constitute the third commonest facial fracture and occasionally involve the temporal bone, frontal bone, and maxil-

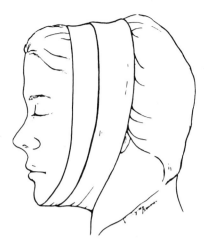

Fig. 20-40. Supporting bandage for fractured jaw (Barton bandage). When applied, it must produce a forward pull so it does not contribute to obstruction of the airway.

lary bone, in which case they are referred to as a triad malar fracture.

Periorbital Fractures

Supraorbital fractures are uncommon, as the orbital ridges are thick and strong. However, blows to this area may result in contusion to the supraorbital nerve, producing anesthesia in a region around the forehead. With significant injuries to the superorbital ridge, there may be some flattening of the contour of the eyebrow, occasionally with downward displacement of the eye and double vision.

Fractures into the frontal or maxillary sinus may result in persistent bleeding or clear discharge from the nose (rhinorrhea). Occasionally, there is some subcutaneous emphysema, which automatically makes one suspicious of communication of the sinuses. It is important to prevent the athlete from blowing the nose to clear the fluid, as it may drive air and mucous from the sinus into the subcutaneous tissues.

A special type of fracture is the blow-out fracture of the orbital floor. This fracture was alluded to earlier in the chapter (Fig. 20-20). The usual cause is a large object striking the front of the eye, normally a ball, which increases intraorbital pressure and deforms the shape of the eyeball. The distorted contour of the eye pushes down into the soft, thin, orbital floor, fracturing the wafer-like bone and frequently communicating with the maxillary sinus. The signs of this fracture include periorbital ecchymosis, often producing a significant black eye, and may be some associated subcutaneous emphysema.

With severe cases it is possible in entrap the inferior rectus muscle in the fracture, which distorts eye movement. Attempted vertical gaze produces diplopia and frequently associated hyperesthesia of the infraorbital nerve as discussed in the section dealing with eye injuries (Fig. 20-19). Occasionally, there is abnormal positioning of the eyeball within the orbit: either excessive protrusion (exophthalmos) or abnormal retraction (enophthalmos). It can also be asso-

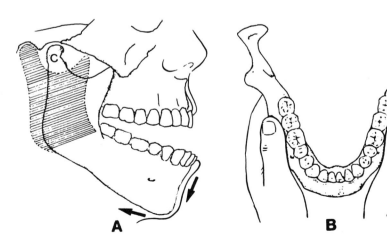

Fig. 20-41. Dislocation of the mandible. **(A)** Condyles are displaced anteriorly from the normal position. **(B)** Reduction is carried out by placing the hands as shown and exerting a downward and backward force to allow the condyles to slip back into their normal relations at the joint.

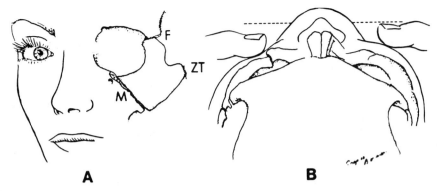

Fig. 20-42. Zygoma trimalleolar fracture. **(A)** Zygoma usually fractures at its attachment to the maxilla (M), frontal bone (F), and zygomatic process of the temporal bone (ZT). **(B)** Evaluation of this fracture is often best done by viewing both cheeks from the top of the patient and palpating to determine and enhance any obvious depression.

ciated with conjunctival hemorrhage. Particularly if the fracture involves the medial wall of the orbit, acute proptosis (fluid bulging of the eye) occurs when the nose is blown. The complications of this type of injury include fever (related to blood in the anterior chamber), inflammation of the iris, damage and subluxation to the lens, and possibly initiation of cataracts secondary to the trauma. Occasionally, glaucoma, intraocular hemorrhage, and retinal detachment occur. These injuries require the prompt attention of an opthalmologist. The first aid measures were outlined earlier in the chapter.

SUMMARY

This chapter has focused on the recognition and treatment of injuries to the head and face. The most common of these injuries is concussion. Because of its frequent occurrence, there has been a tendency to consider it a minor injury. It is now firmly established that concussion must not be taken likely. To do so is to place the athlete at risk. Head injury, along with injuries to the eyes, can be catastrophic. For many the solution is simple, i.e., wearing protective helmets and glasses. All too slowly these guards are being adopted by many of the players. In a similar vein, many injuries to the teeth can be avoided by an adequate mouth guard. At this point in time one of the great mandates of those involved in sports medicine must be an emphasis on prophylaxis. Thus the statistics in favor of wearing the existing protective equipment must be voiced in a convincing fashion at every opportunity.

Because of the delicate nature of many facial struc-

tures specialized knowledge is required to treat many of the injuries. This chapter emphasized recognition and pointed out the need for specialist intervention at an early time. In many instances, treatment outcomes depend on prompt administration of first aid, and rapid transit to a hospital. The more complex principles outlined in each of the sections must be simplified and passed on to the coach and the athlete, as many of these injuries occur in situations that do not have the benefit of a therapist or physician in attendance.

There are no hard and fast rules for the evaluation of head injuries, and a cautious approach is outlined here. Those who wish to gamble gain a certain amount of popularity with players and coaches, but at the same time there is the risk of overlooking significant intracranial injury. The correct judgment can be life-saving in some situations, and decisions must always be based on strict medical and ethical grounds, even in the face of pressure from the players, coach, and crowd. Each sport has its own peculiarities and home remedies. The best advice is to learn the chosen sports well, evaluate the folklore, retain what is good, and discard what is morally and scientifically unsound.

REFERENCES

1. Reif AE: Risk and pain. In Vinger PF, Hoerner EF (eds): Sports Injuries: The Unthwarted Epidemic. 2nd Ed. PSG Publishing, Littleton, Massachusetts, 1986
2. Torg JS: Athletic Injuries to the Head, Face and Neck. 2nd Ed. Lea & Febiger, Philadelphia, 1991

3. Pashby TJ, Bishop PJ, Easterbrook WM: Eye injuries in Canadian racket sports. Can Fam Physician 28:18, 1982

4. Casson I, Siegal O, Sham R et al: Brain damage in modern boxers. JAMA 251:2663, 1984

5. Reid DC, Cuthbertson A, Kelly R: The 1970 World Amateur Wrestling Championships—an injury report. Can Athlet Train Assoc 5:8, 1970

6. Reid DC, Saboe L, Allan G: Off-road vehicle accidents: a survey of cases requiring hospitalization and review of off road recreational deaths. Can J Surg 31:233, 1988

7. Reid DC, Saboe L, Allan G: Spine trauma associated with off-road vehicles. Physician Sports Med 16:143, 1988

8. Reid DC, Saboe LA: Spine fractures in sports and recreation. Clin Sport Med 1:75, 1991

9. Storey MD, Griffi R: Subdural hematoma in a high school football player. Physician Sports Med 11:61, 1983

10. Reid DC: Catastrophic injuries in winter sports. In Torq JS (ed): Athletic Injuries to the Head, Neck and Face. Lea & Febiger, Philadelphia, 1989

11. Lehman LB: Nervous system sports related injuries. Am J Sports Med 15:494, 1987

12. Tator CH, Edmonds VE: National survey of spinal injuries in hockey players. Can Med Assoc J 130:875, 1984

13. Mueller FO, Cantu RC: Catastrophic injuries and fatalities in high school and college sports, fall 1982–spring 1988. Med Sci Sports Exerc 22:737, 1990

14. Fields KB: Head injuries in soccer. Physician Sports Med 17:69, 1989

15. Cantu RC: Guidelines for return to contact sports after a cerebral concussion. Physician Sports Med 14:75, 1986

16. Booker JM, Thibadeau GA: Athletic Injury Assessment. CV Mosby, St. Louis, 1985

17. Hugenholz H, Richard MT: The on-site management of athletes with head injuries. Physician Sports Med 11:71, 1983

18. Gronwall D, Wrightson P: Duration of post-traumatic amnesia after mild head injury. J Clin Neuropsychol 2:51, 1985

19. Symonds C: Concussion and its sequelae. Lancet 1:1, 1962

20. Saunders RL, Harbough RE: The second impact in catastrophic contact-sports head trauma. JAMA 252:583, 1984

21. Hayes RG, Nagle CE: Diagnositc imagings of intercranial trauma. Physician Sports Med 18:69, 1990

22. Schneider RC: Head and Neck Injuries in Football: Mechanisms, Treatment and Prevention. p 77. Williams & Wilkins, Baltimore, 1973

23. Hugenholtz H, Richard MT: Evaluation and resuscitation of head injuries. Mod Med Can 38:843, 1983

24. Miller JD, Becker DP: Secondary insults to the injured brain. J R Coll Surg Edinb 27:292, 1982

25. Rimel RW, Jane JA, Tyson GW: Emergency management of head injuries. Resuscitation 9:75, 1981

26. Roy S, Irvin R: Sports Medicine: Prevention, Evaluation, Management, and Rehabilitation. p 141. Prentice-Hall, Englewood, NJ, 1983

27. Jordan BD, Zimmerman RD, Devinsky O et al: Brain contusion and cervical fracture in a professional boxer. Physician Sports Med 16:85, 1988

28. Jordon BD, Voy RO, Stone J: Amateur boxing injuries at the U.S. Olympic Training Center. Physician Sports Med 18:81, 1990

29. Welch MJ, Sitler M, Kroeten H: Boxing injuries from an instructional program. Physician Sports Med 14:81, 1990

30. Jordon BD, Campbell EA: Acute injuries among professional boxers in New York State: a two-year survey. Physician Sports Med 16:87, 1988

31. Kaste M, Vikki J, Saino K et al: Is chronic brain damage in boxing a hazard of the past? Lancet 2:1168, 1982

32. Lundberg G: Boxing should be banned in civilized countries. JAMA 249:250, 1983

33. Robey JM: Contribution of design and construction of football helmets to the occurrence of injuries. Med Sci Sports 4:170, 1972

34. Garfinkel D: Headache in athletes. Physician Sports Med 11:67, 1983

35. Braker MD, Rothrock JF: Cluster headaches among athletes. Physician Sports Med 17:147, 1989

36. Perry WJ: Exertional headaches. Physician Sports Med 13:95, 1985

37. Martin GJ, Adams SC, Martin MG et al: Prospective evaluation of syncope. Ann Emerg Med 13:449, 1984

38. Rund DA: Syncope. Physician Sports Med 18:141, 1990

39. Vazuka FA: Essentials of the Neurologic Examination. Smith, Kline and French, Montreal, 1970

40. Committee on Trauma: A Guide to Prophylaxis Against Tetanus in Wound Management. Bulletin ACS, 1979

41. Pashby RC: Sports injuries to the eye. Med Clin North Am 33:4672, 1986

42. Vinger PF: How I manage corneal abrasions and lacerations. Physician Sports Med 14:120, 1986

43. Easterbrook M: Eye protection in racket sports: an update. Physician Sports Med 15:180, 1987

44. Briscoe JAD: Sports injuries in adolescent boarding school boys. Br J Sports Med 19:67, 1985

45. Schendel SA: Sports related nasal injuries. Physician Sports Med 18:59, 1990

46. Illum P: Long-term results after treatment of nasal fractures. J Laryngol Otol 100:273, 1986

47. Kelleher JC, Sullivan JG, Gaibak GJ et al: The wrestler's ear. Plast Reconstr Surg 40:541, 1967

48. Reid DC: Assessment and Treatment of the Injured Athlete. Course Manual. University of Alberta Press, Edmonton, 1985

49. Dimeff RJ, Hough DO: Preventing cauliflower ear with a modified tie-through technique. Physician Sports Med 17:169, 1989

50. Kulund DN: The Injured Athlete. 2nd ed. JB Lippincott, London, 1988

51. Eichel BS: How I manage external otitis in competitive swimmers. Physician Sports Med 14:108, 1986

52. Walsh-Healy Act 50-204.10. Occupational noise exposure. Fed Reg 34:790, 1969

53. Bunch CC: Nerve deafness of known pathology or etiology. Laryngoscope 47:615, 1937

54. Castaldi CR: First aid for sports related dental injuries. Physician Sports Med 15:81, 1987

55. Kerr IL: Mouth guards for the prevention of injuries in contact sports. Sports Med 3:415, 1986

56. Keuber WA, Morrow RM, Cohen PA: Do mouth-formed guards meet the NCAA rules? Physician Sports Med 14:69, 1986

57. Rontal E, Rontal M, Wilson K et al: Facial injuries on hockey players. Laryngoscope 87:884, 1977

58. Sanders B: Pediatric Oral and Maxillofacial Surgery. CV Mosby, St. Louis, 1979

59. Van Sickels JE, Timmis DP: How we manage mandibular fractures. Physician Sports Med 14:119, 1986

60. Ellis F, Moos KF, El-Attar A: Ten years of mandibular fractures: an analysis of 2,137 cases. Oral Surg 59:120, 1985

Shoulder Region

21

It is the customary fate of new truths to begin as heresies and to end as superstitions.
— T.H. Huxley

Shoulder girdle pathology is a major concern with swimming, baseball, weightlifting, tennis, and volleyball. Shoulder problems in these sports are common, frequently difficult to manage, and often characterized by chronicity. For the most part they are overuse, inflammatory type lesions, e.g., supraspinatus and bicipital tendinitis or bursitis. Occasionally, capsular and muscular tears are the major presenting complaint with these activities. By contrast, skiing, hockey, and football have a high incidence of fractures and dislocations of the acromioclavicular and glenohumeral joints. For example, major joint and bone trauma constitutes about 5 percent of the total injuries with skiing, 7 percent in football, and 15 percent in hockey. Medical doctors are frequently not present when these injuries occur thus emphasizing the need for therapists and, to some extent coaching staff, to be able to recognize these serious problems so adequate immobilization, transport, and treatment may be arranged.[1]

In the past, inflammatory problems and instability were dealt with as discrete entities. It is now apparent that there is a significant overlap in underlying etiologies, producing a spectrum of clinical conditions that may involve elements of both basic causes. Furthermore, there is increasing emphasis on retraining control of the rotator cuff musculature instead of just strengthening.[2,3]

ANATOMY

Traditionally, the anatomic unit referred to as the shoulder girdle comprises the (1) sternoclavicular joint, (2) acromioclavicular joint, (3) glenohumeral joint, and (4) scapulothoracic articulation (Fig. 21-1). This anatomic unit allows the large functional range of motion that is so critical in activities of daily living as well as sport.

If one considers the pathologic unit instead of just the moving bones, it is necessary to include a new series of structures: (5) biceps tendon, (6) coracoacromial arch, and (7) thoracic outlet and the first costosternal and costovertebral joints.[4] These complex series of soft tissue and bony articulations bear the brunt of direct contact in many of the collision sports, e.g., hockey, rugby, and football, and indirectly during falls on the outstretched hand in most recreational and running activities. Even in the very young, shoulder girdle trauma, frequently in the form of a fractured clavicle, is common. In these instances, the multitude of ossification centers, constantly changing with age, makes radiologic diagnosis challenging and comparison with the sound contralateral limb mandatory (Fig. 21-2).

Most examinations of the shoulder girdle are directed at measuring motion in the plane of the body (Fig. 21-3). However, the scapula rests and moves around the chest wall tangential to these planes, and so some clinical tests and functional measurements may be recorded in the "plane of the scapula."[5]

Sternoclavicular Joint

The sternoclavicular articulation, a variety of saddle joint, represents the only bone-to-bone connection of the upper limb to the trunk. Thus it is surprising that this joint is not more structurally robust and stable. However, as with all of the shoulder girdle units, structural stability has been compromised to allow significant motion, which in turn enables placement of the hand in a wide range of positions, adding to the functional potential of this uniquely versatile anatomic unit.

There is a fibrocartilaginous disc attached superiorly to the clavicle and inferiorly to the manubrium sterni.[6-10] This disc seems to assist absorption of shock transmitted from the arm and shoulder, as well

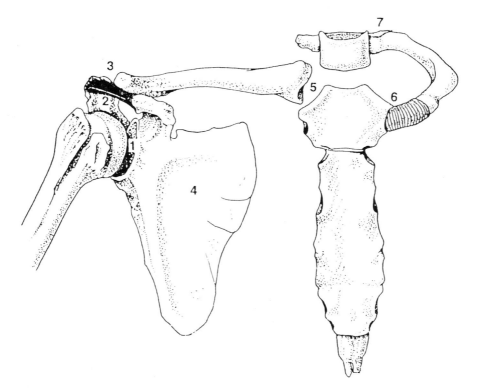

Fig. 21-1. Components of the shoulder girdle and shoulder joint complex: (1) glenohumeral joint; (2) coracoacromial arch; (3) acromioclavicular joint; (4) scapulothoracic articulation; (5) sternoclavicular joint; (6) first costosternal joint; (7) first costovertebral articulation with the body in transverse process. (Adapted from Kaput,[3] with permission.)

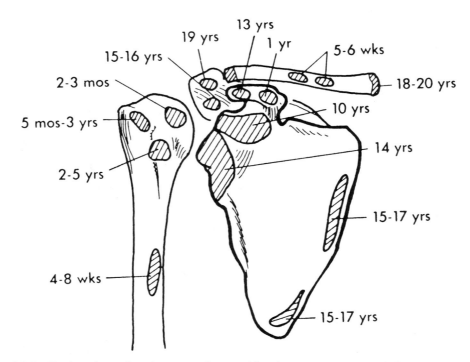

Fig. 21-2. Fusion times for the secondary ossification centers around the shoulder.

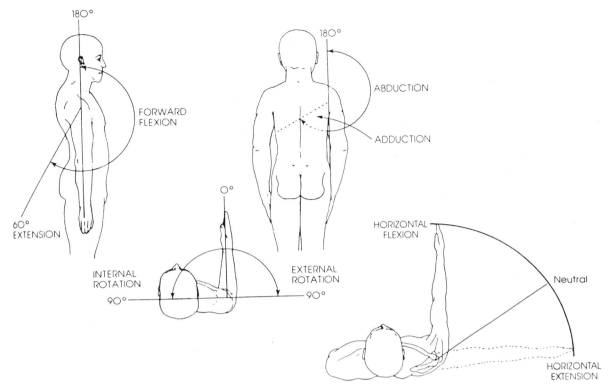

Fig. 21-3. Ranges in motion of the shoulder complex, including forward flexion, internal-external rotation, abduction, adduction, and horizontal or cross flexion. These motions are all shown in the plane of the body. (After Perry,[6] with permission.)

as adding stability to the joint. Further structural strength is provided mainly by the interclavicular and costoclavicular ligaments, as well as the anterior and posterior sternoclavicular ligaments, which primarily serve to reinforce the capsule.

Acromioclavicular Joint

The acromioclavicular joint is essentially a plane joint allowing a limited amount of gliding and rotation between the clavicle and the scapula. The structural integrity of the joint depends on the intrinsic capsular elements, particularly the superior acromioclavicular ligament and, more importantly, the extrinsic conoid and trapezoid bands of the coracoclavicular ligament (Fig. 21-4). The varying shape of the articular surfaces may influence the stability. A rudimentary disk is usually situated in the joint and may cause mechanical symptoms with acromioclavicular joint pathology.[5]

The coracoacromial ligament forms a hood over the interval between the coracoid process and the acromion. Phylogenetically, it is probably the divorced tendon of the pectoralis minor. It is a substantial structure, being 3 to 5 cm in width and up to 2.8 cm in thickness. It is directly confluent with the inferior capsule of the acromioclavicular joint in most cases, although its contribution to this joint is variable, being significant in approximately 60 percent of specimens[8] (Fig. 21-4). Instead of inserting exclusively on the anterolateral edge of the acromion process, as depicted in most anatomy texts, the coracoacromial ligament spreads out to insert on a large area on the inferior acromial surface. These inferior fibers may act as a soft tissue buffer between the rotator cuff and the bony surface of the acromion process.[9] Degenerative changes in the area include attrition and wear of the coracoacromial ligament, osteophyte formation on the inferior edge of the acromion and clavicle, and subsequent rotator cuff thinning or tears.

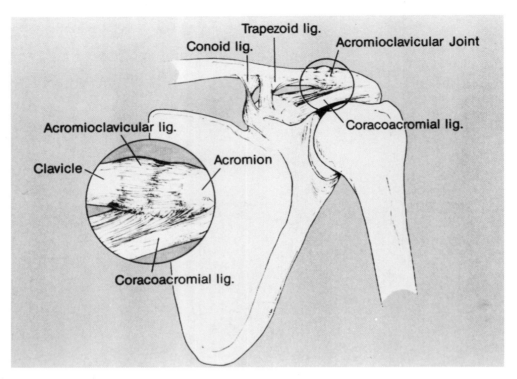

Fig. 21-4. Anteroposterior view of the acromioclavicular joint, showing the contribution of the coracoacromial ligaments to the inferior acromioclavicular joint capsule. (After Salter et al.,[9] with permission.)

Glenohumeral Joint

Bony Structure

The glenohumeral joint is a multiaxial ball and socket joint and the most freely mobile joint in the body. The amount of shoulder abduction varies among individuals, usually 160 to 180 degrees, with 120 to 135 degrees occurring at the glenohumeral joint.[11] Rolling, gliding, and rotation occur at the glenohumeral articulation. *Rolling* occurs when various points on the moving surface contact various points on the stationary one, and *gliding* occurs when one point contacts multiple points on the stationary one. Both of these motions require a significant change in contact area (Fig. 21-5). *Rotation* occurs when there is contact between various points on the moving surface on a single contact area on the stationary surface. There is usually relatively little displacement between the two joint surfaces in rotation; and if it is reduced to its purest form, single points

articulate and the movement is then a *spin.* For the glenohumeral motion rolling or gliding occurs for the first 30 to 60 degrees; above this range the motion is reduced to almost pure rotation.[12] These subtleties of joint play and motion must be restored after an injury.

The humeral head is approximately one-third of a sphere, oriented at 45 degrees from the long axis of the shaft and retroverted 30 degrees.[5] The indistinct anatomic neck contains two important landmarks, the lesser tuberosity anteromedially and the greater tuberosity superolaterally, separated by the bicipital groove. The shallow pear-shaped glenoid cavity is retroverted approximately 7 degrees and inferiorly angulated 5 degrees from the long axis of the scapula.

Labrum

The glenoid labrum, the fibrocartilaginous rim, triangular in cross section and attached along its outer perimeter to the glenoid, increases the available con-

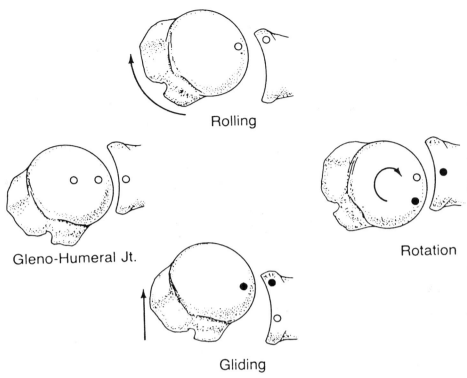

Fig. 21-5. Arthrokinematic motion at the glenohumeral joint includes primarily rolling, rotation, and gliding. (After Kaput,[3] with permission.)

tact area by approximately 70 percent. The importance of this structure to the stability of the joint cannot be overemphasized.[5]

Ligament

The fibrous capsule attaches peripherally to the margins of the glenoid cavity and the anatomic neck of the humerus, close to the articular margins. Superiorly, it extends toward the root of the coracoid process, so it includes the long head of the biceps tendon. The relative laxity of the capsule allows the humeral head to be manually distracted 2 to 3 cm from the glenoid in the relaxed shoulder, an important maneuver for restoring joint range after injury. Three intrinsic capsular ligaments—the glenohumeral ligaments—provide reinforcement to the joint. Anteriorly these ligaments are disposed in a distinct **Z** pattern, with a prominent middle glenohumeral band in nearly 90 percent of shoulders[5,7] (Fig. 21-6). The **Z** pattern includes the coracohumeral ligament, which has an intimate attachment to the superior glenohumeral ligament. The middle glenohumeral ligament,

usually thick and strong in the young, becomes thinner in appearance with age. This finding seems to conflict with the reports of De Palma et al., who thought that the capsule hypertrophied with age.[7] In reality the difference is probably due to viewing the

---

Quick Facts

- Humeral head
  - Approximately one-third sphere
  - Diameter 45 mm $\pm$ 10
  - Head at 45 degrees from long axis of shaft
  - Retroverted 30 degrees
- Glenoid fossa
  - Ovoid shape
  - Average 41 $\times$ 25 mm
  - Tilted inferiorly 5 degrees to long axis of scapula
  - Retroverted 7 degrees

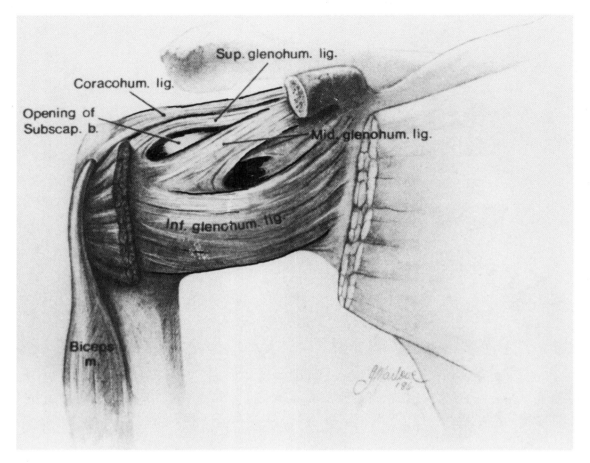

Fig. 21-6. Anterosuperior capsule depicting the distinct **Z** pattern formed by the superior glenohumeral, coracohumeral, middle glenohumeral, and the important inferior glenohumeral ligaments. This pattern is the one seen most frequently. There is a variable opening for the subscapular bursa, which is large in some individuals. (From Ferrari,[14] with permission.)

capsule from its deep surface, where the subscapularis tendon appears to thicken the anterior capsule and masks the defect. A small percentage of individuals are born with a weak or absent glenohumeral ligament, and in others the large capsular defect is developmental.[13]

The coracohumeral ligament appears to assist the capsule in supporting the dependent arm, particularly when pulled in an inferior direction, suggesting that some degree of incompetence must be present before inferior laxity can be demonstrated. It also restrains the amount of external rotation present below 60 degrees of abduction.[14] The coracohumeral

---

Quick Facts

FUNCTIONS OF MIDDLE GLENOHUMERAL LIGAMENT

- Support dependent arm
- Restrain external rotation up to 90 degrees abduction
- Strongest at 45 degrees
- Provide anterosuperior buttress for humeral head

and middle glenohumeral ligaments appear to function together, particularly after 45 degrees of abduction, and they become progressively more important in limiting extensional rotation as the arm is further abducted.

The combination of the shallow ovoid glenoid surface, large convex humeral head, and lax capsule and capsular ligaments allows the joint to assume a relatively noncongruent, loosely packed position for most of its movements. Thus the humeral head is able to spin, roll, and slide over the relatively small glenoid surface, increasing the available range. In external rotation and abduction the joint surfaces obtain greater congruency, the ligaments spiral taut, and the joint is closely packed. Any additional motion beyond this point is compensated for by thoracic spine and trunk motion or, in pathologic situations, by subluxation, dislocation, or fracture.

Rotator Cuff

Four interrelated muscles originating from the scapula provide the much needed dynamic stability of the glenohumeral joint. Their tendons are intimately associated with the joint capsule and are in sufficient proximity to form a tendinous cuff around the head and upper half of the anatomic neck of the humerus. The term "rotator cuff", although describing the structure and gross function, does not do justice to the more subtle role of controlling and adjusting the position of the head within the glenoid during movements of the upper limb. Fine adjustments of the head during both powerful and rapid motion required in the overhead throwing motions of many sports or the repetitive pulling action of activities of swimming, demand intricate control of the small swings and glides on a moving scapular surface (Fig. 21-7). *Thus the emphasis of many rehabilitation programs is leaning toward the development of control and balance of strength between elements of the cuff and away from pure strengthening activities.*[3,6]

Hilton's law indicates that a joint is innervated by the same nerves that supply the muscles crossing it; hence controlling the joint is an efficient neuromotor arrangement for fine control and protection of the joint. Three nerves in particular affect the glenohumeral joint, rotator cuff, and deltoid muscle: the suprascapular nerve (supraspinatus and infraspinatus), the subscapular nerve (subscapularis and teres major), and the axillary nerve (deltoid and teres

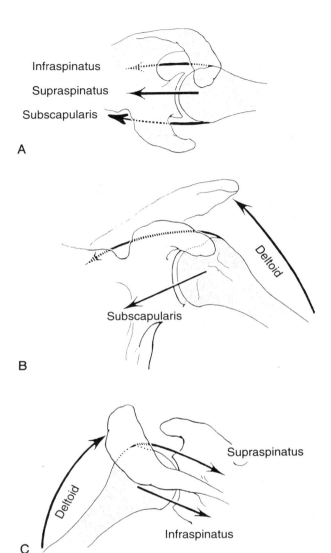

Fig. 21-7. Fine adjustments of the humeral head within the glenoid is achieved by the coordinated action of the rotator cuff muscles. In the movement of abduction: Supraspinatus steadies the head from above. Infraspinatus depresses the head. Subscapularis steadies the head in front, paralleling the action of the infraspinatus. This combined action allows the deltoid muscle to swing up the arm from a steady fulcrum irrespective of the position of the scapula. (**A**) Superior view; (**B**) anterior; (**C**) posterior.

TABLE 21-1. Muscles Controlling Scapular Motion, Nerve Supply, and Innervation

Scapular Motion	Muscle	Nerve Supply	Segment Level
Lateral rotation of inferior angle	Trapezius (upper and lower fibers)[a]	Accessory	Cranial XI; C3,4
	Serratus anterior[b]	Long thoracic	C5,6 (7)
	Levator scapulae[a]	Dorsal scapula	C3,4 (5) (roots)
Elevation	Trapezius (upper fibers)	Accessory	Cranial XI; C3,4
	Levator scapulae	Dorsal scapula	C3,4 (5) (roots)
	Rhomboid major	Dorsal scapula	(C4) C5 (roots)
	Rhomboid minor	Dorsal scapula	(C4) C5 (roots)
Depression	Serratus anterior	Long thoracic	C5,6 (7)
	Pectoralis major[c]	Lateral pectoral	C5,6 (lateral cord)
	Pectoralis minor	Medial pectoral	C8, T1 (medial cord)
	Latissimus dorsi	Thoracodorsal	C6,7,8 (posterior cord)
	Trapezius lower fibers	Accessory	Cranial XI; C3,4
Protraction	Serratus anterior	Long thoracic	C5,6 (7)
	Pectoralis minor	Medial pectoral	C8,T1
	Latissimus dorsi	Thoracodorsal	C6,7,8
Retraction	Trapezius	Accessory	Cranial XI; (C3,4)
	Rhomboid major	Dorsal scapula	(C4) C5
	Rhomboid minor	Dorsal scapula	(C4) C5
Medial (downward) rotation	Rhomboid major	Dorsal scapula	(C4) C5
	Rhomboid minor	Dorsal scapula	(C4) C5
	Levator scapulae	Dorsal scapula	C3,4 (C5)

[a] Acting as force couples.
[b] Mainly lower four digitations.
[c] Acting through the clavicle.
( ) = Subsidiary segments.

minor). All of these nerves arise from the brachial plexus at the anterior primary rami of cervical segments 5 and 6 (Tables 21-1 and 21-2).

The tendon of the long head of the biceps may assist in strengthening the upper capsule as well as contracting synergically with the deltoid, latissimus dorsi, and pectoralis major to stabilize the humeral head. This action is particularly obvious with climbing, pulling, and throwing activities.

Bursae

There are numerous bursal structures around the shoulder, but it is the large subdeltoid bursa, with its subacromial component, that is mostly involved with clinical symptoms. It functions in allowing the smooth gliding of the deltoid over the rotator cuff tendons and the cuff and capsular structures under the acromion and coracoacromial arch. With contusion or overuse it may become inflamed and symptomatic. With the vascular, metabolic, and structural changes, the bursal walls thicken and with aging calcific deposits, inflammation, or adhesions may develop. There

may even exist communications between the joint and the bursa if sufficient degenerative attrition has taken place.

Scapulothoracic Articulation

Except for its attachment to the axial skeleton at the acromioclavicular joint, the scapula could be almost thought of as a sesamoid bone developed in the rhomboids, levator scapulae, trapezius, serratus anterior, and the teres major and minor muscles.[3,6] Underneath these muscles and the scapula is a shearing plane of loose areolar tissue that facilitates the gliding of this whole unit around the chest wall.

Although not a true anatomic joint, the importance of scapulothoracic motion cannot be overlooked. *The scapula serves as a mobile platform from which the upper limb operates.* In the resting position, the scapula lies between the second and seventh ribs, and for any given arm position the scapula aligns itself to allow the glenoid cavity to be in the best position to receive the head of the humerus.[15] The apparently simple motion of the scapula is neurologically complex be-

TABLE 21-2. Glenohumeral Muscle Action and Innervation

Motion	Muscle	Nerve Supply	Segmental Innervation
Abduction	Deltoid[a]	Axillary	C5,6 (posterior cord)
	Supraspinatus[a]	Suprascapular	C5,6 (trunk)
	Infraspinatus[b]	Suprascapular	C5,6 (trunk)
	Subscapularis[b]	Subscapular	C5,6 (posterior cord)
	Teres minor[b]	Axillary	C5,6 (posterior cord)
	Biceps (long head)	Musculocutaneous	C5,6 (7) (lateral cord
Adduction	Pectoralis major[a]	Lateral pectoral	C5,6 (lateral)
	Latissimus dorsi[a]	Thoracodorsal	C6,7,8 (posterior cord)
	Teres major	Subscapular	C5,6 (posterior cord)
	Subscapularis	Subscapular	C5,6 (posterior cord)
Flexion	Deltoid (anterior fibers)[a]	Axillary	C5,6
	Pectoralis major (clavicular lateral pectoral fibers)	Lateral pectoral	C5,6
	Coracorbrachialis	Musculocutaneous	C5,6 (7)
	Biceps (against significant resistance)	Musculocutaneous	C5,6 (7)
Extension	Deltoid (posterior fibers)[a]	Axillary	C5,6
	Latissimus dorsi[a]	Thoracodorsal	C6,7,8
	Teres major	Subscapular	C5,6
	Teres minor	Axillary	C5,6
	Triceps (long head)	Radial	(C5) C6,7,8 (T1) posterior cord
Horizontal adduction	Pectoralis major[a]	Lateral pectoral	C5,6
	Deltoid (ant. fibers)[a]	Axillary	C5,6
Horizontal abduction	Deltoid (post. fibers)[a]	Axillary	C5,6
	Teres major[b]	Subscapular	C5,6
	Teres minor[b]	Axillary	C5,6
	Infraspinatus[b]	Suprascapular	C5,6
Medial (internal) rotation	Pectoralis major[a]	Lateral pectoral	C5,6
	Latissimus dorsi	Thoracodorsal	C6,7,8
	Deltoid (anerior fibers)	Axillary	C5,6
	Teres major	Subscapular	C5,6
	Subscapularis (when arm is adducted)	Subscapular	C5,6
Lateral (external) rotation	Infraspinatus[a]	Suprascapular	C5,6
	Teres minor	Axillary	C5,6
	Deltoid (posterior fibers)	Axillary	C5,6

Actions are described in the plane of the body.
[a] Prime movers.
[b] Control and centralize position of the head of the humerus in the glenoid.

cause there is relatively little direct muscle action. Many of the motions are controlled by prime movers with antagonistic actions that work around an extrinsic fulcrum to produce movements via "force couples." Thus it is not surprising that pain, weakness, or atrophy from immobilization may affect these complicated motions, and they require specific attention during rehabilitation of most proximal upper limb problems.

Motion of Abduction

Abduction in varying degrees of flexion is the key to all overhead motion. For it to take place, a complicated series of events must unfold involving all of the elements of the shoulder girdle.

The initial phase of shoulder abduction requires scapular stabilization. During this phase the scapula may move slightly toward the vertebral column as it is

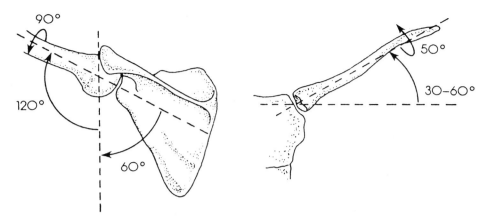

Fig. 21-8. Movement of the scapula, humerus, and clavicle are necessary for normal scapulohumeral abduction. During the movement of abduction, the glenohumeral joint moves 120 degrees as the scapula swings about 60 degrees around the chest wall in a smooth 2:1 ratio.

stabilized by the rhomboids against the action of the rotator cuff, which centralizes the humeral head in preparation for motion[5,6] (Fig. 21-8).

The second phase is the initiation of glenohumeral abduction with the combined action of the supraspinatus and the deltoid. The vertically oriented deltoid becomes increasingly efficient as abduction proceeds past 15 to 20 degrees. Further abduction involves lateral rotation of the humerus, which avoids the impact of the greater tuberosity under the coracoacromial arch that would occur at 60 degrees in the neutral position. It requires fine control and adjustment by the rotator cuff muscles.

As abduction progresses, the 2:1 ratio of motion between glenohumeral and scapulothoracic motion is established. This normal synchrony is referred to as glenohumeral rhythm and is disturbed in pain syndromes. Full abduction requires 60 degrees of scapular motion and 120 degrees of glenohumeral movement; above 90 degrees, the conjoint motion of medial rotation of the humerus, the so-called Codman's paradox, brings the hand into the most useful functional position.

In order for scapular rotation to occur in the smooth manner that is seen during functional abduction motions, approximately 50 degrees of clavicular elevation and 30 degrees of rotation are necessary, which obviously require movement at both the sternoclavicular and acromioclavicular joints (Fig. 21-8). Most of this motion occurs with more than 90 degrees of elevation. Extension and rotation of the thoracic spine increase the range and versatility of overhead motion. This fact, along with the knowledge that the huge prime movers, the trapezius and latissimus dorsi, link the motion through the spine to the pelvis, means that attention must be paid to movement patterns and posture throughout the trunk in recalcitrant cases of upper quadrant dysfunction.

Practice Point

Attention must be paid to thoracic spine motion in cases of recalcitrant upper quadrant dysfunction.

Clinical Point

REVERSED GLENOHUMERAL RHYTHM

Pain or stiffness disturbs the normal synergy of motion between the scapula and the glenohumeral joint, causing abnormal elevation of the shoulder on attempted abduction.

Strength Parameters

In fit athletic individuals, there is usually little difference in power between the dominant and nondominant limbs. The exceptions are obviously those individuals engaging in occupations or sports that require predominantly one-arm skills, e.g., tennis players, pitchers, bowlers, and quarterbacks. Males usually test about twice as strong as females unless the latter have engaged in prolonged intensive strengthening programs (Fig. 21-9). The strongest muscle group is the adductors, having approximately twice the power of the abductors. If the strength of the adductors is designated 100 percent, the normal strengths for the other muscle groups are approximately as follows: abductors 50 percent; internal rotators 45 percent; external rotators 30 percent when the arm is elevated to 90 degrees and 45 percent when the arm is by the side in the neutral position. The external/internal rotation ratio is approximately 80 percent.[2,16] A similar ratio for the abducted arm was reported by Fowler, but he suggested an external/internal rotator ratio of 65 percent with the arm in neutral.[17] Because of the important role of the infraspinatus in preventing excessive forward glide of the humeral head during overhead actions, the higher ratio is probably more desirable. These ratios are im-

portant rehabilitation goals for the upper limb in much the same way as the quadriceps/hamstring ratios are used at the knee.

PRINCIPLES OF EXAMINATION

Shoulder pathology is characterized by a feeling of instability, stiffness, or pain on use. These characteristics help distinguish it from cervical pain, which is often present even at rest and is generally aggravated by chronic postural positions, e.g., sitting, reading, or studying at a desk. However, the two areas are not always easily distinguished, as occasionally neck pathology causes shoulder problems, e.g., C5 root impingement generating an associated frozen shoulder. Furthermore, in the older age groups (55 years plus), about 20 percent of individuals have coexisting shoulder and cervical spinal pathololgy.

Thus the key to diagnosing shoulder pain is to appreciate the common patterns of cervical disease referring to the C5–C6 area, as well as the sites of

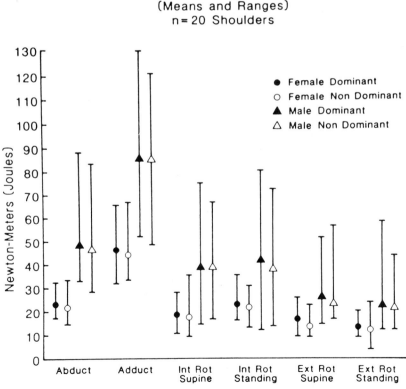

Fig. 21-9. Peak torques (newton-meters) of shoulder girdle motion (*n* = 20 shoulders). Ranges on either side of the mean are shown.

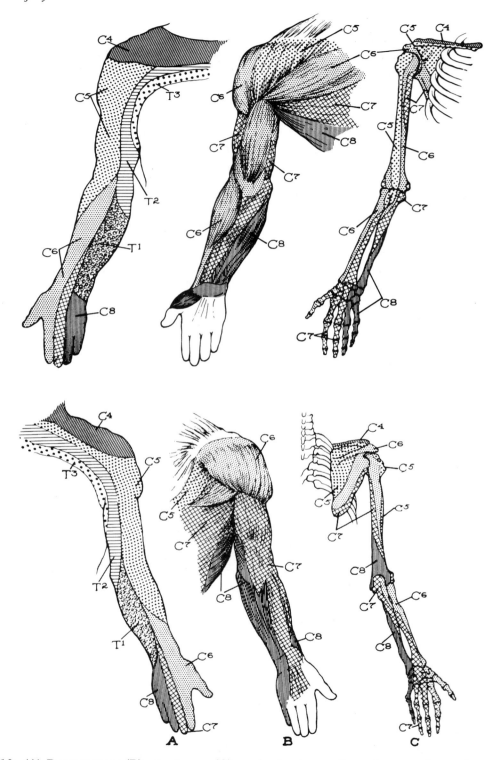

Fig. 21-10. **(A)** Dermatomes **(B)**, myotomes **(C)**, and scleratomes from the anterior and posterior views. These areas show the segmental links between the various layers of tissue and the possible mechanisms for referred pain. (After Inman VT and Saunders JB. Referred pain from skeletal structures. J Nerv Mental Dis 99:660, 1944. Williams & Wilkins, Baltimore.)

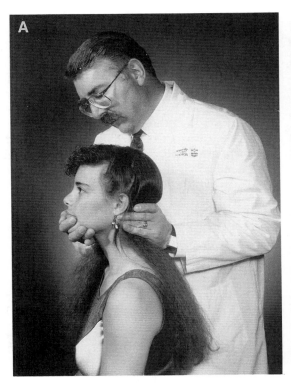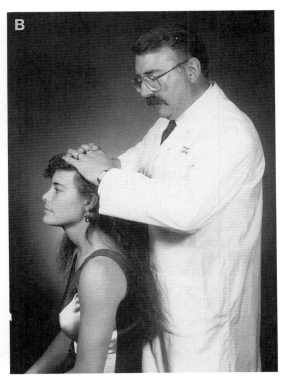

Fig. 21-11. **(A)** Cervical distraction. **(B)** Axial compression used as part of an upper quadrant screen to rule out cervical radicular impingement as part of shoulder pain.

radiation and trigger points along the medial border of the scapula generated from inflamed tendinous insertions of the periscapular muscles. These patterns of radiation are probably related to embryonic and neural segmental links of the muscles, ligaments, connective tissue, and skin, the so-called myotomes, sclerotomes, and dermatomes (Fig. 21-10). Although distal radiation is frequently shown in the anatomic charts, in clinical practice it is unusual.

It is important to be aware of the common deformities occurring secondary to congenital skeletal variations, trauma, and muscle wasting and the distinct reactions of impingement or instability. Only a methodical approach allows familiarity with these

---

Clinical Point

PROBABLE SPINAL ORIGIN OF PAIN

- Absence of shoulder tenderness
- Cervical spinal movements guarded
- Biceps reflex decreased
- Biceps weak
- Root compression tests positive
- Postural aggravation of symptoms

Clinical Point

PAIN PATTERNS ASSOCIATED WITH SHOULDER PATHOLOGY

- Most common pattern
  -Shoulder to deltoid insertion
- Less common pattern
  -Shoulder to scapula
  -Shoulder to elbow
- Infrequent pattern
  -Past elbow
- Almost never
  -Into hand

clinical pictures and ensures that the clinician does not overlook systemic disease, neoplasia, and more remote medical conditions such as heart disease and upper abdominal problems. A detailed history, methodical palpation, and a thorough test of motion usually reveals a specific diagnosis with the associated degree of severity. Furthermore, failure to respond to therapy or fit into a specific pain pattern prompts an efficient and logical sequence of investigative tests.

History

All data concerning the chief complaint should be related to the patient's age, occupation, recreational goals, and side of dominance. Specifically, the complaint of pain should be distinguished from that of weakness. The mode of onset, whether single or repetitive trauma, overuse, occupation aggravated by recreation or vice versa, and the precipitating factors for the current episode of a recurrent problem are important details.

The family history of joint disease, the absence of other joint symptoms and inquiry regarding heart

disease or gastrointestinal problems help identify referred pain and systemic disease. In the age group 45 and over, left shoulder pain related to activity must always raise some suspicion of cardiac symptoms and should prompt questions as to its cessation with rest, association with chest or neck pain, and the presence of shortness of breath. Neck pain and dysesthesia radiating past the elbow tend to implicate the cervical spine as a source of the problem. Lastly, the nature and response to previous physical and drug therapy are germane, along with some idea of the patient's compliance to such regimens.

Practice Point

Left shoulder pain with activity in the over 45 age group should always prompt a more detailed history to unmask possible cardiac disease.

Observation

Adequate exposure of the patient is essential so the initial examination can encompass the thorax, spine, and shoulder girdle. The size and shape of scars or stretch marks should be noted to supplement the history of surgery and the subsequent overall impression of ligamentous laxity.

Viewing from behind allows an impression of wasting in the supraspinatus fossa, the trapezius, and the deltoid region. Deformity of the shoulder girdle or spine may be enhanced by neck or shoulder motion or the forward bending scoliosis screening test.

Viewing from the side allows assessment of kyphosis and neck–head posture. The anterior inspection is useful for detecting muscle wasting, head posture, and thoracic deformity. In each case, the nature of the deformity triggers the need for roentgenograms.

Range of Motion

It is reasonable to start the range of motion examination with the cervical spine, as it can indicate a possible need for further investigation of this area. Any pain or restriction of range should prompt at least a rotation and axial distraction and compression test to attempt to exacerbate or relieve the symptoms (Fig. 21-11).

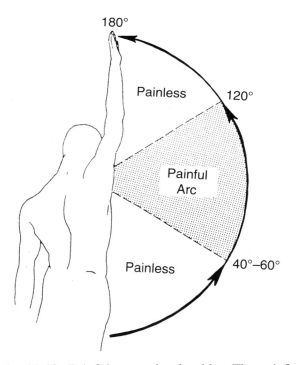

Fig. 21-12. Painful arc at the shoulder. The painful arc increases with the severity of the pain and is indicative of the amount of impingement. (After Hawkins and Hobeika,[19] with permission.)

Clinical Point
SHOULDER GIRDLE ASSESSMENT

History	• Pain versus weakness
	• Trauma versus slow onset
	• Precipitating factors
	• Cardiac history age 45 years plus
Observation	• Obvious wasting
	• Obvious deformity
	• Check spine
ROM	• Cervical spine with compression and distraction
	• Painful arc or reverse glenohumeral rhythm
	• Presence of capsular pattern
	• Ability to do functional motions
	• End feel: contracture, pain inhibition
Strength	• Isolate muscle groups
	• Weakness versus pain
Special tests	• Impingement positions
	• Instability, local or general
	• Thoracic outlet
	• Neurologic, sensory, reflexes
Palpation	• Isolate specific anatomic entity
	• Record radiation of pain
Investigation	• Roentgenogram with special views, shoulder, neck, or chest
	• Blood and biochemical analysis, ECG
	• Arthrogram
	• CT, MRI, bone scan, sonography
	• Nerve conduction and electromyography
	• Selected injections of local anesthetic
	• Arthroscopy
	• Isokinetic muscle testing

Quick Facts
RANGE OF MOTION

Range	Degrees	Plane
Extension	50	Sagittal
Flexion	180	
Abduction	180	Frontal
Adduction	75	
Horizontal extension	30	Transverse
Horizontal flexion	135	
With arm at side		
Ext. rotation	65	
Int. rotation	80	
With arm 90 degrees abduction		Sagittal
Ext. rotation	90	
Int. rotation	70	

Shoulder girdle motion is initially done actively; and if there is restriction or pain, passive tests help delineate the source of the problem using Cyriax's selective stress tests. These principles generally are accurate, although with the acutely painful shoulder all tests are uncomfortable. A painful arc, reverse glenohumeral rhythm, and capsular pattern of restricted range are used to guide subsequent palpation and direct special tests at distinguishing pain, weakness, or contracture as a cause of the symptoms (Figs. 21-12 and 21-13). Experience leads to an accurate interpretation of the end feel of each motion, whether spasm, a springy or bony block, or an empty or unusual sensation. A special note should be made of any discrepancy between active and passive range of motion.

Specific range of motion may be measured with a goniometer, and such isolated motion measurements

Clinical Point
DISCREPANCY BETWEEN ACTIVE AND PASSIVE ROM

Usually secondary to:
- Muscle weakness
- Nerve injury
- Tendon rupture
- Volitional action

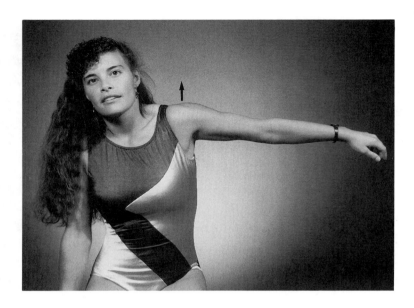

Fig. 21-13. Reversed glenohumeral rhythm. As the discomfort increases, the patient tries to limit the amount of glenohumeral joint motion, resulting in abnormal elevation of the scapula.

should be supplemented by functional tests of activities of daily living or sport-specific positions and maneuvers (Fig. 21-14). Knowledge of training regimens and the arm and shoulder action in selected sport skills are necessary to utilize this knowledge to its fullest.

Strength

Some idea of strength is gained from selective stressing of structures when the chief complaint is pain. However, when weakness is a feature of the condition or for the athlete preparing to return to competitive sport, specific testing of the major muscle groups is important. Weakness of the deltoid after dislocation, supraspinatus weakness after a rotator cuff tear, serratus anterior weakness secondary to

---

Clinical Point

CYRIAX SELECTIVE STRESS TESTS

- Active ROM
  - Tests patient's willingness
  - Allows observation of capsular and noncapsular patterns
  - Gives overall impression of range
- Passive ROM
  - Selective stressing of noncontractile elements
  - Pain in capsule, ligaments, bursa
- Isometric strength
  - Selective stressing of contractile elements (muscles and tendons)
  - Overall impression of strength and pain inhibition

Quick Facts

OXFORD (MRC) MANUAL MUSCLE TESTING SCALE

0	No voluntary contraction
1	Muscle flicker—no movement
2	Muscle contraction—movement if gravity eliminated
3	Contraction—movement against gravity
4	Contraction—movement against some resistance
5	Normal contraction against normal resistance

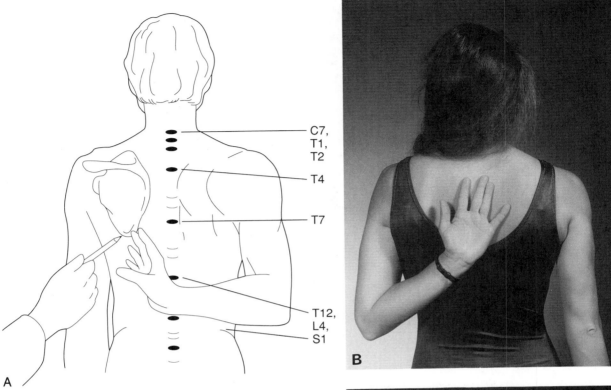

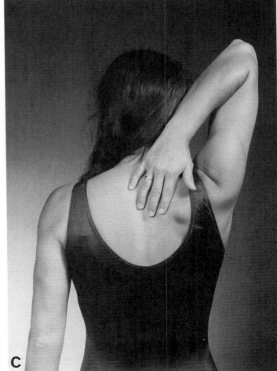

Fig. 21-14. Measured range of motion should be supplemented by functional assessment (Aply's scratch test). **(A)** Palpable landmarks used as an alternative to tape measurements. Vertebra prominens C7, T1; superior angle of scapula T2; base of scapula spine T4; inferior angle of scapula T7; lowest rib T12, iliac crest L4; dimples at posterior superior iliac spines S1,2. **(B)** Patient is asked to put the hand in the pocket, on the hip, and the small of the back, and then slide it up as high as possible on the thoracic spine (testing abduction and internal rotation). **(C)** Patient can be asked to touch the opposite shoulder, the mouth, and the top of the head and then to slide the hand down the back of the neck to reach as low as possible (testing abduction and external rotation).

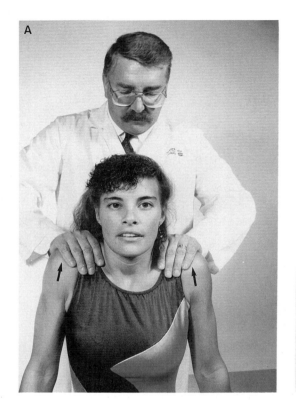

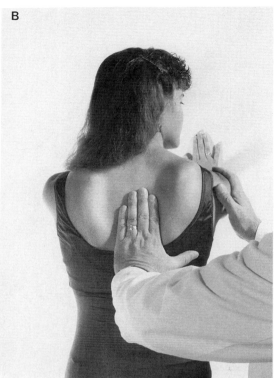

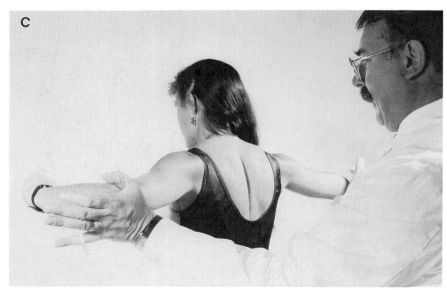

Fig. 21-15. Screen of the prime movers of the scapula is carried out prior to specific muscle testing of the glenohumeral joint. **(A)** Shoulder shrug for trapezius (C2–C4). **(B)** Protraction and pressure against a resistance (wall), for serratus anterior and **(C)** retraction of the shoulders for rhomboids (C5–C7).

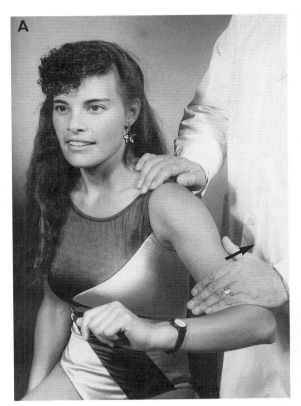

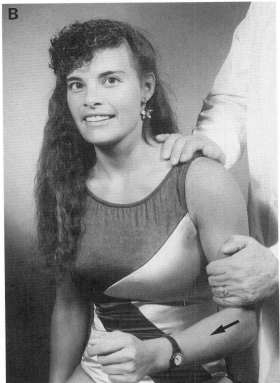

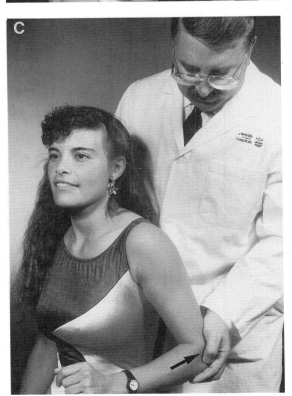

Fig. 21-16. Manual resistance tests for deltoid strength (C5–C6). **(A)** Abduction. **(B)** Forward flexion for anterior fibers. **(C)** Shoulder extension for posterior fibers.

nerve palsy, and muscle wasting after surgical procedures are common examples of conditions requiring assessment of strength. In the latter example, isokinetic testing may allow documentation of postoperative progress of rehabilitation so that safe resumption of activity may be gauged. In most situations manual testing is adequate and sensitive enough for diagnostic purposes, and it is certainly the best method for distinguishing pain inhibition from lack of effort or actual weakness (Table 21-3).

A hand-held dynamometer or computerized isokinetic testing may be used to supplement this information when specific figures are deemed important. The key to muscle testing is an accurate knowledge of muscle action and the ability to fix the proximal segment and isolate the movement (Figs. 21-15 through 21-18). The Oxford (Medical Research Council, MRC) scale is the simplest way to record recovery from nerve injury.

Special Tests

The object of special tests is to isolate inflammation and impingement syndromes from instability and to ensure exclusion of neurologic problems of the peripheral or central nervous system.

Impingement

Impingement may be associated with varying degrees of inflammation. In the chronic situation the inflammatory component is minimal, and hence response to anti-inflammatory medication and modalities is poor. The indication of impingement as the source of the problem is the presence of a painful arc during abduction. Cross flexion stresses the acromioclavicular joint and is painful with acute first and second degree injuries as well as inflammatory and degenerative conditions of the joint (Fig. 21-19). An-

TABLE 21-3. Clinical Muscle Testing Positions

Muscle	Innervation	Myotomes	Technique for Testing
Trapezius	Spinal accessory	C2–C4	Patient shrugs shoulders against resistance.
Sternomastoid	Spinal accessory	C2–C4	Patient turns head to one side with resistance over opposite temporal area.
Serratus anterior	Long thoracic	C5–C7	Patient pushes against wall with outstretched arm. Scapular winging is observed.
Latissimus dorsi	Thoracodorsal	C7–C8	Downward/backward pressure of arm against resistance. Muscle palpable at inferior angle of scapula during cough.
Rhomboids	Dorsal scapula	(C4) C5	Hands on hips pushing elbows backward against resistance.
Levator scapulae	Dorsal scapula		
Subclavius	Nerve to subclavius	C5–C6	None
Teres major	Subscapular (lower)	C5–C6	Similar to latissimus dorsi; muscle palpable at lower border of scapula
Deltoid	Axillary	C5–C6 (C7)	With arm abducted 90°, downward pressure is applied. Anterior and posterior fibers may be tested in slight flexion and extension.
Subscapularis	Subscapular (upper)	C5	Arm at side with elbow flexed to 90°. Examiner resists internal rotation.
Supraspinatus	Suprascapular	C5 (C6)	Arm abducted against resistance (not isolated). With arm pronated and elevated 90° in plane of scapula, downward pressure is applied.
Infraspinatus	Suprascapular	C5 (C6)	Arm at side with elbow flexed 90°. Examiner resists external rotation.
Teres minor	Axillary	C5–C6 (C7)	Same as for infraspinatus.
Pectoralis major	Medial and lateral pectoral	C5–T1	With arm flexed 30° in front of body, patient adducts against resistance.
Pectoralis minor	Medial pectoral	C8,T1	None
Coracobrachialis	Musculocutaneous	(C4) C5–C6 (C7)	None
Biceps brachii	Musculocutaneous	(C4) C5–C6	Flexion of the supinated forearm against resistance.
Triceps	Radial	(C5) C6–C8	Resistance to extension of elbow from varying position of flexion

Numbers in parentheses indicate a variable but not rare contribution.
(From Rasch and Burke,[15] with permission.)

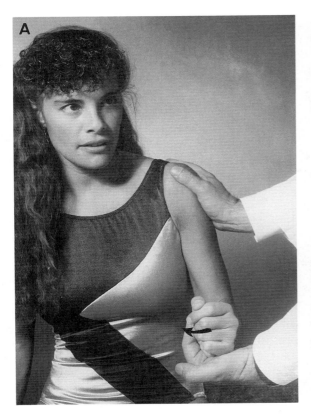 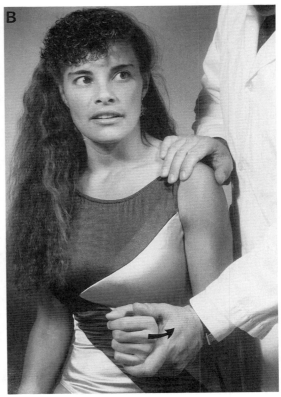

Fig. 21-17. **(A)** Resisted internal rotation (C5). **(B)** Resisted external rotation in the neutral position (C5,6).

terior impingement underneath the coracoacromial arch is elicited by supplementing the painful arc abduction test by feeling for subacromial crepitus while passively fully abducting the arm. When the patient gently lowers the fully abducted limb, the discomfort through the painful arc is usually increased. The symptoms may be further exacerbated by gently putting pressure on the arm and asking the patient to resist while passing through the painful range. Usually pain is exacerbated if the contractile structures are involved. Furthermore, an acute onset of sharp pain may make the patient suddenly stop or catch, or even let the arm fall rapidly to the side. These results constitute a positive Codman's "drop arm test." Further evidence of anterior impingement is pain elicited by forceful abduction of the internally rotated arm against the acromion[19,20] (Fig. 21-20).

By testing for pain in the nonimpingement position for each specific structure, it is possible to distinguish an isolated inflammatory response from simple im-

pingement. However, when significant inflammation is present, there may be false-positive impingement tests, as all positions of testing are uncomfortable. Inflamed tissue is uncomfortable on a passive stretch as well as when put under tension by contracting the associated muscle.

Clinical Point

With significant inflammation of tissues, impingement tests may be falsely positive.

A positive impingement injection test is relief of at least 50 percent of the patient's pain, through the painful arc or impingement position, by 5–10 ml of 1 percent lidocaine (Xylocaine) placed in the suba-

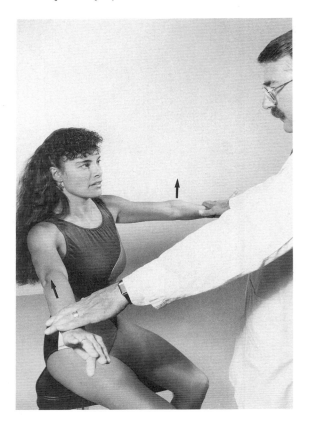

Fig. 21-18. Specific test for the supraspinatus. The arms are abducted to 90 degrees, brought forward into 30 degrees of flexion, and internally rotated pointing the thumbs toward the floor. Manual resistance in this position often reveals weakness of the supraspinatus. The test is positive in presence of rotator cuff tears.

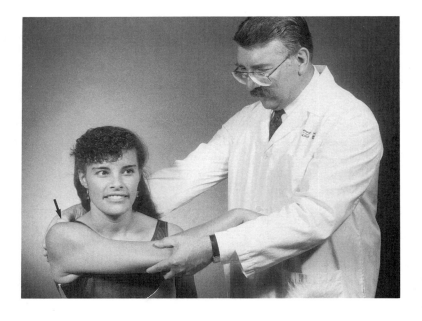

Fig. 21-19. Forced cross flexion of the arms in the 90 degree position is most likely to exacerbate symptoms from the acromioclavicular joint. The examiner palpates the acromioclavicular joint to confirm the source of the pain.

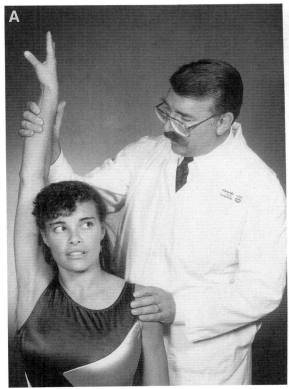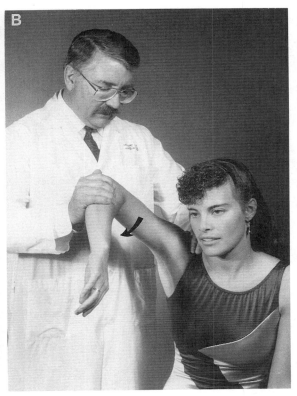

Fig. 21-20. Anterior impingement tests. **(A)** With the arm fully abducted, overpressure is put on the internally rotated shoulder. Positive test is exacerbation of anterior should pain. **(B)** Hawkins sign. Positive impingement test generated by forward flexion and internal rotation. In this internally rotated position, the pain increases with either further overpressuring to internal rotation, abduction, or cross flexion. Resisting forward flexion by applying pressure at the elbow may also exacerbate the signs.

cromial space. This test is not specific, as it relieves pain in the subacromial bursa, the acromioclavicular joint, the biceps tendon, and the superior and anterior rotator cuff. In individuals with a painful cuff tear, it may relieve pain sufficiently to allow muscle testing. A partial tear is often compatible with normal strength, but a full-thickness tear should still cause obvious weakness, even when the pain is alleviated.

Pain located mainly in an inflamed long head of the biceps tendon may be exacerbated by asking the athlete to flex the shoulder with the elbow extended and the forearm supinated against the examiner's resistance. A positive test is pain in the region of the intertubercular groove (Fig. 21-21). This test is more frequently positive than the classic Yergason's test of flexion and supination with the arm in the neutral position.

> ### Clinical Point
>
> If stiffness is present, many of the impingement and range of motion tests for inflammation are frequently invalid, as a stiff shoulder may be painful.

Instability

A series of specific clinical tests help unmask instability.[20-22] In the sitting position the humeral head may be grasped through the deltoid and attempts made to glide it anteriorly or posteriorly (Fig. 21-22). Excessive anterior glide leaves a void under the posterior acromion, and posterior subluxation is considered abnormal when more than 50 percent of the

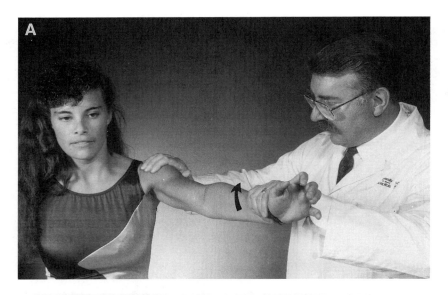

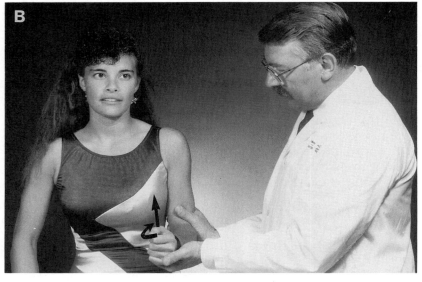

Fig. 21-21. Test for biceps tendon impingement. **(A)** Speed's test, resisted flexion adduction and supination with the elbows extended. **(B)** Yergason's test, resisted elbow flexion and supination with the arm in the neutral position. The addition of attempted external rotation may make the test more sensitive.

humeral head can be translated off the glenoid in a posterior direction. Anteriorly, the shift is recorded as grade I (mild, less than a third), grade II (moderate, head riding on the edge of the glenoid), grade III (severe, dislocated head). Complete relaxation is necessary. This test is difficult to perform in athletes with large deltoid muscles. In individuals with significant laxity, these displacements may be produced voluntarily.

Perhaps the easiest test to perform is the sitting apprehension test of anterior instability. The abducted arm is firmly rotated externally while anterior pressure is exerted on the proximal humerus (Fig. 21-23). A positive test is signaled by a sudden uneasi-

ness, tensing of the muscles, or a feeling of impending or actual subluxation.

Further confirmation of direction and magnitude of instability is obtained by two other maneuvers while sitting. The examiner may demonstrate posterior subluxation by positioning the athlete's arm in forward flexion and internal rotation and directing a posterior force along the axis of the humerus. An athlete with a lax capsule and recurrent posterior subluxation frequently subluxes merely with forward flexion. The diagnosis is confirmed by feeling the reduction of the humeral head, often with a quick snap, as the arm is taken back to the neutral position. (The posterior subluxation flexion test.)

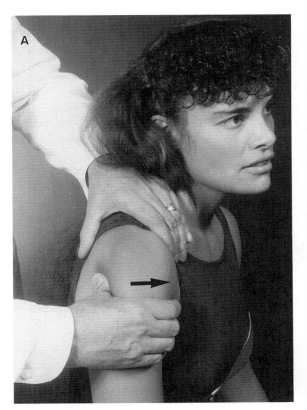 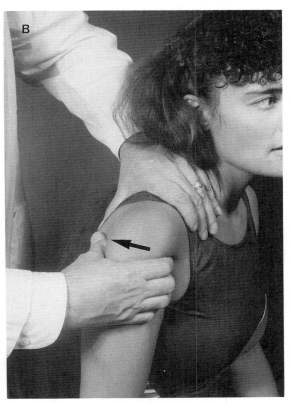

Fig. 21-22. Anteroposterior gliding of the glenohumeral joint (load and shift test). The scapula is stabilized with one hand and an anterior glide (**A**) and a posterior glide (**B**) is performed by pressure over the humeral head to test for excessive mobility. Clinical grading of translation of the humeral head is somewhat inaccurate but by frequent use of the load and shift test, experience allows assessment of the degree of motion. For some clinicians this is the single best test of posterior subluxation.

Fig. 21-23. Apprehension test. Positive test is indicated by contraction of the muscle with inability to relax as the elbow is brought into further extension or the amount of external rotation is increased. Exaggerated by forward pressure over the proximal humerus.

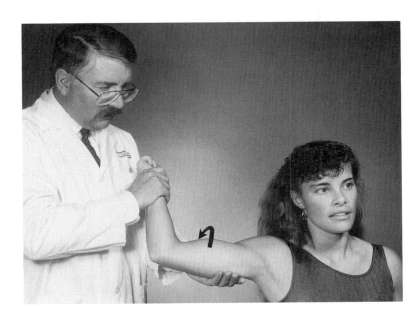

Anterior inferior instability is reproduced with the Feagin maneuver.[21] The athlete's arm is at 90 degrees with the elbow supported on the examiner's shoulder. Then, with both hands over the top of the proximal humerus, the arm is pushed down (inferiorly) with a quick motion. Reproduction of the subluxation or palpable bounce is considered a positive finding.

At the completion of these tests while sitting, the athlete may be examined in a lying position. Anterior capsular laxity is confirmed by either externally rotating or extending the abducted shoulder (Fig. 21-24).

The glenoid labrum grind or clunk test is performed with the athlete's shoulder fully abducted and internally rotated. Forward pressure is exerted over the humeral head as the elbow is grasped and the shoulder circumducted or taken from flexion to extension (Fig. 21-25). During these maneuvers the patient may experience the apprehension of instability,

or there may be a popping or clunking sensation with or without pain, which indicates the possibility of a glenoid labral lesion.

Suspected posterior laxity is tested by direct posterior pressure over the proximal humerus of the abducted arm, while the shoulder is taken into varying degrees of cross flexion (Fig. 21-26). This is usually only positive with gross laxity. Inferior laxity and multidirectional instability are confirmed by direct longitudinal traction in the long axis of the humerus. The positive "sulcus" sign is the appearance of a palpable defect underneath the acromion (Fig. 21-27). Occasionally in the lax individual, as the traction is released the joint reduces with a "clunk". This may be done in sitting or lying.

These tests for instability may be followed by specific maneuvers to unmask compression in the thoracic outlet, such as the Adson test and the hyperabduction test. Sensory testing and elicitation of reflexes completes this section of the examination.

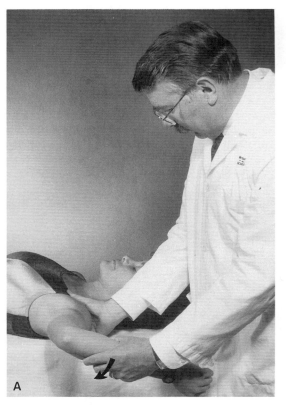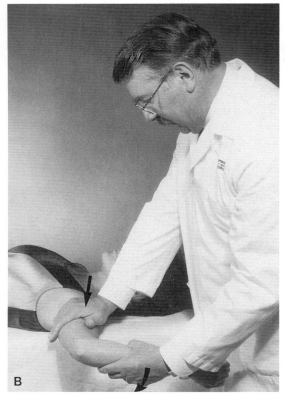

Fig. 21-24. Confirmation of anterior instability by external rotation and extension in abduction. **(A)** As the elbow is taken into further extension, there is a feeling of apprehension and instability. **(B)** Counterpressure directed posteriorly over the proximal humerus and humeral head gives the patient a feeling of confidence, and further rotation or extension is possible. (Fowler's sign.)

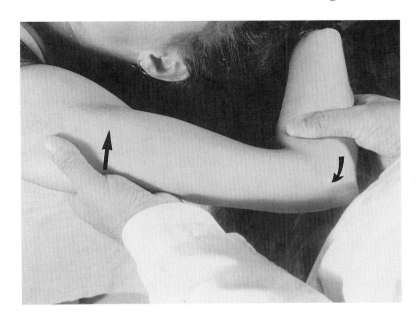

Fig. 21-25. Glenoid labrum clunk test. Circumduction of the shoulder in full abduction may produce a positive clunk or grinding sensation with a positive test, which may be indicative of internal derangement of the shoulder.

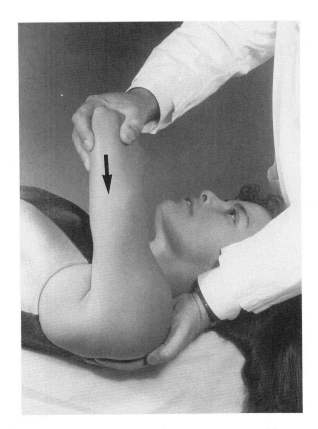

Fig. 21-26. Pressure through the long axis of the arm may reproduce the feeling of posterior subluxation or laxity. This is not a very sensitive test.

Palpation

Many clinicians prefer to palpate early in their examination, but because it may be an uncomfortable experience, particularly with acute tendinitis, it is frequently better left until the end. By this time, the history and examination have given a high index of suspicion as to the diagnosis, and the palpation may be used to confirm and isolate the pathologic structure. It is an exercise in careful surface anatomy techniques (Fig. 21-28). If neoplasia or infection is considered, care must be taken to include the supraclavicular triangles and the axilla. If the inflamed structure is under the bony projection of the acromion, internal rotation, with the athlete's hand placed in the small of the back, can deliver the supraspinatus and subacromial bursa anteriorly. The presence of grinding, snapping, or clunking is recorded. Trigger points, pain radiation, and size and consistency of any unusual swelling are important. The emphasis of the palpation is dictated by the findings to this point. Finally, confirmation of the degree of scapula versus glenohumeral motion may be achieved by fixation of the scapula while abducting the shoulder.

Laboratory Investigations

Usually the clinical examination is sufficient to give an excellent working diagnosis. However, when systemic disease is suspected, surgery contemplated, or

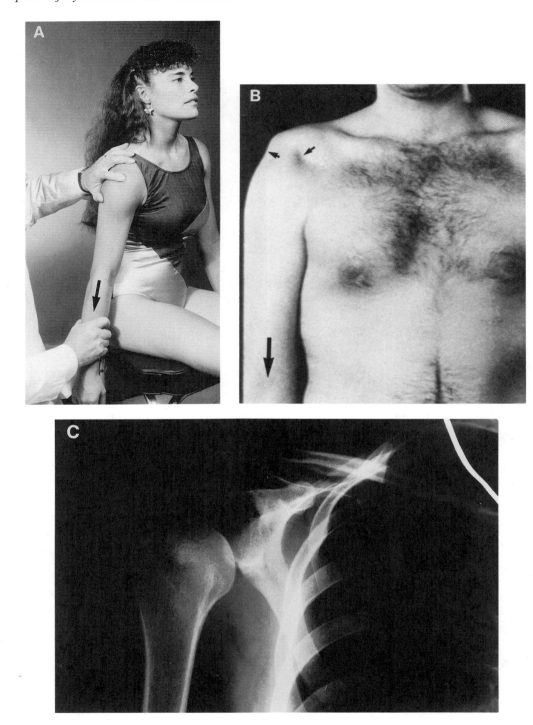

Fig. 21-27. Long axis glenoid traction on the arm helps confirm inferior subluxation and multidirectional instability. **(A)** This test can be done sitting or lying, and the area underneath the acromion is palpated for a detectable gap. **(B)** With excessive inferior instability, the visible sulcus sign is one of depression anteriorly and laterally in the subacromial region. **(C)** Roentgenogram demonstrates the inferior subluxation with longitudinal traction.

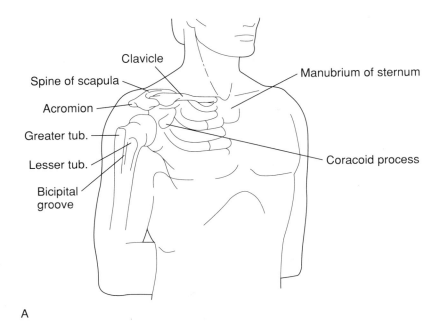

A

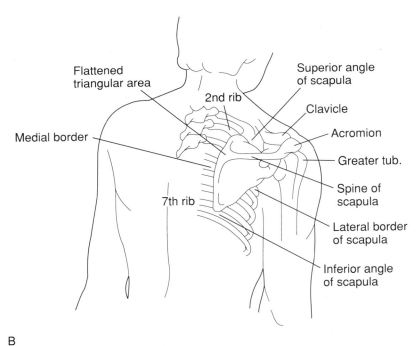

B

Fig. 21-28. Palpable surface landmarks that should be examined either at the beginning or end of the physical examination. In addition to the bony points, the supraclavicular fossa, the supraspinatus, biceps and infraspinatus tendons, and the parascapular soft tissues for trigger points are important. **(A)** Anterior. **(B)** Posterior.

the diagnosis difficult, the disease entity may be further clarified, classified, graded, or delineated by special tests, including plain roentgenograms, arthrograms, bone scans, CT, and MRI. Blood and biochemical analyses, electrocardiography (ECG), and electromyography (EMG) have a role in confirming the diagnosis and following the progress of treatment. It is easy to get into a spiraling web of investigations with common shoulder problems because of their tendency to chronicity and recurrence. This practice frustrates the physician and leads to a chain of expensive and frequently unnecessary tests. Such tests should not be used to replace careful clinical examination, and their indications should be kept clearly in mind for each athlete and diagnostic entity.

STERNOCLAVICULAR INJURY

The strength of the sternoclavicular joint depends mainly on its capsule, supraclavicular ligaments, and disc. Structurally, it is still one of the most unstable joints in the body. Because ultimately all forces through the upper limb must resolve to some degree at this articulation it is little wonder that this joint occasionally dislocates. Such injury is, however, rare, comprising about 3 percent of all shoulder girdle dislocations. Nearly all major injuries are due to a direct blow; vehicle accidents cause two-thirds of the dislocations, and about one-third are due to sporting activities.[23]

First degree injuries are characterized by pain centered around the joint that is aggravated by stressing the medial end of the clavicle; there is no obvious associated instability. Second degree injuries suggest stretching or rupturing of the sternoclavicular and costoclavicular ligaments and obviously comprise a broad spectrum of injuries. There is usually bruising, swelling, and significant pain. Care should be taken to relieve the joint of stress for 3 to 6 weeks, depending on the severity of injury, because there is a tendency to heal with increased mobility, which on occasion leads to a painful subluxation. Diagnosis may be confirmed with cephalic tilt roentgenograms (Fig. 21-29). Treated carefully these second degree injuries usually resolve; and even though there is sometimes excessive permanent swelling around the joint, they do not produce symptoms.

The third degree injury with dislocation is a serious injury on two counts. The first is of immediate concern and involves potential pressure of adjacent vital structures; the second is the propensity for recurrent subluxation.

Posterior dislocation with pressure on the trachea, subclavian artery, and esophagus occurs in about 30 percent of these unusual injuries. Pressure on the trachea may almost totally obstruct the airway, producing a gasping, snorting type of breathing. In milder cases the athlete mentions some difficulty breathing, perhaps shortness of breath, and extreme pain over the sternoclavicular area. It is important not to overlook this situation. With pressure on the major vessels, symptoms range from claudication of the upper limb to an absent pulse or ischemic changes.

The emergency care of this critical clinical situation requires that the athlete lie on the back, preferably with a bolster, sandbag, or pillow between the shoulder blades. Traction is applied in the long axis of the abducted affected limb, with some posterior pull (extension) to allow retraction of the shoulder (Fig. 21-30). This distraction of the joint often allows it to reduce spontaneously, with a "pop." Reduction into the anterior position usually brings immediate relief of symptoms. Occasionally, it is necessary to pull the clavicle forward manually or with a "towel clip." If the asphyxia is sufficient to cause unconsciousness, the situation requires speedy resolution, and anesthesia is not required. A particularly rare complication is tearing of a major vessel with hemorrhage.

Quick Facts

STERNOCLAVICULAR INJURY COMPLICATIONS

- Early posterior dislocation
  - Pressure on trachea
  - Asphyxia
  - Pressure on major vessels
  - Decreased circulation to upper limb
  - Pressure on plexus
  - Dysesthesia
- Late dislocation
  - Chronic pain with activity
  - Recurrent subluxation
  - Recurrent dislocation
  - Muscle wasting
  - Cold intolerance

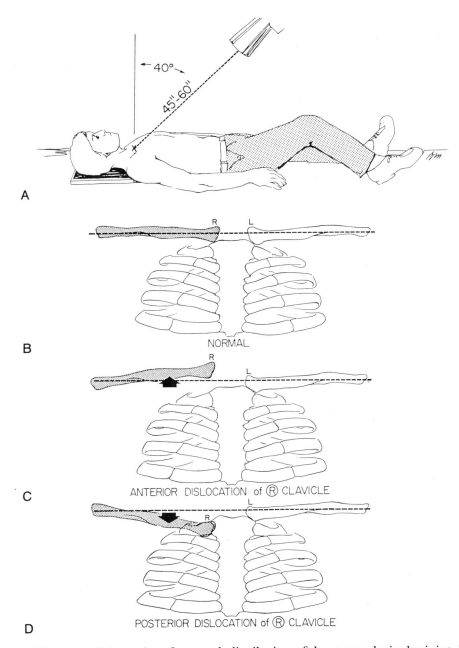

Fig. 21-29. **(A)** Position of the patient for a cephalic tilt view of the sternoclavicular joint. In children the true distance should be approximately 45 inches; with thick-chested athletes the distance should be increased to 60 inches. **(B)** In the normal individual the posterior clavicle should appear on the same imaginary line going horizontally across the film. **(C)** With anterior dislocation, the medial end of the clavicle projects above this line. **(D)** With posterior dislocation, the medial half of the clavicle is displaced below this imaginary line. (Adapted from Rockwood and Green,[23] with permission.)

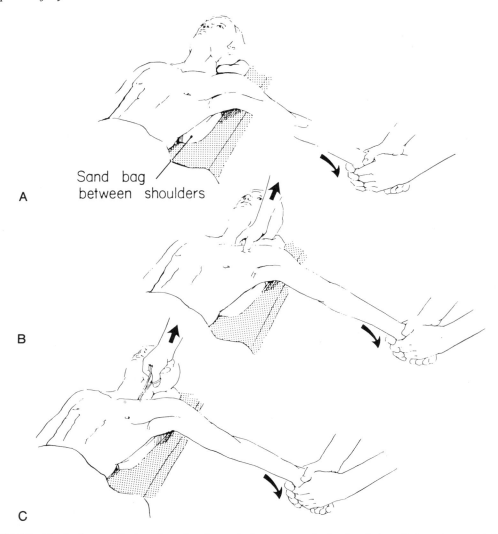

Sand bag between shoulders

A

B

C

Fig. 21-30. Technique of closed reduction of the sternoclavicular joint dislocation. **(A)** With the thorax elevated enough to facilitate a cantilever effect, traction and extension are placed through the arm. **(B)** If it is not sufficient, additional leverage is gained by grasping the clavicle with the fingers. **(C)** If this maneuver does not affect the reduction, a sterile towel clip can be used to grasp the clavicle and lift it anteriorly and laterally. (Adapted from Rockwood and Green,[23] with permission.)

Hence the therapist or physician should be prepared to treat shock. Fortunately, few practititioners have to deal with this injury.

It has been mentioned that the second problem relates to the fact that these tears and subluxations do not heal well and a chronic subluxing sternoclavicular joint may result. Occasionally, it is particularly painful and may take months to become asymptomatic.

Surgical repairs of this joint are difficult and often unsatisfactory. For this reason, although the subluxation and dislocation of the sternoclavicular joint is not a common injury, it is certainly a serious one. Fortunately, the anterior dislocations are not associated with life-threatening complications, but are more common, and have a greater propensity for late recurrent instability.

ACROMIOCLAVICULAR JOINT INJURY

Acute Tears

Acute tears are seen frequently in injured joints in hockey, rugby, football, equestrian accidents, and the martial arts.

Mechanism and Classification

The stability of the acromioclavicular joint is influenced to some extent by the slope and size of the articular surfaces, These anatomic variations make some individuals more vulnerable to subluxation and dislocation than others. The mechanism of injury is most frequently a direct blow or a fall, with the impact taken on the point of the shoulder and occasionally with the force transmitted through the arm during a fall on the outstretched hand. A separated shoulder should be suspected when the following signs and symptoms are present.

1. Pain over the superior aspect of the acromioclavicular joint
2. Tenderness over the acromioclavicular joint
3. Pain on all motion of the shoulder
4. Abnormal prominence of the clavicle (Fig. 21-31)

As has been pointed out before, these injuries are divided into first, second, and third degree injuries. The first degree (type I) injury is signified by swelling and occasionally bruising of the joint itself. The joint may be exquisitely tender to move or touch, but there is no obvious deformity. There is some microscopic tearing of the ligament and minimal instability. Treatment for this type of injury is mainly conservative, with early mobilization and activities within the tolerance of pain.

The second degree (type II) injury suggests more extensive tearing of the joint capsule with some subluxation of the joint surfaces. There may be detectable increased anteroposterior mobility, some bleeding, and some tearing of the fibers of the deltoid. The ligaments attaching the coracoid process to the clavicle should be intact. For this reason, there is some intrinsic stability, although this injury is painful. Radiologically, it is characterized by joint space widening rather than significant upward displacement. It can be treated adequately in a conservative fashion, but the severe nature of this injury must be recognized as further insult to the shoulder while it is in this condition may convert it to a third degree injury, or complete disruption of the joint. For this reason, the joint must be carefully inspected, and athletes such as rugby, football, or hockey players should not be allowed to resume playing until all tenderness is gone from the joint, a full range of motion has been established, and deltoid strength is restored.

The third degree injury suggests there is complete tearing of both ligaments of the acromioclavicular joint itself and the ligaments connecting the clavicle to the coracoid process. There is usually considerable deformity, excessive mobility, and often significant tearing of the deltoid muscle attachment to the distal end of the clavicle. Because of the differing opinions

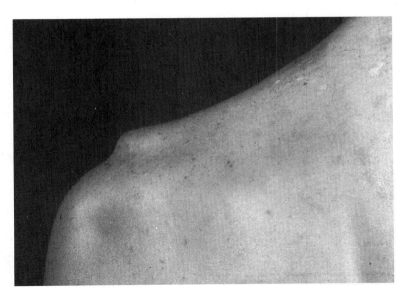

Fig. 21-31. Typical deformity produced with a third-degree acromioclavicular separation.

Clinical Point

ACROMIOCLAVICULAR SPRAINS

First Degree (Type I)
- Incomplete tear of acromioclavicular ligament
- No deformity
- No instability
- Point tenderness over acromioclavicular joint
- Pain on elevation and abduction past 90 degrees
- Pain on cross-flexion spasm

Second Degree (Type II)
- Tear of acromioclavicular (AC) ligament
- Partial tear of coracoclavicular (CC) ligament
- Widening of joint to palpation
- Palpable gap or minor step
- Swelling, bruising, some instability
- Demonstrable instability

Third Degree (Types III, IV, V, VI)
- Complete tear of AC and CC ligaments
- Swelling, bruising, and step deformity
- Demonstrable instability
- Tearing of deltoid and trapezius
- Wider area of tenderness

21–32). This system is modified slightly from that offered by Rockwood and Matsen.[18] With this classification, the type III disruption is characterized by a relative upward displacement of the outer end of the clavicle, increasing the coracoclavicular space by 25 to 100 percent.[18]

Type IV is a severe version of type III, with the coracoclavicular space increased 100 to 300 percent. There is detachment of the deltoid and trapezius for at least one-third, and frequently to the middle, of the clavicle.

Type V separations are produced by posterior dislocation of the distal clavicle into the trapezius, with significant tearing of deltoid and trapezius muscle from the outer end. Furthermore, the clavicle may be incarcerated within the fibers of the trapezius.

Type VI, a much rarer injury, is usually accompanied by complete disruption of both sets of ligaments, although occasionally the coracoclavicular ligaments remain intact. The clavicle is dislocated inferiorly, frequently locked under the acromion or coracoid process.

Children below the age of 13 years rarely sustain a complete acromioclavicular joint dislocation, as the mechanism of injury results in a fracture of the distal clavicle with an intact acromioclavicular joint.[24] Usually good to excellent results are anticipated with closed methods of treatment. Associated epiphyseal separation should be carefully ruled out by scrutiny of the roentgenogram, with comparison to the opposite side. If older than 13 years, the patient should be treated as an adult, following the principles outlined in the following sections.

Radiologic Findings

A fairly accurate clinical diagnosis is possible at the playing area, but definitive treatment sometimes requires radiologic confirmation. The occasional fracture of the distal end of the clavicle, epiphyseal separation of the distal clavicular epiphysis in the skeletally immature patient, and avulsion of the tip of the coracoid process may be ruled out. An anterior view comparing the two joints helps to establish a pathologic joint width in a relatively undisplaced second degree tear. Any displacement frequently may be enhanced by taking films with and without distraction of the joint with 10 to 15 pounds of weights held in the athlete's hands or hanging from the wrists. Ensuring relaxation gains the maximum value from this technique. The normal coracoclavicular space is less

regarding management of third degree injuries, there has evolved a grading system that divides complete disruption of the joint into types III, IV, V, and VI depending on the amount of associated damage and position of the displaced lateral end of clavicle (Fig.

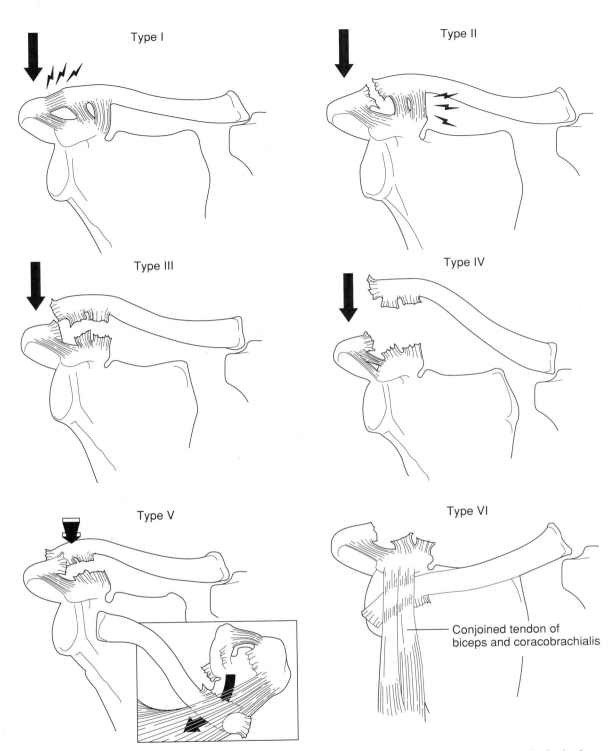

Fig. 21-32. Classic description of first, second, and third degree separations of the acromioclavicular joint can be expanded to include a type IV separation, which is a severe version of the type III with the coracoclavicular space increased over 100 percent. It signifies significant disruption of the deltoid and trapezius fibers. With type V there is posterior dislocation of the distal clavicle which incarcerates into the trapezius muscle. Type VI is an unusual situation of a subcorticoid dislocation. (This system has reversed the sequence of grade IV and V offered by Rockwood and Matsen[18] to facilitate an easily recalled progression.

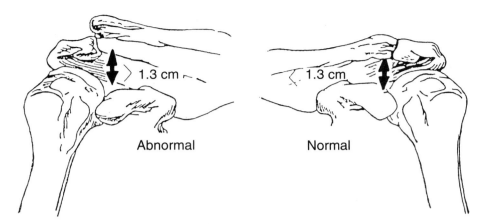

Fig. 21-33. One hundred percent displacement or more than 1.3 cm between the coracoid silhouette and the distal clavicle usually indicate a third degree acromioclavicular joint sprain.

than 1.3 cm, so values larger than 1.3 cm are usually abnormal (Fig. 21-33).

Treatment

First Degree Injury

Treatment of first and second degree injuries is usually symptomatic. First degree injuries require support for comfort if there is significant pain. NSAIDs, initial therapy with ice, and later ultrasound, laser, hot packs, or interferential therapy may assist early recovery. Range of motion is progressed as tolerated. As soon as the swelling is resolved and approximately 75 percent of range is restored pain-free, the emphasis switches to strengthening exercises for the shoulder girdle. Dips between bars, heavy dead lifts, wide grip bench press and dumbbell bench presses are avoided for at least 6 weeks, as it is possible to stress the joint unduly and provoke pain and inflammation. Depending on the sport, rapid return to full activity is anticipated. A custom-made shoulder pad or doughnut is frequently helpful for reducing discomfort in contact sports.

Second Degree Injury

Second degree sprains require slightly more intensive administration of the above protocol. A sling or modified Kinney-Howard brace may be worn for up to 2 weeks. With contact sports where the joint is at risk of further disruption, e.g., hockey, rugby, and football, the return to activity is usually delayed for about 3 weeks. A full range of motion relatively pain-free and approximately 90 percent return of strength are the criteria. With the professional athlete this time period is frequently shortened, but not without the risk of reinjury.

Complete Disruptions

The acromioclavicular joint enjoys the dubious distinction of being one of the few joints in which total dislocation is routinely treated by simply leaving the joint dislocated.[25] Since Cooper (1861) first operated on a acromioclavicular dislocation, there have been conflicting opinions about management.[26] The operative approach has frequently been advocated for manual workers, sportsmen, and members of the armed forces. Residual shoulder weakness, deformity, and pain are cited as the rationale for surgery.[27,28] Nevertheless, comparable results have been reported after conservative management.[24,29–32] This nonoperative management usually involves the use of a Velpeau bandage (sling and swath) or modified Kinney-Howard sling to support the joint, which minimizes the deformity and allows some early healing (Fig. 21-34).

In Bannister's study conservatively treated patients regained movement significantly more rapidly and fully, returned to work and sport earlier, and had fewer unsatisfactory results than those having early operations.[31] The surgical group were fixed with a clavicular-coracoid screw, and the nonoperative group had 2 weeks' rest in a broad arm sling followed by rehabilitation. In severe acromioclavicular dislocation (grades IV, V, and VI, with acromioclavicular

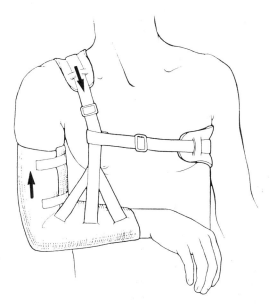

Fig. 21-34. Severe second and third degrees injuries may be treated by a modified Kinney-Howard shoulder harness. The strap that runs over the top of the shoulder and under the elbow is tightened sufficiently to reduce the clavicle to the acromion. A halter strap around the trunk keeps the pad from slipping off the shoulder.

separation of more than 2 cm and significant muscle detachment), the younger active patients may have benefited from operative repair. This series reflects our own experience in which initial anatomic reduction is achieved in most patients but lost in up to 35 percent of cases. Usually the patients who do well are those who maintain a relatively anatomic alignment at the joint and those who lose complete apposition of the bones. The patients who ultimately have partial apposition frequently suffer from pain during vigorous activity. This latter fact may explain why many individuals with grade II separation have pain and muscle weakness at late follow-up. Strength deficits up to 25 percent, particularly with horizontal adduction, may occur with both grade II and III injuries, irrespective of method of treatment. For the athlete these injuries are frequently incompletely rehabilitated, and pain with resisted motion above the level of the shoulder is often a contributing feature.

In summary, we recommend nonoperative treatment for grade I, II, and III separations and consideration of an operative approach with grades IV, V,

Clinical Point
ACROMIOCLAVICULAR SEPARATIONS

- First Degree (type I): no radiologic changes
  - Confirm accurate diagnosis
  - Early motion and strengthening
  - Pain control paces progress
  - Return to contact activities when full range of motion and little or no pain on resisted abduction
- Second Degree (type II): widening of joint space; coracoclavicular (CC) space slightly increased <25%
  - May require sling
  - Allow 3 weeks for capsular healing where possible for contact sports
  - Spectrum of injury; thus the degree of displacement indicates relative risk of early reinjury
- Third Degree (type III); marked widening of acromioclavicular (AC) joint space; CC space increased by 25–100%
  - May require sling
  - Allow 3 weeks for capsular healing where possible for contact sports
  - Spectrum of injury
- Type IV: distal clavicle space increased 100–300%
  - Significant muscle disruption
  - Consider surgery
- Type V: posterior dislocation distal clavicle into trapezius
  - Significant muscle disruption
  - Surgery usually indicated
- Type VI: clavicle dislocated inferiorly
  - Clavicle may be trapped under acromion or coracoid
  - Surgery usually indicated

and VI. This treatment obviously leaves the operative group with an increased risk of infection, an unsightly scar, and the frequent need for removal of the internal fixation device. Nevertheless, in highly competitive individuals it may offer the best solution in the long run. In those situations where the elevated clavicle threatens to button-hole through the skin, early surgical reduction is mandatory. In all cases, the best surgical result is achieved by perfect reduction, which requires meticulous repair of damaged muscle, as well as of the capsule and coracoclavicular ligaments when possible. Six weeks of relative immobilization is necessary to allow good soft tissue healing. Compromising this time period frequently leads to some loss of reduction. Intensive early rehabilitation must be followed by a well taught home program, which should be progressed for at least 6 months to gain optimal strength parameters.

Degenerative Changes

Traumatic Osteolysis

Repetitive contusions and impacts to the acromioclavicular joint or repeated stresses to a slightly unstable joint with a previous second degree separation may result in traumatic osteolysis of the distal end of the clavicle. This condition is particularly prevalent in professional hockey players and rugby players, who may present with varying degrees of pain. The radiographic changes are reminiscent of rheumatoid arthritis or hyperparathyroidism, with cyst formation and resorption. However, unlike these diseases, the rest of the clavicle and other bones are not osteopenic.[10,33]

Osteoarthrosis

The acromioclavicular joint is a frequent site of arthrosis, which is the result of repetitive minor stresses, previous grade I or II separations, clavicular fractures, or some more generalized condition that produces degenerative changes. Subchondral sclerosis, cysts, and osteophyte formation are the obvious radiologic changes. There are a wide range of symptoms, from minor aching with repetitive throwing or resisted exercises, to pain with most activity, discomfort only when there is pressure on the joint such as lying in bed, or even fairly continual pain with daily activities. There may be painful or painless crepitus or snapping and tenderness, which is usually localized specifically in the joint, with little radiation of pain. Occasionally, there is referral of pain to the acromion and anterior deltoid. Cross flexion in 90 degrees elevation is the most specific test for acromioclavicular symptoms (Fig. 21-19).

Treatment may be as simple as analyzing the activity pattern and avoidance of certain exercises or maneuvers. If episodes of pain are intermittent, courses of NSAIDs usually help. Severe symptoms may be alleviated with an occasional injection of steroid. When protracted, severe, and interfering with important recreational activities or activities of daily living, excision of the distal clavicle, the Mumford procedure, may be considered.

Mumford Procedure

During the 1940s Mumford and Gurd described resection of the distal clavicle for symptomatic grade II and III acromioclavicular separations, respectively.[34,35] This operation is not advised for the acute injury but is excellent for treating late symptoms that do not respond to nonoperative measures. As much bone is removed as possible while leaving the coracoacromial ligaments or their remnants intact. Additional space may be achieved by removing part of the acromion. Great care is required to reattach securely the fascia of the trapezius and deltoid over the gap. Long-term follow-up of competitive athletes indicates excellent functional results. Cybex testing showed minimal deficits, particularly with rapid motion.[36] It is surprising how well some throwing athletes do with this procedure, but significant patience is required for it to be successful, as at least 12 weeks is necessary before vigorous exercise and training are progressed. This interval allows firm healing of the muscle attachment and some maturation of the collagen. Weight-lifting athletes may continue to have difficulty with maximal bench pressing activities and should be warned about this possibility.

GLENOHUMERAL JOINT PROBLEMS

Formerly shoulder instability and impingement syndromes were considered distinct entities. In reality, there are two overlapping spectrums (Fig. 21-35). The stability of the joint ranges from the most structurally secure to a lax, poorly controlled joint with multidirectional instability. Added to this picture are the results of trauma, which range from mild repetitive overuse, to single significant forms of stress, e.g., a blow or a fall. Problems of the glenohumeral joint are discussed under the headings of impingement, adhesive capsulitis (frozen shoulder), bicipital syndromes, and subacromial bursitis (subdeltoid bursitis).

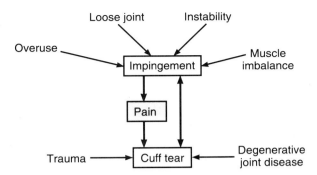

Fig. 21-35. Relations between impingement, pain, and cuff tears.

Clinical Point

ANTERIOR IMPINGEMENT SYNDROME

- Young athlete
  - Tendinitis
  - Mainly overuse
  - Occasionally trauma
- Older individual
  - Tendinitis or bursitis
  - May be related to overuse
  - Also consider osteophytes
- All ages
  - Consider cuff tears

Impingement

Anatomic Considerations

Impingement occurs underneath the coracoacromial arch. This arch is formed by the acromion as far back as the acromioclavicular joint and anteriorly by the coracoacromial ligament (Fig. 21-4). Formerly most impingements were thought to be laterally underneath the acromion, but usually the major site of compression is slightly anterior underneath the angle of the acromion and the coracoacromial ligament. In the past there has been a suggestion that the anatomic shape of the acromion, in particular those with an anterior beak, leaves an individual congenitally susceptible to impingement. Although impingement undoubtably exists, and the term anterior impingement syndrome is reasonable to use, it should not detract from the major source of problems in the young athlete, which is tendinitis. This tendinitis is generated by overuse, poor training techniques, inappropriate selection of exercises, and trauma. In many young athletes the impingement is secondary to chronic soft tissue inflammation, swelling, and thickening. In some situations, particularly in the older individual where significant osteophytes develop under the surface of the acromion or in a degenerative acromioclavicular joint, impingement occurs either laterally or medially in relation to the latter structures. This fact may ultimately affect important surgical decisions in intractable cases. The most vulnerable structures for impingement are the greater tuberosity and the overlying supraspinatus tendon, the subdeltoid (subacromial) bursa, and the long head of the biceps tendon.

The biceps tendon may be important for supporting the superior aspect of the glenohumeral joint. In particular, during the motion of abduction and flexion, the biceps tendon slides through the bicipital groove. Sometimes it is preferable to think of the biceps tendon being static in this situation and the grooves sliding over the tendon. Hitchcock and Bechtol in 1948 pointed out that the bicipital groove is not in the direct line of pull of the biceps tendon. In fact, the tendon turns abruptly over the head of the humerus to run in the groove and angles about another 30 to 40 degrees medially.[37] Inflammation of this tendon is one of the most common entities causing shoulder disability in the swimmer and in the throwing arm of the baseball pitcher, quarterback, and javelin thrower. The stress on this tendon during throwing motions is incredible. In addition, there are some anatomic variations of this bicipital groove. In some individuals the groove is narrow, leading to increased friction during the movements of rotation and abduction and flexion, whereas in others the groove is shallow allowing the tendon to sublux up and down in the groove, which may eventually lead to tendinitis of the shoulder. This subject is discussed in the section on bicipital syndromes (see below). Bicipital tendinitis is one of the entities included under the heading swimmer's shoulder.

The rotator cuff muscles are the deep rotator muscles of the shoulder girdle, and they become confluent as their tendons insert around the head of the humerus (Fig. 21-36). These muscles work indirectly with the other muscles of the shoulder to produce the large movements that are present. In addition, they make fine adjustments of the position of the humeral head in the glenoid fossa (Fig. 21-7). It has been dem-

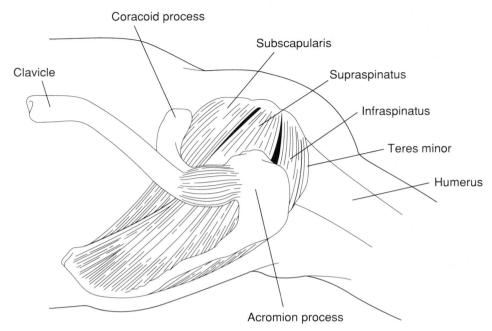

Fig. 21-36. Muscles of the rotator cuff reinforce the glenohumeral joint capsule. They include the subscapularis, supraspinatus, and teres minor muscles (viewed from above).

onstrated by McNab that there is a poor blood supply to this tendon, particularly while the arm is in the dependent position.[38] For this reason there is often degeneration of the tendon with age, and the cuff is susceptible to inflammation and tearing. Both entities may heal slowly and cause considerable problems during abduction.[39]

Clinical Entities

Although the spectrum of pathologic changes within the soft tissues underneath the coracoacromial arch may occur at any age, frequently the time course and basic pathophysiology are such that, classically, three major clinical subgroups may be identified (Table 21-4). The emphasis on either bicipital or supraspinatus tendinitis as a distinct entity has shifted, as invariably both structures are involved to a lesser or greater degree. Hence there is a tendency just to use the term anterior impingement syndrome.

Grade I Impingement

Grade I is the commonest impingement in young athletes. It usually occurs between the ages of 16 and 30 but is often seen in the early teens in young swimmers and gymnasts. The main etiologic factor is over-

stress of the area by prolonged repetitive overhead activity, frequently in the impingement position. For example, the young high level competitive swimmer who has trained up to 7,000 meters per day has experienced approximately 750,000 shoulder rotations a year. If a 7- or 8-year-old competes for 5 years, he or she will have performed about 4 million shoulder rotations.[40] As a result, many of these individuals have developed significant cuff and bicipital tendon inflammation at the age of 13 and 14 years. A specific subgroup among these young athletes are those with varying degrees of instability at the shoulder and hence poor control and positioning of the humeral head in the glenoid. Some have sufficient instability to experience subluxation. This aspect must be detected because the treatment not only involves modification of activity but greatly emphasizes control of the humeral head.

There is usually a reversible inflammation and edema of either the long head of biceps or supraspinatus tendon. There is pain with activity, initially only in the impingement position, but ultimately through a larger range as the inflammation and edema become more severe and more of the cuff is involved. The result is an increasingly broader painful arc. One of the prime responsibilities of the rotator cuff ten-

TABLE 21-4. Pathologic Changes Underneath the Coracoacromial Arch

Impingement	Common Age Group (years)	Main Etiologic Factors	Diagnosis	Treatment
Grade I	18–30	Overstress Repetitive circumduction activities Joint laxity	Clinical Impingement tests	Activity modification Analysis of techniques Modification of style Decrease stresses of weight training Correct muscle imbalance Selective stretching Ultrasound, laser, ice If long-standing, transverse friction NSAIDs, steroid injection
Grade II	30–45	Overuse Sudden increase in activity Fall or subluxation Some early degenerative changes in cuff Occasionally calcification	Clinical impingement tests X-ray films to reveal dystrophic calcification or osteophytic lipping Occasionally osteolysis of distal clavicle	Restrict aggravating activities Treat as above Early consideration of steroid injection Decompressive surgery
Grade III	45+	Occupational Falls Sudden increase in activity Atrophic and degenerative changes in cuff Occasionally acute tear	Clinical Impingement tests External rotation weakness X-ray plain films May be superior migration of humeral head Consider arthrogram (CT)	As above Greater restriction of activity May need surgical decompression or rotator cuff repair

dons is to hold the humeral head in the fossa. With inflammation comes reflex weakness and atrophy, and the cuff may then fail to stabilize the head. Hence the deltoid may pull the humeral head tighter under the coracoacromial arch, developing further aggravation and impingement. The specific impingement tests are then positive for either the biceps tendon, the supraspinatus, or both.

Treatment depends on the severity, acuteness, and duration of the inflammatory response, as well as the activity goals of the individual. Complete restriction of motion through the painful range allows the earliest resolution of symptoms. An analysis of aggravating exercises and motions can direct the advice on modification of training programs. When the condition is severe and long-standing, all activities should be carefully itemized by the athlete and put in three columns with the following headings: painless, mildly uncomfortable, and painful. The latter two columns are rank-ordered as to the severity of the discomfort (Table 21-5). In this fashion a logical approach to restriction of activity, activity modification, and eventually gradual resumption of activity may be carried out. Activities from the "painful" column should not

be reintroduced until the individual is pain-free during all movements in the "mildly uncomfortable" column. With early mild but acute conditions, the activity sequence may be progressed after 2 weeks of being completely free of symptoms. With chronic, severe cases, a minimum of 6 weeks pain-free is desirable before starting to add activities from the formally "mildly uncomfortable" and subsequently the "painful" column. More rapid resumption of activity may be possible but frequently runs the risk of flaring up the symptoms or prolonging the treatment due to repetitive minor setbacks. This system is referred to as the "activity progression protocol" for brevity in further discussions of the impingement syndrome (Table 21-5). It is a good system to adopt with most cases of tendinitis throughout the body.

Anti-inflammatory medication and the judicious use of the occasional cortisone injections are useful supplements to the physiotherapy modalities of ultrasound, laser, interferential therapy, ice, and heat. When the history of inflammation and pain is longer than 12 weeks and there is an element of chronicity, transverse frictions are a reasonably initial approach. If the latter is considered part of the therapy, it

TABLE 21-5. Preparation of an Activity Progression Protocol

Step I	List all activities performed by the athlete during a workout.

Step II	Categorize activities and list in columns
	   1. Painless
	   2. Mildly uncomfortable
	   3. Painful

Step III	Rank order items in columns 2 and 3 worst to least severe.
Step IV	Devise workout from item in column 1. Consider strength, flexibility, cardiovascular requirements of sport. Consider skills required for activity.

Step V	Early mild cases of inflammation.
	   Start adding sequentially higher items from column 2 one at a time after a 2-week pain-free period.
	   Do not add items from column 3 until all column 2 items have been substituted and no flare-up of
	      symptoms is seen.
	   Increase intensity and duration carefully with each item.
	Chronic or severe symptoms of inflammation.
	   Do not add items from column 2 until athlete is pain-free for 6 weeks.

Step VI	As appropriate skills are gained, add frequency and intensity, allowing gradual resumption and integration
	   into sport.
	If symptoms start to flare up, back up one or two items from the appropriate column and keep doing it
	   until a pain-free level of activity achieved.
	Reassess diagnosis, and alter medication or physical therapy as needed.

should precede the use of NSAIDs or injections, which are best timed to coincide with the completion of the course of "transverse frictions." Although injections into the subacromial space is perhaps safer and assumes dispersal throughout the involved area of the cuff, a more direct approach is usually efficacious (Fig. 21–37).

The active component of therapy involves setting out the activity progression protocol and then assessing the role of hypermobility of the glenohumeral joint versus normal or decreased motion. Any contributing cervical pathology is attended to, along with an analysis of thoracic motion and thoracolumbar integration in movement patterns. These peripheral contributing elements are treated pari passu with the shoulder inflammation. Exercises for the shoulder must be in the pain-free range, concentrating on the deep rotators and aiming at restoring control during rotation and elevation rather than pure strengthening (Figs. 21-38 and 21-39). Biofeedback may be appropriate if there is excessive laxity of the humeral head or if the athlete is unable to gain control of the rotators. When good control is achieved and pain has resolved, the emphasis may be switched to include more specific strengthening. An isokinetic evaluation may unmask strength deficits or strength ratio disproportion. Ultimately, a careful analysis of contrib-

uting factors, e.g., the style of the swimming strokes, throwing techniques, the serving style at tennis, or the performance of special aggravating weight training exercises or stretching maneuvers, is the key to preventing recurrence. Therapy culminates with the introduction of specific functional exercises and usually, with competitive athletes, some dialogue with the coach to ensure an appropriate buildup to preinjury levels of training.

On occasion, failure to respond to therapy promotes further investigation of contributing factors by plain roentgenograms, an arthrogram, CT scan, and arthroscopy. Resection of the coracoacromial ligament is appropriate in a small number of young athletes. These principles are applicable to some degree to all of the subsequent clinical subgroups described.

Grade II Impingement

Individuals with grade II impingement are invariably in a slightly older age group, between 30 and 45 years. Again, the history is one of overuse; and middle-aged athletes doing excessive weight training, tennis, squash, or swimming for triathlons comprise the major group of physically active individuals. The condition is also frequently seen as the result of occupational stress, subsequent to large bouts of episodic

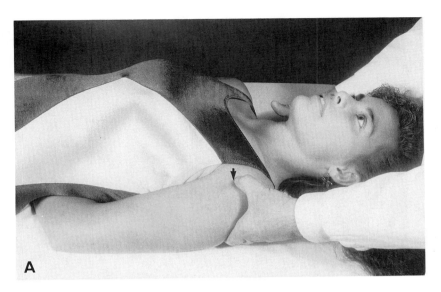

Fig. 21-37. Injection for anterior impingement syndrome. **(A)** Patient is positioned lying with the arm internally rotated and placed in the small of the back. The tender point is confirmed. **(B)** This positioning delivers the supraspinatus and biceps tendon to the anterior aspect of the joint, where it is easily accessible. The needle is introduced with approximately 1 ml of steroid suspension mixed with 1–2 ml of 1 percent lidocaine hydrochloride. The needle is advanced until it reaches the resistance of bone and is then withdrawn slightly. It then can be "walked" across the most tender area with a series of half withdrawals and reinsertions. This technique may be more effective if it is supplemented by placing half of the solution into the subacromial bursa area.

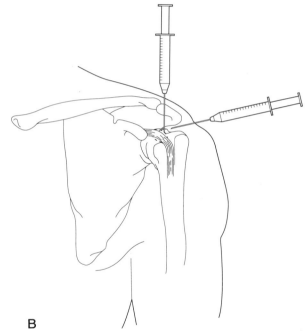

activities such as weekend gardening or wood chopping, and occasionally following single bouts of trauma such as a fall or a subluxation-dislocation of the shoulder.

The basic pathophysiology is inflammation superimposed on fraying or thinning of the cuff. In some individuals it is complicated by varying degrees of calcification or even early osteophytic lipping from the edge of the acromion.

The athlete presents with a fairly broad area of anterior tenderness, sometimes with exquisite point pain to palpation over either the biceps or the supraspinatus tendon. Occasionally, there is associated subacromial bursitis. There is a decreased range of motion largely due to pain and a positive impingement test. Radiologic studies may show some calcification or early osteophyte formation.

Treatment usually involves significant early restriction of specific aggravating motions and activity modification. NSAIDs are frequently necessary to allow

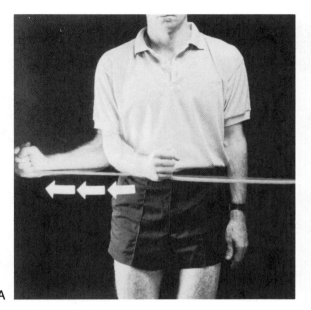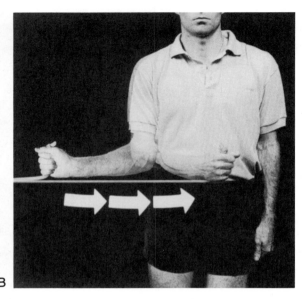

A   B

Fig. 21-38. **(A)** External rotation using elastic tubing for resistance. It is important to keep the elbow well tucked into the waist so the rotation is isolated at the shoulder. **(B)** Internal rotation.

resolution, often in association with a corticosteroid injection. After initial local therapy with ultrasound or laser, emphasis is on restoring range of motion and stretching tight structures. Restoration of strength and balance of strength between muscle groups, as well as an activity progression protocol, are required to allow resumption of sport. Because the infraspinatus is the only muscle in a position to generate a significant inferior vector on the humeral head, attention to specific strengthening of this muscle may help reduce the dynamic impingement in abduction. For some individuals the symptoms fail to resolve, or they have repeated "flare-ups"; in these cases arthroscopy, surgical decompression, or possibly permanent adjustment and modification of activity is a solution.

Grade III Impingement

By age 45 most individuals have some quality change in the collagen of the rotator cuff and perhaps some subtle alteration in the vascular supply. MacNab illustrated well a watershed area in the cuff where the microvasculature is diminished, perhaps leaving a vulnerable critical zone that is susceptible to trauma and less able to heal itself efficiently after damage.[38] Grade III changes in the cuff include thinning and fraying, degenerative changes, even full-thickness de-

fects and tearing in the region of the supraspinatus, and occasionally rupture of the biceps tendon.

There is usually a history of long usage in the individual's occupation or sport, although an acute tear may follow a specific episode of trauma or violent activity. Radiologic studies may show osteophytes from the inferior and anterior edge of the acromion and occasionally from the inferior surface of the distal clavicle at the acromioclavicular joint (Fig. 21-40). There may be a decreased distance between the humeral head and the acromion. Special studies such as arthrograms, CT scans, or MRI may reveal a defect.

Clinical Point

INDICATIONS FOR ARTHROGRAPHY

- Unresponsive impingement syndrome (>40 years of age)
- Sudden weakness after trauma
- Bicipital tendon rupture
- Glenohumeral instability (>40 years of age)

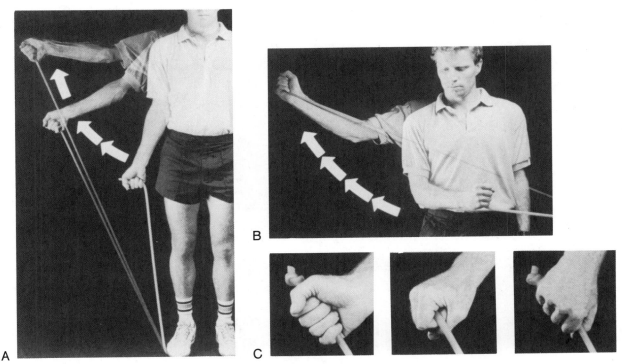

Fig. 21-39. Abduction using tubing resistance. It can be done in the plane of the body, **(A)** or in a diagonal pattern **(B)**, which amalgamates flexion and rotation, and is a more physiologic motion in the plane of the scapula. **(C)** Hand positions adopted for pure abduction exercises.

Examination is characterized by finding a painful area, frequently a reversed glenohumeral rhythm and tenderness over a wide area. There is a varying amount of weakness, particularly in abduction and internal rotation. It is more pronounced, and usually accompanied by wasting, if there is a rotator cuff tear.

The therapy is much the same as in a grade II situation, but the need for surgical decompression and possible repair of the cuff tear is more likely.

Glenohumeral Joint Arthropathy

Glenohumeral joint arthropathy is usually seen after the age of 65. The pathophysiology includes varying degrees of degenerative change of the joint, osteophyte formation, and often an associated rotator cuff arthropathy characterized by a large defect in the cuff and superior migration of the humeral head (Figs. 21-40 and 21-41).

The history is one of long-standing shoulder pain, weakness, and decreased range. Activity and usage of the shoulder has been curtailed and trick compensatory motions adopted. Examination reveals a broad area of tenderness, often referred pain into the neck and posterior shoulder area, and weakness and muscle wasting. Adduction and external rotation are particularly affected, and a reverse glenohumeral rhythm invariably is present.

Treatment involves the use of NSAIDs and occasionally an injection of corticosteroid. An attempt is made to restore a functional range of motion. A careful assessment of activity patterns is necessary. Frequently the recreational goals in this age group entails golf, tennis, and swimming; and advice regarding the degree of participation in these areas must be considered in light of the magnitude of the problem. For the less severe cases, decompression by excision and division of the tip of the acromion and coracoacromial ligament and possible excision of the distal clavicle with removal of associated acromial osteophytes may be satisfactory, along with a cuff repair. Usually the damage is more extensive, and the edges of the defect

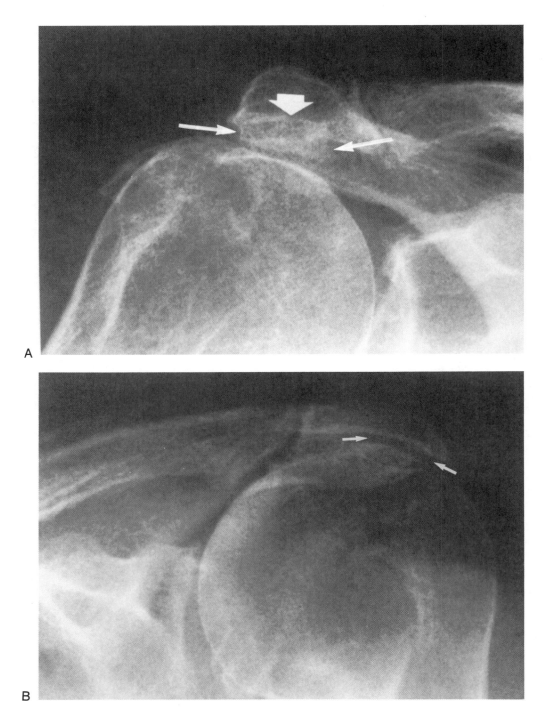

Fig. 21-40. Rotator cuff degeneration and impingement. **(A)** Sclerosis of the greater tuberosity and the acromion process with hypertrophic changes, osteophytes, and lipping at the margin, which contributes to the painful inflammatory response. **(B)** Superior migration of the humeral head. The anterior acromion process and the distal clavicle frequently develop a concave appearance as a result of pressure over a long period of time by the humeral head. Long-standing cuff disease is often associated with subcortical cystic erosion at the angle of the cuff insertion and greater tuberosity; frequently it is seen with degenerative changes in the acromioclavicular joint. This problem contributes to the impingement picture.

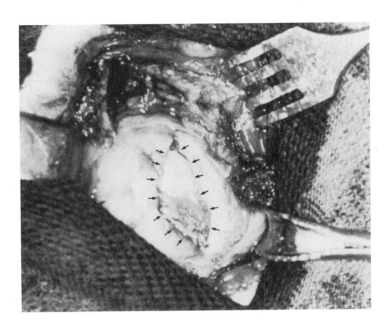

Fig. 21-41. Large tear in the rotator cuff mainly in the supraspinatus muscle (outlined by arrows). Articular surface of the humeral head is visible through the defect.

are debrided with no repair attempted. This treatment is compatible with remarkably good function because it relieves much of the pain. When advanced and end-stage glenohumeral arthritis is present, the only surgical treatment may be a shoulder arthroplasty, but it is reserved for selected cases.

Rotator Cuff Tears

Rotator cuff tears have been dealt with in the previous paragraphs. There are two main groups: traumatic and degenerative. The two merge imperceptibly into each other, but obviously the trauma required to rupture a healthy strong cuff in a young individual is dramatically different from that required to injure the thin atrophic cuff of the elderly.[39]

Clinical Point

Cuff tears are frequently overlooked.

The main purpose of the discussion is to raise the level of awareness of the possibility of a cuff injury, as this entity is frequently overlooked.[40] In the age group 25 and over, the possibility of a cuff tear must always be entertained when an impingement syndrome exists that is intractable to treatment.

In the young athlete, a cuff tear should be considered when an impingement syndrome develops after a traumatic episode and the pain is accompanied by significant weakness and wasting in the supraspinatus fossa. A decrease in external rotation strength is highly suggestive of a partial or complete tear if the history and the remaining physical findings are compatible.

Clinical Point

EXTERNAL ROTATION STRENGTH

- Decrease in external rotation power frequently is related to size and location of cuff tears.
- Isolated supraspinatus tear may present with weakness of external rotation

---

Special tests such as arthrography, CT, or MRI can confirm the presence, location, and size of the defect. Severe tears are usually easy to diagnose clinically, have significant functional deficits, and require early surgery. Small tears are treated with respect to their size, functional implications, the aims and goals of the individual. They have some capacity to heal, and it may be appropriate to carry out a nonoperative rehabilitation regimen for 6 months before deciding on surgical repair. It should be recalled that a C5–C6 disc lesion may result in weakness similar to that demonstrated by an individual with a cuff tear.

Initially the treatment is directed at reducing pain and allowing early healing. At first range of motion is emphasized, and then by 6 weeks the strengthening is increased and slowly progressed. If recovery is nearly full at 6 months and most symptoms have resolved, it is appropriate to wait until nine month post injury before deciding on the need for a surgical course. Significant symptoms at 6 months invariably indicate lack of healing, and surgical cuff repair is the treatment of choice in those individuals who have an active life style (Fig. 21–41).

Adhesive Capsulitis (Frozen Shoulder)

The term "frozen shoulder" describes a syndrome rather than a diagnosis. It is the adverse outcome of several clinical entities, usually within the shoulder complex although sometimes remote. It is characterized by painful restriction of active and passive motion of the glenohumeral joint, with no significant improvement after corticosteroid injection and a demonstrable contracted capsule on the arthrogram.[41] It is an uncommon entity in athletes, but when it does occur it is usually the result of excessive immobilization following trauma or in association with tendinitis or bursitis in the age group 40 years and over. There seems to be an individual predisposition to develop the entity, and frequently it merges imperceptibly into the syndrome of reflex sympathetic dystrophy, in which case there should be swelling, skin changes, vasomotor instability, and excessive resorption of calcium from the humeral head. In the full-blown picture the entire upper limb is involved in the "shoulder-hand syndrome."

Duplay is credited with the initial description in 1872, referring to it as humeroscapular periarthritis. Codman (1934) coined the term "frozen shoulder."[39] Neviaser in 1945 surgically explored the lesion noting capsular thickening, contraction, adhesions, and decreased synovial fluid. Thus arose the term adhesive capsulitis.[42,43] The degree of capsular adhesion and inflammation is subject to much debate and may depend on the precipitating etiologic factor and the stage of evolution of the condition. Whatever the pathology, it appears that both inert and contractile elements are involved, and there is usually a global or capsular pattern of stiffness in which exter-

nal rotation is limited most, followed by abduction, then forward flexion and internal rotation.

Clinical Point

SHOULDER CAPSULAR PATTERN OF RESTRICTION

- External rotation loss
    greater than
- Abduction loss
    greater than
- Forward flexion

- Internal rotation least affected

The gradual evolution from a primary contractile element inflammation may confuse the picture until the syndrome is well established. However, this entity should be suspected whenever the usual favorable clinical response to therapy of a bursitis or tendinitis is replaced by increasing generalized discomfort and a tendency to lose range of motion. It is possible that aggressive intervention at the earliest possible stages may thwart the usual protracted clinical course of the fully developed frozen shoulder. Wiley and Older brought our attention to the findings of internal derangement in the form of labral lesions, cuff tears, and obliterated subscapular bursa as potential triggering factors in the development of this syndrome. These lesions were identified by arthroscopy even in the presence of a normal arthrogram.[42] These causes must be considered in the young athlete and the possible use of early arthroscopy considered. Reeves described three overlapping phases: pain, stiffness, and recovery.[44]

Phase I (Pain)

The early painful period lasts 10 to 36 weeks. Arthrographic findings include decreased joint volume and obliteration of the subscapularis bursa and sometimes the biceps sheath. By the end of this stage, as the pain starts to decline the capsular capacity is at its smallest.

Treatment during phase I includes encouraging active range of motion within the pain-free range, gentle joint mobilization and a trial of NSAIDs. Usually a one-per-day preparation is most practical, as these NSAIDs may have to be continued for a protracted period of time to allow the most comfort and maintain maximal function. Aggravating factors must be discontinued, and there is an emphasis on rest and support.

It is worthwhile attempting a distension injection of the joint with 10 to 30 ml of sterile saline mixed with some injectable steroid preparation. The normal joint has a capacity of 25 to 35 ml, and as much fluid is forced into the joint as the patient can tolerate. It is important to allow time for the local anesthetic to have effect and often as little as 3 ml can be administered, followed by gradual instillation up to 10 ml. After this point, instillation may be easier. With respect to needle placement, the best and most reproducible point of entry is the lateral margin of the coracoid process, with the arm at the side and externally rotated.[41] This procedure may be supplemented with a posterior subacromial distension, which may be repeated two or three times at 6-week intervals. It may abort a full-blown frozen shoulder syndrome. It may be helpful to consider a manipulation under anesthesia, but there are few guidelines to the best timing of this procedure.

Phase II (Stiffness)

Phase II is characterized by stiffness for a duration of approximately 4 to 12 months. The condition seems to become static. Although attempts to increase motion must be encouraged, great care is necessary not to increase pain. It is tempting to consider that manipulation under anesthesia would help these individuals and that after an initial acute flare-up of pain and inflammation the range gained at operation could be regained by intensive therapy. The efficacy and role of this type of forceful, gross manipulation is uncertain. The timing and indications are equally obtuse. Results at any stage are unpredictable. The best results are probably obtained if the manipulation is performed during the first 12 to 20 weeks, after which the trauma involved becomes more dangerous, fracture of the weakened bone a reality, and capsular tearing and dislocation well documented. Nevertheless, there are advocates for this therapy at all stages and enough success to make condemnation of this approach inappropriate.

By contrast, mobilization techniques to restore joint play are important adjuncts to treatment (Figs. 21-42 and 21-43). The classic techniques illustrated may have to be modified to adjust for the amount of restriction present. The use of heat, ice, ultrasound,

transcutaneous electrical nerve stimulation (TENS), and acupuncture have their advocates, and their use should be gauged according to their success with each patient. Similarly, even the NSAIDs are idiosyncratic in terms of efficacy with the frozen shoulder syndrome.

Phase III (Recovery)

Phase III is the recovery period and lasts 6 months to 2 years. It is heralded by a gradual increase in the amount of external rotation obtainable. Previous studies have shown it to coincide with the reappearance of the subscapular bursa. Exercise, activity, and the use of modalities should fit the changing clinical condition (Figs. 21-44 and 21-45).

Essentially, the goal in this extraordinary, ill-understood condition is to be alert for the earliest signs of its development, and then to treat aggressively. Whenever possible, avoid prolonged immobilization with painful, inflammatory conditions, thereby reducing the risk of the syndrome. For the most part the length of recovery correlates well with the duration of the early painful phase; thus reduction of this component has the greatest impact on early and late morbidity.

Bicipital Syndromes

This section deals with three basic pathologic processes that involve the long head of the biceps: inflammation, instability, and rupture. Although an incredibly important component of the anterior impingement syndrome, biceps tendinitis has received relatively little attention in the sports medicine literature.

The tendon is stressed during all rapid overhead motions, and thus bicipital pathology is frequently seen in baseball pitchers, football quarterbacks, swimmers, javelin throwers, and shot-putters.

The tendon of the long head of the biceps has its origin at the supraglenoid tubercle and adjacent glenoid labrum. It passes intracapsularly into and through the osseofibrous tunnel formed by the bicipital groove and the transverse ligament. The transverse ligament is composed of specialized transverse fibers of the capsule extending between the two tubercles. Within the capsule the long head arises as a round tendon, becomes flattened coursing through the shoulder joint, and narrows in the intertubercular area.[45] Hitchcock and Bechtol pointed out that the

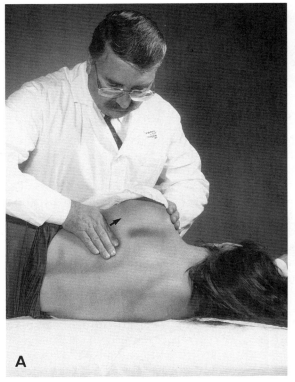

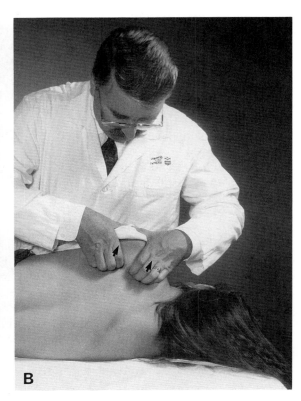

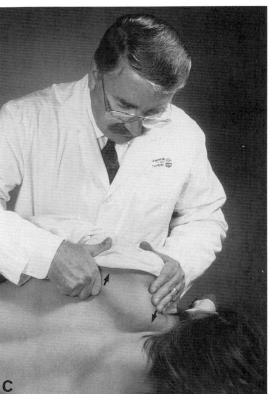

Fig. 21-42. Mobilization techniques for the scapula on the chest wall. **(A)** Superior and inferior motion. **(B)** Elevation and protraction. **(C)** Rotation of the superior and inferior angle.

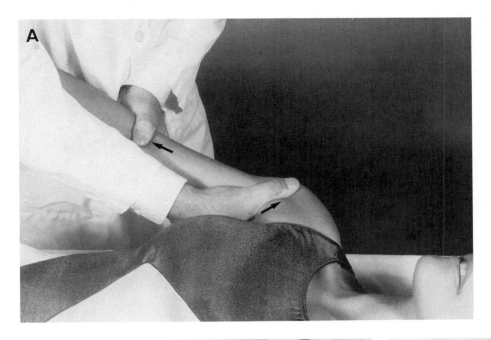

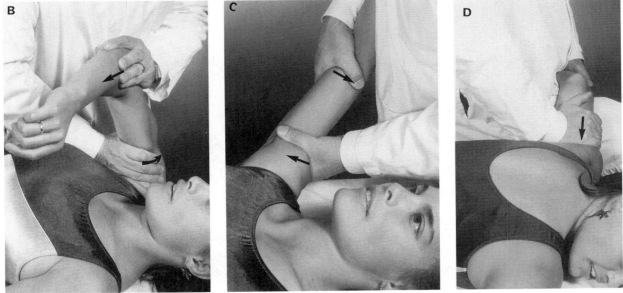

Fig. 21-43. Mobilization of the glenohumeral articulation. **(A)** Longitudinal distraction levering over the proximal hand to produce an inferior glide of the humerus with lateral distraction. **(B)** Lateral distraction in cross flexion. **(C)** Glenoid gliding done at various positions of abduction and flexion. **(D)** Anterior glide using the therapist's knee as a fulcrum and the patient in the prone position. All of these mobilizations **(A–D)** can be done with two hands much nearer the fulcrum, producing smaller movements initially. Occasionally a strap is used to stabilize the chest and scapula.

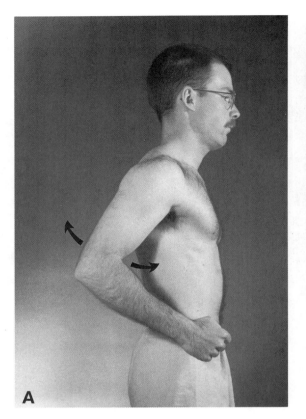
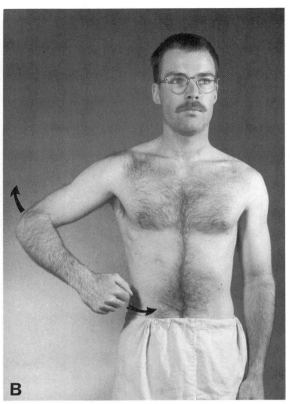

Fig. 21-44. Gentle active mobilizing exercises for the shoulder. **(A)** Flexion extension saw exercises. **(B)** Cross body saw exercises, start position. These movements added to pendular exercises are increased in magnitude as range is gained. (See Fig. 21-65.)

biceps tendon does not so much slide in the bicipital groove but, rather, the groove slides over the tendon.[37] Indeed, the relative motion of the osseous groove with the tendon is approximately 1.5 to 3.8 cm.

Apart from the biceps' well established function of flexion and supination at the elbow, the long head is active during flexion of the shoulder if the forearm is supinated and during abduction when the arm is externally rotated. It also apparently assists in stabilization of the glenohumeral joint, possibly by controlling upward and forward motion of the head, but in a subsidiary manner to the cuff.

Bicipital Tendinitis

In the young athlete overuse is the outstanding etiologic factor for bicipital tendinitis and it usually forms part of the etiology of the anterior impinge-

ment syndrome. De Palma noted that the synovial sheath was inflamed, swollen, frequently hemorrhagic, and bulged proximally and distally to the transverse ligament. The tendon may become stenotic and rest within a meshwork of adhesions.[47] Approximately two-thirds of clinically localized inflammation involved the biceps tendon alone, with the remaining cases showing pathology of the adjacent rotator cuff or subacromial bursa.

Clinically, like most tendinitis, the syndrome goes through stages of discomfort and may ultimately preclude all activity if not treated. Symptoms are noticed during: (1) the serve and overhead strokes of tennis; (2) the follow-through stages of the golf swing as the shoulder flexes and externally rotates; (3) the catch and pull-through phases of many of the swimming strokes; and (4) many overhead motions of other sports activities.[48] Local tenderness in the groove, an increasingly sensitive painful arc, and positive im-

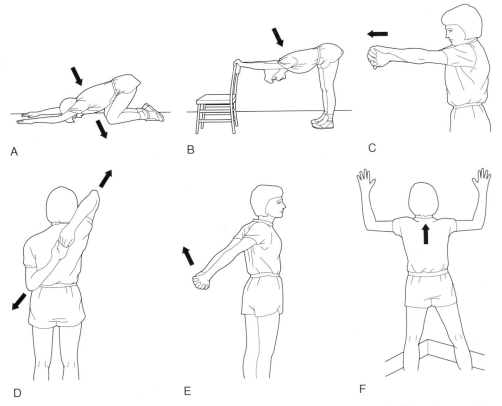

Fig. 21-45. Advanced shoulder flexibility exercises. **(A)** Kneeling stretch. Kneeing on the mat and leaning forward with the arms extended in front of the head. The chest is lowered to the mat and held for a few seconds. The stretch is felt on the upper chest and anterior shoulder girdle. **(B)** Progression of the anterior stretch to a standing position. Start by flexing at the waist and lowering the head between the arms as far as possible, then hold the stretch position. **(C)** Posterior scapular and shoulder girdle stretch. The hands are clasped with thumbs pointing to the floor, and forearms are crisscrossed. The stretch is performed by reaching as far forward as possible and holding. **(D)** Back-hand pull. Initially this exercise can be done with a towel or a piece of rope between the hands until extra range is gained. The hands are held as close together as possible, and a pull and hold position is maintained. The exercise is repeated by reversing hands. **(E)** Back-arm lift. This exercise stretches the anterior shoulder girdle. The arms are slowly raised as far as possible behind and held for a few seconds. Initially the exercise can be commenced by holding a small pillow between the hands until greater flexibility is achieved. **(F)** Anterior capsular stretch in corner of room.

pingement tests are present if the inflammation is sufficient. Other tests that have varying degrees of efficacy and sensitivity are the Yergason's supination test and Speed's test. Although frequently associated with bicipital tendinitis, none is pathognomonic.

Yergason's test involves the patient attempting to supinate the flexed elbow while externally rotating the shoulder. The examiner makes sure the elbow remains stabilized against the trunk (Fig. 21-21). Pain in the bicipital groove constitutes a positive test.[49]

Speed's test involves forward shoulder flexion of the extended, supinated elbow.[50] A positive test is marked by pain in the region of the bicipital groove. Because of the relative motion of the tendon, this test is frequently more sensitive than Yergason's test (Fig. 21-21).

Treatment is along the lines described for grade I impingement syndromes. In the early stages, activity modification and an activity progression protocol are important, along with NSAIDs, ultrasound, laser, or interferential therapy. Adequate pre- and post-activity icing followed by warm-up and stretching help to contain the symptoms. The judicious use of injections of corticosteroid, carefully infiltrated around the tendon or in the subacromial space and repeated at 6-week intervals on one to three occasions, may resolve protracted cases. Often patients must be counseled to realistically evaluate their aspirations and goals if the problem is unresponsive to the usual treatment approaches. When sufficiently protracted, or if athletes are unwilling to give up their activity goals, consideration should be given to surgical decompression of the coracoacromial arch. Tenolysis of the tendon in its groove or even transfer of the tendon to the tip of the coracoid may be considered in recalcitrant cases.[50]

Tendon Instability (Subluxation and Dislocation)

The first reported case of dislocation of the long head of the biceps was in 1694 by William Cowper, who reported on such a lesion manifested when wringing out clothes.[45] Sporadic reports appeared after that, but it was O'Donoghue who brought attention to the lesion in athletes, noting that it was not rare in baseball pitchers, quarterbacks, javelin throwers, and shot-putters.[51]

The transverse humeral ligament is classically offered as the most important restraining structure, holding the long head of the biceps tendon in its groove. This concept is contested by others, however, who believe that the coracohumeral ligament is equally, if not more, important. The coracohumeral ligament is a thickening in the fibrous capsule that arises from the lateral edge of the coracoid process; it blends with the capsule and inserts into the lesser and greater tuberosities. Slatis and Alato resected the transverse ligament in cadavers and noted that the biceps tendon did not displace until the coracohumeral ligament was also divided.[52] Thus it seems both structures play a role.

There are several factors that may predispose to subluxation and dislocation, including the angle of the medial wall of the groove, the depth of the groove, and the presence of a supratubercular ridge. The normal medial wall angle is approximately 60 to 70 degrees, and angles less than 30 degrees are frequently associated with a shallow groove and predispose to subluxation.[37,51]

Quick Facts

UNSTABLE LONG HEAD OF THE BICEPS

- Normal bicipital groove 60 to 70 degrees
- Less than 30 degrees associated with instability
- Shallow groove associated with instability
- Coracohumeral and transverse ligament important
- Presence of supratubercular ridge predisposes tendon to attrition and subluxation
- Repetitive forceful abduction in external rotation may precipitate pathology
- Single traumatic episode may be triggering factor particularly with a cuff tear

---

The presence of a supratubercular ridge may be associated with tendon attrition, degeneration, or even instability. This ridge of bone extends proximally, continuous with the medial wall of the groove on the lesser tuberosity in 55 percent of the population but is well developed in only approximately 18 percent.[7] It possibly forces the biceps tendon against the transverse ligament, increasing the tension. Furthermore, spur formation on the lesser tuberosity is seen more frequently with this ridge, which may aggravate the tendon and its sheath.

Peterson has illustrated that the dislocating tendon frequently slips over the medial wall of the groove and lesser tuberosity, under the subscapularis muscle,[53] which lends support to the notion that the mechanism is associated with either a traumatic cuff tear, as would occur with glenohumeral subluxation or dislocation, or a chronic stretching secondary to repetitive forceful throwing activities (Fig. 21-46).

Clinically the athlete may complain of anterior shoulder pain during and after activity. Occasionally, with violent overhead motion, the "dead arm syndrome" is experienced—a feeling of transient weakness and the shoulder "going out." In these circumstances the diagnosis may be overlooked and the symptoms attributed to glenohumeral instability. When the athlete describes snapping in the region of the tendon, the diagnosis is more obvious. Pain over

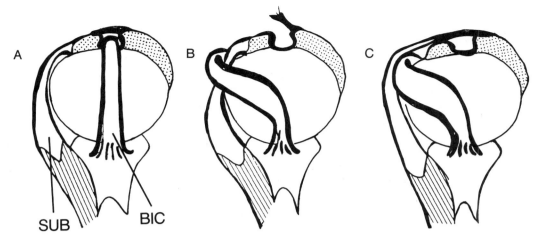

Fig. 21-46. Relation between the tendinous long head of the biceps (BIC) and the subscapularis (SUB). **(A)** Normal relation. **(B)** Medial dislocation of the biceps tendon riding over subscapularis with either rupture or stretching of the transverse ligament. **(C)** Medial dislocation where the tendon has slid medially to the bicipital groove, deep to the subscapular tendon.

the tendon to palpation and a click during internal-external rotation maneuvers help confirm the diagnosis. Sometimes the instability of the tendon is better demonstrated with the Yergason's or Speed's test (Fig. 21-21). The snapping may be enhanced by asking the athlete to hold a 5 pound weight in each arm and bringing the extended, externally rotated limbs above the head through abduction. When the examiner stands behind and palpates the biceps tendon, a palpable, frequently audible snap may be experienced, often with associated sharp pain, in the range 90 to 110 degrees.

Radiologic tests may help supplement the clinical diagnosis. Plain roentgenograms of the bicipital groove may help evaluate its shape and depth, and they may record the presence of a supratubercular ridge and osteophyte formation. Arthrograms may demonstrate a displaced tendon.

Nonoperative treatment is commenced along the lines of that for any anterior impingement syndrome. It is directed at reducing repetitive stress, reducing inflammation, alleviating pain, and restoring strength, balance of power, and range of motion. If this regimen fails to resolve the problem, the contribution of the tendon instability versus simple impingement to the symptoms must be assessed. Finally, if surgery is to be contemplated, any associated cuff tear should be identified. The definitive surgical treatment may therefore include plication of the tendon to the floor of the groove and removal of the

proximal extension into the joint, decompression of the coracoacromial arch, or repair of the rotator cuff.[37,51,54]

Tendon Rupture

Ninety percent of biceps ruptures involve the proximal portion of the tendon of the long head, with 10 percent occurring more distally. Midsubstance rupture of a tendon is unusual. McMaster recognized that normal tendons rarely rupture but, rather, the tendon insertion or musculotendinous junction gives way.[55] In his experiments, he had to sever at least one-half of the tendon before rupture occurred. He estimated that up to 75 percent division of the tendon would still be compatible with the stresses of normal everyday activity.

Probably most biceps tendon ruptures are caused by subacromial impingement with tendon degeneration. With severe degenerative change, the rupture may be almost asymptomatic. Usually, however, a sudden forceful lifting effort or a fall causes the disruption. For the athletic individual over age 50, the precipitating event may be a tennis or golf swing. In younger individuals, a significant history of bicipital tendinitis and usually steroid injection feature in the story. Even so, rupture in the young person is rare, although it has been recorded in weight lifters on anabolic steroid supplementation.

The clinical picture may vary as described above,

from a vague feeling of discomfort and weakness to a dramatic painful snap. Ecchymosis and swelling appear, and the classic bunching of the tendon may take several days to develop, as adhesions stretch or remaining tendon fibers give way (Fig. 21-47).

Treatment is somewhat controversial. Most advocate surgical repair in the young athletic individual. Mariani and Cofield summarized the results of the respective surgical versus nonsurgical approaches following rupture.[56]

1. There is no difference in residual pain.
2. There are no differences in elbow motion.
3. The surgical scar is usually acceptable cosmetically.
4. The nonsurgical group were aware of the arm deformity.
5. The nonsurgical group usually returned to activities and work more rapidly, but initially at a reduced intensity.
6. There was no difference in strength of elbow extension, forearm pronation, or grip strength.

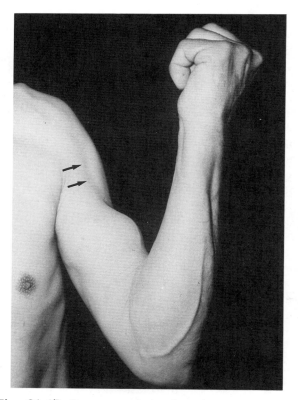

Fig. 21-47. Rupture of the long-head of biceps, showing a depression near the groove in the subdeltoid region and bunching up of the muscle distally.

7. There is usually approximately 10 percent loss of elbow flexion strength and 20 percent of supination in the nonsurgical group, although with intensive work these losses may possibly be reduced.
8. Subjectively, many individuals were aware of this weakness.

These findings confirm the advisability of the operative approach in the young, competitive individual. In the older, less competitive or sedentary individual a nonoperative approach is acceptable provided the presence of an associated cuff tear is ruled out.

Practice Point

RUPTURED BICEPS TENDON

- Complete tear in young competitive individual best treated operatively
- Nonoperative treatment acceptable
- May be loss of 10% flexion power and 20% supination power
- Ensure no associated cuff tear

When repair is carried out, there does not appear to be a clear superiority of any one procedure, but associated coracoacromial arch decompression should be considered. The rehabilitation should be tailored to fit the surgical technique and requirements of the patient.

Subacromial Bursitis (Subdeltoid Bursitis)

Acute subacromial bursitis is often generated by direct trauma in the young athletic individual, particularly a fall on the point of the shoulder. In the middle-aged and older individual this bursitis is more frequently associated with some degenerative changes in the cuff or overuse.

The athlete complains of pain in the region of the shoulder often referring to the point of the deltoid insertion. It is aggravated by motion and is frequently worse during the night and first thing in the morning. There may be a period of relief as the shoulder warms up and some of the edema is disbursed. Then during the day, with increasing activity, the pain becomes worse again. There may initially be a painful arc; and although the other movements are limited, this is not usually in a capsular pattern. With an acute, intense inflammatory response in the bursa, the patient may lose almost all capacity to abduct the arm, and the pain may refer even as far as the elbow or wrist. Whereas abduction is still painful passively, other passive movements often retain nearly full range. Resisted movements in the nonimpinged position are often free of discomfort, and palpation around the acromion process is uncomfortable.

Treatment consists in local physiotherapy, rest as indicated, and, if the condition is acute, an injection of steroid into the area.[56] The injection should be into the subacromial space; and if there is any specific uncomfortable point, a supplementary injection can be placed in that area (Fig. 21-48). Sometimes an anterior injection underneath the acromioclavicular joint as well as in the subdeltoid bursa from the lateral approach is efficacious.

In situations where the acute bursitis is associated with a calcific deposit, it is occasionally possible to aspirate some of the deposited calcific crystals with a large needle. This procedure, along with an injection of lidocaine and steroid, brings dramatic relief to what is sometimes an intense, painful condition.

After resolution of the acute syndrome, restoration of range and strength is essential. Moreover, if this condition recurs frequently, the underlying cause must be sought, e.g., degenerative changes in the cuff or acromioclavicular joint or simply overuse.

Infraspinatus Tendinitis

Infraspinatus tendinitis is seen in throwing sports, tennis, and boxing. Although the onset of this pain may be global, there is usually some localization to the infraspinatus tendon just adjacent to the joint line, approximately comparable to the musculotendinous junction. Pain on resisted lateral rotation tends to incriminate the infraspinatus tendon, but when different components of the tendon are involved, the physical signs may change subtly. When major inflammation occurs at the insertion around the posterior aspect of the greater tuberosity, a painful arc is part of the syndrome. Palpation helps locate tenderness situated near the musculotendinous junction, but it has to be distinguished from inflammation of the insertion of the long head of triceps. There is no capsular pattern with infraspinatus tendinitis.

Treatment consists in activity modification, reducing the sudden movements of follow-through or impact, and applying laser, ultrasound, or one of the heating modalities to the area. If this method fails to resolve the problem promptly, an injection of corticosteroid into the area may be helpful[55] (Fig. 21-49). A word of caution is appropriate, as the axillary nerve is situated reasonably near the tendon insertion in the quadrilateral space, and ill-advised placement of the corticosteroid injection has been reported to result in permanent axillary palsy.[57]

As is discussed in considerable detail in the section on instability (see below), the infraspinatus muscle is the key in shoulder stabilization. It is essential to follow up with treatment directed at relief of symptoms by an intensive, carefully progressed strengthening program for the external rotators and the infraspinatus in particular.

Sprains of the Shoulder (Glenohumeral) Joint

As with most joints, three degrees of severity of sprain occur at the glenohumeral joint. The mechanism is essentially the same but involves forces of increasing magnitude.

Anterior Capsular Sprain

Mild Sprains

The fibers of the capsule and capsular ligament remain intact with mild sprains, as the damage does not structurally weaken the joint. The major clinical complaint is pain. The anterior shoulder is diffusely uncomfortable to palpation. External rotation with abduction aggravates the pain, but the range should be full on passive motion; there might be slight restriction of active range. Swelling and hemorrhage are absent.

Treatment depends on the severity of the pain and restriction of active and resisted motion. Ice and possibly NSAIDs are given during the initial 12 to 24 hours followed by heating modalities if pain persists. Rarely, a sling is used for comfort. Depending on the sport, resumption of activity is dictated by a return to full range of motion and the ability to generate a significantly strong contraction of the deltoid and rotator cuff without discomfort.

Moderate Sprains

Moderate sprains produce some mechanical disruption of the capsule and hence have some potential for residual capsular laxity. In reality, this lesion, produced by a direct posterior blow or more frequently forced external rotation in abduction, is usually a traumatic subluxation. Pain is usually se-

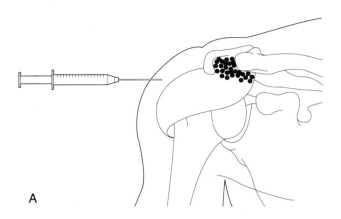

A

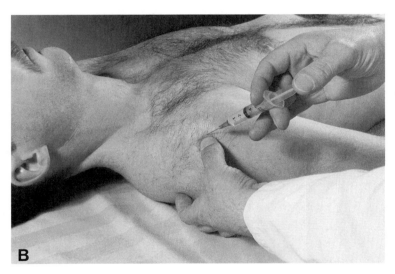

B

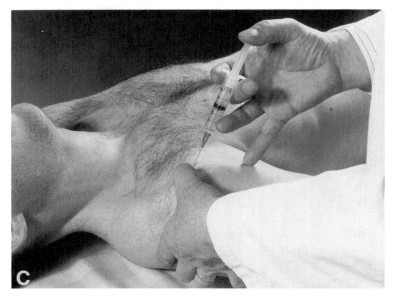

C

Fig. 21-48. Injection of the subacromion (subdeltoid bursa). **(A)** Location of the bursa just under the arch of the acromion. **(B)** Initial injection of 0.5 ml sliding under the lateral extent of the acromion. **(C)** Another 0.5 ml is injected through the accessible anterior extent of the bursa adjacent to the acromioclavicular ligament. By injecting 1 cm medial and proximal to the tip of the coracoid process, the needle is usually placed safely into the joint space. (Sterile technique and the use of gloves is important.)

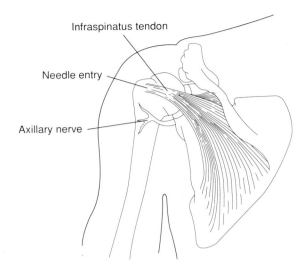

Infraspinatus tendon

Needle entry

Axillary nerve

A

Fig. 21-49. Injection of the infraspinatus tendon. **(A)** Anatomic landmark. **(B)** Best position for maximizing the accessibility of the tendon. The elbows should be tucked in slightly, under the chest. Injection of 1 ml into the tendon is achieved by inserting the needle down to bone and withdrawing it slightly, followed by multiple withdrawals and advancing the needle in a circular area of about 1.5 cm. This injection technique is difficult, and the structure is often very deep in a heavily muscled individual. Care should be taken to avoid the axillary nerve. (Sterile technique is essential, gloves should be worn.)

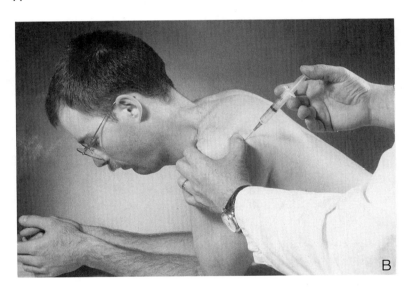

vere; active and passive range of motion, particularly abduction, are limited; and there may be swelling or bruising. Occasionally, there is labral damage along with the capsular tear. The problem with this injury is that a significant percentage of young athletes, particularly those in throwing sports, develop a progressive functional instability based on subluxation or labral damage that may become more incapacitating than are intermittent episodes of dislocation.

Treatment of moderately severe sprains should be cautious and conservative because of the natural history as outlined above. Adequate time is required for capsular healing, (approximately 3 weeks), before emphasis is placed on restoring full external rotation and abduction. Modalities and NSAIDs are used as indicated, and wherever possible the young athlete should be protected from violent, unexpected stresses on the shoulder for the duration of healing. The early emphasis is on strengthening in the pain-free and restricted range. Motion is usually restored easily by 3 weeks.

Like many second degree injuries to major joints, this injury has a broad spectrum of trauma. It requires considerable clinical skill and experience to judge the pace of rehabilitation that will result in the fewest long-term functional problems. Particularly

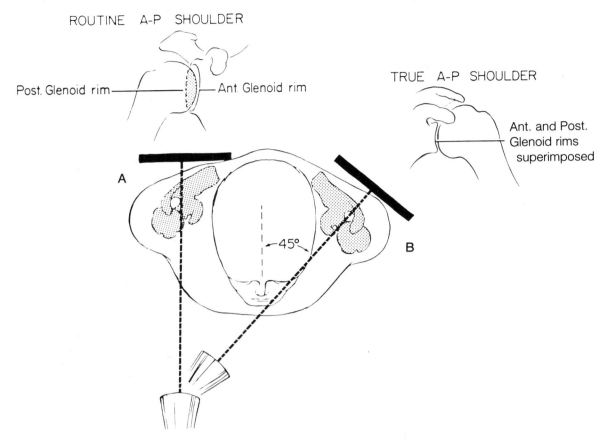

ROUTINE A-P SHOULDER

Post. Glenoid rim——————Ant. Glenoid rim

TRUE A-P SHOULDER

Ant. and Post. Glenoid rims superimposed

A

45°

B

Fig. 21-50. Routine and true anteroposterior (A-P) views of the shoulder. **(A)** Because the scapula sits at an angle in the chest wall, a routine A-P view obtains an oblique silhouette of the joint. There should be an overlap of the humeral head with the glenoid. **(B)** Forty-five degree view minimizes the superimposition and allows a view of the glenoid margin and the joint space.

for the amateur and recreational athlete, return to function should be guided at a conservative pace.

Severe Sprains

The capsule and capsular ligaments and usually the glenoid labrum have been significantly damaged with the severe sprain. The injury may have completely displaced the head from the glenoid fossa. Management of traumatic first time or recurrent dislocation is discussed on page 963.

Posterior Shoulder Sprains

Posterior shoulder sprains have a different mechanism of injury than anterior sprains, but the clinical course is similar. Failure to recognize and treat this injury adequately can cause long-term disability and complications. The usual mechanism of this injury in sport is an indirect force applied through the shoul-

der via a fall on the outstretched hands or elbow. The limb is usually flexed, medially rotated and adducted.

Grade I (mild) and II (moderate) sprains involve increasing damage to the posterior capsule and ligaments. The grade II injury, even though the result of

---

Practice Point

ACUTE TRAUMATIC SHOULDER SUBLUXATION (MODERATE SPRAIN)

- Present with early loss of motion and pain
- Frequently associated with chronic symptoms, including subluxation and pain
- Treat conservatively
- Allow for capsular healing (3 weeks)

a subluxation, usually heals without residual problems if adequately treated.[23,57] The type III injury is frequently a posterior dislocation and requires protection from forward flexion and adduction movements until capsular healing takes place. If chronic attenuation of the posterior capsular structures occurs as the result of an acute sprain, recurrent posterior subluxation or dislocation may result, usually with internal rotation adduction maneuvers. Fortunately, it is not a common entity and should be distinguished from the atraumatic voluntary or habitual dislocation, which is not associated with an initial traumatic episode.

Reduction of the acute (grade III) dislocation, is usually successfully accomplished by longitudinal traction, with adequate anesthesia, in the direction of the adducted limb. Either direct posterior pressure over the proximal humerus or slight internal rotation disengages the impinged head. Provided there are no operative indications, e.g., a locked dislocation, large bone fragments, or associated fractures, a standard sling and swath immobilization with the arm adducted by the side is adequate. As has been previously emphasized, sufficient time for capsular healing is mandatory. Before this course of treatment is utilized, however, the stability of the reduction should be ascertained.

The major concern with posterior shoulder dislocation is that the injury is frequently overlooked. Indeed, McLaughlin in 1952 said that posterior dislocations of the shoulder are misdiagnosed, misinterpreted, mistreated, and misunderstood—comments that, to some degree, are true today.[58] Whereas subglenoid and subspinous dislocations are readily apparent on routine plain films, axillary and trans-scapular views help delineate the subacromial posterior dislocation (Figs. 21-50, 21-51, 21-52). Furthermore, careful clinical examination nearly always reveals some cardinal signs, including (1) an altered contour of the affected versus the normal shoulder, (2) the patient supporting the arm tightly against the chest and the forearm across the front of the trunk, and (3) any attempt at abduction or external rotation produces an inordinate degree of pain (Table 21-6).

The method of treatment was suggested in previous paragraphs.

Other shoulder instabilities are discussed in the next section. The main emphasis has been to alert the clinicians to distinguish between minor shoulder sprains and the more significant subluxations and dislocations, which require a cautious approach and, despite treatment, may eventually be associated with a

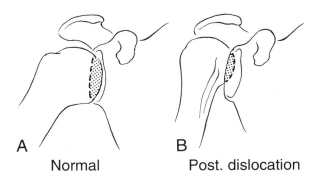

Fig. 21-51. Normal and posterior dislocated shoulder. **(A)** With the normal view there should be considerable overlap of the shadow of the head in the glenoid. **(B)** With a posterior dislocation there may be an ''empty glenoid'' sign with no overlap of the humeral head or, alternately, minimal overlap in the subspinous position. With this dislocation the inferior one-third of the glenoid is empty of overlapping shadow.

high complication rate. Furthermore, the danger of overlooking the more uncommon acute posterior dislocation stresses the importance of being alert and provides a lesson in careful clinical observation.

SHOULDER INSTABILITY

The broad spectrum of minor asymptomatic subluxation to frank dislocation is all too common in sport. Many of the entities overlap and have been alluded to earlier in the chapter; functional instability, muscle imbalance, and painful impingement may be closely associated. It is helpful to consider the type, direction, and etiology in the classification of shoulder problems. In this way the classic entities may be defined and treatment strategies outlined. With this knowledge firmly in mind, the subtle associations between pain and functional instability and the blurring of the margins between injuries that do not fit easily into this compartmentalization may be better understood. Only the most common entities encountered in the athletic population are described here in any detail, including subluxations, anterior dislocation, and multidirectional instability.

There has been considerable debate over the importance of the various anatomic structures that play a role in stability. Turkel et al. performed selective cutting experiments of the capsule with the arm in a variety of positions.[54] At 45 degrees of abduction, the subscapularis, middle glenohumeral, and the supe-

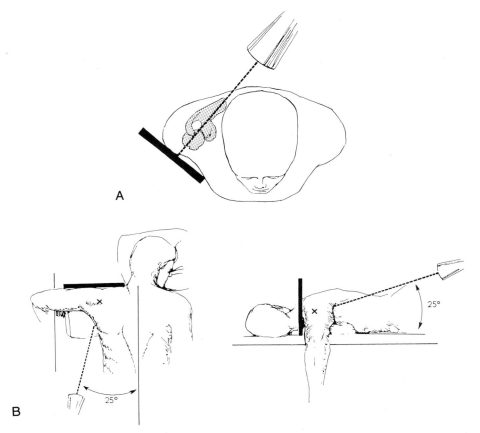

Fig. 21-52. Extra views for evaluating shoulder trauma and dislocations. **(A)** True lateral or transscapular view. **(B)** The west-point view, which visualizes well the antero-inferior rim of the glenoid. With an acute dislocation, it may not be possible to abduct the arm sufficiently to get this view, and a more modified accessory view can be used.

rior portion of the inferior glenohumeral ligament were important. At 90 degrees, with associated external rotation, anterior dislocation would not occur unless the entire anterior capsular ligaments, including the posterior half of the inferior glenohumeral ligament, which is way past the six o'clock position of the glenoid margin, was disrupted.

Warren's study on the static restraints to posterior dislocation with the shoulder internally rotated and flexed to 90 degrees illustrated that, in addition to removing posterior capsular integrity from the twelve o'clock to the six o'clock position, it was necessary to make an incision through the capsule and superior glenohumeral ligament from one to three o'clock to produce posterior dislocation.[59] Thus both these studies showed that usually some damage must occur at both sides of the circle for instability to occur. This

concept is different from true multidirectional instability, where there is significant capsular laxity, usually with generalized loose joints, frequently an intact labrum, and a degree of abnormal inferior motion.

Subluxation

Shoulder subluxation refers to increased humeral head excursion in the glenoid fossa and need not necessarily be accompanied by pain. Indeed, no precise definition of subluxation exists, as the limits of normal excursion on the glenoid are still not fully agreed on and, in the heavily muscled individual, are clinically often difficult to record accurately. Many sports activities, e.g., throwing, serving at tennis, swimming, and gymnastics, may result in increased shoulder motion. Hence marked increased excursion

TABLE 21-6. Pathology and Clinical Signs of Acute Posterior Dislocation[a]

Pathology
  Stretched posterior capsule
  Detached posterior glenoid and capsule
  Fracture of posterior glenoid
  Stretched subscapularis muscle or tendon anteriorly
  Avulsion of subscapularis tendon
  Avulsion of lesser tuberosity by subscapularis
Clinical signs
  Arm positioned in adduction and internal rotation
  External rotation blocked
  Abduction limited
  Posterior aspect of shoulder more prominent
  Anterior shoulder flatter
  Occasionally visible coracoid process anteriorly
Radiologic
  Empty (vacant) glenoid in AP view with subacromial
    dish
  Subspinous or subglenoid position in axillary or
    transcapsular view

[a] Depending on severity.
(After Rockwood and Green,[23] with permission.)

of the humeral head, even to the point of mild sub-luxation, becomes a common, essentially asymptomatic accompaniment.[59]

When symptoms do occur they may be associated with impingement due to abnormal motion and over-use or to mechanical internal derangement, such as labral tears due to trauma. In addition, subluxation may occur after a previous dislocation, as described earlier; or, conversely, subluxation may progress to dislocation. Frequently recurrent subluxation episodes may be more functionally disabling than periodic relatively predictable dislocation.[59,60]

Anterior Subluxation

Many athletes who present with anterior shoulder subluxation have been seen by a wide range of physicians with a complaint of shoulder pain but without having obtained a specific diagnosis.[60,61] Indeed, it is the patient whose main symptom is a vague persistent glenohumeral ache or intermittent flare-up of anterior impingement syndrome who is most difficult to diagnose.

Clinical Presentation

A careful history, specifically with attention to the relation of the pain to the sport activity, helps shed light on the true cause. Sharp exacerbation of the pain during the acceleration phase of the throw, while reaching overhead for a rebound, or while reaching out widely to the side to make a tackle in rugby or football or to prevent an opponent driving for the basket is a common complaint. Usually with closer questioning, many patients admit that they have felt the sensation of the shoulder moving or slipping "in

---

Quick Facts

CLASSIFICATION OF SHOULDER INSTABILITY

- Type
  - Subluxation
  - Dislocation
- Direction
  - Anterior
  - Posterior
  - Multidirectional
  - Luxatio erecta
  - Intrathoracic
- Etiology
  - Traumatic
  - Post-traumatic recurrent
  - Atraumatic voluntary (habitual, developmental, congenital)
  - Persistent (unreduced, locked, fixed)
  - Neuromuscular (stroke, seizures)

Practice Point

ATRAUMATIC SUBLUXATION

- Acquired or congenital ligament laxity
- Intermittent symptoms
- Usually overhead throwing activities
- May produce dead arm syndrome
- May be mechanical, clicking, clunking, or pseudolocking
- May present as impingement
- Anterior shoulder pain only
- Reflex weakness and wasting of cuff muscles
- Primary treatment: rehabilitation
- Consider arthroscopy
- May need surgical stabilization

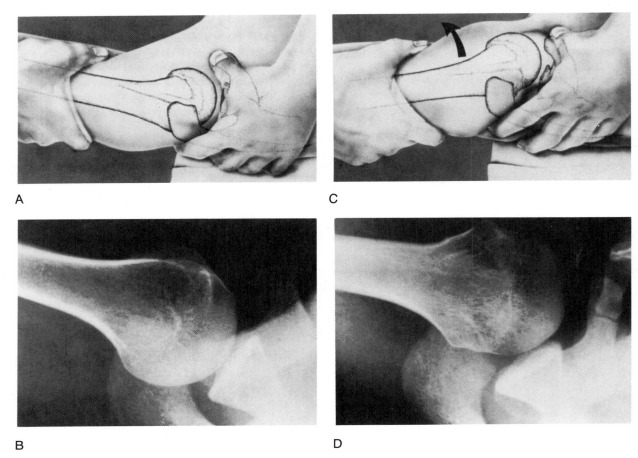

Fig. 21-53. Anterior drawer test of the shoulder. **(A)** Fixation of the scapula and proximal humerus. **(B)** Accompanying roentgenogram shows normal position. **(C)** Extension with an anterior gliding pressure subluxes an unstable shoulder. **(D)** Radiographic confirmation. This test is a modification of the load and shift test and can be graded in a similar fashion (p. 918). (After Gerber and Ganz,[22] with permission.)

and out" of joint. Sometimes the pain is in the joint on the opposite side to the instability; such pain is due to inflammation within the cuff as the result of recurrent traction on these tissues during episodes of subluxation.

Some athletes describe intermittent, paralyzing, transient pain over the shoulder or down the entire arm when performing ballistic-type activities. This intense pain may be followed by a sensation of numbness, which quickly goes away but may leave a vague feeling of weakness that remains for a varying period of time but is rarely protracted. The latter is the "dead arm" syndrome and is almost pathognomonic of shoulder instability. It is probably due to transient stretching of the plexus.

Occasionally, labral lesions contribute to glenohumeral instability. They may be shoulder clicks, catches, locking, or a clunking sensation with or without a feeling of instability. Sometimes athletes describe having to shake their shoulder in order to "get it in place." The anterior drawer test may unmask the underlying instability (Fig. 21-53). The anterior subluxation may create a void under the posterior acromion and a slight bulge below the coracoid process.

Treatment

Treatment depends on making a presumptive diagnosis. Occasionally, roentgenograms in association with special studies such as arthrography or CT reveal post-traumatic abnormalities. We have experimented with a biofeedback program designed to assist in controlling the position of the humeral head during overhead activities.

When the arm is overhead, the subscapularis, the main dynamic support, is not able to control the humeral head effectively because it has moved superiorly with external rotation. The angle of the humeral head with the shaft and the pull of the large prime movers, e.g., the deltoid and pectoralis major, tend to produce forces that glide the humeral head anteriorly. The integrity of the anterior capsular ligaments is the major static resistance to subluxation. Only infraspinatus can produce an effective dynamic support by pulling the head back in the glenoid[5,62] (Fig. 21-54). Thus a targeted biofeedback program to perfect motor skills, particularly control of the infraspinatus, was evolved in 1988.[63] By electronically monitoring and amplifying activity of the external rotators during an apprehensive motion, with immediate visual and auditory feedback, the performance is changed or shaped. *This program emphasizes muscle control, rather than strength,* and requires motivation, dedication to training, and a prolonged home program to maintain the established engrams that control shoulder instability. A protocol is described

using a MyoTrac biofeedback unit, but the system may be adopted easily for other units following these principles (Fig. 21-55).

Single Channel Biofeedback Treatment Protocol

Step 1. Electrode placement is critical. Attach the sensor electrode below the scapular spine. *Do not* place it over the posterior deltoid, as increased activity in this muscle would drive the humeral head anteriorly. The patient remains connected to the biofeedback unit during training and must practice at home with and without the unit. For home practice the therapist might wish to place an indelible mark on the skin for electrode placement.

Step 2. Have the patient flex the shoulder forward to 70 degrees and establish a baseline reading for muscle activity.

Step 3. Ensure that the shoulder is in a pain-free neutral position and set the machine to give an audio or visual feedback. Instruct the patient to use this visual and audio EMG biofeedback to increase EMG activity well above the baseline level. It is done by tightening rotator cuff muscles in the neutral position in order to glide and hold the humeral head posteriorly. This step is a key component and must be

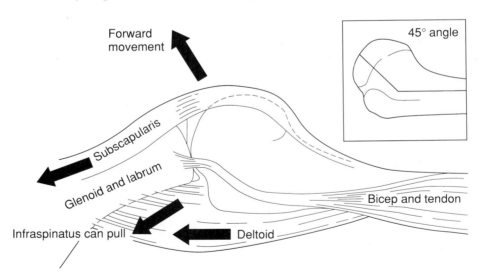

Fig. 21-54. With the arm abducted and externally rotated, the humeral head tends to slide anteriorly in the glenoid. The normal restraints are the labrum, capsule, subscapularis muscle, and biceps tendon. With further abduction and external rotation, both biceps and the subscapularis move superiorly, leaving only the capsule to protect the head. With traumatic dislocations the capsule becomes stretched and the glenoid damaged; and it is easy for the head to slip out in this vulnerable position. Only a posterior pull by the infraspinatus is capable of dynamically restoring the head to the central position.

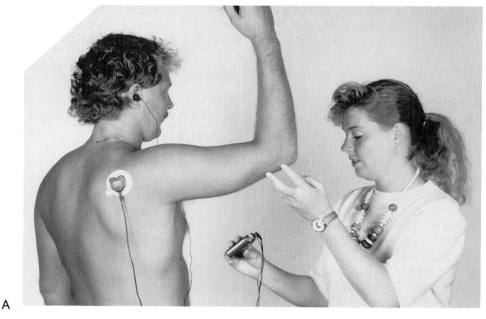

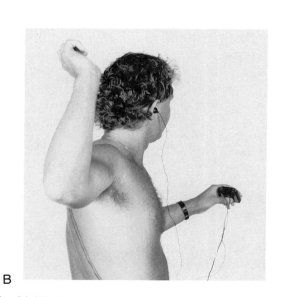

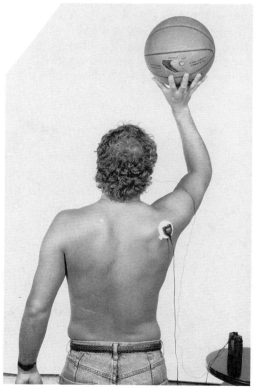

Fig. 21-55. For biofeedback training, placement of the electrode underneath the spine of the scapula is critical. It should be as close to the deltoid as possible without going under that muscle. **(A)** After effecting contraction in the neutral position, the arm is taken to forward flexion at 70 degrees. **(B)** Functional positions are then duplicated, e.g., throwing and shooting **(C)** in basketball.

successfully performed 100 times (ten sets of ten) prior to progressing to active movement. The use of many repetitions builds endurance. This procedure is fatiguing, and it may require several sessions before the patient can progress to step 4.

Step 4. With the threshold set at twice the value achieved in step 2, instruct the patient to forward-flex the adducted and neutral rotated shoulder to 90 to 100 degrees, with elbow in flexion. As the shoulder is flexed, have the patient tighten the rotator cuff and achieve the threshold setting between 70 and 90 degrees, trying to push the biofeedback readings as high as possible. If pain or a sense of subluxation is experienced, stop, rest, and start again through a smaller arc of movement or with altered threshold settings (or both). When the patient can successfully perform 100 consecutive repetitions, progress by altering the threshold or the movement (or both).

Step 5. Movement progression comprises this phase. As the patient masters each level, progress through the following exercises:

1. Forward flexion with a straight elbow.
2. Forward flexion with increasing external rotation.
3. Abduction with flexion, progressing to elbow extension.
4. Abduction with elbow extension with increasing external rotation.
5. Abduction from flexion.
6. Abduction from flexion with increasing external rotation.
7. Reaching for objects behind the back or overhead.

Clinical Point

BIOFEEDBACK TRAINING

- Program emphasizing muscle control
- Strength acquisition important but secondary
- Electrode placement critical
- Biofeedback physically and mentally demanding
- Appropriate rest intervals allowed
- Slow careful progression planned
- Long-term commitment necessary to ensure continued effectiveness of new engrams

---

When this progression of increasingly difficult tasks has been completed, progress to the activities specific to the sport or the position that caused difficulty (Fig. 21-55). Break the movement down into component parts and introduce catching or throwing activities in preparation for a gradual return to the sport.

Step 6. If general weakness exists, instruct the patient in appropriate progressive resistance exercises. These exercises should emphasize scapular control. Include pushups for the serratus anterior with the arms adducted (elbows kept close to the body) and external rotation exercises resisted with surgical tubing or dental dam. *Avoid* resisted exercises that load in an impingement position. All pain-free activities are allowed and encouraged. The patient requires 2 to 3 weeks of supervised physiotherapy but must undertake a life-long home program to maintain the engram. It might be desirable for patients to return for occasional brief refresher courses.

Comment. The early results of our follow-up on patients who have completed this program is promising. However, it does not overcome some of the mechanical symptoms due to labral damage, and it may not be as effective for a significant functional instability in the throwing athlete.

If therapy directed at the pain and potential muscle weakness is not successful, arthroscopy may be considered for débridement or, when appropriate, glenoid resuturing. This treatment is particularly useful when mechanical symptoms, suggesting a glenoid lesion, predominate.[61,64] It also provides the opportunity to examine the shoulder under anesthesia. Garth et al. pointed out that attritional changes in the anteroinferior capsule and developmental hypertrophy of the internal rotators of the throwing shoulder may result in excessive anterior displacement of the humeral head during the early acceleration phase of throwing.[61] Such displacement may result in excessive traction on the biceps tendon anterosuperior labrum complex, resulting in labral lesions or avulsions. Frequently, rehabilitation of the infraspinatus teres minor complex after arthroscopic débridement of these labral lesions leads to resolution of pain and may allow correction of the dynamic imbalance, thereby allowing return to sport.[65] If nonoperative treatment is unsuccessful and arthroscopy (when indicated) has not alleviated the instability, surgical stabilization of the shoulder should be considered.

Posterior Subluxation

Complete posterior dislocation occurs rarely in the athlete.[66] The instability is usually subluxation rather than dislocation, and it seldom requires reduction.[67] Whereas many patients with posterior instability are active with no difficulties, many complain of pain.[67,68] The diagnosis is easy when the individual can demonstrate the posterior subluxation voluntarily; frequently, however, posterior instability is a difficult diagnosis. The posterior drawer test may unmask lesser degrees of instability (Fig. 21-56).

Clinical Point

VOLUNTARY POSTERIOR SUBLUXATION — DISLOCATION

- As the humeral head moves back, the coracoid process often becomes visible.
- It is best seen from above and behind the patient.

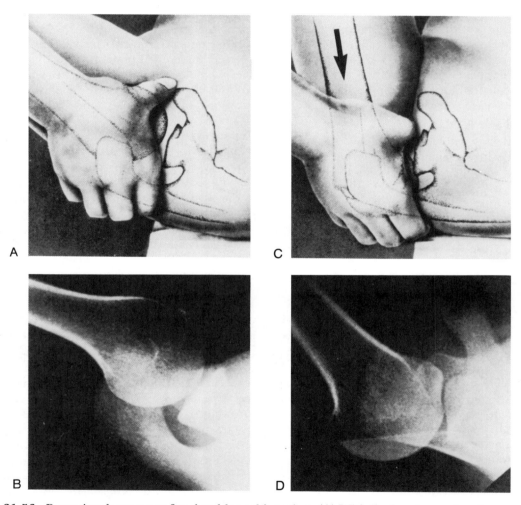

Fig. 21-56. Posterior drawer test for shoulder subluxation. **(A)** With the hand grasping the proximal shoulder and the thumb firmly over the humeral head, the elbow is supported with the other hand of examiner. **(B)** Roentgenogram of the located position. **(C)** Arm is brought into adduction and posterior pressure exerted with both the supporting hand at the elbow and the proximal hand over the humeral head. The thumb slides along the lateral aspect of the coracoid process as the head of the humerus is pushed backward. **(D)** Subluxated position is confirmed radiographically. (After Gerber and Ganz,[22] with permission.)

Anatomic changes are often subtle, with redundancy of the posterior part of the capsule as the main finding rather than a torn or detached labrum (as would be anticipated with the anterior instability). The bones are rarely abnormal, and no single pathologic change has been found to explain posterior instability of the shoulder. It is sometimes part of a multidirectional instability syndrome. In the athletic population posterior subluxation may be generated by a single traumatic episode, but it more frequently follows a pattern of chronic overstress. *Only a small percentage of this subpopulation are habitual dislocators with an abnormal psychological profile.*[68]

Treatment of this chronic instability is controversial, and many approaches have been suggested. A thorough attempt at nonoperative treatment should be undertaken, with special attention to rotator cuff strength and normal muscle balance. This regimen may include a biofeedback program with emphasis on controlling the subluxation in the vulnerable position.

If surgery is attempted, simple approaches such as posterior capsular stapling are successful in only a small number of individuals.[66] In a few instances, excessive retroversion of the glenoid cavity is noted. Usually, to be significant this angle should approach 10 degrees more than the normal side, which, on average, retroverts approximately 7 to 10 degrees. In this instance, an opening wedge with bone graft to correct the angulation may supplement other procedures.[69] Because of the high association with multidirectional instability, particularly inferiorly, capsular infraspinatus shortening and a posterior inferior capsular shift is probably the most reasonable surgical approach.[59,67,68]

Dislocation

Acute traumatic anterior dislocation, recurrent post-traumatic anterior dislocation, and multidirectional instability are discussed here because of their prevalence in the athletic population.

Acute Traumatic Anterior Dislocation

Anterior shoulder dislocation, both primary and recurrent, are disabling for the athlete, a situation made worse by the uncertainty about the best method of treatment and the probable long-term outcome of such treatments. The injury is common in ice hockey, wrestling, rugby, football, basketball, baseball, and gymnastics. Initial traumatic anterior dislocations may be due to a force applied directly to the posterior aspect of the humeral head, driving it anteriorly. However, the more common mechanism in sport is an indirect force via the externally rotated and abducted limb, such as would be seen in a football player attempting to block a high pass or a hockey player sliding head first into the boards.

Matsen has clearly defined two major groups of dislocations, which have been given the eponymous designations TUBS and AMBRI.[99] The traumatic group (TUBS) is described here. The other group occurs with relatively little trauma in a predisposed individual.

Clinical Point

TUBS

- **T**raumatic etiology
- **U**nidirectional
- **B**ankart labral lesion present
- **S**urgical treatment indicated for specific cases initially, or as the treatment of subsequent recurrent instability

---

Recognition and Reduction

The diagnosis of anterior dislocations is usually not difficult. There is a characteristic hollow underneath the acromion, and the athlete supports the arm adducted and across the trunk. Attempts at internally or externally rotating the shoulder produce exquisite pain. Unfortunately, the padding and equipment of sports such as hockey and football may lead to unnecessary discomfort and manipulation unless the significance of this inability to move the limb is recognized. The clothing must be removed for visual inspection or the shoulder area carefully palpated for the loss of deltoid contour in order to confirm the diagnosis, although the athlete invariably tells the therapist or physician that the "shoulder is out."

Careful examination for loss of ability to statically contract deltoid and biceps, as well as the detection of any dysesthesia in the distribution of the axillary, musculocutaneous, or ulnar nerves is important in order to establish a baseline immediately before and after reduction (Fig. 21-57). When practical, an initial roentgenogram is obtained to confirm the diagnosis. Particularly useful is an axillary view, which can

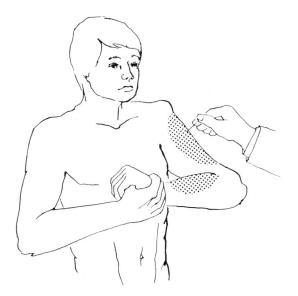

Fig. 21-57. Testing skin sensation for damage to the axillary nerve at the shoulder and the musculocutaneous nerve in the forearm before relocation. Although not always accurate, it is important to perform and document the results. (After Rockwood and Green,[23] with permission.)

rule out major associated fractures. An immediate post-reduction film gives further information regarding injury to the greater and lesser tuberosities and anteroinferior glenoid and hence the possible need for specialized studies such as the CT scan or even surgical therapy.[70]

Reduction is achieved using adequate anesthesia

designed to reduce pain as well as the protective reflex muscle spasm, so that minimal trauma and discomfort are produced. A safe method for the less experienced, or where medication is not advisable or available, is the modified Stimson technique of traction through the limb, which is hanging over the edge of a table (Fig. 21-58). This procedure may require additional manipulation, although frequently spontaneous reduction occurs. This position may be adopted while awaiting transport or the arrival of more experienced medical help if the diagnosis is certain. A successful method is longitudinal traction into slight abduction. Careful positioning of the patient allows the pull to be adjusted into flexion and also some gentle external, then internal, rotation (Fig. 21-58). The clinician should wear rubber gloves to prevent the hands from slipping on the athlete's skin. With adequate anesthesia and good positioning, most of the traction may be delivered by the clinician leaning back and using the effect of their own body weight. Slow, prolonged traction is required to allow relaxation of the athlete's muscles before reduction can be anticipated. The usual cause for failure is poor positioning, inadequate anesthesia, insufficient time for muscle relaxation, and poor body mechanics. If the conditions are correct and reduction is not achieved after a couple of good efforts, general anesthesia is indicated and the possibility of an open reduction considered. Other primary indications for open reduction of glenohumeral dislocations are large bony glenoid fragments, fractured humerus, vascular lesions, or a sudden severe deterioration in neurologic status after reduction, which may indicate incarceration of the nerve. The latter circumstance is rare.

Clinical Point

ACUTE TRAUMATIC ANTERIOR DISLOCATION

- First episode or repeat after long stable interval
- Capsular injury 30% versus labrum lesion 60%
- Reduce promptly
- Check for complications
- Immobilize 3 weeks
- Relative immobilization for another 3 weeks
- Intensive rehabilitation
- Know indications for surgical intervention

Clinical Point

INDICATIONS FOR POSSIBLE OPEN REDUCTION IN FIRST TIME DISLOCATION

- Irreducible
- Large glenoid fragment displaced
- Instability after reduction
- Fractured humerus
- Vascular damage
- Appearance of significant peripheral nerve injury immediately after reduction

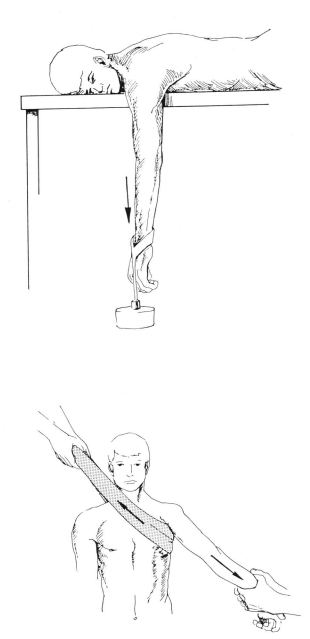

Fig. 21-58. Methods of reducing an anterior dislocation. **(A)** Modified Stimson technique. Gentle traction on the arm over a period of time allows muscle fatigue and relaxation. Either reduction occurs spontaneously or gentle rotation of the limb allows the shoulder to relocate. **(B)** Longitudinal traction in abduction and increasing angles of flexion with a slow, steady pull over a period of 30 to 60 seconds usually effects reduction even in the most stubborn shoulder. (After Rockwood and Green,[23] with permission.)

Treatment After Reduction

The orthopaedic literature reflects confusion as to the correct management of first dislocations.[71–73] The length of strict immobilization after reduction varies considerably, from 2 days to 8 weeks.[71,74] The result of these haphazard approaches is reflected in the subsequent redislocation rate, which is 80 to 90 percent in persons less than 20 years of age at the time of their first dislocation, approximately 60 percent for those 20 to 30 years of age, and 20 to 40 percent for those who are more than 40 years of age.[23] These figures have left most practitioners with a feeling of inevitability; hence many physicians and therapists believe that because there is a great chance of redislocation, whatever the treatment, it is better to opt for early mobilization, early strengthening, and rapid return to sport, activity, or occupation—a rather fatalistic approach based on poor control of early treatment, low patient compliance, and inadequate therapy.

A more careful review of the literature reveals an important underlying concept, first suggested by Watson-Jones in 1940, that the initial period of immobilization is important for prevention of recurrence.[75] This perspective has been adopted by several groups and is gaining acceptance.[76] In one report of 50 individuals less than 30 years of age, the recurrence rate was reduced to less than 20 percent after treatment of 6 weeks of strict immobilization.[2] With this regimen isometric exercises are taught to the individual by the therapist at an early stage while the arm is immobilized in a sling and swath; the exercises are then performed twice daily for the first 3 weeks (Fig. 21-59). Axillary hygiene is performed by moving the arm into a small but adequate amount of abduction. The elbow is removed from the sling several times a day to allow flexion and extension, which assists comfort and prevents stiffness. Care is taken to avoid all external rotation (Table 21-7). For the second 3-week period, gentle pendular exercises are continued, mainly with the arm in a sling, and external rotation is allowed just short of neutral with the arm kept adducted against the body. External rotation is not permitted with the arm away from the side. Abduction with the arm internally rotated is permitted to 45 degrees. After this period, from 6 weeks on, the emphasis is on strengthening for about 4 weeks, allowing range of motion to resume with gentle, active motion (Figs. 21-38 and 21-39). After this time, range of motion can be actively pursued and becomes

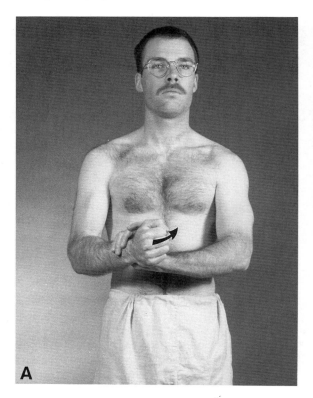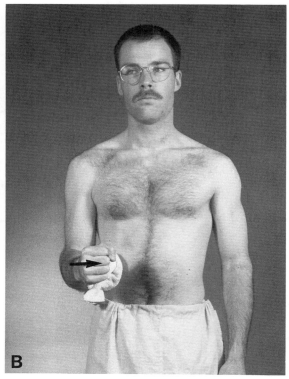

Fig. 21-59. Early isometric exercises that do not jeopardize the stability of the joint. **(A)** Isometric internal rotation keeping the elbow close to the body and using resistance offered by the uninjured side. **(B)** Isometric adduction exercises with a towel or pillow placed between the trunk and the arm. Similarly isometric flexion, extension and abduction, using the wall as a resistance, may be performed.

a major rehabilitation goal. Passive stretching should be avoided during the first 12 weeks after dislocation. In a few instances in which the shoulder appears particularly stiff, mobilization can be pursued more aggressively and slightly earlier, but only 6 weeks after dislocation. Ultimately, normal muscle strength and balance of strength must be restored.

Smith and Brunoll recorded proprioception deficits in individuals who had dislocated their shoul-

Clinical Point

PROPRIOCEPTIVE DEFICITS

- It is possible that residual proprioceptive deficits after shoulder dislocation may add to functional instability.
- At some point this should be addressed in the rehabilitation.

ders.[77] They included angular reproduction tests, threshold to sensation of movement, and end range reproduction tests (Table 21-8). The implication of this study is that more attention should be paid to proprioception training during rehabilitation of shoulder instability. This concept has been established for knee ligament rehabilitation but is not well recognized at the shoulder. Perhaps the biofeedback training outlined for subluxing shoulders could be integrated with a proprioceptive program to enhance muscle control.

Kuriyama et al., in 1984, gave us a better insight as to the pathology of anterior dislocations by performing arthrograms on 143 first dislocations.[78] This group noted that there were two main types of dislocation: two-thirds were capsular tears (i.e., the humeral head ripped out through the capsule), and one-third were capsular detachments (i.e., the glenoid labrum or adjacent capsule was detached from the glenoid margin). The importance of this observation is that capsular tears have a great propensity for heal-

TABLE 21-7. Protocol for Initial Traumatic Anterior Dislocation

Immediate post reduction
    X-ray film to establish reduction
    Rule out associated fractures
    Test for neurologic deficit
    Sling and swath
    Keep arm adducted except for axillary hygiene
    Remove elbow regularly to prevent stiffness
    Ice and NSAIDs
    Progress when pain subsides

Early Post-reduction (up to 3 weeks)
    Avoid abduction past 45°
    Avoid external rotation past 45°
    Gentle pendular exercises with arm in sling
    Isometric internal rotators in neutral[a]
    Isometric abductors and adductors, arm at side
    Isometric flexion-extension, arm at side
    Progress at 3 weeks when sufficient capsular healing

Early capsular healing (approx. 3 weeks)
    Supervised rehabilitation
    Continue pendular exercise
    Tube exercises for internal rotation
    External rotation to neutral: tube exercise
    Still no abduction past 45°: tube exercise
    Exercise rest of upper body
    Maintain fitness
    Progress at 5–6 weeks

Intermediate rehabilitation
    Progress all exercises
    Commence resisted work on equipment
    Do not resist external rotation past neutral
    Abduction resisted to 90°
    Avoid external rotation with abduction until 8 weeks
    Do not work range of motion unless signs of stiffness

Final rehabilitation
    Isokinetic values 75% of normal
    Progress full range resisted work
    Return to full contact sports when isokinetic values
        85% plus

[a] Isometrics: hold 8 to 10 seconds in sets of 10 to 15 repetitions. They should be pain-free

ing, which is not as obvious with the labrum detachments. This concept is reinforced by the fact that of those shoulders that later redislocated, 90 percent were of the capsular detachment type—the danger group for redislocation. More importantly, those persons who were strictly immobilized for 3 weeks had a redislocation rate that was amazingly low: 3.4 percent versus 47.7 percent for those who were immobilized for a shorter period.[78] Kuriyama et al. also showed, with follow-up arthrograms, that capsular healing could be demonstrated at 3 weeks but not before.[78] This finding underlines the importance of early immobilization during this vulnerable 3-week period.

These findings have been substantiated by Baker and Uribe, who arthroscopically evaluated a series of first time dislocations and noted that those with capsular tears and no labral lesions were stable under anesthesia and exhibited no or minimal hemarthrosis.[79] A second group of patients had a capsular tear in association with partial labrum detachment, and these injuries were mildly unstable to stressing and had mild to moderate hemarthrosis. The third group of patients had capsular tears with labrum detachment, and these injuries were grossly unstable to examination under anesthesia and arthroscopically had large hemarthroses. These observations reinforce the important concept of allowing capsular healing when feasible and considering alternate treatment, perhaps operative, in selected cases of traumatic dislocation where the chance of redislocation is high.[79] These investigators stressed the fact that the type of initial traumatic lesion is related to both the age of the patient and the force of the injury, which has bearing on the subsequent redislocation rate.

With these data as a background, every effort should be made to obtain patient compliance for early immobilization with a sling and swath supple-

TABLE 21-8. Kinesthetic Deficits After Shoulder Dislocation

Shoulder Group	Angular Reproduction (°)			Threshold to Sensation (°)			End Range Reproduction (°)		
	$\overline{X}$	S	Range	$\overline{X}$	S	Range	$\overline{X}$	S	Range
Normal dominant arm	1.50	0.63	0.33–2.33	1.18	0.77	0.33–2.33	1.40	0.64	0.67–2.67
Normal nondominant arm	1.40	0.60	0.33–2.33	1.04	0.46	0.50–2.00	1.05	0.58	0.00–2.00
Dislocator uninvolved side	1.08	0.64	0.33–2.33	0.91	0.65	0.33–2.17	0.98	0.59	0.00–2.00
Dislocator involved side	2.75	1.22	1.00–3.67	2.58	0.93	1.00–3.67	3.00	0.81	1.67–4.33

All values are significantly different, normal and uninvolved shoulder, to previously dislocated shoulder. (From Smith and Brunoll,[77] with permission.)

mented by carefully taught isometric exercises. The outlined regimen provides excellent functional outcomes and reduces the devastatingly high redislocation rate that has come to be accepted as inevitable.[80-82]

Complications

The major complication of traumatic anterior dislocation is the tendency to recurrence. However, an unusual but dramatic association with tearing or thrombosis of the axillary artery or vein must be borne in mine. Suspicion is aroused when there is a rapidly expanding hematoma, excessive ecchymosis, marked pain in the axilla, diminished or absent radial pulse, and numbness or paralysis of the whole limb. The extremity may be cold and the hand pale or cyanotic, and with severe disruption the patient may show signs of shock.

The most common neural injury is damage to the axillary nerve (Fig. 21-60). Fortunately, these injuries are mostly mild neuropraxic type lesions. There is subclinical involvement in as many as 30 percent of individuals, but significant damage occurs fewer than 5 percent.[80] Most of these athletes recover full function even if there is residual EMG evidence of denervation at 1 year. Because many of the injuries do not clinically involve the sensory component of the nerve, there is a tendency to overlook the injury initially.

Fractures of the neck of the humerus are more common in the elderly, but avulsions of the greater tuberosity or fractures of the glenoid are more common in the young athlete. The need for open reduction is assessed on a case by case basis, and the discussion includes the potential block to motion, the size and displacement of any intra-articular fragment, and the residual instability after reduction.

Hawkins et al. made some observations that apply to traumatic dislocations in the older athlete.[82] They confirmed that the redislocation rate is low, but a large number of patients sustained rotator cuff tears that did not heal and caused persistent symptoms. Whether these tears are due to pre-existing degener-

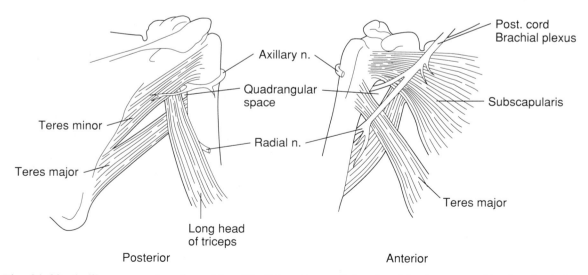

Fig. 21-60. Axillary nerve is vulnerable with dislocations of the shoulder because of its fixed origin from the posterior cord of the brachial plexus and its entrapment in the quadrilateral space when dislocation occurs.

ative changes in the cuff or solely to the trauma of the dislocation is unsure. Thus Hawkins et al. recommended that patients over 40 years of age who present with a primary shoulder dislocation should undergo a more aggressive rehabilitation program after reduction.[82]

Active patients who fail to progress should have an arthrogram, preferably within 4 weeks, and be considered for decompressive anterior acromioplasty and rotator cuff repair if the defect is demonstrated. Less active individuals may choose to accept their disability but when symptoms persist may elect to have surgery at a later date. This problem of associated cuff tear should be considered in cases of persistent pain when the individual is referred late and appropriate investigations initiated. Furthermore, if recurrent instability does result from the initial dislocation in the older patient, it should not be addressed surgically until the presence and magnitude of any associated cuff tear is delineated. If none is found, standard stabilizing techniques are appropriate. When significant cuff tears are found, the emphasis should be on cuff reconstruction.[82]

Clinical Point

TRAUMATIC DISLOCATION IN ACTIVE INDIVIDUALS 40 YEARS PLUS

- There is a high incidence of nerve and vascular injury.
- There is a close association with cuff tears.
- Early aggressive rehabilitation is required.
- Failure to progress at 4 weeks is an indication for arthrography.
- Consider early cuff repair.
- If recurrent instability and cuff tear coexists, the latter takes priority.
- If no cuff tear, standard stabilizing techniques are adequate.

Recurrent Anterior Dislocations

Recurrent anterior dislocation of the glenohumeral joint is a common phenomenon accounting for more than 80 percent of dislocations of the upper extremity.[15] In some individuals the dislocation is predictable and can be avoided for the most part by modification of activity. In others the unpredictabil-

ity makes it a disabling problem. The usual mechanism of dislocation in day-to-day activities is external rotation in the abducted position. However, in sporting activities another situation is frequently described that involves simple abduction and adduction. For the volleyball player it may occur during spiking or blocking, for the swimmer during touching for the turn, and for the tennis player during the serve. Little discussion has related to this particular mechanism. Furthermore, the role and efficacy of exercise in the prevention of dislocation is poorly understood. It is to this group of individuals that Matsen has given the eponym TUBS: The mechanism of the first episode was *t*raumatic; the injuries are *u*nidirectional and invariably anterior; *B*ankart and and Hill-Sachs lesions are common; and usually *s*urgery is the eventual treatment required[99] (Fig. 21-61). Surgery, however, should not be contemplated without an adequate trial of nonoperative therapy.

Quick Facts

RECURRENT TRAUMATIC DISLOCATION (TUBS)

- Frequently younger athlete
- Traumatic etiology originally
- Unidirectional (anterior)
- Bankart or Hill-Sachs lesion with time
- Surgery required if rehabilitation fails

Rehabilitation

Isokinetic testing of 40 subjects who had dislocated their shoulder a minimum of three times and had symptoms sufficient to cause them to consider operative repair revealed some interesting results.[1] As would be anticipated, these subjects could not generate significant torque in the position of apprehension, i.e., external rotation in abduction. Surprisingly, however, the abductor and adductor groups reflected most weakness throughout the range, more so than the rotators.

Some individuals dislocated their unstable shoulders while being tested. It did not occur while they were actively going into the abduction externally rotated position but as they started to return from the fully abducted position. In other words, as they contracted their adductors to bring their arm down to

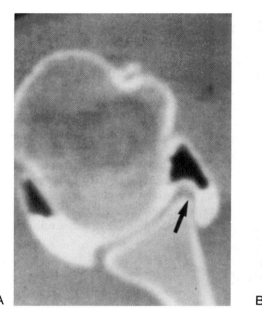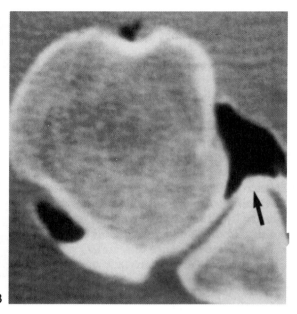

Fig. 21-61. CT arthrograms of the shoulder with recurrent dislocation. **(A)** Normal CT showing the anterior capsule forming a smooth reflexion on the scapula, ultimately blending with the anterior glenoid labrum (arrow). **(B)** CT of the recurrent dislocating shoulder showing a disintegrated anterior glenoid labrum with a thin, irregular surface (arrow) and a thickened capsular reflexion.

their sides, their unstable shoulders dislocated. This point may explain a mechanism of dislocation frequently seen in sport. Furthermore, it emphasizes the concept that once someone has developed sufficient capsular laxity to allow recurrent dislocation, muscle strengthening may do little to alleviate the situation. Indeed, the muscles that keep the humeral head securely in place, in the so-called safe positions of the joint, may actively dislocate the head from the glenoid in the abducted position. That is, recurrent dislocation frequently tends to be an active process and not simply a passive phenomenon accompanying abduction with external rotation.

The statements summerized in the box do not deny the usefulness of shoulder rehabilitation when muscle weakness exists but explain why muscle strengthening alone rarely prevents recurrent redislocations if there is sufficient capsular laxity. Thus many active individuals require surgical treatment for capsular laxity and instability after failure of an intensive rehabilitation protocol designed to correct all detectable muscle strength deficits and imbalances. If the sport's activity is compatible with restriction of abduction, some form of harness may allow play with a reduced chance of dislocation (Fig. 21-62).

Surgical Treatment

If surgery is to be considered, the diagnosis must be refined to make absolutely certain that the problem is unidirectional and anterior. A complete history and documentation of direction during prior episodes of dislocation are helpful. Plain roentgenograms dem-

---

Practice Point

RECURRENT ANTERIOR DISLOCATION

- Once capsular laxity and labral damage is established, redislocation may occur passively or actively in abduction and external rotation.
- The active method (closed kinematic chain) is assisted by the same muscles that help stabilize the shoulder in the neutral position.
- Rehabilitation must be directed at control, not just strength.

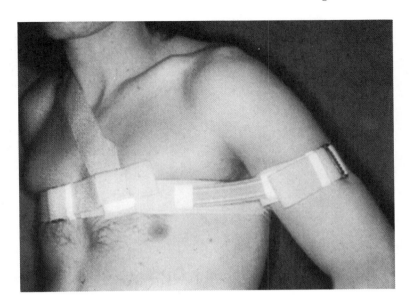

Fig. 21-62. Chest-arm harness used to limit abduction. Some form of elasticized connection with some "give" between the chest and the arm allows restriction of abduction. The new range can be adjusted according to the propensity for dislocation of the athlete and the tasks to be performed.

onstrating the presence of a Hill-Sachs lesion and glenoid rim fractures may be supplemented by special views (e.g., Stryker notch view, West Point modified axillary view), arthrography, and CT arthrography (Figs. 21-61 and 21-63). These data, along with the needs of the individual, assist in selecting the appropriate surgical procedure.

The difficulty of managing the unstable shoulder is not a new problem. Hippocrates, some 400 years BC, recognized instability, described reduction with the fist or the heel as a fulcrum in the axilla, speculated on loose ligaments as a cause of recurrent dislocation, and is credited with devising the first surgery to help stabilization.[18,39,46] He proscribed the use of cautery or "red hot irons" inserted into the anteroinferior shoulder to produce a cicatrix (scar). He did not report on complications but warned of the anatomic structures in the area.

Further delineation of the pathologic anatomy came with Eve's identification of a posterolateral defect in the head of the humerus associated with dislocation in 1880.[84] Five years later Caird linked the lesion to subcoracoid dislocation; and with the evolution of radiographic techniques, Hill and Sachs reported on an impaction fracture that left a posterolateral defect in the humeral head[85,86] (Fig. 21-63). This lesion was ultimately to bear their names. Broca and Hartman in 1890 were the first surgeons since Hippocrates to attempt a surgical repair.[87,88] They based their capsulorrhaphy approach on a detailed discussion of the detachment of the anterior glenoid

labrum from the periosteum of the scapular neck, acknowledging the role of the humeral head defect, thus pre-empting Bankart. By 1906 Perthes had suggested reattachment of the separated labrum and capsule to the glenoid rim using drill holes, an operation Bankart popularized in 1923.[89,90]

Currently, three techniques are commonly used for stabilizing the recurrently dislocating shoulder: the Putti-Platt, Magnuson-Stack, and Bristow repairs.[82,83,85] These three repairs are based on different principles. In 1943 Magnuson and Stack proposed a method for converting the subscapularis muscle into a protective sling across the anterior inferior aspect of the joint.[91] The Magnuson-Stack operation is a relatively simple type of repair, taking either the subscapularis alone or all layers—capsule, cuff, and subscapularis tendon—and overlapping them as one, frequently fixing them with a staple inferolaterally while taking care to avoid the long head of the biceps.[92,93] Although using all layers is a more secure method, it may unduly restrict external rotation. Thus using only the subscapularis tendon may be preferable in selected athletes.

Redislocation rates range from 0 to 7.5 percent (average 3.8 percent).[23] Sir Harry Platt, disturbed by noting that the occasional patient with recurrent dislocation did not have a Bankart lesion, devised a procedure of shortening and plicating the subscapularis and capsule. Originally performing the operation in 1925, he was unaware that Victorio Putti had described the same procedure. Neither of these men

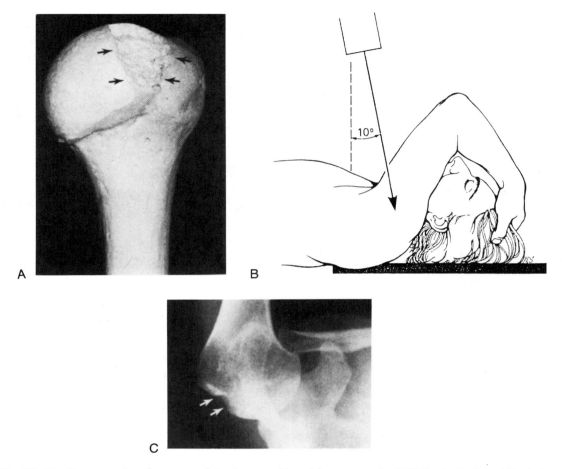

Fig. 21-63. Compression fracture of the humeral head known as the Hill-Sachs lesion. **(A)** Cadaver specimen. **(B)** Technique of the Stryker notch. **(C)** Clinical large Hill-Sachs defect (arrows). (From Danzig et al.,[88] with permission.)

reported their experience, and in 1948 Osmond-Clarke assigned the eponym and wrote up the procedure.[94] Essentially the capsule is taken in one layer and the subscapularis in another, and then they are plicated over each other independently. This technique tends to produce a tight repair, limiting external rotation; hence it may be less than ideal for the treatment of athletes in some sports. The redislocation rate ranges from 0 to 7.3 percent (average 3.4 percent).[23] Redislocation in athletes often occurs in individuals who have re-established a greater than normal range of motion in the affected shoulder.

In 1958 Helfet reported utilizing the principle of a dynamic sling provided by the conjoint tendon of the coracobrachialis and the short head of the biceps, crediting the idea to his mentor Rowley Bristow. He

appreciated that in abduction and external rotation the dynamic support normally provided by the subscapularis, biceps, and coracobrachialis moves superiorly. Thus, these structures do not reinforce the joint anteriorly in this vulnerable position.

The Bristow repair is based on transfer of the tip of the coracoid process with the conjoint tendon to the neck of the scapula (Fig. 21-64). As such, a dynamic sling is formed in the position of abduction and external rotation when these tendons tighten across the front of the neck of the scapula.[94-96] Although there is some debate as to whether the bone block forms a static impediment to dislocation, in many cases it is able to do so, sitting as it does in the fossa that may be occupied by a dislocating humeral head. It may be the preferred operation for athletes because of the possi-

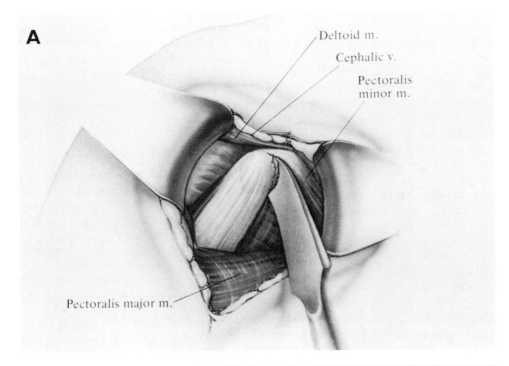

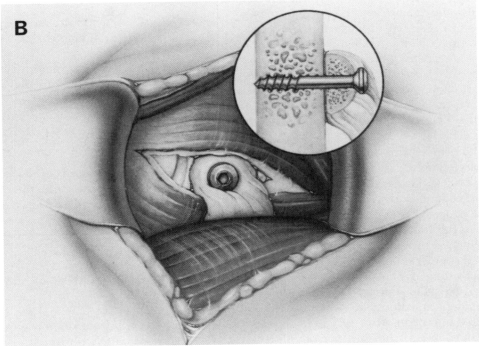

Fig. 21-64. Bristow procedure. **(A)** Tip of the coracoid process is osteotomized, along with the conjoint tendon of the short head of the biceps and the coracobrachialis. **(B)** It is transferred to the glenoid neck so that during the process of abduction the conjoint tendon pulls across the front of the joint, dynamically supporting it.

bility of early restoration of nearly full range of motion. The redislocation rates range from 0 to 3 percent (average 1.9 percent), making it an effective procedure.

The decision for one operation over another has largely been based on complication and redislocation rates, and there is little information about functional outcomes.[2,23] Our data are incomplete on the functional endpoint of these three classes of operation. Our study so far includes 40 patients with the Putti-Platt procedure and a preliminary series with other procedures; patients have been followed 1 to 11 years (mean 6 years). Present information indicates that adequate rehabilitation provides normal strength on the operated side with all repairs. Furthermore, full range of motion or minimally limited external rotation and abduction is also possible. Occasionally, individuals with a Putti-Platt or Bristow repair have an unacceptable range for a few selected sports, but the incidence is low. Range of motion is usually achieved more rapidly with the Bristow repair. However, external rotation in abduction is usually limited to some degree unless special attention is paid to it during rehabilitation. Conversely, we have several athlete-patients with these repairs who have regained the excessive motion required to perform their sports and have re-established a subluxing or dislocating shoulder. It is anticipated that passive restriction may be in the range of 15 to 20 degrees of extended rotation in abduction and dynamic range against resistance slightly more.[97] If return to a throwing sport is the goal, earlier emphasis on gaining range is necessary and usually achievable.

Based on this information, the type of operation should be selected according to the desired activity, the surgeon's skill and experience in performing the particular procedure, and its known complication rates. All the procedures are more compatible with early return to full function if coupled with an adequate rehabilitation protocol.

The known complications include redislocation, pain, vascular and neural compromise, loose or migrating internal fixation devices, interference with the biceps tendon, infection, and, with the Bristow repair, possible nonunion. Most of these complications are uncommon, with the exception of redislocation rates. A literature review reveals that after the Magnuson-Stack procedure there is a redislocation rate of 0 to 17 percent (average approximately 4 percent). The Putti-Platt repair has a redislocation rate of 0 to 8 percent (average 4 percent); finally, the

Bristow procedure is reported as having an average of slightly more than 2 percent redislocation, with a range of 0 to 3 percent.[23,80,81,94,95] Thus with care taken to obtain an adequate bone block and good screw fixation, and with well planned rehabilitation therapy, the Bristow procedure is likely to provide the earliest return to normal function and the lowest redislocation rate.[85]

Rehabilitation Protocol

The following protocol is outlined for the postoperative care of an athlete who has undergone a Bristow repair. It assumes an adequately harvested and secured bone block from the tip of the coracoid. It may be modified to be suitable for the other procedures. The program is organized along the four stages of recovery.

Practice Point

STAGES OF REHABILITATION AFTER BRISTOW REPAIR

- *Stage I*   Early postoperative period: relative immobilization (first 10–14 days)
- *Stage II*   Limited range of motion and early strengthening (2–6 weeks)
- *Stage III* Progressive range of motion strengthening (6–12 weeks)
- *Stage IV*   Return to activity (12–24 weeks)

Stage I: Relative Immobilization (Early Postoperative Period). Immediately after operation the arm is immobilized in a Velpeau bandage (commercial sling

---

Clinical Point

EARLY AIMS OF TREATMENT (POST–OP)

- Decrease pain
- Decrease inflammation response
- Restore muscle control
- Allow healing of soft tissue or bone block
- Prevent undue stiffness
- Maintain cardiovascular fitness
- Maintain general strength

---

and swath). From day 1, the sling may be removed for showering and bathing, but the shoulder motion should be just sufficient to permit adequate axillary hygiene. The patient is encouraged to straighten and bend the elbow in order to avoid stiffness and ulnar nerve symptoms. The goal is to allow wound and muscle healing. Gentle isometric exercises, for the deltoid only, are performed within the tolerance of discomfort. The aim is to minimize wasting rather than aggressive hypertrophy.

Stage II: Limited Range of Motion (2 to 6 Weeks). It is assumed that capsular and bone block healing are incomplete. The sling is worn at all times, but the swath (harness) may be removed during the day. The patient is encouraged to wear both at night to prevent unguarded motion. Careful instruction concerning the exercise progression is given by the therapist so misunderstanding is minimized. The sling is removed four times a day for Codman's pendular exercises in all directions with a goal of 90 degrees of flexion and abduction by the end of 6 weeks after operation (Fig. 21-65). At no point during this stage should external rotation past neutral be encouraged, although some individuals obtain and pass this point easily without effort. External rotation in abduction is contraindicated. Light isotonic resisted exercises for deltoid, triceps, and scapular muscles can be added to the isometric program. Resisted biceps work is not started during this phase, as direct stressing of the healing bone block should be avoided. Furthermore, it tends to flare up a bicipital tendinitis.

Stage III: Progressive Range of Motion and Strengthening (6 to 12 Weeks). At 6 weeks it is assumed that bone healing is well under way and that the capsular repair is sound. Subsequent rehabilitation is guided by pain. If there is evidence of a bicipital tendinitis NSAIDs may be considered. Emphasis is on regaining the extremes of motion and functional levels of strength. Only active and resisted external rotation is performed, and at no point during this phase is passive stretching of this motion entertained. Once full range of motion is achieved with good control and strength, higher velocity exercises and endurance work are important.

Stage IV: Return to Activity (12 to 24 Weeks). Return to activity usually requires 85 percent plus return to strength in all muscles and 90 percent plus range of motion. Heavy resisted work is commenced during this phase to attain preoperative levels of power (Fig. 21-66). Care is taken not to precipitate a tendinitis or capsulitis by too rapid progression.

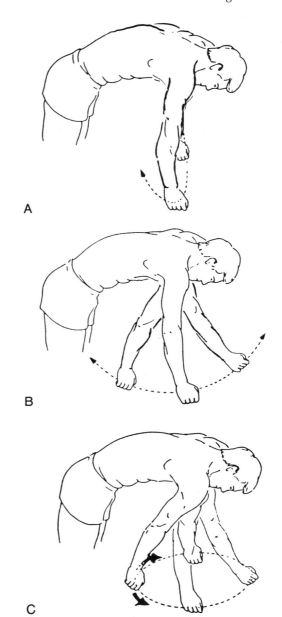

Fig. 21-65. Codman's pendular exercises. **(A)** Horizontal arm swing. **(B)** Vertical arm swing. **(C)** Circle exercises. The aim is to allow a loose, gentle swinging motion, encouraging a comfortable gain in range.

There should be an element of proprioceptive training through this phase to assist in fine control of joint motion.

By 12 to 16 weeks, most athletes can return to their sports, at least in a modified way, unless the activity

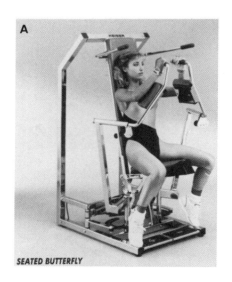

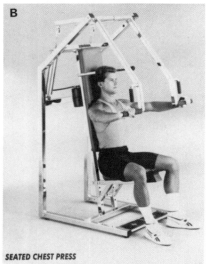

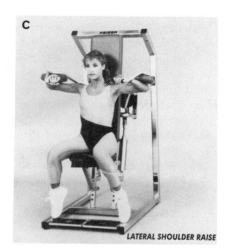

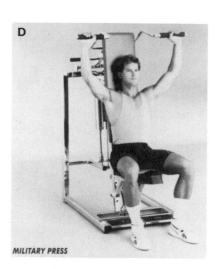

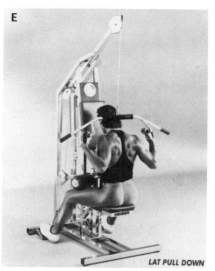

Fig. 21-66. Sequence of advanced shoulder strengthening exercises using hydraulic equipment. **(A)** Seated butterfly for pectorals and anterior deltoid. **(B)** Seated chest press for triceps, anterior deltoid, and pectorals. **(C)** Lateral shoulder raise for all fibers of the deltoid and trapezius. **(D)** Military press for anterior deltoid and triceps. **(E)** LAT pull-down for latissimus dorsi, rhomboids, and posterior deltoid.

involves overhead throwing and striking or heavy contact. By 16 to 24 weeks, if there are no complications, all sports are allowed, but there still needs to be considerable individual advice.

Clinicians frequently assume that the uninjured extremity may be used as a predicator of preinjury strength. This assumption of bilateral equivalency is usually valid so far as rehabilitation goals are concerned. However, for some groups of athletes, e.g.,

pitchers, it is not so, and the issue of handedness must be addressed.[98]

Multidirectional Instability

Neer and Foster emphasized the concept of multidirectional instability in 1980.[68] The shoulder subluxes in more than one direction with a combination of inferior and anterior or inferior and posterior motion, and more rarely all three.[67] In contrast to the generally loose-jointed individuals described by Neer and Foster, athletes who have sustained a traumatic dislocation in one direction occasionally develop a subluxation in the opposite direction. Furthermore, athletes who repetitively use their shoulders in a stressful situation may also develop subluxation in more than one plane, although many of them have a predisposition to such a problem because of lax tissue structures around the shoulder (Fig. 21-67). Many of these athletes fit Matsen and Thomas's AMBRI group, who have relatively atraumatic findings.[99] In most of these individuals, who use their arms for competitive activities such as swimming, throwing, or tennis, pain is a major component of their complaints. Although plain roentgenograms show normal location, inferior subluxation is usually present on

stress views. The presence of a sulcus sign with longitudinal traction and a positive Feagin maneuver help confirm the diagnosis (Fig. 21-27). Excessive translation is present to anteroposterior stressing. The major pathology is failure of the inferior glenohumeral ligament to support the humeral head; which shows up as an enlarged inferior capsular pouch on arthrography.

A nonoperative approach is usually directed at resolving the tendinitis, restoring strength particularly of the rotators, ensuring a reasonable balance of strength between the muscle groups, and stretching any specific structures that may be paradoxically tight, e.g., the pectoralis major. Proprioceptive training, biofeedback, activity modification, and bracing are considered and, when practical, attempted. Nevertheless, for competitive individuals this injury causes signiciant disability, and surgical therapy must be contemplated.

Operative management of these patients is difficult. The diagnosis must be ensured, which may require arthrography, CT arthrograms, or even fluoroscopic visualization of manipulation while the patient is anesthetized. Occasionally, arthroscopy enables visualization of the joint structures, correction of internal derangement, and confirmation of the direction of instability. With gross labral and capsular detachment surgery may be necessary from both anterior and posterior directions. Usually, however, the major pathology dictates either an anterior or a posterior inferior capsular shift procedure. A definite posterior dislocation associated with inferior subluxation is better approached posteriorly (Fig. 21-68). Otherwise, an anteroinferior capsule shift is usually more appropriate (Fig. 21-69). Despite the disability, the inferior capsular shift procedure produces satisfactory results in a large number of athletes. Occasionally, the outcome is an excessively stiff shoulder, with return to full function not possible. The postoperative immobilization should fit the procedure; likewise the speed of progression of the rehabilitation must be tailored to the patient's needs and the surgeon's concerns.

PECTORALIS MAJOR SYNDROMES

Tendinitis of Pectoralis Major

Tendinitis of the pectoralis major insertion is an uncommon entity even in sports where large forces are generated by the upper limb.[100] Nevertheless, it is

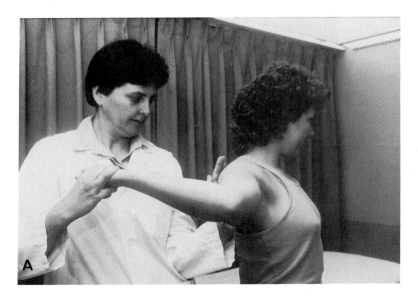

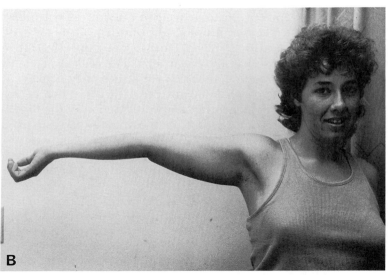

Fig. 21-67. Generalized ligamentous laxity in an athlete with multidirectional instability. **(A)** Excessive external rotation in abduction. **(B)** Hyperextending elbows. *(Figure continues.)*

occasionally encountered and presents with aching and tenderness around the region of the humeral insertion. Often it goes undiagnosed for a long time; and in these instances it may be associated with reactive changes to underlying humerus or calcific deposits within the tendon. These calcific deposits are particularly likely to occur after partial rupture. Occasionally, these changes are confused with aggressive lesions involving primarily the humerus. In these instances of patients who have been referred for exploratory surgery, biopsy specimens obtained during operation have revealed extensive inflammatory changes within the tendon of the pectoralis major muscle.

Essentially these problems are treated like any other case of tendinitis—with local modalities such as ultrasound, laser, or interferential therapy. NSAIDs or even injections of cortisone may be considered. After resolution of the symptoms, an effort should be made to ensure that the pectoralis major muscle has been adequately stretched and is not unduly tight. A progressive strengthening exercise for the muscle is necessary when the condition has been long standing.

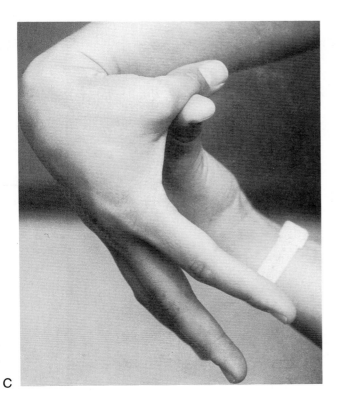

C

Fig. 21-67. *(Continued).* **(C)** Generalized flexibility shown by the hypermobility of the thumb.

Rupture of Pectoralis Major

Pectoral major rupture is discussed in detail in Chapter 18. This lesion is seen in sport, particularly with weight lifting, wrestling, judo, boxing, parachuting, ice hockey, swimming, and football. Previously considered a rare entity, the incidence is rising possibly in association with anabolic steroid abuse. The usual mechanism is sudden exertion against a heavy weight, sudden stretching with co-contraction of the pectoralis major, as would be seen in a clothes-lining maneuver in football, the sudden exertion of bench pressing, or punching in boxing.

The patient usually describes the sudden stress or direct blow applied to the shoulder region while the arm is abducted and extended. The most common symptom is a sharp pain in the shoulder and upper arm, and frequently the athlete reports feeling a snap or "pop" at the time of the injury. Physical findings depend on the site of the injury and the extent of the rupture. Usually the rupture site is close to the musculotendinous junction, although it may be near the attachment to the humerus.[101] The ecchymosis and swelling can extend throughout the axilla and track down the arm past the elbow. Occasionally, with extensive hemorrhage, the ecchymosis and swelling extend over the entire anterior chest wall. Initially, ad-

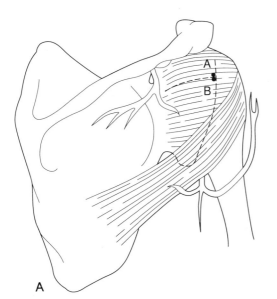

A

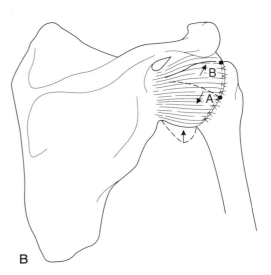

B

Fig. 21-68. Posteroinferior capsular shift. **(A)** Capsule incision is marked out. Care is taken to stay away from the axillary nerve. **(B)** Inferior flap B is advanced superiorly and laterally and the superior flap A is advanced inferiorly and laterally. Thus the redundant inferior capsule is eliminated.

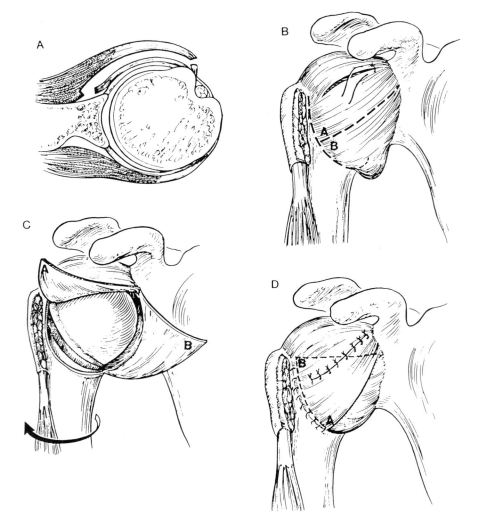

Fig. 21-69. Anteroinferior capsular shift. **(A)** Tendon of the subscapularis is divided, leaving the deep portion to reinforce the weakened inferior capsule. **(B)** Proposed capsular incision. **(C)** Superior flap is advanced inferiorly; and **(D)** the inferior flap is advanced superiorly and laterally, tightening up the whole capsular structure. (After Matsen and Thomas,[99] with permission.)

duction, flexion, and internal rotation are painful, and the muscle is noticeably weaker when compared to that on the opposite side. Depending on the extent of the lesion, there may be a palpable defect.

Treatment of this problem depends on the goals and the sport the athlete wishes to pursue. For top class athletes who depend on chest and shoulder strength, e.g., weight lifters, hockey players, throwers, and football players, surgery is probably the best choice.[102] It ensures return of full strength after adequate rehabilitation. For many individuals, nonoperative treatment is acceptable, particularly with partial ruptures. Most long-term follow-up stud-

ies of nonoperative treatment report some slight defect in strength in adduction and occasionally flexion, but only competitive athletes report significant interference with their function. Partial tears are probably well treated nonoperatively. Surprisingly, many of these individuals present with a delayed diagnosis; in these instances, although operative treatment is technically more difficult it should be attempted in the highly competitive individual.[103]

Late deformity from muscle rupture must be distinguished from congenital partial absence of the pectoralis major, or complete absence of pectoralis minor.

THORACIC OUTLET SYNDROME

Thoracic outlet or inlet syndrome is a complex of signs and symptoms that result from compression of the neurovascular bundle as it emerges from the thorax and enters the upper limb. Depending on the site of compression and the structure involved, there are a variety of clinical manifestations. The presentation may be confusing, and the complaints and physical findings are often vague. Indeed there is debate as to the existence of such a syndrome; and as a result, the attitude of the clinician dictates whether this syndrome is diagnosed with regularity or not at all.

There are two major components to the syndrome, the first relating to problems with the major vessels and the second to pressure on the nerves. If there is thrombosis of the subclavian artery or vein, it is a clearly defined entity that is easily confirmed and usually presents with dramatic clinical signs. There is no speculation regarding this problem. By contrast, the neural signs and symptoms are more difficult to pin down, even with sophisticated electrophysiologic tests.

Relevant Anatomy

The narrow confines of the thoracic outlet may be considered the space between the relatively fixed immobile thorax, particularly the first rib, and the clavicle. Traditionally, this space is extended to include the triangle between the scalenus muscles, which border the roots and trunks of the brachial plexus, en route to the upper limb, within the axillary sheath (Fig. 21-70). During normal development of the human shoulder girdle, the scapula descends from a relatively high position at birth to a low one during adolescence and maturation. These relations are affected by hypertrophy or atrophy of muscles and chronic postural positions. Thus as the configuration of this area changes throughout life, the possibility of a dynamic pathogenesis is possible.

The first potential site of compression is within the interscalene interval (triangle) between the scalene anterior muscle anteriorly and the middle scalene posteriorly. Both are attached to the first rib and serve as a framework for the brachial plexus. This triangle can be compromised by accessory muscles, hypertrophy of the existing muscles, the presence of a bony first rib, or fibrous bands. Accessory ribs are found in approximately 0.5 percent of the general population.[104]

The second major area of potential compression is between the mobile clavicle and the relatively fixed first rib. Fractures of the clavicle with large callus, congenitally bifid clavicles, a changing posture, a postfixed plexus, or thickened, tight clavipectoral fascia may compromise this space. As has been previously emphasized, many of the problems are congenital rather than acquired, but they are in a dynamic state of changing relations; thus true thoracic outlet compression is rarely found before puberty. The scapula tends to descend more in females than males, which may partly explain the greater incidence of thoracic outlet syndrome in women. With increasing age and changing shoulder posture, particularly in association with excessive body weight and large breasts, this problem may become more manifest. It is worthwhile recalling that the suspension of the mobile scapula is virtually entirely muscular in nature; and the strength and tone of the trapezius muscles, rhomboids, and levator scapulae are particularly important to the possible pathogenesis of the problem as well as when considering treatment. Direct and indirect trauma — a single blow or repetitive, excessive use of the upper limb — may trigger this syndrome. Furthermore, in the young athlete it is often the particularly heavy muscled individual, with huge trapezius and neck development, who runs into difficulty.

Quick Facts

POTENTIAL SITES OF NEUROVASCULAR COMPRESSION

- Supraclavicular — scalene triangle

- Subclavicular — between clavicle and first rib
- Infraclavicular — subcoracoid and costo-coracoid membrane

The third potential area of compression for the neurovascular structures is in the subcoracoid region adjacent to the tendon pectoralis minor. Here the thickened clavipectoral fascia, often referred to as the costocoracoid membrane, forms a dense line of fascia. With full circumduction of the arm, the coracoid process almost forms a fulcrum for the subclavian vessels and the neurovascular structures.

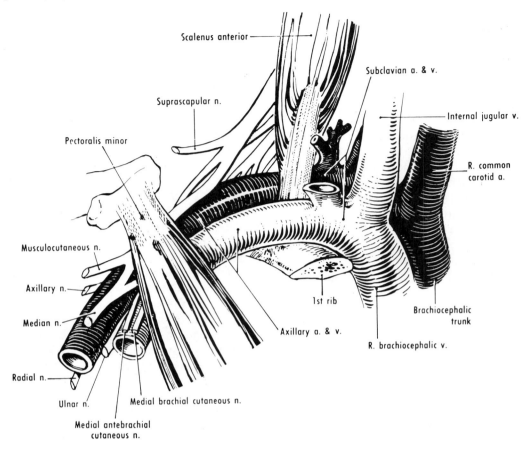

Scalenus anterior

Subclavian a. & v.

Suprascapular n.

Internal jugular v.

Pectoralis minor

R. common carotid a.

Musculocutaneous n.

Axillary n.

Median n.

1st rib

Brachiocephalic trunk

Axillary a. & v.

R. brachiocephalic v.

Radial n.

Ulnar n.

Medial brachial cutaneous n.

Medial antebrachial cutaneous n.

Fig. 21-70. Anatomic relation of the nerves of the plexus and the axillary artery and vein to the first rib, the scalene, and the pectoralis minor muscle at the thoracic outlet. The scalene triangle may be further compromised by accessory muscle, rib or fibrous band.

Clinical Presentation

Neural Compression

Because of the various potential anatomic areas of compression and the variety of structures that can be involved, the clinical manifestations can be inconsistent in nature. The most common clear presenting symptom of the thoracic outlet syndrome arises from compression of the lower trunk of the brachial plexus. The pain extends from the root of the neck to the shoulder and then down the arm in a diffuse fashion. It may be accompanied by paresthesias involving the medial aspect of the hand, particularly the little finger and ring finger, but it may involve the whole of the medial aspect of the arm, particularly from the shoulder to the elbow. Less commonly patients complain of weakness of the affected hand, and there may be detectable wasting.[103,105] Tennis or baseball players may find difficulty gripping the racket or bat. Occasionally there is only painless intrinsic atrophy of the hand. Ultimately the whole of the hand may be involved, but it usually starts on the ulnar side. Some patients complain mainly of neck and shoulder pain, with vague discomfort extending into the trapezius and suboccipital region, which they may describe as a headache-type sensation. During the history it is important to elicit that the athlete relates the symptoms to upper limb motion in the arc where the nerves are either stretched or compressed. Adopting the posture that either narrows the costoclavicular interval or allows compression of the underlying structures should reproduce the symptoms. Numbness and tingling in the hand with overhead movements must be distinguished from the dead arm syndrome of shoulder instability, where rapid movements are involved. Some patients complain of nocturnal paresthesias, waking to find that they have slept with their arms in an overhead position.

Arterial Compression

Symptoms of arterial compression are usually related to numbness of the whole arm with rapid fatigue during overhead exercises. These symptoms may be an isolated finding or occur in association with some neural symptoms. When there is significant arterial compression, the hand may be obviously cool and pale compared to that on the contralateral side when both are held above the head. In addition, the radial pulse may disappear only to return when the arm is replaced at the side. However, this phenomena is frequently seen in the general population, and so great care should be taken when drawing any conclusions from a weakening or a disappearing pulse with the arms above the level of the shoulder. Rarely there are signs of acute arterial insufficiency with major vascular compromise to the hand or even the entire limb.

Venous Compression

When venous compression in the thoracic outlet is the presenting problem, the patient may arrive with a swollen, discolored limb several hours after a bout of intense exercise. In the general population unaccustomed activity such as a building project may cause the problem, but with the athlete it is usually a sudden change in exercise pattern, either different activity or an intense increase in volume of a specific overhead movement. Occasionally, this obvious swelling and color change disappears over several hours so by the time the patient is examined by the physician there is little to see; thus a careful history is important. When venous compromise is sufficiently severe or there is also occlusion of the subclavian vein, a visible venous collateral pattern may become evident across the patient's shoulder, chest, and ipsilateral breast (see Chapter 18).

Clinical Point

CLINICAL MANIFESTATION

It may have a neural or vascular origin.

- Vascular
  - Dull aching
  - Venous distension
  - Peripheral edema
  - Occasional ulceration
- Neural
  - Intermittent
  - Usually ulnar dysesthesia (T1)
  - Aggravated by overhead activity
  - Generalized upper limb ache

Diagnostic Tests

In addition to a detailed history, it is essential to evaluate the cervical spine, shoulder, elbow, and hand for evidence of neural compression. It is mandatory to distinguish the classic ulnar and median nerve compression syndromes and cervical radicular signs. Instability of the shoulder should be ruled out and posture evaluated. Inasmuch as the diagnosis of the thoracic outlet compression is usually one of exclusion, this initial screening is mandatory.

The *hyperabduction test* is performed by taking the arm into gradual abduction and extension of the shoulder while monitoring the pulse. This test is considered positive only if it reproduces all the clinical signs; it is also helpful if there is confirmatory bruit over the subclavian arterial at the time of pulse diminution and reproduction of the symptoms[103] (Fig. 21-71).

The *overhead exercise test* is performed by having the patient take the arms into full elevation and then rapidly flex and extend the fingers. In susceptible individuals a feeling of fatigue or even cramping of the forearm muscles may be experienced within about 20 seconds. The elevated arm may also become pale compared to the normal side, and the obliteration or diminishing of a pulse assists in confirming the diagnosis. A variation of this test is the 3-minute elevated arm exercise test (Fig. 21-71).

The classic provocative maneuvers for thoracic outlet compression produce many false-positive findings. *Adson's maneuver* — with the arm at the side and

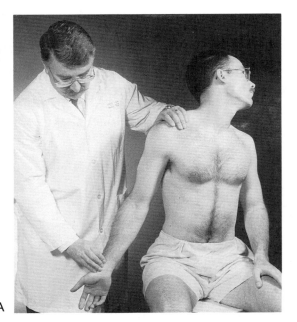

Fig. 21-71. (A) Wright's maneuver, in which the head is rotated and the chin elevated in a forceful manner away from the side to be tested. A deep breath is taken, and held. A positive test is aggravation or precipitation of symptoms or obliteration of the pulse. **(B)** Hyperabduction test includes abduction and extension of the shoulder, which should obliterate the pulse or exacerbate the symptoms. **(C)** Three-minute elevated arm exercise test. Patient opens and closes the fists slowly for full 3 minutes. A positive test is reproduction of the symptoms, undue fatigue, forearm cramping, or inability to continue.

A

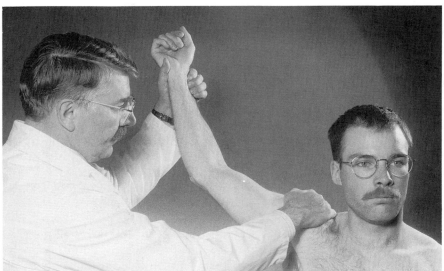

B

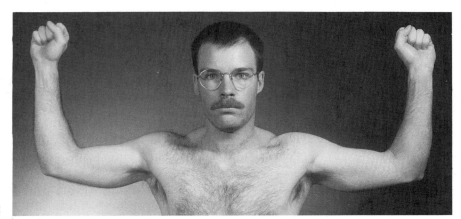

C

externally rotated and the examiner monitoring the pulse while the individual rotates the head toward the involved side, elevates the chin, pushes into full rotation, and takes a deep breath to fix the upper rib — is mildly positive in a large percentage of the population.[105]

With *Wright's maneuver,* the pulse of the abducted and laterally rotated arm is monitored while the neck is rotated to the opposite side. The patient takes a deep breath while adopting the so-called military brace position with the shoulders retracted and pulled down (Fig. 21-71).

Plain cervical spinal roentgenograms may help to rule out certain intrinsic conditions, e.g., cervical spondylosis, narrowed intervertebral discs, and osteophytic impingement. The presence of cervical ribs or long C7 transverse processes may fit in with the findings of thoracic outlet compression. All patients should have adequate studies of the apex of the lung on the affected side.

There is a discrepancy of opinion regarding the value of *electrodiagnostic studies.* There is considerable difficulty accurately determining the nerve conduction velocity through the thoracic outlet. In many ways, the biggest value of electrodiagnostic studies is to rule out peripheral entrapment, e.g., ulnar neuropathy at the elbow or hand or carpal tunnel syndrome of the median nerve at the wrist.

If there is significant evidence of arterial venous involvement suggesting either thrombosis, aneurysm or compression, it may be prudent to obtain *Doppler, Angiographic,* or *venographic studies.*

Differential Diagnosis

Because there are few definite indicators of the thoracic outlet syndrome, its diagnosis is one of exclusion. Thus the differential diagnosis assumes significance.

Practice Point

THORACIC OUTLET SYNDROME

- It is usually a diagnosis of exclusion.
- Make sure cervical pathology is excluded.
- Surgical treatment should not be carried out unless electrophysiologic tests rule out peripheral entrapment.

Cervical Spine

Cervical spinal pathology is the most common cause of paresthesia in the upper limb, and efforts should be made to distinguish radicular pain in the C8 and T1 distribution. Most disc diseases affect the C5–C6 level and to somewhat lesser extent the C7 level. Thus paresthesias in the ulnar side of the hand are more likely to be of distal origin.

Supraclavicular Fossa

Any space-occupying lesion within the thoracic outlet, particularly the Pancoast's tumor at the apex of the lungs, may mimic the symptoms of the thoracic outlet syndrome. Although it is believed that the pursuit of health and fitness is not compatible with smoking, a large number of athletes do indeed smoke on a regular basis. The incidence of lung cancer parallels this habit, and so the middle-aged and elderly athlete is not immune from lung tumors.

Peripheral Neuritis

Peripheral entrapment of the ulnar nerve at the elbow and in the cubital tunnel, or in the hand in Guyon's canal, can produce typical dysesthesia in the ring and little fingers. Similarly, compression of the median nerve and the carpal tunnel may produce paresthesias in the distribution of that nerve, typically in the thumb and index and middle fingers, with wasting of the hyperthenar eminence. In previously reported series of cervical rib resection for thoracic outlet, there was an uncomfortably large percentage of individuals who subsequently required release of the ulnar or medial nerve peripherally. It is tempting to postulate a double-crush syndrome, with irritation at a subclinical level in both sites, combining to produce a significant clinical entity. One should remain pragmatic, however, and assume that in many of these instances an incorrect diagnosis has been made.

Reflex Sympathetic Dystrophy

Like the thoracic outlet syndrome, reflex sympathetic dystrophy presents as a constellation of peripheral symptoms, including dysesthesias, hypersensitivity, and muscle wasting. The key to diagnosing reflex sympathetic dystrophy is awareness of the possibility of this syndrome. A key feature is the disassociation between the sensations of touch, pressure, and pain. It may be particularly difficult to distinguish the two syndromes if there is appreciable swelling within the hand. The presence of a "hot" bone scan helps to differentiate them.

Management of Thoracic Outlet Syndrome

With the exception of patients who present with an impending vascular catastrophe, the initial thrust of treatment should be nonoperative. Thorough assessment of muscle strength and posture leads to establishment of an adequate retraining program for the muscles of the scapula and shoulder girdle. In the slightly overweight person or in those with large breasts, the choice of appropriate sporting underwear is part of the treatment program. In situations where there has been a sudden change in activity pattern, treatment with anti-inflammatory medication, modification of activity, thorough investigation into past exercise habits, and a proposed direction of future training plans should be carefully examined.

When nonoperative treatment has failed and the diagnosis is firmly established, consideration of *operative* treatment is appropriate. The first rib resection is the usual, most effective treatment, as it deals with both the supraclavicular and the infraclavicular etiologic factors in this syndrome. The surgery may be well achieved through an axillary approach, as described by Roos and Owens in 1966, and allows fairly rapid resumption of physical activity.[103] Complications of this surgery include pneumothorax and occasional transient damage to the long thoracic nerve and winging of the scapula. Return to full activity should follow an adequate rehabilitation program designed to provide full strengthening of the shoulder girdle muscle, to re-establish the range of motion of the shoulder, and a plan of exercise progression for the ensuing season.

FRACTURES AROUND THE SHOULDER

With the exception of fractures of the clavicle, fractures of the shoulder girdle and proximal humerus are uncommon in sport (Fig. 21-72).

Fractures of the Clavicle

Most fractures of the clavicle are caused by direct blows sustained by a fall on the point of the shoulder, although occasionally forces transmitted through the

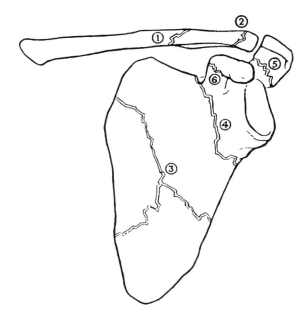

Fig. 21-72. Classification of fractures of the shoulder girdle: (1) fracture of the clavicle; (2) fracture adjacent to the acromioclavicular joint; (3) fracture of the body of the scapula; (4) fracture of the neck of the scapula; (5) fracture of the acromion process; (6) fracture of the coracoid process.

outstretched hand are responsible. The usual site is the junction of the middle and outer thirds.

Treatment depends on the amount of displacement. Undisplaced and minimally displaced fractures are adequately treated with a sling, which is used primarily for comfort. Significantly displaced and overlapping fractures may require a figure-of-eight bandage to retract the shoulder girdle, minimize the overlap, and allow more anatomic healing; the efficacy of this technique for altering displacement, however, is doubtful. If the fragment is threatening to pierce the skin, the figure-of-eight bandage may be supplemented by a sling and some plaster wrap to make it more secure. If there is significant jeopardy of the bone end piercing the skin, it might be construed as an indication to open the fracture and reduce the bone ends. Essentially, there are few indications for open reduction and internal fixation of a fractured clavicle.

An exception to the above rules is the fracture near the distal end of the clavicle. Such fractures act similar to acromioclavicular separations and should be reduced and pinned in much the same way. Furthermore, in the skeletally immature, this distal fracture often is a shoulder epiphyseal separation and likewise should be reduced appropriately.

Having outlined these principles, it must be said that the aim of bringing fragments back into apposition by figure-of-eight bandages is seldom realized. Moreover, this method has the distinct disadvantage that if the bandage is applied too firmly venous return from the upper limb is obstructed. Furthermore, constant pressure over the axilla may generate neuropraxia of the nerve. For this reason, nearly all of these fractures are often treated with some form of sling despite an imperfect reduction.

Healing in the young is usually well under way within 2 to 3 weeks; even in the adult it seldom is longer than 6 to 8 weeks. The complications of this fracture are a mild deformity and occasionally, because of displacement, disruption of the adjacent acromioclavicular joint with chronic symptoms in that joint. Non union is uncommon. There is a rare but theoretic risk of the fracture bone end piercing the subclavian artery and some care should be exercised with early return to activity.

Fractures of the Scapula

Most scapular injuries are generated by direct blows, with the exception of glenoid rim fractures, which are usually in association with dislocations. They are divided into fractures of the body of the scapula, fractures of the neck, fractures of the acro-

mion process, and fractures of the coracoid process (Fig. 21-72).

Fractures of the body of the scapula rarely require treatment except for support and immobilization to relieve pain. Because of the investing muscles around this area, displacement is usually minimal, and healing usually occurs uneventfully. Early motion should be encouraged.

Fractures of the neck of the scapula are, for the most part, treatable with nonoperative means. If there is significant displacement or if the fracture extends onto the glenoid margin and involves the joint, some consideration must be given to glenohumeral stability (discussed in the section on dislocations). Treatment again focuses on pain relief and early mobilization.

Fractures of the Acromion Process

Acromion process fractures are caused by direct blows. If the fracture is a simple crack without displacement, a sling is worn for comfort followed by early motion. If the acromion fracture is comminuted and markedly depressed, surgery is usually advised because of the potential interruption of abduction in the young athletic person. Depending on the amount of acromion involved, the fragment may be either excised or fixed with small pins. A period of immobilization depends more on the ability of the muscles to be reattached and heal securely than on the fracture itself.

Fractures of the Coracoid Process

Fractures of the coracoid process have been reported on several occasions in the sports medicine literature. They are related to avulsions by the conjoined tendon or pectoralis minor. For the most part, these fractures are best ignored and usually heal uneventfully.

Humeral Head and Neck Fractures

Humeral head fractures involve some key anatomic structures including the joint surface itself and the attachments of the supraspinatus and subscapularis. Furthermore, the bicipital groove between the greater and lesser tuberosity allows smooth passage of the biceps tendon. The large range of motion that is so necessary at the glenohumeral joint is jeopardized after injury, frequently by the formation of adhesions. Therefore it is important to institute motion

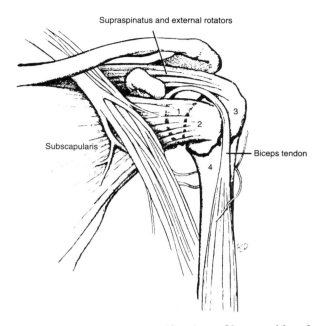

Fig. 21-73. Four-part classification of humeral head and neck fractures: (1) humeral head; (2) lesser tuberosity with attached subscapularis, which may generate a deforming force; (3) greater tuberosity with supraspinatus, which may displace the fracture; (4) humeral shaft.

prior to the maturation of these inherent adhesions whenever possible. In some cases it influences the decision of whether to treat the fractures by closed or open means. In the case of most fractures with minimal displacement, early gentle, active assisted exercises are the treatment of choice. The large amount of cancellous bone in the area allows satisfactory union of the fracture. Nevertheless, nonimpacted fractures do require a period of immobilization or surgical repair.

It is helpful to divide the humeral head into the four major segments that are involved either in isolation or in combination with trauma to this region (Fig. 21-73). These segments are the articular area of the head back to the anatomic neck level, the greater tuberosity to which the supraspinatus attaches, the lesser tuberosity to which the subscapularis attaches, and the remaining shaft of the humerus from the surgical neck down.[106] The relations of each of these four major segments must be carefully analyzed and identified on the initial roentgenograms in order to plan treatment. Essentially, when any of the four segments are displaced more than 1 cm or angulated more than 45 degrees, the fracture is considered to be displaced. Usually displaced fragments must be reduced and fixed. Occasionally, these fractures are associated with dislocation, which is nearly always an indication for open reduction (Table 21-9). Whatever

TABLE 21-9.   Fractures of the Proximal Humerus

Type	Approx. Incidence (%)	Major Problem	Usual Treatment
Minimally displaced	80	Adhesions	Initial support Early passive exercises Progress to active as union advances
Two-part	10	Adhesions	Closed treatment except for displaced greater tuberosity or widely displaced shaft
Three-part	3	Rotary forces of muscles prevent acceptable reduction	Frequently need open reduction Buried wire fixation Repair of rotator cuff
Four-part	4	High incidence of avascular necrosis	Attempt open reduction in young Consider prosthesis in older individual
Articular surface	3	Late degenerative changes; difficult to stabilize	Attempt reduction if possible May require prosthesis

(After Rockwood and Matsen,[18] with permission.)

the method of treatment, the ultimate aim is to restore range of motion in the short term, unimpaired by either the displacement or the internal fixation device, before adhesions form and mature.

Fractures of the Proximal Humerus

Fractures of the proximal humerus start just below the level of the surgical neck and extend to approximately the midshaft. The displacement of these fractures depends on their level and the relation to the supraspinatus, pectoralis major, deltoid, coracobrachialis and short head of the biceps (Fig. 21-74). Fortunately, a large number of these fractures are impacted, which facilitates closed treatment and relatively early mobilization. Provided the alignment of the fragments is good, it is usually not necessary to secure perfect end-to-end apposition. Nevertheless, it is important to have contact of about one-fourth to one-third of the area of the fracture to expedite reasonable healing. Although many of these fractures are capable of being treated by closed means, the circumstances of the particular athlete should be taken into account. Open reduction and internal fix-

ation are considered when they offer distinct advantages in terms of timing and the ability to keep the joints and muscles healthy.

One of the major concerns with fractures of the humerus is the relation of the axillary nerve proximally and the radial nerve in the middle third as it passes through the spiral groove. However, the nerve is seldom divided, and so the lesion is one of continuity, with excellent recovery anticipated. It should be recalled that whereas fresh fractures of the humeral shaft heal well and rapidly, nonunion of the humerus can be difficult to treat and may require intermedullary nailing and bone grafting. Thus every effort should be made to provide optimal conditions for the early healing of the initial fracture.

NERVE INJURIES

Most of the nerve injuries that occur in sport are transient in nature, usually neuropraxic. Nevertheless there are a series of upper limb nerve injuries that are indicative of a more serious injury of the axonotmesis variety. Transection of a nerve occurs rarely.

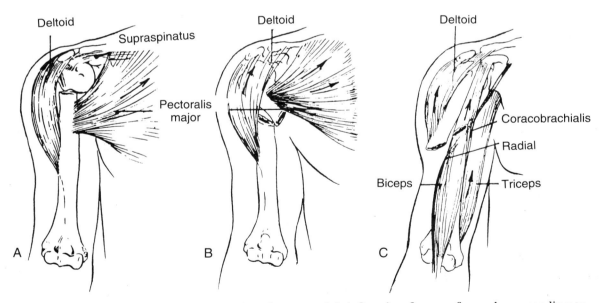

Fig. 21-74. Proximal humerus illustrating the potential deforming forces of muscles according to fracture level. **(A)** Between the rotator cuff and the pectoralis major, gives relative abduction of the proximal fragment. **(B)** Between pectoralis major and the deltoid, leading to adduction of the proximal fragment. **(C)** Below the deltoid insertion, producing shortening and abduction of the proximal fragment.

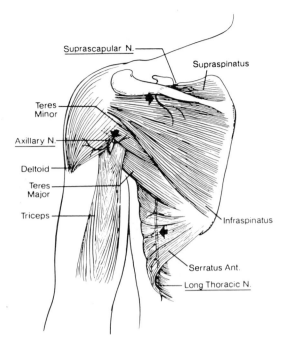

Fig. 21-75. Axillary, suprascapular, and long thoracic nerves. Arrows indicate possible sites of entrapment. (After Goodman,[108] with permission.)

The etiology of such nerve injuries is frequently an acute episode of traction or a direct blow, crushing the nerve against the underlying bony structures. More rarely repetitive minor crushing, traction, or pressure results in dysesthesia or paralysis. For this reason excellent functional recovery is usually anticipated, and surgical exploration is rarely needed. This section deals with nerve injuries to the suprascapular nerve, the nerve to the serratus anterior, the musculocutaneous nerve, and the axillary (circumflex) nerve (Fig. 21-75).

Suprascapular Nerve Injuries

The largest series of suprascapular nerve injuries involve volleyball players, but these lesions are also seen in baseball pitchers, weight lifters, swimmers, and exponents of the martial arts.[107] The suprascapular nerve consistently originates from either the distal portion of the root of C5 or from the upper trunk of the brachial plexus. It passes across the scalenus medius and under the trapezius, entering the supraspinatus fossa by obliquely passing through the suprascapular notch, underneath the transverse scapular ligament when it is present. Occasionally, this ligament is ossified, forming a small bony frame. The nerve divides in the suprascapular notch, sending a branch to the supraspinatus muscle. The main nerve continues with the suprascapular artery and vein, curling around the blunt base of the spinous process of the scapula (Fig. 21-76).

In many individuals there is an osseous fibrous canal formed by the spinoglenoid ligament, which is in an aponeurotic band that separates the supraspinatus and infraspinatus muscle. At this point the nerve frequently heads medially to break up and supply the infraspinatus muscle. From this description it may be seen that the nerve is relatively fixed at its origin and within the muscle of infraspinatus, and it has two potentially critical areas of impingement or pressure along its course. The first is in the suprascapular notch, and the second is just by its termination as it courses around the base of the spine of the scapula. With repetitive circling and overhead motions of the upper limb, there may be repetitive minor

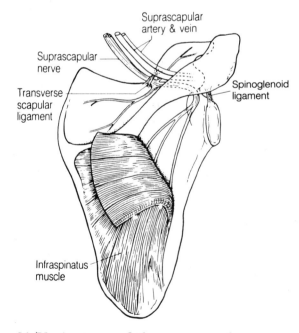

Fig. 21-76. Anatomy of the suprascapular nerve. Spinoglenoid ligament is present in approximately 50 percent of individuals. Occasionally the nerve takes a sharp turn around the base of the spinal scapula and runs parallel before breaking up into the muscle. It is possible that this configuration makes the nerve more susceptible to traction.

traction on this nerve, thus generating an injury. The suprascapular nerve is particularly stretched when the arm is taken across the body into adduction in forward flexion.[107–110]

Making the diagnosis of suprascapular nerve injury is not always easy, and indeed the athlete may present simply with a complaint of shoulder pain.[109] Many present with an anterior impingement syndrome that is probably related to the dyssynergy of shoulder function. The etiology of the pain in others is not fully understood. There may be weakness in abduction, and adaptive mechanisms may evolve for initiating abduction. Wasting of the muscle belly may be apparent in the supraspinus fossa (Fig. 21-77).

Isolated paralysis of the infraspinatus, which suggests that the distal part of the nerve is involved subsequent to passing around the base of the spinous process, has been reported in volleyball players, weight lifters, and baseball pitchers.[111]

In some instances the presentation is benign, but once again the athlete may present with shoulder pain because paralysis of the infraspinatus causes loss of function of the major humeral head depressor and therefore results in potential imbalance in the force couples formed by the deltoid and shoulder rotators. However, this situation may not entirely explain the pain. Most of the athletes complain of shoulder weakness, and there may be wasting in the infraspinous area of the scapula (Fig. 21-78). A CT scan of the area can confirm the atrophy.

The nerve has been reported to be compressed secondary to a ganglion cyst, and usually this lesion resolves with nonoperative treatment. Considerable improvement may occur in 1 to 2 months, but it frequently takes 6 months to a year to fully resolve and allow full return to function. When there is failure to improve, EMG may help make a decision about the advisability of surgical exploration.

One of the major problems is the differential diagnosis between rotator cuff tear and suprascapular nerve palsy in instances where direct trauma is the immediate cause of the weakness. Shoulder arthrograms or EMG help solve this problem. Once recovery is well under way, the weakness is easily compensated for by specific and progressive rehabilitation programs.

Nerve to Serratus Anterior (Backpack Palsy)

The serratus anterior muscle is a powerful stabilizer and protractor of the shoulder, and it is essential for strong, smooth abduction particularly when done against resistance. It is supplied by the long thoracic nerve, and this nerve appears to be vulnerable as it passes from the plexus across the root of the neck, and then again more distally as it applies itself to the chest wall (Fig. 21-75). A blow across the top of the shoulder or, more usually, chronic compression or traction due to wearing an asymmetric backpack re-

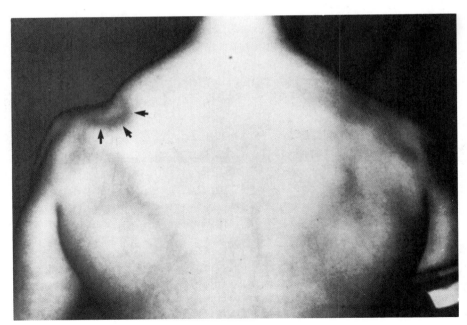

Fig. 21-77. Atrophy of the left supraspinatus subsequent to suprascapular nerve palsy. Wasting is seen in the supraspinus fossa.

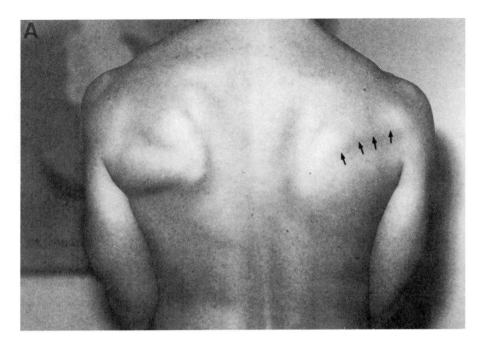

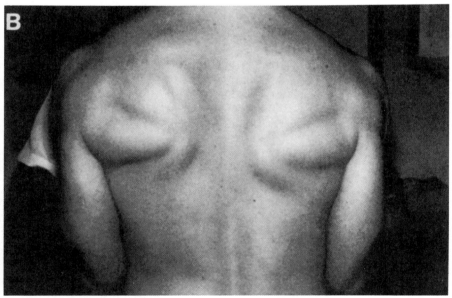

Fig. 21-78. Isolated palsy of the infraspinatus muscle. **(A)** Wasting is obvious with resisted external rotation. **(B)** Subsequent to recovery, the normal contour is once again seen on the right shoulder.

sults in transient or even semipermanent paralysis of this muscle. The patient may present complaining of pain in the neck area or shoulder girdle or simply a weakness and heavy feeling of the arm when attempting to do overhead movements. Examination reveals scapular winging with resisted protraction when the amount of nerve involvement is significant. This winging becomes more obvious after a few weeks

as the parascapular muscles become stretched out. When attempting to elevate the arm, only glenohumeral motion takes place, and abduction is always limited (Fig. 21-79). Once again, relieving the nerve of stress usually allows total recovery over a period of several months to a year. Many of these individuals do have some residual EMG evidence of permanent change within the muscle and nerve; but because of

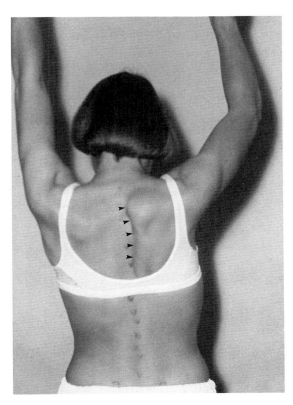

Fig. 21-79. Paralysis of serratus anterior with some winging on elevation of the shoulder. Full range of motion is not possible. The failure of the scapula to rotate is obvious (arrows).

the huge size of the muscle it is usually possible to rehabilitate the remaining fibers to overcome the strength deficits.

Musculocutaneous Nerve

The musculocutaneous nerve arises from the lateral cord of the brachial plexus opposite the lower border of the pectoralis minor. The fibers are derived from the fifth, sixth and seventh cervical nerves. The nerve pierces the coracobrachialis and runs between the biceps and the brachialis to reach the lateral side of the arm. A major nerve trunk running right through the middle of a muscle is an unusual arrangement and probably stems from the fact that phylogenetically the coracobrachialis was a muscle with three heads in the lower primates. Subsequently, these heads have either recessed or fused to form a single muscle in humans. It is possible that this arrangement restricts the mobility of the nerve in some individuals. The most common cause of damage to

the musculocutaneous nerve is its association with anterior dislocations of the shoulder. Many cases have been noted in weight lifters, either secondary to traction or after intense bouts of upper body work for the biceps and brachialis.[112]

It is possible that this nerve is involved in an exercise-induced anterior compartment syndrome of the arm, secondary to delayed muscle soreness and edematous reaction following an intense exercise bout. The nerve supplies the flexors of the arm, including the coracobrachialis, biceps, and brachialis. It continues as the lateral cutaneous nerve of the forearm, supplying lateral skin and the area adjacent to the base of the thumb. Sensation is usually altered in this area with involvement of the nerve. Once again this injury usually resolves spontaneously.

Axillary Nerve (Circumflex Nerve) Injury

The axillary nerve arises from the posterior cord of the brachial plexus, its fibers being derived from the fifth and sixth cervical nerve roots. At first it lies on the lateral side of the radial nerve behind the axillary artery and just in front of the subscapularis muscle. At the lower border of the subscapularis it winds backward in close relation to the lower part of the articular capsule of the shoulder joint, accompanied by the posterior circumflex vessels. It passes through the quadrilateral space, bounded above by scapulae, in front by teres minor, behind by the teres major, medially by the long head of triceps, and laterally by the surgical neck of the humerus (Fig. 21-60). The nerve then ends by dividing into anterior and posterior branches. The anterior branch runs deep to the deltoid as far as the anterior border of muscle, supplying it and giving off a few cutaneous twigs. The posterior branch supplies the teres minor and the posterior part of deltoid, as well as forming the upper lateral cutaneous branch, which supplies an area of skin over the deltoid. When damaged it obviously causes weakness of the deltoid and therefore affects abduction as well as all of the other movements of the shoulder girdle. In addition, there is a small area of sensory loss over the deltoid muscle.

In athletes, this nerve is most frequently damaged secondary to dislocations of the shoulder (discussed earlier in the chapter). Occasionally, athletes have the nerve damaged during surgical procedures, particularly the inferior capsular shift for recurrent multidirectional instability. Inadvertently injecting the nerve with corticosteroid when treating tendinitis of the long head of triceps or the infraspinatus may also result in paralysis.

Essentially, the lesion has a good prognosis except when there is complete involvement of the nerve. Recovery takes 6 to 12 months if a major portion of the nerve is involved. Some of the return to function is via the branching and formation of large motor units. Although there is usually some residual weakness with incomplete recovery, as detected by isokinetic testing, a functional shoulder is often achieved. For many individuals with lesser involvement, recovery is usually complete.

TUMORS

The proximal humerus is a fairly common site of bone tumor. Whenever a painful soft tissue lesion is not responding in the traditional fashion, repeat roentgenograms are advised, as many cases of bone tumor to the shoulder present as pain and are initially diagnosed as capsulitis, bursitis, or muscle injury.

Benign Tumors

Simple (Unicameral) Cysts

Simple bone cysts are common in the proximal humerus and probably represent an area of altered growth plate activity. They are seen as a lytic lesion on plain films and are usually fluid-filled cysts. Treatment depends on their size and activity of the person involved. The decision to operate depends on the certainty of the diagnosis based on the classic appearance on the roentgenogram and the degree of potential mechanical weakening due to the size of the lesion. Stress fractures through these lesions are common.

Chondroblastoma

Chondroblastomas are rare primary, usually benign, bone tumors of immature cartilage cell derivation. Chondroblastomas comprise less than 1 percent of all primary bone tumors. Codman's description in 1931 pointed out its affinity for the shoulder. This tumor has subsequently been referred to as Codman's tumor. However, the most frequent site is around the knee, followed by the pelvis, and then the shoulder region. The peak age at onset is between 10 and 30 years. These lesions form within the epiphyseal area of long bones, an occasional extension to the adjacent metaphysis. Radiographically, they appear as a more or less lytic, round or oval area of bone destruction. Histologically, they are locally aggressive; they tend to recur and in rare cases metastasize. The location of the lesion brings up a differential diagnosis of giant cell tumor and even aneurysmal bone cysts. Thus biopsy is frequently mandatory.

Malignant Tumors

The shoulder can be a site of osteosarcoma and Ewing's tumor, but by far the greatest number of malignant lesions are secondary, particularly from carcinoma of the breast. Thus in the young and middle-aged female athlete presenting with a lytic lesion in the proximal humerus or shoulder, the question of it being a secondary lesion must always be entertained; even prior to biopsy, a search must be made for a primary source.

SUMMARY

This chapter has stressed the interrelations between impingement, muscle imbalance, and instability. Dislocation of the shoulder occurs frequently in sport and has often received less attention than it deserves. A careful approach to treatment of the acute first time lesion may affect its natural history and reduce recurrence rates.

The entity of multidirectional instability is a difficult one with which to deal, and a clear diagnosis is mandatory if surgical therapy is entertained. Overlooking this pattern of laxity leads to unsuccessful nonoperative and surgical treatment. Coaches must be made aware of the danger of routinely putting all athletes on stretching programs in an unselective fashion. In those individuals with a propensity to shoulder laxity, stretching may lead to pathology.

Nerve injury to some of the rotator cuff muscles is relatively frequent and not always obvious. The presenting complaint for many is pain. A careful physical examination should unmask the weakness.

Lastly, benign and malignant tumors are found at the shoulder at a frequency exceeded only by tumors of the distal femur and proximal tibia. Thus when apparently simple lesions fail to resolve, a repeat roentgenogram is often in order.

The modalities of CT, MRI, and arthroscopy have begun to lead to a new understanding of many shoulder disorders in the athlete. However, even a greater understanding does not always make treatment of the complex articulations of the shoulder girdle easy. For many athletes, the fact that they must reduce or curtail the activities that cause the stress or provocation is an unpalatable truth.

REFERENCES

1. Reid DC, Saboe L, Burnham R: Common shoulder problems in the athlete. In Donatelo R (ed): Physical Therapy of the Shoulder. 2nd Ed. Churchill Livingstone, New York, 1991

2. Reid DC: Functional Anatomy and Joint Mobilization. University of Alberta Press, Edmonton, 1970

3. Kaput M: Anatomy and biomechanics of the shoulder. In Donatelli R (ed.): Physical Therapy of the Shoulder. Churchill Livingstone, New York, 1987

4. Reid DC: The shoulder girdle: its structure and function as a unit in abduction. Physiotherapy February 1969.

5. Reid DC: Assessment and Treatment of the Injured Athlete. Teaching Manual. University of Alberta, Edmonton, 1989

6. Perry J: Anatomy and biomechanics of the shoulder in throwing, swimming, gymnastics and tennis. Clin Sports Med 2:247, 1983

7. De Palma AF, Callery G, Bennett GA: Variational anatomy and degenerative lesions of the shoulder joint. Instruct Course Lect 6:255, 1949

8. Warwick R, Williams PL (eds): Gray's Anatomy. 35th Ed. Longman, Edinburgh, 1973

9. Salter EG, Nasca RJ, Shelley BS: Anatomic observations on the acromioclavicular joint and supporting ligaments. Am J Sports Med 15:199, 1987

10. Petersson CJ: Degeneration of the acromioclavicular joint. Acta Scand 54:434, 1983

11. Freedman L, Munro RR: Abduction of the arm in the scapula plane: scapular and glenohumeral movements: a roentgenographic study. J Bone Joint Surg [Am] 48:1503, 1966

12. Poppen NK, Walker PS: Normal and abnormal motion of the shoulder. J Bone Joint Surg [Am] 58:195, 1976

13. Rowe CR, Zarins B: Recurrent transient subluxation of the shoulder. J Bone Joint Surg [Am] 63:863, 1981

14. Ferrari DA: Capsular ligaments of the shoulder: anatomical and functional study of the anterior superior capsule. Am J Sports Med 18:20, 1990

15. Rasch PJ, Burke RK: Kinesiology and Applied Anatomy. 2nd Ed. Lea & Febiger, Philadelphia, 1963

16. Reid DC, Oedekoven G, Kramer JF, Saboe LA: Isokinetic strength parameters for shoulder movements. Clin Biomech 4:97, 1989

17. Fowler P: Swimmer's problems. Am J Sports Med: 7:141, 1979

18. Rockwood CA, Matsen FA: The Shoulder. WB Saunders, Philadelphia, 1990

19. Hawkins RJ, Hobeika PE: Impingement syndrome in the athletic shoulder. Clin Sports Med 2:391, 1983

20. Hawkins RJ, Kennedy JC: Impingement syndrome in athletes. Am J Sports Med 8:151, 1980

21. Norris TR: History and physical examination of the shoulder. In Nicholas JA, Hershman EB (eds): The Upper Extremity in Sports Medicine. CV Mosby, St. Louis, 1990

22. Gerber C, Ganz R: Clinical assessment of instability of the shoulder with special reference to anterior and posterior drawer tests. J Bone Joint Surg [Br] 66:551, 1984

23. Rockwood C, Green D: Fractures in Adults. 2nd Ed. JB Lippincott, Philadelphia, 1984

24. Eidman DK, Sift SJ, Tullos HS: Acromioclavicular lesions in children. Am J Sports Med 9:150, 1981

25. Walsh MW, Peterson DA, Shelton G et al: Shoulder strength following acromioclavicular injury. Am J Sports Med 13:153, 1985

26. Cooper ES: New method of treating long standing dislocations of the scapulo-clavicular articulation. Am J Med Sci 41:389, 1961

27. Horn JS: The traumatic anatomy and treatment of acute acromioclavicular dislocation. J Bone Joint Surg [Br] 36:194, 1954

28. Kennedy JC, Cameron H: Complete dislocation of the acromioclavicular joint. J Bone Joint Surg [Br] 36:202, 1954

29. Larsen E, Bjerg-Nielson A, Christensen P: Conservative or surgical treatment of acromioclavicular dislocation: a prospective controlled, randomized study. J Bone Joint Surg [Am] 68:552, 1986

30. Urist MR: Complete dislocations of the acromioclavicular joint: the nature of the traumatic lesion and effective methods of treatment with an analysis of forty-one cases. J Bone Joint Surg 28:813, 1946

31. Bannister GC, Wallace WA, Stableforth PG, Hutson MA: The management of acute acromioclavicular dislocation: a randomized prospective controlled trial. J Bone Joint Surg [Br] 71:848, 1989

32. MacDonald PB, Alexander MJ, Frejuk J et al: Comprehensive functional analysis of shoulders following complete acromioclavicular separation. Am J Sports Med 16:475, 1988

33. Tehranzadeh J, Serafina AN, Pais MJ (eds): Avulsion and Stress Injuries of the Musculoskeletal System. Karger, Basel, 1989

34. Mumford EB: Acromioclavicular dislocation: a new operative treatment. J Bone Joint Surg 23:799, 1947

35. Gurd FB: The treatment of complete dislocation of the outer end of the clavicle: a hitherto undescribed operation. Ann Surg 63:1094, 1941

36. Cook FF: The Mumford procedure in athletes: an objective analysis of function. Am J Sports Med 16:97, 1988

37. Hitchcock H, Bechtol CO: Painful shoulder: observations on the role of the tendon of the long head of biceps brachii in its causation. J Bone Joint Surg [Am] 30:263, 1948

38. McNab I: Rotator cuff tendinitis. Ann R Coll Surg Engl 53:271, 1973

39. Codman EA: The Shoulder. Robert E. Krieger, Malabar, Florida, 1934

40. Nash HL: Rotator cuff damage: reexamining the causes and treatment. Physician Sports Med 16:129, 1988

41. Fareed DO, Gallivan WR: Office management of frozen shoulder syndrome: treatment of hydraulic distension under local anaesthesia. Clin Orthop 242:177, 1989

42. Wiley AM, Older MWJ: Shoulder arthroscopy: investigation with a fibro-optic instrument. Am J Sports Med 8:31, 1980

43. Neviaser JS: Adhesive capsulitis of the shoulder: study of pathological findings in periarthritis of the shoulder. J Bone Joint Surg 27:211, 1945

44. Reeves B: The natural history of the frozen shoulder syndrome. Scand J Rhematol 4:193, 1975

45. Mariani EM, Cofield RH: The tendon of the long head of biceps brachii: instability, tendinitis, and rupture. Adv Orthop Surg 11:262, 1988

46. Furlani J: Electromyographic study of m. biceps brachii in movements of the glenohumeral joint. Acta Anat (Basel) 96:270, 1976

47. De Palma AF: Surgery of the Shoulder. 2nd Ed. JB Lippincott, Philadelphia, 1973

48. Penny JN, Welsh RP: Shoulder impingement syndromes in athletes and their surgical management. Am J Sports Med 9:11, 1981

49. Yergason RM: Supination sign. J Bone Joint Surg 13:160, 1931

50. Crenshaw AH, Kilgore WE: Surgical treatment of bicipital tenosynovitis. J Bone Joint Surg [Am] 48:1496, 1966

51. O'Donoghue DH: Subluxing biceps tendon in the athlete. J Sports Med 1:20, 1973

52. Slatis P, Alato K: Medial dislocation of the tendon of the long head of biceps brachii. Acta Orthop Scand 50:73, 1979

53. Peterson CJ: Spontaneous medial dislocation of the tendon of the long biceps brachii: an anatomic study of prevalence and pathomechanics. Clin Orthop 211:224, 1986

54. Turkel SJ, Panio MW, Marshall JL et al: Stabilizing mechanisms preventing anterior dislocation of the glenohumeral joint. J Bone Joint Surg [Am] 63:1208, 1981

55. McMaster PE: Tendon and muscle ruptures: clinical and experimental studies on the causes and location of subcutaneous ruptures. J Bone Joint Surg 15:705, 1933

56. Mariani EM, Cofield RH: Rupture of the tendon of the long head of biceps brachii: surgical versus non-surgical treatment. Clin Orthop 228:233, 1983

57. McFarland R, Dugdale TW, Gerbino P et al: Neurovascular complications resulting from corticosteroid injections. Physician Sports/Med 18:89, 1990

58. McLaughlin HL: Posterior dislocation of the shoulder. J Bone Joint Surg [Am] 34:584, 1952

59. Warren RF: Subluxation of the shoulder in athletes. Clin Sports Med 2:339, 1983

60. Zarins B, Rowe CR: Current concepts in the diagnosis and treatment of shoulder instability in athletes. Med Sci Sports Exerc 16:444, 1984

61. Garth WP, Allman FL, Armstrong WS: Occult anterior subluxations of the shoulder in non-contact sports. Am J Sports Med 15:579, 1987

62. Jobe F, Tibone J, Perry J et al: An EMG analysis of the shoulder in throwing and pitching. Am J Sports Med 11:3, 1983

63. Saboe L, Chapeha J, Reid DC et al: The Unstable Shoulder Electromyography: Applications in Physical Therapy. Thought Technology, Montreal, 1990

64. Hastings DE, Coughlin LP: Recurrent subluxation of the glenohumeral joint. Am J Sports Med 9:352, 1981

65. Cain PR, Mutschler TA, Fu FH et al: Anterior stability of the glenohumeral joint: a dynamic model. Am J Sports Med 15:144, 1987

66. Tibone J, Ting A: Capsulorrhaphy with a staple for recurrent posterior subluxation of the shoulder. J Bone Joint Surg [Am] 72:999, 1990

67. Hawkins RJ, Bell RH: Shoulder instability: diagnosis and management. Can J Sports Sci 12:67, 1987

68. Neer CS, Foster CR: Inferior capsular shift for involuntary inferior and multidirectional instability of the shoulder. J Bone Joint Surg [Am] 62:897, 1980

69. Brewer BJ, Wubben RC, Carrera GF: Excessive retroversion of the glenoid cavity: a cause of non-traumatic posterior dislocation of the shoulders. J Bone Joint Surg [Am] 68:724, 1986

70. Rafii M, Minkoff J, DeStefano VJ: Diagnostic imaging of the shoulder. In Nicholas JA, Hershman EB (eds): The Upper Extremity in Sports Medicine. CV Mosby, Philadelphia, 1990

71. Rowe CR: Factors related to recurrences of ante-

rior dislocation of the shoulders. Clin Orthop 20:21, 1961

72. Hovelius L: Anterior dislocation of the shoulder in teen-agers and young adults. J Bone Joint Surg [Am] 69:393, 1987

73. Henry JH, Genung JA: Natural history of glenohumeral dislocation—revisited. Am J Sports Med 10:135, 1982

74. Simonet WT, Cofield RH: Prognosis in anterior shoulder dislocation. Am J Sports Med 12:19, 1984

75. Watson-Jones R: Fractures and Joint Injuries. E & S Livingstone, Edinburgh, 1940

76. Aronen JG, Regan K: Decreasing the incidence of recurrence of first time anterior shoulder dislocation with rehabilitation. Am J Sports Med 12:283, 1984

77. Smith RL, Brunoll J: Shoulder kinesiology after anterior glenohumeral joint dislocation. J Orthop Sports Phys Ther 11:507, 1990

78. Kuriyama S, Fujimaki E, Katagiri T et al: Anterior dislocation of the shoulder joint sustained through skiing. Am J Sports Med 12:339, 1984

79. Baker CL, Uribe JW: Arthroscopic evaluation of acute initial anterior shoulder dislocations. Am J Sports Med 18:25, 1990

80. Blom S, Dahlback LO: Nerve injuries in dislocations of the shoulder joint and fractures of the neck of humerus. Acta Chir Scand 136:461, 1970

81. Shields CL: Manual of Sports Surgery. Springer-Verlag, New York, 1987

82. Hawkins RJ, Bell RH, Hawkinds RH et al: Anterior dislocation of the shoulder in the older patient. Clin Orthop 206:195, 1986

83. Hall RH, Isaac F, Booth CR: Dislocation of the shoulder with special reference to accompanying small fractures. J Bone Joint Surg [Am] 41:489, 1959

84. Eve FS: A case of subcoracoid dislocation of the humerus with the formation of an indentation on the posterior surface of the head. Med Chir Trans Soc (Lond) 63:317, 1880

85. Caird FM: The shoulder joint in relation to certain dislocations and fractures. Edinb Med J 32:708, 1887.

86. Hull HA, Sachs MD: The groove defect of the humeral head: a frequent unrecognized complication of dislocations of the shoulder joint. Radiology 35:690, 1940

87. Broca A, Hartman H: Contribution a l'étude des luxations de l'épaule (luxations anciennes, luxations recidivantes) Bull Soc Anat Paris 65:416, 1890

88. Danzig LA, Greenway G, Resnick D: The Hill-Sachs lesion. Am J Sports Med 8:328, 1980

89. Perthes G: Über Operationen bei labitueller Shulterluxation. Dtsch Z Chir 85:199, 1906

90. Bankart ASB: Recurrent or habitual dislocation of the shoulder joint. Br Med J 2:1132, 1923

91. Magnuson PB, Stack JK: Recurrent dislocation of the shoulder. JAMA 123:889, 1943

92. Aamoth GM, O'Phalen EH: Recurrent anterior dislocation of the shoulder: a review of 40 athletes treated by subscapularis transfer. Am J Sports Med 5:188, 1977

93. Miller LS, Donahue JR, Good RP et al: The Magnuson-Stack procedure for treatment of recurrent glenohumeral dislocations. Am J Sports Med 12:133, 1984

94. Osmond-Clarke H: Habitual dislocation of the shoulder: the Putti-Platt operation. J Bone Joint Surg [Br] 30:19, 1948

95. Halley DK, Olix MD: A review of the Bristow operation for recurrent anterior shoulder dislocation in athletes. Clin Orthop 106:175, 1979

96. Braly WG, Tullos H: A modification of the Bristow procedure for recurrent anterior dislocation of the shoulder. Am J Sports Med 13:81, 1985

97. Bonci CM, Hensal FJ, Torg JS: A preliminary study on the measurement of static and dynamic motion at the glenohumeral joint. Am J Sports Med 14:12, 1986

98. Perrin DH, Robertson RJ, Ray RL: Bilat isokinetic peak torque; torque acceleration energy, power and work relationships in athletes and nonathletes. J Orthop Sports Phys Ther 9:184, 1987

99. Matsen FA, Thomas SC: Glenohumeral instability. In Everts CM (ed): Surgery of the Musculoskeletal System. 2nd Ed. Churchill Livingstone, New York, 1989

100. Zeman SC, Rosenfeld RT, Lipscomb PR: Tears of the pectoralis major muscle. Am J Sports Med 7:343, 1979

101. Roi GS, Respizzi S, Dworzak F: Partial rupture of the pectoralis major muscle in athletes. Int J Sports Med 11:85, 1990

102. McEntire, JE, Hess WE, Coleman SS: Rupture of the pectoralis major muscle: a report of eleven injuries and review of fifty-six cases. J Bone Joint Surg [Am] 54:1040, 1972

103. Roos DB, Owens JC: Thoracic outlet syndrome. Arch Surg 93:71, 1966

104. Lord JW, Rosati LM: Thoracic outlet syndromes. Clin Symp, Ciba Geigy 24:3, 1972

105. Adson AW: Surgical treatment for symptoms produced by cervical ribs and the scalene anticus muscle. Surg Gynecol Obstet 85:687, 1947

106. Neer CS: Displaced proximal humerus fractures. I. Classifications and evaluation. J Bone Joint Surg 52:1077, 1970

107. Ferretti A, Cerullo G, Russo G: Suprascapular neuropathy in volleyball players. J Bone Joint Surg [Am] 69:260, 1987

108. Goodman CE: Unusual nerve injuries in recreational activities. Am J Sports Med 11:224, 1983

109. Black KP, Lombardo JA: Suprascapular nerve injuries with isolated paralysis of the infraspinatus. Am J Sports Med 18:225, 1990

110. Bryan WJ, Wild JJ: Isolated infraspinatus atrophy.

a common cause of posterior shoulder pain and weakness in throwing athletes? Am J Sports Med 17:130, 1989

111. Drez D: Suprascapular neuropathy in the differential diagnosis of rotator cuff injuries. Am J Sports Med 4:43, 1976

112. Hirasawa Y, Sakakida K: Sports and peripheral nerve injury. Am J Sports Med 11:420, 1983

Elbow Region

22

From the sublime to the ridiculous is but a single step.
— *Napoleon Bonaparte*

Traumatic injuries to the elbow joint occur frequently in sport and recreation. They comprise approximately 7 percent of gymnastics, 6 percent of wrestling, 5 percent of handball, and 4 percent of hockey injuries. The incidence is even higher for recreational activities, with roller skating (11 percent), skateboarding (8 percent), cycling (7 percent), ice skating (6 percent), and surfing (5 percent) predominating. In contact sports and activities where there is frequent falling, the subcutaneous bony surfaces, particularly the olecranon process, are vulnerable to contusion, as is the ulnar nerve. However, the number of nontraumatic, overstress elbow injuries seen in a sports medicine practice, particularly those due to tennis, squash, baseball, and weight training, probably equal the above problems. Unfortunately, despite being common, they are not always treated well.[1] There is a tendency to consider overuse elbow injuries trivial because the athlete frequently continues to participate, even with significant symptoms. It leads to delay in diagnosis, difficulty in resolving the pathology, and long-standing or even permanent disability.

ANATOMY

The elbow joint is a unique multifaceted articulation between the capitellum and trochlea of the distal end of the humerus, and the radial head and olecranon of the proximal radius and ulna. Nevertheless, it is classically considered a uniaxial hinge joint, which belies its complexity because it is also closely related to the superior radioulnar joint (Fig. 22-1). These two articulations share the same joint capsule, and the joint spaces are continuous.[2] If this unusual arrangement of three articulations within one joint space is appreciated, it is easier to understand why the response of the elbow joint to trauma, exercise, heat, and massage is sometimes surprising, often unusual, and unfortunately not always good.[1-4]

Capsule and Ligaments

The capsule is reinforced and thickened by the lateral (radial) and medial (ulnar) collateral ligaments, which resist and prevent excessive abduction and adduction stresses and movements (Fig. 22-2). These

---

Quick Facts

JOINT STABILITY FACTORS[a]

In Extension

- Valgus stability
  -Anterior and oblique bands of medial lig. (31%)
  -Anterior capsule (38%)
  -Bony contact (31%)
- Varus stability
  -Anterior capsule (32%)
  -Bony contact (55%)
  -Lateral ligament (14%)

At 90 Degrees Flexion

- Valgus stability
  -Anterior and posterior oblique bands of medial ligament (54%)
  -Bony contact (33%)
- Varus stability
  -Anterior capsule (13%)
  -Lateral ligament (9%)
  -Bony contact (75%)

Distraction in extension 85% medial ligament and anterior capsule combined; in flexion 78% medial ligament

[a]Figures vary with different studies.

999

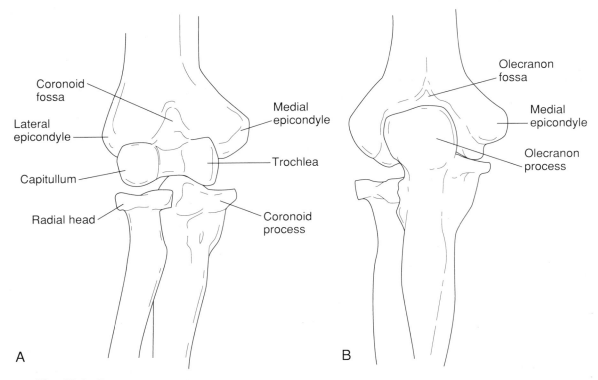

Fig. 22-1. Bony contours involved in the elbow joint. **(A)** Anterior view. **(B)** Posterior view.

ligaments do not, however, impede pronation and supination.[5]

Valgus stability is provided equally by the medial collateral ligament, anterior capsule, and bony configuration in extension, whereas at 90 degrees of flexion the contribution of the anterior capsule is assumed by the medial collateral ligament.[6,7] (Fig. 22-2). Varus stress is resisted primarily by the bony configuration supplemented by the anterior capsule, with only a minor contribution from the lateral collateral ligament. This arrangement changes little throughout the range.[6]

Distraction stresses, which are most significant during high velocity throwing maneuvers, are resisted primarily by the medial collateral and anterior capsule combined in extension and the ulnar collateral ligament in flexion.[4]

Data from cadaver studies (see box), of necessity, underscore the considerable contribution to stability made by muscle in the living state.[8] Furthermore, careful dissection reveals that many of the fibers of the so-called collateral ligaments of the elbow are continuous with the collagenous septa of the muscles crossing the joint. It is this intimate association of the

connective tissue of ligaments and overlying muscle that renders pathology at the site of the tendon insertion, versus the noncontractile portion of the joint, sometimes difficult to isolate. These important fibrous strands, blending into the ligament, provide a basis for considering a single musculoligamentous unit contributing to the dynamic stability of many joints.[2,5,8]

Practice Point

There is a continuous structural relation between the muscles attaching near the elbow joint and the collagen of the ligaments. They constitute a musculoligamentous unit.

Arthrology

Classification

The elbow joint is a compound paracondylar joint, as one bone, the humerus, articulates with two others

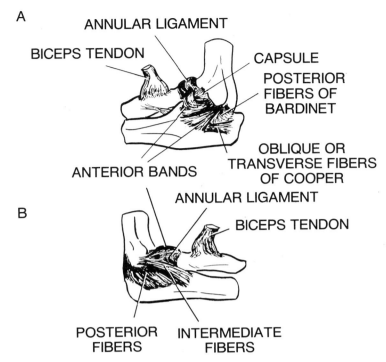

Fig. 22-2. (A) Medial (ulnar collateral) ligament consists of strong anterior fibers in two bundles that reinforce the annular ligament and some less impressive oblique or transverse fibers. **(B)** Similarly, the lateral (radial collateral) ligament reinforces the annular ligament. Although shown as three discrete bands, in reality the collagenous connections with the overlying intermuscular septa form a musculotendinous unit. (After Reid and Kushner,[2] with permission.)

that are side by side by way of two distinct facets. The humeroulnar component is a modified sellar articulation (convex in one direction and concave at right angles to the first plane). The humeroradial component is an unmodified ovoid (convex or concave in all planes). The proximal radioulnar articulation, by contrast, is a modified ovoid (Fig 22-1).[9]

Resting, Closed Packed Positions, and Capsular Pattern

The joint capsule is most relaxed in the *resting position,* and the greatest amount of joint play is then possible. With pathologic states, the maximum intra-articular volume is present, and the joint adopts the position best able to minimize capsular tension secondary to effusion and thus reduce pain. This information is central to the concept of joint mobilization procedures, which are ideally performed in the resting position (which may be specific for each articulation). However, pathology seldom isolates each joint component so specifically. Generally with synovitis of

---

> **Quick Facts**
>
> **RESTING POSITIONS**
>
> - Superior radioulnar joint—70 degrees flexion 35 degrees supination
> - Humeroulnar joint—70 degrees flexion 10 degrees supination
> - Humeroradial joint—near extension, some supination

the elbow, the joint is held in 70 degrees of flexion and 10 degrees of supination.[3]

In the *closed packed position* the capsule and ligaments are tight or maximally tensed. There is usually maximal contact between articular surfaces, and the surfaces cannot be separated by distractive forces. Obviously, testing and mobilization cannot and should not be performed in this position.[10–12]

Quick Facts

CLOSED PACKED POSITION

Humeroulnar joint: extension and supination

Humeroradial joint: 90 degrees flexion and 5 degrees supination

---

The *capsular pattern* is a proportional pattern of limitation of movement at a joint. Initially triggered by pain, synovial irritation, or effusion, it is subsequently reinforced by capsular shortening and contractures. It is usually accepted as an indication of capsular or intra-articular disease. For the elbow, flexion is usually more restricted than extension, but with time they may be equally affected. Once marked limitation of flexion and extension are present, pronation and supination may become restricted equally. There are many extrinsic factors that can produce the significant degree of individual variation common at the elbow.

Range of Motion

The lower end of the humerus is offset in two planes. The angulation in the coronal plane, the carrying angle, alters the axis of flexion and extension so that the forearm sweeps through an arc, facilitating hand to mouth movement (Fig. 22-3). The humeral trochlear groove is spiral and is the main factor that dictates the arthrokinematics.[3] Anteriorly, the groove is vertical and parallel to the longitudinal humeral axis; and posteriorly the groove runs obliquely, forming the carrying angle of 5 to 20 degrees.[10]

The radiohumeral articular pathway follows the axis dictated by the anatomy of the humeroulnar joint surfaces. Restoration of these angles after fracture allows resumption of normal range of motion. Fortunately, the most frequent fractures in this area occur in children; and although they present the potential problem of injury to the growth plates, they usually heal satisfactorily with restoration of the delicate anatomy through remodeling provided adequate initial reduction is achieved.

The normal range of flexion-extension is approximately 150 to 160 degrees with about 10 degrees of hyperextension commonly present, particularly in

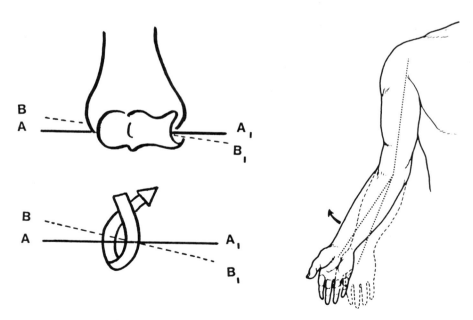

Fig. 22-3. Owing to the configuration of the trochlea, the axis of movement changes progressively from horizontal A–A₁ in flexion to oblique B–B₁ in extension. This movement results in midline movement during flexion and the carrying angle during extension in most individuals. The angle is usually greater in females. (After Kapandji,[5] with permission.)

women (Fig. 22-4). Active flexion is usually limited by opposition of the soft parts but occasionally by bone on bone.[13] Passive flexion is limited by tension of the posterior capsule and passive tension of the triceps. Extension is limited by contact of the tip of the olecranon in its contiguous fossa in the posterior lower humerus. At about the time of apposition, the anterior capsule tightens and tension develops in the elbow flexors so that bony impact is attenuated.[3,13]

When treating elbow pathology with splinting, flexion is usually chosen as the resting position; therefore loss of extension is a common feature after immobilization. The anterior band of the ulnar collateral ligament has been implicated as one of the prime limiting factors in humeroulnar motion.[14,15] Studies have failed to support this concept, however, and it is more likely that in pathologic states adhesions and adaptive shortening of the adjacent anterior capsule is more important.[16] When normal range is possible, active extension is some 5 to 10 degrees short of that obtainable by forced extension. This finding reflects the contribution of the muscle, as demonstrated by experiments using myoneural blocking agents.[17] The unwillingness of living subjects to allow terminal extension reflects MacConaill's statement

that, in living subjects, positions just short of the closed packed state are used functionally rather than the full closed packed position.[10]

Supination and pronation occur at both the radiohumeral and the proximal radioulnar joints. The superior radioulnar joint highlights the subtle differences in anatomy that make the elbow joint difficult to treat. In this case, 80 percent of the articular surface is made up by the annular ligaments rather than articular cartilage. This ligament is tough and coneshaped, and it usually prevents dislocation in the adult. The imperfectly formed radial head of the young child, by contrast, may be easily dislocated by excessive traction with rotation.

The axis for pronation and supination passes from the center of the radial head to the pit adjacent to the styloid process of the ulna distally. This compound movement, involving the three articulations at the elbow as well as the distal radioulnar joint and radiocarpal articulation, can obviously be compromised by pathology at any of these joints. Normal range encompasses approximately 90 degrees of both pronation and supination.

The elbow is a highly congruous joint but nevertheless depends significantly on its soft tissue re-

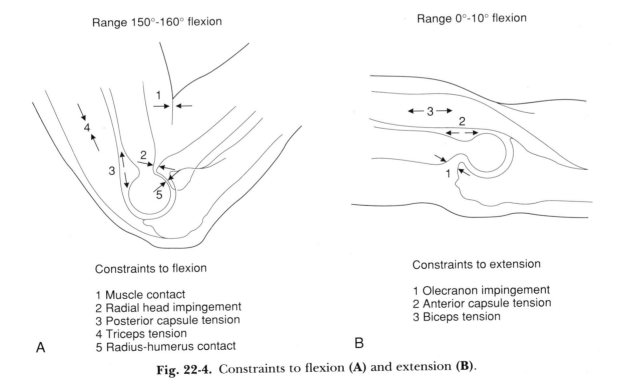

Range 150°-160° flexion

Range 0°-10° flexion

Constraints to flexion

1 Muscle contact
2 Radial head impingement
3 Posterior capsule tension
4 Triceps tension
5 Radius-humerus contact

Constraints to extension

1 Olecranon impingement
2 Anterior capsule tension
3 Biceps tension

A

B

Fig. 22-4. Constraints to flexion (**A**) and extension (**B**).

straints during its complex motions. Indeed, these ligaments have to resist considerable valgus and, to a lesser degree, varus stresses, that accompany rapid flexion and extension. In many throwing activities for instance, elbow motion exceeds 300 degrees per second and it is of little wonder that chronic overuse syndromes manifest at this joint.[18]

Muscle Action

During flexion there is considerable interplay between biceps, brachialis, and brachioradialis, with these three muscles working to various degrees at different ranges, speeds, and among individuals (Fig. 22-5). Hence it is not surprising that many studies on their actions appear, at first glance, to be contradictory.[3,19] The following main points emerge.

1. Biceps and brachialis are muscles of considerable bulk; they add power and are the prime movers of flexion.[20,21]
2. The body tends toward economy; therefore slow movements, without added resistance, may be performed by one or other of these muscles or by a diminished amount of work by both.
3. Biceps may actively supinate the arm while flexion is taking place unless it is counteracted.
4. With rapid movements the brachioradialis may act

in two ways. Initially it serves as a shunt muscle, overcoming centrifugal forces acting at the elbow; subsequently it adds power to increase the speed of flexion. It does it most efficiently in the midprone position.[21]

5. The common flexor mass from the medial epicondyle may weakly assist the prime movers or be hypertrophied to assist flexion in cases of paralysis of the proximal muscles (Table 22-1).

Of the three heads of the triceps, the medial head seems to be most consistent in its action over the extensor mechanism of the elbow[19,20] (Fig. 22-6). The long and lateral heads provide extra strength for this motion but electrically may be relatively silent for slow, low power movements. The triceps is most powerful when the elbow and shoulder are extended simultaneously. Deep extensions from the triceps insert into the capsule of the posterior recess of the elbow joint and help pull the redundant synovium away during extension, thereby avoiding impingement.[1] This action is similar to the articularis genu mechanism over the suprapatellar pouch at the knee.

The pronator quadratus needs the power offered by the pronator teres for most everyday motions and all resisted pronation activities.[3] Similarly, the biceps, for most actions, supplements the power of the supinator, particularly for high speed motion.[19]

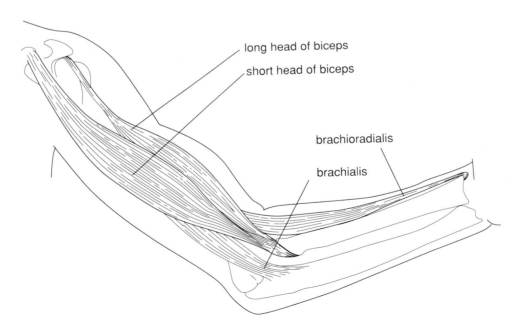

Fig. 22-5. Main elbow flexors.

TABLE 22-1. Muscles Producing Elbow Motion

Motion	Muscle[a]	Nerve Supply	Segmental Innervation[b]
Flexion (elbow joint)	*Biceps*	Musculocutaneous	C5,6
	Brachialis	Musculocutaneous	C5,6
	Brachioradialis	Radial	C6
	Pronator teres	Median	C7
	Muscles from common flexor origin	Median	C7,8
Extension (elbow joint)	*Triceps*	Radial	C7,8
	Anconeus	Radial	C7,8
	Muscles from common extensor origin	Posterior interosseous branch	
Supination[c] (radioulnar joint)	*Biceps*	Musculocutaneous	C5,6
	Supination	Radial	C5,6
Pronation[c] (radioulnar joint)	*Pronator teres*	Median	C7
	Pronator quadratus	Median (anterior interosseous branch)	C7,8

[a] Prime movers, supplying most power, are in italics.
[b] Major segments only.
[c] Brachioradialis returns forearm to midposition from either full pronation or supination.

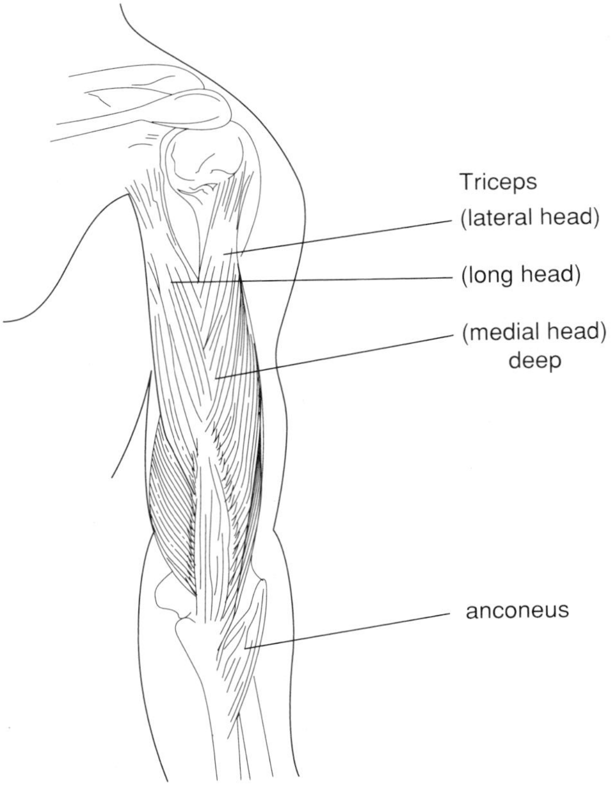

Triceps
(lateral head)
(long head)
(medial head) deep

anconeus

Fig. 22-6. Main elbow extensors.

ASSESSMENT

History

An adequate history assists in ruling out cervical spine and shoulder pathology, as both may refer pain to the elbow (Figs. 22-7 and 22-8). Conversely, trauma to the vulnerable ulnar nerve at the elbow may cause only distal symptoms. Asking athletes to re-enact the mechanism of injury with the opposite limb allows them to clarify their explanation of what happened and provides more information on what structures might have been stressed. If the examiners are not fully familiar with the sport or recreational activity involved, including the equipment, they should use the athlete as a source of education. Questions about the weight of the bat, the speed of the puck, the action of the serve, and the location of equipment padding allow a more exact diagnosis and a better formulated treatment plan. This approach usually ensures a more productive athlete-clinician relationship.

Practice Point

Use the experienced athlete as a source of information on the subtleties of the sport, injury patterns, and protective equipment.

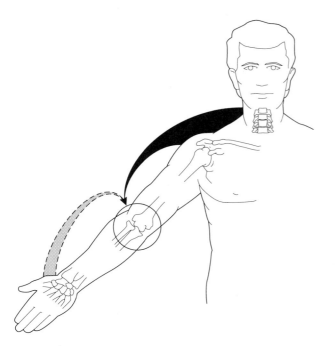

Fig. 22-7. Cervical and shoulder pathology may refer to the elbow. Wrist problems less frequently refer pain proximally, although wrist pathology may affect proximal radioulnar motion and thus produce elbow pain.

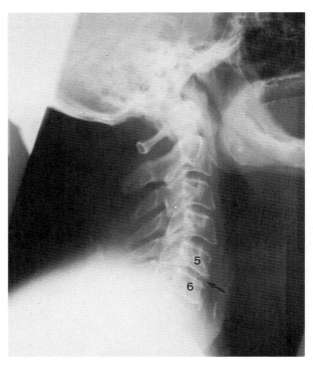

Fig. 22-8. This patient complained of symptoms compatible with lateral epicondylitis. Interrogation and examination unmasked cervical pathology. The roentgenogram confirmed C5–C6 degenerative changes. Local injection resolved the elbow problem, but recurrence is likely unless the neck dysfunction is also attended to.

Specific points in the history, e.g., age, occupation, recreational pursuits, pattern of pain, and functional difficulties, should be used to focus the examiner on the diagnostic probabilities. For example, the complaint of intermittent locking suggests loose bodies in a pitcher or boxer. Family history is particularly important because the elbow may be involved in collagen disorders, e.g., rheumatoid arthritis, early in the disease process.

The degree of pain is not always a good indicator of the severity of an injury. For example, complete ligament disruptions may cause little discomfort, whereas even minor periosteal inflammation may generate severe pain. Furthermore, the degree of discomfort may be related to swelling, which is greater if the joint capsule is intact. The mode of onset of the symptoms may be helpful: Immediate severe pain is usually related to tearing or pinching of a structure; pain of gradual onset during activity is usually related to microtrauma and overuse; and delayed pain and stiffness about 6 to 12 hours after activity may signify effusion, bursitis, or biochemical changes associated with joint disorders, tendinitis, or muscle microtrauma.

Observation

The elbow joint is particularly difficult to examine because many of the changes are frequently subtle; only careful comparison with the sound limb can reveal the discrepancy. The patient's elbow is observed for swelling, contours, color, and carrying angle. The carrying angle is normally 5 to 10 degrees in males and 10 to 15 degrees in most females. If the carrying angle is more than 20 degrees, cubitus valgus exists; and when it is less than 5 degrees, there is cubitus varus. The patient is told to place the arms at 90 degrees of forward flexion at the shoulder, and the elbow–wrist relation is then observed while the arm is in pronation and supination. These relations may be altered after trauma.

Palpation

Palpation should be systematic and include all bony points, tendons, and ligaments with attention to crepitus, pain, boggy edematous changes, and abnormal contours. It should always be commenced by asking the athlete to place "one" finger exactly on the most painful spot. The main landmarks are the medial and lateral epicondyles, the olecranon, and the radial head.

Range of Motion

Lack of supination and pronation is easily masked by shoulder motion. Conversely, distal radioulnar and wrist disease restrict these motions at the elbow. Thus careful isolation of the movement and examination of the shoulder and wrist are part of elbow assessment. Restricted flexion of the elbow cannot be adequately compensated for either proximally or distally. The functional implication of loss of range is

profound, interfering with many activities of daily living, e.g., feeding, dressing, shaving, and combing hair. By contrast, significant loss of elbow extension prohibits the throwing action and interferes with many recreational activities. Thus special attention to recording these parameters is crucial to any treatment plan.

Active Range

Flexion is tested in supination and is normally 150 degrees. Extension is normally to 0 degrees for men and up to 5 degrees in women, although 15 degrees of hyperextension in females or children is not uncommon. Supination and pronation are tested with the shoulder adducted and the elbow against the trunk to rule out shoulder rotation. These movements range from 0 degrees at the neutral position to 80 or 90 degrees (Fig. 22-9). Most activities of daily living are accomplished in the arc from 30 to 130 degrees of flexion and between 50 degrees of pronation and 50 degrees of supination. However, for many athletic endeavors, particularly throwing, a full range is imperative.

Passive Range

The movements are tested with particular attention to the end feel. The flexion end feel is one of soft tissue approximation; extension is bone to bone; pronation and supination are soft tissue stretches. The forearm should be held proximal to the wrist to rule out problems in this joint.

Muscle Tests

Resisted movements are tested isometrically in a neutral position. The test is best repeated for five contractions in order to uncover subtle weakness caused by neurologic conditions such as nerve root palsies. Minimal to maximal resistance is applied (Fig. 22-10).

Minimal isometric resistance causing pain is indicative of a contractile lesion, whereas if pain is elicited only with maximal resistance one must also consider the possibility that the discomfort in inert structures is due to increased articular pressure.

Primary selective tissue tension tests determine the muscle group involved; secondary tests assist in pointing to the specific muscle. For example, if resisted elbow flexion is painful, the biceps, brachioradialis, or brachialis muscle may be involved. If with

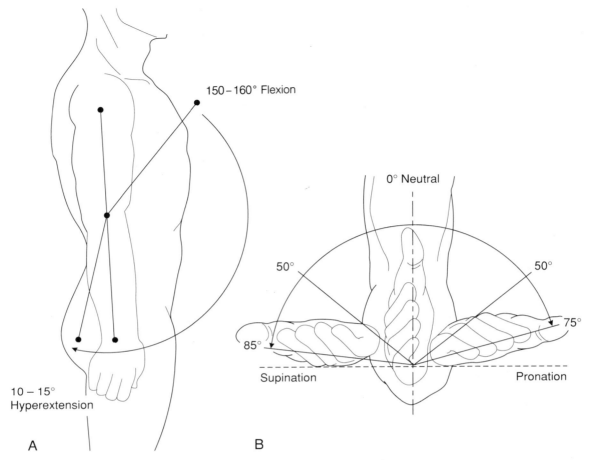

Fig. 22-9. (A) Flexion is about 150 to 160 degrees, limited by soft tissue apposition or in some cases bone against bone. Hyperextension is recorded as the degrees past neutral. **(B)** Pronation and supination are measured from the midposition. The elbow must be kept fixed at the side to prevent shoulder rotation and abduction affecting motion. Most daily functions may be performed with 50 degrees of each motion; sport activities frequently require more.

Quick Facts

RESISTED MOTION

- Pain on minimal isometric resistance probably indicates a lesion in the contractile elements.
- Pain in maximal isometric resistance may also be from inert structures.
- Distinguish pain inhibition from true weakness.

---

further testing resisted supination from neutral position increases the pain, the biceps is probably the source. Testing of wrist flexor and extensor strength must be included because of their proximal insertions of the forearm musculature on the epicondyles and supracondylar ridges.

Ligamentous Tests

The collateral ligaments should be tested 15 to 30 degrees short of full extension. They may also be tested in midflexion, as with moderate pathology there may be signs only in selected positions where tension is maximal.

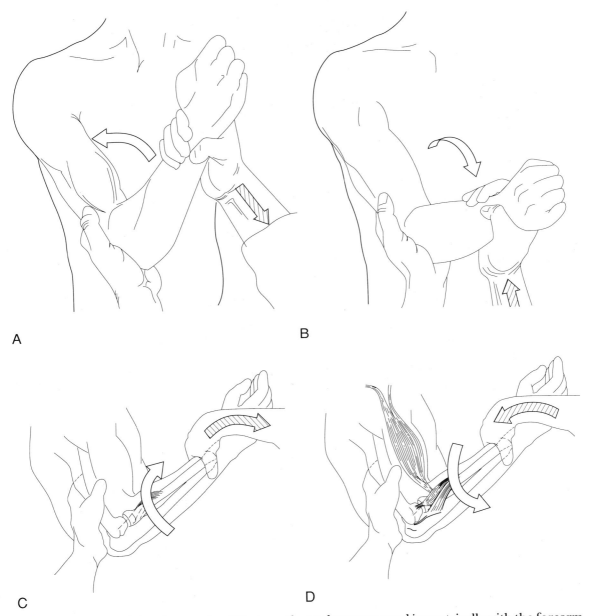

A

B

C

D

Fig. 22-10. Flexion (**A**) and extension (**B**) strengths are best measured isometrically with the forearm in neutral and approximately 90 degree position. Pronation (**C**) and supination (**D**) are also tested in this position. Arrows represent direction of patient's effort and examiner's resistance.

Accessory Movement Tests

Frequently an experienced therapist or physician with special training can obtain additional information on the condition of the joint or progress of treatment by evaluating accessory joint motions. The involved elbow is compared to the normal one, with special attention to the end feel. These tests are as follows.[11,12]

1. Lateral and medial glide of the ulna on the humerus is tested just short of full extension (Fig. 22-11A).

2. Distraction of the ulna on the humerus is carried

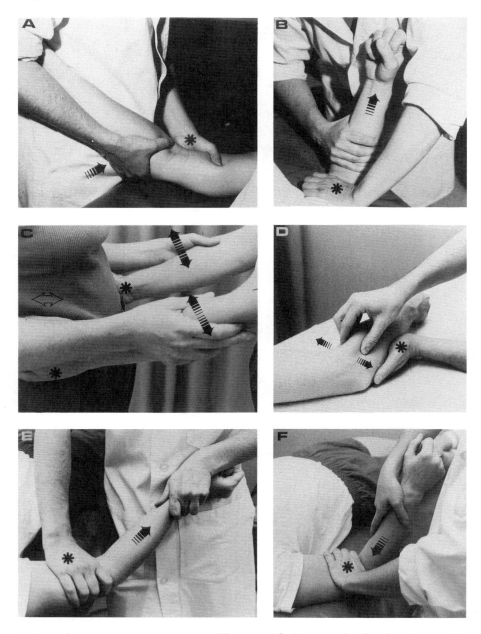

Fig. 22-11. Tests for accessory movements. The asterisk denotes the fixed point and the arrow the movement direction. **(A)** Lateral and medial ulnar glide. **(B)** Ulnar distraction. **(C)** Flexion and extension of the radial head while the patient's hands are fixed on the therapist's hips. Forward and backward motion helps produce flexion and extension at the patient's elbow. **(D)** Dorsal and ventral glide of the radial head. **(E)** Distraction of the radial head. **(F)** Compression of the radial head. (After Reid and Kushner,[2] with permission.)

out with 70 degrees flexion and 35 degrees supination (Fig. 22-11B).

3. Flexion and extension of the radial head on the humerus is performed while passively flexing and extending the elbow while standing (Fig. 22-11C).

4. Dorsal and ventral glide of radial head on the ulna is performed in 70 degrees elbow flexion and 35 degrees supination (Fig. 22-11D).

5. Distraction of the radial head on the humerus is performed in 70 degrees flexion and 35 degrees supination (Fig. 22-11E).

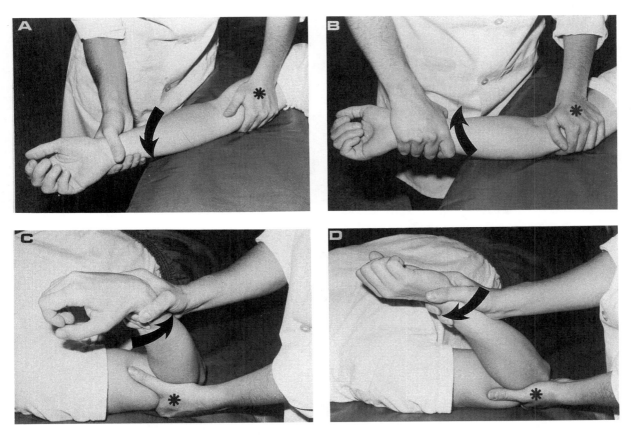

Fig. 22-12. Accessory movement tests. Asterisk denotes the fixed point. **(A)** Extension adduction quadrant. **(B)** Extension abduction quadrant. **(C)** Flexion abduction quadrant. **(D)** Flexion adduction quadrant. (After Reid and Kushner,[2] with permission.)

6. Compression of radial head on humerus is performed in 70 degrees flexion and 35 degrees supination (Fig. 22-11F).
7. Extension adduction quadrant 10 degrees from full extension (Fig. 22-12A).
8. Extension abduction quadrant 10 degrees from full extension (Fig. 22-12B).
9. Flexion abduction quadrant 10 degrees from full flexion and supination (Fig. 22-12C).
10. Flexion adduction quadrant 10 degrees from full flexion and pronation (Fig. 22-12D).

Other Tests

Reflexes are usually tested during the cervical scan and include the biceps (C5), brachioradialis (C6), and triceps (C7). These results are compared to those on the other side and listed as hyperreflexic, normal, hyporeflexic, or absent (Fig. 22-13). Dermatomes are also tested with the cervical scan. Generally, the lateral elbow is C5, the anterior elbow C6, the posterior elbow C7, and the medial elbow T1 and T2. The dermatomes at the elbow, however, are nonspecific, and there are considerable individual variations and overlaps (Fig. 22-14).

Special tests that detect pathologic entities conclude the examination and are discussed with the appropriate conditions. Occasionally, there is a question of intra- versus extra-articular pathology. In this case, an intra-articular injection of lidocaine (Xylocaine) hydrochloride is given through the lateral triangle (Fig. 22-15). This injection is particularly easy if an effusion is present, as the bulging capsule allows ready access of the needle into the joint. A sample should be aspirated if present and sent for appropriate laboratory studies.

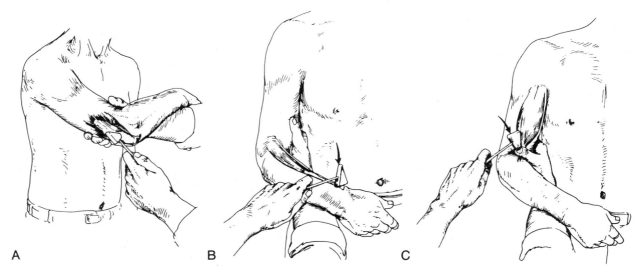

Fig. 22-13. **(A)** Triceps reflex (C7). The elbow should be supported and relaxes. **(B)** Brachioradialis reflex (C6). **(C)** Biceps reflex (C5). (Adapted from Hoppenfeld S: Physical Examination of the Spine and Extremities. Appleton-Century-Crofts, New York, 1976. With permission.)

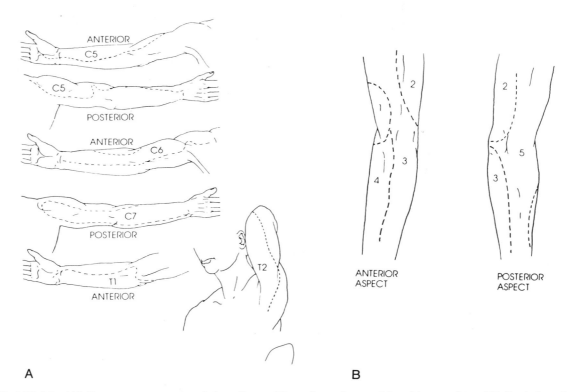

Fig. 22-14. **(A)** Dermatomes around the elbow. Note there is considerable overlap. **(B)** Peripheral nerve sensory distribution: (1) lower lateral cutaneous nerve of arm (radial); (2) medial cutaneous nerve of arm; (3) medial cutaneous nerve of forearm; (4) lateral cutaneous nerve of forearm (musculocutaneous); (5) posterior cutaneous nerve of forearm (radial). (After Magee,[7] with permission.)

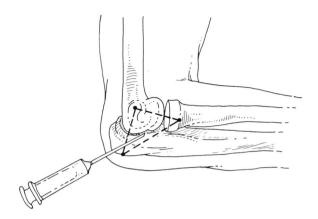

Fig. 22-15. Palpation of three prominant landmarks on the lateral aspect of the elbow—lateral epicondyle, head of the radius, and tip of olecranon—provides accurate landmarks for aspiration or injection of the joint. (From Morrey BF: The Elbow and Its Disorders. WB Saunders, Philadelphia, 1985. With permission.)

CONDITIONS AND TREATMENT

Tennis Elbow Syndrome (Lateral Epicondylitis, Lateral Stress Syndrome)

Lateral epicondylitis has been recognized for about a century. First distinguishd from writer's cramp by Runge in 1873, it was named "lawn tennis arm" by Morris shortly thereafter.[22,23] There have been numerous reports implicating a wide variety of etiologic and anatomic factors, and even now some of the subtleties of the condition are controversial.[24-28] There are more than 20 million tennis players in North America, and as many as one-third, or possibly more, suffer from elbow problems at some time, particularly if they are over age 35.

Definition

By definition, tennis elbow is a lesion affecting the tendinous origin of the wrist extensors. Like many eponyms, the term is used loosely and is often ill-defined; thus it tends to have different meanings for different people (Table 22-2). The term "tennis elbow" has been used to encompass posterior and medial symptoms which have been referred to as posterior and medial tennis elbow, respectively, adding

TABLE 22-2. Pathology of Lateral Tennis Elbow[a]

Proximal
  Periostitis
  Common extensor origin
      Tendinitis
      Microtearing with painful granulation
      Degenerative changes in tendon
  Lateral epicondyle epiphysis sprain or separation (in child)
Joint
  Lateral ligament sprain
  Radiohumeral bursitis
  Inflammation of annular ligament
  Hypertrophic synovial fringe
  Degenerative changes, radial head cartilage
  Panner's osteochondrosis (in child)
Neural
  Cervical radiculopathy
  Posterior interosseous nerve entrapment

[a] These causes of elbow pain have all been implicated in the tennis elbow syndrome.

confusion to an already complicated topic.[22,23,29-31] Tennis elbow in the context of this section refers only to lateral epicondylitis and associated common extensor origin tendinitis. Thus the definition includes local tenderness over the common extensor origin, at

---

Quick Facts

LOCATION OF ELBOW PAIN WITH "TENNIS ELBOW"[a]

- Lateral epicondyle — Attachment of common extensor muscles — 75%
- Lateral muscle mass — Musculotendinous junction of common extensors just proximal to radial head — 17%
- Medial epicondyle — Attachment of common flexor origin — 10%
- Posterior — Around margins of olecranon process — 8%

[a] More than 100 percent because individuals may experience pain at more than one site. Classic tennis elbow refers only to lateral symptoms.

the lateral epicondyle, exacerbated by continual use and resisted elbow extension, and frequently producing aching and pain down the back of the forearm into the extensor muscle mass.

Pathology and Symptoms

The exact pathology at the common extensor origin is open to question, and it is likely that several basic etiologic entities with slightly different pathologic changes in the tissue may produce a similar clinical picture[26,28] (Table 22-2). The three major sites of pathology are the common extensor origin, the radiocapitellar joint, and the radioulnar joint with fibrillation and chondromalacic changes. Furthermore, neurogenic causes such as C6 radiculopathy and, more locally, radial tunnel entrapment of the posterior interosseous nerve must be considered. This subject is discussed under a separate heading later in the chapter. With C6 root involvement secondary to dysfunction at the C5–C6 segment, there may be weakness of the radial wrist extensors, leaving them prone to injury. The patient's clinical picture resembles a true tennis elbow resistant to treatment (Fig. 22-8). While the elbow is being treated, simultaneous attention must be given to the cervical spine. Only then will the patient respond.[2] The "culprit" must be treated, not only the "victim." In skeletally immature patients, sprains and minor separations of the lateral epicondylar epiphysis and fragmentation of the capitellum (Panner's disease) must be considered in the differential diagnosis. By contrast, elbow joint arthrosis in the older individual is a distinct possibility.

In view of the high success rate of local limited release of the common extensor origin, and recovery at surgery of granulation tissue and scar from this area, this site of pathology probably accounts for most cases.

Whatever the etiology, there is generally an element of overuse or overstress, and 45 percent of tennis players with daily games or practices experience problems.[30,31] Furthermore, the tennis elbow syndrome is a frequent occupational hazard in individuals carrying out forceful pronation and supination motions, heavy lifting, or repetitive hammering type activities.

Quick Facts

PLAYING FREQUENCY AND LATERAL EPICONDYLITIS[24]

Frequency of Play	% With Elbow Pain
Daily	45
3–4 Times weekly	33
1–2 Times weekly	26
2–3 Times per month	7
Once per month or less	9

Clinical Tests

There is local tenderness on the outside of the elbow at the common extensor origin with aching and pain in the back of the forearm (Fig. 22-16). The condition is aggravated by continual use. Special tests include resisted wrist extension, which precipitates pain at the extensor origin (Fig. 22-17). Performing the test in full elbow extension decreases the number of false-negative results. Painful resisted extension of the middle and ring fingers implicates the extensor digitorum communis, and painful resistance of wrist extension and radial deviation points to extensor carpi radialis longus and brevis. Another test for tennis elbow is performed by holding the elbow in extension and performing passive wrist flexion and

---

Practice Point

POSSIBLE PATHOPHYSIOLOGY AND RELATED SYMPTOMS

- Stage I
  -Acute inflammation
  -No angioblastic invasion
  -Pain during activity
  -Minor aching, usually after activity
- Stage II
  -Chronic inflammation and scar
  -Some angioblastic invasion
  -Pain during activity and at rest
- Stage III
  -Extensive angioblastic invasion and scar
  -May be microruptures of tendon
  -Sometimes partial (macro) rupture
  -Pain at rest, sometimes night pain
  -Hurts during numerous activities of daily living

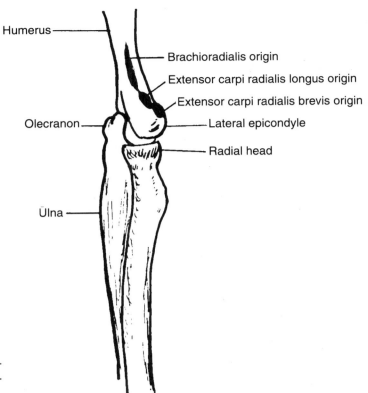

Humerus
Brachioradialis origin
Extensor carpi radialis longus origin
Extensor carpi radialis brevis origin
Olecranon
Lateral epicondyle
Radial head
Ulna

Fig. 22-16. Palpable structures attaching to the supracondyle ridge and lateral epicondyle.

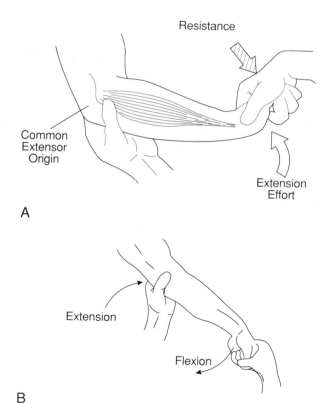

Resistance
Common Extensor Origin
Extension Effort

A

Extension
Flexion

B

Fig. 22-17. (A) Palpation over the common extensor origin while resisting extension elicits symptoms of lateral epicondylitis. The test may be even more sensitive when done in full extension. **(B)** Passive extension of the elbow with forced flexion of the wrist may precipitate pain at the lateral epicondyle.

pronation, thereby stretching the tendinous insertion. A positive test elicits pain at the common origin.

Etiology and Treatment

Treatment is outlined in detail for the tennis player, but many of the principles may be exrapolated to other situations. Both sexes are affected equally, and it rarely occurs under the age of 20 years. Less experienced players with poor stroke technique, but who play frequently, are in the high risk group. The average age of players developing tennis elbow is 40 years, reflecting (1) typical microcirculatory changes in the blood supply at the myotendinous junction of the extensor muscles at the elbow and (2) perhaps an increasing number of joint symptoms, but not true tennis elbow. Even so, in a study of world class tennis players, about 13 percent had current symptoms, and more than half had suffered from tennis elbow at one time or other.[24]

The etiology and treatment of this condition can be considered under three headings: playing style, anatomic factors, and equipment. An understanding of these etiologic features leads to a logical approach to therapy.

Playing Style

The poorly executed backhand stroke in tennis is mainly implicated. The forearm is used as the power source instead of utilizing the kinetics of the body and weight transfer from the body to the shoulder (Fig. 22-18). It frequently reflects the inability to anticipate and assume a satisfactory position for the return stroke.

A typical faulty backhand has no forward weight transfer, and the front shoulder is usually elevated. The trunk leans away from the net at the time of impact and the racquet head is down. The elbow and wrist extend prior to impact, and the power source is forearm extension in the pronated position. It is usually a nonrhythmic, jerky movement with sharp pronation in the follow-through. When the ball is hit incorrectly, the forces are transmitted as an acute strain along the muscle mass to the extensor origin at the elbow.[33] Repetitive stress may eventually cause small tears and inflammation, which are reflected in the pain associated with tennis elbow.

Anatomic studies confirm that the extensor carpi radialis brevis (ECRB) is under maximum tension

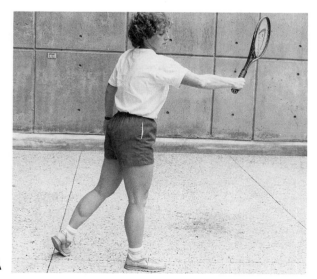 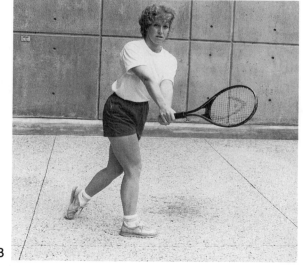

A   B

Fig. 22-18. Poor technique unduly stresses the elbow. **(A)** Common faults include poor body positioning, leading with the elbow and failure to use trunk and shoulder power. **(B)** Two-handed backhand ensures a more proximal source of power and de-emphasizes the elbow and wrist extensors.

Practice Point
MOST PAINFUL STROKES

Stroke	%
Backhand	38
Serve	25
Forehand	23
Backhand volley	7
Overhead smash	4
Forehand volley	3

when contracting while the forearm is pronated, the wrist flexed, and the ulna deviated.[26] Furthermore, the head of the radius rotates anteriorly against the ECRB during pronation, where a bursa is frequently located, which may account for some individuals who experience pain at the head of the radius, perhaps secondarily to inflammation of the bursa.[26]

The backhand grip is usually the main precipitating factor even with relatively good technique. The use of a backhand grip forces the arm into a hyperpronated position, thereby stressing the extensor origin. Second, some tennis players who have played seriously for many years have increased the bulk of their extensor muscles considerably but may have lost full flexibility. Therefore they have increased stresses at the completion of the stroke.[26]

A frequent error is an exaggerated effort to hit the ball hard. Maximum speed is imparted to the ball by good style, keeping the eye on the ball and hitting it on the "sweet spot" in the center of the racquet. Little is to be gained by sacrificing style for power. Usually the result of overpowering the stroke is failure to transfer the body weight, thus relying on the forearm as the main source of strength, often aggravating a preexisting condition further.

Therefore so far as technique is concerned, the stroke most implicated in tennis elbow is firmly established as the backhand. Investment in a few tennis lessons to improve technique should be considered. The development of a two-handed backhand stroke also alleviates the problem for some players with chronic repetitive symptoms.

Many of the more experienced players run into trouble with the forehand and top spin. The common fault is to roll the racquet head over the ball in an attempt to produce topspin. This action produces excessive strain, as the impact is sustained at the hy-

perpronated position. Supination follows, with the ball only on the strings for 0.004 second, not long enough to impart adequate top spin. The more correct long stroking maneuver, starting low and ending high, with a good followthrough, is more effective and produces less stress.[33,34]

During the serve, the racquet head travels 300 to 350 mph before ball impact, at which time it slows abruptly to about 150 mph. With poor use of trunk and legs, the forearm once again absorbs too much stress.[30] Indeed, hitting a tennis ball traveling at 30 mph may be equivalent to lifting a 50 lb weight.

When recovering from tennis elbow, the patient should commence with the easiest strokes, try not to be too competitive, and play only with people who are willing to have an easy game.

Anatomy

Many individuals play tennis with less than optimal grip strength. Indeed, the average woman has a forearm girth of 9 inches and a grip strength of about 50 lb, and the average man has a forearm girth of 11 inches and a grip strength of approximately 80 lb. By contrast, the professional tennis player has a forearm girth of about 12 inches and a grip strength of 105 lb.[33] The normal wrist extensors should be about 45 to 50 percent of the flexor strength.[29] Wrist flexors have been found to be the strongest group, followed by radial deviators, ulnar deviators, and then extensors. The supinators are normally stronger than pronators.[10] In regular tennis players, the extensor muscles may need to be strengthened, so they are at least 50 percent and perhaps as much as 70 to 75 percent of the flexor strength. An even grip, taking care not to allow the thumb to be placed along the line of the shaft assists in arranging an even distribution of forces.

Equipment

In individuals with incipient or established symptoms, the racquet should be strung to 52 to 55 lb.[35] This tension allows the impact to be spread over slightly more time and decreases the forces into the forearm muscles.[34] Sixteen gauge catgut is more resilient than nylon and has the ability to lessen the shock of the impact of the ball. However, gut is expensive and loses resilience quickly; probably 16 gauge nylon is the best compromise.

A racquet handle that is too large or too small may produce an uneven force distribution across the hand

and hence to the muscles. This point is particularly applicable to women whose average hand size is about 4⅛ inches. Measurement taken from the distal hand crease to the tip of the ring finger along its radial border gives an indication of grip size[33,37] (Fig. 22-19).

Heavy duty or rubber-centered balls impart more concentrated moments of force and may aggravate the symptoms. Regular duty balls are recommended. Furthermore, playing with balls soaked from hitting puddles after the rain may trigger problems.[30]

It is difficult to give advice with regard to the racquet itself. Both wooden and metal racquets have merits and disadvantages. The heavy wooden racquets should be avoided by all but the most experienced players. Nirschl advised a midsize, graphite racquet weighing only 12.0 to 12.5 ounces. The graphite absorbs the shock better than wood, and the midsize racket has a larger "benevolent" or "sweet" zone, the area on the strings where minimal torque is produced on impact.[31] The lighter racquet allows players to position it more quickly and lessens the chance of hitting late.[36] Balanced weight, hand size, and stringing are all factors. Most of all, good style, hitting the ball in the sweet spot in the center of the racquet, can do more to reduce stress on the forearm than does any change of racquet.

General Treatment

Treatment is aimed at relief of inflammation, promotion of healing, reducing the overload forces, and increasing upper extremity strength, endurance and

---

Quick Facts

CONTRIBUTING FACTORS TO TENNIS ELBOW

- Little playing experience: novice player frequently at risk
- More stress if consistently miss "sweet spot" when hitting
- Poor stroke technique, use of arm instead of body
- Inadequate power, flexibility, or endurance
- Heavier, stiffer racquets increase stress (12.0 to 12.5 oz best)
- Lighter racquet enables player to position quicker
- Large handle size (>4⅜) may generate symptoms
- Too tight racquet stringing (string 2 to 3 lb less than normal)
- 16-gauge gut more resilient than nylon
- Heavy duty or wet balls cause greater stress
- Playing surface: balls bounce quicker off cement

---

flexibility.[21,25] Some points important in the prevention treatment of tennis elbow are as follows.

1. Before practicing, warm up slowly and do adequate stretching exercises for the forearm and hand.

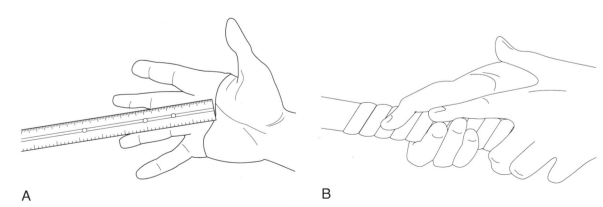

A   B

Fig. 22-19. Proper grip size may be determined by **(A)** measuring along the radial side of the ring finger from the distal palmar crease to the finger tip; **(B)** alternatively, hold the racquet and see if a finger fits into the gap between the thumb and fingers. (From Liu,[34] with permission.)

Sometimes it helps to rub ice onto the common extensor origin before playing.

2. Wearing a tennis arm band (epicondylar splint) of nonelastic fabric lined with foam rubber to prevent slipping, may reduce stress on the common extensor origin. By limiting muscle expansion, the contraction force is reduced, decreasing irritation of the muscle. This tennis elbow band must be wide enough, i.e., 3.0 to 3.5 inches. The narrower widths are usually not as effective.[38] The band should be applied by tensing the muscles of the arm and then placing the band tightly. If this elbow band is applied while the muscles are relaxed it may cut off the circulation. The band should be comfortable with the forearm relaxed. The band should not be put too proximally but, rather, over the major muscle belly, about two fingers' breadth distal to the elbow flexor crease. A pneumatic splint may be more comfortable, with the air bag centered over the extensor muscle mass (Fig. 22-20). The efficacy of these straps in decreasing pain during numerous activities has been well documented.[39-41]

3. Occasionally, a wrist resting splint can be made and adapted to suit the occupation or sport

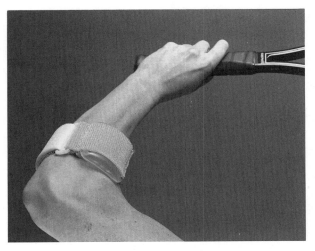

Fig. 22-20. Pneumatic device (air splint) for functional decompression of extensor stresses.

of the individual. This moderate defunctioning of some of the wrist extensor contraction may slowly allow a resistant clinical problem to resolve with considerable comfort during the activities of daily living.

4. Physiotherapy treatment initially consists in assessment, modification of activity, and application of ice and selected modalities.[28,42]

Grip strength correlates well with visual pain scales and thus may be used to objectively assess the severity of the clinical complaints. Even measuring grip strength with the aid of a simple sphygmomanometer cuff, preinflated to 20 mg Hg, can give a reasonable assessment of the pain threshold and progress of treatment.[43-45] Electrotherapy modalities such as laser, ultrasound phonophoresis with 10 percent hydrocortisone, interferential therapy, high voltage galvanic stimulation, and transcutaneous electrical nerve stimulation (TENS) have all been advocated to relieve pain and inflammation. Cure rates have been reported from 55 to 90 percent.[43]

Topical application of dimethylsulfoxide (DMSO) has also been suggested,[32,33] but it is not recommended. A better combined approach might be the application of cortisone–lidocaine–thixotropic gel and ultrasound or simply the use of a dermal preparation of NSAIDs, which seems able to permeate through to tissues in a subcutaneous location. Manual therapy techniques, e.g., transverse frictions, joint

---

Quick Facts

SIGNIFICANT RELIEF OF SYMPTOMS OF LATERAL EPICONDYLITIS[a]

Treatment	% Relief
Changing tennis stroke or getting lessons	92
Stretching and strengthening exercises	84
Wearing forearm splint or brace	83
Use of medication	
Aspirin	70
NSAIDs	85
Steroid injection	88
Modalities	
Heat	73
Cold	63
Ultrasound	53
Rest > 1 month	72

[a] Complete relief (lack of recurrence) requires combined, intensive therapy.[35]

TABLE 22-3. Comparison of Manipulation Techniques

Parameter	Mills[48]	Cyriax I[46]	Cyriax II (Mills)[46]	Kaltenborn[49]	Mennell[50]	Stoddard[51]
Lesion	Frayed or detached ligament in acute cases. Adhesions in chronic cases.	Partial tear at tenoperiosteal junction of extensor carpi radialis brevis.	Inadequate healing. Scar in extensor carpi radialis brevis at tenoperiosteal junction.	Lateral epicondylitis.	Painful scar in common extensor tendon.	Adhesions binding origin or extensor digitorum communis to radial collateral ligament.
Position	Lying. General anesthetic	Sitting. No anesthetic. After 5–10 minutes of deep friction.	Sitting. After 10–15 minutes deep friction.	Sitting or supine. No anesthetic.	Standing. Prior injection of local anesthetic.	Supine.
Manipulation	Forced extension of elbow. Wrist and fingers flexed. Forearm pronated.	Elbow fully extended. Forearm supinated. Fixation at medial elbow. Varus thrust at lateral wrist.	Shoulder abducted and medially rotated. Forearm pronated, wrist flexed. Fixated at wrist. Extensor thrust at elbow.	Fixation at wrist. Varus thrust at extended elbow.	Fully flexed and pronated wrist and elbow. Elbow extension with forced over pressure.	Shoulder abducted 90°. Pronate and supinate to identify maximum tension in extensor digitorum communis. Varus thrust at elbow by forearm adduction.
Indication	Minimal loss of range of motion of elbow extension. Tested with full wrist and finger flexion in pronation. Local epicondylar or radiohumeral joint tenderness.	Pain over lateral epicondyle or common extensor tendon origin.	Tenoperiosteal variety. Pain on resisted wrist extension and radial deviation.	Lateral epicondylitis. Restricted movement of radial head.	Painful area at common extensor origin on palpation.	Chronic cases. No response to hydrocortisone injection. Pain on gripping.
Contraindication	Gross limitation of extension. Full range of motion.		Loss of full elbow extension. Osteoarthrosis. Loose bodies, traumatic arthritis.	Inability to fully extend.		Acute condition. Rest pain. Restriction of elbow extension.
Frequency	Usually one manipulation.	Three times per week. Average four treatments (range one to nine).	Two or three times per week until cure. Range 4–12 sessions.			

(From Kushner and Reid,[47] with permission.)

mobilization and manipulation, myofascial release, and strain and counterstrain techniques may be used[46,47] (Table 22-3).

Whatever the treatment employed, as resolution occurs and the patient returns to the sport or occupation, exercise is a mainstay of the treatment. Complete rest is seldom indicated (Table 22-4). Reduced physical activity leads to reduction in strength. Thus on resuming the activity recurrence of the injury may be precipitated by stresses of lesser magnitude than those causing the initial insult unless a strengthening program is instituted.

Isometric exercises for the wrist extensors with the elbow in flexion, moving closer to extension as pain relief permits, can be used during the acute phase.[47] In addition, the patient can be instructed to carry out passive and active stretching of the extensor muscle during the day. The latter may initially flare up the symptoms, but it is an important step in regaining pain-free functional contraction (Fig. 22-21).

As pain permits, concentric and then eccentric strengthening using free weights or surgical tubing is undertaken. Isokinetic strengthening eccentrically and concentrically may also be used. Not only are the flexors and extensors strengthened, but also the radial and ulnar deviators, pronators, and supinators (Figs. 22-22 and 22-23).

Curwin and Stannish have developed a program to combine stretching and eccentric strengthening of the wrist extensors.[47,52] Exercising the muscle eccentrically may allow it to withstand greater resistance and prevent injury that occurs by eccentrically loading an inflexible muscle. The patient warms up with local heat or general exercise. The wrist extensors are stretched passively three times for 30 seconds each time. Three sets of ten eccentric contractions are performed with a weight of 1 to 5 pounds. Alternatively, surgical tubing may be an effective way of applying resistance. The stretches are repeated, and ice is then applied. This 20-minute session is undertaken daily for about 3 weeks.

Prior to returning to the sport or occupation, the

TABLE 22-4. Exercise Progression for Lateral Epicondylitis

Stage	Exercise
I	Prepare for exercise with heat, ice, or ultrasound Isometrics progressed through 　　Elbow flexion 　　Neutral 　　Elbow extension Progress when maximal isometric contraction possible in extension with no pain
II	Prepare for exercise with heat and stretching Isotonic exercise through a full range of motion Start with small resistance Build up to 5 lb Progress when pain-free through full range
III	Isotonic exercises full range Work up to 15–20 lb resistance Start adding sequentially tubing exercises and then other resistance apparatus Add wrist flexor and extensor stretches Ice down common extensor origin after each session Progress if no pain
IV	Ensure adequate warm-up Commence functional exercises with a partner, no opponent Hit ball against wall for 1 minute Build up speed or power of stroke Practice forehand only; work on technique Build up time When pain-free, start backhand
V	Ensure adequate warm-up Commence practice Build up intensity and time slowly Continue home strengthening and stretching program Ice after heavy workouts

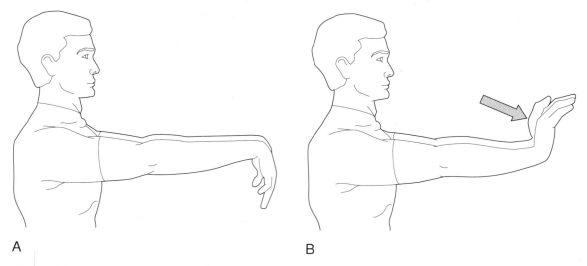

A   B

Fig. 22-21. Wrist extensor stretch. **(A)** Performed passively with the other hand. **(B)** Dynamic. The athlete generates the strongest isometric hold compatible with the symptoms and holds for 10 seconds. This exercise is repeated numerous times throughout the day, and in different ranges.

patient mimics the backhand, forehand, and serve or specific tasks using surgical tubing or pulleys for resistance. Throughout the physiotherapy, shoulder and trunk strength and range of motion are maintained. Particular attention should be given to correcting range of motion deficits in shoulder rotation and any weakness in shoulder external rotation and abduction.[53] The goal is to restore the flexibility, strength, endurance, and coordination of the whole upper limb needed for the patient's specific activity. In addition, where appropriate cardiovascular fitness must be maintained.

5. Injection of a steroid preparation can be effective, provided the lesion is well localized.[43] This treatment is best supplemented with oral anti-inflammatory medication and may be repeated at 1-month intervals for up to 3 months or until the patient is asymptomatic. Certainly no more than three injec-

tions should be used. Considerable care is needed with the injection technique to avoid skin atrophy. In the series of Calvert et al. 17 percent of patients receiving two to five injections developed either depigmentation and/or subcutaneous fat necrosis and atrophy.[32] It must be stressed that simply injecting the elbow does not constitute complete treatment. Assessment and modification of precipitating factors, as well as exercise therapy, is usually necessary.

6. Whenever a therapy is successful in removing the symptoms of epicondylitis, education of the patient to ensure adequate warm-up, stretching, and perhaps icing prior to activity is essential to reduce the possibility of recurrence.

7. When nonoperative management fails, surgery may be considered. The indications for surgery include (1) documented adequate nonoperative treatment including injection; (2) adequate time, which

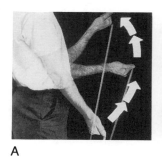   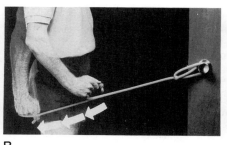   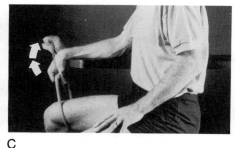

A   B   C

Fig. 22-22. Tubing exercises for **(A)** elbow flexors, **(B)** elbow extensors, **(C)** wrist extensors.

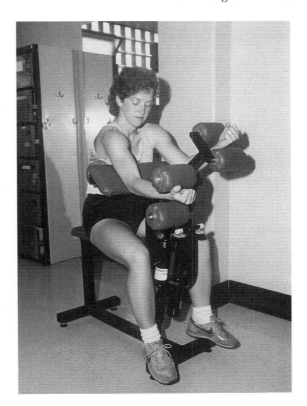

Fig. 22-23. Resisted work for biceps and triceps using a variety of equipment ensures sufficient proximal strength.

should be up to a year where practical; and (3) a level of residual pain that interferes with activities of daily living, employment, or in the case of a serious tennis player the ability to continue competing.[25] Usually release of the fascia and part of the common extensor origin is sufficient and gives excellent short- and long-term results (Table 22-5). Variations of this procedure involve increasingly radical releases, to include part of the annular ligament of the superior radio-ulnar joint, and extensor capri radialis brevis or the fascial band at the proximal edge of supinator.[55,57,58] The variation in the extent of the procedure reflects the confusion as to the exact site of the pathology.[59]

Postoperative rehabilitation involves a short period of gentle active motion and, at 3 weeks, increasing range of motion, strengthening, and stretching exercises. The recovery period ranges from approximately 4 weeks to 3 months in most series.[33,35,55,56]

Medial Epicondylitis (Epitrochleitis, Golfer's Elbow, Medial Tennis Elbow)

Etiology

Medial epicondylitis is probably a tendinopathy of the common flexor origin including the pronator teres. Pain is located over the medial epicondyle and is exacerbated by resisted wrist flexion and ulnar deviation. Pain is also elicited on passive elbow and wrist extension in supination. It is an overuse syndrome seen in (1) throwing sports, where it may be related to repetitive valgus stresses along with pronation and wrist flexion; (2) golfing with excessive driving, or brought on acutely by mishitting the ground; (3) and racquet sports due to the wrist action. Chronic symptoms may eventually lead to contractures with inability to fully extend or supinate.[60]

Treatment

Prevention and restoration of lost range of motion are important parts of the treatment. In the acute phase, ice, ultrasound, and other physical modalities may be used in conjunction with anti-inflammatory medication. Any course of treatment must culminate in a strengthening program. The stretching and strengthening routine described under tennis elbow is used, but the direction of motion is reversed.[61] Injection into the area of a steroid preparation is done with care because of the propensity for skin atrophy in this area as well as the proximity of the ulnar nerve. In recalcitrant cases, a release of the

TABLE 22-5.   Outcome of Surgical Intervention for Tennis Elbow, 1973–1988

Study	Response Rate[a] (%)	Follow-Up Period	Duration Before Surgery (months)	Good Result[b] (%)	Operative Complications (%)	Recovery Period[c]
Conrad & Hopper[54]	100	1–9 years	7–12	100	Nil	3–12 months
Boyd & McLeod[55]	92	5 months to 6 years	6–96	100	3[d]	2–4 months
Posch et al.[56]	52	8 years	3	86	5[e]	3–4 months
Murtagh (reported by Cameron et al.[57]	100	4–15 months	8	70	5[f]	1 week
Nirschl & Pettrone[33]	87	1–7 years	21–51	85	3[e,d]	2–4 months
Berahang[27]	100	15 months	15	90	10[d]	3 mo
Cameron et al.[57]	90	2 years	6–48	93	Nil	<2 weeks
Yerger & Turner[58]	73	1–11 years	Not stated	93	4[e,g]	3–12 months
Calvert et al.[32]	86	6 years	24	89	3[h]	4–8 weeks
Goldberg et al.[59]	90	4 years	6–60	73	Nil	5 weeks

[a] Percent follow-up.
[b] No pain or loss of function.
[c] Time to full use of elbow.
[d] Loss of full extension.
[e] Infection.
[f] Hematoma.
[g] Synovial fistula.
[h] Painful scar.
(Data from Kamien,[25] with permission.)

common origin is possible with surprisingly little measurable loss of functional strength.

Injuries to the Throwing Arm (Medial Tension Overload Syndrome)

Throwing Action

The throwing mechanisms adapted in various sports have more mechanical similarities than differences. The baseball throwing action is frequently used to demonstrate these principles and their effect on the supporting anatomy. Three stages are defined: the cocking phase or wind-up, the acceleration phase (early and late), and the follow-through[62–65] (Fig. 22-24). They are discussed here only in relation to stress on the elbow.

1. *Cocking phase.* The shoulder is abducted to around 90 degrees and simultaneously taken into extreme external rotation with extension. The elbow is flexed to approximately 45 degrees and the wrist extended. There is a distractive force applied to the medial elbow.

2. *Early acceleration phase.* During this phase the

Quick Facts

COCKING PHASE

- Distractive force to medial elbow
  -Stress on medial collateral ligament structures
  -Stretching of ulnar nerve
  -May eventually encourage traction spurs into ulnar collateral ligament

---

body and shoulder are brought rapidly forward, leaving the forearm and hand behind, prestressing all the structures at the elbow, in particular the ulnar collateral ligament.

3. *Late acceleration phase.* As vigorous contraction of the shoulder flexors and internal rotators takes place, with early co-contraction of the elbow extensors and wrist flexors, the forearm and wrist are accelerated to add speed to the throw. The maneuver results in a whipping action, placing significant additional stress on the medial elbow.

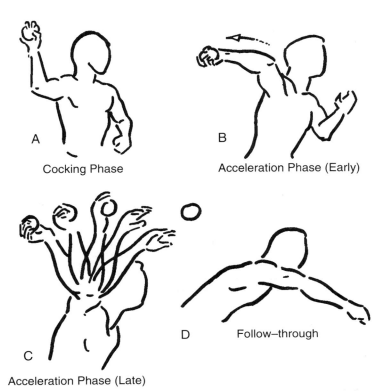

A Cocking Phase

B Acceleration Phase (Early)

C Acceleration Phase (Late)

D Follow–through

Fig. 22-24. Throwing mechanism is common to many sports, initially putting stress on the shoulder and elbow, with a final distraction force largely dampened by muscle and ligamentous structures at the elbow.

Quick Facts

ACCELERATION PHASE

- Extreme valgus tensile stress on medial elbow
  -Strain of flexor muscle origin
  -Medial collateral ligament stress
  -Spurs on ulnar coronoid process
  -Ulnar nerve traction symptoms
- Simultaneous compressive forces laterally
  -Lateral epicondylitis
  -Radial head injury
  -Capitellar osteochondral injuries
  -Loose body formation

Quick Facts

FOLLOW THROUGH

- Olecranon jams into fossa giving posterior stresses
  -Triceps strain
  -Synovial impingement
  -Olecranon fractures
  -Loose bodies and degenerative changes

---

4. *Follow through phase.* This phase begins with the missile release and varies somewhat with the type of throw. It is characterized by stress on the structures around the olecranon as the forearm pronates and the olecranon jams into its fossa.

Injuries

The sequence of events described above and repeated multiple times may result in a series of pathologic changes, best considered under the headings of acute and chronic (Table 22-6). The lateral joint line experiences compressive forces during throwing, while shear forces are generated posteriorly in the olecranon fossa and tensile forces develop along the medial joint line.[18,66-69]

**TABLE 22-6.   Throwing Injuries
of the Elbow**

Medial tension overload
   Muscular
      Overuse
      Fascial compression syndrome
   Ligamentous and capsular
      Ulnar traction spur
      Loose bodies
      Medial epicondylitis
      Joint degeneration

Lateral compression injuries
   Osteochondritis dissecans
   Capitellar fractures
   Loose bodies
   Lateral epicondylitis
   Joint degeneration

Extensor overload
   Acute
      Triceps strain
      Olecranon fracture
   Chronic
      Bony hypertrophy
      Stress fracture
      Olecranon fossa loose bodies
      Joint degeneration

(From Slocum,[62] with permission.)

Acute Injuries

Musculotendinous Strains. Minor muscular strains are common, presenting with point tenderness to palpation and pain with resisted contraction. These injuries, usually to the common flexor group, are frequently self-limiting and require only modified rest, ice, treatment by modalities, and gentle stretching. With healing, progressive strengthening is added to ensure adequate ability to return to function without reinjury. Flexion contractures, which predispose to muscle strains, are present in more than one-half of professional pitchers.[18]

Major tears or ruptures, usually of the forearm flexors, must be recognized, as surgery may be required (Fig. 22-25). Usually deformity, a palpable defect, and considerable ecchymosis alert the practitioner to the correct diagnosis. In the muscular individual, a transverse sulcus may be present at the anterior border of the lacertus fibrosis (bicipital aponeurosis), and this normal groove should not be confused with a rupture of the pronator teres or common flexor muscle belly. Rarely, the biceps tendon ruptures distally. This injury is compatible with acceptable function in the noncompetitive individual, al-

though surgical repair gives the best results in the heavy manual laborer and the athlete.

Medial Collateral Ligament Sprains. Repetitive valgus stress in pitchers and javelin throwers (javelin thrower's elbow) may cause acute inflammation of the medial collateral ligament. Point tenderness over the medial joint line and the absence of instability help to make this diagnosis. Treatment is the same as muscular strains.

Avulsion of the Medial Epicondyle. Prior to epiphyseal closure, rapid strong contraction of the forearm flexors is capable of avulsing the medial epicondyle[68-70] (Fig. 22-25). Tenderness in the region of the medial condyle in an adolescent should arouse suspicion of this injury. Failure to detect it may lead to increasing varus deformity. With extreme tenderness and minimal or no displacement, prophylactic splinting of the elbow for 2 weeks is a safe precaution. A repeat roentgenogram at this time may show callus. A widely displaced fragment may require surgical reattachment. These injuries are discussed again under the section on fractures around the elbow.

Practice Point

**MEDIAL EPICONDYLAR
EPIPHYSEAL INJURY**

Grade I	• No roentgenographic changes • Local tenderness • Symptoms only with stress • Treat by reducing activity
Grade II	• May be widening or quality changes on roentgenograms • Up to 4 mm of displacement • Significant symptoms • Treat by rest and possibly splinting
Grade III	• 5 mm or more displacement • Immediate withdrawal from activity • Probably needs surgical treatment

---

Chronic Injuries

The effects of repeated valgus stress of the elbow are most pronounced in the professional pitcher, particularly if this individual commenced his career at

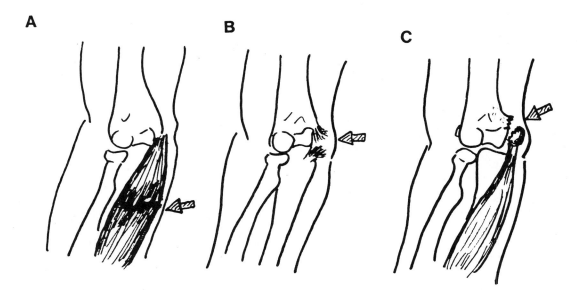

Fig. 22-25. Acute stress to the medial elbow may result in: **(A)** a muscle belly tear; **(B)** a ligament sprain; or **(C)** an avulsion fracture, which, in the skeletally immature athlete, may be an epiphyseal injury. (From Reid and Kushner,[2] with permission.)

an early age. These injuries were alluded to in the description of the throwing mechanism. Clinically, elbow flexion contractures occur in up to 50 percent of professional pitchers, and an increased carrying angle is seen in about 3 percent.[64,65,67,69] Repeated stress results in attenuation of the medial collateral ligament with laxity (Fig. 22-26). Pain and swelling, catching, and locking are often manifestations of additional bony and joint surface changes. X-ray films

may reveal loose bodies, particularly in the olecranon fossa, hyperostotic changes and osteophytes around the posteromedial olecranon process, and traction spurs at the attachment of the medial collateral ligament to the ulna. Oblique views and tomograms may be necessary to elucidate all these changes. Occasionally, the joint symptoms are accompanied by associated ulnar nerve neuritis or neuropathy secondary to repeated minor traction stresses or chronic scar-

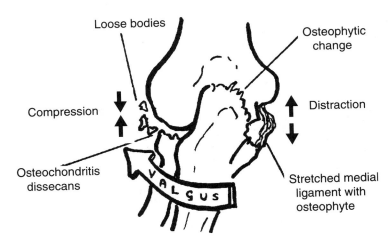

Fig. 22-26. Repetitive valgus stresses associated with throwing produce stretching and instability on the medial side, with shearing forces on the olecranon. The result is growth defects in the young and degenerative changes in the adult. (From Reid and Kushner,[2] with permission.)

ring. Surgical excision of osteophytes and removal of loose fragments may be necessary to restore range of motion and a fully functional elbow.

Little Leaguer's Elbow

The young pitcher is exposed to the same risks as those already outlined, and there is the additional risk of epiphyseal injury. The original concept of "little leaguer's elbow" referred to an epiphysitis of the medial epicondylar epiphysis related to the repeated trauma of pitching.[66-70] This stress is greatly increased by throwing "curve balls" and other breaking pitches, which require forceful pronation of the wrist. The clinical features of little leaguer's elbow include pain and tenderness with loss of full extension. Characteristic changes are accelerated growth of the medial side as well as fragmentation of the medial epicondylar epiphysis.[65,71] Subsequently, the term "little leaguer's elbow" has encompassed all of the stress changes involved in pitching that occur in the skeletally immature athlete.

Such changes include compression of the lateral joint, which may trigger changes of osteochondritis dissecans of both the capitellum and radial head. It is important to recognize this condition early, as adequate rest from repeated stress may allow resolution of the problems. Failure to protect the joint may result in the formation of loose fragments, pain, deformity, and possibly arthrosis. The incidence of this problem is unknown, varying widely in reported series.[72]

In 1972, before major rule changes were adopted to protect the youngsters, accelerated growth and separation of the medial epicondylar epiphysis was present in up to 90 percent of Little League pitchers between the ages of 9 and 14 in southern California. These same changes were seen in fewer than 10 percent of children of the same age who did not play baseball.[72]

Osteochondritis dissecans, particularly of the capitellum, is reported in other sports, notably gymnastics, where the arm frequently functions as a weight-bearing extremity under stress.[72-75]

Treatment

Treatment is initially aimed at decreasing inflammation with ice and rest, as dictated by the signs and symptoms. Electrical modalities to decrease pain and inflammation may be used, including TENS, high-voltage galvanic stimulation, ultrasound, interferential current, and laser.

If splinting or immobilization has been used, the initial emphasis is on gentle active range of motion as soon as it is discontinued. Gentle resisted isometric exercises within the patient's pain tolerance are added and then progressed to strengthening with surgical tubing or free weights. Isokinetic strengthening such as push-ups and pull-ups and use of special apparatus are directed at gaining full strength. Shoulder range of motion and isometric exercises are performed throughout the rehabilitation period.

Injuries in throwing sports may be reduced and prevented by attention to flexibility, decreasing muscle imbalances, and correcting the throwing technique. Proper use of body mechanics alters the stress on the elbow. Overhead throws rather than side arm and curve ball shots should be taught. Whipping and snapping of the elbow should be discouraged. The frequency and length of time each player is allowed to pitch should be decreased. Javelin throwers may have to change their technique or hold in order to reduce the stress of the medial joint.[73-75]

Prophylactic taping to prevent hyperextension and decrease valgus stresses may be used when the individual returns to practice. Care of the throwing arm includes the following.[75,76]

1. Gently stretching and massage of the elbow and shoulder before throwing
2. Performing throwing actions without the ball
3. Commencing with gentle throwing, wearing a warm-up jacket
4. Gradually increasing the velocity of the throw
5. After throwing, replacing the warm-up jacket, performing gentle stretching, allowing a period of time to cool down
6. Applying ice after each throwing session

Osteochondrosis of the Capitellum (Panner's Disease, Osteochondrosis Deformans, Osteochondritis)

Etiology

Osteochondrosis of the capitellum may be directly related to trauma, or it may be due to changes in the circulation. It is referred to as Panner's disease, or aseptic or avascular necrosis.[75,77,78]

There has been much debate as to the etiology of this condition; cartilage rests, bacterial infection, vascular insufficiency, primary fracture with separation, and hereditary factors have been implicated.[75-79] However, the evidence always seems to lead back to some form of disordered endochondral ossification in association with trauma or vascular impairment. Certain common features prevail. More than 90 percent of the lesions occur in males, fewer than 5 percent are bilateral, and the dominant arm is virtually always involved in unilateral cases. In children below the age of 8 years, the lesions are similar to those described by Panner, with changes in density and fragmentation of the capitellum; whereas in older children and adolescents, loose bodies are more frequent.

Osteochondritis is rarely seen before the age of 5 years when the chondroepiphysis of the capitellum has an abundant nutrient vascular supply.[77] The lesion usually manifests clinically when the capitellar nucleus is supplied only by one or two discrete vessels with no obvious anastomosis.[72] The path of these vessels from the posterior surface of the chondroepiphysis is through unossified epiphyseal cartilage to the capitellum, and they are therefore situated, at least part of the way, in compressible cartilage.

There is a vulnerable period so far as the circulation is concerned until fusion of the ossific nucleus during the late teens. Repeated minor trauma may damage the tenuous vasculature and may account for the prevalence of this condition in young baseball pitchers, gymnasts, and javelin throwers. Whatever the underlying etiology, the ultimate outcome may be healing, nonhealing, or loose body formation. Frequently the symptoms do not occur until the end of the growing period at age 13 to 17 and even later.

The major presenting symptoms are usually pain, swelling, limitation of range of motion in a non-capsular pattern, and sometimes clicking and locking. The fragments may or may not separate. If they remain in situ, there may be spontaneous recovery. If they fail to heal, they may separate into the joint as fragments (joint mice).[46] The diagnosis can usually be made from plain roentgenograms.

Treatment

Nonoperative treatment requires rest from stress and, rarely, a short period of immobilization with a splint. Treatment is as outlined for the throwing injuries.

The indications for surgery include a locked elbow, loose fragments, or failure of conservative therapy to relieve symptoms. Surgical treatment may include re-

---

> ## Practice Point
>
> ### TREATMENT AIMS
>
> - Prevent progression of pathology by reducing stresses appropriately
> - Resolve present symptoms
> - Restore range of motion
> - If separating fragment visible, attempt to keep it "in situ"
> - If symptoms mainly synovitis: NSAIDs, modalities, rest
> - If loose bodies or osteophytes present: possibly surgical removal or excision

moval of loose fragments, excision of the capitellar lesions, and curettage down to bleeding bone.[79] Usually, joint motion is restored or improved with manual therapy, a graduated strengthening and stretching program. A return to organized competitive sport is possible provided there are no excessive joint changes.[79] If the condition occurs in young children before epiphyseal closure, the prognosis for recovery is good. Continued rigorous activities in the face of symptoms or progression of the pathology after epiphyseal closure is likely to lead to degenerative changes and possible chronic restriction of motion and symptoms with activity.

Ligament Ruptures and Dislocations

Acute Ligament Tears

Acute ligament tears without dislocation are relatively rare but occasionally occur secondary to valgus or varus stresses in sport or recreation. The medial collateral ligament appears to be more vulnerable, and this injury is surprisingly easy to overlook in the acute stage unless there is an index of suspicion and careful valgus and varus stressing is carried out with the elbow flexed at 15 degrees[80,81] (Fig. 22-27). Often acute medial collateral ruptures are associated with some ulnar nerve paresthesias. Disability, restriction of range of motion, and minimizing of adhesions can be achieved by early protected range of motion in minor cases. Surgical repair may be considered for more significant tears. For some individuals, a functional brace eliminating valgus or varus stress allows resumption of strenuous activities moderately early.

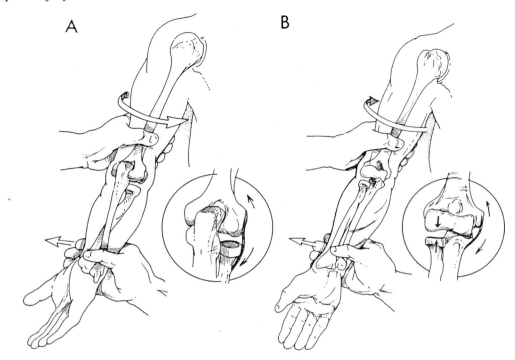

Fig. 22-27. Varus valgus stressing is done in 15 to 20 degrees of flexion. **(A)** Varus instability measured with the humerus in full internal rotation. **(B)** Valgus instability with the humerus in neutral and the forearm supinated. (After Morrey GF: The Elbow and Its Disorders. WB Saunders, Philadelphia, 1985. With permission.)

Dislocations

Radius and Ulna

A fall on the outstretched hand may result in elbow dislocation frequently with an associated fracture of the olecranon or coronoid process. After reduction, careful examination of the ulnar nerve is necessary and then immobilization with a sling for about 3 weeks. At this time gentle range of motion can be commenced.[82] The main danger of this injury is the potential for vascular damage to the brachial artery and incipient acute forearm compartment syndrome.

In those situations where there is considerable post-reduction instability, there may be a role for ligament repair.

Radial Head

In the adult dislocation of the radial head has a significant tendency to recurrence. Careful scrutiny of the lateral and anteroposterior films after reduction is mandatory.

Immobilization for 3 to 6 weeks in flexion is usually necessary. Any evidence of imperfect reduction is an indication for operative intervention.

Radial Head in Children (Pulled Elbow, Nursemaid's Elbow)

The imperfectly formed radial head may allow subluxation or dislocation in association with damage and unfolding of the immature annular ligament (Fig. 22-28). The common age of occurrence is 2 to 4 years. Distraction with rotation of the radius caused by swinging the child by the arms gives rise to one of the eponyms. Reduction is usually easily accomplished by elbow flexion and rotation of the forearm, or it may occur spontaneously. The major features of successful treatment are demonstration of the reduction by a normal roentgenogram, restoration of range of motion, and prompt resolution of pain. An inadequately reduced radial head progresses to significant overgrowth and deformity, culminating in serious disability of the elbow joint (Fig. 22-29).

Fractures About the Elbow

Supracondylar Fracture

Supracondylar fractures largely occur in children and, like most elbow fractures are fraught with difficulties at every stage—difficulties of diagnosis and

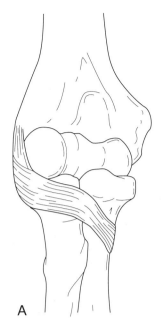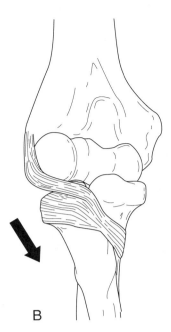

Fig. 22-28. Pulled elbow produced by distraction-rotation forces damages the annular ligament, allowing all or part of it to be carried into the joint. **(A)** Normal, **(B)** entrapped ligament.

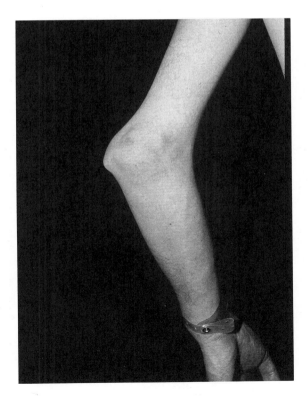

Fig. 22-29. Late deformity at the elbow as the result of an undiagnosed radial head dislocation during childhood.

reduction, neurovascular complications, loss of reduction in the cast, malunion, and stiffness.[83] Many of these injuries are greenstick or minimally displaced fractures with a tough medial periosteal hinge. If the fracture is angulated more than 20 degrees, it is best to reduce the fracture with adequate anesthesia and flex just above right angles to stabilize. Roentgenograms should be obtained before application of the cast in order to check reduction. The long-term problem with underestimated initial displacement is significant cubitus varus deformity.

Practice Point

SUPRACONDYLAR FRACTURES IN CHILDREN

- Unquestionable orthopaedic emergency
- Best reduction achieved before significant swelling
- Should be treated by practitioner with experience
- Must be admitted to hospital
- Frequent checks on adequacy of circulation

With the classic displaced supracondylar fracture, initial care involves looking for signs of ischemia and nerve palsy. Median nerve injury may result only in loss of flexion of the distal interphalangeal joint of the thumb and numbness of the tip of the index finger. The initial emergency splint should be with the arm extended to maximum comfort, as this position is less likely to jeopardize circulation. Initial roentgenograms should be obtained in the splint to prevent the radiology technician from rotating the arm at the fracture site. The quicker the reduction, the easier it is achieved, as the rapidly accumulating edema and hemorrhage add to the difficulty. Usually closed reduction is successful (Fig. 22-30). There are four steps to reduction: (1) Apply traction with the arm at 10 degrees to attempt to restore the fragment to its periosteal sleeve. (2) Correct any displacement; usually the correction is a medial shift. (3) Flex the elbow and press anteriorly over the olecranon for the common extension type posteriorly displaced fracture. (4) Externally rotate to correct the usual internal rotation deformity; if the initial displacement was medial, pronate to lock the fracture (Fig. 22-31). The real dilemma lies in balancing the added stability of increased elbow flexion with the decreasing perfu-

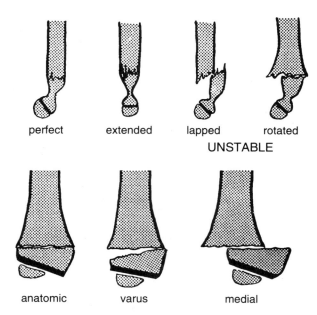

perfect   extended   lapped   rotated
UNSTABLE

anatomic   varus   medial

Fig. 22-30. Appearance of the anteroposterior and lateral roentgenograms assists in determining the adequacy of reduction. The thick black line of the supracondylar epiphysis should be at 70 degrees to the humeral shaft (Baumann's angle).

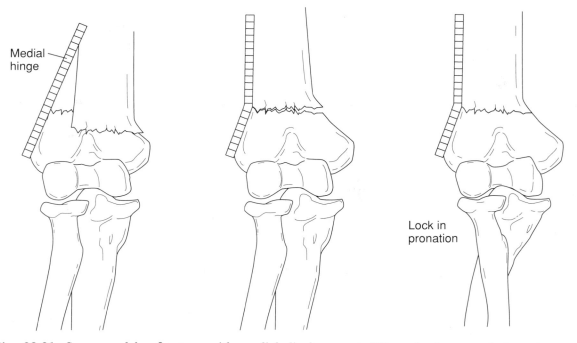

Medial hinge

Lock in pronation

Fig. 22-31. Supracondylar fracture with medial displacement. When the bone ends have been brought into contact, rotation of the forearm into pronation often secures the fracture by tightening the medial periosteal hinge.

sion. The circulation takes preference; and if there is an absent or decreased pulse or any other evidence of circulatory impairment, further extension of the arm is required. If adequate reduction is not achieved, or lost, or if there is neurovascular compromise, it is usually wise to consider a percutaneous wire or interosseous screw for traction. For the older child or in cases where there is inadequate reduction, percutaneous pinning or even open reduction with K-wires or plates may be considered. Whatever the case, good healing is usually well under way at 3 weeks, and gentle mobilization is usually possible soon after this point to prevent long-term stiffness.

Condylar and Epicondylar Fractures

Knowledge of the secondary growth centers around the elbow is necessary to judge the frequently subtle injuries to the condyles and epicondyles (Fig. 22-32). Roentgenographic comparison with the uninjured opposite side is usually mandatory. The rarer fracture patterns—transcondylar fractures and comminuted injuries—are not discussed.

Medial Epicondyle Fractures. These fractures are mainly avulsion injuries of the medial epicondyle via the ulnar collateral ligament and common flexor mass and have been described earlier. There is a varying degree of associated ligament and capsular damage. The displacement and fracture line depend on the presence or absence of the epicondylar apophysis.

In children between the ages of 5 and 15, the clinical signs of a medial hematoma may be more obvious than the radiographic clues. Associated radial neck fractures and ulnar nerve damage should be sought. In children under 5 years of age the epiphysis may not be visible, and until the age of 12 years separation of the whole medial condyle may masquerade as an epicondylar separation.[83] With significant clinical signs, it is safer to examine the child's elbow under general anesthesia. Instability is a possible indication for exploration. When there is good radiographic evidence

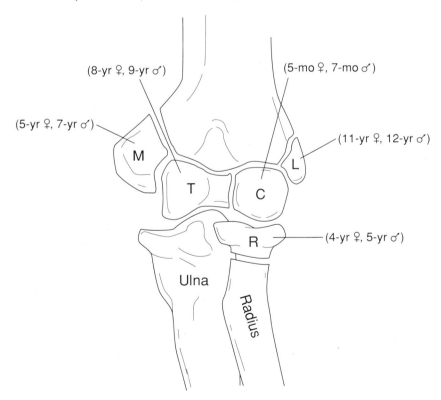

Fig. 22-32. Key secondary growth centers that may focus fracture lines or be avulsed with trauma. The average age of appearance. M = medial epicondyle; I = trochlea; C = capitellum; L = lateral epicondyle; and R = radial head. Age of appearance is in brackets. Most fuse at 14 and 17 years in females and males, respectively.

of the position, treatment depends on the displacement (Fig. 22-33).

Practice Point

MEDIAL EPICONDYLAR FRACTURE

- Minimally displaced and stable — treat with immobilization
- Definite displacement — may need open or closed pinning
- Trapped or dislocated — treat with open reduction and pin fixation

---

Lateral Epicondyle Fracture. This fracture is similar to the medial epicondylar fracture and probably represents an avulsion injury. The secondary center for the lateral epicondyle appears at the age of 12 years and fuses with the lateral condyle at the age of 14 years. The center is often irregular and hence confused with a fracture when in reality only a minor soft tissue injury or contusion exists. It is an unusual injury, and frequently the only treatment necessary is immobilization with a sling.

Lateral Condyle Fracture. Undisplaced, recognized, and treated by a sling or back slab for 3 weeks, lateral condyle fractures do well. Displaced and unrecognized they may go on to nonunion and cause valgus deformity, an ugly elbow, and potentially ulnar nerve damage. There is no place for a trial of conservative therapy with displaced fractures. Immediate open reduction and fixation provides excellent results (Fig. 22-34).

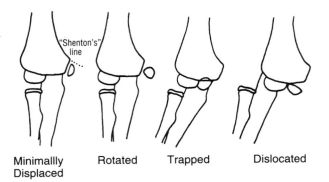

Minimallly Displaced   Rotated   Trapped   Dislocated

Fig. 22-33. Varieties of medial epicondylar fracture in the skeletally immature.

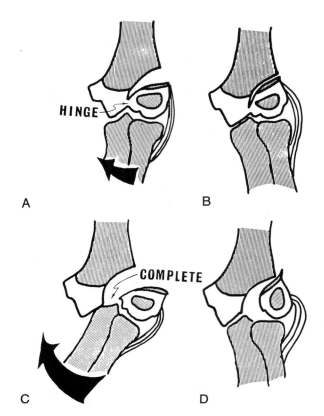

Fig. 22-34. Undisplaced fractures of the lateral condyle have an excellent prognosis. **(A)** Initial varus stress separates through the epiphyseal lines **(B)**, reduces when stress is relieved **(C)**, further varus stress, elbow subluxation, or dislocation separates the fragment **(D)**, and this does not reduce but rotates and is associated with a poor prognosis unless recognized and fixed anatomically.

Radial Head Fractures. Radial head fractures in the adult are mostly treated by gentle early motion to prevent joint stiffness, with protection from further stresses. If more than one-third of the articular surface is involved, if there is more than 30 degrees angulation, or if there is 3 mm or more of fracture gap, open reduction can probably improve the functional outcome. If significant long-term symptoms persist, excision of the radial head may help, but migration of the radius can cause wrist pain in the competitive athlete.

In the child, the radial head injury is frequently a Salter II epiphyseal separation. Up to the age of 5 years, angulations as large as 45 to 50 degrees will remodel. By age 10 years, 30 degrees is acceptable; greater angulation should be manipulated in an attempt to reduce the magnitude. By age 15 years, only about 15 degrees of angulation is acceptable. Greater degrees of displacement should be manipulated or openly reduced. Usually longitudinal traction and direct pressure over the head accomplish closed reduction.

Olecranon Fractures. Stress fractures of the olecranon in the baseball pitcher are discussed under the section on olecranon pathology. In the adult the displaced olecranon fracture is usually a significant injury with associated instability. Because the fractures are intra-articular, they require open reduction and internal fixation unless absolutely anatomic. Tension band wiring is the most effective treatment, having the advantage of allowing relatively early elbow motion (Fig. 22-35).

Monteggia Fracture-Dislocation. Falls on the outstretched hand may result in the combined injury of dislocation of the radial head and fracture of the olecranon (Fig. 22-36). The importance of the Monteggia fracture is that the radial head dislocation may be overlooked. Careful scrutiny of the roentgenograms after reduction of the ulna establishes if the radial head is in apposition with the capitellum. Any displacement usually constitutes an indication for open reduction.

Myositis Ossificans

The proximity of attachment of the fleshy brachialis and triceps to the joint and the complex nature of the three articulations in one capsule give the elbow a propensity for stiffness and myositis ossificans after trauma. Usually a fracture or dislocation is involved, but occasionally direct contusion is the precipitating

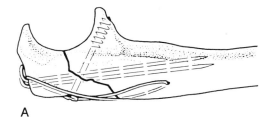

A

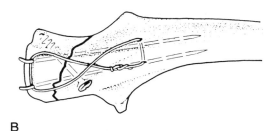

B

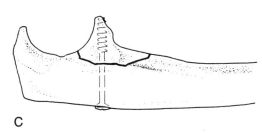

C

Fig. 22-35. Proximal ulnar fractures. Olecranon fractures are intra-articular and must be reduced automatically. **(A & B)** Tension band wire supplemented by screw fixation. **(C)** Screw fixation of an isolated coronoid process fracture.

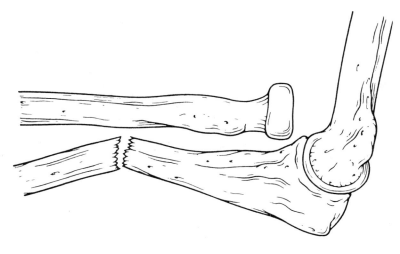

Fig. 22-36. Monteggia fracture. Proximal ulnar fracture is in association with a radial head dislocation. This picture shows the usual anterior dislocation.

factor. Therapists treating elbow trauma must be constantly aware of the syndrome of increasing pain and decreasing range during rehabilitation, as they are frequently in a position to recognize the evolution of this condition by detecting a subtle difference in the feel of the motion or by an increasingly firm mass in the muscle. At the first sign of this problem, soft tissue roentgenograms should be obtained as a baseline and repeated at 2-week intervals if the elbow fails to improve. Heat should be discontinued, anti-inflammatory medication commenced, and rest (with the exception of gentle, active range of motion) instituted. No resisted exercises should be performed. With stabilization of the condition, as evidenced by decreasing inflammation, bone mass, and pain, gentle therapy is reinstituted; the latter plays an important role in safely pacing the return to full activity. More often, with fractures around the elbow, the myositic ectopic bone is present concurrent with removal of the cast after 3 to 6 weeks of immobilization (Fig.

22-37). With maturity of the ectopic bone, as evidenced by bone scan, surgical excision may be the best treatment to restore a significant loss of range of motion.

Compartment Syndromes

Volkman's Ischemic Contracture

Classic Volkman's ischemic contracture is associated with supracondylar fractures in children (Fig. 22-38). It is useful to recall, however, that it may also occur with severe bleeding due to trauma to the forearm, crushing injuries, or a tight cast or bandage for any reason. Awareness of the impending disastrous situation and prompt attention to complaints of numbness, swelling, and discoloration of the fingers with increasing pain avert an unhappy outcome.

Compartment Syndromes

Traditionally, compartment syndromes of the forearm have become synonymous with the more dramatic Volkman's ischemic contracture secondary to dislocation of the elbow or supracondylar fractures as described above. However, in 1959 Bennett described a fascial compartment compression syndrome secondary to overuse.[82,83] Repetitive pitching for example, could lead to a syndrome of medial

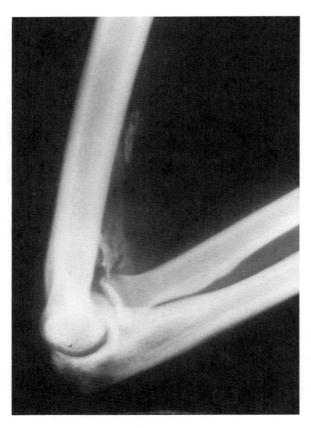

Fig. 22-37. Myositis ossificans after elbow dislocation.

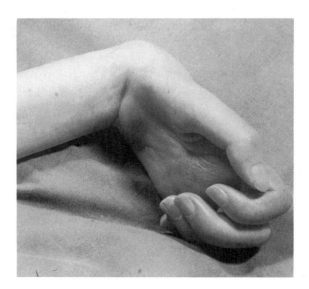

Fig. 22-38. Volkman's ischemic contracture. This classic deformity is due to scarring and contractures of the flexor muscle mass and ulnar and median nerve paralysis.

elbow and forearm pain secondary to swelling and edema within the tight forearm compartments. Recognition of the problem allows resolution with adequate rest. On resumption of activity, sufficient warm-up and carefully spaced and graduated work is usually successful, although in recalcitrant cases fasciotomy may be required.[61]

Nerve Entrapment, Neuritis, and Neuropathies

Ulnar Nerve Neuropathy

Site of Injury

The ulnar nerve is well protected by the bulk of the medial head of the triceps above the elbow and is rarely involved in humeral shaft fractures. However, it is more susceptible to damage in connection with supracondylar and epicondylar fractures (Table 22-7). When passing from the anterior to the posterior compartment of the arm, the ulnar nerve may be involved in fibrous compression or adhesion to the medial intermuscular septum. This septum slopes from a wide base at the medial epicondyle, where it is thick and unyielding, to a weak thin edge at varying distances more proximally on the humeral shaft. If the nerve is rerouted by surgery to the anterior aspect of the elbow, it may be drawn across or compressed on the firm edge of the septum unless mobilized sufficiently proximally, which may explain some surgical failures with anterior transposition of the ulnar nerve.[83]

Behind the epicondyle the ulnar nerve is superficial and is particularly vulnerable to direct injury. Dislocations, contusions, traction injuries, fractures of the epicondyle, callus, osteophytes from the radiocapitellar articulation and olecranon, or subluxation of the nerve with flexion and extension may contribute to neuritis or neuropathy.[84] Simple ganglia and benign tumors such as lipomas also have been implicated in neural compression (Table 22-7).

Cubital Tunnel

The cubital tunnel, as traditionally described by Feindel and Stratford, is an osseoaponeuritic canal behind the medial epicondyle.[85] It is formed by the epicondyle, olecranon, medial collateral ligament, and an aponeurotic arch, giving origin to and formed by the two heads of flexor carpi ulnaris. This tunnel may be considered to extend distally to varying degrees between the two heads of the flexor carpi ul-

TABLE 22-7. Factors Contributing to Ulnar Nerve Compression Symptoms

Neuritis
  Tension through repetitive elbow flexion
  Subluxing nerve

Neural pressure
  Perineural adhesions
  Congenital variations—bifid nerve
  Exostosis and osteophytes
  Sharp border of medial intermuscular septum
  Flexor carpi ulnaris, superficial and deep aponeurosis

Trauma
  Fractures
  Dislocations
  Callus
  Progressive valgus deformity
  Prolonged bed rest
  Leaning on elbow (repetitive minor trauma)
  Saturday night palsy (prolonged traction or pressure)

Predisposing conditions
  Peripheral neuritis
  Anatomy
  Rheumatoid arthritis
  Osteoarthritis

naris. This fibrous arch, the arcuate ligament, is slack in extension and becomes progressively more taut in flexion, thus potentially contributing to ulnar nerve compression. This arch must be released to ensure adequate surgical decompression in resistant cases of tardy ulnar palsy[1,84,86] (Fig. 22-39). Prolonged flexion, with its associated mild traction on the nerve, may cause sufficient pressure to cause transient paresis in the absence of external pressure. In addition, repeated rapid movements of the elbow, as with pitching or serving in volleyball, may also irritate the nerve. Contraction of the flexor carpi ulnaris may narrow the tunnel by pulling on the aponeurotic portion and narrowing the interval between the two heads.[1,84]

Signs and Symptoms

In sport the commonest malady involving the nerve at the elbow is a frictional neuritis with mainly sensory symptoms of pain and numbness in the classic ulnar distribution of the little finger and contiguous side of the ring finger. The nerve may be hypersensitive to tapping behind the elbow, which exacerbates the distal symptoms (Tinel's sign) (Fig. 22-40). In many patients the elbow flexion test is positive. The elbow is fully flexed for 5 minutes, and a positive test is aggra-

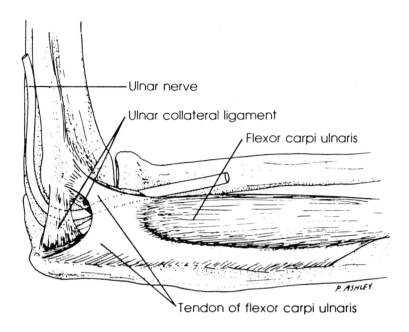

Fig. 22-39. Cubital tunnel. The two heads of the flexor carpi ulnaris are connected by a fibrous arch, the arcuate ligament, which forms a roof over the ulnar nerve. It is slack during extension and becomes progressively more taut during flexion, contributing to ulnar nerve symptoms.

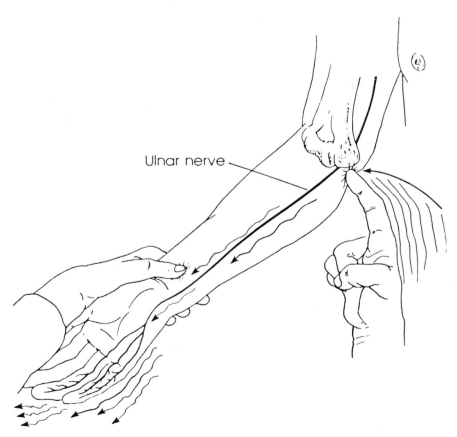

Fig. 22-40. Tinel's sign is produced by tapping the ulnar nerve at the elbow. Pain or tingling is felt in the ulnar-innervated portion of the hand.

vation of numbness or paresthesia (or both) in the ulnar nerve distribution (Fig. 22-41).

Untreated, the symptoms may progress. The signs of wasting of the intrinsic muscles of the hand, often most noticeable as atrophy of the first dorsal interosseous muscle reducing the bulk of the web space may become evident. Soon weakness of grip starts to accompany the increasing clumsiness in fine prehension, which was initially due to poor stereognosis. Sensation is decreased at the palmar and dorsal surfaces of the little finger and ulnar half of the ring finger. Two-point discrimination, which can be measured and recorded, deteriorates with increasing pathology. In the normal hand, compass points set 3 to 4 mm apart are clearly distinguished as separate stimuli (Fig. 22-42). Testing of the adductor pollicis reveals weakness, a positive Froment sign. Weakness of the interossei causes an inability to squeeze the little finger to the rest of the hand, a positive Wartenburg sign.[13]

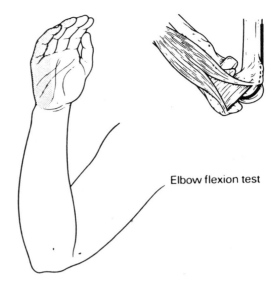

Fig. 22-41. Elbow flexion test. Reproduction of ulnar nerve dysesthesia or numbness within 5 minutes constitutes a positive test. (After Wadsworth,[13] with permission.)

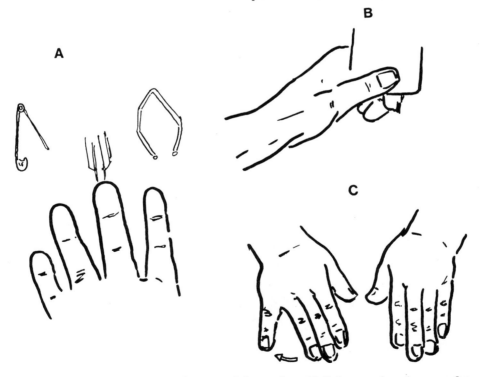

Fig. 22-42. **(A)** Sensory function may be tested for pain and light touch using a safety pin and two-point discrimination (normal 3 to 4 mm on the fingertip) with calipers or a paper clip. **(B)** Weakness of the adductor pollicis is detected by the presence of Froment's sign. Weakness is compensated for by flexing the thumb tip as the paper is pulled away. **(C)** A positive Wartenburg sign is the inability to obtain close adduction of all fingers. (From Reid and Kushner,[2] with permission.)

Treatment

Treatment depends on frequency, duration, intensity, magnitude, and etiology of the symptoms. If the neuritis is secondary to repeated blows, as in wrestling, or pressure, as with a student studying and writing, a well constructed pad may help. If the neuritis is frictional, it may be sufficient to block terminal extension for a period of time by initially taping the elbow. Persistent symptoms should not be allowed to continue or progress. Complete rest from the offending activity supplemented by anti-inflammatory medication usually helps the acute case. In more chronic situations the diagnosis and exact location is confirmed by roentgenography and nerve conduction studies, and surgical treatment is considered.

Practice Point

ULNAR NERVE NEUROPATHY

- Persistent severe symptoms
- Significant electrophysiologic changes
- Obvious muscle wasting

Surgical decompression is required if irreversible changes are to be avoided.

Decompression and transposition of the ulnar nerve are the major alternatives, and exact knowledge of the anatomy is needed if success is to be achieved.[87] With tumors or stenosis of the cubital tunnel, usually decompression is adequate; however, sufficient distal release is mandatory to ensure division of both the superficial and deep aponeuroses[86] (Fig. 22-43). If there are large osteophytes, callus, a subluxing nerve, significant nerve changes, and severe clinical signs, or a situation of repeated local trauma, transposition may be a better alternative to relieve minimal continued tension on the nerve. Adequate proximal release is necessary to avoid tension across the medial intermuscular septum.[86] If transposition is desirable but would entail devascularization of too great a section of nerve, medial epicondylectomy with nerve decompression may be the most suitable alternative. This technique is particularly useful in athletes with large arm girths and in whom more than 20 cm of nerve would have to be mobilized for adequate transposition.[87,88] Removal of the condyle does not appear to significantly alter grip strength or elbow flexor power after adequate rehabilitation.[55,84]

Median Nerve Neuropathy

Median nerve entrapment about the elbow is a rare phenomenon, although cases have been reported following posterior dislocation. When it does occur it is usually in children, and recognition of the problem is usually delayed.[89] Furthermore, progressive involvement of the nerve in developing callus following distal humeral fractures has also been recorded.[89] Rarely, the nerve becomes compressed above the elbow as it

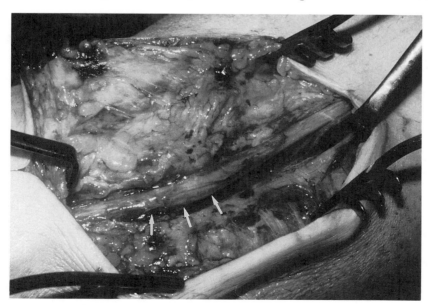

Fig. 22-43. Severely irritated, inflamed ulnar nerve at surgery. Release or frequently transposition is necessary when symptoms persist.

passes under the anomalous ligament of Struthers, which attaches to a spur (the supracondylar process) in the lower third of the humerus. This supracondylar process is found in only about 7 of every 1,000 individuals. Because of its anterior location, the median nerve may be subjected to direct blows, particularly in some sports. However, the result is generally neuropraxia or infrequently axonotmesis, and patients usually recover without surgical intervention.

There may be decreased sensation to the lateral three digits and palm, as well as decreased motor and sensory conduction. Careful initial neurologic assessment and meticulous assessment of pinch and grip strength and two-point discrimination during the early rehabilitation phase allow diagnosis of a persistent defect or progressive median nerve function deterioration. It also indicates the need for electro-myographic (EMG) evaluation and the potential advisability of nerve exploration.

Anterior Interosseous Nerve Neuropathy (Kiloh-Nevin Syndrome)

Entrapment or damage of the anterior interosseous branch of the median nerve is more frequent than injury to the main nerve. Several causes of entrapment of the anterior interosseous nerve have been described, including tendinitis of the deep head of the pronator teres origin due to repetitive heavy lifting and pressure from accessory or anomalous muscle bellies, the more frequent of which are an accessory head of the flexor pollicis longus (Ganser's muscle) and an accessory muscle from the flexor digitorum superficialis. The nerve may also be involved in scar after trauma or fracture usually as the nerve passes between the two heads of the pronator teres (Fig. 22-44). Fractures and dislocation of the radius and ulna may also precipitate injury. Infrequently, ganglia or soft tissue tumors such as lipomas compress the nerve.

The deficit is purely motor, involving the flexor pollicis longus and flexor digitorum profundus to the index and middle fingers and the pronator quadratus. The inability to carry out a tip-to-tip pinch is the diagnostic sign. Attempts at pinching paper or a card between the thumb and index finger results in pulp-to-pulp apposition (Fig. 22-45). Moreover, the pa-

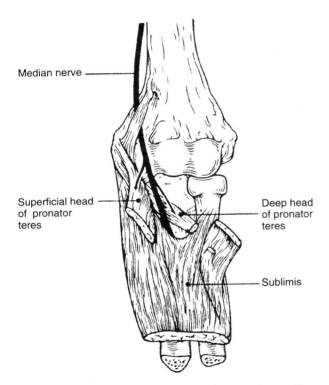

Median nerve

Superficial head
of pronator
teres

Deep head
of pronator
teres

Sublimis

Fig. 22-44. With the pronator syndrome, the median nerve may be kinked against the sublimis muscle or compressed by the forceful action or structural hypertrophy of the deep head of the pronator teres. Compression of the nerve above the elbow leads to weakness of the pronator teres, whereas this muscle is spared in the pronator syndrome as the branches to the two heads of the pronator teres arise proximal to the muscle. (From Wadsworth,[13] with permission.)

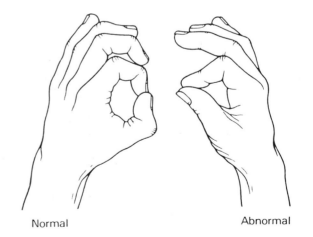

Normal

Abnormal

Fig. 22-45. Characteristic attitude of pinch in the anterior interosseous nerve compression syndrome. Tip-to-tip pinch is lost and only pulp-to-pulp is possible due to weakness of the flexor digitum profundus to the index finger and flexor pollicis longus.

tient may have some difficulty pronating with a flexed elbow. In the flexed position the functional pronator teres action is reduced by 75 percent, allowing detection of subtle weakness due to paralysis of the pronator quadratus.

When making a diagnosis it is well to remember that in 15 percent of limbs there is a Martin-Gruber type anastomosis or communication between the median and ulnar nerves. The motor fibers of the median nerve may proceed to the ulnar nerve from either the main nerve itself or the anterior interosseous branch. These neurologic malformations may cause confusion in diagnosis. Recovery spontaneously, or after surgical release is to be anticipated. Rehabilitation is directed at strengthening grip.[90]

Radial and Posterior Interosseous Nerve Neuropathy

The radial nerve is most vulnerable in the spiral groove of the humerus. Midshaft humeral fractures always jeopardize the nerve, first during the initial trauma and subsequently through callus production. Less frequently the nerve is damaged by direct blows on the lateral aspect of the distal arm as it dives into the bulk of the brachioradialis and extensor carpi radialis longus. The most common site of pathology in the forearm is at the point at which the main motor branches of the radial nerve continue as the posterior interosseous nerve (Fig. 22-46).

Posterior interosseous entrapment, or radial tunnel syndrome, is a compression neuropathy of the radial nerve from the radial head proximally to the supinator muscle distally. There are four possible sites of compression.[91-93] The first is by either a ganglion or fibrous band lying anterior to the radial head. The second is by the leash of vessels (leash of Henry) accompanying the radial recurrent artery, which lie across the radial nerve underneath the brachioradialis. The third is the tendinous margin of the extensor carpi radialis brevis. The fourth, and perhaps most frequently discussed, is the ligamentous band over the deep radial nerve (posterior interosseous branch) as it enters between the two heads of the supinator. (This area is the arcade of Frohse.[91])

This syndrome is probably relatively uncommon. During extension and pronation, the extensor carpi radialis brevis and the fibrous edge of the superficial

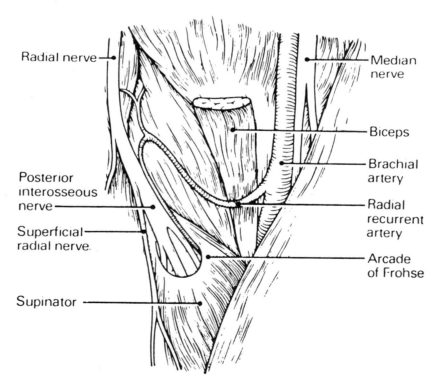

Fig. 22-46. Possible site of entrapment of the posterior interosseous nerve at the level of the arcade of Frohse.

part of supinator are seen to tighten around the nerve. This entrapment (radial tunnel syndrome) is thought to be important in the differential diagnosis of resistant tennis elbow.

In a series reported by Roles and Maudsley the clinical findings were fairly uniform.[91] At the onset the patient usually complained of the classic signs and symptoms of lateral epicondylitis, i.e., tenderness over the common extensor origin, pain on passive stretching of the extensor muscles, and pain on resisted extension of the wrist and fingers. However, maximal tenderness should be over the supinator muscle, four fingers' breadth distal to the lateral epicondyle.[92] After the usual therapies these patients are often left with pain radiating up and down the arm, weakness of grip, tenderness over the radial nerve, and pain on resisted extension of the middle finger, which tightens the fascial origin of the extensor carpi radialis brevis.[93] It has also been suggested that resisted supination is generally much more painful than resisted wrist extension owing to the contraction of the supinator muscle.[28] Nerve conduction studies should show significant delay in motor latencies measured from the spiral groove to the medial portion of extensor digitorum communis, although in most published series electrophysiologic changes are present in only about 20 percent of the cases.

Clinical Point

POSTERIOR INTEROSSEOUS NERVE ENTRAPMENT

Differentiate as a cause of tennis elbow by:

- Significant muscle belly tenderness
- Failure to relieve symptoms with lidocaine injection into common extensor origin
- Occasionally, electrophysiologic changes

In the absence of positive EMG studies, diagnostic local anesthetic blocks may be used. An injection of 1 to 2 ml of lidocaine in the common extensor origin at the lateral epicondyle should eliminate the discomfort of classic lateral epicondylitis (tennis elbow) but not that of radial nerve entrapment. Confirmation by further injection of lidocaine about four to five fingers' breadth distal to the epicondyle over the point of maximum tenderness is possible, but it usu-

ally also produces transient radial nerve palsy. Recognition of the few but significant resistant cases of tennis elbow allows prompt effective treatment by surgical release of the entrapment.

Olecranon Pathology

Pain around the olecranon is common and may be the result of olecranon bursitis, triceps tendinitis, intra-articular loose bodies, synovial pinching, or stress fractures of the olecranon[69] (Fig. 22-47). Some of these entities are considered under the heading of posterior impingement syndrome and have been discussed under the heading of lesions to the throwing arm.

Posterior Impingement Syndrome

The most common mechanism of posterior impingement syndrome is extension overload during pitching, although a similar sequence of events results from repetitive punching, the so-called boxer's elbow. Anterior traction on the coronoid process and posterior compression between the olecranon trochlea and fossa may generate synovitis, hypertrophic changes, degenerative and destructive joint changes, and even loose bodies.

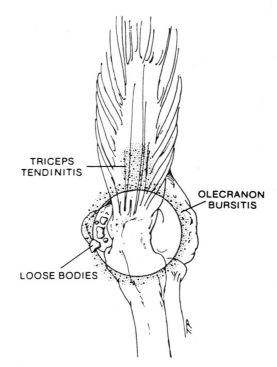

Fig. 22-47. Posterior impingement syndrome.

Depending on the pathology, the athlete may complain of sudden sharp pain at the end of rapid elbow extension, with reproducible discomfort produced by overpressure of extension during examination. The pain is usually posterior but may be difficult to localize. Untreated there is usually a gradual loss of terminal extension. If there are loose bodies, they may cause sudden pinching or locking at different points in the range, and the symptoms can be intermittent. Occasionally, it is possible to palpate loose chips.

Roentgenograms can confirm the degree of osteophyte formation, bony hypertrophy, and degenerative change. Sometimes loose bodies are easily visualized. However, if the clinical picture is highly suggestive of loose bodies and the plain films are negative, tomograms, arthrograms, or computed tomography (CT) may delineate small bony or cartilaginous fragments.

Therapy is directed at restoring range, restrengthening muscles, and gradually reintroducing the athlete to increasingly strenuous activity. NSAIDs are helpful, and occasionally an intra-articular injection of steroids is useful. When the main symptom is synovial pinching, resistant to the above treatment, an orthosis limiting full extension may allow continuation of activity until associated therapy resolves the pathology (Fig. 22-48).

When the main problem is bony impingement or loose fragments, surgical exploration is sometimes

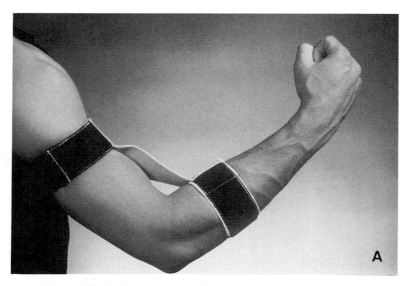

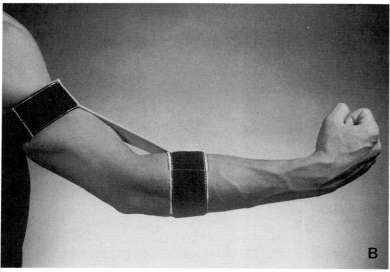

Fig. 22-48. Orthosis for limiting extension. **(A)** Full flexion possible. **(B)** Extension block. A similar effect may be achieved by taping.

the definitive treatment to retrieve the loose fragments, remove osteophytes, or débride the joint. In some situations arthroscopy has an advantage, although many individuals require a lateral arthrotomy.

Snapping Elbow

An unusual cause of triceps tendinitis is the "snapping elbow" syndrome.[81] During flexion the medial head of the triceps subluxes over the medial epicondyle, producing a snap. It usually occurs in the presence of an anomalous separated medial belly of the muscle. It may become painful, either during the snapping or more constantly with triceps work if a tendinitis results.

Treatment consists in rest, if painful, to resolve the symptoms. Ice, ultrasound, and NSAIDs may be helpful. Gradual reintegration to activity with stretching and strengthening exercises may be successful. Rarely, surgery is necessary to stabilize the subluxing head. The syndrome must be distinguished from snapping of the ulnar nerve out of its groove. Subluxation of the ulnar nerve may be seen to some degree in 16 percent of the population as the arm moves from full extension to full flexion, but it is rarely a problem.[86] A dislocating nerve however, may become irritated and painful, with distal symptoms of dysesthesia or numbness. In this situation transposition of the nerve may be considered.

It is worth mentioning that the elbow, like most joints, may produce frequent nonpainful joint sounds such as "popping" or "snapping." These noises should be ignored, for the most part, once significant pathology has been ruled out.

Triceps Tendinitis

Triceps tendinitis is seen in boxers, javelin throwers, shot-putters, pitchers, and weight lifters. In many ways the pathology may be likened to that of patellar tendinitis in "jumper's knee"; the treatment principles are the same.[7] Inflammation and microtrauma occurs at the triceps insertion to the olecranon process.

Treatment involves reducing activity to the point of eliminating symptoms. Local application of ice, ultrasound, or laser may be helpful, complemented by NSAIDs. Occasionally, in chronic situations, cross (transverse) frictional massage is indicated. Good training habits, involving adequate warm-up and cool down along with an icing routine, is stressed.

Eventual return to activity must be graduated. For throwing, a set distance, usually 30 feet, and only half speed are used. Distance and speed are progressed independently up to 60 feet with three-quarter speed, always increasing speed before distance. Eventually reintegration to full training is allowed. These principles must be extrapolated to fit the appropriate sport and situation.

Olecranon Bursitis

The olecranon bursa, lying as it does superficial to the insertion of the triceps tendon and distally over the olecranon, can be irritated by a single episode of trauma, e.g., a fall on the point of the elbow, or by repetitive grazing and weight-bearing as is often seen in wrestling. Acute bursitis may present as a swelling over the olecranon process, varying in size from slight distension to a swelling that can be the size of a small chicken egg (Fig. 22-49). Depending on the acuteness of the inflammatory reaction, there is a variable amount of heat and redness associated with this swelling.

The important diagnostic differential here is between simple post-traumatic bursitis and an infected olecranon bursa. The former may be treated with ice, elastic wrap, and various forms of well fitting protective pads and it usually, with time, disappears spontaneously. The infected bursa, however, must be brought to prompt medical attention so appropriate antibiotic therapy can be started and drainage instituted if necessary. Failure to do it may lead to spreading cellulitis and an infection that involves a large part of the forearm or upper arm. The proximity of the

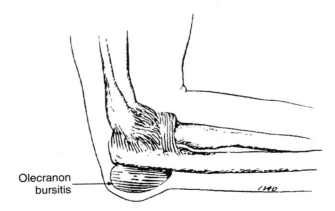

Fig. 22-49. Olecranon bursitis with typical enlargement. (From O'Donaghue DH: Treatment of Injuries to Athletes. WB Saunders, Philadelphia. With permission.)

bursa to the elbow joint makes treatment all the more urgent.

Repeated post-traumatic bursitis may lead to fibrin deposits in the bursa. These fragments may eventually metaplase into a cartilage-like material and form tiny seeds within the bursa itself. They then form a source of aggravation even with minor friction, and a perpetual painful bursitis may be established. In these instances, conservative treatment is no longer warranted, and surgical excision of the bursa should be considered.

Stress Fractures of the Olecranon

The valgus and varus overload during forceful throwing action has been dealt with under the title of pitcher's or javelin thrower's elbow. Stress fractures of the olecranon, although uncommon, must be borne in mind as part of the differential diagnosis.[94] Individuals usually experience pain in the elbow of the throwing arm for some weeks or months before the lesion is obvious on roentgenograms. The etiology is linked to the explosive forces applied to the olecranon during the final phases of delivery and perhaps impingement of the olecranon process against the base and medial wall of the olecranon fossa.[95] These injuries are disastrous for competitive athletes because if ignored they may complete themselves during a throw; and if the fracture line is sufficiently distal, dislocation may occur.

If the lesion is treated early, throwing may be resumed in 8 to 12 weeks. However, significant stress fractures or complete fractures may take up to 4 months to heal sufficiently for resumption of throwing. If internal fixation is used splinting or casting is usually not required. Excision of a proximal stress fracture of the tip of the olecranon, the most frequent site, allows resumption of throwing at 8 weeks. Fractures treated conservatively may take up to 18 months before throwing is resumed successfully if the lesion is well established.[89]

A similar lesion is a fracture-separation of the olecranon epiphysis in children, and an even more rare situation is fracture-separation of an incompletely fused olecranon physis in adults.[96] The proximal ulnar ossification center appears at age 8 years in females and age 10 in males. It usually unites with the ulnar shaft at ages 14 and 16 years, respectively. Variations exist in the size of the olecranon ossification center, varying from a small flake to up to 25 percent of the olecranon.[97] The secondary ossification center may also be bipartite. Usually the physis closes from deep to superficial, with rarely a deep posterior cleft

persisting. It is this cleft that may form the start of a stress fracture or a weakened area that may give secondary to a direct blow. The etiology is usually a direct blow from a fall, frequently in football players. These injuries are difficult to treat and may require bone grafting as well as open reduction and internal fixation, as there is a propensity to fibrous union.[96]

Tendon Avulsions and Ruptures

Triceps Tendon

Injuries involving avulsion or rupture of the triceps tendon are among the least frequent of tendon injuries, and major ruptures of the belly of the triceps are even more uncommon.[97,98] The mechanism is essentially the same for both sites, i.e., decelerating stress superimposed on the contracting triceps muscle due to a fall on the outstretched hand or to sudden contact during an extension maneuver such as a karate chop. Significant tears of the tendon must be recognized immediately, as a successful functional outcome depends on early surgical repair (Fig. 22-50). Delayed repair is possible, but it is technically more difficult and has less chance of an excellent result. Recognition is through loss of active extension, a palpable gap, pain, and a large hematoma that develops into diffuse swelling and echymosis.[99] In the case of tendon avulsion, a small fleck of olecranon is often seen on the plain roentgenogram. When there is doubt as to the diagnosis, computed tomography accurately visualizes the pathology. Muscle belly tears usually involve only the medial head, and usually nonoperative treatment results in a satisfactory outcome.[100]

It is well to recall that normal tendon must sustain considerable force before it ruptures; hence avulsion of the insertion is an expected event when the trauma is sufficient. For this reason, rupture of the substance of the tendon should lead to a search for associated pathology. Conditions such as rheumatoid arthritis, systemic lupus erythematosus, hyperparathyroidism, xanthomatous degeneration, and hemangioepithelioma, as well as use of systemic steroids and local steroid injections, may predispose to rupture of the tendon.

Biceps Tendon

Biceps ruptures at the elbow are rare. Although the injury is compatible with normal function in a relatively sedentary individual, surgical repair is probably best carried out early in the young or the active individual. Diagnosis is made by the inability to palpate

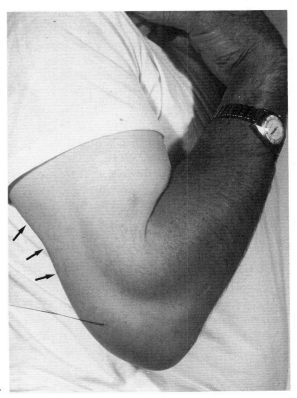

Fig. 22-50. Complete triceps rupture. **(A)** Defect in the tendon is visible. **(B)** Rupture site is filled with hematoma, visualized at surgery.

A

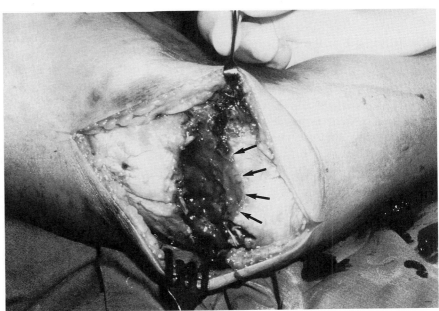

B

the tendon and the altered muscle delineation. Hemorrhage is often considerable and may obscure the diagnosis unless an adequate index of suspicion is maintained. This injury is sometimes associated with a radial head dislocation; both injuries require therapy.

Brachialis Tendon

Most tears of the brachialis tendon are partial, but infrequently isolated complete tears may occur. Dislocation of the elbow is the commonest associated injury. The major significance of brachialis rupture is the propensity to myositis ossificans or delayed instability of an associated unrecognized elbow dislocation.

Extensor or Flexor Muscle Mass

Rapid, violent contraction in association with a blow to the forearm may lead to rupture of the flexor or extensor muscle mass. Usually this injury is compatible with excellent function when treated nonoperatively. Treatment includes splinting and gentle range of motion, muscle strengthening, and functional exercises. Avulsion of the muscles from their tendons at the musculotendinous junction should be repaired operatively, and these injuries are usually associated with an excellent surgical outcome. Early mobilization and therapy are the keys to success.

Systemic Conditions

Systemic conditions are mentioned only to emphasize the need for constant awareness of the broad differential diagnosis of elbow pain. Treatment is not outlined.

Mainly Monoarticular Conditions

Osteoarthrosis

Osteoarthrosis of the elbow may be the result of repeated minor trauma in such occupations as mining and working with compressed air hammers and with recreation and sports that involve repetitive throwing. Mild osteoarthritis may be relatively painless, although it may be accompanied by loss of extension and occasionally ulnar nerve symptoms.

Chrondromatosis

The elbow is a site of predilection for synovial chondromatosis (synovial chondrometaplasia) along with the knee and shoulder. The presentation may be pain, limitation of motion, or more often catching and locking. Synovectomy may be necessary to restore function to the joint.

Pigmented Villinodular Synovitis

Pigmented villinodular synovitis is an uncommon disease of synovium that occurs primarily at the knee. The elbow and ankle are the next most frequently involved joints. Repeated hemarthrosis may be the presenting sign. Treatment involves synovectomy

with persistent physiotherapy postoperatively if joint range is to be maintained.[69]

Diseases of the Blood and Arthropathies

The elbow is probably the second most frequently involved joint in hemophiliacs, second only to the knees.[100] Repeated joint bleeds may destroy the synovium and joint surface. Normal growth is disturbed; marginal overgrowth of the radial head, early loss of joint range, deformity, and sometimes ankylosis are possible sequelae of the disease.[100] Similarly, though less commonly, the elbow may be involved in hemoglobinopathies such as sickle cell anemia and thalassemia. In contrast to most elbow pathology, contractures due to severe, advanced hemophilia may respond to prolonged stretching techniques using slings and pulleys or spring-loaded splints. For these specialized techniques, the reader is referred to the classic articles by Duthie et al. and Dickson.[101,102]

Mainly Polyarticular Conditions

Rheumatoid Arthritis

In only about 3 percent of cases does rheumatoid arthritis present for the first time with elbow symptoms. However, after 3 years of the disease, almost 50 percent have elbow involvement, and this percentage increases with time. These prevalence figures are also probably accurate for juvenile chronic arthritis as well. About 20 percent of rheumatoid patients have rheumatoid nodules, which classically develop on the extensor surface of the olecranon and proximal ulna. Nodules in association with seropositive disease often indicate a poor clinical course.[97,103] The adult disease is characterized by severe painful synovitis and ultimately much joint destruction whereas bony ankylosis is more common in children with juvenile chronic arthritis.

Seronegative Arthropathies

The seronegative arthropathies include ankylosing spondylitis, Reiter's syndrome, and the reactive arthropathies. In this seronegative group also are the arthropathies that complicate Crohn's disease and ulcerative colitis, Bechçet's syndrome, and Whipple's disease. Generally, the elbow is involved only in patients in whom the disease is widespread and chronic; and usually only one side is affected. The exception is the destructive psoriatic arthropathy in which both elbows are frequently involved.[103]

Gout

It is rare for gout to present initially with elbow involvement; but with severe gout, almost one-third of individuals eventually have involvement of the joint. The extensor surface of the forearm and olecranon are the commonest sites of gouty tophi.

Chondrocalcinosis

Chondrocalcinosis is a roentgenographic diagnosis based on visualization of calcification in the joint capsule or cartilage. Chondrocalcinosis of the elbow joint is frequently indicative of hyperparathyroidism, but it may be seen with ochronosis, hemochromatosis, gout, and Wilson's disease. Elbow involvement is seen in approximately one-third of patients with calcium pyrophosphate deposition disease (pseudogout), where the deposit is often in the capsule.

Tumors and Infections

Neoplasms around the elbow are rare with both primary and metastatic disease. Nevertheless, it is an important consideration in situations where the pain and swelling do not resolve in response to normal treatment regimens and the radiologic appearance is abnormal. Similarly, although infection is rare, local extension of infection due to intravenous therapy may involve the elbow.

CONCLUSIONS

A superficial discussion of the elbow joint underestimates the complexity of the anatomy. Arising out of the subtle biomechanics, the proximity of muscle belly attachments, and multiple articulation is the propensity for loss of range and myositis ossificans. Furthermore, loss of function at this joint seriously impairs the versatility of the hand and compromises the useful range of the whole upper limb segment because, unlike the shoulder, wrist, and fingers, little compensatory adjustments are possible. For this reason, early diagnosis and careful, well planned, meticulous therapy is essential to successful treatment. Failure to pick up subtleties of diagnosis or a changing pathologic state and the institution of mistimed or inappropriate therapy have the potential to result in permanent significant disability. The exclusion of C5, C6, and C7 pathology must always be kept in mind with elbow pain syndromes.

The late appearance of multiple secondary ossification centers around the elbow adds to the difficulty of detecting fractures and assessing the magnitude of displacement. Bilateral roentgenograms are mandatory with trauma in the growing individual. Furthermore, the frequent association of supracondylar fractures and elbow dislocation with catastrophic neurovascular impairment provides an indication for admission to hospital, at least overnight, and is prudent with many of these injuries. Lastly, the frequent involvement of the elbow with systemic collagen diseases should alert the physician to an early diagnosis, particularly when symptoms are bilateral.

REFERENCES

1. Reid DC: Assessment and Treatment of the Injured Athlete. University of Alberta Press, Edmonton, 1985
2. Reid DC, Kushner S: The elbow region. In Donatelli R, Wooden MJ (ed): Orthopaedic Physical Therapy. Churchill Livingstone, New York, 1989
3. Reid DC: Functional Anatomy and Joint Mobilization. 2nd Ed. University of Alberta Press, Edmonton, 1975
4. Thompson HC, Garcia A: Myositis ossificans: aftermath of elbow injuries. Clin Orthop 50:129, 1967
5. Kapandji IA: The Physiology of the Joints. 5th Ed. Vol. 1. Churchill Livingstone, Edinburgh, 1982
6. Morrey BF, Kai-Nan A: Articular and ligamentous contributions to the stability of the elbow joint. Am J Sports Med 11:315, 1983
7. Magee DJ: Orthopaedic Physical Assessment. WB Saunders, Toronto, 1987
8. Van Mameren H, Drukker J: A functional anatomical basis of injuries to the ligamentous and other soft tissues around the elbow joint: transmission of tensile and compressive loads. Int J Sports Med, suppl. 5:88, 1984
9. MacConaill MA: A structurofunctional classification of articular units. Ir J Med Sci 142:19, 1973
10. MacConaill MA: Arthrology. In Warwick R, Williams PL (eds): Gray's Anatomy. 35th Ed. WB Saunders, Philadelphia, 1975
11. Maitland G: Peripheral Manipulation. 2nd Ed. Butterworth, Boston, 1977
12. Kaltenborn F: Mobilization of the Extremity Joints. 3rd Ed. Olaf Norlis Bokhandel, Oslo, 1980
13. Wadsworth TG: The Elbow. Churchill Livingstone, New York, 1982
14. Schwab G, Bennett, J, Woods G et al: Biomechanics of elbow instability; the role of the medial collateral ligament. Clin Orthop 146:42, 1980
15. Gutieriez L: A contribution to the study of limiting

factors of elbow extension. Acta Anat (Basel) 56:145, 1964

16. Schuit D, McPoil TG, Knecht HG: Effect of tightened anterior band of the ulnar collateral ligament on arthrokinematics at the humeroulnar joint. J Orthop Sports Phys Ther 8:123, 1986

17. Cummings GS: Comparison of muscle to other soft tissue in limiting elbow extension. J Orthop Sports Phys Ther 5:170, 1984

18. Jobe FW, Nuber G: Throwing injuries of the elbow. p. 621. In McCue FC (ed): Clinics in Sports Medicine. Vol. 5. No. 4. WB Saunders, Philadelphia, 1986

19. Basmajian JV: Muscles Alive: Their Function Revealed by Electromyography. 2nd Ed. Williams & Wilkins, Baltimore, 1967

20. Pauly JE, Rushing JL, Schering LE: An electromyographic study of some muscles crossing the elbow joint. Anat Rec 1:42, 1967

21. Rasch PI: Effect of position of the forearm on strength of elbow flexion. Res Q 27:333, 1956

22. Runge F: Zur genese und behandlung des schreibekrampfes.`Berl Lin Wochenschr 10:245, 1973

23. Morris H: The Rider's sprain. Lancet 133:29, 1882

24. Nirschl RP: The etiology and treatment of tennis elbow. Am J Sports Med 2:308, 1974

25. Kamien M: A rational management of tennis elbow. Sports Med 9:173, 1990

26. Briggs CA, Elliott BG: Lateral epicondylitis: a review of structures associated with tennis elbow. Anat Clin 7:149, 1985

27. Berahang AM: The many causes of tennis elbow. NY State J Med 79:1363, 1979

28. Regan WD: Lateral elbow pain in the athlete: a clinical review. Clin J Sports Med 1:53, 1991

29. Van Swearingen JM: Measuring wrist muscle strength. J Orthop Sports Phys Ther 4:217, 1983

30. Leach RE, Miller JK: Lateral and medial epicondylitis of the elbow. Clin Sports Med 6:259, 1987

31. Nirschl RP: Soft tissue injuries about the elbow. Clin Sports Med 5:637, 1986

32. Calvert PT, Allum RL, Macpherson IS et al: Simple lateral release in treatment of tennis elbow. J R Soc Med 78:912, 1985

33. Nirschl RP, Pettrone FA: Tennis elbow: the surgical treatment of lateral epicondylitis. J Bone Joint Surg [Am] 61:832, 1979

34. Liu YK: Mechanical analysis of racquet and ball during impact. Med Sci Sports Exer 15:388, 1983

35. Legwold G: Tennis elbow: joint resolution by conservative treatment and improved technique. Physician Sports Med 12:168, 1984

36. Elliot BC: Tennis: the influence of grip tightness on reaction impulse and rebound velocity. Med Sci Sports Exerc 14:348, 1982

37. Kuland DN, McCue FC, Rockwell DA et al: Tennis injuries: prevention and treatment—a review. Am J Sports Med 7:249, 1979

38. Froimson AI: Treatment of tennis elbow with forearm support band. J Bone Joint Surg [Am] 53a:183, 1971

39. Groppel JL, Nirschl RP: A mechanical and electromyographical analysis of the effects of various joint counterforce braces on the tennis player. Am J Sports Med 14:195, 1986

40. Burton AK: Grip strength and forearm straps in tennis elbow. Br J Sports Med 19:37, 1985

41. Burton AK, Edwards VA: Electromyography and tennis elbow straps. Br Osteopath J 14:83, 1982

42. Priest JD, Braden V, Gerberlich SG: The elbow and tennis. Part 2. A study of players with pain. Physician Sports Med 8:77, 1980

43. Halle JS, Franklin RJ, Karalfa BL: Comparison of four treatment approaches for lateral epicondylitis of the elbow. J Orthop Sports Phys Ther 8:62, 1986

44. Percy EC, Carson JD: The use of DMSO in tennis elbow and rotator cuff tendinitis: a double blind study. Med Sci Sports Exerc 13:215, 1981

45. Burton K: Grip strength as an objective clinical assessment in tennis elbow. Br Osteopath J 16:6, 1984

46. Cyriax J: Textbook of Orthopaedic Medicine. Diagnosis of Soft Tissue Lesions. 5th Ed. Vol. 1. Williams & Wilkins, Baltimore, 1970

47. Kushner S. Reid DC: Manipulation in the treatment of tennis elbow. J Orthop Sports Phys Ther 7:264, 1986

48. Mills GP: Treatment of tennis elbow. Br Med J 2:212, 1937

49. Kaltenborn FM: Manual Therapy for the Extremity Joints. 2nd Ed. Olaf Noris Bokhandel, Oslo, 1976

50. Mennell JM: Joint Pain—Diagnosis and Treatment Using Manipulative Techniques. Little, Brown, Boston, 1964

51. Stoddard A: Manipulation of the elbow joint. Physiotherapy 57:259, 1971

52. Curwin S. Stanish WD: Tendinitis: Its Etiology and Treatment. Collamore Press, Lexington, MA, 1984

53. Dilorenzo CE, Parkes JC, Chmelar RD: The importance of shoulder and cervical dysfunction in the etiology and treatment of athlete elbow injuries. J Orthop Sports Phys Ther 11:402, 1990

54. Conrad RW, Hopper WR: Tennis elbow, its course, natural history, conservative and surgical management. J Bone Joint Surg [Am] 53a:117, 1973

55. Boyd HB, McLeod AC: Tennis elbow. J Bone Joint Surg [Am] 55a:1183, 1973

56. Posch JN, Goldberg VM, Larrey R: Extensor fasciotomy for tennis elbow: a long term follow-up study. Clin Orthop 135:179, 1978

57. Cameron HU, Proctor M, Fornaiser VL: Tennis elbow. Can Family Physician 29:2177, 1983

58. Yerger B, Turner T: Percutaneous extensor tenotomy for chronic tennis elbow: an office procedure. Orthopade 8:1261, 1985

59. Goldberg EJ, Abraham E, Siegel I: The surgical treatment of lateral humeral epicondylitis by common extensor release. Clin Orthop 233:208, 1988

60. Cabrera JM, McCue FC: Non-osseous athletic injuries of the elbow, forearm and hand. Clin Sports Med 5:681, 1986

61. Woods GW, Tullos HS, King JW: The throwing arm: elbow injuries. J Sports Med 1:43, 1973

62. Slocum DB: Classification of the elbow injuries from baseball pitching. Tex Med 64:48, 1968

63. Wilson FD, Andrews JR, Blackburn TA et al: Valgus extension overload in the pitching elbow. Am J Sports Med 11:83, 1983

64. Russotti GM, Cooney WP: Throwing injuries in baseball pitchers: a review. Adv Orthop Surg 10:247, 1987

65. Albright JA, Jokl P, Shaw R et al: Clinical study of baseball pitchers: correlation of injury to the throwing arm with method of delivery. Am J Sports Med 6:15, 1987

66. Indelicato PA, Jobe FW, Kerlan RK et al: Correctable elbow lesions in professional baseball players: a review of 25 cases. Am J Sports Med 7:72, 1979

67. Torg JS, Pollack H. Sweeterlitsch P: The effect of competitive pitching on the shoulder and elbows of preadolescent baseball players. Pediatrics 49:267, 1972

68. Grana WA, Rashkin A: Pitcher's elbow in adolescents. Am J Sports Med 8:333, 1980

69. Bennett JB, Tullos HS: Acute injuries to the elbow. In Nicholas JA, Hershman EB (ed): The Upper Extremity in Sports Medicine. CV Mosby, St. Louis, 1990

70. Grenier R, Rouleau C: Boxer's elbow: an extension and hyperextension injury. Am J Sports Med 3:282, 1976

71. Adams JE: Injuries to the throwing arm—a study of traumatic changes in the elbow joints of boy baseball pitchers. Calif Med 102:127, 1965

72. DeHaven KE, Everts CM: Throwing injuries of the elbow in athletes. Orthop Clin North Am 4:801, 1973

73. Singer KM, Roy SP: Osteochondrosis of the humeral capitellum. Am J Sports Med 12:351, 1984

74. Pappas AM: Osteochondrosis dissecans. Clin Orthop 158:59, 1981

75. Roy S, Irvin R: Sports Medicine Prevention Evaluation, Management and Rehabilitation. Prentice-Hall, Englewood Cliffs, NJ, 1983

76. Panner JH: A peculiar affection of the capitellum humeri resembling Calve-Perthes' disease of the hip. Acta Radiol (Stockh) 10:234, 1929

77. Haraldsson S: On osteochondrosis deformans juvinelis capituli including investigation of intraosseous vasculature in distal humerus. Acta Orthop Scand 38; [Suppl], 1959

78. Lindholm TS, Osterman K, Vankka E: Osteochondritis dissecans of the elbow, ankle and hip: a comparative study. Clin Orthop 148:245, 1980

79. McManama GB, Micheli LT, Berry MV et al: The surgical treatment of osteochondritis of the capitellum. Am J Sports Med 13:11, 1985

80. Norwood LA, Shook JA, Andrews JR: Acute medial elbow ruptures. Am J Sports Med 9:16, 1981

81. Dreyfuss U, Kessler I: Snapping elbow due to dislocation of the medial head of triceps. J Bone Joint Surg [Br] 60B:56, 1978

82. Rockward CA, Green DP: Fractures. JB Lippincott, Toronto, 1975

83. Rang M: Children's Fractures. JB Lippincott, Philadelphia, 1974

84. Dangles CJ, Bibs JZ: Ulnar nerve neuritis in a world champion weightlifter. Am J Sports Med 8:443, 1980

85. Feindel W, Stratford J: The role of the cubital tunnel in tardy ulnar palsy. Can J Surg 1:287, 1958

86. Wojtys EM, Smith PA, Hankin FM: A cause of neuropathy in a baseball pitcher. Am J Sports Med 14:422, 1986

87. Broudy A, Leffert R, Smith R: Technical problems with ulnar nerve transposition at the elbow: findings and results of re-operation. J Hand Surg 3:85, 1978

88. Neblett C, Elini G: Medial epicondylectomy for ulnar nerve palsy. J Neurosurg 32:55, 1970

89. Rappaport NH, Clark GL, Bara WF: Medial nerve entrapment about the elbow. Adv Orthop Surg 9:270, 1985

90. Van Der Wuff P, Hagmeyer RH, Rijnders W: Case study: isolated anterior interosseous nerve paralysis: the Kilohnevin syndrome. J Orthop Sports Phys Ther 6:178, 1984

91. Roles NC, Maudsley RH; Radial tunnel syndrome. J Bone Joint Surg. [Br] 54b:499, 1972

92. Regan WD: Lateral elbow pain in the athlete: a clinical review. Clin J Sports Med 1:53, 1991

93. Spinner M: The arcade of Frohse and its relationship to posterior interosseous nerve paralysis. J Bone Joint Surg [Br] 50:809, 1968

94. Hulkko A, Orava S, Nikula P: Stress fractures of the olecranon in javelin throwers. Int J Sports Med 7:210, 1968

95. London JT: Kinematics of the elbow. J Bone Joint Surg [Am] 63a:529, 1981

96. Kovac J, Baker BE, Mosher JF: Fracture separation

of the olecranon ossification centre in adults. Am J Sports Med 13:105, 1985

97. Kohler A: Roentgenology: The Borderlands of the Normal and Early Pathology in the Skeleton. William Wood, New York, 1928

98. Kunichi A, Torisu T: Muscle belly tear of the triceps. Am J Sports Med 12:485, 1984

99. Sherman O, Snyder ST, Fox JM: Triceps tendon avulsion in a professional body builder. Am J Sports Med 12:328, 1984

100. Bach BR, Warren RF, Wickiewicz TL: Triceps rupture — a case report and literature review. Am J Sports Med 15:285, 1987

101. Duthie RB, Matthews JM, Rizza CR et al: The management of musculoskeletal problems in hemophiliacs. Blackwell Scientific Publications, Oxford, 1972

102. Dickson RA: Reversed dynamic slings — a new concept in the treatment of post-traumatic elbow flexion contractures. Injury 8:35, 1976

103. Rodnan GP (ed): Primer on the Rheumatic Disease. 7th Ed. Reprinted from JAMA, Suppl. 224:5, 1973

Forearm, Wrist, and Hand

23

*Errors of judgement must occur in the practice of an art
which consists largely in balancing probabilities.*
—*William Ostler, 1984*

The forearm, wrist, and hand are vulnerable in many sports, and protective equipment is somewhat difficult to design in view of the requirements for speed of movement and dexterity. The ball in cricket, basketball, baseball, and volleyball is a formidable missile, capable of directly contusing the hand or even fracturing or dislocating the digits. In rugby, boxing, martial arts, football, and hockey the hand and forearm often form the initial point of contact or collision, adding to its vulnerability. In reality the relatively low incidence of hand injuries is surprising and attests to the strength and flexibility of this segment of the upper limb. Nevertheless, activities with a particularly high incidence of hand trauma show some interesting features. For example, with skiing, 60 percent of upper limb injuries are to the thumb and usually the direct result of leverage across the handle of the ski-pole. In hockey, 80 percent of hand injuries are the result of infringement of the rules, i.e., slashing or fighting, when the gloves are discarded.[1] In wheelchair sports, blisters and abrasions comprise more than 80 percent of the total injuries, and protective handwear is primitive and frequently ineffective.[2] Furthermore, most of the nerve injuries involving the wrist and hand are due to poor training techniques or inadequate adaptation of equipment, e.g., ulnar nerve entrapment in road racing cyclists.[3]

Despite the obvious importance of the subtle control and sensitivity of the hand in so many occupations and activities of daily living, hand injuries are frequently underdiagnosed and inadequately treated. Indeed there is a tendency to shrug off a major injury to the finger as inconsequential and treat it with abuse and neglect. This situation has given rise to the eponym "coaches' fingers," which is applied to the

sequel of stiffness, pain, and deformity following dislocation or intra-articular fractures in football, basketball, and volleyball players.

Thus we see a spectrum of largely preventable injuries, frequently underdiagnosed and all too often neglected, that ultimately may have significant impact on hand function. This chapter serves as a guide, as well as a warning, emphasizing diagnostic clues to severity and indicating where referral to a more experienced practitioner is the safe and sensible course of action. Lastly, this book is not devoted to all the nuances of fracture care, and mere guidelines are suggested. Further details should be obtained from more definitive texts.[4,5]

ANATOMY

Specialization is the differentiation of an organ or part for a special function. According to this definition, the human hand is not a specialized unit. In fact, it is a generalized organ, one of the most generalized in the primates. The human hand has lost virtually nothing in its development from that of its most primitive ancestors. It has kept the five-digit arrangement of the first tetrapods and, except for the thumb, the mammalian three segments to each finger[3] (Fig. 23-1).

Evolution has just modified, broadened, and refined the anatomy for the flexibility, movement, and delicacy of grasp that is so characteristic of the human hand. These movements are made possible by such features as rotation of the radius on the ulna, the development of flat nails instead of claws, the ability to oppose the thumb to the other fingers, and the

BONES   JOINTS

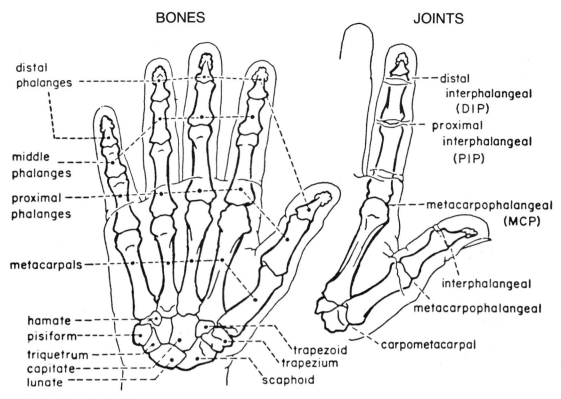

Fig. 23-1. Correlation between cutaneous landmarks and underlining bones and joints. (After Burton et al.,[23] with permission.)

increasing flexibility of the digits, which makes them capable of independent movement.

All primates have prehensile hands. That is, they have the ability to enclose an object by grasping movements in which the thumb or some other digit is opposed to the remaining digits. Only in humans, however, do we have the precise movements needed for such activities as surgery or putting the spin on a fastball. Although there is a tendency to concentrate on the hand, precision evolved through the development of the voluntary control of each digit by the brain. The increase in manual dexterity and eye to hand coordination has required enlargement of the motor cortex and cerebellum. Manual dexterity, then, is the result of elaboration of the central nervous system, not just specialization of the hand.[4–6]

Wrist

Joints of the Wrist

The apparently simple movements of flexion, extension, and radial and ulnar deviation at the wrist are in fact complex movements. The joints involved are the radiocarpal, midcarpal, and intercarpal joints. The middle finger, the third metacarpal, and the capitate are the axial bones of the hand (Fig. 23-2). The ligaments tend to absorb stress and condense forces toward the large central capitate.[7] The midcarpal joint tends to act mainly as a hinge joint, allowing flexion and extension; however, there are many small joint play movements taking place in radial and ulnar deviation that are necessary for full range.

Movements of the Wrist and Intercarpal Joints

Flexion and Extension

The movements of flexion and extension occur at the radiocarpal and midcarpal joints, flexion occurring mainly at the midcarpal joint and extension at the radiocarpal joint (Table 23-1). The limitation of both flexion and extension is mainly due to tension in the antagonistic muscle group, and the close-packed position for the wrist joint is that of full extension.

The synergic action of the wrist flexor and extensor groups in functional activities have been well docu-

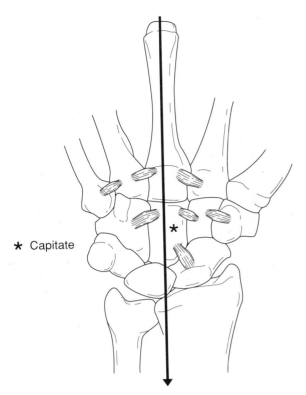

* Capitate

Fig. 23-2. Direction of the intraosseous ligaments tends to condense stresses and forces through the centrally located capitate. (Adapted from MacConnaill and Basmajian,[5] with permission.)

mented, but the large variation among people makes a detailed account of individual and group muscle action impractical.[7,8] The position of function is extension of the wrist joint, although the range from 30 degrees of extension through to the neutral position still allows full strength of pinch and grasp. Standard tests of dexterity, e.g., eating, writing, and hair combing, can be accomplished well in this range. By contrast, if the wrist is fixed in as little as 15 degrees of flexion, all of the above mentioned movements and many functional grips in sport are impaired. This fact has obvious implications for casting and immobilization.

Ulnar Deviation (Adduction)

There is a much greater range of ulnar than radial deviation owing to shortness of the ulnar styloid process. Most of the movement occurs at the radiocarpal joint. The lunate moves entirely onto the radius, and the triquetrum comes into contact with the articular disc.

TABLE 23-1. Major Muscles Producing Wrist Motion

Movement	Muscles	Peripheral Nerve	Cord Segment
Flexion (mainly at midcarpal joint)	Flexor carpi radialis	Median nerve	C6,C7
	Flexor carpi ulnaris	Ulnar nerve	C7,C8,T1
	Palmaris longus	Median nerve	C7,C8,T1
	Flexor digitorum superficialis	Median nerve	C7,C8,T1
	Flexor digitorum profundus	Median nerve and ulnar nerve	C7,C8,T1
Extension (mainly at radiocarpal joint)	Extensor carpi radialis longus	Radial nerve	C6,C7
	Extensor carpi radialis brevis	Post. interosseous branch	C6,C7
	Extensor carpi ulnaris	Post. interosseous branch	C6,C7,C8
	Extensor digitorum	Post. interosseous branch	C6,C7,C8
Adductors (ulna deviation)	Flexor carpi ulnaris	Ulnar nerve	C7,C8,T1
	Extensor carpi ulnaris	Post. interosseous branch. of radial nerve	C6,C7,C8
Abductors (radial deviation)	Extensor carpi radialis longus	Radial nerve	C6,C7
	Flexor carpi radialis	Median nerve	C6,C7
	Extensor pollicis brevis	Post. interosseous branch. of radial nerve	C6,C7
	Abductor pollicis longus	Post. interosseous branch. of radial nerve	C6,C7

Quick Facts

WRIST RADIAL AND ULNAR DEVIATION

- Depends on position of elbow
- Radial deviation 20 degrees (15 to 30 degrees)
- Ulnar deviation 30 degrees (30 to 50 degrees)
- Axis of movement arbitrarily designated as center of radiocarpal joint line.

Radial Deviation (Abduction)

Radial deviation occurs almost entirely at the midcarpal joint. The capitate rotates around a horizontal axis, so the head moves medially. As a result, the distance between lunate and hamate is greatly increased.

Metacarpals and Phalanges

Movement of the Metacarpals

The metacarpals articulate with the carpals proximally and the phalanges distally, where they are anchored by the tough intermetacarpal ligaments. The arrangement is such that the lateral side of the palm is kept mobile, allowing adaptation to all surfaces when gripping and more efficient opposition of the thumb to the fifth finger during fine movements.[9,10] The second and third metacarpals are relatively restricted and thus form an efficient post for the thumb to work against.

Movement of the Fingers

The metacarpophalangeal (MCP) joints are condyloid biaxial synovial joints that allow the important movements of abduction and adduction as well as flexion and extension. The interphalangeal joints permit only flexion and extension.[11]

It is essential to realize that in all of these joints of the functional unit we refer to as the hand there is considerable "joint play," which is necessary for full normal range. Moreover, because these joints are synovial, they are vulnerable to a great deal of pathology.

The flexor tendons continually rub the anterior aspects of their respective MCP joints, so the capsule becomes locally thickened to form a strong, dense collagen plate referred to as the palmar plate or palmar ligament (Fig. 23-3). Each palmar plate is firmly attached to the anterior edge of the base of its respective phalanx, whereas its attachment to the metacar-

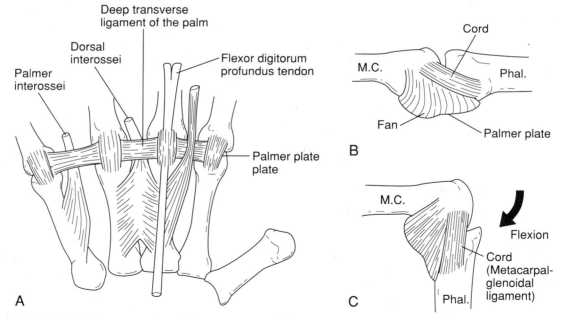

Fig. 23-3. (A) Palmar aspect of the metacarpophalangeal (MCP) joint showing the relation to the deep transverse ligaments, palmar plate, lumbrical muscles, and palmar and dorsal interossei. **(B)** Extension. Collateral MCP ligaments and condensation of the palmar capsule. It makes up the palmar plate. **(C)** Note how the cord part of the collateral ligament becomes taut as the joint goes into its closely packed position of flexion.

pal head is loose. In consequence, it tends to move with the phalanx.

The side of each plate is attached to its neighbor by a square ligament known as the deep transverse ligament of the palm (intermetacarpal ligament). The tautness of the MCP ligaments make abduction and adduction impossible in flexion, and yet their laxity in extension permits free movement.[12] Flexion of the MCP joints, then, is the close-packed position. In fact, part of the function of the MCP collateral ligaments is to guide or bring the fingers together to make a fist, as they gradually become taut[13] (Fig. 23-4). This arrangement ensures that the joints are well supported when they are being maximally stressed.

Muscle Action During Finger Movement

Extensor digitorum, flexor digitorum profundus, and flexor digitorum superficialis, as well as the long flexors and extensors of the thumb add considerable power to the hand.[14] In most cases they act as prime movers; however, there are many fine adjustments and isolated movements they alone cannot perform. These movements are made possible by the intrinsic muscles of the hand, i.e., the muscles of the thenar and hypothenar eminence, the lumbricals, and the interossei.

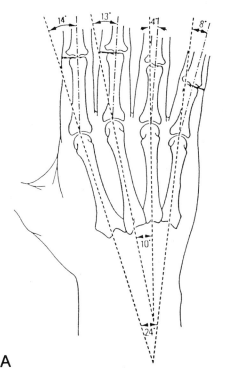

A

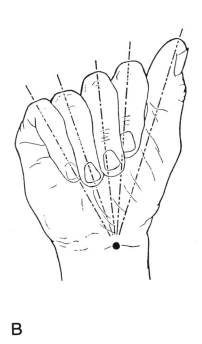

B

Fig. 23-4. (A) Normal alignment with the fingers in extension. The loose packed position allows abduction and adduction, increasing the versatility of the grip. The digits are in relative ulnar deviation to the long axis of the metacarpals. **(B)** As the fingers flex to the palm, only the index flexes toward the median axis; the other MCP and interphalangeal joints converge toward the scaphoid tubercle. The gradual tightening of the ligaments into the close packed position help guide this motion. This economic arrangement for gripping may easily be disturbed by the malrotation of fractures. (After Tubiana,[13] with permission.)

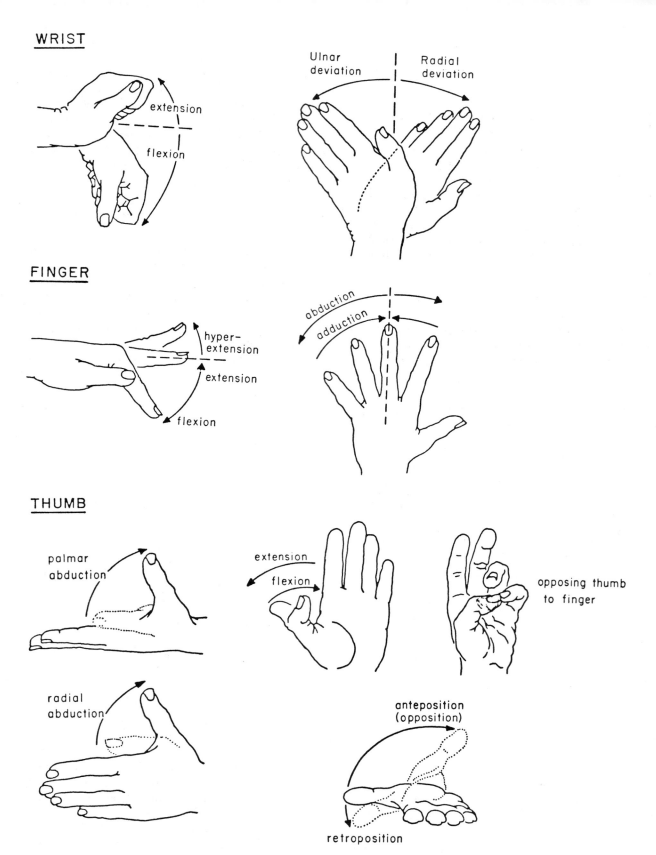

Fig. 23-5. Terminology of hand and digit motions. (After Burton et al.,[23] with permission.)

The extrinsic musculature serves with little assistance to provide the gross motion of opening and closing of all the joints of the hand simultaneously, but for any goal-oriented function the intrinsics are immediately called into play. The extensor digitorum is the sole extensor of the MCP joint.[15-17]

The flexor digitorum profundus and flexor digitorum superficialis are composed of separate bundles of fibers that may be used to activate the long flexor tendons of the four fingers individually. In addition, the ulnar and median nerves innervate the respective lumbricals, which are attached to the appropriate long flexor tendons they supply.[18] Intricate movements of the hand depend on learning these individual adjustments. The extensor digitorum is unable to move the fingers individually to the same degree because of the fibrous bands that interconnect the extensor tendons on the back of the hand. The ring finger is especially limited; however, the index and little fingers are provided with their own small extensor muscles: the extensor indicis and extensor digiti minimi, respectively. This knowledge is used when clinically testing tendon integrity.[19,20]

To summarize, at any instance, the balance between intrinsic and extrinsic muscles depends not on the position of the several joints involved but on their direction of movement. The palmar interossei and lumbricals act as MCP joint flexors only when their other action of extending the interphalangeal joint does not conflict with the intended action of the extrinsic musculature.

Thumb Movements

Opposition of the thumb to the fingers is a unique movement in which the opponens pollicis is the key muscle. Although it is aided by the adductor and flexor pollicis brevis, true opposition is absent with paralysis of the opponens.[21,22] By definition, opposition is a movement that takes place at the carpometacarpal joint of the thumb; however, with nearly all functional activities, opposition is accompanied by varying degrees of flexion at the MCP and interphalangeal joints (Fig. 23-5).

The muscles of the thumb function so similarly in many activities that they are difficult to distinguish

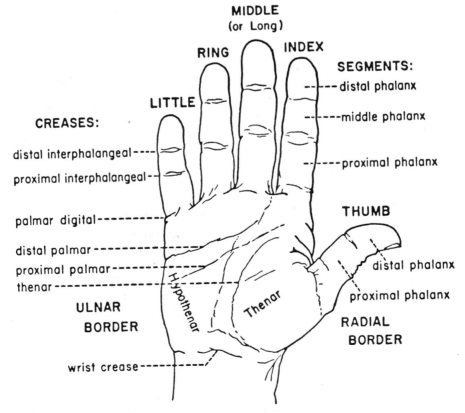

Fig. 23-6. Standard terminology of the fingers and cutaneous creases. (After Burton et al., with permission.)

electromyographically. For many motions, muscles that might not be expected to function show definite activity, presumably acting to stabilize and adjust the movement. A good example is the strong activity of the abductor pollicis brevis throughout opposition as well as during abduction.[21,22]

Terminology relating to movements of the thumb suffer the same unfortunate confusion as other areas of the body. For the sake of classification, some of these terms are explained (Fig. 23-5).

Slight adjustments of the position of the thumb make possible the variety of movements needed for the various grips. Insurance companies estimate the value of the thumb as half that of the whole hand. Because of this large contribution, the traumatic loss of a thumb function has serious consequences.

Grips

Perhaps it would be as well at this point to mention that the misuse of and changes in anatomic nomenclature have been a source of constant confusion to both student and expert alike. The latest revisions and standardizations by the American Academy of Orthopedic Surgeons suggests that the digits be named from the radial side and referred to as the pollex or thumb, index finger, long or middle finger, ring finger, and little or baby finger[23] (Fig. 23-6).

Although the prehensile functions of the hand are discussed in detail, it should be realized that there are a multitude of everyday and sporting functions during which the hand is used as a shovel or probe and during which there is no prehensile motion. Here the object is pushed or lifted, but no seizing is involved. These grips are used for functional testing during hand assessment after injury and during recovery.[3] Napier defined two basic grips: the power grip and the prehension grip[6] (Fig. 23-7).

Power Grip

The power grip is achieved by flexion of the fingers with marked ulnar deviation and rotation. This action brings the fingers into apposition with the thenar eminence. The thumb then wraps around the object or, if the object is small, around the adjacent fingers. Synergic wrist extension is an obvious accompaniment.

The power and prehension grips can be further subdivided into hook, cylindrical, fist, and spherical grasps.

Hook Grasp

With the hook grasp the fingers are used as a hook, as when carrying a dumbbell or a briefcase. The thumb is not necessarily active. The hook grasp may involve only the interphalangeal joints or the MCP joints, depending on the weight of the object being handled. This grasp requires relatively little muscular effort and is employed when precision requirements are minimum and when power must be exerted continuously for a long period (Fig. 23-7).

Fist and Cylindrical Grasp

For the fist grasp the fist closes over a comparatively narrow object, and the grip is secured by the thumb over the other digits, as when grasping a hockey stick or a golf club. When used to secure a larger object it may be referred to as a cylindrical grip. It allows maximum use of the palmar gutter to enhance control of the object being held. As a simple closed fist it is used for punching.

Spherical Grasp

For the spherical grasp the grasp is adjusted to the size of the object, e.g., a ball, by utilizing the mobility of the medial side of the palm and the spread of the fingers.

Prehension Precision Grips

Precision grips involve pad-to-pad contact between the thumb and fingers. The thumb opposes the fingers, which are actively flexed, rotated, and ulnar-deviated at the MCP joint. These precision grips include tip-to-tip, pulp-to-pulp, lateral prehension, and some variations that add versatility to the hand.

Palmar Prehension (Palmar Pinch)

The pulp-to-pulp, or palmar pinch is the one most frequently used because it allows fine precision handling and brings the most sensitive parts of the fingers in contact with the object. Thumb opposition makes it possible. Frequently, pulp-to-pulp contact is used as a chuck, involving the thumb and index and middle fingers (Fig. 23-7).

Lateral Prehension (Key Pinch)

A wide object, e.g., a card, is grasped between the thumb and the lateral side of the index finger. This side-to-side pinch does not require thumb opposition. It is used in some cases of paralysis or weakness

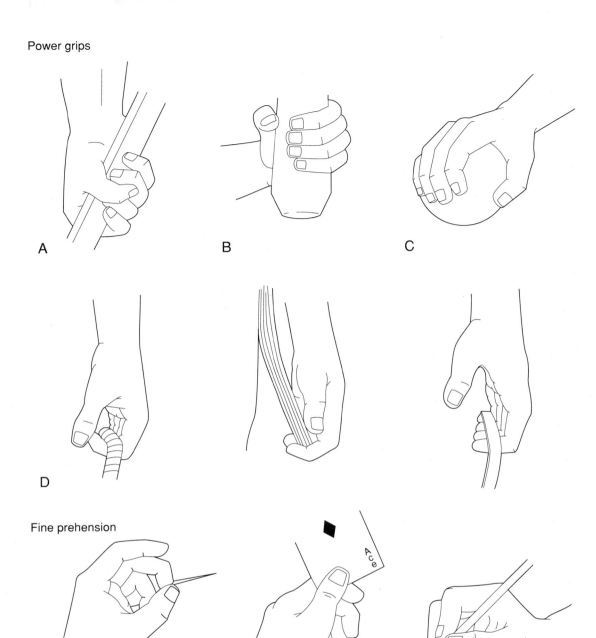

Fig. 23-7. Hand function is tested by evaluating the standard power and fine prehension grasps. Power grips: **(A)** Fist grasp that may be totally closed, as with punching or slightly open around a small object as illustrated. **(B)** Cylindrical is a further modification of the first grip. **(C)** Spherical in which the fingers splay around a spherical object. **(D)** Three modifications of the efficient hook-grasp using only the fingertips. A more secure grip for heavy objects uses all of the fingers and possibly the body as counterpressure. Alternatively the object is supported in a fully hooked position, and the thumb may or may not supply some assistance locking in the object, e.g., a barbell. Fine prehension: **(E)** pulp; **(F)** lateral; **(G)** palmar prehension. This latter grip is a physiologic analogue of the mechanical chuck and is a modification of the standard pulp to pulp grip.

of the intrinsic muscles, and also when there is loss of stability of the joints at the base of the thumb. Although it does not permit fine manipulation, significant power may be generated.

Tip Prehension

The tip of the thumb may be used against the tip on one of the other digits, an action that can be refined for picking up small objects, e.g., a pin. However, it does not permit the working surfaces of the pads of the fingers to grasp the object, and so it lacks some stability and sensitivity.

In summary, these power and precision grips require the fingers and thumb to be put through a wide and complete range of motion and thus should be included when functionally assessing the hand.

Skin and Fascia of the Hand

There is a natural tendency to devote time to the spectacular, and consequently muscle and joint movement assume a prime spot in any anatomic discussion. However, fascia, fat, sweat glands, and papillary ridges contribute to the successful working of the hand.

The superficial fascia is fat-bearing, particularly over the palm where condensations facilitate grip by molding the surface of the hand to the object held in it. The major skin folds are devoid of fat owing to septa from the deep fascia, which tends to anchor the superficial fat pads and fascia on the palm preventing displacement. It enables a firmer grip by aiding the development of friction. The multiple retinacula pass from the deep fascia and the palmaris longus to the palmar surface, carrying its blood supply. This arrangement of having the vessels enter the skin from deep in the palm avoids the necessity of having multiple vessels crossing a surface that is constantly exposed to pressure and trauma. For this reason, surgical procedures on the palm often interfere with the blood supply and present problems of healing and mobilization. The dorsal superficial fascia is loose, and it moves with movement of the hand. It also provides a potential space for the collection of edema fluid.

The deep fascia forms the flexor retinaculum and the digital sheaths, which harness the contractile potential of the muscles by channeling the line of pull of the tendons and preventing bowstringing. When passing through or under these retinacula, the tendons are provided with synovial sheaths that minimize friction and aid in nutrition. However, this same re-

markable mechanism is also the cause and site of much of the pathology of the hand, particularly in reference to tendinitis and carpal tunnel syndrome.

Quick Facts
SKIN AND FASCIA

- These structures are loose on the dorsal surface, allowing accumulation of post-traumatic edema.
- Multiple septa pass from the deep fascia to the palmar surface to the skin, facilitating grip.
- Vessels pass to the skin with these multiple retinacula, and care is necessary with palmar incisions.
- Deep fascia forms flexor retinaculum and digital sheaths channeling tendinous line of pull.
- Surrounding synovium may be vulnerable to inflammatory overuse syndromes.

The papillary ridges provide a roughened surface to increase the coefficient of friction during manipulative movements. Perhaps equally important is their sensory role.[24] They provide multiple points of contact in which pressure-sensitive endings are situated. In particular, there are numerous Meissner's corpuscles that lie in the dermal papillae. The arrangement of the dermal papillae is genetically determined and, in addition to being of interest to the police for purposes of identification, there is a correlation between certain dermal patterns and some genetically determined diseases.[25]

Perhaps it is an opportune time to stress the importance of the sensory function of the hand. Impulses from the skin, joints, ligaments, and tendons produce a veritable maelstrom of electrical activity that allows the in-progress modification of movement. Hilton in 1863 brought attention to the fact that sensory innervation reaches the hand and finger joints from the same nerves that supply muscles acting over these joints, and that these nerves also supply the overlying skin.[26] Think how this arrangement must facilitate central integration. Without its sensory component, the hand is a crude, inept tool. As Harty (1971) pointed out, nowhere are the vivid delicacies of digital sensibilities more fully developed, realized, and appreciated than in the dark domain of the blind.[27]

Traditionally, the palmaris brevis is described as being a quadrilaterally shaped muscle arising from the palmar aponeurosis and flexor retinaculum and inserting into the skin of the ulnar aspect of the hypothenar eminence. It is rarely absent, although it may vary in size and thickness.[25] William Cheselden in 1713 outlined the function of the palmaris brevis, a description that is still used in most anatomic textbooks today.[28] He stated that the palmaris brevis deepens the cupping of the palm of the hand by displacing the skin and fascia of the hypothenar eminence, thereby facilitating grasp. In addition, the supporting fascia on the dorsal surface of the muscle bundle forms the anterior wall of the pisohamate tunnel of Guyon.[29,30]

Handedness

Handedness is the tendency to use one hand in preference to the other. Those whose right hand is dominant are called *dextrals;* left-handers are *sinistrals* or "southpaws." Rarely, individuals are equally proficient with both — hence the term *ambidextrous.*[31] However, true ambidexterity is rare in sports, even with the professional athlete. Most have a side of preference for both the hand and arm in upper limb sports, e.g., throwing or shooting, or with lower limb sports for kicking or take-off.

The dominant speech area is mainly in the left frontal lobe, and in those cases that do not follow the rule there is not necessarily a correlation with handedness. There is, by contrast, a strong correlation between handedness and ocular dominance, which may be an additional factor in skill acquisition. Dominance leads to unilateral hypertrophy of the particular limb, noticeable in both bone and muscle in some sports. Hence it must be borne in mind when comparing normal and affected sides during functional assessment for return to game fitness.

ASSESSMENT OF HAND AND WRIST

Full function of the hand depends on mobility, strength, adequate sensation, and neural control. Hence examination of the wrist and hand must include the following.

1. History of the mechanism of injury from the athlete or an observer
2. Comparison with the opposite limb or noticeable deformity, swelling, tenderness, and discoloration
3. Passive and active tests of the affected part of the hand to establish range of motion
4. Palpation of bony and soft tissue contours particularly noting areas of inflammation
5. Testing for numbness or dullness of sensation in the affected area
6. Checking grip strength of the injured side and comparing it with that of the uninjured limb

History

Because most sports-related hand problems are traumatic in nature, the history focuses on the when, where, what, and why of the injury.

When

Knowledge of the duration between injury and assessment helps to assess the implication of the degree of swelling and the impact of the contamination of an open wound on potential infection. If there is an infection without an open wound, a sore throat, or recent visit to the dentist may point to the origin of the organism, suggesting an appropriate antibiotic. Immediate swelling suggests a more severe injury or hemorrhage. Swelling at 6 to 12 hours after the injury or activity may be a slow accumulating synovitis. Continuous and fluctuating swelling may be related to an arthritic joint problem.

Where and What

The nature of the trauma may provide insight into the likely course and prognosis. An abrasion on the hand made by a tooth during a fight, a deep scratch due to a fall from a bike, a compound wound from a dislocation, and a laceration from a skate blade have potentially different implications for infection of the tendon sheath and spaces of the hand, the likelihood of contamination with gram-negative organism, the need for tetanus prophylaxis, and the possible associated vessel, nerve, and tendon injury. The possibility of embedded foreign material must also be considered.

Why

With acute and chronic injuries, the question "why" may produce an answer that suggests both treatment and prophylaxis against recurrence of a similar problem. For instance, tendinitis may be triggered by poor technique of poling when skiing, carpal tunnel syndrome by sudden excessive increases in training over a period of a few days, and lacerations by engaging in fighting during a hockey game, or wearing inadequate protective equipment, as with a wheelchair athlete.

Quick Facts

WRIST AND HAND EXAMINATION

- History
  -Establish chief complaint
  -When, where, what, why
- Observations
  -Swelling, color, deformity, nails
- Examination
  -Active movements
  - Pronation and supination
  - Wrist flexion, extension, radial and ulnar deviation
  - Finger flexion and extension — MCP, PIP, DIP
  - Thumb motion
  -Functional grips: power and precision
  -Passive motion if indicated
  -Coordination if indicated
  -Resisted movements as for active motion
  -Tests of tendon integrity (prn)
  -Reflexes and skin sensation
  - Pin prick: two-point discrimination
  -Palpation
  -Joint play motion (prn)
- Special tests
  -Roentgenography
  -Bone scan
  -CT and MRI
  -Arthroscopy

Examination

Observation and Palpation

The initial observation assesses the magnitude of the deformity, swelling, general posture of the wrist and hand, and, if an open wound or crush injury exists, the need or advisability of cleansing it prior to further examination. If a fracture is suspected, and there is an associated wound, rapid complete, thorough débridement becomes urgent, as all open fractures constitute surgical emergencies. Failure to attend to these injuries appropriately increases the chance of soft tissue infection and possibly osteomye-

litis. At 4 hours after the injury, the complication rate starts to rise exponentially.

After the initial screen, a more careful second scan is carried out. There may be the characteristic deformity of a specific dislocation or a nerve or tendon injury. Note is made of the pattern of any swelling. Generalized swelling collects on the dorsum of the hand where the skin is more loosely attached and cannot be considered specific when localizing the injury. Local swelling around joints with sprains must be distinguished by history and pattern from the synovitis of rheumatoid disease, which presents classically at the MCP joints. The swelling and deformity around the distal interphalangeal joints (Heberden's nodes) in the older individual must be distinguished from the local swelling and deformity of tendon avulsions or phalangeal fractures.

Other common swelling includes the localized, smooth, slightly mobile swelling of the classic dorsal wrist ganglion and the firm nodular swelling that moves with the flexor tendon, situated at the base of the thumb or second digit, which probably represents the fibrous nodule of a trigger finger. Lastly, there is the diffuse, sometimes boggy, usually painful swelling that may be palpated along the involved tendon; it represents a synovitis. Swelling of the wrist joint itself is difficult to detect and is usually manifested only by stiff, painful motion and swelling of the overlying structures.

After a significant hand injury, tense edema may delay healing and increase residual fibrosis and the risk of infection. It is even possible to get sufficient pressure within the spaces of the forearm and hand to generate a compartment syndrome. One technique of evaluating impending ischemia is the use of a 256 Hz turning fork applied over the autonomous sensory areas of the fingers or thumb.[32] This test is affected early with sensory impairment. If there is sufficient clinical concern, pressure may have to be monitored by introducing a catheter or manometer.

With crush injuries, the degree of damage or loss of skin prompts referral to a hand specialist in case grafting is required. A contaminated ragged laceration may require a preliminary scrub with Ivory soap or pHisoHex for a few minutes. Soaking in a basin of provodine-iodine for 20 to 30 minutes is a common practice but has the disadvantage that the iodophors and detergents emulsify or break down the protective mantle that holds resident bacteria in the skin recesses. Transient, newly introduced bacteria are usually effectively stripped off with a short preparation with bland soap.[33] Knowledge of the surface landmarks of the underlying major nerves and vessels assists in assessing those structures in jeopardy.

Sensation

The sensory supply to the hand is particularly rich, and normal function requires normal sensation. The skin may change in texture, and sensation may be abnormal in cases where the limb has been immobilized for any length of time.[34] Re-education of sensation may therefore be part of the consideration in an exercise program.

Sensation is a specific indicator of nerve integrity that usually follows a distinct pattern in the hand. There are known areas of relatively isolated skin supply. For the radial nerve, the autonomous zone is over the dorsal web space between the thumb and index finger. For the median nerve, the isolated innervation is the volar distal phalanx of the index finger, and for the ulnar nerve it is the volar distal phalanx of the little finger (Fig. 23-8). However, when testing and treating patients with nerve injuries, it is important to bear in mind that anomalous innervation in the hand is common, with all possible combinations and permutations of ulnar and median nerve innervation appearing. It extends from complete ulnar dominance to complete median dominance. Anomalies of the radial nerve are less common.

The pattern of dysesthesia or sensory loss also assists in locating the level of the lesion, as cervical pathology, peripheral nerve entrapment at the elbow and wrist, and systemic conditions such as diabetes leading to peripheral neuritis may produce hand symptoms as the presenting, chief complaint (Table 23-2). Clinically the sensations are divided into pain, temperature, touch, stereognosis, and joint sensation. There are tests for vibration sense and two-point discrimination. The following points may be helpful.

1. *Pain.* If pain is present at rest or with function, inquire as to the nature of the pain and its distribution. Occasionally, the specific elements of sensation must be distinguished to aid in the diagnosis of central nervous system disorders or to assess the progress of peripheral nerve recovery. In these cases, temperature, touch, stereognosis and joint position senses are evaluated (Table 23-2).

2. *Temperature.* Hot and cold are tested by water in test tubes. Make the temperature realistically different. Keep the sides of the tubes dry. Allow the patient to experience the warm and cold before the test is

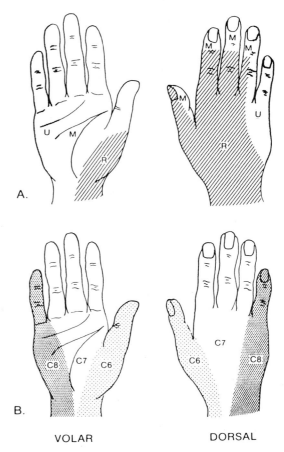

Fig. 23-8. (A) Cutaneous distribution of the radius (R), median (M), and ulnar (U) nerves. **(B)** Dermatomes of the hand.

conducted. The patient should not watch the procedure.

3. *Touch, pressure, pain.* Light touch is evaluated with a bristle or hair, pressure by normal contact, and pain by pinprick.

4. *Stereognosis.* A series of objects may be placed in patients' hands and they are asked to identify them without looking. The type of object usually includes keys, buttons, pins, money. Note the accuracy of description, hesitancy, and time taken to respond.

5. *Joint sensation.* The joint is moved passively by the examiner. Patients close their eyes and are asked to report the position of the limb in space, the direction of movement, and the joint involved.

From a more practical point of view, sensation is usually tested using either soft touch or pinprick. It may be supplemented by an assessment of two-point

TABLE 23-2. Patterns of Altered Sensation on the Hand and Clinical Implications

Location: Dysesthesia or Anesthesia	Implication
All four limbs	Diabetes, anemia, vascular occlusive disease, neuritis
Thumb alone	Numbness only—occupational pressure on digital nerves to thumb
Thumb and index finger	Fifth cervical disc lesion
Thumb, index, and middle fingers	Fifth cervical disc lesion or thoracic outlet syndrome
Thumb, index, and middle fingers, adjacent side of ring finger	Palmar surface—median nerve in carpal tunnel Dorsal surface—radial nerve
All five digits of one or both hands	Thoracic outlet syndrome Cervical disc protrusion
Index, middle, and ring fingers	Sixth cervical disc lesion or carpal tunnel syndrome
Index and middle fingers	Sixth cervical disc lesion
All four fingers	Sixth cervical disc lesion
Middle finger alone	Sixth cervical disc lesion
Middle and ring fingers	Sixth cervical disc lesion
Middle, ring, and little fingers	Seventh cervical disc lesion
Ring and fifth fingers	Ulnar nerve lesion, seventh cervical disc lesion, thoracic outlet syndrome

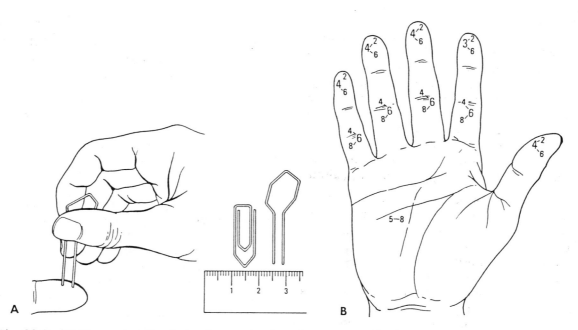

Fig. 23-9. (A) Two-point discrimination testing by using a paper clip. (B) Values of discrimination in the Webber's test in the zones of the hand. The largest figure (millimeters) represents the mean for the area along with the minimum and maximum values in smaller print. (From Tubiana,[13] with permission.)

discrimination. Normal sensibility in the hand is capable of distinguishing the two points as close as 3 mm apart. An inability to distinguish one from two points until they are 8 to 10 mm apart is clearly abnormal. This test may be done simply with a paper clip bent with the two ends about 8 mm apart or, more precisely, with calipers.[32,34] If the integrity of the digital nerve is being tested, it is important to test along the side of the pulp, as testing transversely may test an area of overlap of the two nerves (Fig. 23-9).

If there is sensory loss over the pulp of the little finger secondary to ulnar nerve involvement, the athlete should not be able to cross the long finger over the index finger because the interossei are also ulnar-innervated.

If there is sensory loss over the dorsal web space between the thumb and index finger due to a proximal radial nerve injury, the patient should not be able to give the "thumbs up" or "hitch-hiker's sign," as the extensor pollicis longus is radial-innervated.

The simplest gross test of motor and nerve function is to ask the athlete to bring the tips of the thumb and all of the fingers together to form a small circle. It is impossible to perform this maneuver if the radial, median and ulnar nerve, and the intrinsics they supply are not intact. This test may form part of a "2-minute screening examination," which rules out major pathology or focuses an in-depth examination in situations where time is limited[33,35] (Fig. 23-10).

Testing Strength

To evaluate muscle strength it is necessary to have a clear idea of the specific action of each muscle and the particular point of differentiation. It is not within the scope of this book to discuss muscle testing; however, the actions are outlined in the anatomy review at the beginning of this chapter (Table 23-1).

When testing grip and dexterity, attempt to make the assessment realistic. Grip strength may be assessed by either special dynamometers or by squeezing a sphygmomanometer and recording the pressure change. This index is crude but useful as a screening test. The most important part of this section of the examination is to relate the findings to the athlete's sport. Is the strength sufficient, and is the athlete able to utilize the strength demonstrated in the static isolated test in the dynamic situation of the specific sport?

Range of Motion

Measurement of joint range in the hand is difficult because of the size of the part involved and the great complexity of movement taking place in the various components. Furthermore, the movements of the thumb are defined in a plane different from that of the rest of the hand. However, there is a need for accuracy of measurement if this method is to be useful for evaluating the effectiveness of a particular treatment program and the progress of a condition. Particularly important is the establishment of a goal for the patient and the incentive that can be produced by an overt display of gain in range. Stiffness after trauma to the tendons or joints is a major problem in the hand, and early mobilization is the rule whenever possible.

Wrist flexion is approximately 80 degrees, and extension is 70 degrees. The axis of motion is taken as the radial styloid process. The range of ulnar and radial deviation is controversial because of the wide range of methods used. Using an arbitrary point in the center of the radiocarpal joint line, there is approximately 30 degrees of ulnar deviation and 20 degrees of radial deviation.

Finger motion is even more difficult to record. There are small plastic or metal goniometers that may be suitable if the therapist has enough skill and has had sufficient practice. It is usually simpler to use other equipment, e.g., a tape measure, pipe cleaner, pencil outlines on paper, and hand-prints. The MCP joints normally extend actively no more than 20 degrees and flex to 90 degrees. Passive range may be greater. The proximal interphalangeal joint flexes to about 100 degrees and the distal joint 90 degrees (Fig. 23-11).

Essentially, these motions are best tested functionally by having the athlete assume all of the strength and precision grips outlined in the previous section. These maneuvers ensure flexibility of the mobile ulnar side of the hand, stability of the radial half including the base of the thumb, and the ability to both

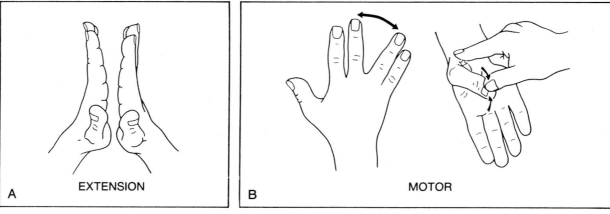

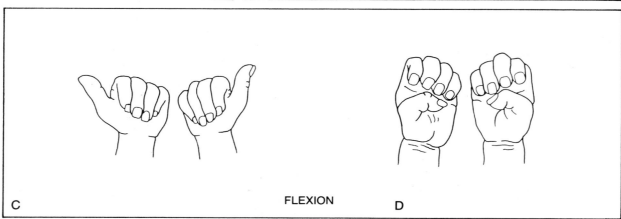

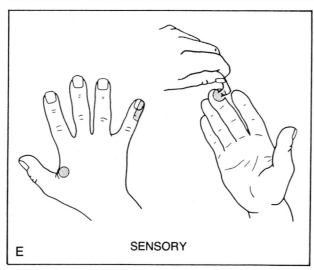

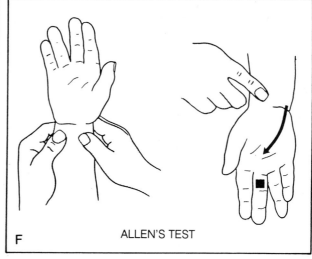

Fig. 23-10. Two-minute screening and examination of the injured hand. **(A)** Extension of the fingers and thumb evaluates radial nerve function and the extrinsic extensors of the digits. **(B)** Abduction and adduction of the fingers and thumb test ulnar and median nerve function and intrinsic musculature. **(C & D)** Flexion of the fingers and thumb tests ulnar and median function and long finger and thumb flexors. **(E)** Sensory testing of the isolated areas for radial, ulnar, and median nerves. **(F)** Allen's test for patency of circulation. Normal testing of all these functions rules out most of the significant injuries to the hand. (After Zondervan JH, Continuing Medical Education Newsletter. University of Saskatchewan. Nov, 1985, with permission.)

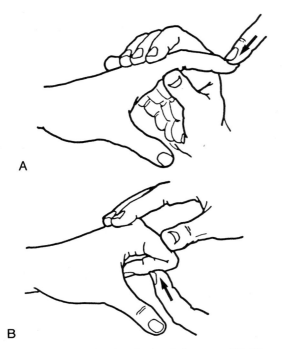

Fig. 23-11. Test for intrinsic tightness. **(A)** Finger held with MCP joint in extension. The PIP joint is passively flexed. **(B)** If this movement is not possible in the extended position but possible in the flexed position, the test is positive for tight intrinsics. (After Burton et al., with permission.)

spread the fingers into abduction as well as flex fully into the palm. Pulp-to-pulp and tip-to-tip capability ensures dexterity along with an adequate range of finger flexion and thumb opposition[3] (Fig. 23-7).

Whenever there has been a significant laceration to the wrist or fingers, specific tests must be carried out to ensure that the tendons have not been divided. These special examinations are described within the sections on the respective tendon and nerve injuries.

Circulation

The arterial supply of the hand is principally from the radial and ulnar arteries. Patency of both arteries is assessed by the Allen's test.[36] The radial and ulnar arteries are tested individually by asking the patient to make a tight fist, forcing the blood out of the palm and giving it a pale appearance. Before the fingers are uncurled, pressure is placed on the appropriate artery. Failure of rapid capillary circulation return when the hand is opened indicates that there is insufficient collateral flow entering the hand from the vessel not being compressed. Each artery is tested in turn (Fig. 23-12).

With sufficient practice and skill, the accessory and joint play motions of the carpus and digits may be assessed. This assessment does not form a routine part of a hand examination, but for the therapist it may be built in as an integral part of the ongoing

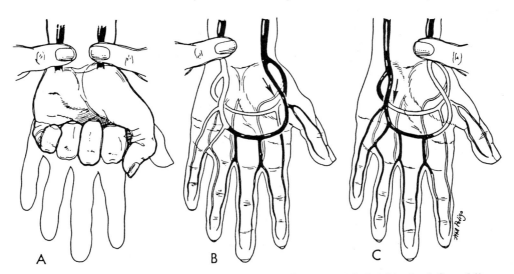

Fig. 23-12. Allen's test for patency of the digit arteries. **(A)** Tightly clenched fist obliterates the patency of the capillary beds of the palmar surface. **(B)** Pressure of the ulnar artery reveals if there is adequate filling through the anastamosis with the radial artery. **(C)** After further clenching of the fist, patency of the circulation through the ulnar–palmar arteries is tested by obliterating the radial artery. (After Post,[93] with permission.)

assessment and therapy. Thus the same maneuvers that evaluate the joint play and end feel may be adapted to restore absent or insufficient motion after trauma (Figs. 23-13 and 23-14).

FRACTURES AND LIGAMENT INJURIES

Fractures of the forearm are characterized by nonunion should the initial treatment fail to control the stresses of pronation and supination. With the carpus, the major concern is avascular necrosis, carpal instability, and late degenerative changes, and with the phalanges, joint stiffness, pain, and mal-

union. Thus all these fractures are thwart with problems unless treated aggressively, promptly, and effectively by the physician. Many require an experienced orthopaedic or plastic surgeon to be involved in the initial care. It is not a crime nor a sign of failure to know one's limitation in the treatment of hand injuries. It is, however, negligence to treat these delicate anatomic structure with inadequate knowledge or experience.

Radius and Ulna

Thin bones such as the radius and ulna may be fractured singly or in combination, frequently secondary to a fall on the outstretched hand or a direct

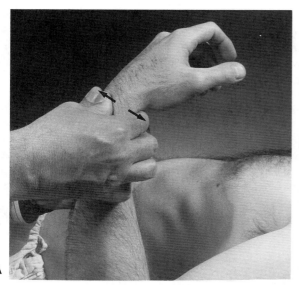

A

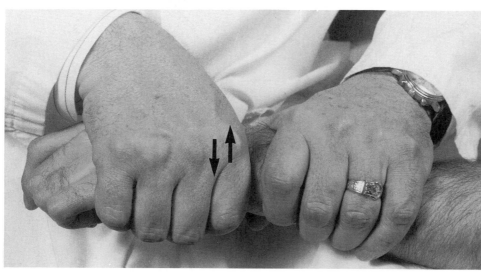

B

Fig. 23-13. Assessment of accessory movements and restoration of joint play by mobilization techniques. **(A)** Distal radial-ulnar joint and anterior posterior glide of the radius. The ulna is stabilized with the thenar grasp, and the radius is mobilized with the thumb and forefinger. **(B)** Radiocarpal joints. Volar and dorsal radiocarpal glides. The thumb, index finger, and first web space stabilize the radius and ulna dorsally while the other hand grasps the proximal carpal row to produce the glide. (*Figure continues.*)

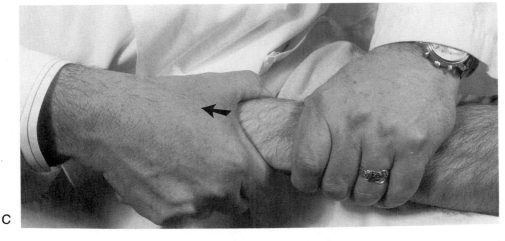

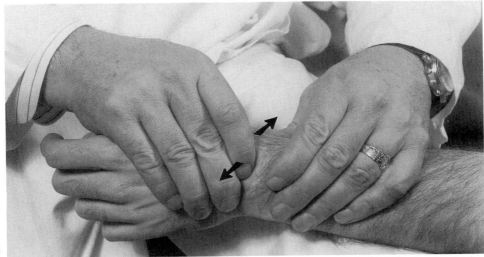

Fig. 23-13. *(Continued).* **(C)** Distraction of the radiocarpal joint and carpal bones distally. **(D)** Isolation of the various intercarpal and carpometacarpal joints with anteroposterior gliding. These are precise mobilizations and require exact fixation of one carpal bone while exerting very localized pressure over the desired carpal bone to be moved.

blow such as slashing in hockey or during a tackle in football.

Treatment depends on whether one or both bones are fractured, on skeletal maturity, whether the fracture is open or closed, if there is associated dislocation, and the degree of displacement. There is a tendency to significant displacement when both bones are fractured in the adult.

If one bone is fractured, great care is taken to rule out a dislocated radial head in the case of a fractured ulna (Monteggia) and a dislocated distal ulna in the case of a fractured radius (Galeazzi) (Fig. 23-15). Thus initial roentgenograms must include both elbow and wrist, and particular attention is paid to obtaining

Quick Facts

FRACTURES OF FOREARM

Consider

- Skeletal maturity
- One or both bones
- Open or closed
- Displacement
- Possible associated dislocation

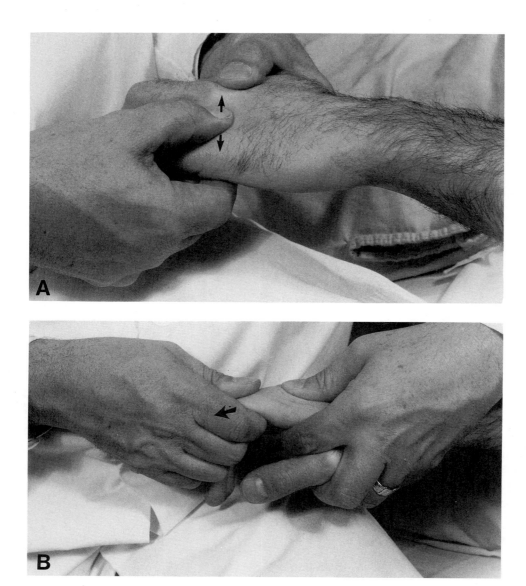

Fig. 23-14. Accessory movements and mobilization of the joints of the hand. **(A)** Intermetacarpal glide. One hand stabilizes the head of metacarpal while the other hand grasps the contiguous bone and glides it into an anteroposterior direction. **(B)** Metacarpophalangeal distraction. Similar technique can be used progressively more distally for each interphalangeal joint. *(Figure continues.)*

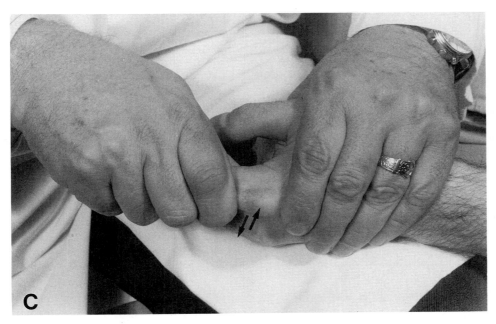

Fig. 23-14. *(Continued).* **(C)** Anteroposterior gliding of the MCP joint. Successive distal stabilization allows mobilization of the interphalangeal joints.

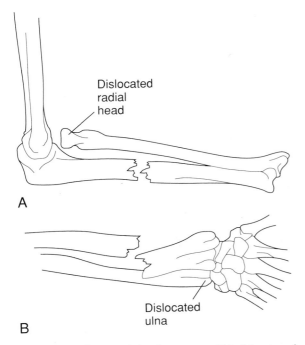

Fig. 23-15. Monteggia's fracture. **(A)** Monteggia fracture that includes the fractured shaft of the ulna and the dislocated radial head. **(B)** Galeazzi's fracture with a fractured distal radius and a dislocated ulna. In both situations **(A & B)** the dislocation is frequently overlooked and is usually an unstable injury, often necessitating open reduction.

> **Practice Point**
>
> **FRACTURE OF SINGLE BONE OF FOREARM**
>
> - Rule out dislocation of radial head or distal ulna
> - Need good lateral views of elbow and wrist

good lateral views and carefully inspecting them against films of the uninjured side if necessary.

The radial head should have good alignment with the capitellum and the distal ulna with the carpus. Most Monteggia and nearly all Galeazzi fracture-dislocations require open reduction and internal fixation, sometimes with soft tissue repair of ligaments.[37]

Greenstick Fracture

In the skeletally immature patient the fracture frequently involves both bones and is incomplete (greenstick fracture). These fractures usually heal well in 6 to 8 weeks. If both bones are "greensticked," a below-elbow cast is sufficient. If they are displaced, an above-elbow cast is required until callus is visible. Reduction is required if: (1) the angulation gives an

---

Practice Point

FRACTURE-DISLOCATIONS: TREATMENT PRINCIPLES

- Monteggia
  -Fracture proximal one-third of ulna
  -Dislocated radial head
- Galeazzi
  -Fracture of distal radius
  -Dislocation distal ulnar
- Ensure ends of both bones are included in screening roentgenograms.
- Both fractures probably need open reduction and internal fixation.

---

unacceptable deformity; (2) the bowing is likely to impede pronation or supination; or (3) there is a rotational deformity. In these three circumstances, remodeling will not be sufficient. To reduce the bones adequately, an incomplete fracture may have to be completed by initially increasing the deformity. With 100 percent displacement or shortening, open reduction is required.

Open Fractures

Open fractures, no matter how small, require formal débridement and prophylactic antibiotics. If they are unstable, an external fixator is used when practical.

Radius and Ulna (Adult)

In the adult some relatively undisplaced or minimally angulated fractures may be treated closed. There is little remodeling potential in the forearm. Malrotation or an obvious block to pronation or supination requires reduction. When closed treatment is elected, the cast must initially extend above the elbow. Only when good callus is visible should the cast be reduced to allow elbow motion. This is necessary because usually the ulna heals rapidly and the torque of pronation and supination tends to stress the radial fracture site, leading to delayed union or nonunion. If open reduction is performed, substantial plates and at least three screws on either side of the fracture is desirable. This method allows earlier motion without metal failure or loss of fixation.

Stress Fracture

Stress fractures of the forearm are rare, although they have been reported in weight-lifters, tennis players, and athletes involved in some throwing sports. Particularly in gymnasts, with significant unremitting forearm pain often referred to as "pommelitis," the possibility of radius and ulnar stress reaction or fracture should be entertained.

Distal Radial Fractures

Distal radial fractures historically occur in two groups. One is the more common low velocity fracture of older individuals, usually the result of trying to reduce the impact of a fall, where the osteoporotic bone crumbles. In the young, it is usually a high energy injury, frequently shattering the bone and producing a complex intra-articular fracture. The distal radio-ulnar joint or associated ulnar styloid process may also be disrupted. Other than the common fracture pattern of the Colles' variety, occasionally a reversed Colles' or Smith's fracture, with predominantly volar displacement, may occur. It is easy to overlook a minimally displaced transverse fracture in a young person and diagnose a severe wrist sprain, unless the exact site of maximal tenderness is noted and roentgenograms are obtained.

The Colles' injury classically involves a dorsally angulated and displaced, and a radially angulated and displaced fracture within approximately 1.5 inches of the wrist joint (Fig. 23-16). There may be additional avulsion or fracture of the tip of the ulnar styloid. Initially, the bones are usually impacted, and so there is an element of shortening. Classically, it produces the so-called dinner-fork deformity.

Treatment decisions depend on the age, quality of bone and severity of the displacement. Increasingly severe distal radial fractures involve intra-articular extensions and fragmentation as well as disruption of the distal radius and ulnar joint, with or without the ulnar styloid avulsion or the fibrocartilaginous disc damage. Open reduction and internal fixation of the more severe Colles' fractures is a difficult undertaking but must be considered for the more complicated and displaced intra-articular varieties.[37] Frequently, a combined approach is used, with an external fixator for distraction and maintaining length plus the option of percutaneous reduction and perhaps bone grafting. The bottom line is that this common fracture is a spectrum of injuries and treatment must be individualized.[38] As a guideline, the most important

Colles fracture (A)

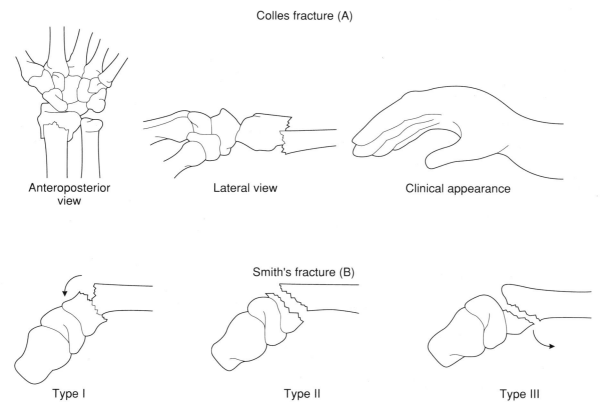

Anteroposterior view

Lateral view

Clinical appearance

Smith's fracture (B)

Type I

Type II

Type III

Fig. 23-16. (A) Classic Colles' fracture with radial and dorsal angulation and deviation and clinically dinner-fork deformity. **(B)** Smith's fracture with volar displacement and angulation. Type I is transverse, type II is oblique, and type III is intra-articular (Barton's type). These are progressively more unstable injuries, and they must be distinguished from the Colles' fracture.

predictive factor for significant disability and likely failure of closed techniques is radial shortening of more than 4 mm.[39]

Simple fracture lines with minimal displacement are well handled by the family physician by closed

---

Practice Point

CONSIDERATIONS FOR OPERATIVE TREATMENT OF COLLES' FRACTURE

- Radial shortening > 4 mm
- Displaced intra-articular fragment
- Wide disruption of distal radio-ulnar joint
- Failure to maintain acceptable reduction of the dorsal angulation
- Young individual

---

means; however, care should be taken to monitor median nerve function, as carpal tunnel syndrome is a common complication. The nerve may require decompression. Furthermore, loss of reduction frequently occurs at 10 to 14 days as the cast loosens and the fracture ends resorb; thus meticulous follow-up is essential. In the young, active person, careful restoration of the distal radius-shaft angle and specific attention to intra-articular displacement are necessary. Frequently, open reduction is necessary, and this procedure should be done only by an experienced person: It is always more difficult than it appears, and specialized internal fixation is often required.

The complications of this injury include (1) the early problem of impaired circulation caused by swelling and (2) damage to the median nerve in the carpal tunnel. The former requires careful assessment and consideration of bivalving the cast; and the latter may require release of the carpal tunnel. Intermediate complications are related to loss of reduction and continuation of the carpal tunnel syndrome. The late complications include loss of joint range, malunion, nerve impingement, and occasional tendon rupture of the long extensor to the thumb.

Smith's Fracture

The mechanism of injury for the Smith's fracture is similar to that for Colles' fracture, but the fracture pattern is such that there tends to be either volar angulation or displacement, and hence the reduction technique required is different (Fig. 23-16). Type I is usually fairly stable and readily treated closed. Type II is more unstable and must be carefully followed if treated closed. Consideration is given to open reduction. Type III, also called the Barton's fracture, is intra-articular and thus frequently requires open reduction. The importance of the Smith's fracture is recognizing and distinguishing it from the Colles' injury.

Pronator Quadratus Fracture

In the skeletally immature individual the distal radial epiphysis is in the anatomic location usually disrupted by the Colles' type fracture in the adult. A dorsal epiphyseal separation may occur with a strong intact dorsal periosteal hinge. This periosteum prevents reduction by straight traction. Repositioning can be effected only by significantly increasing the deformity, hooking the fragment over the edge of the proximal dorsal fracture site, and correcting the angulation using the periosteum as a hinge. This type of fracture is seen while the epiphysis is widely open, up to the age of 10 to 12.

As the epiphysis starts to narrow and becomes stronger, the fracture occurs just proximally, under the pronator quadratus muscle, giving it its designa-

tion. Reduction is usually effected the same way as for the epiphyseal injury in younger individuals or as for a Colles' fracture in the older athlete. There are a wide range of possible combinations and fractures, and only the most common injuries are outlined.[39]

Carpal Fractures and Dislocations

Fractures or dislocation of the carpus frequently result from a fall on the outstretched hand or a mistimed landing in gymnastics. They are frequently misdiagnosed and are characterized by early avascular necrosis and later carpal instability and arthrosis,

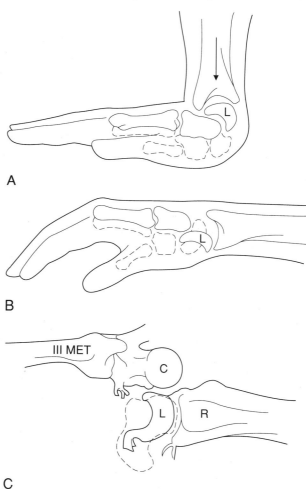

Fig. 23-17. (A) Falling on the outstretched hand opens up the volar surface of the carpus and results in **(B)** a dislocated lunate or **(C)** a perilunar dislocation. The latter injury is often seen in association with a fractured scaphoid. L = lunate; R = radius; C = capitate, S = scaphoid; III Met = third metacarpal.

which is difficult to treat satisfactorily in the athlete. Hence prompt and correct treatment is mandatory in order to give a reasonable chance of a satisfactory outcome. Also, the lack of callus makes judgment about the progress of union difficult without experience.[40-42]

Dislocated Lunate and Perilunar Dislocation

Lunate and perilunar dislocations account for a significant percentage (8 to 10 percent) of carpal dislocations. A forced extension injury to the wrist allows disruption of the ligaments and volar subluxation or *dislocation of the lunate* (Fig. 23-17). There may be associated median nerve symptoms. Reduction is effected by extending the wrist with direct pressure over the lunate or by traction and direct pressure. The wrist is then splinted in slight flexion for 3 weeks and no extension is allowed for 5 to 6 weeks. Frequently, open reduction is required and, if still unstable, transection with a small Kirschner wire until the ligaments have healed. Because so much of the lunate surface is articular, there is a high frequency of avascular necrosis, even if the injury is treated promptly

and well (Fig. 23-18). This dislocation should be managed by an experienced surgeon.

Occasionally the same mechanism of injury results in rupture of the ligaments between the lunate and triquetrum, and the carpal bones dislocate off the lunate. Thus the radiolunate relation is preserved. This injury is called a *perilunar dislocation*. This diagnosis is frequently missed, particularly the highly associated scaphoid fracture (transscaphoid-perilunar dislocation). This complex injury needs to be referred to, and treated by, an expert, as late carpal instability and wrist arthrosis are common accompaniments and may be reduced to a minimum by optimal treatment (Fig. 23-19).

Frequently there is partial or complete tearing of the interosseous ligaments without dislocation. Usually this problem resolves after a brief period of support or immobilization followed by progressive rehabilitation. However, occasionally there is persistent instability. Local tenderness, crepitus, and a "jump" or click with radial and ulnar deviation are suggestive of instability. A positive ballottement test adds confirmation (Fig. 23-20): The triquetrum is grasped be-

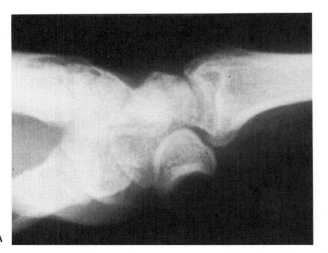

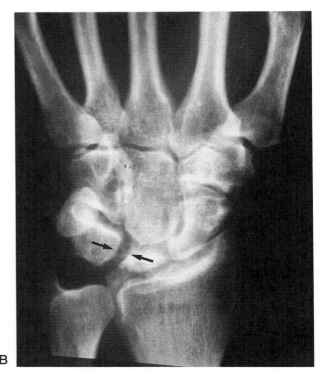

A   B

Fig. 23-18. **(A)** Roentgenogram of a volar dislocation of the lunate. **(B)** Subsequent avascular necrosis and collapse of the carpus (arrows). The collapse is manifested by an increased scapholunate distance > 2 mm.

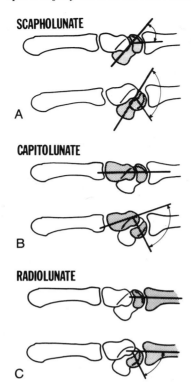

SCAPHOLUNATE

A

CAPITOLUNATE

B

RADIOLUNATE

C

Fig. 23-19. Carpal instability may be assessed from a lateral roentgenogram of the carpal bones. In each illustration, the normal is shown above in comparison to the abnormal angle seen in the instability pattern. **(A)** In the scapholunate, disassociation an angle of more than 80 degrees is evidence of dorsiflexion instability. **(B)** Capitolunate angle should normally be 0 degrees with the wrist in neutral; it is considered abnormal if it is in excess of 15 degrees. **(C)** Similarly, the radiolunate angle is abnormal if it exceeds 15 degrees. (Adapted from Green,[40] with permission.)

tween the thumb and forefinger of one hand, and the lunate similarly by the other hand. Forward and back-back displacement generating laxity, crepitus, and pain constitute a positive test.

Kienböck's Disease

Occasionally, spontaneous avascular necrosis develops without an obvious associated major traumatic episode or displacement.[43] This idiopathic avascular necrosis (Kienböck's disease) may be related to repeated minor trauma. Initially, the avascularity is noted by an apparent density of the affected lunate, as the surrounding bones are slightly demineralized. Subsequently, if the bone collapses, the lunate ap-

pears truly dense and deformed. Initially cold on bone scan, the bone becomes hot during the revascularization phase. Early diagnosis may be difficult, as the athlete presents only with wrist pain and synovitis. When diagnosed early, the lunate must be protected from repetitive stress in the hope that revascularization will occur without the accompanying collapse. Occasionally osteotomy of the radius with lengthening, is the treatment in cases of a negative ulnar variance (slightly shortened ulna).

Fractured Scaphoid

Accounting for 70 percent of carpal injuries, the scaphoid is the most commonly fractured carpal bone. In athletes these fractures frequently occur in contact sports, particularly football, soccer, and basketball. The scaphoid is unique, connecting both the proximal and the distal carpal rows, and thus is subjected to significant torque during falls where the weight is thrust through the carpus. In addition, the styloid process of the radius may impinge with sudden force against the midscaphoid, helping to initiate the fracture line.

The vascular arrangement is such that the main vessel enters the distal pole of the scaphoid and then runs back through the waist of the scaphoid to the

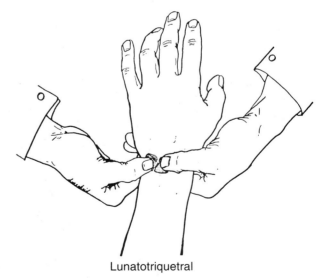

Lunatotriquetral

Ballottement Test

Fig. 23-20. Ballottement test (anteroposterior gliding of the triquetrum). The lunate is the fixed bone. A positive test is excessive laxity or crepitus and pain with this maneuver. It may signify damage to the intraosseous ligaments.

proximal pole. Hence with waist and proximal pole fractures, union is slow and the incidence of avascular necrosis high. Early attention and meticulous treatment are necessary to avoid an unacceptable complication rate. Normal healing times for scaphoid fractures are at least 8 to 12 weeks, and a 12 to 20 week period is common in many series.[44]

Quick Facts

SCAPHOID INJURIES

- Blood supply mainly from distal pole in approximately 30 percent
- High incidence of avascular necrosis
- Fracture management
  -Suspected: cast and check again
  -Nondisplaced: Prognosis good; cast treatment
  -Angulated: One periosteal surface intact; delayed healing
  -gap > 2 mm; consider surgery
  -Displaced: Ligamentous disruption; late instability of carpus; nonunion high (50 percent); osteoarthrosis and pain common; consider open reduction

---

Without displacement, the crack may be invisible or difficult to distinguish. Several clinical tests have been described.

1. Axial compression along the index and middle fingers, which press indirectly on the scaphoid
2. Percussion on the top of the thumb
3. Forced dorsiflexion of the hand
4. Active pronation of the hand against manual resistance

Probably the most reliable sign is the scaphoid fracture test, described by Powell et al.[44,45] (Fig. 23-21). The patient's hand is pronated and gently stressed by ulnar deviation. A positive test is an indication by the patient that there is maximum pain generated in the "anatomic snuffbox." Probably with fracturing, the integrity of the volar stabilizing ligaments is disrupted and this maneuver places stress across the fracture line. This test has a 52 percent positive predictive value, and there were no false negatives in the only series reported.[45] Thus if an athlete presents with a positive scaphoid fracture test, as described above, combined with point tenderness in the anatomic snuffbox (the interval between the abduc-

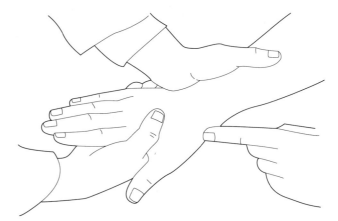

Fig. 23-21. Scaphoid fracture test. Patient's hand is pronated and gently stressed in the ulnar plane. Usually the patient indicates the anatomic snuffbox as the area of maximal tenderness. This is supplemented by directed palpation.

tors and long extensors of the thumb), particularly if associated with swelling, the presumptive diagnosis is a scaphoid fracture and the wrist is protected. Immobilization is usually with a forearm cast, incorporating the proximal interphalangeal joint of the thumb, for 10 to 14 days.

At this point the cast is removed and a repeat roentgenogram of the wrist obtained, out of the cast, with a scaphoid series. These six views of the carpus allow careful inspection of the scaphoid.[46] Usually if no obvious fracture is seen, even with the demineralization at this point, it is safe to treat the injury as a sprain provided there is minimal local tenderness and most symptoms have resolved. Although it is a safe approach, it results in about 60 percent of individuals with suspected scaphoid fractures being cast unnecessarily.[40]

Dias et al. showed that interpretation errors made with the 2- to 3-week films were comparable to those made with the initial films. Indeed most observers are unable to reproduce their opinions consistently when shown the films "blind." The mean percentage error at 2 to 3 weeks is about 40 percent.[44] Thus in view of the potential morbidity and long-term catastrophic sequelae of displaced nonunion, a conservative approach that relies heavily on clinical findings of symptoms is still the wisest approach. Rarely, if the individual is put back into intensive competition, e.g., volleyball, a stress reaction added to the initial injury may lead to a fracture line appearing, even after 3 weeks. This situation is unusual and should be suspected when there is increasing pain and tenderness despite treatment.

Practice Point

SCAPHOID FRACTURES (INITIAL CASE)

- Fracture may not show up on initial film.
- Treat according to symptoms.
- Repeat roentgenogram at 10 to 14 days.
- If still excessively painful re-cast.

The other injury that is frequently misdiagnosed is the perilunar transscaphoid dislocation. Here the fractured scaphoid is associated with a dislocation of the wrist (capitate) off the lunate. Careful examination of the lateral roentgenographic view is the key to this diagnosis. Treatment is usually surgical. Failure to detect it leads to avascular necrosis, carpal collapse, stiffness, pain, and arthrosis.

Depending on circumstances, it is prudent to openly reduce and fix scaphoid fractures in athletes when there is a special demand or time constraint. It is difficult to make hard and fast rules about the possibility and progress of union. In athletes it is best to make definitive decisions early and not wait too long for slowly healing fractures that might result in established, displaced nonunions.[42–44]

Practice Point

SCAPHOID FRACTURES (TREATMENT)

- If undisplaced, cast it, including thumb.
- If displaced, consider manipulation.
- If still step in joint line, openly reduce.
- If union slow, consider early bone grafting ± internal fixation.

The following rules are a reasonable guide to the treatment of the fractured scaphoid.

1. If fracture is undisplaced, use cast immobilization for 8 to 12 weeks. Obtain roentgenogram out of cast at 2 to 6 weeks and 12 weeks. If progressing to union, apply further immobilization and reassess in 4 weeks. If healed, gradually increase mobilization and stress out of cast. May need initial protection for sport.

2. If no obvious sign of union or progress, consider internal fixation and bone grafting.

3. For a displaced fracture, refer to an orthopaedic or hand surgeon, as these injuries usually require open reduction. Permanent displacement disrupts the carpus, causing instability, pain, and arthrosis (Fig. 23-22). This instability is sometimes possible to pick up on clinical examination because, in addition to pain on palpation, passive ulnar and radial deviation may cause crepitus or even a "clunk" (Fig. 23-23).

4. If there is a late diagnosis with proximal pole avascular necrosis, with or without carpal collapse, bone grafting or fusion may be needed depending on the time frame since the initial injury, the type of sport and occupation of the athlete, the symptoms experienced, and the associated carpal instability and arthrosis.

Flake or Avulsion Injuries

Minor ligamentous avulsion of the various dorsal and volar processes are usually treated in proportion to the symptoms they produce; the splinting and activity are progressed accordingly. These injuries should be distinguished from the common anatomic

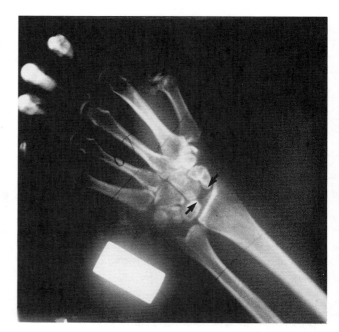

Fig. 23-22. Late carpal collapse with widening of the scaphoid lunate gap (arrows) in the anteroposterior roentgenogram. (Terry Thomas sign). Normal interval is less than 2 mm.

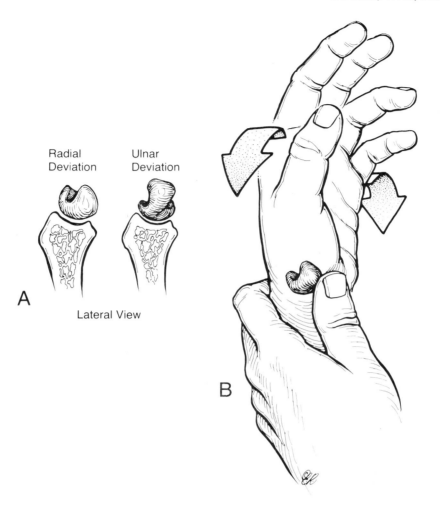

Radial
Deviation

Ulnar
Deviation

A

Lateral View

B

Fig. 23-23. Watson described a clinical test for scaphoid lunate disassociation. It requires experience to interpret correctly. The patient's radius is stabilized by the examiner's hand while the thumb presses firmly against the tubercle of the scaphoid. The wrist is passively moved from ulnar to radial deviation. A positive test is pain, crepitus, and sometimes an audible clunk. (From Green,[40] with permission.)

variations seen in the carpus. On the volar surface, contusion of the pisiform and fracture of the hook of hamate are the commonest. They usually occur during a fall, but may be the result of direct impact from the butt of the handle in tennis, squash, racquetball, golf, and baseball.[49] It is thought that fractures of the hook of hamate may also be the result of violent contraction of the flexor carpi ulnaris. The signs and symptoms usually include tenderness to direct palpation. Gripping and swinging a bat produce pain, but there is usually minimal discomfort on gripping alone or finger and wrist motion. Unless there are symptoms relating to the ulnar nerve, these fractures are generally treated symptomatically.

Wrist Ligament Sprains

Falls and contusions to the wrist are common. Overloading the wrist is seen in weight lifting and contact sports such as football. In one study 55 percent of the gymnasts surveyed had experienced significant episodes of wrist pain.[50]

Acute Sprains

Most acute wrist ligament sprains respond well to initial ice and nonsteroidal anti-inflammatory drugs (NSAIDs), support by bandage, tape, or splint, and progressive activity (Fig. 23-24). However, during the initial assessment it is important to rule out fracture

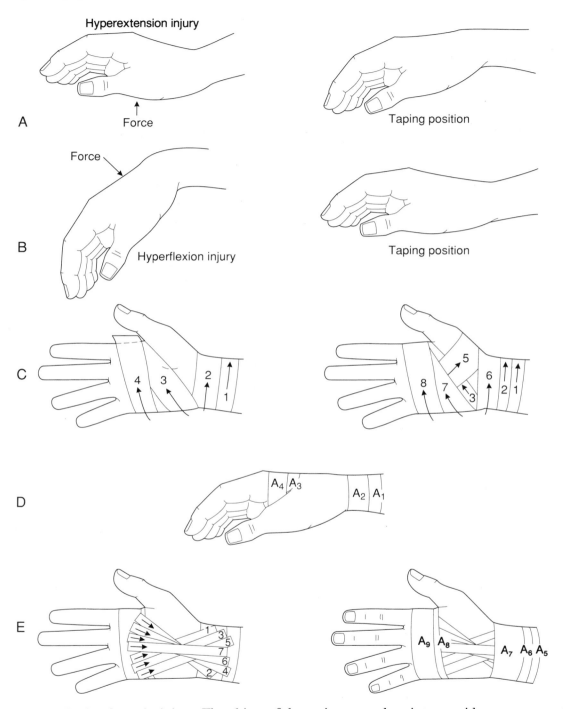

Fig. 23-24. Taping for wrist injury. The object of the taping procedure is to provide some support and perhaps limit the range slightly. **(A)** If the initial injury has damaged the ligaments of the volar surface, the wrist is held slightly flexed. **(B)** By contrast, if the dorsal ligament is sprained, slight extension is usually the position that protects it the most. **(C)** Strapping with 1.5 inch tape. **(D–F)** Alternate method using reinforcing tape — on the volar or dorsal surface to limit excessive extension or flexion as described. (Adapted from Roy and Irvin,[101] with permission.)

and possibly instability, which may require flexion-extension views, with comparison to the opposite side. If symptoms fail to resolve, an alternative diagnosis should be considered, including stress fracture, avascular necrosis, intra-articular chip of bone, synovitis, or benign tumor. A bone scan is helpful for localizing discrete areas of increased uptake or a generalized synovitis pattern (Fig. 23-25). Tomograms with or without arthrography help delineate normally radiolucent chips within the joint. Forced flexion, extension, and ulnar and radial deviation views may unmask abnormal movement patterns of the carpus.

Chronic Injuries

The fibrocartilaginous disc of the wrist acts as a powerful intra-articular ligament, stabilizing the joint and perhaps cushioning the forces transmitted through the lunate and triquetrum[51] (Fig. 23-26). The repetitive "drilling" effect of the ulna on this intra-articular disc during loaded or forced supination and pronation may generate tears or perforation.[52] Studies have linked a positive ulnar variance with perforation of the triangular fibrocartilage disc complex. Over the short term this abnormality may

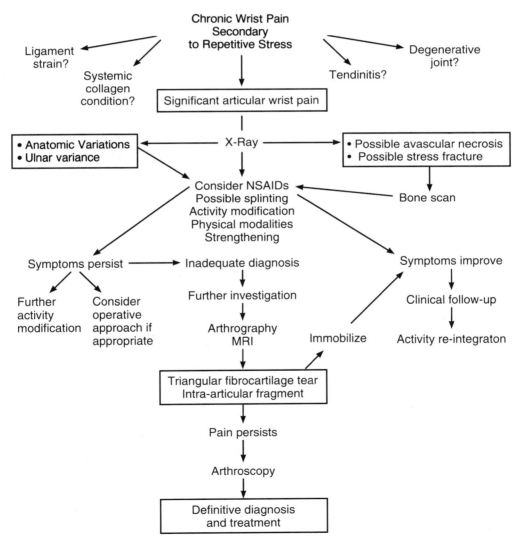

Fig. 23-25. Flow chart of assessment and management of chronic wrist pain.

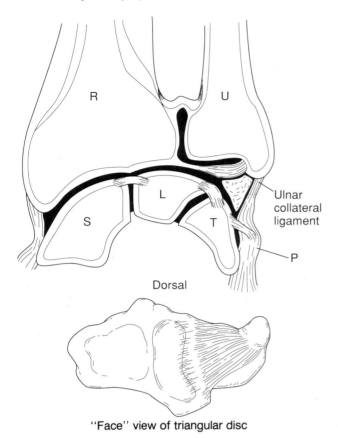

Dorsal

"Face" view of triangular disc

Fig. 23-26. Distal radial ulnar joint, showing separation of that joint by the triangular disc. R = radius; U = ulna; S = scaphoid; L = lunate; T = triquetrum; P = pisiform. (Adapted from Vesely,[51] with permission.)

produce localized tenderness dorsally over the inferior radio-ulnar joint that may be aggravated by pronation and supination. Occasionally, there is a painful or painless click, and sometimes swelling of the wrist. In the long term, chondromalacia and degenerative changes may develop around the lunate and triquetrum.

Evidence of these changes was found in the classic report of Mendelbaum et al. They also emphasized that in gymnasts repetitive compressive impacts of significant duration, frequency, and intensity during development may be important.[50] Particularly the repetitive impact on the epiphyseal structures during certain routines on the pommel horse may have a cumulative negative effect on the normal growth mechanisms. This problem has been referred to as the scaphoid impaction syndrome. If detected early,

these findings suggest a need to modify or limit specific routines in the young gymnast.

There is a variation of this chronic overload syndrome called the radial styloid impingement syndrome, produced by repetitive forced radial deviation. The radial styloid process becomes tender, causing pain in the anatomic snuff box. It is seen mostly in golfers, generated by decelerating the club during backswing.

Treatment

Treatment of these chronic overload syndromes in the wrist consists in modification of activity and splinting or taping according to the symptoms. Ultrasound, ice, and as improvement occurs, gradual strengthening and ultimately functional exercises are added (Fig. 23-27); NSAIDs and intra-articular steroid injections are helpful. If the wrist symptoms are persistent and seriously interfere with activity, surgical exploration and sometimes complete or partial excision of the disk may be indicated.[53] Prior to

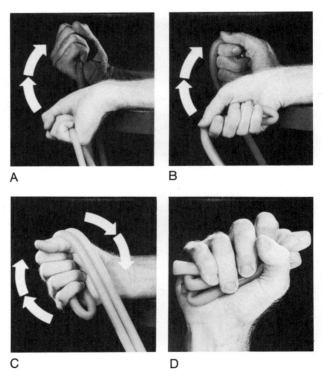

Fig. 23-27. Exercises for the wrist and hand using rubber tubing. **(A)** Wrist flexion. **(B)** Radial deviation. **(C)** Supination or pronation depending on line of pull. **(D)** Grip strength exercise.

this action, the diagnosis is confirmed by arthrogram with or without CT, and in some cases the use of arthroscopy, in which case the surgical correction may be achieved at the same time the diagnosis is confirmed. It requires a small arthroscope and special training and experience.

Fractures and Sprains of the Hand

This section includes fractures of the metacarpals and phalanges of the fingers and thumb, as well as associated joint injuries. They are a common occurrence in hockey, football, boxing, volleyball, cricket, and basketball.

Metacarpal Injuries (Excluding Thumb)

There are five common metacarpal fractures: (1) compacted fractures through the metacarpal neck (boxer's or punch fracture); (2) intra-articular fractures of the MCP joint; (3) transverse or short oblique fractures of the shaft; (4) spiral fractures of the shaft; (5) proximal fracture and fracture dislocation of the metacarpals (Fig. 23-28). The thumb metacarpal fractures and dislocations are discussed separately. Conservative treatment is preferable for most injuries of the hand. However, with some injuries surgical therapy is required for a reasonable outcome, and it is important to recognize these situations. Some sports regulate whether a cast may be worn during competition. Therefore imaginative splinting devices sometimes provide a reasonable compromise.[54,55]

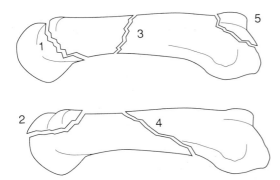

Fig. 23-28. Common fracture patterns of the metacarpals. (1) Neck; (2) intra-articular head fracture; (3) transversal short oblique of the midshaft; (4) unstable spiral fracture; (5) intra-articular fracture of the base to metacarpal and fracture locations.

Principles

1. The intermetacarpal ligaments between the second and third metacarpal heads allow only limited motion and allow the radial side of the hand to form a stable post for the thumb to work against.
2. These same ligaments often prevent wide displacement of fractures.
3. Fractures causing angulation of the midshaft area, particularly the second and third metacarpals, generate significant deformity and are often chronically painful to direct blows. They are subcutaneous, and hence there is little soft tissue padding or masking of the deformity. These injuries should be reduced relatively anatomically.
4. Fractures near the metacarpal neck produce relatively less deformity and interruption of function, particularly the fourth and fifth metacarpal necks. Hence more angulation may be accepted.
5. Rotational deformities do not remodel and therefore cause significant functional problems. Thus a careful inspection for malrotation is important and, if found, it must be corrected.
6. Only limited varus and valgus angulation is acceptable, as it causes functional deficits such as finger crossing with flexion.
7. Widely displaced or multiple metacarpal fractures may require open reduction and some form of internal fixation.
8. Intra-articular fractures may require open reduction or percutaneous fixation unless compatible with treatment by early motion without fixation.
9. If an appreciable percentage of the articular surface is displaced, open reduction is necessary.
10. There is a tendency to overlook these injuries. Therefore careful clinical examination should lead to appropriate roentgenography so the correct treatment may be given at the correct time.
11. Optimal results cannot be achieved without early, active, aggressive rehabilitation.
12. The complications and subsequent disability caused by the mode of treatment and length of immobilization should not exceed the functional loss anticipated from the injury.
13. The hand may need protection for practice and games in contact sports, even after healing, in order to avoid early refracture.

Fractured Metacarpal Neck (Boxer's or Punch Fracture)

Fracture of the metacarpal neck is produced by striking something with a closed fist or by being struck on the hand with direct force. Classically, the term "boxer's fracture" alludes to the neck fracture of the fifth metacarpal. However, the principles are similar across the hand, and the term is frequently used generically to include all metacarpal neck fractures. Interestingly, in the series of Jordan et al., who studied boxing injuries, there were no boxer's fractures even though upper extremity injuries accounted for 32.9 percent of the problems and two-thirds of them were wrist and hand injuries.[56] Unfortunately, a large proportion are the result of fighting at sports or during drunken brawls in other situations. Hence there is merit in the eponym "idiot's" fracture. In any event, the injury is common and frequently overtreated.[57,58]

The deformity is one of dorsal angulation at the fracture site, leaving a depression where the knuckle should be. It may be masked initially by swelling and hemorrhage. A careful inspection is made for associated rotation.

The treatment options include (1) protection of the injured extremity, (2) closed reduction of the fracture, and (3) percutaneous pinning or open reduction and internal fixation. The usual guidelines are as follows.

1. Accept the position and splint the injury if volar displacement produces angles of less than 20 degrees at the second and third metacarpal neck, 30 degrees at the fourth, and 45 degrees at the fifth.[59] It should be stressed that these values pertain only to angulation at the neck. The more proximal the fractures down the shaft, the less is the angular deformity that can be accepted.[60]

2. Manipulation is required if there is any significant rotational deformity or angulation greater than the above values. It is best accomplished by flexing the appropriate MCP joint to tighten the collateral ligaments and reducing via counterpressures through the phalanx and metacarpal shaft. Usually a local or regional block is adequate (Fig. 23-29).

Both of these methods of reduction are well treated by either a gutter splint or hand cast that extends to at least the neck of the proximal phalanx. Padded taping to adjacent fingers helps control rotation. It is not necessary, or desirable, to control the MCP and proximal interphalangeal (PID) joint in flexion,[61] as it would only result in skin problems, stiff joints, and a disability greater than an untreated fracture.

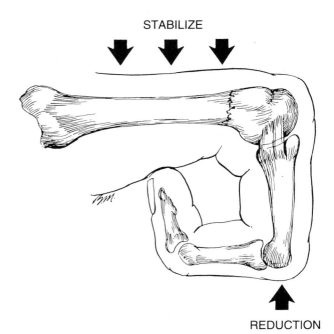

STABILIZE

REDUCTION

Fig. 23-29. Reduction of a volarly displaced metacarpal neck fracture via the 90–90 method. Although an acceptable technique of reduction, this position should not be used for the eventual mobilization because of the possible stiffness of the proximal interphalangeal joints and the potential for ultimate dorsal skin damage. (After Rockwood and Green,[37] with permission.)

3. Occasionally, instability or failure to reduce angulation to an acceptable level necessitates percutaneous pinning with Kirschner wires. Rarely, open reduction with internal fixation is required when percutaneous pinning is not successful or possible, or if there is an extension of the fracture into the joint with displacement.

Intra-articular Fractures

Open reduction is required if a significant percentage of the articular surface is displaced either as a step or a wide fracture gap. Small peripheral fractures are probably better left alone and the principle of early motion used to establish the best functional outcome. To justify open reduction and internal fixation the surgeon must be firmly convinced that: (1) the fracture fragment is large enough for fixation; (2) technically the situation may be improved; and (3) prolonged immobilization will not result because of the choice of fixation. It is a wise surgeon who remembers that a situation can always be made worse by operative interference. Rarely, with gross comminution or an unsatisfactory outcome of previous treatment, consideration must be given to arthroplasty with or without a Silastic prothesis.[54]

Transverse and Short Oblique Shaft Fractures

Transverse and short oblique shaft fractures are best controlled with a well molded short arm cast if minimally displaced. The associated finger is taped (with padding to prevent maceration) to the adjacent finger. Usually a cast change is needed at 7 to 10 days as the edema subsides. Incomplete or undisplaced fractures, particularly of the second and third metacarpals, may not require casting if they are not stressed during activity. Usually, if casting is required, the fracture is stable at 4 to 6 weeks but may need longer protection during games and practice in contact sports. A well padded silicone cast, or some variation thereof, may be safe for the injured athlete and the opponent.[50,60,61]

Long Oblique or Spiral Fractures

Long oblique or spiral fractures frequently have a sharp spike that tents and jeopardizes the skin. They also have a propensity to shortening and of producing a rotational deformity. Hence although closed treatment using a short arm cast and finger taping is possible, more of these fractures require percutaneous pinning or open reduction. Carefully planned surgery and rehabilitation can reduce the tendency to compromised blood supply, adherence of extensor tendons, fibrosis of the interosseous muscles, and infection.[58]

Proximal Fracture and Fracture-Dislocations

Proximal fractures and fracture-dislocations are uncommon and usually are sustained only after considerable trauma. The base of the fifth metacarpal is usually involved. They generally require manipulation and fixation with percutaneous Kirschner wiring, although occasionally open reduction is necessary.

Thumb Injuries

Fractures of the First Metacarpal

The first metacarpal is a particularly frequent site of fracture. The usual mechanism of fracture, particularly intra-articular injuries, is axial compression, as with a punch. However, a twisting injury may produce the same effect. Because the only stabilizing factor is the intrinsic musculature, there is frequently wide displacement of these fracture fragments.

Midshaft fractures, if displaced, are managed by traction, manipulation, and percutaneous transfixion of the fracture site if they are unstable.

Basal fractures of the first metacarpal require accurate diagnosis because they may involve the metacarpal triquetral joint.[62] This joint is the key to thumb mobility.

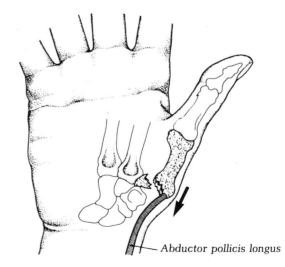

— *Abductor pollicis longus*

Fig. 23-30. Classic Bennett's fracture being displaced proximally by the pull of the abductor pollicis longus.

The Bennett's fracture-dislocation of the first metacarpal is a trans-articular fracture in which a small fragment of the joint remains in its anatomic position held by the strong volar ligament. The whole shaft of the first metacarpal is subluxed proximodorsally by the action of the abductor pollicis longus muscle (Fig. 23-30). Anatomic reduction of the articular surface is mandatory to avoid post-traumatic arthritis with decreased function and chronic pain. The reduction is easy to achieve but difficult to maintain. Thus cast treatment is frequently inadequate, and internal fixation or percutaneous fixation with wire is necessary.

Transverse fractures of the base require only manipulation and immobilization, but any fracture entering the joint, the so-called Rolando fractures, may need some form of percutaneous pin fixation to keep them in reasonable alignment. The choice of treat-

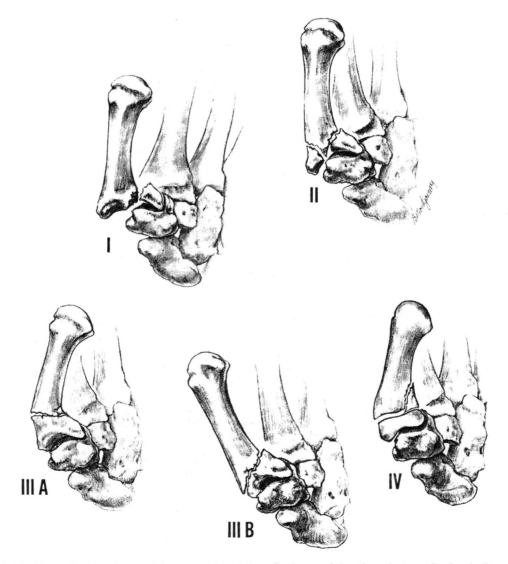

Fig. 23-31. Four distinct fracture patterns involving the base of the thumb: type I, classic Bennett's fracture dislocation; type II, comminuted intra-articular fracture of Rolando. These two are differentiated from type III, an extra-articular fracture whose stability depends on whether the fracture is transverse or oblique. Type IV, epiphyseal separation in the skeletally immature patient. (Adapted from Green and O'Brien,[62] with permission.)

ment depends on the amount of comminution and the degree of displacement[62] (Fig. 23-31).

Ulnar Collateral Ligament Injuries (Gamekeeper's Thumb; Skier's Thumb)

The ulnar collateral ligaments at the base of the thumb stabilize the MCP joint. Integrity of this liga-ment is vitally important, as it stabilizes the joint as the thumb is pushed against the index and middle fingers while performing many gripping motions.[63,64] If the thumb is jammed back, as is commonly seen with line-men in football or hockey players who have thrown their gloves on the ice in order to engage in fighting, this ligament can be severely torn.[64] This injury makes up 60 percent of the upper limb problems associated

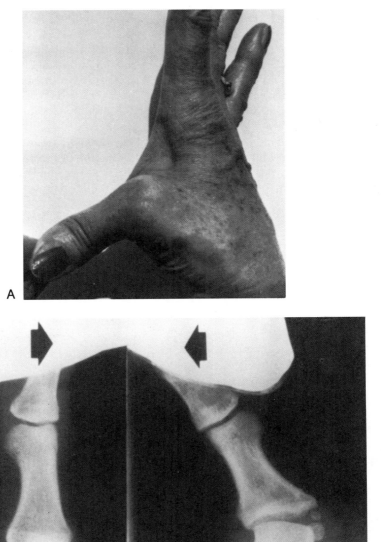

Fig. 23-32. **(A)** Stress view of the first MCP joint showing excessive motion. **(B)** Roentgenogram shows normal stress test, but reveals an angle of more than 35 degrees and a small articular chip, both signifying rupture of the ulnar collateral ligament with valgus stressing.

with skiing and is due to falling with the pole in the hand.[65] Unfortunately, it is frequently overlooked or underdiagnosed, and the result may be chronic instability and severe functional impairment of activities of daily living.

Anatomy. The MCP joint of the thumb allows flexion, extension, and a limited degree of rotation. The range of motion varies considerably among individuals, and even different sides within the same individual; and this variation makes interpreting clinical stress tests difficult.[66] The average abduction motion to valgus stressing of the MCP joint is 20 degrees in men and 25 degrees in women.[66] If stress views show ulnar collateral instability of more than 35 degrees, a ligament rupture is almost certain (Fig. 23-32).

The ulnar collateral ligament is lax in extension and taut in flexion (Fig. 23-33). It has an accessory portion that supports the volar plate. Even if the ulnar collateral ligament proper is completely torn, the accessory portion can support the joint in extension to some degree.

The cartilaginous portion of the volar plate pre-vents impingement of the volar structure during flexion. It also contains the sesamoids. With dislocation of the joint and incarceration of the volar plate, as may occur with a complex dislocation, these sesamoids may be seen within the joint space radiologically, providing a clue to the seriousness of the disruption.

Passive stabilization of the thumb MCP joint is via the capsuloligamentous apparatus provided by the collateral ligaments and volar plate. Dynamic stabilization is generated by the insertion of the adductor pollicis muscle. In particular, it is via insertion through the ulnar sesamoid and hence the volar plate as well as dorsally via the adductor aponeurosis (Fig. 23-34). With disruptions of the ulnar collateral ligament, the proximal end may flip outside the margin of the aponeurosis and hence not re-establish healing to bone, which in turn may lead to chronic instability.

Diagnosis. The history of jamming the thumb into abduction or extension is easily obtained for the acute injury. The ulnar aspect of the MCP joint is swollen and tender, and often there is visible bruising. Insta-

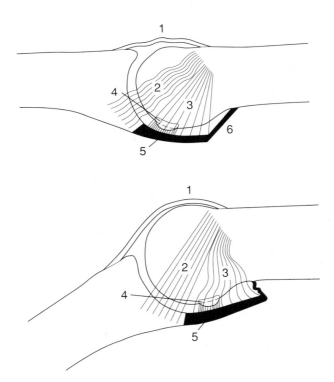

Fig. 23-33. Anatomy of the ulnar collateral ligaments and the associated volar plate. (1) Dorsal capsule; (2) ulnar collateral ligament proper; (3) accessory ulnar collateral ligament; (4) ulna sesamoid; (5) volar plate (cartilaginous portion); (6) volar plate (pars flaccida).

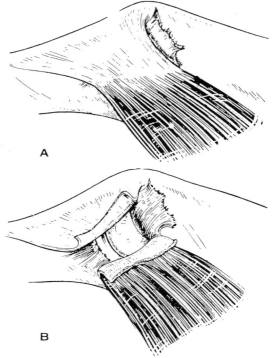

Fig. 23-34. **(A)** Intact adductor aponeurosis prevents reduction of the torn and dislocated ulnar collateral ligament. **(B)** Disruption of the aponeurosis may allow reapposition of the ligament. This structure is usually divided surgically for ligament repair.

bility is detected by carefully fixing the metacarpal, which in itself can present difficulty, and applying radial or abduction stress to the proximal phalanx. The abduction stress should be applied in both extension and flexion, as the MCP joint may be stable in extension with just the ulnar collateral ligament proper involved because the accessory ligament may fix the joint. The application of this abduction (radial) stress is frequently relatively painless in complete disruption.

When the magnitude of abnormal motion is in doubt, the examination may be repeated using a stress roentgenogram. Angulation of more than 35 degrees is abnormal. In any event, films are needed to rule out bony avulsion or, if present, to assess the magnitude of the intra-articular fragment. If stress is generated on the MCP joint for the roentgenogram by the patient opposing the thumb and index finger, there should be a careful check to make sure the force is applied in the correct line to produce optimal abduction stress. The chronic injury is recognized by the instability and functional difficulty.

Treatment. There is some controversy as to the best treatment for the more severe ligamentous disruptions of the first MCP joint. Treatment decisions may

> ### Practice Point
>
> #### ULNAR COLLATERAL LIGAMENT DISRUPTION (SKIER'S THUMB)
>
> - It is frequently underdiagnosed.
> - Make sure ligaments are adequately tested.
> - Stress views with an opening of more than 35 degrees signify complete tear.
> - Stress is applied in both extension and slight flexion to ensure integrity of both bands of the ligament.
> - Look for small bony avulsion.
> - Second degree injuries require support or immobilization.
> - Third degree injuries may require surgery.

be modified by the occupation, sport, recreation, goals, and time of season for the individual concerned.[63,64]

For the mild but painful first degree injury with no detectable instability and the less severe second degree injury, early mobilization and adjunctive treat-

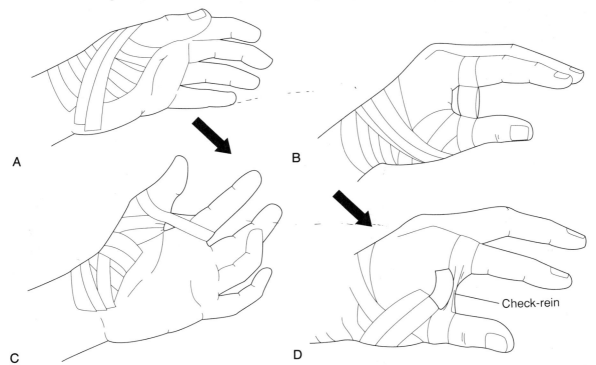

Fig. 23-35. Thumb taping techniques with the addition of a check-rein, which protects the ulnar collateral ligament. **(A)** Thumb spica **(B)** and **(C)** strip of tape connecting proximal phalanx of thumb and index finger. **(D)** Check-rein folded to give additional strength.

ment with therapy in the form of contrast baths, NSAIDs, ice, and ultrasound are compatible with an excellent outcome. The thumb should be protected by strapping or taping for practice and games if further injury risk is deemed likely[67] (Fig. 23-35).

Those with more severe second degree injuries and athletes with third degree tears for whom, for some reason, surgery is not advised may be given some form of modified thumb spica for 3 to 6 weeks. This therapy is compatible with a good outcome in many instances. Further cast or taping protection is continued during risk activities for another 3 to 6 weeks. Depending on the magnitude of the disruption, as the ligament gains strength and heals, the spica may be removed for hygiene and controlled motion by adapting it with Velcro fasteners[68,69] (Fig. 23-36). Small avulsions with little or no articular surface, along with undisplaced larger fragments, are also amenable to nonoperative treatment. The spica may or may not include the wrist and can be positioned to allow the specific function of the sport, provided the MCP joint is in an optimal healing position (Fig. 23-37).

Surgical repair is indicated for severe third degree tears of this ligament because it is most compatible with a stable functional outcome. Furthermore, if roentgenography reveals a significantly displaced bony fragment large enough to support pin fixation, open reduction guarantees the best outcome.

Dislocations: Normal and Complex

First MCP Joint Dislocation. Dislocation of the first MCP joint is an uncommon injury but is particularly seen in football linemen. Usually the deformity makes the diagnosis obvious, and for the most part reduction is easily achieved with long axis traction. If the alignment is satisfactory, a thumb spica cast for 4 weeks, with protection from significant stress for another 4 weeks is reasonable treatment. Late instability may require surgery to correct the specific ligament problem.

The importance of this lesion, as was alluded to in the section on skier's thumb, is to distinguish it from the MCP joint dislocation in which the volar plate invaginates into the joint. This lesion rarely reduces

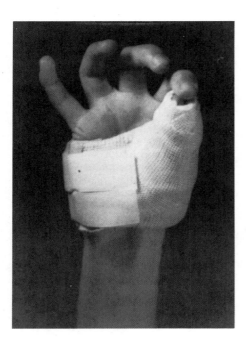

Fig. 23-36. Mobilization of the base of the thumb with the spica cast, which is adapted for functional considerations. It can be brought above the wrist. Alternatively, with a less severe injury or one further along in the healing process, it can be positioned below the wrist as shown with Velcro straps for ease of removal for therapy of hygiene.

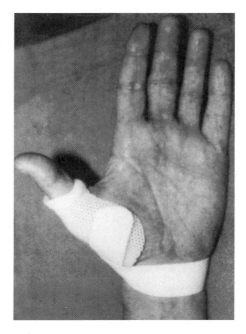

Fig. 23-37. Molded thumb splints for painful first and second degree sprains or recovering third degree injuries. They can be worn during participation and removed subsequently. They are small enough that they may even fit in hockey gloves. (After Nicholas. The Upper Extremity in Sport. C.V. Mosby. St. Louis, 1990.)

by simple traction. Clinically, there may be a dimple over the joint due to the invaginated tissue, and roentgenograms may show the incarcerated sesamoid bone. Thus for all dislocations, failure to reduce with one or two ample efforts at traction, with anesthesia if necessary, should indicate that open reduction with the option for ligament repair and repair of the volar plate is reasonable.

First Interphalangeal Joint Dislocations. Dislocation of the first interphalangeal (IP) joint of the thumb is rare and requires significant disruption of soft tissue. Thus after reduction, adequate splinting is necessary to allow healing. The initial displacement may be sufficient to tear the skin, with dislocation of any of the MCP and IP joints (Fig. 23-38). Adequate débridement, cleaning, testing of tendon function, and confirming integrity of the digital nerves comprise the initial care.

Injuries to the Phalanges

The range of injuries to the phalanges includes contusion, sprains, dislocations, intra-articular fractures, and shaft fractures. The overall principles outlined for metacarpal injuries essentially apply to these injuries. Unfortunately, the magnitude of these inju-

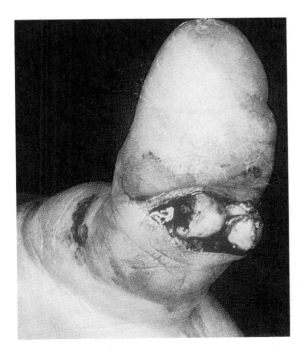

Fig. 23-38. Dislocation of the interphalangeal joint of the thumb sufficient to disrupt the skin and expose the bone.

ries, particularly those involving dislocation, is frequently overlooked because of the ease of reduction and the lack of radiographic evidence of damage. Thus the outcome may be either disabling instability or stiffness, both included under the eponym "coach's finger." "Coach's finger" is a manifestation of a careless approach to a common injury, usually accompanied by the philosophy of: "Reduce quickly, tape it, and let's get on with the game." The basic principles for safe care include the following.

1. Never jeopardize the final results. Although some injuries are compatible with continued play, if there is any question as to the diagnosis or outcome, protect the hand.
2. Never isolate a finger. An injured finger separated from the rest of the hand is more liable to injury. Fractures are subjected to angulatory and rotary stress. These problems may be largely avoided by "buddy taping," i.e., splinting or taping to the adjacent finger.
3. When in doubt, obtain a roentgenogram. The distinction between contusion, sprain, and fracture, particularly intra-articular, may be subtle. When motion is jeopardized, swelling significant, or pain considerable, it is usually worthwhile to obtain a roentgenogram of the injured digit.
4. After initial immobilization there is usually a period of protected motion followed by further splinting or taping to minimize the risk of reinjury during practice and competition (Table 23-3).

MCP and IP Joint Injuries and Dislocations

Joint injuries range from contusion to collateral ligament sprains to dislocations.

Contusion and Collateral Ligament Sprain. Direct blows, particularly to the end of the fingertips, or torsional injuries to the fingers may result in contusion or sprains to the collateral ligaments. These injuries are fairly common, and the main concern is to establish the integrity of the collateral ligaments. If the joint is unstable, usually some form of buddy taping is a reasonable treatment so movement can be instituted early. If the joint is stable, early motion is encouraged. There is often a large component of subperiosteal and joint bruising, and contrast baths are a useful method of reducing discomfort prior to exercise.

Two bowls of water are procured, one filled with ice chips or flakes of ice and the other with fairly warm water. The individual places the hand in the warm water for 45 seconds while moving the fingers actively

TABLE 23-3.   Immobilization and Splinting of Finger Injuries[a]

Injury	Position for Healing	Complete Immobilization (weeks)	Protected Motion (weeks)	Splinting During Competition (weeks)[b]
Fractures				
Metacarpal	Neutral	0–3	3	+6
MCP joint	30° Flexion	3	3	+6
Phalanageal	Depends on stability	4–6	4	+3
PIP and DIP joints	30° Flexion	6	6	+3
Dislocations				
DIP and PIP	30° Flexion	3	3	+3
Tendons and ligaments				
Boutonnière deformity	Isolated PIP in extension	6	6–8	6
Volar plate injury	30° Flexion	3	3	3
Collateral ligament (3°)	30° Flexion	3	3	3
FDP avulsion repair	Slight flexion DIP, PIP	3	3	3
Mallet finger (ED)	Slight DIP hyperextension	6	6	6

MCP = metacarpophalangeal; PIP = proximal interphalangeal; DIP = distal interphalangeal; FDP = flexor digitorum profundus; ED = extensor digitorum.

[a] Guidelines only. Must be adjusted for individual circumstances—"The personality of the injury."

[b] If contact sport or risk activity for hand.

and then places the hand in the cold water for 15 seconds. This 1-minute cycle is repeated 10 to 15 times, and during this period a fair amount of exercise is achieved. During the early postinjury period it can be repeated several times in the evening and even over the course of the day when convenient. Other methods of mobilizing the hand consist in the use of wax baths or ultrasound under water to the small joints.

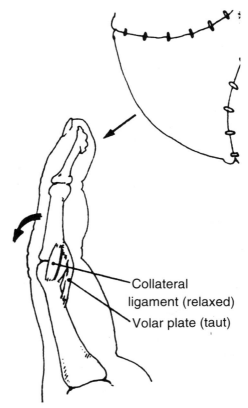

Fig. 23-39. Hyperextension injury with damage to the vulnerable collateral ligaments of the volar plate. This injury may present clinically as either a jammed finger, subluxation, or dislocation.

Practice Point

CONTRAST BATHS FOR FINGER INJURIES

- Obtain bowls of warm and cold (ice chips) water.
- Immerse in warm water for 45 seconds.
- Exercise by active or passive range of motion.
- Place in cold water for 15 seconds.
- Repeat sequence ten times.

Dislocation and Volar Plate Injuries. Dislocations of the small joints of the hand signify major ligamentous disruptions. Frequently, the mechanism of injury is forced hyperextension (Fig. 23-39). Thus the deformity is one of the distal bone moving dorsally or laterally. Usually the injury is readily reduced with steady traction, after which the degree of injury must be assessed. This injury is often dismissed as a simple "jammed" finger if dislocation is not apparent or has spontaneously reduced. It must be recalled, however, that there is no "insignificant" hand or finger injury, as each blow that produces tissue damage has the

potential to limit permanently even the simplest functions.[70] Specifically, an inadequately treated volar plate injury may result in a "swan neck" deformity. A roentgenogram should be obtained at the earliest possible time to rule out intra-articular fractures in association with a dislocation (Fig. 23-40).

Soon after injury, the athletes complain of pain in

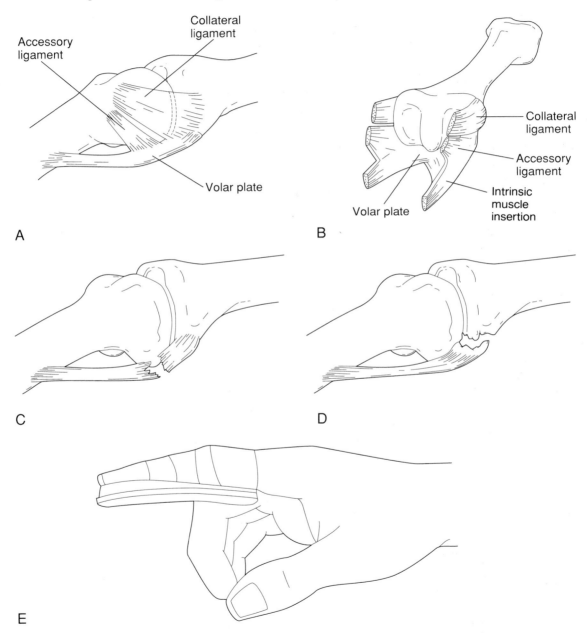

Fig. 23-40. Extension injury to the PIP joint. **(A)** Anatomy of the collateral ligament. **(B)** Volar plate. **(C)** Rupture of the volar plate. **(D)** Avulsion fracture of the base of the middle phalanx. **(E)** Correct splinting technique at 25 to 30 degrees of flexion.

the proximal (PIP) or distal (DIP) interphalangeal joint area. They hold the finger in a mildly flexed posture if there has been spontaneous reduction. The degree of swelling and dislocation vary depending on the amount of damage and the time since injury. If there is a volar plate injury, careful examination can establish the degree of stability. If both the volar plate and collateral ligaments are damaged at the PIP joint, the instability is considerable. A small volar chip is further evidence of the hyperextension mechanism. If the chip involves a significant amount of the articular surface (25 to 30 percent) with volar displacement, surgery may be indicated; this possibility is best evaluated and carried out by an experienced hand surgeon.[70]

Dislocations of the MCP joint may be more difficult to reduce if the volar structures become incarcerated within the joint. If a single, well applied technique of traction fails to reduce the finger, roentgenograms can be obtained to rule out fractures and then consideration given to either another attempt at reduction under more adequate anesthesia or even open reduction to ensure that the soft tissues have been restored to their normal alignment.

Usually the MCP joint is reasonably stable following reduction after wound healing. For best protection the initial treatment for this injury is "buddy taping." The definitive care usually involves splinting the finger at about 20 degrees of flexion at the involved joint. It should be left for 7 to 10 days, after

---

TABLE 23-4.   Finger Injury with Suspected Volar Plate Trauma or Dislocation

Examination
1. Athlete complains of pain in the PIP joint area with or without motion and holds the affected finger slightly flexed.
2. The physician should get a complete history including:
   a. Mechanism of injury.
   b. Right- or left-handed.
   c. Current or planned occupation.
   d. What tasks he does with his hands.
3. The physician should begin the examination by looking for other hand and finger injuries.
   a. Note pattern of swelling and amount of discoloration at the joint (which depends on the degree of injury and the length of time after the injury).
   b. Note patient's ability to actively move the MCP, PIP, and DIP joints.
   c. Check for pain during flexion and local tenderness at the volar aspect of the PIP joint. Palpation can help differentiate which structures are involved.
   d. Examine the integrity of the collateral ligaments to assess PIP joint stability.

Radiology
1. Most finger injuries with swelling and bruising require roentgenograms.
2. A "negative for fracture" roentgenogram does not eliminate the likelihood of ligamentous injury or volar plate rupture.
3. Check for a chip fracture (a small fragment of bone avulsed from the volar aspect of the middle phalanx). It is often present with volar plate injuries and alerts the clinician to the serious nature of the injury.
4. If the x-ray film shows an avulsion fracture that constitutes a significant portion of the articular surface (25 to 30%) with volar displacement of the fragment, the injury may require surgery and should be evaluated by a hand surgeon. The mechanism that usually produces this injury is a severe direct blow to the finger rather than simple hyperextension.

Early treatment
1. Immediate application of ice is always helpful to decrease swelling and discomfort.
2. After the diagnosis is made, the finger should be splinted with the PIP joint in approximately 20° of flexion.
3. Apply the splint with nonallergenic paper tape from the fingertip to the MCP joint, with the tape completely covering the finger so a tourniquet effect is avoided.
4. The splint should be left on for 7 to 10 days. After this period it may be removed three or four times each day for the next 2 weeks for active range of motion exercises. It should be worn at all other times.

Rehabilitation
1. As movement increases and the joint returns to a near-normal, comfortable range of motion, the splint need not be used, although the finger may remain swollen for many weeks.
2. Giving the athlete an idea of what will take place during rehabilitation alleviates anxiety.
3. Significant improvement in range of motion usually occurs within a week of resuming activity.
4. Protect the finger by buddy-taping or splinting for 6 to 8 weeks after injury.

(Adapted from Melchionda and Linberg,[70] with permission.)

which time the splint may be removed three to four times each day for the next 2 weeks for range of motion exercises. The finger must be protected during sports participation for at least 6 weeks. Unfortunately, the finger is usually sensitive or uncomfortable for up to 3 to 6 months, and it must be protected during this period. In addition, a follow-up examination should be arranged to ensure that the joint has not become unduly stiff and that the home rehabilitation program is being followed (Table 23-4).

Fractures

Intra-articular Fractures. Intra-articular fractures of the MCP or IP joint are treated much along the same line as any intra-articular injury. Whenever there is significant displacement or a large fragment, attempts must be made to reduce the anatomic configuration of the joint surface. When the articular fracture involves the volar fragment, there is a tendency for subluxation and dislocation of the more distal bone dorsally (Fig. 23-41).

Phalangeal Shaft Fractures. These fractures are essentially divided into stable and unstable lesions, and the major concern is shortening and rotation (Fig. 23-42). The degree of deformity due to any angula-

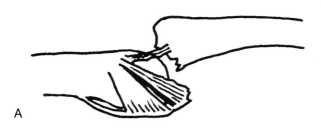

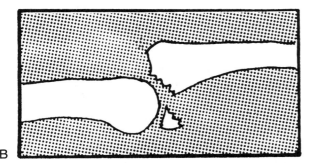

Fig. 23-41. Unstable fracture of the PIP joint. **(A)** It is frequently a ligamentous disruption that allows dorsal displacement. **(B)** A lateral roentgenogram would reveal the position of the fragment as well as the degree of subluxation.

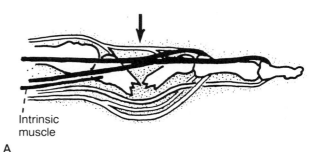

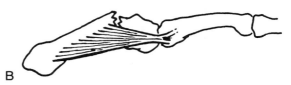

Fig. 23-42. Deforming forces acting on an unstable fracture. **(A)** Intrinsics flex the proximal fragment of a midshaft or basal proximal phalangeal fracture. **(B)** Intrinsics conversely produce dorsal angulation with a base–neck metacarpal fracture. (After Burton et al.,[23] with permission.)

tion is assessed, and when necessary reduction is carried out. In instances where there is a long oblique fracture line with shortening and rotation, internal fixation is required. Usually postfracture or postoperative immobilization consists in a molded splint for 2 to 4 weeks with the institution of gentle motion at the earliest possible time compatible with stability of the fracture.

NERVE INJURIES

Nerve injuries to the hand are not common in sport, but they do occur frequently enough in association with tendon inflammation or secondary to trauma that they warrant discussion. Clinical diagnosis and assessment demands a knowledge of anatomy, particularly muscle innervation (Fig. 23-43).

Median Nerve Entrapment (Carpal Tunnel Syndrome)

Median nerve entrapment syndrome at the wrist (carpal tunnel syndrome) was first described by Sir James Paget in 1854.[71] In athletes it is seen in association with flexor tendinitis as part of an overuse syndrome, particularly in weight trainers, rowers, and skiers. In pitchers and catchers it is possibly secondary to repeated pounding of an inadequately padded

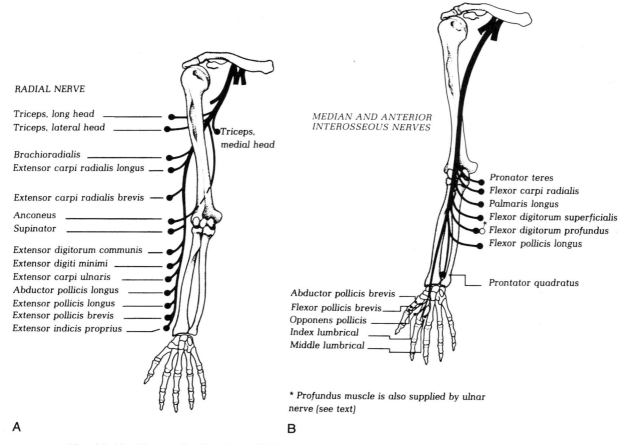

RADIAL NERVE

Triceps, long head _____
Triceps, lateral head _____
•Triceps, medial head

Brachioradialis _____
Extensor carpi radialis longus ___

Extensor carpi radialis brevis ___

Anconeus _____
Supinator _____

Extensor digitorum communis ___
Extensor digiti minimi _____
Extensor carpi ulnaris _____
Abductor pollicis longus _____
Extensor pollicis longus _____
Extensor pollicis brevis _____
Extensor indicis proprius _____

MEDIAN AND ANTERIOR
INTEROSSEOUS NERVES

Pronator teres
Flexor carpi radialis
Palmaris longus
Flexor digitorum superficialis
Flexor digitorum profundus
Flexor pollicis longus

Prontator quadratus

Abductor pollicis brevis
Flexor pollicis brevis
Opponens pollicis
Index lumbrical
Middle lumbrical

* Profundus muscle is also supplied by ulnar
nerve (see text)

A   B

Fig. 23-43. Motor distribution of **(A)** radial nerve, **(B)** median nerve. *(Figure continues.)*

glove. It is also common in the wheelchair athlete for obvious reasons. In many circumstances recreational activity exacerbates an occupationally induced syndrome. Most affected individuals perform tasks daily that demand repetitive digital manipulations.

Anatomy

The carpal tunnel is bounded by bone on three sides and connective tissue on the superficial (roof) surface. The floor is an osseous arch of the carpal bones and the roof; the transverse carpal ligament (flexor retinaculum) attaches to the pisiform and hook of the hamate medially and the tubercle of the scaphoid and ridge on the trapezium medially. The tunnel accommodates the tendons of the flexor digitorum profundus and superficialis in a common sheath and the tendon of the flexor pollicis longus in

an independent synovial sheath. Thus synovitis, or thickening of the synovial covering of these tendons, can generate pressure on the median nerve trapped in this nonexpandable tunnel. The motor fibers of the mixed median nerve supply the first and second lumbricals and almost the entire musculature of the thenar eminence. The exception is the deep head of the flexor pollicis brevis. It also contains the sensory fibers to the skin of the palmar surface, and the extensor surface of the terminal phalange of the radial three and one-half digits provided there is normal distribution of the nerves within the hand. Even in normal circumstances repetitive flexion and extension of the fingers produces increased pressure within the tunnel. There is also a suspected hormonal influence on carpal tunnel syndrome, accounting for the flare-up of symptoms during pregnancy and the prevalence of women in all series.

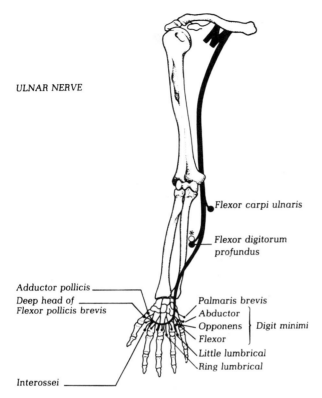

ULNAR NERVE

Flexor carpi ulnaris

Flexor digitorum profundus

Adductor pollicis
Deep head of
Flexor pollicis brevis

Palmaris brevis
Abductor
Opponens } Digit minimi
Flexor
Little lumbrical
Ring lumbrical

Interossei

Profundus muscle is also supplied by median nerve (see text)

C

Fig. 23-43 *(Continued).* **(C)** Ulnar nerve.

Clinical Picture

Pain is usually the presenting complaint, and frequently the initial symptoms are nocturnal. They may wake the patient, and the discomfort is often relieved at first by shaking and letting the hands dangle out of bed. There may be associated morning stiffness, which is also alleviated by movement. The pain may be widespread in distribution, even affecting proximal sites. Daytime exacerbation is related to activity.

The pain of carpal tunnel syndrome is often associated with the occurrence of paresthesia and dysesthesia, which unlike the pain are limited to the areas supplied by the median nerve, initially only the fingertips. As the syndrome progresses, the sensory disturbance may progress to almost analgesia. There is gradually detectable widening of two-point discrimination. The numbness manifests as distinct clumsiness with motor function.

Motor disturbance is a manifestation of more se-

Practice Point

CLINICAL STAGES OF CARPAL TUNNEL SYNDROME

- Stage I
  - Uncharacteristic discomfort in hand
  - No precise localization to median nerve
- Stage II
  - Symptoms localized to territory supplied by the median nerve
- Stage III
  - Impairment of digital function
  - Usually complaints of clumsiness
- Stage IV
  - Sensory loss in median nerve distribution
  - Obvious wasting of thenar eminence

vere compression or prolonged symptoms. Weakness and difficulty with time coordination precede obvious thenar atrophy. The median innervated muscles may be tested by asking the patient to touch the thumb and little finger together so the nails are parallel (Fig. 23-44).

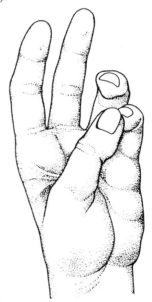

Fig. 23-44. Opposition of the tips of the thumb and little finger tests the integrity of the median innervated hyperthenar eminence. By contrast inability to achieve tip to tip pinch with the thumb and index finger signifies involvement of the anterior interosseus branch of the median nerve.

Autonomic dysfunction occurs less frequently even though 80 percent of the sympathetic fibers to the hand are contained in the median nerve. Hyperhidrosis, skin temperature alterations, erythema and discoloration, and diffuse hypersensitivity to touch may herald the onset of reflex sympathetic dystrophy and should prompt early treatment.

Differential Diagnosis

The differential diagnosis is large because it includes all pain syndromes involving the hand, either in isolation or in combination with motor and sensory loss. Thus a systematic review of proximal to distal sites of potential pathology combined with a consideration of the various tissues prevents overlooking obvious primary or coexisting disease (Table 23-5).

In addition to conditions that may present with hand pain, carpal tunnel syndrome may be a secondary manifestation of a large variety of conditions including trauma (e.g., Colles' fracture), tenosynovitis, metabolic conditions, pregnancy, endocrine disorders, and degenerative changes in the bones of the carpus.

Clinical Tests

The provocative clinical tests for carpal tunnel syndrome include the wrist flexion (Phalen's) test,[72] tourniquet test,[73] median nerve (Tinel's) percussion test,[74] and median nerve compression test. These tests are important screening devices for, and as adjuncts to, electrophysiologic testing.

TABLE 23-5.   Differential Diagnosis of Carpal Tunnel Syndrome

Site	Possible Diagnoses
Nervous system	
Spinal cord	Tumors, syringomyelia, amyotrophic lateral sclerosis
Spinal roots	Disc protrusion, spondyloarthrosis
Plexus	Cervical ribs, Pancoast's tumor, thoracic outlet syndrome
Peripheral nerves	Neuropathy, pronator teres syndrome, tumor (ganglion)
Locomotor system	
Muscles	Dystrophy, myalgia
Tendons	Tenosynovitis, spondylitis, bursitis, periarthropathy
Joints	Rheumatoid arthritis, osteoarthritis

Quick Facts

PRIMARY DISORDERS ASSOCIATED WITH CARPAL TUNNEL SYNDROME

- Trauma
  -Colles' fracture
  -Wrist contusion or hematoma
- Inflammation
  -Tenosynovitis secondary to overuse or other disease
- Endocrine disorders
  -Pregnancy
  -Hypothyroidism
  -Diabetes mellitus
  -Menopause
- Metabolic disorders
  -Gouty tophi
- Others
  -Anatomic variants (accessory muscle belly)
  -Ganglion in carpal region
  -Osteoarthrosis of carpal bones

Wrist Flexion (Phalen's) Test

For the Phalen's test, the patient actively places the wrist in complete but unforced flexion (Fig. 23-45). If numbness and tingling are produced or exaggerated in the median nerve distribution of the hand within 60 seconds, the test is positive. This test is the most sensitive and useful of the provocative tests. A positive reaction is easily elicited in 70 to 80 percent of individuals with proved carpal tunnel syndrome, and it has a specificity of 80 percent and a 20 percent false-positive result rate.[75]

Tourniquet Test

For the tourniquet test a pneumatic blood pressure cuff is applied proximal to the elbow and inflated higher than the patient's systolic pressure. It should provoke paresthesia or numbness in the thumb or index or long finger within 60 seconds to be positive. This test is the least reliable, with only 65 percent of patients with proved carpal tunnel syndrome testing positive. There is a 40 percent false-positive rate among normal individuals, and its specificity in patients with positive electrophysiologic tests is 60 percent.[75]

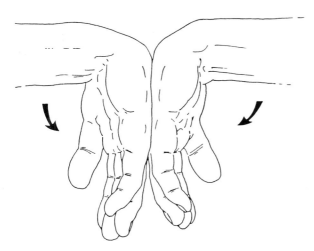

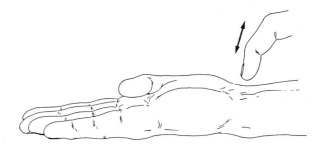

Fig. 23-46. Median nerve percussion test (Tinel's sign). Tapping over the center of the carpal tunnel at the wrist may produce tingling or paresthesia distal to the point of pressure (positive test).

Fig. 23-45. Wrist flexion (Phalen's) test. Positive test is the onset of tingling or numbness in the thumb or index or middle finger within 60 seconds. (After Magee,[20] with permission.)

Median Nerve Percussion Test

In the median nerve percussion test the examiner gently taps the area over the median nerve at the wrist (Fig. 23-46). A positive test induces tingling in the fingers. This test is the least sensitive of the three provocative tests, with only 44 percent of patients with proved carpal tunnel syndrome testing positive. However, it is also the most specific in that it only has a 6 percent false-positive rate in the control group.[75]

Median Nerve Compression Test

For the median nerve compression test the examiner sits opposite the patient and grasps the patient's median nerve (Fig. 23-47). The direct pressure at the proximal end of the carpal tunnel (distal flexor wrist crease) is exerted equally over both wrists. The first phase is the time taken for symptoms to appear (15 seconds to 2 minutes). The second phase is the time taken for the symptoms to disappear after release of pressure.[76] This test is usually specific for carpal tunnel syndrome, but the sensitivity is unknown.

Two-point discrimination allows some determination of peripheral nerve function but does not localize the lesion sufficiently that it can be used alone. Approximately one-third of individuals with carpal

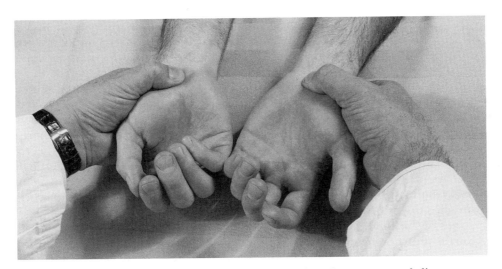

Fig. 23-47. Median nerve compression test. Examiner's thumb exerts equal direct pressure at the proximal end of the carpal tunnel over the median nerve of both hands. A positive test is the appearance of symptoms (paresthesia or numbness) within 15 to 120 seconds.

tunnel syndrome have an abnormal test (6 mm or more).

Electrophysiologic Testing

Electrodiagnostic tests are not infallible, and a small percentage (8 to 10 percent) of individuals with carpal tunnel syndrome have normal values. Usually the first abnormality to be noted is a decrease in sensory amplitude. Increased distal latencies are diagnostic.

Practice Point

ELECTROPHYSIOLOGIC TESTS

- Verification of diagnosis
- Ruling out proximal disease
- Recognition of diffuse polyneuropathy
- Assist in assessing magnitude of compression
- Assessing outcome of therapy

Currently accepted limits of abnormality include (1) motor terminal latency in excess of 4.5 ms; (2) sensory antidromic terminal latency in excess of 3.5 ms; or (3) a differential of 1 ms or more between hands regardless of absolute values if the clinical symptoms fit. In addition, a conduction latency in excess of 6 ms or the presence of fibrillations indicates advanced compression and should prompt early surgical decompression.[77]

Treatment

Nonoperative treatment starts with making sure all associated medical conditions are optimally controlled. When there is an element of tenosynovitis, NSAIDs may be used; and if the response is partial or symptoms quickly recur after suppression, a course of prednisone over 8 days may be given, starting with 40 mg for 2 days and tapering by 10 mg every 2 days. However, the protracted use of NSAIDs just to allay some of the symptoms of the condition is not advisable. They are probably functioning as analgesics in this situation and thus allow continuing nerve damage. In some situations a short course of diuretics may help terminate an acute onset of edema around the wrist.

If the sensory symptoms are intermittent in nature and less than a year in duration, a single injection of cortisone combined with neutral splinting for 3 weeks is worth trying. There should be no evidence of thenar muscle atrophy. There is usually a transient response to this regimen in 80 percent of individuals, and about half of them have permanent relief.[78]

Practice Point

INDICATIONS FOR INJECTION

- Symptoms mainly intermittent
- Less than a year's duration
- Severe sensory deficit not present
- No marked thenar atrophy

If injection is used, the technique is important. The safest method is to identify the tendons of flexor digitorum superficialis to the long finger (the ulnar side of palmaris longus when present) at the distal flexor crease by asking the patient to move the digit. The needle is then inserted with the finger held in flexion until contact is made with the tendon. The patient is then asked to extend those fingers so the needle is carried into the midportion of the carpal tunnel to the ulnar side of the median nerve. The needle is then slightly withdrawn and the corticosteroid injected.

This therapy should be supplemented by the use of neutral position resting splints, sometimes ultrasound making sure to avoid direct sonation of the nerve, and gentle stretching of the wrist area, provided it does not exacerbate the symptoms. Patients likely to fail this regimen include those over age 50 years with associated stenosing tenosynovitis, constant severe paresthesia and atrophy at the thenar eminence, and measurable sensory deficits.[78]

Surgical therapy is indicated if there is a failure of nonoperative treatment, or if there is significant thenar atrophy or sensory loss in the distribution of the median nerve, and if the lesion is demonstrated to be in the carpal tunnel.[78] Most published series report over 85 percent near-complete resolution of symptoms; however, there are complications of the procedure, including further damage to the nerve, inadequate release, neuroma in the palmar sensory branch, and reflex dystrophy.[79,80] With long-standing symptoms and muscle wasting, it may be wise to add neurolysis to the release of the carpal tunnel.[81]

Ulnar Nerve Entrapment (Guyon's Canal)

The ulnar nerve may be damaged in the region of the hypothenar eminence owing to repetitive blows, as is seen with baseball catchers, or chronic pressure, as is seen in cyclists who ride long distances leaning on the handle bars. The pathology is one of pressure on the ulnar nerve as it passes into the hand through the pisohamate, or Guyon's canal (Fig. 23-48). Occasionally a ganglion in the proximity of the canal presses on the ulnar nerve.

Guyon's canal is a fibro-osseous tunnel, the floor of which is formed by the pisohamate ligament, an extension of the flexor carpal ulnar tendon. The passage is obliquely orientated between the pisiform bone and the hamate, and through it passes the ulnar nerve and artery. The roof is provided by the fascia underlying the palmaris brevis. It may be that the contraction of the palmaris brevis, by tightening its fascia, protects the underlying nerve and artery against prolonged overlying compression or traumatic insults associated with prehensile maneuvers.

The signs and symptoms of ulnar nerve problems include altered sensation in the area of the little finger and, with continued trauma or pressure, atrophy and progressive paralysis of the muscles of the hypothenar eminence as well the interossei and the medial two lumbricals. Thumb adduction may be tested by having the patient pinch a piece of paper between the thumb pad and the radial side of the index proximal phalanx (Fig. 23-49). The muscle that powers this maneuver is the adductor pollicis; and when it is weak, usually signifying ulnar nerve involvement, the thumb interphalangeal joint flexes in an attempt to hold onto the paper (Froment's sign). This action allows use of the long thumb flexor, which is innervated by the median nerve and is thus spared with ulnar paresis. Using this evaluation the hands are compared.[23]

The interossei abduct and adduct the fingers and thus may be tested by asking the patient to spread the fingers. This movement may be resisted. A refinement is to ask the athlete to place the hand flat on the table, elevate the middle finger, and then deviate it radially and ulnarly. This movement tends to eliminate use of the extrinsic extensors, which may mimic this action.[23] Finally, the hypothenar muscles—the abductor digiti minimi, flexor digiti minimi, and opponens digiti minimi—which are ulnar-innervated, are evaluated as a group by asking the patient

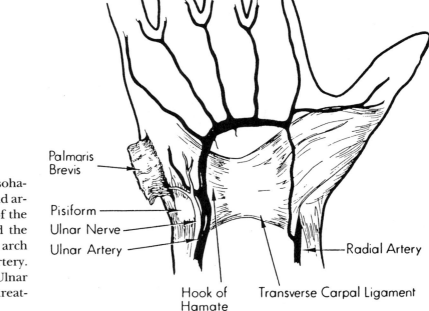

Fig. 23-48. Anatomy of the pisohamate canal with the ulnar nerve and artery. Also depicted is the course of the ulnar artery within the hand and the anastomotic superficial palmar arch with its connection to the radial artery. (After Koman LA, Urbaniak JR: Ulnar artery insufficiency: a guide to treatment. J Hand Surg 6:16, 1981.)

Palmaris Brevis

Pisiform

Ulnar Nerve

Ulnar Artery

Hook of Hamate

Transverse Carpal Ligament

Radial Artery

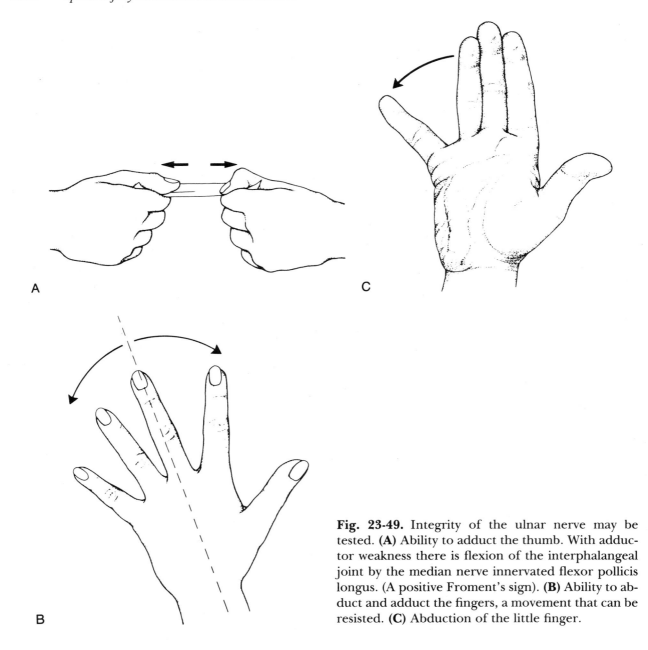

A

B

C

Fig. 23-49. Integrity of the ulnar nerve may be tested. **(A)** Ability to adduct the thumb. With adductor weakness there is flexion of the interphalangeal joint by the median nerve innervated flexor pollicis longus. (A positive Froment's sign). **(B)** Ability to abduct and adduct the fingers, a movement that can be resisted. **(C)** Abduction of the little finger.

to bring the little finger away from the other fingers (Fig. 23-49). It is usual to palpate the contraction of the muscle mass simultaneously. With chronic severe ulnar palsy there may be sufficient wasting and secondary intrinsic contracture to give the classic clawing of the ring and little finger (Fig. 23-50).

Frequently the symptoms are mild and resolve when pressure is relieved. For the cyclist in particular,

change in grip from the top to the sides of the handlebars as well as the use of additional padding is usually sufficient to prevent this problem from recurring. If the symptoms persist, it is important to differentiate pressure in Guyon's canal from that of the cubital tunnel syndrome with involvement of the ulnar nerve at the elbow. Lower cervical root pathology must also be eliminated as a cause of the dysesthesia in the

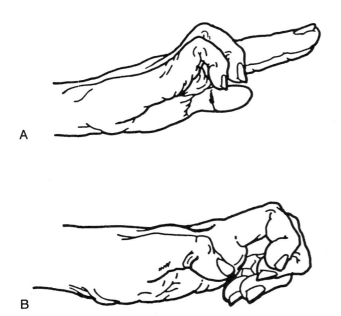

Fig. 23-50. Late deformity in ulnar nerve paralysis. **(A)** Contractures due to wasting of the intrinsics of the ring and little fingers. **(B)** Associated median nerve paralysis produces the classic claw hand with involvement of all fingers in the hyperthenar eminence.

hand. Rarely, when this syndrome fails to resolve after relief from the precipitating causes, surgical exploration of the canal is required with decompression of the ulnar nerve.

CIRCULATORY DISORDERS

Circulation to the hand in athletes is altered in a variety of circumstances that basically fall into four categories: (1) digital ischemia syndrome; (2) ulnar artery thrombosis; (3) aneurysms; and (4) Raynaud's phenomenon. The more general problems of compartment syndrome to the forearm and sudex dystrophy, as it involves the hand, are also mentioned.

Digital Ischemia Syndrome (White Finger Disease)

The signs and symptoms of digital ischemia syndrome include numbness, stiffness, cyanosis, pallor, and often a positive digital Allen's test (Fig. 23-12). This condition, seen most often in baseball pitchers and catchers, handball players, volleyball players, and

exponents of the martial arts, frequently involves the index finger.[82-84]

> **Practice Point**
>
> **WHITE FINGER DISEASE PRESENTATION**
>
> - Intermittent white painful finger
> - Usually the index finger
> - Aching and numbness
> - Often positive digital Allen's test
> - Delayed healing of wounds on finger
> - May even have ulceration
> - Decreased digital perfusion possible on arteriogram

The etiology is probably one of repeated trauma producing episodes of spasm of the ulnar artery or more permanent diminution of perfusion due to secondary changes. In most of these individuals the digital vessels are compressed within the lumbrical canal. Hypertrophy of the lumbrical muscles or thickening of the palmar aponeurosis is responsible for the compression. In pitchers it is aggravated by the prolonged hyperextension of the PIP joint to increase speed and spin of the ball.

Treatment includes additional padding to gloves, reducing the amount of direct trauma, prewarming the hand prior to activity, and applying physiotherapy to restore range of motion. If these measures fail or the condition is severe, the vessel within the digit may be decompressed by resecting Cleland's ligaments or the palmar aponeurosis.

Ulnar Artery Thrombosis (Hypothenar Hammer Syndrome)

Thrombosis of the ulnar artery and the superficial palmar arch, first recognized by Von Rosen[85] in 1934, is found most frequently in the laboring population who use the hand as a hammer or utilize pneumatic tools. In sport it is most frequently seen in baseball, karate, judo, and handball where there is repetitive blunt trauma to the hand, touring cyclists with prolonged pressure from the handlebars, and occasionally with a single episode of severe blunt trauma.

The ulnar artery is most vulnerable to injury immediately distal to the volar carpal ligament (Fig. 23-48). At this point the relatively exposed distal ulnar artery and superficial arch may be repeatedly traumatized by being struck against the hook of the hamate. The ulnar artery, vein, and nerve are also predisposed to trauma within the confines of the relatively inflexible Guyon's canal. Trauma may lead to episodes of spasm, which if prolonged may allow distal vessel occlusion.[86] Further ischemia may increase sympathetic tone, leading to more spasm. Distal ischemia can result from embolization of the ulnar artery thrombosis. The thrombosis may be generated by intimal damage.

The common symptoms are pain, cold intolerance, and numbness.[87] The pain is associated with repetitive hand activity and direct contact with the hypothenar eminence. Rest pain and night pain occur in severe cases, where even ulceration and gangrene may be seen. Pain, numbness, and tingling can be precipitated by exposure to cold, smoking, or emotional upsets. More than half of the patients have associated ulnar nerve symptoms of decreased sensitivity, paresthesias, or hyperesthesias. Weakness or stiffness of the hand may be present in the involved fingers.[88]

Physical findings include those of both ulnar artery and ulnar nerve origin. The area of Guyon's canal may be tender. There may be a palpable difference in the temperature of the digits involved, the ulnar side of the hand usually being cool. There may be cyanosis or paleness of the fingers and a positive Allen's test.[89] If the ulnar nerve is affected, there may be a positive Tinel's sign and perhaps sensory changes to testing.

If the history and clinical examination lead to a suspicion of ulnar artery thrombosis, confirmation is achieved by arteriography or thermography. Arteriography reveals evidence of spasm, intimal damage, or thrombosis.

Treatment includes cessation of the precipitating activity and of smoking where applicable. Steroids, anticoagulants, vasodilators, sympathetic blocks, and sympathectomy have been advocated. In cases of significant occlusion by thrombosis, resection of the thrombosed segment with possibility of vein grafting is the treatment of choice.[88,89]

Ulnar Artery Aneurysms

In sports ulnar artery aneurysms are usually due to nonpenetrating injuries, either single or repetitive blows. Damage to the tunica intima and media leads to true arterial aneurysm.[89,90] There is usually a gradual dilatation of the vessel over several days to several months.

The clinical presentation includes an initial ecchymosis, eventually a pulsatile mass, sometimes a palpable thrill, and symptoms relating to compression of the adjacent ulnar nerve. Diagnosis is confirmed by increased uptake during the angiographic phase of a three-phase nuclide screening. Treatment includes early surgery to resect the aneurysm. Decision for restitution of vessel flow versus vascular ligation is based on careful evaluation of the distal circulation.[90]

Raynaud's Phenomenon

Raynaud's phenomena includes painful vasoconstriction followed by vasodilation. The digits go from a white or bluish hue to a reddened postconstrictive phase. This vasospastic phenomenon is most commonly triggered by cold, but may also be initiated by repeated trauma. There is particular sensitivity to cigarette smoke. The vasospastic response may be part of the previously described thrombosis or aneurysmal conditions.

Treatment may include vasodilatory drugs or, if of sufficient severity, surgical sympathectomy. For the most part, desisting from the triggering activities, stopping smoking, and protecting the hand from cold reduce the number of episodes and their severity to the point that they may be tolerated.

Compartment Syndrome

Classically, forearm compartment pressure elevation is secondary to elbow fractures and dislocations or crush injuries and fractures to the forearm. Frequently there is some involvement of the brachial artery. It nearly always has an acute onset and is recognized by its classic symptoms: swelling, discoloration, pain not responding to adequate analgesia, decreased or absent pulse, and subsequent onset of sensory change and paralysis. Early diagnosis and aggressive surgical intervention are usually required to achieve a functional outcome.

A chronic or acute exercise-induced compartment syndrome of the forearm is occasionally seen after heavy repetitive upper limb activities, e.g., weight lifting or baseball pitching. Prompt recognition may allow resolution by the use of rest, NSAIDs, and perhaps cooling with ice. However, delay in diagnosis, or the failure of prompt resolution of symptoms makes early surgical decompression essential.

Reflex Sympathetic Dystrophy (Sudex Dystrophy, Shoulder-Hand Syndrome)

Reflex sympathetic dystrophy is a vasomotor dysfunction characterized by hyperesthesia, burning pain, edema, discoloration, and stiffness in the extremities. There are many triggering factors, but the most common in sport is varying degrees of trauma to the hand, particularly if the injury has required significant immobilization. This condition has been described in previous chapters and is mentioned here because of the frequent involvement of the hand.

In the older population, the single most common cause is after a Colles' fracture and in the younger population after an injury to the peripheral nerves. However, in the latter situation, the diagnosis is usually causalgia because of the associated nerve injury. Causalgia, which may be resistant to treatment, produces intractable pain and dysfunction. Similarly, the reflex dystrophy of the hand may be associated with a frozen shoulder and involvement of the whole upper limb. In this wider context, it is referred to as the shoulder-hand syndrome.

The most successful treatment is that which is instituted early in the evolution of this condition, before the symptoms have fully evolved. Usually analgesics are not efficacious, but occasionally NSAIDs help. However, because the edema is associated with alteration in blood flow rather than peripheral inflammatory mechanisms, their success is limited. The early mainstay of the treatment is gentle but firm encouragement to increase the use of the hand. Desensitization techniques and TENS may be effective. The judicious use of splinting and support with elevation of the limb and a sling to minimize edema is sometimes helpful. If there appears to be progression of the syndrome despite early treatment, consideration to the use of α- and β-adrenergic blocking drugs, e.g., phenoxybenzamine 10 to 40 mg four times a day or propranolol 10 to 40 mg four times a day, respectively, may manipulate the peripheral circulation sufficiently to relieve the intense vasoconstriction. Calcium channel blocking drugs (nifedipine 10 to 20 mg tid) have also been used, as they tend to produce vasodilatation and may interrupt the painful discharges from the injured extremity that serve to retrigger the exaggerated response and the associated increased sympathetic tone.

TENDON INJURIES

This section deals with a miscellaneous group of tendon problems, including avulsions, tendinitis, infection, Dupuytren's contracture, and trigger finger. There is a frequent association between phalangeal dislocations, intra-articular fractures, and tendon injuries; and hence this aspect must always be considered in the assessment of these joint and bone injuries.

Tendon Anatomy

Although most tendons are surrounded by a loose areolar paratenon, the flexor tendons of the fingers and thumb are surrounded by a special condensation of fibroareolar tissue known as the digital sheath. The sheath consists of an inner synovial layer and an outer fibrous layer. The synovial layer has a visceral portion that intimately surrounds the flexor tendons and a parietal portion that lines the undersurface of the fibrous layer. The fibrous layer itself is condensed into a series of annular and cruciate pulleys that keep the tendon applied to the bone during flexion movements. The tendon sheath receives its blood supply from segmental perforating vessels that arise from the digital arteries in the palm and within the digit itself through a variable number of fine suspensory structures called vincula, which form as anchors for the tendon as well as a passageway for the vessels (Fig. 23-51).

By holding the flexor tendons close to the axis of motion of the finger joints, the pulley system commits a maximum amount of angular motion at the joint for a minimum amount of excursion of the tendon. Thus a total of only 3 cm of tendon excursion is necessary for a full 270 degrees of total finger joint angular motion. To achieve this efficiency, the pulleys must be spaced far enough apart that they can "accordion" as the finger flexes yet be strategically placed to avoid bowstringing.[91] Proper pulley balance is important and is easily disrupted with surgery to the finger. Whenever possible the system is preserved with primary tendon repair or grafting.

Tendon forces are usually a reflection of the load applied to the fingers during varying pinch and grasp maneuvers. Theoretic tendon forces in the flexor digitorum profundus and superficialis tendons are 2.5 to 3.5 times the pinch or grasp loads. Thus with precision maneuvers using pinch forces of up to 10 kg and sometimes more, tendon forces can reach 25 to

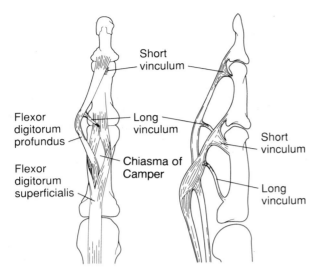

Fig. 23-51. Anatomy of the flexor tendon system. The flexor digitorum profundus (FDP) passes through the split in the flexor digitorum superficialis (FDS) on its way to insert on the base of the distal phalanx. Short and long vincula act as anchors and serve as a passageway for the vascular supply to the tendon.

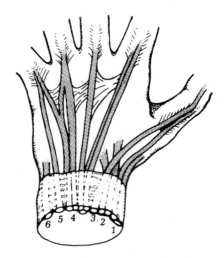

Fig. 23-52. Extensor tendons on the dorsum of the wrist with the six tendon sheath compartments.

35 kg. Power grips of 50 to 60 kg or more can obviously produce even greater values even though the force is usually distributed among all the fingers of the hand.[92] Thus it should be borne in mind that these forces exceed the tendon holding force for the various sutures after tendon repairs. Passive flexion and active exercises without extrinsic loading usually generate less than 0.5 kg of tensor force and therefore are considered more acceptable methods of maintaining tendon gliding during the repairative process.

Testing Tendon Functions

Tendons on the Dorsum of the Wrist

The tendons of the large extrinsic extensor muscles of the forearm cross the dorsum of the wrist in six tendon sheath compartments (Fig. 23-52). After trauma, nerve injury, or suspected tendon rupture, the tendons passing through each compartment are systematically checked. An established routine is more important than the order. Resisted motion is always accompanied by palpation to confirm tendon action.

The first compartment contains the tendons of the abductor pollicis longus inserting into the base of the thumb metacarpal and those of the extensor pollicis brevis on its way to the base of the proximal phalanx of the thumb. They are evaluated by asking the patient to bring the thumb directly out to the side (Fig. 23-53).

The second compartment contains the tendons of the extensor carpi radialis longus and brevis, which insert at the base of the index and middle metacarpals, respectively. They are tested by asking the patient to make a tight fist and extend the wrist. The examiner resists the lateral side of the dorsal wrist (Fig. 23-54).

The third dorsal compartment contains the extensor pollicis longus tendons, which curve around the dorsal tubercle of Lister to the base of the distal phalanx of the thumb. They are tested by asking the patient to extend the tip of the thumb while lifting it off of a flat surface (Fig. 23-53).

The fourth compartment contains the extensor digitorum indices and communis. The fifth contains the extensor digiti minimi. These tendons as a group are tested by straightening the fingers. The isolated extensors to the index and little fingers are tested by straightening the specific digit while the others are curled under to make a fist (Fig. 23-55).

The sixth dorsal compartment is for the extensor carpal ulnaris, which inserts on the base of the fifth metacarpal. By ulnar deviation with only slight exten-

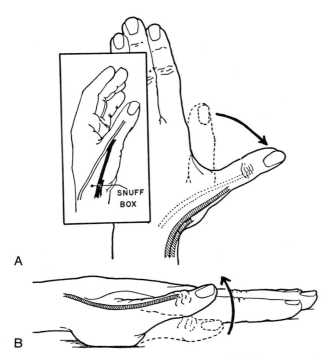

sion, this tendon is fairly well isolated. The patient is asked to push the hand out to the side (Fig. 25-54).

Tendons on the Flexor Surfaces

The flexor tendons to the fingers accompany the median nerve through the carpal tunnel. Flexor digitorum superficialis is individually tested by asking the patient to bend the finger at the middle joint (PIP). The other fingers are stabilized so as to block profundus function (Fig. 23-55).

Flexor digitorum profundus is tested by stabilizing the middle phalanx of each finger in turn and then asking the patient to flex up the tip of the finger. The flexor carpi ulnaris and radialis and palmaris longus are palpated to confirm contraction as a forceful or resisted wrist flexion is performed. Flexor pollicis longus, whose tendon inserts into the distal phalanx of the thumb, is evaluated simply by the ability to bend the tip of the thumb (Fig. 23-56).

Occasionally there is an anomalous tendinous connection between the flexor pollicis longus and the index profundus (10 to 15 percent of hands). Flexing the thumb maximally into the palm may be associated with flexion of the distal phalanx of the index finger (Fig. 23-56). Active stretching of the index finger into extension produces discomfort (Linburg sign). This anomaly may be associated with the clinical picture of discomfort in the palm or wrist with a persistent pinch position.[93]

Fig. 23-53. **(A)** Test for abductor pollicis longus and extensor pollicis brevis. The patient is asked to bring the thumb directly out to the side. **(B)** Test for extensor pollicis longus. The patient is asked to extend the tip of the thumb while lifting it from a flat surface. The rest of the hand must be kept flat on the surface. (After Burton et al.,[23] with permission.)

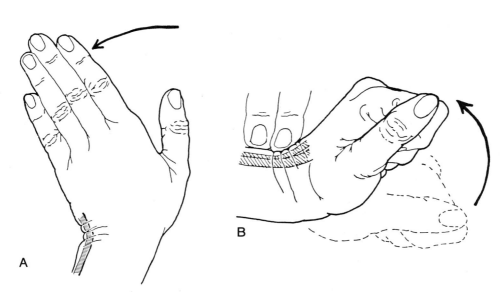

Fig. 23-54. **(A)** Test for extensor carpi ulnaris. **(B)** Test for extensor carpi radialis longus and brevis. (After Burton et al.,[23] with permission.)

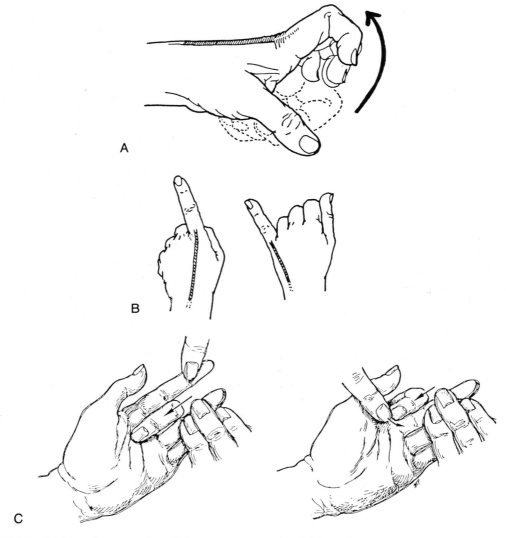

Fig. 23-55. **(A)** Test for extensor digitorum communis. **(B)** Test for extensor indices and extensor digiti minimi. **(C)** Test for the flexor digitorum superficialis. Note that the distal end of the phalangeal joint of the index finger must be lax to confirm the superficialis tendon function to the index.

Principles of Healing and Repair

Tendon Healing

The goal of tendon healing is to allow strong reconstitution of the tendon itself without strong adhesions forming, which would link the healed site on the tendon to the scar tissue response of the surrounding sheath and other tissues. With minimal trauma at the time of surgery, satisfactory nutrition pathways, and early judicious use of motion, it is often possible to allow healing without permanent adhesions.[94] There

is evidence to support the concept that tendons with good vascularization heal with fewer restricting adhesions than those that have impaired vascularity and hence impaired nutrition.

Nutrition is supplied to the tendon via two routes: the previously mentioned vascular nutrition via the vincula system and supplemented by synovial nutrition. This latter synovial route of nutrition is accelerated by active finger motion, which apparently causes pumping of nutrients into the tendon, similar to the mechanism found in the articular cartilage of joints.

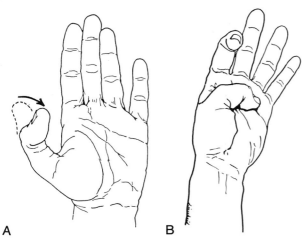

Fig. 23-56. (A) Testing for flexor pollicis longus tendon function. **(B)** Linburg's test for symptomatic interconnections between the flexor pollicis longus and the flexor index profundus. Thumb flexion is associated with flexion of the distal phalanx of the index finger.

These observations lend support to the current concepts that strive for tendon sheath preservation and early mobilization after tendon injuries.

Technique of Tendon Repair

The previous paragraph should lend support and emphasize the importance of minimizing operative trauma and unnecessary injury to tendon sheath integrity. Because special training and constant practice are required to hone surgical skills in this area, it is appropriate that, whenever possible, significant tendon injuries should be treated by surgeons who devote a significant portion of their practice to hand injuries. Whenever possible, direct suturing provides the best outcome. The concept of a "no man's land" for tendon resuturing is not uniformly valid, and surgical decisions should be made to suit the individual injury.[95] Whenever possible, all tendons should be preserved and repaired. Frequently, lacerations into the hand go through both tendons, i.e., flexor digitorum superficialis and profundus, and the practice of excising the superficialis and repairing only the flexor digitorum profundus has been abandoned by most hand surgeons.[96]

Postoperatively the rehabilitation principle should reflect the previously described anatomy and pathophysiology of healing. The main goals are to minimize adhesion, restore active range of motion, prevent

disruption of the repair, and ultimately restore function.

In the past the best position of immobilization for the hand was thought to be with the wrist at 20 degrees of extension, the fingers flexed to 45 degrees at the MCP joints, and slight flexion of the IP joints. The thumb was held in the midabduction, midopposition position. However, it is now believed that a modification of this functional position, the position of "protection or hoe-hand," is better for immobilization after trauma in order to stretch the intrinsic muscles and collateral ligaments. In this position the wrist is extended, the MCP joints are flexed, and the PIP and DIP joints are extended. The thumb is abducted from the plane of the palm. The most frequently encountered complications of hand injuries include adhesions of tendons and stiffened small joints.

Dressings should be applied after completion of assessment and immobilize the hand in the appropriate position, e.g., the position of protection. Dressings should not produce circular constriction. Tight dressings can result in ischemic changes with excessive edema and increased fascial compartment pressure.

Clinical Point

REPAIR OF TENDON INJURIES

- Repair all tendons where possible primarily.
- Initial immobilization:
  -Wrist extension
  -MCP joint flexion 45 degrees
  -PIP and DIP extended
- Movements aid nutrition and reduce adhesions.
- Start with passive-assisted exercise.
- At 6 weeks:
  -Passive stretching of joints
  -Active-resisted work
- At 8 weeks progress strengthening.

Few surgeons permit active flexion of the repaired tendons until 3 weeks after injury. Most then recommend protected active mobilization for 2 to 3 weeks, incorporating some passive-assisted flexion and extension, making sure to avoid forceful extension. At about 6 weeks after the injury or repair, more active resisted flexion can begin, and any residual joint contractures can be passively stretched. Strengthening of the repaired tendon can begin after 8 weeks.[95]

Flexor tendon repair provides results superior to those seen with tendon reconstruction using a tendon graft. Relative contraindications to primary repair includes severe wound contamination, multiple level tendon injury, significant loss of tendon substance by crushing or infection, or associated conditions that render the patient incapable of cooperating with the postoperative therapy program. Although ideally the repair should be performed within a few hours of the injury, delays as long as 2 to 3 weeks are still compatible with a satisfactory outcome subsequent to primary tendon repair. If multiple tendons are lacerated, all should be repaired.

In summary, when tendon lacerations and injuries occur in athletes, prompt efficient treatment by an experienced surgeon yields satisfactory results in about 90 percent of individuals.

Avulsion Injuries

Extensor Tendon Injury (Mallet Finger)

Mallet finger is a common injury usually the result of forced flexion of the distal phalanx while the extensor tendons are actively trying to extend the digit. The baseball catcher, football receiver, basketball player, and blocker at volleyball are all vulnerable. The thin extensor tendon is torn in its substance or

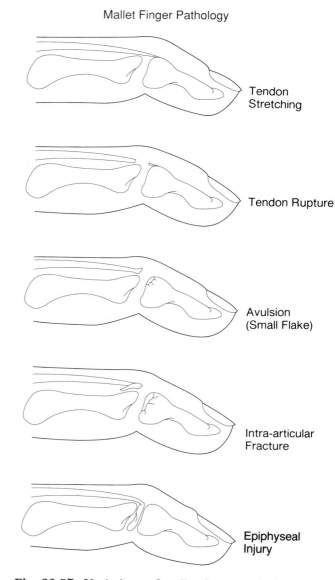

Mallet Finger Pathology

Tendon Stretching

Tendon Rupture

Avulsion (Small Flake)

Intra-articular Fracture

Epiphyseal Injury

Fig. 23-57. Variations of mallet finger pathology.

pulls off a small piece of bone at its insertion. In the young individual with an open growth plate, the injury appears much the same, but the pathology is different because there is an epiphyseal plate injury. The extensor tendon inserts onto the epiphysis proximal to the fracture line, whereas the flexor tendon inserts distally beyond the epiphyseal growth plate (Fig. 23-57).

On examination, there is flexion deformity, which initially may be minimal. There is inability to actively extend the distal joint. Passive extension is usually

---

Quick Facts

MALLET FINGER (CLASSIFICATION)

- Type I
  -Avulsion of tendon from distal phalanx
  -Most common
- Type II
  -Avulsion fracture distal phalanx
  -Less than one-third of articular surface
- Type III
  -Avulsion fracture distal phalanx
  -More than one-third of articular surface
  -DIP joint may be unstable
- Type IV
  -Epiphyseal injury in skeletally immature
  -Usually Salter I or II

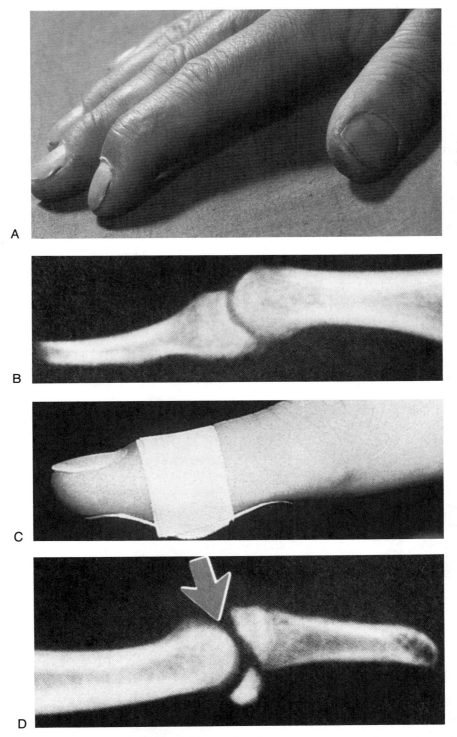

Fig. 23-58. **(A)** Mallet finger deformity. **(B)** Associated roentgenogram rules out bony injury. **(C)** Small volar splint with finger at corrected position. **(D)** Tendon avulsion with associated dorsal chip. Type III involving more than one third of the articular surface. There is potential instability and significant joint disruption.

relatively painless with the acute extensor avulsion. Passive extension with the growth plate injury usually meets some resistance and causes more pain, as in this situation the fracture is being reduced.

Support can be found in the literature for both nonoperative and operative management. Stern and Kastrup reported early complications in 45 percent of nonoperatively treated cases, but most of them had resolved by late follow-up.[97] Furthermore, a significant number of operatively treated individuals developed complications (of which joint incongruity, fixation failure, and infection featured highly) and often had more permanent sequelae.[98,99] Thus it is easy to overtreat this common injury.

Treatment is splinting of the distal end interphalangeal joint in slight extension. It may be achieved with a dorsally or volarly applied splint (Figs. 23-58 and 23-59). It is important to maintain the extended position and avoid further injury. The extension must be sufficient to overcorrect if there is a small chip of bone and allow the tendon to heal in a short position. There is some danger of forcing the extension too much in that it may impair the blood supply to the skin over the joint, and therefore provision must be made for inspecting the area on a regular basis to ensure that maximum extension has been achieved without jeopardizing the circulation. Skin care is an important part of nonoperative treatment. The splint is periodically removed, avoiding flexion, and the skin swabbed with an alcohol sponge or water, allowed to dry, and the splint reapplied. Such splinting must be maintained for approximately 6 to 8 weeks, after which a night splint or protective day splint may be applied for an additional 4 weeks (Fig. 23-60).[100,101]

Practice Point

MALLET FINGER TREATMENT

- Large flake of bone with instability may require fixation.
- Small flake and tendon avulsion are usually treated nonoperatively.
- Immobilize DIP joint only.
- Maintain slight extension 6 to 8 weeks.
- Check skin regularly.
- May remove splint for skin care but maintain in neutral or extended position.
- Day or night splint only for further 4 weeks.

The extensor tendon is relatively thin, and the healing scar is easily stretched by the thicker, stronger flexor tendons. Inadequately treated, this injury results in a mallet finger deformity, with slight flexion of the distal end of the phalangeal joint. For some individuals it presents a functional problem, and so the treatment of this injury should be relatively aggressive, as indicated. Occasionally, the extensor tendon, having lost its connection to the distal phalanx,

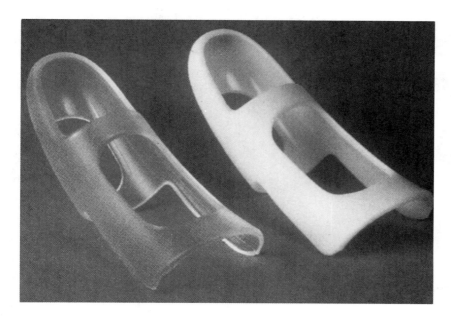

Fig. 23-59. Commercial extension splint for the DIP joint.

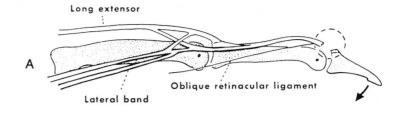

Fig. 23-60. Mallet finger area. **(A)** Avulsion of tendon. **(B)** Small flake of bone. **(C)** One-third of articular surface. Injuries shown in Figs. **A** and **B** are usually treated closed, but that in Fig. **C** may require an open reduction if the joint is unstable.

pulls on the middle joint producing hyperextension (swan neck) deformity (Fig. 23-61).

Should the flake of bone that is avulsed be relatively large and involve one-third or more of the articular surface, it is important to ensure that the fragment is reduced by the extended position and consideration given to fixing the fragment if this reduction is not adequate.[100] The main concerns with the larger fragment are lack of congruity of the articular surface and the tendency of the joint to sublux volarly. It is these considerations that provide an indication for surgical treatment, more than the size of the fragment[102] (Fig. 23-60).

Extensor Tendon Injuries at the PIP Joint

A particularly common closed tendon injury in the athlete is the acute or subacute *boutonnière deformity*. It includes flexion of the PIP joint and hyperextension of the DIP joint. It is the result of disruption of the extensor tendon insertion into the dorsal base of the middle phalanx[23] (Fig. 23-61).

Mechanism

The mechanism may be either a severe flexion force to the PIP joint or a direct blow to the dorsal aspect of the PIP joint with the distal end of the proximal phalanx acting as an anvil against which the central slip is crushed. Frequently, there is a dislocation of the PIP joint, which may or may not reduce spontaneously. Whatever the mechanism, the dorsal ten-

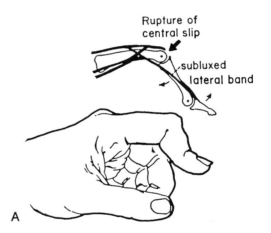

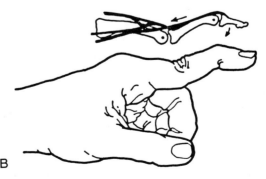

Fig. 23-61. (A) Boutonnière deformity. **(B)** Swan neck deformity.

don is deficient, and the lateral bands slip volarly to the axis of the PIP joint and thus become flexors of this joint. The deformity may not be present immediately after injury but may develop gradually as the lateral bands drift progressively volarly.[23]

Diagnosis

Accurate diagnosis is essential for adequate therapy. Unfortunately, the inability of the athlete to extend the PIP joint completely is attributed to swelling and pain instead of to potential disruption of the tendon.

After appropriate roentgenograms have been obtained to rule out fracture, it may be appropriate to consider a digital block to relieve pain so a more definitive assessment can be made.[63] If after adequate anesthesia the athlete is unable to extend the PIP joint fully and an extension lag of more than 30 degrees persists, serious consideration should be given to diagnosing disruption of the central slip of the extensor mechanism.

Boyes Test. The classic Boyes' test usually is positive only in the chronic stages. If the PIP joint is held passively extended, it is possible for the normal individual to flex the DIP joint in isolation (Fig. 23-62). However, if the central slip has been ruptured, there

is increasing difficulty performing this action. Unfortunately, this test becomes positive only when the proximal part of the ruptured central slip has retracted and become adherent to the surrounding tissues.

Elson's Test. This test has the advantage in that it may be positive immediately after complete rupture of the central slip.[57] The finger to be examined is flexed comfortably at a right angle at the PIP joint, over the edge of a table, and is firmly held in this position by the examiner (Fig. 23-63). The patient is then asked to attempt to gently extend the PIP joint. Any pressure felt by the examiner through extension of the middle phalanx in the posture described can be exerted only by an intact central slip. Final proof is that the DIP joint remains flail during this effort, as

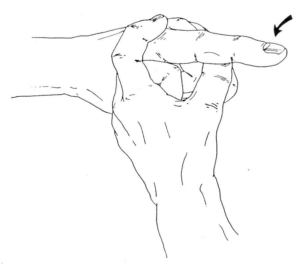

Fig. 23-62. Boyes test. PIP joint is held passively into extension. A normal test is the ability of the individual to flex the DIP joint in isolation. If the central slip has been ruptured, it becomes increasingly difficult to perform this action as the lateral bands become contracted, shortened and adherent. (After Magee,[20] with permission.)

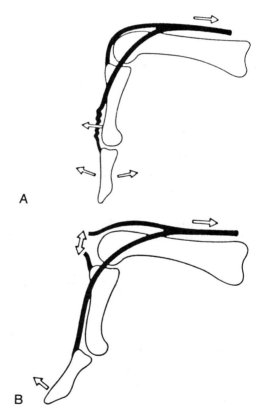

Fig. 23-63. Elson's test. The finger is flexed at right angles at the PIP joint over the edge of a table and stabilized by the examiner. The patient is then asked to extend the PIP joint. **(A)** Extension is achieved at the proximal interphalangeal joint (normal). **(B)** Extension occurs only at the distal joint, through the lateral bands, because the central slip is ruptured (abnormal test).

the competent central slip prevents the lateral bands from acting distally.

In the presence of complete rupture of the central slip, any extension effort perceived by the examiner is accompanied by rigidity at the DIP joint with a tendency to extension. It is produced by the extensor action of the lateral bands alone. This test does not demonstrate partial rupture of the central slip, and its performance may be impeded by pain or by lack of cooperation from the patient. Pain can be relieved, if necessary, by proximal infiltration of the dorsal nerves of the finger. Delayed rupture may occur without significant additional trauma at about 10 to 14 days, and so adequate follow-up is important.

Treatment

Disruption of the central slip or avulsion of a small flake of bone from the base of the middle phalanx in full extension is treated by immobilization in full extension for 6 to 8 weeks. The DIP and MCP joints may be left unsplinted, at least after the first 2 weeks. A night splint, as well as protection during training and competition in "at risk" sports, is necessary for a further 6 to 12 weeks. Unprotected activity should not be allowed until the athlete has full active extension and at least 45 degrees of active flexion.

Practice Point

AVULSION OF CENTRAL SLIP

- Frequently overlooked
- May need local anesthesia to diagnose acutely
- Late deformity—boutonnière
- Splint in extension 6 to 8 weeks
- After first 2 weeks, DIP and MCP joints left out of splint
- Further 4 weeks of night splinting

Flexor Tendon Injury (Sweater or Jersey Finger)

The mechanism of the common flexor tendon injury is almost exclusively one of tackling and grasping a jersey in football or rugby. The sudden marked force exerted on the gripping finger causes avulsion of the strong flexor digitorum profundus tendon from its insertion onto the distal phalanx. Nearly always it is the ring finger that is involved. Sudden pain is experienced but little in the way of deformity. The finger has no characteristic posture, as with the droop of a mallet finger. This diagnosis is missed by casual examination, and the injury is often misdiagnosed as a "sprain" or a "jammed" finger. The functional problem is inability to flex the distal phalanx, which may go unnoticed by the athlete or examiner unless specifically checked (Fig. 23-64). Although athletes may have noticed that the finger was "jammed" or "popped," they frequently ignore it during the excitement of the competition and complain of pain and swelling the next day. Occasionally, a large bone fragment can be pulled off the distal phalanx, producing deformity; and if it does not reduce with the resting position, fixation may be required. For this reason, roentgenography is usually indicated. There is often significant bleeding and swelling within the flexor sheath with the tendon avulsion. The tendon itself may retract.

Usually, splinting in a position of function is adequate treatment; however, when there is a potentially significant functional deficit, consideration must be given to surgical repair of the tendon (Table 23-6). The rare late functional problems may be dealt with by DIP tenodesis or arthrodesis and occasionally by flexor tendon grafting.

Tendinitis

Extensor Tendinitis

Inflammation of the extensor tendons of the wrist and fingers is most commonly seen with cross-country skiing, as an over-use injury, or secondary to a fall in

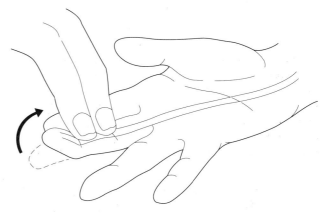

Fig. 23-64. Test for integrity of the flexor digitorum profundus.

TABLE 23-6. Flexor Digitorum Profundus Tendon Avulsion Injuries

Type	Displacement and Pathology	Treatment
I	Avulsion of tendon into the palm. Associated disruption of vincula longa and breva. Disruption of blood supply to tendon.	Surgery during first 5–10 days. Late repair may allow contraction and resorption of tendon.
II	Avulsion of tendon and retraction to the level of the PIP joint. Further retraction prevented by vincula longa. Adequate vascularization of tendon but proximal scarring may interfere with motion of whole finger.	Surgical reattachment of tendon. Late repair acceptable.
III	Avulsion of tendon with an attached osseous fragment. Tendon does not retract past the DIP joint.	If anatomic reduction possible, consider closed treatment. If wide displacement and large fragment, surgical therapy.
IV	Avulsion of small volar flake of bone with some tendon retraction. Associated volar flake of distal phalanx due to infraction during continued forced extension. Roentgenographic diagnosis.	May require open reduction to restore joint continuity. Reinsertion of profundus tendon.

(Adapted from Leddy and Packer,[98] and Buscem and Page,[99] with permission.)

contact sports. Physical examination should attempt to identify the specific tendons involved. Treatment includes modification of activity, ultrasound, laser, and the use of NSAIDs. If this regimen is not sufficient to resolve the problem, consideration of a resting splint and possibly an injection of corticosteroid into the tendon sheath is considered. During the recovery phase there should be specific attention to strengthening the muscles of the forearm, which is probably best started as an isometric or concentric contraction and gradually progresses to eccentric loading, thereby progressively increasing stress on the tendon. Adequate warm-up prior to activity and application of ice during the postactivity phase are important for preventing recurrence.

Flexor Tendinitis

Repetitive bowling and pitching as well as blows and falls, stressing the flexor tendons, may trigger inflammation. There is the additional worry with flexor tendinitis that the increasing volume of the tendon may trigger an associated carpal tunnel syndrome. Essentially, however, in the absence of neurologic findings the treatment parallels that for extensor tendinitis.

DeQuervain's Tenosynovitis (Paddler's Wrist, Hoffman's Disease)

DeQuervain's tenosynovitis is the commonest form of tenosynovitis around the wrist. Originally described by deQuervain in 1895, it involves an inflam-

mation of the tendons of the first dorsal compartment of the wrist, i.e., the abductor pollicis longus and extensor pollicis brevis (Fig. 23-65).

Classically, it presents with pain along the course of the outcropping tendons. Palpation not only elicits tenderness but also occasionally reveals crepitation. All movements of the thumb are usually uncomfortable, but the most dramatic clinical sign is the Finkel-

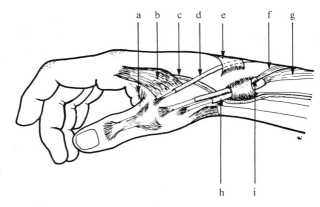

Fig. 23-65. DeQuervain's tenosynovitis involves the sheaths of the long abductor and short extensor tendon of the thumb. (a) adductor; (b) first dorsal interosseous; (c) radial artery; (d) long thumb extensor tendon sheath; (e) dorsal carpal ligament; (f) short thumb extensor; (g) long thumb abductor; (h) long thumb abductor tendon sheath; (i) short thumb extensor tendon sheath.

stein test. The patient positions the thumb within the flexed fingers, and the hand is quickly manipulated into ulnar deviation (Fig. 23-66). Many individuals complain of difficulty when grasping objects firmly.

In many mild cases, simple modification of activity and local therapy in the form of physical modalities supplemented by NSAIDs are sufficient to allow the problem to resolve. When the inflammation is more intense or the duration of the symptoms longer, it is often necessary to consider steroid injection or immobilization with a thumb spica. Combining the latter two therapies is usually successful. The thumb spica is usually applied for about 3 weeks. The injection into the tendon sheath is usually carried out with a 22-gauge needle and a suspension of 1 ml of methylprednisolone (Depo-Medrol) and 1 ml of lidocaine without epinephrine. The needle is introduced 1 cm proximal to the tip of the radial styloid process and angled distally at a 45 degree angle to the longitudinal axis of the long axis of the forearm (Fig. 23-67). Confirmation that the injected material is in the tendon sheath is the observation that the tendon sheath distends distal to the annular ligament of the first dorsal compartment.

The thumb spica extends from the proximal part of the forearm to the IP joint of the thumb and maintains the wrist in 20 degrees of dorsiflexion and the MCP and IP joints of the thumb in midextension. The splint can be removed for bathing and hygiene; once removed permanently, gradual increase in activity is allowed.

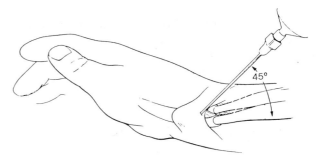

Fig. 23-67. Technique of injecting the tendon sheath in deQuervain's tenosynovitis. (After Witt J, Pess G, Gelberman RH, J Bone Joint Surgery 73A:219, 1991, with permission.)

Trigger Finger or Thumb

A form of stenosing tenosynovitis may occur that manifests as a snapping action of the digit when moving from flexion to extension. It usually occurs in the ring or middle finger and occasionally the thumb. Inflammation, trauma, and congenital variations may generate a discrepancy between the size of the tendon and its pulley at the base of the proximal phalanx. The tendon usually thickens just before it enters the pulley (Fig. 23-68). Apart from the inconvenient "snapping" action, the nodule may be painful to pressure while gripping. If the condition progresses, the finger

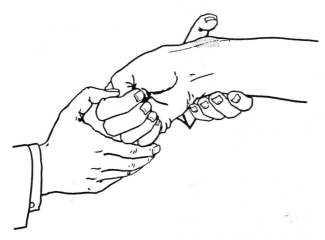

Fig. 23-66. Finkelstein's test for deQuervain's disease. With the thumb held in the palm of the hand, the wrist is ulnar-deviated. A positive test is sharp pain along the tendons of the abductor pollicis longus and extensor pollicis brevis.

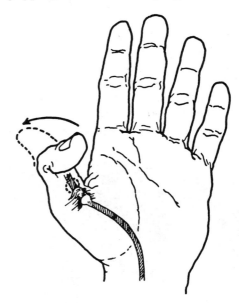

Fig. 23-68. Nodule on the flexor tendon of the thumb producing a triggering action due to relative stenosis of the sheath. (After Burton et al.,[20] with permission.)

may become stuck and have to be moved passively. At an early point, ultrasound, local frictional massage, NSAIDs or steroid injection, and decreased aggravating activities may be effective in relieving symptoms. If the condition progresses, release of the sheath under local or regional anesthesia is usually curative.

Lacerations, Tooth Puncture, Infections, and Ring Injuries

Lacerations

Lacerations to the hand and forearm must be examined with due respect to the possibility of tendon and neural injury (Fig. 23-69). The athlete should be asked to lie down with the hand elevated, preferably with a sterile dressing covering the wound, while gentle direct pressure is applied to help reduce or stop any hemorrhage. The practice of "clamping a bleeder" in the lacerated hand should be avoided because previously undamaged vital structures, e.g., nerve or tendon, may be inadvertently and irreversibly crushed or damaged in what usually amounts to an unnecessary attempt to stem bleeding. Furthermore,

---

Practice Point

DEEP LACERATIONS TO THE HAND

- Stop bleeding by pressure and elevation.
- Clamping bleeders may cause more damage.
- Suspect tendon or nerve injury.
- Confirm integrity by clinical testing, not by probing wound.

---

there is a tendency on the part of inexperienced practitioners to want to look into the wound to see if nerves or tendons have been cut. More can often be learned on the initial examination by covering the wound and performing a gentle, systematic examination of forearm and hand distal to the injury. The areas of sensation should be carefully determined in turn, followed by systematic testing of the functions of the important tendons. Whereas a partially cut tendon may be able to flex the finger, it cannot do so against resistance without causing discomfort.

The position of the unsupported finger should be noted to see if there is a characteristic posture. When the flexor tendon is completely severed, usually the unsupported finger rests in extension. When the extrinsic extensor tendon is completely severed, there is a tendency for the supported finger to remain flexed.

When planning the definitive treatment, the wound should be gently inspected, the depth assessed, and decisions made regarding further treatment: (1) appropriateness of thoroughly cleaning the area and closing with sterile strips or sutures; (2) if débridement is necessary; (3) if a local, regional or general anesthetic is required to explore the wound in an attempt to assess damage and perhaps resuture damaged structures; (4) if there is foreign material within the wound; (5) if the assistance of a specialized surgeon is required because of the extent of the laceration, partial amputation, or nerve and tendon damage; and (6) if a swab should be prepared for culture and sensitivities prior to the possible institution of antibiotic therapy and tetanus immunization.

Roentgenograms of the hand with appropriate views should be obtained to assess associated fractures and to determine if foreign material is present. It should be recalled that some glass, wood, and plastics are not radiopaque, and thus the apparent ab-

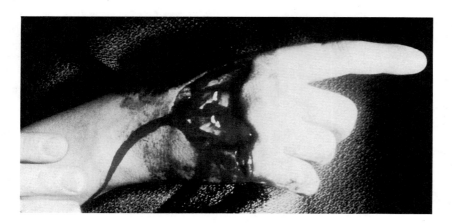

Fig. 23-69. Laceration of the dorsal part of the hand caused by a skate blade. Such wounds must be inspected carefully for tendon and nerve injury. Clamping of bleeders may add to the damage. Usually the most profuse hemorrhage is abated by simple pressure.

sence of these substances on a plain film does not rule out their presence.

Tooth Puncture

Wounds that are caused by a tooth puncture frequently occur over the metacarpal heads where the skin is thin and where often the initial contact of a punch is taken. It should be remembered that the tooth easily penetrates the joint and tendon sheath. Often the wound is relatively small and painless, and it seals over quickly. The organisms in the small wound cavity rapidly multiple and generate a red, hot swollen knuckle. If the wound is seen late, it presents an urgent medical problem necessitating surgical drainage and antibiotics in order to prevent destruction of the joint and spread along the tendon sheaths.

The athlete should be made aware of the seriousness of this injury and be prompt about reporting it. If there is the slightest suspicion that the wound has been caused by a tooth, vigorous washing and rinsing with soap and water should be undertaken, and the wound should not be sutured even if the tendon has been lacerated. Dressing, perhaps buddy taping, and observation may allow rapid return to the sport. Appropriate swabs for culture and sensitivities, followed by antibiotics, should be considered. The wound should be checked within 24 hours, and if there is any evidence of progressive or developing infection, further débridement may be necessary and even admission to hospital for intravenous antibiotics.

Fingertip Injuries

If there is tissue loss at the fingertips, simple direct closure is best when possible. There should be an attempt not to sacrifice length; and if it is not deemed possible, it may be appropriate to apply a small split-thickness skin graft from the lateral side. During wound contraction over the ensuring months, the graft usually shrinks to about 50 percent of its initial size, and the tip of the finger remodels. When bone is exposed, the free graft is a poor choice, and usually more imaginative local pedicles are appropriate. As soon as this treatment goes beyond simple suturing or free graft, it is better to consult a more experienced practitioner.

Ring Injuries

Wedding bands are traditionally worn on the left ring finger, and many people have adopted the style of wearing rings on any or all of their fingers. The medical literature includes many case reports of ring avulsion injuries occurring in sport, on the job, or in the home.[103] They are usually associated with an accidental fall that involves catching the ring on an immovable object while the entire weight of the body is projected forcefully in the direction that pulls the finger out of the ring. The results are variable, but often portions of the finger are avulsed or the finger is completely amputated.

Quick Facts

RING INJURIES

- Class 1
  - Abrasion or bruise to finger
  - Lacerations of skin (minor)
  - No neurovascular impairment
  - No tendon damage
  - No bone or joint damage
- Class 2
  - Extensive lacerations of skin
  - Crushing of soft tissues
  - One neurovascular bundle injured
  - No tendon damage
  - No bone or joint damage
- Class 3
  - Severe crushing of soft tissue
  - Damage to tendons
  - Damage to both neurovascular bundles
  - Bone and joint not damaged
- Class 4
  - Severe crushing of skin
  - Both tendons damaged
  - Both neurovascular bundles damaged
  - Dislocation of joints or fractures

Class 3 and 4 injuries frequently require amputation.

Attempts to salvage a damaged finger are often unsuccessful. Skin, nerves, vessels, tendons, and even bones and joints are disrupted by the extreme force transmitted to a small area of the skin and the underlying structures trapped by the ring. The force often destroys the distal neurovascular structures so that even microsurgical techniques fail to provide a successful outcome.

Fractures and dislocations of the finger are complicated by the presence of rings, which may compromise the circulation with the subsequent swelling. They are difficult to remove, initially because of pain and later because of the swelling.

The dangers of ring injuries are well known in industry, so safety programs forbid the wearing of rings in certain occupations. The dangers of ring injuries are not sufficiently emphasized in sports practice and competition. Routine education of athletes about the dangers of ring injuries is rare. In most sports there is no emphasis on the need to remove rings before participation. Nevertheless, many ring avulsion injuries have been due to individuals catching their rings in volleyball netting, basketball goals, and while rodeo riding. Coaches, therapists, and physicians should be encouraged, if not required, to restrict the wearing of rings in most sports. Likewise, the athlete must be aware of the devastating consequences of ring injuries.[104]

Acute Infections of the Hand

Acute infections of the hand are usually due to the introduction of pyogenic organisms. When pus is present, the common term "Whitlow" is frequently used to describe them. The onset is usually abrupt, and the local manifestations are those of inflammation, i.e., heat, redness, swelling, and pain. Pain may become severe and is worse if the arm is dependent or if there is any pressure on the area. Prompt institution of antibiotic therapy usually aborts an early infection. However, if there is a significant amount of pus with edema and congestion of the hand, often antibiotics are not sufficient to halt the progress of the local infection into the tendon sheath. It may then spread through this system to the rest of the palmar spaces in the hand (Fig. 23-70). Thus, if there is no immediate improvement, it is prudent to admit the patient to hospital and surgically débride the area in order to prevent destruction of the tendons and the tendon sheaths themselves, as well as to try to negate the risk of osteomyelitis.

Paronychia

Paronychia is a troublesome form of subcuticular infection that usually affects the nail folds. It may start during trauma to the corner of the nail or separation and elevation of the eponychium during a manicure (Fig. 23-71). The infection starts on one side of the nail as an acute localized focus but tends to spread rapidly toward the base and around to the opposite side. In some cases the pus burrows deeply toward the bone, as the proximal edge of the nail lies in contact with the phalanx. After a period of time,

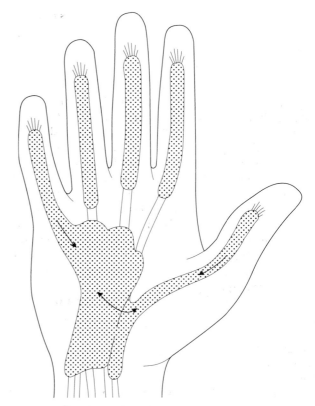

Fig. 23-70. Possible communicating pathways for infection within the hand via the flexor tendon sheaths sometimes referred to as palmar, radial, and ulnar bursas.

pus can be expressed from the various parts of the eponychium. A few weeks later the entire nail may become detached along its base.

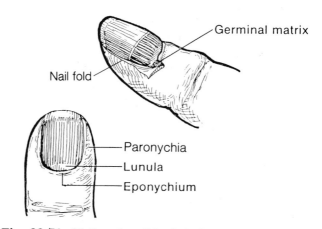

Fig. 23-71. Nail and nail bed. Infection frequently starts in the nail fold, where it is referred to as a paronychia.

Early treatment consists of antibiotics and, if necessary, drainage via a surgical incision. If the infection is long-standing or if progress is not apparent, it is often prudent to remove the nail and treat the infection aggressively in order to preserve a relatively cosmetic digit. Even so, the growing nail may be deformed. Often with the passage of time, if successfully treated, only a small amount of ridging on the nail remains, an acceptable deformity.

Dupuytren's Contracture

The condition first described by Dupuytren in 1834 is not a consequence of athletic activity. It is common enough, however, that it should be mentioned as a deformity of the hand. The condition begins as an insidious onset of thickening and contracture of the palmar fascia. The exact pathophysiology is ill understood, but the earliest manifestations are an isolated nodular thickening usually seen in the line of the flexor tendon of either the ring or little finger, or sometimes both. Later, the nodule may appear in the fascia over the other flexor tendons, but the middle and index fingers are rarely affected. The skin on the distal side of the primary nodule is drawn up into a fold; and after an interval, the finger or fingers become progressively flexed at the MCP and PIP joints. The DIP joint is usually held in extension (Fig. 23-72).

During the early stages, exercise involving hyperextension of the fingers should be prescribed, and the patient should be taught to straighten and contract the fingers themselves at regular intervals. The patient can even be taught to sit on the hands for periods to obtain a prolonged stretching effect. The lesion frequently progresses despite this treatment, and at this point the individual must decide how much the deformity is interfering with day to day function and recreational activities. The surgical treatment is careful radical dissection of the scar and pathologically involved tissue. It is a technically difficult operation and should be performed only by an experienced surgeon.

SKIN AND NAILS

The major skin problems of athletes reflect constant use or friction. Blisters may occur with unaccustomed activity in such sports as rowing and gymnas-

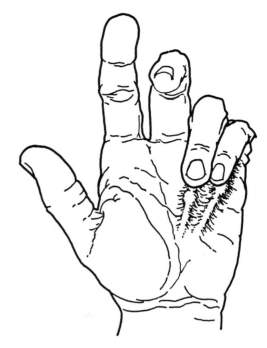

Fig. 23-72. Classic appearance of Dupuytren's contracture involving the ring and little fingers. (After Burton et al.,[23] with permission.)

tics. Usually calluses develop that thicken the palm of the hand, particularly the area over the metacarpal heads. The individual athlete must decide as to the balance between having a thick enough callus to protect the palm versus an excessively thick area that catches on the bar. The latter generates its own trauma and becomes painful owing to secondary edema and bleeding underneath the area. These calluses should be pared at frequent intervals to achieve the optimal thickness.

In many ways the hand is a "mirror" of underlying systemic diseases, and characteristic patterns of deformity and color reflect such problems.[105] This point is particularly true for the nail, where the effects of trauma, disease, aging, and poor nutrition are easily reflected (Table 23-7).

It is not appropriate to cover all of these conditions in a text of this nature, but it must be remembered that the athlete is susceptible to the same spectrum of systemic disorders as any other individual. Thus some specific complaints regarding the hands or nails and the incidental observation of changes during examination for another condition should prompt the appropriate questions in the history, and when necessary, laboratory and radiographic investigation.

TABLE 23-7. Glossary of Selected Nail Pathology

Condition	Description	Occurrence
Beau's lines	Transverse lines of ridges marking repeated disturbances of nail growth	Systemic diseases, toxic or nutritional deficiency states of many types, trauma (from manicuring)
Fragilitas unguium	Friable or brittle nails	Dietary deficiency, local trauma
Hippocratic nails	"Watch-glass nails" associated with "drumstick fingers"	Chronic respiratory and circulatory diseases, especially pulmonary tuberculosis; hepatic cirrhosis
Koilonychia	"Spoon nails"; nails are concave on the outer surface	In dysendocrinisms (acromegaly), trauma, dermatoses, syphilis, nutritional deficiencies, hypothyroidism
Leukonychia	White spots or striations or rarely the whole nail may turn white (congenital type)	Local trauma, hepatic cirrhosis, nutritional deficiencies and many systemic diseases
Mees' lines	Transverse white bands	Hodgkin's granuloma, arsenic and thallium toxicity, high fevers, local nutritional derangement
Moniliasis of nails	Infections (usually paronychial) caused by yeast forms (*Candida albicans*)	Frequently in food-handlers, dentists, dishwashers, gardeners
Onychauxis	Nail plate greatly thickened	Mild persistent trauma; systemic diseases such as peripheral stasis, peripheral neuritis, syphilis, leprosy, hemiplegia; at times congenital
Onychia	Inflammation of the nail matrix causing deformity of the nail plate	Trauma, infection, many systemic diseases
Onychodystrophy	Any deformity of the nail plate, nail bed, or nail matrix	Many diseases; trauma; chemical agents (poisoning, allergy)
Onycholysis	Loosening of the nail plate beginning at the distal or free edge	Trauma, injury by chemical agents, many systemic diseases
Onychoschizia	Lamination and scaling away of nails in thin layers	Dermatoses, nail infections, many systemic diseases, senility, injury by chemical agents, hyperthyroidism
Pterygium unguis	Thinning of the nail fold and spreading of the cuticle over the nail plate	Associated with vasospastic conditions such as Raynaud's phenomenon; occasionally with hypothyroidism

(From Berry,[105] with permission.)

Practice Point

SUBUNGUAL HEMATOMA

- Prompt drainage relieves symptoms and may save nail.
- Minor injury: soak finger in ice water for 10 to 15 minutes.
- Significant bleed: drill hole in nail.
  - Nail drill
  - Hot paperclip
  - Rotating No. 11 surgical blade

The one condition that is frequently related to recreational activity is the subungual hematoma (bleeding under the nail). A hematoma can develop that is exceptionally painful and may incapacitate the person in those sports that require use of the hand. The amount of blood can damage the nail bed itself, and the outcome is loss of a nail, producing further protracted morbidity.

First aid treatment for a nail contusion with a significant subungual hematoma consists in burrowing a hole through the nail to the blood so it can be released, thereby reducing the underlying pressure. The nail should be cleaned with antiseptic solution and a small digital cautery or simply a red hot paper-

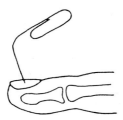

Fig. 23-73. Subungual hematoma relieved by drainage. In this case a hot paperclip is used to develop the channel.

clip can be used to create a channel through the nail, which is insensitive, and into the underlying hematoma (Fig. 23-73). Relief is almost immediate.[101] The procedure should be followed up with an appropriate dressing to protect the wound from exposure to contaminants.

TUMORS OF THE HAND

Stack in 1960 analyzed 300 tumors of the hand and found that 61 percent of them were ganglia over the dorsum of the wrist or in relation to the MCP joints. Ten percent were epidermoid cysts. The nearly 30 percent that remained were more worrisome, and some were frankly aggressive. The latter included tumors of the skin (e.g., fibroma or melanoma), tumors of the tendon sheaths (e.g., synoviomas or fibromas), tumors of blood vessels (e.g., hemangiomas), tumors of the nerves (e.g., neurofibromas), and tumors of bone, particularly enchondromas and osteochondromas. Only the common mucous cyst, glomus tumors, and ganglia are described here.

Mucous Cysts, Epidermoid Cysts, Glomus Tumors

Mucous cysts commonly arise close to the base of the nail, particularly in women after menopause, and accompanying the degenerative arthritic changes of the DIP joints. Although they are easily removed, they have a high recurrence rate.

The epidermoid or implantation dermoid cyst is thought to be related to previous minor injuries with scarring, particularly on the palmar surfaces of the hand or fingers in athletes and manual workers. It is thought that the fragment of skin implanted during the injury develops a cyst consisting of squamous epithelial cells with a fibrous tissue outside this layer; the contents of the cyst are a mixture of proteins and

cholesterols. Alternatively, there may be some epithelialization around a hematoma or inflammatory focus.

The glomus tumor arises from cells that make up the normal neuromyoarterial system, which may regulate temperature and circulation of the digits. These tumors have a predilection for the nail bed and consist of a small reddish mass under the nail that is tender to pressure and even to temperature change. Treatment is usually by excision, which relieves the symptoms dramatically. One of the important features of this tumor is that it must be distinguished from the slightly less common but more important malignant melanoma.

Ganglion

A ganglion is a cystic swelling in the neighborhood of a joint or tendon sheath. It usually contains a clear jelly-like colloid or thick mucinous fluid.

There is usually one large main cyst that is either unilocular or multilocular, but frequently accessory cysts are present. The walls of the cyst contain dense fibrous tissue resembling that of the capsule of the joint. The cyst itself contains the jelly-like colorless fluid of mucin.

The ganglion gives rise to a swelling, occasionally pain, and less commonly impaired function. The swelling can be gradual or sudden in onset, and once established it is often found to fluctuate in size from time to time. The size varies with the local anatomic situation; the largest ganglia usually occur on the dorsal aspect of the wrist. The ganglion is usually tense, although a few are fluctuant. In the hand they are usually found attached to the tendons around the level of the metacarpal heads, and here they are frequently tender and disabling. In the wrist, they most frequently occur on the dorsal surface and are usually found over the articulation between the carpal bones and between the various tendons (Fig. 23-74). Particularly troublesome ones are found lateral to the pisiform bone, where they may press on the ulnar nerve; yet another site is adjacent to the flexor tendons where the ganglion may compress the median nerve in its carpal tunnel.

Treatment of these ganglia is aimed at disrupting the wall and content by direct pressure or by injection followed by aspiration and inoculation with a steroid. However, the tendency for recurrence is high, and the definitive treatment usually includes surgical excision of the ganglion, taking care to reach the base of origin. Obliteration of the defect in the capsule or

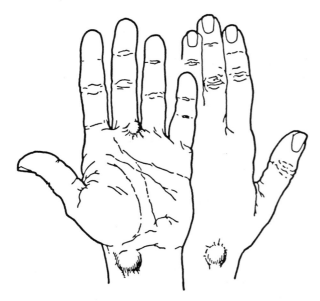

Fig. 23-74. Common locations for ganglia of the wrist and hand. (After Burton et al.,[23] with permission.)

tendon sheath is also helpful for preventing recurrence. Alternatively, the defect in the joint may be left; but for successful surgical treatment, the entire cyst wall must be removed to minimize the chance of recurrence.

SUMMARY

In many respects, the hand is a mirror of disease, as there are numerous pathologic processes that manifest with clinical signs in the hand and nails. For this reason, a chapter of this nature must be highly selective. The emphasis has been on trauma in the athlete, with injury to the small bones of the fingers, associated intra-articular damage, and disruption of the complex tendon and pulley systems, which may lead to long-term disability. There is a tendency to both overlook and undertreat hand injuries. The hand responds poorly to immobilization, and there is a fine line between adequate splinting to permit healing and prevent further deformity, and early mobilization to ensure perfect function. This compromise usually entails a short period of complete immobilization, an intermediate period of restricted motion, and a final period of protected motion during physical activities.

Thorough, intensive, intelligently applied therapy maximizes the successful results of these traumatic disruptions.

Trauma to and dislocation of the carpal bones runs the risk of avascular necrosis because of the tenuous nature of the blood supply. (A large portion of the surface of the carpal bones is articular cartilage, so there is little area available for the passage of blood vessels.) The end result of avascular necrosis can be collapse, instability, and arthritis in the surrounding articulations. Early recognition of this impending problem may allow some measure of protection of the wrist during the healing phases.

There are some unusual conditions directly related to the trauma experienced in some sports. Examples include tearing of the triangular fibrocartilage at the wrist secondary to repetitive loading and pivoting activities, specifically on the pommel horse. Furthermore, these young gymnasts exhibit one of the few documented adverse changes of activity on growing bone when heavy training is pursued relentlessly over a period of years. Early recognition can spare these young gymnasts significant problems.

Lastly, it should be recalled that the final destination of many nerves of the upper limb is the sensitive skin of the fingers and their intricate intrinsic musculature. The repetitive impact and movements of certain sports generate special patterns of nerve injury, particularly that related to the pisohamate canal and the associated ulnar nerve and artery.

The importance of early, meticulous assessment is stressed throughout this chapter. Fortunately, most of the diagnostic tests are easily performed clinically, with a little practice; and most of the sophisticated laboratory work-ups can be used selectively.

It should be recalled that surgery of the hand is a specialized area and there are many intricate yet common problems that require the experience of a surgeon who has been prepared to dedicate a large amount of time to treatment of the hand. Inasmuch as even small anatomic losses can cause huge functional disabilities, and the fact that the hand is relatively unforgiving in terms of allowing a second attempt at correction should the initial treatment fail, each practitioner must be cognizant of the appropriate moment for referral to a more experienced physician. Despite this statement, most hand injuries can be effectively managed with optimal outcome by careful examination and well timed, appropriately progressed therapy.

REFERENCES

1. Reid DC: Selected conditions of the elbow forearm, wrist and hand. J Can Athletic Ther Assoc 10:15, 1983

2. McCormack DAR, Reid DC, Steadward RD et al: Injury profiles in wheelchair athletes: Results of a retrospective survey. Clin J Sport Med 1:35, 1991

3. Reid DC: Functional Anatomy and Joint Mobilization. University of Alberta Press, Edmonton, 1976

4. Reid DC: Assessment and Treatment of the Injured Athlete. Teaching Manual. University of Alberta, Edmonton, 1988

5. MacConnaill MA, Basmajian JV: Muscles and Movements. A Basis for Human Kinesiology. Williams & Wilkins, Baltimore, 1969

6. Napier JR: The prehensile movement of the human hand. J Bone Joint Surg [Br] 38:902, 1956

7. Kaplan EB: Functional and Surgical Anatomy of the Hand. 2nd Ed. JB Lippincott, Philadelphia, 1965

8. Radonjic D, Long C: Kinesiology of the wrist. Am J Phys Med 50:57, 1971

9. Kapandji JA: The physiology of joints: annotated diagrams of the mechanics of the human joints. In Honore LH (translator): Upper Limb. Vol. 1. 2nd Ed. ES Livingstone, London, 1970

10. Hall EA, Long C: Intrinsic hand muscles in power grip. Electromyography 8:397, 1968

11. Kuczynski K: The proximal interphalangeal joint: anatomy and causes of stiffness in the fingers. J Bone Joint Surg [Br] 50:656, 1968

12. Eyler DL, Markee JE: The anatomy and function of the intrinsic musculature of the fingers. J Bone Joint Surg [Am] 26:18, 1954

13. Tubiana R: The Hand. WB Saunders, Philadelphia, 1981

14. Kaplan EB: Guidelines to deep structures and dynamics of intrinsic muscles of the hand. Surg Clin North Am 48:993, 1968

15. Landsmeer JMF: Power grip and precision handling. Am Rheum Dis 21:164, 1962

16. Landsmeer JMF: The coordination of finger joint motions. J Bone Joint Surg [Am] 45:1654, 1963

17. Long C, Brown ME: Electromyographic kinesiology of the hand: muscles moving the long finger. J Bone Joint Surg [Am] 46:1683, 1964

18. Long C, Brown MF, Weiss G: Electromyographic kinesiology of the hand. Part II. Third dorsal interossei and extensor digitorum of the long fingers. Arch Phys Med 42:559, 1961

19. Sunderland S: The actions of the extensor digitorum communis, interosseoius and lumbrical muscles. Am J Anat 77:189, 1945

20. Magee DJ: Orthopaedic Physical Assessment. WB Saunders, Toronto, 1987

21. Tubiana R, Valentin P: Opposition of the thumb. Surg Clin North Am 48:967, 1968

22. Weatherby HT, Sutton LR, Krusen HL: The kinesiology of muscles of the thumb: an electromyographic study. Arch Phys Med Rehabil 44:321, 1963

23. Burton RI, Bayne LG, Bectron JL et al: The Hand. Examination and Diagnosis. American Society for the Surgery of the Hand, Colorado, 1978

24. Von Prince K, Butler B: Measuring sensory function of the hand in peripheral nerve injuries. Am J Occup Ther 21:385, 1967

25. Barron JN: The structure and function of the skin of the hand. Hand 2:93, 1970

26. Hilton J: Rest and Pain. 6th Ed. Bell & Daldy, London, 1863

27. Harty M: The hand of man. Am J Phys Ther 51:777, 1971

28. Cheselden W: The Anatomy of the Human Body. 1st Ed. Privately printed, London, 1713

29. Guyon F: Note sur une disposition anatomique propre a la face anterieure de la region du poignet et non encore decrite. Bull Soc Anat Paris 6:184, 1961

30. Shrewsbury MM, Johnson RK, Ousterhout DK: The palmaris brevis — a reconsideration of its anatomy and possible function. J Bone Joint Surg [Am] 54:334, 1972

31. Reid DC: On handedness, speech and body asymmetry. Can Med Assoc J 107:12, 1172, 1972

32. Dellon AL: Clinical use of vibratory stimuli to evaluate peripheral nerve injury and compression neuropathy. Plast Reconst Surg 65:416, 1980

33. Omer GE: Assessment of hand trauma. Orthop Nurs 4:29, 1985

34. Magee D: Orthopaedic Physical Assessment. WB Saunders, Toronto, 1987

35. Allen EV: Thomboangiitis obliterans: methods of diagnosis of chronic occlusive arterial lesions distal to the wrist with illustrative cases. Am J Med Sci 178:237, 1929

36. Axelrod TS, McMurtry RY: Open reduction and internal fixation of comminuted intra-articular fractures of the distal radius. J Hand Surg [Am] 15:1, 1990

37. Rockwood C, Green D (eds): Fractures. Lippincott, Philadelphia, 1975

38. Leung KS, Shen WY, Tsang HK et al: An effective treatment of comminuted fractures of the distal radius. J Hand Surg [Am] 15:11, 1990

39. Abbaszadegan H, Jonsson U, Sivers K: Prediction of instability of Colles' fractures. Acta Orthop Scand 60:646, 1989

40. Green D: Operative Hand Surgery. 2nd Ed. Churchill Livingstone, New York, 1988
41. Zemel NP, Stark HH: Fractures and dislocations of the carpal bones. Clin Sports Med 5:709, 1986
42. Hill NA: Fractures and dislocation of the carpus. Orthop Clin North Am 1:275, 1970
43. Kuzma GR: Kienbock's disease. Adv Orthop Surg 8:250, 1985
44. Dias JJ, Thompson J, Barton NJ et al: Suspected scaphoid fractures: the value of radiographs. J Bone Joint Surg [Br] 72:98, 1990
45. Powell JM, Lloyd GJ, Rintoul RF: New clinical test for fracture of the scaphoid. Can J Surg 31:237, 1988
46. Leslie IJ, Dickson RA: The fractures carpal scaphoid: natural history and factors influencing outcome. J Bone Joint Surg [Br] 63:225, 1981
47. Hopkins FS: Fractures of the scaphoid in athletes. N Engl J Med 209:687, 1933
48. White SJ, Louis DS, Braunstein EM et al: Capitate-lunate instability: recognition by manipulation under fluroscopy. Adv Orthop Surg 143:361, 1984
49. Parker RD, Berkowitz MS, Brahms MA et al: Hook of the hamate fractures in athletes. Am J Sports Med 14:517, 1986
50. Mendelbaum BR, Bartolozzi AR, Davis CA et al: Wrist pain syndrome in the gymnast: pathogenetic diagnosis and therapeutic consideration. Am J Sports Med 17:305, 1989
51. Vesely DG: The distal radio-ulnar joint. Clin Orthop 51:75, 1967
52. Palmar AK, Werner FW: The triangular fibrocartilage complex of the wrist: anatomy and function. J Hand Surg 6:153, 1981
53. Coleman HM: Injuries of the articular disc at the wrist. J Bone Joint Surg [Br] 42:522, 1980
54. Dobyns JH, Sim FH, Linscheid RL: Sports stress syndromes of the hand and wrist. Am J Sports Med 6:236, 1978
55. McCue FC: How I manage fractured metacarpals in athletes. Physician Sports Med 13:83, 1985
56. Jordan BD, Voy RO, Stone J: Amateur boxing injuries of the US Olympic training centre. Physician Sports Med 18:81, 1990
57. Elson RA: Early test for rupture of the central slip of the extensor hood of the finger. J Bone Joint Surg [Br] 68:229, 1986
58. McCue FC, Andrews JR, Hakala M et al: The coach's finger. J Sports Med 2:270, 1974
59. McKerrell J, Bowen V, Johnston G et al: Boxer's fractures, conservative or operative management? J Trauma 27:486, 1987
60. Bowen V, Hochban T, Johnston G: Angular deformity in fractures of the fifth metacarpal. Adv Orthop Surg 12:214, 1988
61. Bergfeld JA, Weiker GG, Andrisch et al: Soft play-
ing splint for protection of significant hand and wrist injuries in sports. Am J Sports Med 10:293, 1982
62. Green DP, O'Brien ET: Fractures of the thumb metacarpal. South Med J 65:807, 1972
63. Dunn EJ: Gamekeeper's thumb. Orthop Rev 2:52, 1973
64. McCue FC, Hakala MW, Andrews JR et al: Ulna collateral ligament injuries of the thumb in athletes. J Sports Med 2:70, 1974
65. Gerber C, Senn E, Matter P: Skier's thumb. Am J Sports Med 9:171, 1981
66. Coonrad RW, Goldner JL: A study of the pathological findings and treatment in soft tissue injury of the thumb metacarpophalangeal joint. J Bone Joint Surg [Am] 50:439, 1968
67. Frank WE, Dobyns J: Surgical pathology of collateral ligamentous injuries of the thumb. Clin Orthop 83:102, 1972
68. Primiano GA: Functional cast immobilization of thumb metacarpophalangeal joint injuries. Am J Sports Med 14:335, 1986
69. Gerber C, Senn E, Matter P: Skier's thumb: surgical treatment of recent injuries to the ulnar collateral ligament of the thumb's metacarpophalangeal joint. Am J Sports Med 9:171, 1981
70. Melchionda AM, Linburg RM: Volar plate injuries. Physician Sports Med 10:77, 1982
71. Paget J: Lectures on Surgical Pathology. 1st Ed. Lindsay & Bakiston, Philadelphia, 1854
72. Phalen JS: The carpal tunnel syndrome: clinical evaluation of 598 hands. Clin Orthop 83:29, 1972
73. Gilliat RW, Wilson TG: A pneumatic-tourniquet test in the carpal tunnel syndrome. Lancet 2:595, 1953
74. Tinel J: Le signe du "fourmillement" dans les lésions des nerfs periphériques. Presse Med 23:388, 1915
75. Gellman H, Gelberman RH, Ran AM et al: Carpal tunnel syndrome: an evaluation of the provocative diagnostic tests. J Bone Joint Surg [Am] 68:735, 1986
76. Paley D, McMurtry RY: Medial nerve compression test in carpal tunnel syndrome diagnosis: reproducing signs and symptoms in affected wrist. Orthop Rev 14:41, 1985
77. Pellegrini VD, Burton RI: Carpal tunnel syndrome: an approach to evaluation and treatment. Adv Orthop Surg 9:3, 1985
78. Green D: Diagnostic and therapeutic value of carpal tunnel injection. J Hand Surg [Am] 9:850, 1984
79. Kaplan SJ, Glickel SZ, Eaton RG: Predictive factors in the non-surgical treatment of carpal tunnel syndrome. J Hand Surg [Br] 15:106, 1990
80. Eason SY, Belsole RJ, Greene TL: Carpal tunnel

release: analysis of suboptimal results. Adv Orthop Surg 10:298, 1986

81. Phalen GS: Reflections on 21 years' experience with the carpal tunnel syndrome. JAMA 42:1365, 1970

82. Surgawara M, Ogina T, Minami A et al: Digital ischaemia in baseball players. Am J Sports Med 14:329, 1986

83. Buckout BC, Warner MA: Digital perfusion of handball players: effects of repeated ball impact on structures of the hand. Am J Sports Med 8:206, 1980

84. Itoh Y, Wakano K, Takeda T et al: Circulatory distribution in the throwing hand of baseball pitchers. Am J Sports Med 15:264, 1987

85. Von Rosen S: Ein fall von Thrombosis in der Arteria ulnaris nach einwirkung von stumpfer Gewait. Acta Chir Scand 73:500, 1934

86. Conn J, Bergan JJ, Bell JC: Hypothenar hammers syndrome: post-traumatic digital ischaemia. Surgery 68:1122, 1970

87. Gelberman RH, Blasingame JP: The timed Allen test. J Trauma 21:477, 1981

88. Koman LA, Urbaniuk: Ulna artery insufficiency: a guide to treatment. J Hand Surg 6:16, 1981

89. Porubsky GL, Brown SI, Urbaniuk JR: Ulnar artery thrombosis: a sports related injury. Am J Sports Med 14:170, 1986

90. Ho PK, Dellon AL, Wilgis EFS: True aneurysms of the hand resulting from athletic injury: a report of two cases. Am J Sports Med 13:136, 1985

91. Idler RS: Anatomy and biomechanics of digital flexor tendons. Hand Clin 1:3, 1985

92. An KN, Chao EY, Cooney WP et al: Forces in the normal and abnormal hand. J Orthop Res 3:202, 1985

93. Post M: Physical Examination of the Musculoskeletal System. Year book Medical Publishers, Chicago, 1987

94. Amadio PC, Cooney WP: Current concepts in flexor tendon repair. Adv Orthop Surg 10:207, 1987

95. Wadsworth CT: Clinical anatomy and mechanics of the wrist and hand. J Orthop Sports Phys Ther 4:206, 1983

96. Strickland JW: Opinions and preferences in flexor tendon surgery. Hand Clin 1:187, 1985

97. Stern PJ, Kastrop JJ: Complications and prognosis of treatment of mallet finger. J Hand Surg [Am] 13:329, 1988

98. Leddy JP, Packer JW: Avulsion of the profundus insertion in athletes. J Hand Surg 2:66, 1977

99. Buscem MJ, Page BJ: Flexor digitorum profundus avulsions with associated distal phalanx fractures. Am J Sports Med 15:366, 1987

100. Vetter WL: How I manage mallet finger. Physician Sports Med 17:140, 1989

101. Roy S, Irvin R: Sports Medicine. Prevention, Evaluation, Management, and Rehabilitation. Prentice Hall, Englewood Cliffs, NJ, 1983

102. Burton RI, Eaton RG: Common hand injuries in the athlete. Orthop Clin North Am 4:809, 1973

103. Bennett JB: Ring injuries in sports. Physician Sports Med 8:77, 1978

104. MacCollum MS: Protecting upper extremity injuries in sports. Physician Sports Med 8:59, 1980

105. Berry TJ: The Hand as a Mirror of Systemic Diseases. FA Davis, Philadelphia, 1963

Running: Injury Patterns and Prevention 24

No horse ever ran itself to death until they put a rider on its back.
— *George Sheehan*

It is fitting that the last chapter of this book deals with running. Running is a significant component of a large number of sports and is used as a method of aerobic training for countless others. Furthermore, participation in jogging and running forms the main exercise endeavor and recreational pursuit for more than 30 million North Americans and countless others elsewhere. Unfortunately, up to 60 percent of these runners experience an injury severe enough to cause curtailment of their activity at some time.[1] Therefore running injuries comprise a large percentage of most sports medicine practices. When we realize that the average runner strikes his or her foot to the ground 500 to 600 times per kilometer, it should not be surprising that the major cause of running injuries is training errors, sometimes compounded by mechanics of the individual's running style, and perhaps inadequate or poorly chosen equipment. Indeed the forces of running are high and the biomechanics complex. Thus there is a certain morbidity associated with running. There are some individuals whose body type and ligament and tendon structure make jogging an unsuitable pastime.[2]

However, there are rules and methods that enable most runners to minimize the number of injuries incurred, but the guidelines must be understood and strictly observed. Fortunately, the trend is now turning toward reducing training mileage. Few runners are grinding out the "seventy-mile plus weeks" characteristic of the 1980s. The average runner now is more likely to be doing half that mileage and suffering little or no decrease in competitive ability.[3]

Bowerman, a U.S. Olympic track coach, pointed out a decade ago that there was an increasing trend of runners to try and push their training to "100 to 150 miles a week." He had two very firm rebuttals to the 100 miles per week theory of training. First, he said that he had never coached a successful athlete whose regular training included more than 70 miles per week. This statement is significant, as his record of coaching included 17 sub-four-minute milers, five champion three-milers, and two world class marathon runners. Second, he pointed out that among those who insisted on training with longer distances, there were few champions and a high proportion of physical breakdowns. Thus the wheel has turned, and current thinking suggests that these high mileages of the past are unnecessary and even counterproductive. There is no question that they cause a significant incidence of injuries and diminished, rather than enhanced, performance.

The results of poor training techniques include multiple lower limb overuse syndromes, particularly plantar fasciitis, shin splints, stress fractures, patellar tendinitis, peripatellar knee pain, and the iliotibial band syndrome.[4]

One of the main problems with runners is that they are usually their own coach. Although they attempt to educate themselves through running journals and periodicals, they often lack the knowledge base to properly interpret the information they read and transfer it into practical, safe, training regimens. Every running injury should be viewed as a failure of training technique, even if other contributing factors are subsequently identified. If this premise were adopted, injuries would be treated more efficiently, and frequently further recurrences would be prevented. It is no coincidence that the only animals suffering from stress reactions and stress fractures are greyhounds, racehorses, and humans. No horse ever rode itself to death until a rider was put on its back, and for the human this "rider" is usually one's own ego and aspirations or excessive ill-advised coaching pressure. It is not a perfect world, and no one would be foolish enough to claim that injuries can be eliminated. However, the current unacceptably high incidence of musculoskeletal problems may be greatly reduced by adopting the above philosophy.

There are times when intensity of training and distances must be increased in order to compete successfully at high levels. Nevertheless, most training should be based on distances of under 45 miles a week for recreational runners, and even the more seriously competitive individual may not have to spend much of the year training at 50 miles or more a week.[5] Thus it must be stated that individuals' aims and desires must be melded carefully with their physical makeup and ability. For some, running successfully comprises the main recreational activity, whereas for others it should be interspersed liberally with alternate activities, with an emphasis on walking, cycling, and seasonal pursuits such as cross-country skiing. For many the occasional 10-km race represents the zenith of their abilities, whereas for others a successful attempt at a marathon is within their grasp, although only a small percentage of them can actually race that distance. It is mandatory that the physician and therapist who work with large numbers of individuals sustaining running injuries help these athletes to assess their needs, select realistic goals and then with the aid of exercise physiologists and coaching colleagues, to assist them in achieving them.

RUNNING BIOMECHANICS

Walking, running, and sprinting are characterized by a stance phase, commencing when the foot strikes the ground and lasting until it once again loses contact. At this point the leg enters a swing phase as it traverses the air. The "gait cycle" is the period encompassed and all of the biomechanical events that occur, from one heel strike until the foot once again makes contact with the ground. Knowledge of the forces involved, the joint motion, and the muscle action required is essential to adequately analyze running problems and then give logical advice.

Walking, jogging, and running are a continuum in which the legs are the primary mode of locomotion through their direct contact with the surface being traversed. The difference between ordinary walking and running is easily discerned in the body motions

involved, even though a fast walk may cover more ground in a given time, be more vigorous, and have a greater circulatory and respiratory involvement, than a slow run. The differentiation between jogging and running is not simple and actually may not be necessary, as jogging is running. Still, many definitions have been proposed, and the concept of jogging has various meanings. One concept is simply that it is a slow run. The confusion here arises out of deciding at which point a slow run becomes a fast one. However, at whatever point is chosen, the stresses involved usually correlate with body weight, style, and velocity. In a survey of a large number of runners, nearly 40 percent ran three to five times per week and about 45 percent ran 20 to 40 minutes per session[6] (Fig. 24-1). Certainly many more achieve the accepted guidelines for cardiovascular fitness, i.e., a rhythmic exercise that uses large muscle groups at least three days per week for 15 to 60 minutes per session and at an intensity that gives an age-adjusted heart rate of 60 to 90 percent of maximum.

Quick Facts
RUNNER'S CLASSIFICATION

Runner	Miles* Per Week	at Minutes Per Mile
Jogger	2–18	8–16
Sports runner	20–40	8–10
Long distance	30–40	7–8
Elite	40–+	7–

* 1 mile = 1.6 Km

Forces Involved

The biomechanical stresses of running are high. On initial ground contact there is a vertical force of approximately two to three times body weight, a forward shear of 50 percent of body weight, and a medial sheer of about 10 percent of body weight.[7] Furthermore, most of these forces have to be dissipated over a few milliseconds because the whole stance phase of running is compressed into 200 ms (Fig. 24-2). The initial impact forces are due mainly to the deceleration of the lower extremity at first contact. Active forces are mostly determined by the movement of the center of mass of the total body during the stance phase. Thus the forces of running acting on the human body can easily reach up to ten times the body weight.[8]

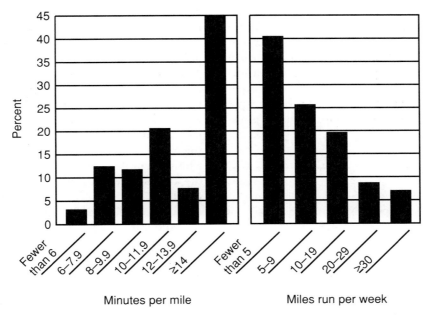

Fig. 24-1. Distribution of runners by time and distance spent in this activity per week. (After Caldwell,[6] with permission.)

To appreciate the magnitude of these forces it can be calculated that if a 150 lb man walks 1 mile, taking an average 2.5 feet per stride, he requires 2,110 steps. Because he absorbs 80 percent of body weight at heel strike, he must ultimately dissipate about 63.5 tons through each foot. By contrast, the same man jogging for a mile, taking on average 4.5 feet strides and approximately 1,175 steps, must dissipate an initial ground contact of 250 percent of body weight, which means that, over the mile, 110 tons of energy would be dissipated through each foot.[9,10] Taken to the extreme, during a marathon the body experiences more than 25,000 impacts with the ground, each equivalent to 2.5 times body weight.

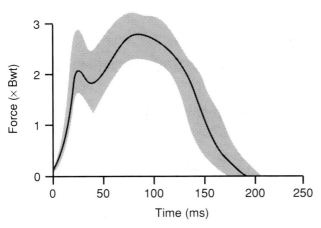

Fig. 24-2. Average vertical component of ground reaction force in subjects running 6.5-minute miles. Shaded area represents the range. Peak force rises to almost three times body weight, and most of it is within the first 20 to 30 ms after foot contact. (Adapted from Cavanagh and LaFortune,[7] with permission.)

Quick Facts

FORCES OF RUNNING HIGH

- Initial ground contact forces.
  - Vertical thrust two to three times body weight
  - Forward shear 50 percent body weight
  - Medial shear 10 percent body weight
- These forces must be dissipated in less than one-third of the time (0.2 second) than available when walking.
- Peak impact forces generally occur during the first 20 to 30 ms after foot contact.

The arch of the running foot depresses about 50 percent more than the walking foot, and the forces are greatest at the medial cuneiform and the base of the first metatarsal.[11] In addition to these vertical forces, a considerable torque occurs with transverse rotations through the leg. There is an internal torque at ground contact and a progressive external torque to foot off. These forces are important and are discussed in the next section.

Quick Facts

STRESS OF RUNNING

- Runner's feet contact ground 800 to 2,000 times per mile.
- Equals 50 to 70 times per minute for each foot.
- Must dissipate more than 100 tons of force for each mile.

Kinematics

The biomechanics of the running gait are complex. Running requires that the foot be stable and yet be able to shock absorb when necessary. It must also be able to convert itself into a rigid lever for the thrust of forward motion. Evolution has made some considerable changes in the human foot to allow bipedal locomotion, but some of these changes are inadequate for repetitive running over long distances.

Walking has been defined as moving at a speed of 5.63 km/hour and is basically divided into two phases: a stance phase, taking up 60 to 65 percent of the cycle; and a swing phase, comprising 35 to 40 percent of the cycle. The whole cycle takes approximately 1 second, and 25 percent of this time is in double support when both feet are on the ground. As the velocity of gait increases, the duration of the cycle decreases.[12]

By contrast, jogging has a cycle lasting only 0.7 seconds (700 ms). There are no periods of double support, and indeed there is some period during which the person is airborne (float phase). The running gait cycle can be divided into (1) a contact, or stance, phase consisting of foot strike, midsupport, and take-off; and (2) the swing phase, consisting of follow-through, forward swing, and foot descent. A pace of more than 200 meters/second is considered

running.[13] The stance phase lasts anywhere from 200 to 600 ms, and the forces through the heel at foot strike are up to two to three times body weight and are affected by style and speed[12] (Fig. 24-3).

A key part of this running motion are the movements that take place at the subtalar and midtarsal joints. As the foot hits the ground, landing usually on the heel posterolaterally, the foot commences the movement of pronation, which effectively unlocks the foot. It is achieved by the heel going into eversion, a movement that can take place because at this point the axis of motion of the talus and the calcaneus are parallel (Fig. 24-4). The initial ground contact force on the posterolateral heel during jogging is relatively low, and it is not until 20 to 30 ms later that the heel or forefoot is flat on the ground.[9] Thus contrary to what is often published, the posterior heel does not take the maximum impact; rather, it is the center of the heel and midfoot at a time when there is maximum support and the foot is most capable of absorbing shock. This point has important implications for running shoe design.

Pronation facilitates shock absorption through the foot by allowing the midtarsal area to yield. Supination takes place during the rest of the gait cycle and locks the foot. Locking occurs because there is a gradual convergence of the axis of motion of the talus and the calcaneus past the midpoint of the range of inversion. The effect of this convergent axis is to lock the bones of the midfoot, and this is assisted by

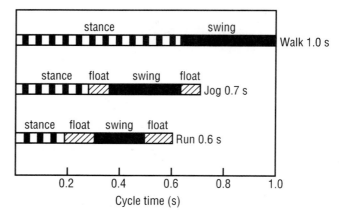

Fig. 24-3. As the speed of gait increases, double support shortens; and ultimately there is a period during which both feet are off the ground, called the float phase. With faster running the length of the stance phase decreases and the period of float phase increases.

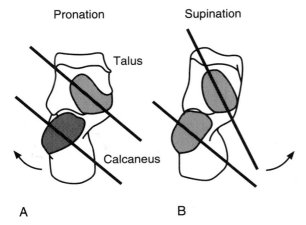

Pronation   Supination

Talus

Calcaneus

A   B

Fig. 24-4. Axis of the subtalar joint. (**A**) As the calcaneus everts, the conjoint axis between the talar navicular and calcaneal cuboid joints are parallel to one another, so increased motion may occur and the foot is allowed to unlock. (**B**) As the calcaneus moves into inversion, and these axes are no longer parallel, there is decreased motion available and increased stability.

muscular action and the ligamentous support (Fig. 24-5).

To summarize the running cycle, it may be divided into the following phases[13,14] (Fig. 24-6).

Float phase. During this time the center of gravity reaches peak elevation and the body maintains its forward lean. During the terminal float phase there is a reversal of the previous hip flexion; and as the hip goes into extension it imparts internal rotation to the limb. There is also rapid knee extension and dorsiflexion at the ankle.

Initial ground contact. This phase requires both joint stabilization and ankle dorsiflexion. The initial contact may be with the posterolateral heel, the whole hindfoot, or almost simultaneous contact of the complete sole, depending on the jogging style. Most joggers run with almost a flat foot for initial ground contact. A few are toe runners, and for them the initial contact is the forefoot. This form is an inefficient jogging and running gait, but with sprinting it is necessary for maximum propulsion during the brief time period of stance.

Shock-absorbing action. This is achieved proximally by flexion of the hip and knee joint. Distally there is ankle dorsiflexion as well as the cushioning by the special fat pad of the heel. In addition, there is the

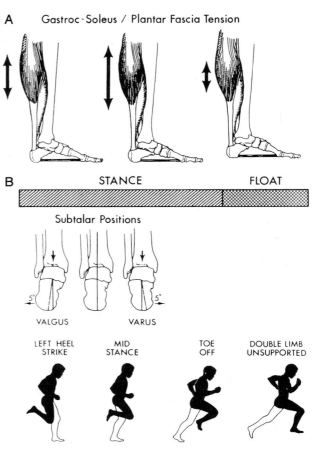

A   Gastroc-Soleus / Plantar Fascia Tension

B   STANCE   FLOAT

Subtalar Positions

5°   5°

VALGUS   VARUS

LEFT HEEL STRIKE   MID STANCE   TOE OFF   DOUBLE LIMB UNSUPPORTED

Fig. 24-5. Changes in the gastrocnemius, plantar fascia, and subtalar joint during the phases of running. (**A**) The gastroc-soleus complex helps control eversion as well as generating plantar flexion forces just prior to toe off. (**B**) Stance and float phases coordinated with subtalar motion and running action. (After Adelaar,[13] with permission.)

most important and subtle mechanism of eversion of the subtalar joint, unlocking the forefoot and allowing foot flexibility. This impact absorption was triggered by the flexion of the limb along with internal rotation of the hip, which in turn imparts internal rotation to the tibia and thus the eversion to the calcaneus and pronation to the foot via the closed kinematic chain. Muscles are used to stabilize this movement.

Midsupport and take-off. This phase of running requires production of a rigid lever. The body's center of gravity passes forward, and there is rapid flexion of the swinging leg on the nonstance side that imparts

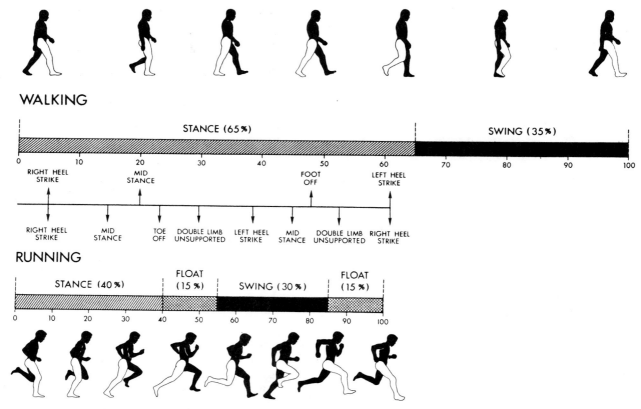

Fig. 24-6. Comparison of the phases of the walking and running cycle. Running introduces a period during which neither foot is in contact with the ground (float phase). (After Adelaar,[13] with permission.)

progressive external rotation on the stance leg through pelvic motion. The proximal external rotation working through the whole lower limb segment on the stance side eventually causes inversion of the calcaneus, making the foot a more rigid lever. In addition, the rapid plantar flexion at the ankle produces a windlass effect through the plantar fascia, helping to stabilize the arch. Naturally, some control is necessary by the posterior tibial muscles. During this phase, the center of gravity is anterior to the base of support, and the key is supination of the foot, locking the midtarsal joints. These events take place within a short time period, and hence the velocities of the limb rotations are phenomenal. The deceleration or reversal of these rotary motions stress the tibia and require considerable muscle control.

When jogging, the average length of stride is about four-fifths of an individual's height. As the runner increases speed, the feet tend to move toward a single center line position to reduce inefficient pelvic sway-

ing. In addition, gradually heel contact is lost, such that in fast running and sprinting, most individuals land and push off mainly from the balls of their feet. The float phase increases simultaneously.[14]

In summary, the complex interactions of the subtalar and midtarsal joints allow eversion shortly after heel strike so the foot becomes a mobile adapter. Eversion is followed by rapid inversion prior to take-off in order to provide stability and a rigid lever (Fig. 24-7).

Muscle Action

When running the muscles work to (1) stabilize the trunk and pelvis and accelerate the limb against gravity and the running surface; (2) decelerate the rapid motion of the swinging leg; and (3) control the rotations down the length of the limb.[10,12]

The gluteus maximus and hamstrings increase their activity 30 to 50 percent over walking levels in order to be able to decelerate the leg. The hip abductors

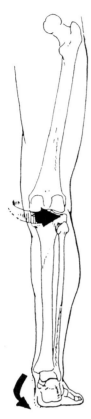

Fig. 24-7. The internal rotation imparted to the leg from the hip is suddenly stopped with foot contact and the subtalar joint acts as a torque converter, generating eversion of the heel. This in turn pronates the whole foot. This motion is controlled by tibialis posterior and to some degree the gastroc nemius-soleus complex. (After Nicholas and Hershman,[15] with permission.)

work throughout the running cycle to help stabilize the pelvis.

The knee extensors are active when walking. They control knee flexion during the swing phase and initiate knee extension during the early stance phase. As a walker increases velocity, the quadriceps activity increases; and there is a greater arc of knee motion needed to clear the foot from the ground. The strength and fatigue capacity of the quadriceps are important because of their prolonged activity in the running cycle.

The foot and ankle intrinsics, plantar flexors, and peroneals work to stabilize the plantar surface and hindfoot during the foot-flat phase and are active during 70 percent of the running cycle. The tibialis

posterior, tibialis anterior, and peroneals are particularly important for controlling the effects of the rapid alternating high velocity rotary torques generated through the tibia and foot. The foot flexors are important for acceleration. This group also assists the intrinsics of the foot, which tend to be active throughout the stance phase. Intrinsics coordinate hindfoot inversion with stabilization of the longitudinal arch and supination of the forefoot.[9,10] This action is also assisted by the windlass action of the plantar fascia, which is an extension of the triceps surae muscle. Specific muscle action in running has been outlined in Chapter 7.

Quick Facts

RUNNING (GAIT) CYCLE

- Early float phase (follow through and forward swing)
  - Initial hip flexion
  - Acceleration of limb
- Terminal float phase (foot descend)
  - Limb into hip extension
  - Deceleration
  - Proximal internal femoral rotation
- Initial ground contact (foot strike to midsupport)
  - Velocity of limb internal rotation rapidly decelerated as heel everts
  - Foot pronates
  - Shock absorption
- Late stance phase (midsupport to take-off)
  - Hip extending, imparts lateral rotation to leg
  - Proximal rotation generates rapid distal rotation
  - Heel inverts
  - Foot supinates and locks
  - Rigid lever for propulsion

The basic cause of overuse injuries is the decreasing duration of the stance phase in running compared to walking—to as little as 200 ms. This decrease necessitates an increase in angular velocities. The effect on muscles is that they are required to increase their power and their speed of contraction, and there is thus an increased whip on the tendons and a decreased rest phase. This situation can account for the evolution of tendinitis and the tibial stress syndromes.

INJURY PATTERNS

In a study of more than 4,000 runners selected from a popular Swiss 16-km race, 45 percent had sustained injuries during the year preceding the race.[5] Despite the "healthy participant" effect, every fifth runner was forced to interrupt training; one of seven (14 percent) had sought medical care; and one of 40 (2.3 percent) had missed work. These figures are comparable to English and North American data.[4,16–20] Although the figure seems high, injuries from most other common recreational activities are probably twice as common; skiing, for example, has about six times the injury rate.

Quick Facts

JOGGING/RUNNING: INCIDENCE, SEVERITY, DURATION

Injury	%	Duration (weeks)
• Grade I—full training with symptoms	28	7.4 (1–40)
• Grade II—reduced training	28	5.7 (1–21)
• Grade III—training interrupted	20	4.8 (2–16)
• Injury sustained in associated activities	9	6.0 (2–20)
• General illness	10	3.9 (2–11)

The most common area of involvement is obviously the lower limbs, and the distribution of injuries varies in different series depending on the type of referral practice of the author, the year of publication, whether the sample is picked from recreational or competitive runners, the percentage of track versus distance runners, and even the definition of an injury.[5] Generally 30 to 40 percent of the injuries are to the knee, 25 percent to the leg, and 15 to 25 percent to the foot and ankle (Table 24-1). From these data emerges a pattern of some of the more frequent diagnoses (Fig. 24-8; Table 24-2).

Unquestionably, the most important etiologic factor is training errors. Indeed Lysholm and Wiklander reported that training errors alone, or in combination with other factors, was implicated in producing injuries in 72 percent of their series of runners.[17] Other contributing factors are age, sex, previous injuries, terrain, competitive training, motivation, experience, inappropriate footwear, and biomechanical and alignment parameters. Medical problems such as hematuria, gastrointestinal complaints, dehydration, exhaustion, hypo- and hyperthermia, and delayed muscle soreness are not dealt with here.

Training Errors

Training errors may be basically divided into excessive mileage and inappropriate progression of intensity or distance. Higher mileage correlates well with occurrence of jogging injury ($p < 0.001$) and more frequent medical consultations. Indeed if one compares injury-free to injury-prone runners, the profile of the latter includes greater weekly mileage, faster 10 km and 16 km running times, a history of a

TABLE 24-1. Incidence of Musculoskeletal Jogging and Running Injuries

Location	Total Injuries No.	Total Injuries %	Men No.	Men %	Men Age (years)	Men Weekly Training Mileage	Women No.	Women %	Women Age (years)	Women Weekly Training Mileage
Lower back	68	4	36	3	32	22	32	4	28	20
Hip	90	5	45	4	31	28	45	6	28	22
Upper leg	66	4	38	4	28	31	28	4	24	27
Knee	761	42	458	43	29	22	303	41	26	18
Lower leg	503	28	292	27	32	30	211	29	25	19
Foot	331	18	212	20	30	25	119	16	27	20
Total	1,819		1,081		—	—	739		—	—
Mean	—		—		30	27	—		26	19

(Adapted from Marti et al.,[5] with permission.)

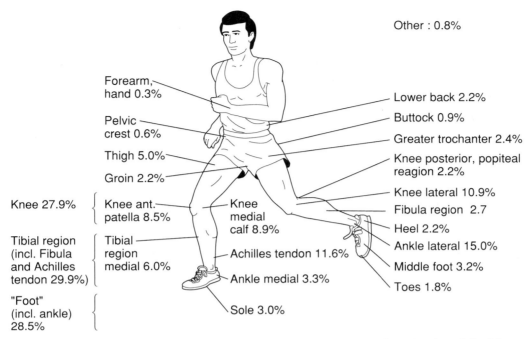

Other : 0.8%

Forearm, hand 0.3%

Pelvic crest 0.6%

Thigh 5.0%

Groin 2.2%

Knee 27.9%

Knee ant. patella 8.5%

Tibial region (incl. Fibula and Achilles tendon 29.9%)

Tibial region medial 6.0%

"Foot" (incl. ankle) 28.5%

Knee medial calf 8.9%

Achilles tendon 11.6%

Ankle medial 3.3%

Sole 3.0%

Lower back 2.2%

Buttock 0.9%

Greater trochanter 2.4%

Knee posterior, popiteal reagion 2.2%

Knee lateral 10.9%

Fibula region 2.7

Heel 2.2%

Ankle lateral 15.0%

Middle foot 3.2%

Toes 1.8%

Fig. 24-8. Body sites of 877 running injuries expressed as percents. (After Marti et al.,[5] with permission.)

previous injury, and more likely to use in-shoe orthotics.

Specifically, there is a sixfold increase in running injuries and medical consultations for individuals who consistently train more than 50 km (30 miles) per week over those who run less than 10 km (6 miles) per week; it is double in those who run 10 to 25 km (6 to 16 miles) per week. In another large series of running injuries, the average distances covered were 43 km (27 miles) per week for men and 30 km (19 miles) for women[5] (Fig. 24-9). It is difficult to show that breaking this mileage up into more frequent sessions, e.g., five rather than three training days, significantly reduces injuries.

It has been suggested that the increased volume of running itself is not the main etiologic factor, but that the individual anatomic and biomechanical predisposition of the runner contributes to chronic overload.[4] Although the latter is undoubtedly true to some degree, it is difficult to prove from the statistical analysis offered in the current literature.

The second component of training errors is the inappropriate progression of intensity or distance. A reasonably *safe figure for increasing mileage is less than 10 percent per week, with a hold pattern every 3 weeks to consolidate gains.* This progression is even more critical when returning from an injury, when the severity and duration of the injury as well as the preinjury mileage must be taken into account. When training toward competition, regular distances of about 50 percent of the race distance with a longer run once per week usually represents a safe training level.[22]

Age and Duration of Jogging/Running

Essentially, as runners get older, the number of injuries decrease; but when injuries do occur, the symptoms tend to persist longer. Part of this statistic may be related to selection bias in that those runners who remain symptom-free have more tendency to continue running. It may also mean that there is intrinsically, or has developed, a better adaptation to the stresses of running on a tissue or biomechanical level in those individuals who have run over many years. There are some injuries that are more prevalent in the older runner: plantar fasciitis, Morton's neuroma, hallux rigidus, Achilles tendinitis, and back and knee pain related to degenerative joint changes.

TABLE 24-2. Fifteen Most Common Overuse Injuries in Running and Jogging

Injury	Marathon		Middle Distance		Recreational		Total 1990	
	Male (n = 279)	Female (n = 99)	Male (n = 56)	Female (n = 37)	Male (n = 2,024)	Female (n = 1,678)	Male (n = 2,359)	Female (n = 7,814)
Patellofemoral pain	17.5	23.2	21.4	18.9	25.3	30.2	24.3	29.6
Iliotibial band friction syndrome	11.8	21.2	3.6	2.7	6.7	7.2	7.2	7.9
Plantar fasciitis	5.7	6.1	1.8	8.1	5.2	3.8	5.2	4.0
Achilles tendinitis	5.7	1.0	5.4	10.8	4.6	2.6	4.7	2.7
Patellar tendinitis	4.7	0.0	5.4	2.7	5.1	3.3	5.1	3.1
Tibia stress syndrome	3.6	3.0	7.2	16.2	4.9	7.2	4.7	7.1
Metatarsal stress syndrome	3.2	3.0	1.8	2.7	3.2	3.9	3.1	3.8
Abductor strain	3.2	2.0	0.0	0.0	1.3	0.4	1.5	0.5
Tibialis posterior tendinitis	2.5	3.0	1.8	2.7	2.1	2.5	2.1	2.5
Gastrocnemius strain	3.6	0.0	1.8	2.7	1.9	1.4	2.1	1.3
Tibial stress fracture	2.5	3.0	10.7	2.7	2.3	4.4	2.5	4.3
Gluteus strain	2.5	2.0	5.4	2.7	0.7	1.5	1.0	1.6
Hamstring strain	2.2	2.0	5.4	2.7	0.1	0.1	0.5	0.2
Quadriceps strain	1.4	1.0	3.6	2.7	0.8	0.5	0.9	0.6
Ankle sprain	1.4	1.0	1.8	5.4	1.9	2.2	1.8	2.2

Results are given as percent of injuries.
(After MacIntyre et al.,[21] with permission.)

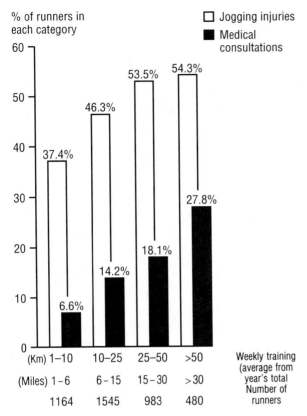

Fig. 24-9. Frequency of jogging injuries and medical consultation expressed according to weekly training averages of kilometers run (After Marti et al.,[5] with permission.)

Flexibility and Strength

Some activities predispose to poor flexibility and altered strength ratios around joints. These factors in turn may expose an underlying vulnerability to injury. In particular, jogging and running predispose the athlete to the development of tight hip flexors, hamstrings, and Achilles tendons. Similarly, hip flexor and gastrocnemius power is often disproportionate to that of other muscle groups. Thus there is a tendency to acute muscle strains of the hamstring, particularly in sprinters. There may be a relation between peripatellar knee pain and inadequate hamstring strength, poor vastus medialis control, and generally tight thigh muscles. Certainly, assessment of these factors should always form part of the evaluation in runners with knee pain; and when appropriate, corrective exercises or stretching should be included in the treatment regimen. There is a

suggestion that gastrocnemius tightness and a mismatch between triceps surae strength and Achilles tendon cross-sectional area may predispose to Achilles tendinitis. Thus eccentric loading exercises and Achilles stretching are an important part of the prophylaxis and treatment of this condition.

Training Surfaces and Shoes

Individuals who run on a regular basis, particularly those whose mileages are high, need to be especially concerned about the surface on which they train. Surfaces that have little or no give force the runner's body to absorb an increasing amount of the impact of foot strike.[23] A good shoe offers some absorption. It must be remembered however, that usually the shock-absorbing qualities wear out relatively quickly. As much as 25 percent is lost after the first 50 miles of running, 33 percent after 100 to 150 miles, and about 40 percent after 250 to 500 miles.[24] The life of the running shoe shortens if there is a lot of running in wet conditions or if the runner perspires excessively into the shoe on a regular basis. Also, depending on the body weight of the individual and the propensity to injury, running shoes should be exchanged when it is calculated that their impact qualities have been significantly reduced, rather than deciding on external features such as the amount of obvious wear to the uppers and contact surface of the heel.

Quick Facts

DETERIORATION OF SHOCK ABSORPTION IN RUNNING SHOES

- 25% Lost after 50 miles (100 Km)
- 33% Lost after 100–150 miles (150–250 Km)
- 40% Lost after 250–500 miles (400–800 Km)

Approximate figures for easy recall

Given the choice, most runners would probably choose asphalt as the ideal surface because it allows good foot control and eliminates the danger of uneven and uncertain terrain.[25] However, the most important feature is to realize that when there is an abrupt change of the quality and type of running surface that is used for training, the injury risk rises considerably. Whenever such changes are made because of the passing seasons or for reasons of reducing boredom or accommodating a travel schedule, some adjustment is necessary for this factor. If the new surface is considerably different from that used on a regular basis, it may be prudent to cut down a 10 mile run by at least 75 percent to eliminate the risk of injury, particularly for someone who has a history of recurrent problems or is recovering from a recent injury.

Practice Point

RUNNING SURFACE

- Injury risk rises with a sudden change in quality and type of running surface.
- Be aware and make the necessary reduction in mileage.

Many acute injuries occur on soft surfaces, e.g., falls on the wobbly support of sand or rock or in potholes and divots in rougher trails. Additionally, for individuals living in cold climates, snow and icy conditions alter the running style. Stance tends to widen, and the stride length shortens, which may throw additional stress on the decelerating muscles (e.g., hamstrings) and the hip stabilizing muscles (e.g., adductors). Sudden slips on ice during a stride may generate hamstring tears. Indeed in the long distance runner, this accident is one of the more common causes of hamstring injuries over the winter months. For others, excessive hill work, running in the camber of the road, and changing to an indoor track with tight corners may precipitate injury.

Alignment Biomechanics

Normal variations in the human body abound, and only a few percent of the population are actually good examples of "normal" (Fig. 24-10). These normal variations occur at all sections of the lower limb, including a large range of ante- and retroversion of the femoral neck, internal and external torsion of the femurs and tibias, different heights of the patella, the degree of hyperextension at the knee, and widely discrepant Q angles. The length of the foot, the shape of the heel and arch, and the length of the toes are also varied. Furthermore, all of these variations are found in world class athletes and seem to produce little ad-

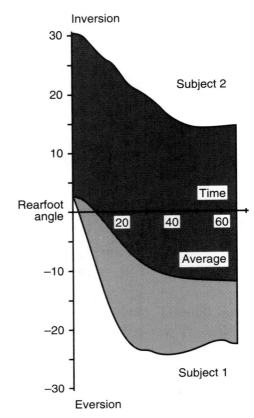

Fig. 24-10. Rear-foot inversion and eversion. The average is expressed along with the two most outlying subjects. On average, the foot starts in slight inversion at foot strike and moves through a range of approximately 16 degrees during the first 40 ms of contact phase. Subject 1 has excessive rear-foot motion. Subject 2 has normal range, but this range occurs entirely in the inversion region of the curve.

verse effect on their ability to perform their sports. Indeed over the years there have been many attempts, usually unsuccessful to define the ideal body build for a particular sport.

The corollary of this enormous variation of body build among enthusiastic amateur and the professional athletes is that there is poor correlation of specific malalignments with specific conditions. Although there is a tendency for certain types of alignment of the lower limbs to be associated with conditions such as chondromalacia, this correlation is generally related more to the fact that a large number of individuals in the active population have this configuration. The evidence to support the fact that certain specific minor malalignments predispose to overuse syndrome is slim indeed.[17-19] However, in Messier and Pittala's study of a limited number of athletes with shin splint-like syndromes, plantar fasciitis, and iliotibial band friction syndrome, there were two significant ($p < 0.05$) discriminators between the control and the shin splint groups: maximum pronation velocity and maximum pronation.[25] Plantar flexion range was a significant discriminator for the plantar fasciitis group. In addition, the injured groups had a nonsignificant trend toward a higher arch and leg length discrepancies of more than 0.5 inch.

Although the physical examination for gross deformities is easy, most of the subtle malalignments in the human body are difficult to discern. Specific roentgenographic views are usually necessary, and even then there is some disagreement among experts as to the interpretation of these radiologic findings. The rather glib statements by many paramedical personnel that they are able to measure subtle malalignments and adjust for them is a gross oversimplification of the clinical situation.[26]

Static Measurements

As indicated in the previous paragraphs; it is important to realize the limitation of these static measurements and the accuracy of recording, as well as the difficulty of establishing a true causal relation between alignment and the many overuse syndromes. Nevertheless, there is a body of literature reasonably arguing that excessive motion in the subtalar region requires excessive muscle action, particularly in tibialis posterior and indirectly the peronei. This situation, in turn, may contribute to the posterior tibial stress syndrome as well as fibular and tibial stress fractures. In addition, the excessive whipping action of the Achilles tendon may precipitate Achilles tendinitis.

Because the acceleration and deceleration of the tibia and perhaps the magnitude of internal-external rotations are linked to the hindfoot inversion and eversion, it is possible that one could link development of the anterior knee pain syndromes to specific alignments when combined with the high stresses of running significant distances each week. Thus a rigid foot, either as pes planus or more frequently as a cavus foot, may inhibit the ability of this unit to efficiently absorb shock. This deficiency in turn may translate into additional stress through the lower limb. Even if one is not prepared to accept variations of alignment as a causative mechanism, it is still reasonable to accept that alteration of the configuration of the foot, and its ability to go through certain ranges of motion may have biomechanical implications which impact on the proximal segments of the limb. Thus alteration of these alignments may be used as a treatment mechanism should painful overuse syndromes arise. In this situation an orthosis may be viewed as a dynamic splint.

When defining these static alignments, however, it is important to realize that the term malalignment should not be used to describe conditions that are within two standard deviations of normal. In all areas of medicine, to be considered abnormal the physiologic parameter must fall on the extremes of the bell curve. Thus throughout this text, the term malalignment has always referred to any degree of alignment that is well outside the normal range; it is certainly not applied to the common minor degrees of variation each side of the norm.

If it is assumed that a neutral alignment of the heel is a desirable feature, a reasonable initial clinical method of assessment is with the athlete lying prone and the feet extended over the end of the table. Subsequently the athlete is asked to stand and the effect of weight-bearing on this alignment is observed.

The initial measurement in the prone or kneeling position is commenced by establishing the neutral position of the subtalar area. This in itself is subjective and there are several different methods proposed. Only one is given here. The examiner grasps the athlete's foot over the fourth and fifth metatarsal heads

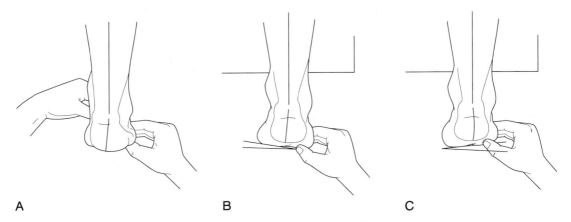

Fig. 24-11. Static measurements of the rearfoot and forefoot while kneeling or lying prone. (**A**) Rearfoot (hindfoot) in approximately 3 degrees of varus. (**B**) Forefoot in slight varus. (**C**) Subtalar joint neutral, forefoot in valgus.

with the index and thumb and then gently dorsiflexes the foot until some resistance is felt. Holding this position, the foot is then moved through an arc of supination and pronation. As the movement is performed, the examiner notes the point at which the foot appears to "fall off" to one side or the other more easily. It is this point that is determined as the neutral position (Fig. 24-11).

Furthermore, the examiner's other hand palpates the recesses medially and laterally just anterior to the smallest: When these medial and lateral talar depressions feel equal to the inversion and eversion motion of the heel, it is assumed that this is the neutral position of congruency of the subtalar joint.

When assessing the leg-heel alignment for rearfoot varus or valgus from this neutral position, a mark is placed over the midline of the calcaneus at the insertion of the Achilles tendon. A second mark is made about 1 cm distal, as near the midline of the calcaneus as possible. These two marks are joined, and two additional marks are made over the midline

of the distal one-third of the leg. These coordinates are meant to represent the longitudinal axis of the tibia. The subtalar joint is then once more repositioned to confirm the neutral position; the position from neutral to as much as 8 degrees of varus is considered normal. Prone measurements of calcaneal inversion/eversion and subtalar joint neutral position have a low to moderate interrater reliability but are significantly better when carried out in the weight-bearing stance[27] (Table 24-3; Fig. 24-12).

The forefoot-heel alignment, which establishes the degree of forefoot varus or valgus, is also established from this position. The alignment is estimated by observing the relation between the vertical axis of the heel and the plane of the forefoot at the second, third, and fourth metatarsal heads.[28] If the medial side of the foot is raised, the forefoot is said to be in varus or supinated. Conversely, if the lateral side of the foot is raised, the forefoot is considered to be in valgus, provided the heel is in neutral position (Fig. 24-11).

TABLE 24-3. Calcaneal Inversion, Eversion, and Palpated Subtalar Joint
in Neutral Position ($n = 20$) Inter-rater Reliability

Examiners	Calcaneal Inversion (Degrees)			Calcaneal Eversion (Degrees)			Palpated Subtalar Joint (Degrees)			Calcaneal Eversion in Stance (Degrees)		
	Mean	SD	ICC[a]	Mean	SD	ICC	Mean	SD	ICC	Mean	SD	ICC
One	14	7		5	4		1	3		6	4	
Two	15	8		7	6		1	.5		6	5	
Three	11	4		8	4		1	6		5	4	
Combined			0.42			0.25			0.60			0.91

[a] Inter-rater reliability correlation coefficients (ICC). Only the measurement taken standing can be considered to have an acceptable reliability.
(After Smith-Oricchio and Harris,[27] with permission.)

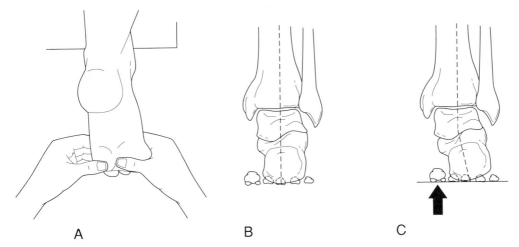

Fig. 24-12. (**A**) Determining the amount of motion at first ray. (**B**) Forefoot non-weight-bearing. Heel is in neutral position. (**C**) With weight-bearing, the first ray fails to support the medial side of the foot, and the heel drops into eversion with the foot pronated.

The static measurements are completed by determining the amount of motion in the first ray. An excessively mobile first ray may fail to support the medial side of the foot, allowing it to fall into a pronated position. Similarly, a rigid plantar-flexed first ray may limit the amount of pronation or indeed even place the foot into slightly varus alignment. Experience allows judgment of the degree of mobility of the first ray (Fig. 24–12). Furthermore, careful examination of the wear pattern of the training shoes enables more confidence to be placed in extrapolating the significance of these static maneuvers (Fig. 24-13).

Dynamic Assessment

Some of the limitations of a static assessment can be overcome by a videotape analysis of the athlete while running (Fig. 24-14). This method is obviously outside the ability of the average physician in the office; but it is perhaps one of the functions that sports medicine clinics and centers can offer. It is reasonable to use a treadmill system, realizing that there may be certain differences in running styles with this apparatus, from the point of view of familiarization and because of the nature of the moving platform. In an ideal system, the athlete can be viewed from above,

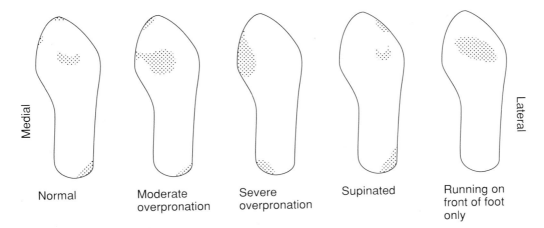

Fig. 24-13. Examination of shoe wear gives some indication of the dynamic alignment and stresses through the foot. (After Arnheim,[29] with permission.)

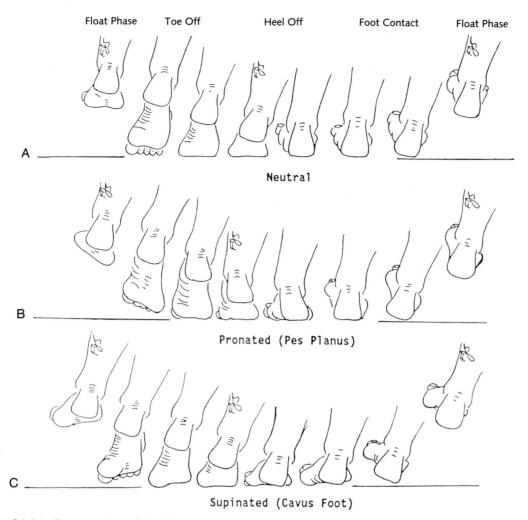

Fig. 24-14. Progression of the foot prior to contact with the floor through to the subsequent float phase. The sequence is read from right to left. (**A**) Neutral heel, normal mobility. (**B**) Flexible foot going into excessive pronation. (**C**) A varus heel with a rigid foot remaining supinated. (After Nicholas and Hershman,[15] with permission.)

the side, and behind, the latter being the most important measurement. Ideally the treadmill should be elevated at least 11 inches off the ground so that the video camera can center over the leg and heel, eliminating a parallax effect.

Depending on the ability of the runner or the presence of an injury, the treadmill is run between 2.5 and 5.0 miles an hour on a level surface. The videotaping may be done with a hand-held camera, and several modifications can be introduced, e.g., placing surface landmarks clearly on the leg or videotaping with or without shoes. In addition, there is some concern about whether the abnormality seen on these treadmill pictures exists during normal running gait. A

hand-held video camera can be used to confirm the presence of these abnormal movements while the individual runs on a normal running surface.

After videotaping, the film is reviewed with the athlete using playback, slow motion, and stop-action. Frequently dynamic idiosyncrasies not obvious in the static examination become plain on this review. The observations from the video tape should then be combined with those points gleaned from a careful inspection of the runner's shoes. For the athlete to learn the most from this interview, a brief discussion of the running action in general is often necessary prior to reviewing the videotape with the individual.

ORTHOSES

It is sometimes uncomfortable to accept the limitations of our knowledge, but it is important to realize that in many ways the use of orthotics is empiric. The exact method by which any orthosis alters biomechanics is challenging to measure.[30] In particular, information is difficult to obtain on the transverse rotations at the subtalar joint during running. Furthermore, movement of the running shoe does not always represent the movement of the foot inside the shoe. Nevertheless, orthotics can be effective, though there is danger that success with treatment is often taken to infer that the etiology is clear. Bearing this point in mind, there are several potential indications for the use of orthotics.

Shock Absorption/Stress Reduction

The first indication is reduction of the load. Of all the functions of orthoses, this one probably has come the closest to be statistically significant in well devised and executed studies. It is one of the advantages of soft systems over rigid systems. However, it is difficult to demonstrate significant in vivo differences between the various viscoelastic materials used for insole orthotics.[26,31,32] Nigg et al. concluded that the use of viscoelastic insoles to replace conventional insoles did not appear to affect the kinetic and kinematic variables during impact in a relevant way.[33] Cinats et al. also reported that the final transmitted stress over the duration of foot strike was not reduced by more than 10 percent by Sorbothane viscoelastic material.[31] Nevertheless, even this small value may be significant with the cumulative stress of running, particularly if customized to incorporate appropriate motion control features when indicated. Furthermore, where areas of the foot take excessive stress, selective unloading may be achieved as with heel pads for painful calcaneal spurs or forefoot pads for metatarsalgia.

Motion Control and Alignment

The second function of orthotics is to attempt to transpose the running surface to the plantar aspect of the foot in a relatively neutral position, thereby maximizing the efficiency of the foot mechanics. Therefore either the medial arch is supported or the range of motion of the hindfoot limited. This function is usually carried out by some external motion control feature in addition to that built into the shoe or by supporting or posting the medial side of the foot. Alternatively, some wedging may be introduced on the outside of the footwear (Fig. 24-15). The latter method is often a more practical consideration for skates and ski boots.

Immobilization and Support

The third function is that of immobilizing or protecting weak, painful, or healing musculoskeletal segments. In this situation the orthosis may extend beyond the confines of the foot.

Correct Deformity

Finally, orthoses can be used to prevent or correct deformity, the most common of which is leg length discrepancy. If it is thought necessary to accommodate for such a discrepancy, approximately 50 percent of the measured inequality between 1 and 3 cm is

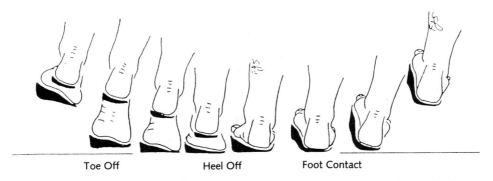

| Toe Off | Heel Off | Foot Contact |

Fig. 24-15. Motion control of a flexible foot with hyperpronation by an orthotic device supporting the medial heel and arch. Sequence is read from right to left through the stance phase. Note that the heel stays in a relatively neutral alignment. (Adapted from Nicholas and Hershman,[15] with permission).

corrected and all of less than 1 cm. An accurate measurement of small discrepancies is not always possible clinically.[26] Moreover, approximately 50 percent compensation is usually adequate for the correction of subtalar and forefoot varus. Exceptions include genu varum and varus bowing of the tibia, where additional correction may be warranted. In individuals who require medial posting but are active in rapid side-to-side sports, e.g., basketball, or who have a history of ankle sprains, less correction is prudent.

Orthoses can be broadly classified into soft, semi-rigid, and rigid. By and large, soft orthoses are more comfortable, have a shorter "break-in" period, are much more easily accepted, and usually impart enough change in the biomechanics to be effective in the treatment of a specific condition. Fitting them to the athlete requires slightly less skill. Some of the commonly used soft materials include sponge, foam, felt, and viscoelastic materials, particularly Sorbothane. The disadvantage of soft orthoses is that they wear out and lose their properties quickly. For a serious runner, they might have to be replaced as often as every 3 to 6 months.

Quick Facts
ORTHOSES

- **Soft** (foam, felt, Sorbothane, Spenco-Second Skin)
  - Protects painful soft tissue
  - Cushions foot
  - Protects prominent areas
  - Correct minor deformities
- **Semirigid** (cork, rubber, plastic, plastozoate, EVA)
  - Shock absorbing
  - Permanent orthosis
  - Correct minor and moderate deformity
- **Rigid** (polypropylene, neoprene, plastics)
  - Accommodate major deformities
  - Must be carefully customized
  - Motion control

Semirigid materials offer much more biomechanical control and are readily adapted to the requirement of extrinsic posting for rearfoot or forefoot variations. They have the disadvantage of being ex-

cessively bulky in certain shoes, particularly if it is the aim of the treatment to allow the individual to wear them in day-to-day footwear. Semirigid materials include cork and ethylene vinyl acetate (EVA). They are more durable than the soft orthoses.

Rigid orthoses obviously offer the promise of more significant biomechanical control. However, there is a limited role for rigid orthoses in the average recreational athlete. These orthoses frequently have little shock-absorbing ability and may require frequent and extensive modification. They leave little margin for error in production and application. Most experienced physicians, when reviewing their patient population, observe that these rigid orthoses have tended to cause as much trouble as they have cured in a significant number of athletes. Furthermore, the desired results can usually be achieved just as well using semirigid materials. Rigid orthoses have the additional disadvantage of being expensive. Probably the most important role of rigid orthoses is in situations where the heel must be contained, there is gross abnormality, or the orthosis can be made an extension of the footwear, as with a ski boot.

It is worth reiterating that the fitting and prescription of orthoses depend on a careful analysis of the foot, the running style, and the footwear. The most important feature of this method of treatment is to supplement the orthotic prescription with attention to the pathophysiology of the condition, advice and alteration of training habits, and evolution of a treatment program. Simply supplying an orthotic device does not constitute treatment. Although it may alleviate the condition, the same problem frequently recurs if the underlying poor training habits are not altered.

FOOTWEAR

There has been a revolution in the development of running shoes. During the late 1960s the running shoe merely provided protection from abrasions. There certainly was no customization for running-related activities such as basketball, volleyball, court games, aerobic dance, and exercise. The use of high speed photography during the 1970s, careful biomechanical analysis of the performance of running shoes, and an increasing demand from the running population led to significant changes. A good running shoe should provide cushioning, support, and stability while still being light and sufficiently flexible.

The design of aesthetic and biomechanically efficient footwear has largely replaced the need for orthotics. However, the insole of the shoe is usually designed in such a way that it can be removed to accommodate customization in the form of an orthotic when necessary.

Practice Point

REQUIREMENTS OF THE RUNNING SHOE

- Be comfortable
- Protect the wearer from injury and environment
- Not be a source of injury
- Facilitate athletic performance
- Be durable and economical

Shoe Components

The main components of the running shoe are the upper and the bottom. The upper is the part of the shoe that surrounds the foot. It includes the heel counter, collar, tongue, lacing, and toe-box. Bottoms include the outer sole, midsole, and inner sole; and it supports the foot and makes contact with the ground (Fig. 24-16).

Upper

Toe Box

The toe-box and vamp provide protection for the toes and forefoot. Ideally, it is a "one-piece" construction with few seams, thereby minimizing any potential irritation. It should be wide enough that the toes are not excessively crowded. A mud guard is often placed around the front of the running shoe. Reinforcements are placed medially and laterally on the vamp to add stability.

Heel Counter

The heel counter is the major stabilizer of the rearfoot and should support and cushion the heel (Fig. 24-16). It may be composed of fiberboard or plastic. It should be balanced with a straight seam that is not excessively prominent. The quarter lining covers the heel counter and is frequently reinforced with a foxing. The heel collar is a padded with a cutout for the Achilles tendon cushion.

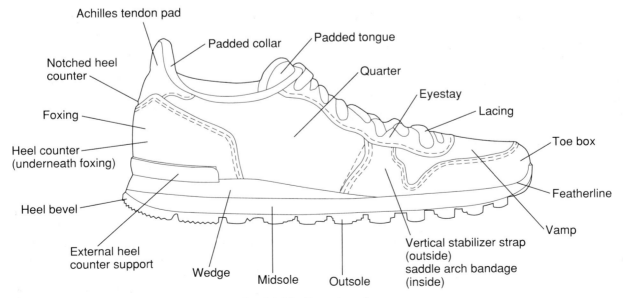

Fig. 24-16. Running shoe.

External Heel Counter (Heel Counter Support)

The external heal counter is usually hard, rigid plastic placed outside of the traditional heel counter to give extra stability to the rearfoot.

Lacing, Tongue, Ankle Collar

The lacing of the shoe is made in such a way that it can be adjusted to accommodate a wide variability in the girth of an individual's forefoot. It forms a vital part of the stability between the foot and the shoe. The tongue should cushion all the seams and reduce lace pressure. The ankle collar is the padding around the uppers that provides a comfortable fit underneath the malleoli.

Bottom

Outsole (Outer Sole)

The outer sole is the part of the shoe that comes into contact with the ground. It is tread-patterned and is made from a material that provides traction, flexibility, and some cushioning. The most common materials are carbon rubber and blown rubber. In the running shoe studs usually provide better traction on dirt surfaces, although low profile bars tend to wear longer on hard surfaces.[34] With special purpose shoes for individual sports, further customization is required. Carbon rubber has the advantage of being hard and durable. It tends to be relatively heavy and may afford less traction on icy surfaces than blown rubber. Blown rubber has air injected into it. Its main disadvantage is its more rapid wear, particularly on abrasive surfaces.

The condition of the outer sole must be checked at regular intervals for excessive localized wear, which might alter the biomechanics at foot strike. The sole on a good shoe is a unit sole (formed as a unit with no break in the material) or, alternately, a vulcanized sole (fused to the upper). In both cases it should be stitched to the upper for additional strength and resistance against torque.

Midsole

The midsole is the part of the shoe between the outsole and the upper, and in many ways it is the most important part of the shoe so far as shock absorption is concerned. In athletic shoes, the midsole replaces the shank and heel seen in nonathletic shoes. It is the part of the shoe that has undergone much research and is often characteristic for the particular brand of shoe. The most common materials are ethylene vinyl acetate (EVA) and polyurethane.

Ethylene vinyl acetate is a firm but highly resilient foam. It is relatively inexpensive to manufacture and may be produced in different densities with varying degrees of stability and cushioning. Its main disadvantage is that it is not durable and breaks down quickly under the stress of running. Compressive-set EVA (compressed and molded under heat) has the advantage over slab EVA in that its life expectancy is about three times greater. Furthermore, it is relatively soft in cold temperatures.

Polyurethane is a more dense and durable foam, and it has the advantage of being more stable and lasting longer. Unfortunately, it is heavier, becomes hard in cold temperatures, and so is less cushioning.

Most shoes have a wedge that gives height to the heel as well as adding absorbing qualities. It begins at the metatarsal area, extends back to the heel, and assists in destressing the Achilles tendon.

The midsole provides shock absorption for the rear-foot during heel strike and rigidity to prevent twisting of the shoe. Medial and lateral flaring of the midsole provide increased stability, but the flaring should be no wider than the ankle. Excessive flaring may generate a fulcrum that predisposes to inappropriately rapid pronation.[35]

Insole

The insole is made up of an insole board, which is an important structure for joining the upper and bottom, and an insole (sock liner), which lies on top of the insole board. The liner is made of nylon, foam, or terrycloth. It usually accounts for minimal cushioning and mainly serves to absorb sweat and protect the insole. In modern shoe designs the insole is removable. Lying on the insole board or as part of the insole is the arch cookie, which supports the medial longitudinal arch. Some of the newest shoes have added foam or Sorbothane heel cushions.[36]

Last

The last is a three-dimensional form, shaped in the outline of a foot, over which the components of the shoe are molded and made. The configuration of the last and the manner in which the shoe is constructed around it obviously determines factors of fit and performance. The extreme shapes of the last are straight (rectus, vector) or curved (abducted).

1. *Straight last.* This mold is used to produce a shoe that forms a straight line from heel to toe, providing maximum support under the longitudinal arches. This last usually forms the basis of motion-control shoes, frequently with boards running along the base of the upper to create both torsional rigidity and lateral support.[37]

2. *Semicurved last.* This last produces a shoe that forms a straight line from heel to midfoot with a slight curve toward the front of the shoe, forming an angle of 4 to 9 degrees.

3. *Curved last.* The shoe has a larger curve forming an angle of more than 9 degrees.

Most running shoes are derived from a combination last, and they provide both stability and shock absorption. Other last shapes and varieties include the wide (Olympic or athletic) last and the female last (usually narrower for fit).

Construction (Lasting)

The construction of the shoe is the manner in which it is fabricated around the last. It naturally influences quality, fit, and biomechanical properties.

1. *Board construction.* The upper is fastened onto the midsole underneath an insole board. This construction makes the shoe relatively rigid and stable.

2. *Slip last (moccasin) construction.* The upper envelopes the entire foot; it is sewn underneath the foot and is glued onto the midsole. This construction allows the shoe to be flexible; and because it surrounds the foot, it probably allows a better fit when the uppers are tightened and pulled up with lacing.

3. *Combination construction.* This method combines the previous two methods. Usually there is slip-last construction in the forefoot and board-last construction in the rearfoot, but it may be the other way around.

Shoe Function

Motion Control

Most control of the foot is achieved by the stability of the heel or the shock-absorbing qualities and height of the medial arch support. Thus much of the refinements center around modifications of the heel. The techniques used to increase rear-foot stability include medial extension of the heel counter, reinforcement of the heel counter, and increased density of the medial half of the midsole. The effectiveness of the heel counter in altering the mechanics of heel strike during running was demonstrated by Jorgensen[38] (Fig. 24-17). Addition of a rigid heel counter decreases the muscle load by a combination of increased shock absorption by heel pad confinement and increased rearfoot stability.[39]

Shock Absorption

Because shock absorption is also a major concern in most athletic footwear, modifications of the midsole have been designed. Frequently the basic material is varying density EVA. However, shoes lose their shock-absorbing qualities relatively quickly, usually at 200 to 400 miles (Figure 24-18). Thus for the serious runner training more than 25 miles per week, it may be necessary to replace the shoes every 3 months.[40] Individuals covering less mileage are usually able to go 4 to 6 months. Even noncompetitive runners should replace their shoes every 6 to 12 months. Shoe models vary as much as 33 percent in their wear characteristics.[24] The look of the tread is not a good guide, although uneven wear may suggest the need for quicker replacement.

There are a variety of specific manufacturer modifications that may give a specific characteristic to a shoe. They evolve frequently, and concepts are added each year.

1. *Asics Gel.* This gel is silicone engulfed in a plastic outer sack to provide cushioning and vibration-reducing qualities.

2. *Avia Counter Lever.* The outsole is concave, allowing it to spread out in a "finger-like" manner at foot contact, potentially adding cushioning.

3. *Arc.* This extension of the cantilever system utilizes a Hytrel plastic skeleton.

4. *Brooks Hydroflow.* A liquid silicone is encased in a bivalved plastic bag. Upon heel (foot) strike the silicone is forced across a pressure gradient, from high to low pressure, with the concept of attenuating forces.

5. *Nike Air.* A gas mixture in a polyurethane bag generates viscoelastic properties and thus cushioning. An extension of this system is the ability to pump varying amounts of air into the shoe, altering the impact qualities.

6. *Reebok ERS (Energy System).* A series of Hytrel tubes within the midsole add cushioning.

7. *Hexalite.* A honeycomb-like construction to the midsole.

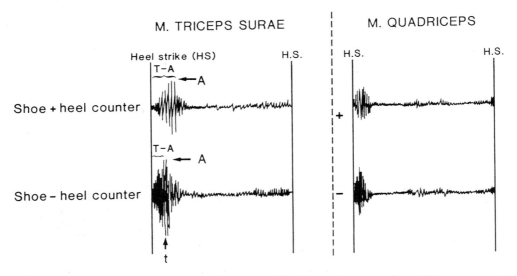

Fig. 24-17. Effects of the heel counter motion control in decreasing muscle activity as recorded in the triceps surae and quadriceps. Recording is done at heel strike. In shoes without heel support, the myographic activity is increased with early activation (T-A), greater amplitude (A), and a greater number of turns (t). (After Jorgensen,[38] with permission.)

8. *Multidensity.* The midsole is composed of materials of more than one density, used in varying combinations to create specific desired stability characteristics. It may be built into the wedge or the main part of the midsole.

9. *Torsion.* The Adidas Company stressed a concept of constructing the shoe in such a way that the rearfoot and forefoot act independently.

Shoe Selection

Selection of appropriate athletic footwear depends on first deciding clearly the function for which it is being purchased: jogging and running on track or cross-country terrains, winter wear, or one of the running-related activities, e.g., field events, basketball, or court sports. Furthermore, there is the concept of training versus competition footwear. There is much customization in each of these designs and hence the need for careful selection (Table 24-4). Obviously, there are specific constructions should cleats or spikes be necessary.

For aerobics a great deal of forefoot cushioning is desirable because of the repetitive jumping. Even the outsole is designed more for shock absorbing than wear characteristics. The shoe should be light for the quick moves but must give adequate torsional sup-port. This property may be partly assessed by grasping the toe and heel and twisting the shoe.

Squash and racquetball require a light shoe for rapid motion. A thin midsole lightens the shoe. The outside should be relatively smooth to allow some sliding on the wood floor.

Tennis shoes need excellent side-to-side support. The shoe should be moderately rigid. Particular attention is paid to the heel counter fit and Achilles and ankle collar cushioning. The sole should bend at the appropriate position on the foot, and durability of the uppers is significant, making leather a good choice. If the individual drags the toe a great deal when serving, look for extra toe cap padding.

Basketball shoes require special attention to ankle stability and shock absorption because of jumping. High tops are more suitable, and a good forefoot fit for side-to-side stability is necessary.

A special walking shoe is a difficult concept to sell. Most exercisers wonder why they have to buy a specific shoe for something they have been doing all their lives. Certainly the need for shock absorbing and stabilizing are not so great as with other activities. However, they are built for comfort. They have a higher wider toe-box that allows good toe movement when walking, and the heel is higher to relieve Achilles tendon stress. Although the outsole should be thick, it

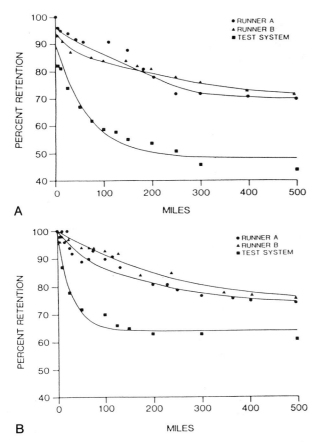

Fig. 24-18. Wear characteristics of different running shoes illustrated by the percent retention of the initial shock absorption as a function of mileage in vivo and in the test system. (**A**) Running shoe 1. (**B**) Running shoe 2, illustrating the different wear characteristics between the two shoes. (After Cook et al.,[24] with permission.)

should not be so stiff that it restricts movement. The flex point should be near the ball of the foot. The type of terrain that is usually covered dictates the need for an increasingly durable walking shoe.

The next consideration is one of understanding the basic foot biomechanics to see if shock absorption or motion control are essential prerequisites. If the addition of an orthotic is desirable, the shoe must be able to accept one. Where there is a tendency to overpronate, a straight last, solid heel counter, and good medial support provide the best chance at motion control. For the neutral foot, a semi-curved last, combination construction, medium to solid heel

TABLE 24-4. Selecting a Running Shoe

1. Clearly visualize the activity for which the shoe is being purchased, e.g., running, basketball, sprinting.
2. It must be appropriate for the conditions under which it will perform.
   a. Wear game socks.
   b. Must fit at end of day when feet are slightly swollen.
3. Choose material.
   a. Leather stretches, nylon does not.
   b. Nylon breathes more.
   c. Nylon is easier to wash.
   d. Leather usually gives better support.
4. Breaking point (bending area) must be correct.
   a. Shoe should break at MTP joint.
   b. Shoe should be sufficient flexible. To test: hold heel and use index finger of other hand to flex up toe. Should be approximately 10 lb (4.5 kg). *OR* test on bathroom scale; should bend before scale reads 10 lb.
5. Ensure adequate length.
   a. Allow 0.5 inch (1.3 cm), or one thumbnail between longest toe and end of toe cap.
   b. Always fit to larger foot.
6. Width must be sufficient.
   a. Test with full weight on shoefoot.
   b. Place thumb and finger around forefoot.
   c. Should not overhang sole.
   d. Should not have obvious large wrinkles when laced up (too wide).
7. Lacing is important.
   a. Eyelets should be parallel from top to bottom.
8. General workmanship is assessed.
   a. Look for flaws in stiching and seams
9. Take time to break in the new shoe to avoid blisters and injury.

counter, and moderate shock-absorbing qualities are adequate. For those who supinate, with a tendency to increased rigidity, a curved last construction with an adequate arch support and an emphasis on shock absorption is usually desirable.[32] When the athlete has a history of or current symptoms due to lower limb injuries, they should also be taken into account when deciding on the desirable qualities of the shoe (Table 24-5).

Lastly, whatever shoe is chosen, it must be comfortable. The toe-box should be of adequate height and width so it does not cause friction on the toes or the toenails (Fig. 24-19). It should extend approximately 0.25 to 0.50 inch beyond the longest toe to prevent jamming and nail injury. The flexibility of the shoe should be maximal at the ball of the foot to coordinate with the axis of the metatarsophalangeal joints. Whereas excessive flexibility causes instability, too little flexibility contributes to arch fatigue and

TABLE 24-5.   Suggested Features of Running Shoes Relative to Foot Type

Cavus Foot[a]	Pes Planus[b]
Curved last	Straight last
Slip last	Board last
Softer EVA	Motion control heel counter
Air sole	Additional medial support
Narrow flare	Wider flare
	Higher density EVA on medial insole
Modifications	
Neoprene sole	Increased medial wedging on insole
Sorbothane insole	
Akton and Zekon insole	Soft orthotic
Soft orthotic	Semirigid orthotic

[a] Usually considered a rigid foot, frequently the heel in supination.

[b] Frequently associated with increased static and dynamic pronation.

Practice Point

GENERAL GUIDELINES FOR FOOTWEAR NEED[a]

Needs	Pronator	Neutral Foot	Supinator
Needs	Stability Arch support	Good fit Adequate arch Shock absorbing	Flexibility Maximum shock absorbing
Features	Straight last Combination construction Solid supportive heel counter Extra support on medial side	Semicurved last Combination or slip last Extra cushioning Medium heel counter	Semicurved or curved last Slip last construction Maximum cushioning

[a]Preferably based on dynamic analysis and static weight-bearing measurements in combination with review of wear pattern of old shoes and past or present history of lower limb problems.

strain on the Achilles tendon. The lateral flare of the heel should be no more than 0.25 inch because if it is excessive it may create an inappropriate lever arm.

Athletic Footwear and Perceptual Illusions

The preceding section presented the traditional concepts of shoe function and biomechanical implication. This information can be summed up as emphasis on motion control, protection, and shock absorption. However, it is essential to realize that there is a totally different perspective that brings well established dogma into question.

The vertical component of plantar impact with running and jumping results in significant propagation of shock waves, which have been shown to produce chronic overloading of bone and connective tissue in various mammals.[41,42] It is possible that under some circumstances these stresses are equally destructive in man.[20,42,43] The high incidence of activity-acquired injury, presumably in response to chronic overloading, suggested to footwear designers that the lower extremity may be fragile. Hence athletic footwear is designed to protect and shield the foot, similar to delicate merchandise being shipped, by the use of soft, shock-absorbing materials. The more recent models have the most packaging, hence the greatest compliance and comfort. Prices have also increased proportionately. Although certain successes are apparent, the story is far from clear. There is some evidence that any decrease in running-related injuries is due more to athlete education, modified training techniques, and mileage adjustment than to improved footwear.

In response to this suggestion, Robbins and Gouw intriguingly hypothesized that the lower extremity is inherently durable and is made susceptible to injury by footwear use.[44] Essentially, they believed that there are efficient shock-absorbing mechanisms and reflexes built into the lower limb kinematic chain. They suggested that modern athletic footwear is unsafe because it attenuates the plantar sensations, which trigger the feedback control circuits necessary to induce the behavior required to prevent injury (Fig. 24-20). In short, they believed that excessively shock-absorbing footwear may generate perceptual illusions that inhibit the triggering of natural shock-absorbing systems within the limbs. These investigators cited several arguments to support the discomfort-impact illusions theory.[44]

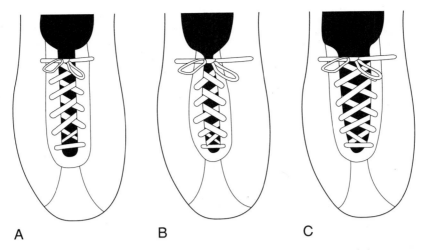

Fig. 24-19. Alignment of the eye stays and lacing, may give an indication of the correct fitting of the shoe. (**A**) Correct fitting with 2 to 3 cm separation and parallel sides. (**B**) Shoe is too wide, the eyelets come too close together and the shoe will probably wrinkle. (**C**) Shoe is too narrow, and the eyelets diverge. This will give less support.

1. Wearers of expensive running shoes having additional features that protect them (e.g., more cushioning, pronation correction) but are injured significantly more frequently than runners wearing inexpensive shoes (costing less than $40 US).[5] These data may simply reflect excessive training mileage.
2. When runners unaccustomed to barefoot running run barefoot, the mean impact is no higher than when shod, and in some cases is lower.[45]
3. Running injuries in barefoot populations are rare.[46]
4. Material tests fail to predict actual impact while running. The more compliant shoe, which according to material tests should attenuate shock more effectively, fails to do so. This fact is possibly related to greater plantar comfort, reducing the need for impact-moderating behavior.[24,47]
5. Gymnasts landing from 0.69 meter high generated less impact when landing on hard surfaces than on yielding mats.[44] To appreciate the magnitude of this perceptual illusion, these subjects reduced their impact moderating behavior so that they delivered peak impacts to the landing surface that were 20 to 25 percent higher than that generated landing on the hard floor. Despite this fact, they retained the impression of lower impact when landing on the mats. This perception is obviously a discomfort perception illusion.

Further experiments by Robbin's group revealed that induced plantar discomfort by barefoot walking or by surface irregularities in footwear are capable of producing impact modification.

These studies are presented because acceptance of the dogma of impact protection by running shoes leads to spiraling assumptions about orthotics. It is obvious that there is still much to learn before pragmatic prescription advice can be given regarding the "best" running shoe for any given individual. The issue is further complicated by the assumptions made concerning the ability and necessity of motion control by footwear. It is important to keep an open mind

---

Practice Point

RUNNING SHOES

- People have different running styles and thus may be more suited for one shoe over another.
- Consider needs, protection versus performance.
- Comfort is the key.
- In the face of injury, training modification is more important than footwear.

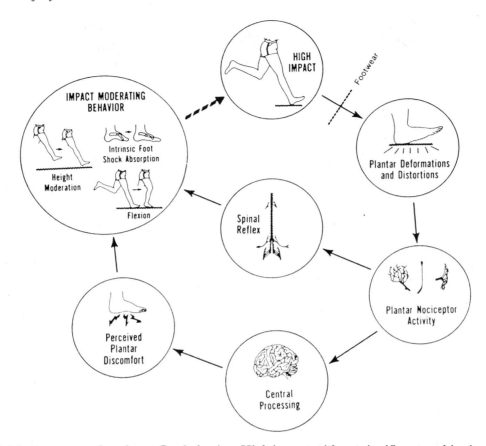

Fig. 24-20. Impact-moderating reflex behavior. High impact without significant cushioning by footwear stimulates plantar nociceptor activity, triggering spinal reflexes that generate impact-moderating behavior. This reaction may be supplemented by central processing and perceived plantar discomfort. Excessive cushioning of impacts may fail to trigger these impact-moderating behaviors, sometimes resulting in higher stresses through the lower limb. (Adapted from Robbins and Gouw,[44] with permission.)

regarding the role of athletic footwear. Most of all, Robbins' work indirectly lent support to and emphasized the major tool of injury prevention and treatment, i.e., careful training techniques for prophylaxis and systemic activity analysis and modification.

All athletic footwear should fulfill two basic functions: protection and performance enhancement. The obvious functional adaptations are the cleats of soccer and baseball shoes. This change, in turn, may generate the risk of excessively efficient traction, producing a propensity for knee injury. Thus the merits of traction must be weighed against increased injury risk. Similarly, the need for protection may outweigh the need for performance. With high-cut shoes for basketball, for example, the player accepts the added weight to obtain support around the ankle.

The marathon runner may opt for a heavier, more shock-absorbing, and supportive shoe in the face of previous injuries.

Although most sports medicine exponents are comfortable with the current rationale and approach to prescription of running shoes, the work of Robbins has introduced healthy suspicion into the system. It further emphasizes the importance of training principles and activity modification.

SUMMARY

Running is often the common link between many recreational and sporting activities. However, despite it being a natural activity, the forces involved are high, the biomechanics complex, and the potential for injury significant. It seems apparent that specific alignments within the lower limb segments may predispose to certain overuse syndromes. Nevertheless, this relation is not as clear as one would hope, and the major theme of all well controlled studies is the relation between excessive mileage, poor training techniques, and inappropriate progression to injury. Undoubtedly, alignment of the lower limb has an influence but not in a simple way. The evolving running shoe has replaced the need for orthotics among many runners. For treatment of running-acquired injuries, it may be necessary to select more appropriate footwear or modify lower limb biomechanics by the use of orthotics.

It has been stressed that cure does not infer etiology, and unless attention is paid to poor training techniques, recurrence is a likely outcome. The relations between foot sensation and impact-attenuating reflexes have been explored, which should stimulate further examination of the relation between footwear and stress through the lower limb joints. Whatever emphasis is placed on the various components of alignment, biomechanics, flexibility, strength, shoes, orthoses, and training techniques, only a thorough understanding of running biomechanics allows an appropriate approach to treatment of the various activity-acquired syndromes.

REFERENCES

1. Koplan JP, Powell KE, Sikes RK et al: An epidemiologic study of the benefits and risk of running. JAMA 248:3118, 1982
2. Reid DC: Assessment and Treatment of the Injured Athlete. Course Manual. University of Alberta Press, Edmonton, 1985
3. Sheehan G: Less is more. Physician Sports Med 19:21, 1991
4. Clement DB, Taunton JE, Smart GW et al: A survey of overuse running injuries. Physician Sports Med 9:47, 1981
5. Marti B, Vader JP, Minder CE et al: On the epidemiology of running injuries: the 1984 Bera Grand Prix study. Am J Sports Med 16:285, 1988
6. Caldwell F: Millions of runners? A matter of definition. Physician Sports Med 13:50, 1985
7. Cavanagh PR, LaFortune MA: Ground reaction forces during distance running. J Biomech 13:397, 1980
8. Nigg BM: Biomechanics, load analysis and sports injuries in the lower extremities. Sports Med 2:317, 1985
9. Bateman JE, Trott A: The Foot and Ankle. Theime-Stratton, New York, 1980
10. Mann RA: Biomechanics of running. In: AAOS Symposium on the Foot and Leg in Running Sports. CV Mosby, St. Louis, 1982
11. Subotnick SI: The biomechanics of running: implications for the prevention of foot injuries. Sports Med 2:144, 1985
12. Mann RA, Hagy J: Biomechanics of walking, running and sprinting. Am J Sports Med 8:345, 1980
13. Adelaar RS: The practical biomechanics of running. Am J Sports Med 14:497, 1986
14. James SL, Brubaker CE: Biomechanics of running. Orthop Clin North Am 4:605, 1973
15. Nicholas JA, Hershman EB (eds): The Lower Extremity in Sports Medicine. Vol. 2. CV Mosby, St. Louis, 1990
16. Corrigan B: Musculoskeletal complications of jogging. Br J Sports Med 14:37, 1980
17. Lysholm J, Wiklander J: Injuries in runners. Am J Sports Med 15:168, 1987
18. Jacobs SJ, Berson BL: Injuries to runners: a study of entrants to a 10,000 meter race. Am J Sports Med 14:151, 1986
19. McQuade KJ: A case-control study of running injuries: comparison of patterns of runners with and without running injuries. J Orthop Sports Phys Ther 8:81, 1986
20. Goodyear NN, Blair SN: Incidence rates and risk of orthopaedic injuries in healthy middle aged runners and non-runners. Med Sci Sports Exerc 16:114, 1984
21. MacIntyre JG, Taunton JE, Clement DB et al: Running injuries: a clinical study of 4,173 cases. Clin J Sports Med 1:81, 1991
22. Stamford B: Training distance and injury in runners. Physician Sports Med 12:160, 1984
23. Chadbourne RD: A hard look at running surfaces. Physician Sports Med 18:103, 1990
24. Cook SD, Kester MA, Brunet ME: Shock absorption characteristics of running shoes. Am J Sports Med 13:248, 1985
25. Messier SP, Pittala KA: Etiologic factors associated with selected running injuries. Med Sci Sports Exerc 20:501, 1988
26. Reid DC, Smith B: Leg length inequality: a review of etiology and management. Physiother Can 35:177, 1984
27. Smith-Oricchio K, Harris BA: Interrater reliability of subtalar, neutral, calcaneal inversion and eversion. J Orthop Sports Phys Ther 12:10, 1990
28. Roy S, Irvin R: Sports Medicine Prevention Evaluation, Management and Rehabilitation. Prentice-Hall, Englewood Cliffs, NJ, 1983

29. Arnheim D: Modern Principles of Athletic Training. 7th Ed. Times Mirror/Mosby, St. Louis, 1989

30. McKenzie DC, Clement DB, Taunton JE: Running shoes, orthotics and injuries. Sports Med 2:334, 1985

31. Cinats J, Reid DC, Haddow J: A biomechanical evaluation of Sorbothane. Clin Orthop 222:15, 1987

32. Rodgers MM, Leveau BF: Effectiveness of foot orthotic devices used to modify pronation in runners. J Orthop Sports Phys Ther 4:86, 1982

33. Nigg BM, Herzog W, Read LJ: Effects of viscoelastic shoe insoles on vertical impact forces in heel-toe running. Am J Sports Med 16:20, 1988

34. Clarke TE, Frederick EC, Hamill CC: The effect of shoe design parameters on rear foot control in running. Med Sci Sports Exerc 15:376, 1983

36. Horbal R: Running footwear. Can Physiother Assoc, Sports Physiother Division, Newslett 11:23, 1986

37. Moore PM, Kelly P: Understanding athletic footwear. Sports Med Info 9:1, 1991 [Sport Medicine Council of Canada]

38. Jorgensen U: Body load in heel-strike running: the effect of a firm heel counter. Am J Sports Med 18:177, 1990

39. Jorgensen U, Ekstrand J: Significance of heel pad confinement for the shock absorption at heel strike. Int J Sports Med 9:468, 1988

40. Cook SD, Brinker MR, Poche M: Running shoes: their relationship to running injuries. Sports Med 10:1, 1990

41. Dekel S, Weissman SL: Joint changes after over-use and peak overloading of rabbit knees in vivo. Acta Orthop Scand 49:519, 1978

42. Radin EL, Orr RB, Kelman JL et al: Effect of prolonged walking on concrete on the knees of sheep. J Biomech 15:487, 1982

43. Dyck PJ, Classen SM, Stevens JC et al: Assessment of nerve damage in the feet of long distance runners. Mayo Clin Proc 62:568, 1987

44. Robbins SE, Gouw GJ: Athletic footwear: unsafe due to perceptual illusions. Med Sci Sports Exerc 23:217, 1991

45. Dickenson JA, Cook SD, Leinhardt TM: The measurement of shock waves following heel strike while running. J Biomech 18:1, 1985

46. Robbins SE, Hanna AM: Running related injury prevention through barefoot adaptations. Med Sci Sports Exerc 19:148, 1987

47. Light LH, McLellan GE, Klenerman L: Skeletal transients on heel strike in normal walking with different footwear. J Biomech 13:477, 1980

APPENDICES

APPENDIX I
Banned and Restricted Doping Classes and Methods*

The only reason an athlete should be taking any drug is for a justified clinical condition that is being treated by a doctor. The International Olympic Committee (IOC) and other international sports organizations started drug testing to protect athletes from (1) the potential unfair advantage that might be gained by those athletes who take drugs to enhance performance and (2) the potential harmful side effects some drugs produce.

Some helpful hints include the following.

1. If there is *any* doubt, do not take the medicine or drug.
2. Some so-called vitamin preparations contain banned drugs.
3. Some medicines have similar brand names. One may contain a banned drug, the other may not. For example, Robitussin is permitted, whereas Robitussin PS contains a banned substance.
4. Remember that medications on the banned list are not all oral (liquid or tablet) medications. Some of them are injectable or suppositories.

Banned drugs fall into several classes: stimulants, narcotics, anabolic steroids, β-blockers, diuretics, peptide hormones, and analogues. Although the categories and examples of drugs listed below are taken from the IOC medical controls brochure, they *do not* include all banned drugs. No list can be considered complete. Different sport associations may ban different drugs. Check with your organization.

Restricted drugs are permitted under specific medically indicated circumstances in appropriate dosages or nonmedically in small quantities. Their use requires judgment on the part of the physician and athlete. Restricted drugs fall into several classes: injectable local anesthetics, asthma and respiratory ailment drugs, corticosteroids, caffeine, alcohol, and marijuana. The categories and examples of these drugs are periodically revised, so this appendix forms the basis of a dynamic list that must be continuously updated. New drugs should be prescribed with caution or after consultation with national sports governing bodies.

SECTION I

IOC-Banned Drugs

Stimulants

Amfetaminil
Amfepramone (Tenuate)
Amiphenazole (Amphisol, Daptazole)
Amphetamine (Benzedrine, Dexedrin, Dexamphetamine, Obetrol)
Benzphetamine (Didrex)
Caffeine (see Restricted Drugs)
Cathine (Amorphen, Reduform)
Chlorprenaline (Asthone, Isoprophenamine)
Clobenzorex
Cocaine
Cropropamide — contained in Micoren
Crotethamide — contained in Micoren
Dimethylamphetamine (Phenopane)
Ephedrine (present in many over-the-counter cold or cough syrups)
Etafedrine
Ethamivan (Emivan, Vandid)
Ethylamphetamine (Apetinil)
Femcamfamine (Altimine, Phencamine, Reactivan)

* This material is reprinted with permission of the Sports Medicine Council of Canada and Sport Canada. Cat. No. #93-103/1989.

Fenetylline
Femproporex
Furfenorex
Mefenorex
Methoxyphenamine (present in Orthoxicol cough syrup)
Methylphenidate
Methylephedrine (present in some European cold tablets and syrups)
Methylamphetamine (Dosoxyn, Methampex, Methedrin)
Monazone
Nikethamide (Coramine)
Norpseudoephedrine Cathine (Amorphan, Reduform)
Pemoline (Cylert, Deltamine, Stimul)
Pentebrazol (Leptazol, Cardiazol, Metrazol, Pentrasol)
Phendimetrazine (Dietrol)
Phenmetrazine (Preludin)
Phentermine (Fastin, Ionamin)
Phenylpropanolamine
Pipradol (Meratran)
Prolintane (Promotil, Katovit)
Propylhexedrine
Pyrovalerone
Strychnine
and related compounds

Narcotic Analgesics

Alphaprodine (Nisentil)
Anileridine (Apodol, Leritine)
Buprenorphine (Buprenex)
Codeine (present in over-the-counter pain relievers, cough and cold tablets and syrups)
Dextromoramide (D-Moramid, Dimorlin)
Dextropropoxyphene (Darvon)
Dihydrocodeine (Paracodin)
Dipipanone (Diconal, Pipadone, Wellconal)
Ethoheptazine (Panalgin, Equagesic)
Ethylmorphine (Terpo-Dionin)
Heroin (Diamorphine)
Levorphanol (Levo-Dromoran)
Methadone (Amidom, Dolophine)
Morphine (M.O.S., Statex)
Nalbuphine (Nubain)
Pentazocine (Talwin)
Pethidine or Meperidine (Demerol)
Phenazocine (Narphen, Prinadol)
Trimeperidine (analgesic in Eastern Europe)

Anabolic Steroids

Bolasterone (Myagen)
Boldenone (Boldane, Parenabol)
Clostebol (Steranabol)
Dehydrochlormethyltestosterone (Turinabol)
Fluoxymesterone (Halotestin, Ora-Testryl, Ultrandren)
Mesterolone (Androviron, Pro-viron)
Methenolone (Primobolan, Primonabol-Depot)
Methandienone (several brand names)
Nandrolone or 19-nortestosterone (Durabolin, Deca-Durabolin, Anabol)
Nethyltestosterone
Norethandrolone (Nilevar)
Oxandrolone (Anavar, Lonovar)
Oxymesterone (Oranabol, Theranabol)
Oxymetholone (Anapolon 50, Adroyd)
Stanozolol (Winstrol, Stromba)
Testosterone* (Malogen, Malogex, Delatestryl, Oreton)
and related compounds

β-Blockers

Acebutolol (Sectral)
Alprenolol (Aptin)
Atenolol (Tenormin)
Labetalol (Trandate)
Metoprolol (Lopresor, Betaloc)
Nadolol (Corgard)
Oxprenolol (Inderal)
Sotalol (Sotacor)
Timolol (Blocadren)
and related compounds

Diuretics

Acetazolamide (Apotex, Diamox)
Amiloride (Midamor)
Bendrofluazide (Naturetin)
Benoroflumethiazide
Benzthiazide
Bumetanide
Canrenone (Phanurane)

---

* For testosterone, the definition of a positive test result depends upon the following: the administration of testosterone or the *use of any other manipulation* having the result of increasing the ratio in urine of testosterone/epitestosterone to above six (6).

Chlormerodrin (Neohydrin, Percapyl)
Chlorthalidone (Hygroton, Uridon)
Dichlorphenamide (Oratrol)
Ethacrynic acid (Edecrin)
Frusemide (Furosemide, Lasix)
Hydrochlorothiazide (HydroDiuril, HCT)
Mersalyl (Salygan)
Spironolactone (Aldactone)
Triamterene (Dyrenium)
  and related compounds

Peptide Hormones and Analogues

Chorionic gonadotropin (hCG — human chorionic gonadotropin)
  Corticotropin (ACTH)
  Growth hormone (hGH, somatotropin)
All of the respective releasing factors of the above mentioned substances are also banned.

Banned Methods

Blood doping:

Blood or red blood cell transfusion or reinfusion

Pharmacologic, chemical, and physical manipulations:

Methods and/or substances that alter the integrity and validity of urine samples used in doping controls are banned.

SECTION II

Restricted Drugs

Injectable Local Anesthetics

Injectable local anesthetics are permitted only under the following conditions.

1. Procaine, lidocaine, carbocaine, etc. can be used but *not cocaine.*
2. Local injections can be used (*intravenous injections are not permitted*).
3. *Vasoconstrictors must not be present* (e.g., epinephrine).

4. When medically justified; the details must be submitted in writing to the Medical Commission.

Asthma and Respiratory Ailments Drugs (β-agonists)

1. The choice of medication for the treatment of asthma and respiratory ailments has posed many problems. Some years ago, ephedrine and related substances were administered frequently. These substances are now prohibited because they are classed in the category of sympathomimetic amines or stimulants and have been in the subject of abuse.
2. The use of corticosteroids by inhalation is permitted for asthma therapy.
3. The use of the β-agonist drugs terbutaline, salbutamol, bitolterol, orcipenaline, and rimiterol for the treatment of asthma is permitted in aerosol form *only. The oral use of β-agonists is still prohibited. Fenetorol is banned for all uses.*
4. Theophylline is *not* prohibited, *but* it is often combined with an ephedrine-type drug in preparations.

Corticosteroids

Stronger restrictions of corticosteroid usage have been required owing to their increasing nontherapeutic use. The use of corticosteroids therefore is now banned *except for* topical use (ear, eye, and skin), inhalation therapy (asthma, allergic rhinitis), and local or intra-articular injections.* Thus the use of corticosteroids orally, intramuscularly, or intravenously is *not permitted.*

Caffeine

A urine specimen is considered positive if the concentration of caffeine exceeds 12 μg/ml. Normal ingestion of coffee, tea, and many caffeine-based drinks (e.g., colas) does not cause this limit to be exceeded or even remotely approached. However, the ingestion of caffeine tablets or the use of caffeine suppositories or injections may result in a positive doping test.

---

* Also, any team doctor wishing to administer corticosteroids intra-articularly or locally to a competitor must give written notification to the IOC or competition medical commission in advance.

Alcohol

Alcohol is not prohibited. However, blood or breath alcohol levels may be determined at the request of an international federation, as has already been the case in fencing and shooting events in the modern pentathalon. Thus it is necessary for athletes competing in these events to abstain from alcoholic beverages for at least 12 hours before the event.

Marijuana

Marijuana is not prohibited. However, tests may be carried out at the request of an international federation.

SECTION II

Permitted Drugs (Drugs not Currently Banned)

It is important to be aware that *most drugs are not banned* and therefore are available if needed to treat a justifiable condition. Drugs in the "permitted drugs" category may be prescription or nonprescription drugs. The list in the following table is not complete but gives some idea of what is not banned. It should not be taken as a recommendation of the relative efficacy of various substances.

Drugs (By Therapeutic Class)	Examples of Permitted Drugs (Canadian Trade Names)	Examples of Banned or Restricted Drugs
Analgesics	Aspirin Atasol Bufferin (plain) Ecotrin Entrophen Exedrin (plain) Feldene Motrin Nalfon Panadol Ponstan Tylenol	Demerol 222's 282's 292's *Beware* of preparations containing codeine, morphine, or heroin (e.g., Darvon-N, Empracet-30, Exdol-30, Exdol-8, Tylenol #1, #2, #3)
Antianginal drugs		Corgard
Antacids	Amphojel Diovol Gelusil Maalox Mylanta Riopan	
Antibiotics (penicillins, tetracyclines, sulfonamides)	Amoxil Bactrim Erythrocyn Gantrisin Keflex Mandelamine Penbritin Penicillin Septra Vibramycin	
Antiasthmatics	Alupent[a] Atrovent Aminophyline Beclovent Bricanyl[a]	See text: Section III, Asthma and Respiratory Ailments Drugs Adrenalin Berotec inhaler

(Continued)

Drugs (By Therapeutic Class)	Examples of Permitted Drugs (Canadian Trade Names)	Examples of Banned or Restricted Drugs
	Choledyl[a] (tablets) Fivent Intal[a] Rynacrom[a] Theo-Dur[a] (tablets) Theolair[a] (tablets) Theophylline Ventolin[a] **[a] β-Agonists allowable by inhalation only**	Fenoterol Ventolin *tablets* Medihaler-ISO *Beware:* Permitted in aerosol (inhalation) form *only* Bitolterol Orciprenaline Rimiterol Salbutamol Terbutaline
Anticonvulsants	Dilantin Mysoline Phenobarbital Tegretol Valium	
Antidepressants	Desyrel (trazodone HCl) Norpramin (desipramine HCl)	
Antidiabetics	Diabinese Dimelor Glucophage Insulin Orinase Tolinase	
Antidiarrheals	Cantil Chloroquin Diphenoxylate Hydrochloride Donnagel (plain) Imodium Kao-Can Kaomycin Kaopectate Lomotil Pepto-Bismol	Diban Donnagel-PG *Beware* of preparations containing codeine
Antifungals	Canesten Desenex Fulvicin Grisactin Loprox Monistat Mycostatin Tinactin	
Antihistamines	Benadryl Chlor-Tripolon Dimetane Hismanal Phenergan Pyribenzamine Seldane	Chlor-tripolon decongestant Dimetapp Elexir Dimetapp Extentabs Drixtab Naldecon Ornade Trinalin

Drugs (By Therapeutic Class)	Examples of Permitted Drugs (Canadian Trade Names)	Examples of Banned or Restricted Drugs
		Beware: Use only plain preparations; combinations often contain banned drugs.

Anti-inflammatories (some have analgesic, antipyretic, and antiarthritic properties)	Anaprox
	Clinoril (Sulindac)
	Diflunisal (Dolobid)
	Feldene
	Idarac
	Indomethacin (Indocid)
	Ketoprofen (Orudis)
	Motrin
	Nalfon
	Naprosyn
	Tandearil
	Voltaren
	All nonsteroidal anti-inflammatories are permitted (topical administration, aural, ophthalmologic, and dermatologic preparations)
		Beware:
		    Use of corticosteroid anti-inflammatories by injection (intra-articular and local) requires notification.
		    Oral and parenteral corticosteroids are prohibited.

Antinauseants	Antivert Bonamine Dramamine Gravol Marzine Stemetil Transderm	
Antiulcer agents	Reglan Tagamet Zantac	
Antivirals	Zovirax	
Contraceptives	All birth control pills, e.g., Ovral, Ortho 1/150	

Cough syrups/lozenges	Syrups
	    Benylin (plain)
	    Benadryl (plain)
	    Neocitran-A
	    Robitussin (plain)
	    (Dextromethorphan)
	
	Tablets
	    Tesalon
		Syrups
		    Actified
		    Coricidin-D
		    Dimetane Expectorant
		    Ornade
		    Robitussin PS
		    Sinutab
		    Tussionex
		    Vicks Nyquil
		    Neocitran-plain
		    neocitran-DM
		Beware: Most cough medicines contain banned drugs.

(Continued)

Drugs (By Therapeutic Class)	Examples of Permitted Drugs (Canadian Trade Names)	Examples of Banned or Restricted Drugs

	Lozenges
	    Benylin Koffettes
	    Bionet
	    Bradosol
	    Cepacol
	    Coricidin
	    Dequadin
	    Sept T red
	    Sept T orange
	    Strepsils
		Spec T green

Decongestants: nose drops/sprays	Beconase Nafrine Otrivin Privine Sustain Tyzine	Naldecon SineAid Sinutab Sudafed Triaminic
Eye/ear drops	Albalon Liquifilm Albalon A Albalon A-Liquifilm Auralgan Cerumenex Collyrium Cortisporin Metimyd Neosporin Polysporin Sodium Sulmyd Visine	
Gonadotropins		Human chorionic gonadotropin and compounds with related activity
Hemorrhoidal preparations	Anugesic-HC Anusol Nupercainal Proctosedyl	
Laxatives	Colace Dulcolax Doxidan Fleet enema Metamucil Milk of magnesia	
Migraine medication	Cafergot Ergomar Fiorinal (plain)	Fiorinal with codeine
Muscle relaxants	Equanil Flexeril Norflex Robaxin	
Ointments/cream/lotions	All topical, antifungal, antihistaminic, anti-infective, antipruritic,	

Drugs (By Therapeutic Class)	Examples of Permitted Drugs (Canadian Trade Names)	Examples of Banned or Restricted Drugs
	coaltar, and protective preparations are safe, e.g., Baciguent, Neosporin, Keri	
Sedatives	Ativan Dalmane Halcion Librium Valium	*Beware* of any preparations containing codeine
Tranquilizers	Xanax	
Uricosuric agents		Probenecid and related compounds
Vaginal preparations	AVC Betadine Canesten Flagyl Flagystatin Monistat Mycostatin Ovoquinol	

APPENDIX II
Travel with Athletes

OBJECTIVE: Allow athletes to compete as effectively as possible by minimizing adverse effects of travel.

BEFORE DEPARTURE

Obtain the following information from the coach, team manager, athlete, or athlete's physician.

1. Who
   a. Number of players traveling, staff, other personnel
   b. Age range
   c. Significant past medical history, medications, allergies
   d. Previous problems with travel
2. Where
   a. Location of competition
   b. Climate, altitude, local endemic medical problems
   c. Accommodation, playing venues
   d. Food and water supplies
3. When
   a. Length of stay
   b. Travel plans, potential for acclimatization
   c. Schedule of practice, games, internal travel

Medical Resources

1. Composition of medical team, therapists, physicians
2. Supplies and budget
3. Local facilities available
4. Provisions for evacuation
5. Drug testing
6. Need for immunization (hepatitis, globulin, tetanus, malaria)
7. Requirements for health insurance.

Medications

1. If crossing international borders, make sure all medications carried can be clearly identified.
2. Carry nonprescription and prescription drugs in the containers as they were dispensed, with labels intact.
3. Ensure appropriate emergency drugs if it is anticipated there will be minimal medical backup.
4. Include provisions for motion sickness.
5. Traveler's diarrhea (see Appendix III).
6. Carry specific medication for athletes and officials with known problems.
7. Include antihistamine and nasal decongestant spray to treat respiratory ailments developed prior to return, specifically to reduce in-flight ear blockage.

IN FLIGHT

Decreased Atmospheric Pressure

1. Aircraft cabin pressures are kept at an equivalent to an altitude of 1,600 to 2,500 meters (5,000 to 8,000 feet).
2. Reduction in atmospheric pressure results in a minimal decrease in oxygen saturation of 3 to 4 percent.
3. It should not affect healthy individuals.
4. It may be a problem in those with unstable angina, chronic obstructive airway disease, or a hemoglobinopathy.
5. Main problem with athletes is expansion of gases trapped in body cavities (dysbarism).
   a. Usually inability to equalize middle ear pressure.
   b. Aggravated by respiratory tract ailments.
   c. Symptoms mainly with flight descent.
   d. Initial feeling of fullness, decreased hearing, and discomfort; may progress to severe pain.
   e. Alleviate by Valsalva maneuver.
   f. Individuals who have been diving for long periods at a depth of 10 meters should not fly for 12 hours—and at greater depths for 24 hours.
   g. Athletes who have recently undergone surgery or invasive tests may experience increased symptoms transiently if air is trapped in body cavities (i.e., arthroscopy or arthrogram).

Humidity and Cabin Environment

1. While cruising, ambient air humidity rapidly drops to between 5 and 10 percent.
2. Dry skin and eye irritation may be a problem.
3. Contact lens wearers may have to use eyedrops frequently.
4. Drink plenty of fluids.
5. Consider taking own bottled water.
6. Use no alcohol.
7. Use no caffeine.
8. Cabin air is renewed every 3 to 4 minutes. However, there may be some contamination from cigarette smoke. Sit as far away from the smoking section as possible.

Motion, Turbulence, and Fear

1. Susceptible athletes can be protected by antiemetics such as Gravol (dimenhydrinate).
2. Alcohol should be avoided with motion sickness tablets (MSTs).
3. Take MSTs 30 minutes before departure.
4. MSTs may produce drowsiness for several hours.
5. Transdermal scopolamine (Transderm-V) may give prolonged side effects and is not recommended for athletes.
6. For anxiety and fear, sublingual lorazepam (Ativan) is effective; 1 mg sublingually produces a peak concentration 60 minutes after administration.

Combating Jet Lag (Circadian Dysrhythmia)

Jet lag is a demonstrable physical, physiologic or psychological deficit associated with internal circadian rhythm dissociation. It requires a period of time for adaptation to the new time area following transmeridian flight across several time zones. There is considerable variation in the individual's ability to adjust their circadian rhythms; and with a transfer across six time zones complete adaptation may take 1.7 to 17.0 days. It is uncertain how much this disruption may influence physical performance, and every effort should be made to minimize the effect and expedite acclimatization to the new time zone. The symptoms are usually worse when traveling east, as the body seems less capable of adapting quickly to a shortening day versus a lengthening one. The following points are helpful.

1. Prior to leaving
   a. Consider partially adapting the anticipated time zone schedule a few days before start of trip.
   b. Do not board the plane too early.
   c. Set watch on new time zone on departure.
2. During flight
   a. Take no alcohol or coffee during flight.
   b. Drink plenty of fluids.
   c. Eat light meals.
   d. Consider support hose.
   e. Otherwise wear loose clothing.
   f. Try to sit on aisle seat to facilitate getting up frequently.
   g. Stretch legs regularly.
   h. Loosen and tighten abdominal and glutei muscles periodically.
   i. Walk up and down aisle hourly.
   j. Cat-nap if possible.

ON ARRIVAL

Further adjustment to jet lag may be made using the following measures.

1. Do some light exercise soon after arrival, preferably outdoors. (Hotel concierge will have information on nearby facilities, parks, jogging trails.)
2. When possible, keep training light for a few days.
3. Train at the time of day of the event.
4. Occasionally methylxanthines are indicated for the early part of the day.
5. Maintain appropriate nutrition and hydration.

SPECIAL CONSIDERATIONS

1. Altitude adjustment
   a. Begin exposure below 2,500 meters.
   b. Have minimal exertion during first 24 hours.
   c. Avoid alcohol for first 24 hours.
   d. Keep daily rate of ascent to less than 300 meters.
   e. Keep well hydrated and avoid sedatives.
2. Heat acclimatization
   a. Do prior training in heat.
   b. Train at the time of day of the event.
   c. Take adequate fluid replacement before, during, and after activity.
   d. Wear appropriate clothing.

3. Medications
   a. Generally take medication at the usual time each day based on local time at destination.
   b. Birth control pills: take at usual time according to local time. If a dose is missed or there is a prolonged layover with further time zone change within the same pill cycle, it may be wise to use an additional form of contraception.
   c. Insulin: diabetic athletes should carry their medication on the flight because even cabin level altitude may result in a lower blood glucose level.
   d. Eastward-traveling diabetics on a twice-daily routine should use a normal morning injection and reduce the evening dose by 10 percent.
   e. Westward-bound diabetics may need to take an extra dose 6 hours after their normal one if they are still active and eating on arrival in the new time zone.
   f. Individuals should consult their own physician for advice prior to departure.

SUGGESTED READINGS

Skjenna DW, Evans JF, Stewart-Moore M et al: Helping patients travel by air. Can Med Assoc J 144:287, 1991

Winget CM, DeRoshia CW, Holley DC: Circadian rhythms and athletic performance. Med Sci Sports Exerc 17:498, 1985

APPENDIX III
Traveler's Diarrhea
(Emporiatric Enteritis)

1. Common eponyms: Delhi belly, Hong Kong dog, Tiki trots, Thai tummy, Rauzom runs, Montezuma's revenge, Rangoon runs, Casablanca crud, Tourista, Aztec two-step, Kowloon crud, seeping sickness, Trotsky's, or Ho Chi Ming's.
2. Syndrome: characterized by a twofold or more increase in frequency of unformed bowel movements and by a number of associated symptoms including fever, malaise, abdominal cramps, nausea, bloating, and urgency. High fever, bloody stools, and dehydration occur in only a small percentage, but a significant number of athletes have sufficient symptoms to interfere with their performance.
3. Etiology
   a. Mostly bacterial, usually enteropathic *Escherichia coli* (40 percent).
   b. If gastroenteritis with bloody, mucus-containing, small-volume stool, think *Salmonella*.
   c. *Shigella* may be responsible in India, Pakistan, or Africa.
   d. Other less frequent bacterial causes is *Campylobacter jejuni*.
   e. Viruses include rotavirus and Norwalk agent.
   f. Parasites include *Entamoeba histolytic* and *Giardia lamblia*.
   g. More than 20 percent of cases of traveler's diarrhea are caused by an unknown pathogen.
4. Prevention
   a. Avoid uncooked vegetables, undercooked meat, raw shellfish, and fruits with broken skins.
   b. Peel fruit before eating.
   c. Do not use ice cubes or drinks made from unpure (untreated) water.
   d. Drink sealed carbonated beverages or bottled water.
   e. Clean the part of the bottle or can that will contact the mouth.
   f. If bottled water is not available, boil local water for at least 20 minutes (30 minutes at high altitude).
   g. Treat unboiled water.
      (1) Iodine: Add 5 drops of 20 percent solution to 1 quart of clear water or 10 drops to 1 quart of cloudy water. Let stand for 30 minutes. This process should kill bacteria as well as ova and cysts of amebae and *Giardia*.
      (2) Tetraglycine hydroperiodide (Globaline, Portable Agua, Coghlan's): Check manufacturer's recommendations. Usually if water is cloudy double the number of tablets.
5. Treatment
   a. Adults who have persistent diarrhea, bloody stools, or fever and chills should seek medical attention.
   b. All athletes should notify team physician immediately if they have problems in order to counteract dehydration and institute early therapy.
   c. Children under 5 years of age should be seen by a physician immediately.
   d. Avoid solid foods and all milk products.
   e. Drink purified water with 0.25 teaspoon of baking soda added per 8 ounce glass. Alternate with fruit juice mixed with honey or sugar and a pinch of salt.
   f. Supplement with carbonated beverages, tea, or purified water.
   g. When diarrhea stops, commence eating light solid food starting with canned apple sauce, cooked rice, and crackers.
   h. Athletes returning home with significant fever should be investigated for malaria.

Clinical Point

MEDICATIONS[a]

Drug	Dosage	Special Features
Diphenoxylate (Lomotil) Loperamide (Imodium)	One tablet with each occurrence of diarrhea bowel movement; no more than 6 every 24 hours	Discontinue if symptoms persist after 48 hours.
Bismuth subsalicylate (Pepto-Bismol)	60 mg (4 tsp or 4 tablets) 4 times daily	Stools and tongue may turn black. Should not be used by persons allergic to aspirin.
Trimethoprim-sulfamethoxazole (Bactrim DS or Septra DS tablets)	160 mg trimethoprim, 800 mg sulfamethoxazole 2 times daily	Do not use if allergic to sulfa.
Trimethoprim (Proloprim, Trimpex)	200 mg 2 times daily	Less effective than trimethoprim-sulfamethoxazole with same rate of side effects for patients allergic to sulfa.
Doxycycline (Vibramycin)	200 mg on day 1, then 100 mg daily	Small incidence of sun-sensitive rash. May cause gastrointestinal upset or alteration of normal gut flora with potential risk of more serious infection. Not to be taken by children or pregnant women.

[a]Prophylactic use not recommended because of side effects unless athlete is in a high risk group.

SUGGESTED READING

Bracker MD: How I manage traveller's diarrhea. Physician Sports Med 13:63, 1985

APPENDIX IV
Temperature Control: Heat-Induced Injury

THERMAL REGULATION

Muscle contraction of exercise generates a 20-fold increase in metabolic rate. Conditioned athletes may produce 1,033 kcal of heat per hour safely for up to 3 hours. It requires a highly efficient heat-dissipating mechanism. Early during exercise, heat production exceeds heat loss, producing a rise in core temperature. Temperature sensors in the hypothalamus, spinal cord, and limb muscles generate adaptive responses, which include increased skin blood flow and sweating.

When the ambient temperature is less than 20°C (68°F), most heat loss is by convection and radiation from the skin. Above this temperature, sweating with evaporative cooling is the major mechanism. One to two liters per hour may be lost by sweating during intense exercise.

The core temperature may rise to 40°C (104°F), where it may plateau without compromising performance. Excessive continued activity, high ambient temperature, and insufficient fluid replacement may generate a dangerous rise in core temperature. There are four common syndromes of exercise-induced heat illness: heat cramps, heat syncope, heat exhaustion, and heat stroke.

HEAT CRAMPS

Heat cramps are a form of muscle spasm and tightening that occur as the result of prolonged or intense exercise, usually in a hot environment, although they occur in cool ambient temperatures as well. The etiology is not clearly defined, but hyponatremia has been implicated. Excessive sweating with sodium loss and large volume water replacement with a dilutional hyponatremia in poorly acclimatized athletes is a common theme. It may also occur with athletes using diuretics.

Treatment includes the following.

1. Rest.
2. Cooling down if in a hot environment.
3. Gentle stretching.
4. Oral hypotonic salt solutions (1 teaspoon of salt to 1 quart of water).
5. If relief not prompt, 1 liter of intravenous normal saline.
6. Failure of sodium replenishment to relieve cramps requires evaluation of potassium, calcium, and magnesium levels.

HEAT SYNCOPE

Heat syncope occurs in an athlete who is maximally vasodilated, possibly dehydrated, and suddenly ceases exercising. With pooling in the extremities, venous return decreases, and blood pressure temporarily drops resulting in light-headedness or fainting.

Prevention and treatment include the following measures.

1. Adequate hydration.
2. Slowly terminating activity.
3. Acclimatization to exercise.
4. Have athlete lie down with feet elevated, resting in a cool place. Prescribe fluid replacement and rest to treat current episode.

HEAT EXHAUSTION

Heat exhaustion is generated by prolonged periods of fluid loss through activity in high ambient temperatures. It is characterized by extreme weakness, exhaustion, profuse sweating, normal or slightly elevated temperature (39.5°C/103°F or less), thirst, decreased urinary output, and an altered mental state that ranges from giddiness to delirium. There may also be simultaneous heat cramps, headaches, tachycardia, and orthostatic hypotension. Myalgia, vomiting, or diarrhea may occur.

Treatment includes the following.

1. Rest.
2. Rapid cooling (fans, ice packs).
3. Hypotonic oral fluids.
4. Intravenous administration of 1 liter of dextrose 5 percent in 0.5 N saline over 30 to 60 minutes if no response.
5. Monitor electrolytes. If serum sodium markedly elevated, continue hydration cautiously to avoid iatrogenic cerebral edema.

HEAT STROKE

Heat stroke is a medical emergency. It indicates failure of the thermoregulatory mechanism. The individual no longer sweats. Diagnosis is confirmed by an elevated temperature (rectal temperature >40.0°C/105°F). The athlete is hot, flushed, and frequently dry. Central nervous system (CNS) impairment ranges from confusion, disorientation, and agitation to hysterical behavior, delirium, or coma. Prompt treatment averts cardiovascular and CNS collapse.

Treatment involves the following.

1. Emergency intervention.
2. External cooling (ice, fans, wetting down, remove clothing).
3. Arrangements for evacuation.
4. Monitor core temperature (until rectal temperature is <38.9°C/102°F).
5. Systemic support, including airway management, oxygenation, intravenous access, careful fluid and electrolyte administration, cardiac and metabolic monitoring.

PREVENTION

American College of Sports Medicine have taken a position stand on the prevention of thermal injuries during distance running. It is the position of the American College of Sports Medicine that the following *recommendations* be employed by directors of distance runs or community fun runs.

Medical Director

A medical director knowledgeable in exercise physiology and sports medicine should coordinate the preventive and therapeutic aspects of the running event and work closely with the race director.

Race Organization

1. Races should be organized to avoid the hottest summer months and the hottest part of the day. As there are great regional variations in environmental conditions, the local weather history is helpful when scheduling an event to avoid times when an unacceptable level of heat stress is likely to prevail. Organizers should be cautious of unseasonably hot days during the early spring, as entrants almost certainly are not heat acclimatized.
2. The environmental heat stress prediction for the day should be obtained from the meterologic service. It can be measured as wet bulb globe temperature (WBGT), which is a temperature/humidity/radiation index. If WBGT is above 28°C (82°F), consideration should be given to rescheduling or delaying the race until safer conditions prevail. If below 28°C, participants may be alerted to the degree of heat stress by using color-coded flags at the start of the race and at key positions along the course.
3. All summer events should be scheduled for the early morning (ideally before 8:00 a.m.) or in the evening after 6:00 p.m. to minimize solar radiation.
4. An adequate supply of water should be available before the race and every 2 to 3 km during the race. Runners should be encouraged to consume 100 to 200 ml at each station.
5. Race officials should be educated as to the warning signs of an impending collapse. Each official should wear an identifiable arm band or badge and should warn runners to stop if they appear to be in difficulty.
6. Adequate traffic and crowd control must be maintained at all times.
7. There should be a ready source of radio communications from various points on the course to a central organizing point to coordinate responses to emergencies.

Medical Support

1. Medical organization
   a. The medical director should alert local hospitals and ambulance services to the event and make prior arrangements with medical personnel for the care of casualties, especially those suffering from heat injury.
   b. The mere fact that an entrant signs a waiver in no way absolves the organizers of moral and legal responsibility.
2. Medical facilities
   a. Medical support staff and facilities should be available at the race site.
   b. The facilities should be staffed with personnel capable of instituting immediate and appropriate resuscitation measures. Apart from the routine resuscitation equipment, ice packs and fans for cooling are required.
   c. Persons trained in first aid, appropriately identified with an arm band and badge should be stationed along the course to warn runners to stop if they exhibit signs of impending heat injury.
   d. Ambulances or vans with accompanying medical personnel should be available along the course.
   e. The emphasis in this appendix is on the management of hyperthermia. However, on cold, wet, and windy days athletes may be chilled and require blankets and warm drinks at the finish to prevent or treat hypothermia.

Competitor Education

The knowledge of runners has increased greatly in recent years, but race organizers must not assume that all participants are well informed or prepared. Distributing guidelines at the preregistration gathering, publicity in the press, and holding clinics or seminars before runs are valuable.

The following persons are particularly prone to heat illness: the obese, unfit, dehydrated, those unacclimatized to the heat, those with a previous history of heat stroke, and anyone who runs while ill. Children perspire less than adults and have a lower heat tolerance. Based on the above information, all participants should be advised of the following.

1. Adequate training and fitness are important for full enjoyment of the run and to prevent heat-related injuries.
2. Prior training in the heat promotes heat acclimatization and thereby reduces the risk of heat injury. It is wise to do as much training as possible at the time of day at which the race will be held.
3. Fluid consumption before and during the race reduces the risk of heat injury, particularly in long runs such as marathons.
4. Illness prior to or at the time of the event should preclude competition.
5. Participants should be advised of the early symptoms of heat injury, including clumsiness, stumbling, excessive sweating (and cessation of sweating), headache, nausea, dizziness, apathy, and any gradual impairment of consciousness.
6. Participants should be advised to choose a comfortable speed and not to run faster than conditions warrant.
7. Participants are advised to run with a partner, each being responsible for the other's well-being.

MEASUREMENT OF ENVIRONMENTAL HEAT STRESS

Ambient temperature is only one component of environmental heat stress; others are humidity, wind velocity, and radiant heat. Therefore measurement of ambient temperature, dry bulb alone, is inadequate. The most useful and widely applied approach is wet bulb globe temperature (WBGT).

$$WBGT = (0.7\ Twb) + (0.2\ Tg) + (0.1\ Tdb)$$

where Twb = temperature (wet bulb thermometer); Tg = temperature (black globe thermometer); and Tdb = temperature (dry bulb thermometer).

The importance of the wet bulb temperature can be readily appreciated, as it accounts for 70 percent of the index, whereas dry bulb temperature accounts for only 10 percent. A simple portable heat stress monitor that gives direct WBGT in degrees Centigrade or degrees Fahrenheit to monitor conditions during fun runs has proved useful. Alternatively, if a means for readily assessing WBGT is not available from wet bulb, globe, and dry bulb temperatures, one can use the following equation.

$$WBGT = (0.567\ Tdb) + (0.393\ Pa) + 3.94$$

where Tdb = temperature (dry bulb thermometer);

and Pa = environmental water vapor pressure. These environmental variables should be readily available from local weather or radio stations.

Instruments to measure WBGT are available commercially. Additional information may be obtained from the American College of Sports Medicine.

USE OF COLOR-CODED FLAGS TO INDICATE THE RISK OF THERMAL STRESS*

1. *Red flag:* high risk—WBGT = 23° to 28°C (73° to 82°F)
   This signal would indicate that all runners should be aware that heat injury is possible, and any person particularly sensitive to heat or humidity should probably not run.
2. *Amber flag:* moderate risk; WBGT = 18° to 23°C (65° to 73°F)
   It should be remembered that the air temperature, probably the humidity, and almost certainly the radiant heat at the beginning of the race increases during the course of the race if conducted in the morning or early afternoon.
3. *Green flag:* low risk; WBGT = 10°C to 18°C (50° to 65°F)
   This guideline in no way guarantees that heat injury will not occur; it indicates only that the risk is low.
4. *White flag:* low risk for hyperthermia but possible risk for hypothermia; WBGT = <10°C (50°F)
   Hypothermia may occur, especially in slow runners during long races and under wet and windy conditions.

ROAD RACE CHECKLIST

1. Medical personnel
   a. Have aid personnel available if the race is 10 km (6.2 miles) or longer, and run in warm or cold weather.
   b. Recruit back-up personnel from existing emergency medical services (police, fire rescue, emergency medical service).

* This scale is determined for runners clad in running shorts, shoes, and a T-shirt (in warm weather, the less clothing the better). For males, wearing no shirt or a mesh top is better than wearing a T-shirt because the surface for evaporation is increased. However, in areas where radiant heat is excessive, a light top may be helpful.

   c. Notify local hospitals of the time and place of the road race.
2. Aid stations
   a. Provide major aid station at the finish point, which is cordoned off from public access.
   b. Equip the major aid station with the following supplies.
   Tent
   Cots
   Bath towels
   Water in large containers
   Ice in bag or ice chest or quick-cold packs
   Hose with spray nozzle
   Tables for medical supplies and equipment
   Stethoscopes
   Blood pressure cuffs
   Rectal thermometers (range up to 43°C)
   Dressings
   Blankets
   Aluminum thermal sheets ("space blankets")
   Elastic bandages
   Splints
   Skin disinfectants
   Intravenous fluids (supervision by a physician is required)
   c. Position aid stations along the route at 4 km (2.5 mile) intervals for races over 10 km and at the halfway point for shorter races.
   d. Stock each aid station with enough fluid (cool water is best) for each runner to have 300 to 360 ml (10 to 12 ounces) at each aid station. A margin of 25 percent additional cups should be available to account for spillage and double usage.
3. Communications/surveillance
   a. Set up communication between the medical personnel and the major aid station.
   b. Arrange for a radio-equipped car or van to follow the race course and provide radio contact with director.
4. Instructions to runners
   a. Apprise the race participants of potential medical problems in advance of the race, so precautions may be followed.
   b. Advise the race director to announce the following information by loudspeaker immediately prior to the race.
      (1) Flag color, indicating the risks for hyperthermia or hypothermia
      (2) Location of aid stations and type of fluid available

(3) Reinforcement of warm weather or cold weather self care

c. Advise the race participants to print their names, addresses, and any medical problems on the back of their registration number.

MEDICAL STATIONS: GENERAL GUIDELINES

1. Staff for large races
   a. Physician, podiatrist, nurse, or emergency medical technologist: teams of 3 per 1,000 runners. Double or triple this number at the finish area.

   b. One ambulance per 3,000 runners at finish area; once cruising vehicle.
   c. One physician to act as triage officer at finish.
2. Water
   a. Estimate 1 liter (0.26 gallon) per runner per 16 km (10 miles) or roughly per 60 to 90 minutes' running time, depending on the number of stations.
   b. For 10 km, the above rule is recommended as well.
   c. Cups = (number of entrants × number of stations) + 25 percent additional per station. Double this total if the course is out and back.
   d. In cold weather, an equivalent amount of warm drinks should be available.
3. Equipment. See Table A-1.

TABLE A-1. Equipment Needed at Aid Stations and the Field Hospital (Per 1,000 Runners)

Item	No.
Aid Stations	
Ice in small plastic bags or quick-cold packs	
Stretchers (10 at 10 km and beyond)	5
Blankets (10 at 10 km and beyond)	5
Elastic bandages, 6 and 4 inch	6 each
Gauze pads, 4 × 4 inch	½ case
Tape, 1.5 inch	½ case
Surgical soap	½ case
Small instrument kits	
Small instrument kits	
Adhesive strips	
Moleskin	
Petroleum jelly	½ case
Inflatable arm and leg splints	2 each
Field hospital	
Stretchers	10
Sawhorses	4
Blankets (depending on environmental conditions)	10–20
Intravenous setups	10
Inflatable arm and leg splints	2 each
Tape, 1.5 inch	2 cases
Elastic bandages, 2, 4, and 6 inch	2 cases each
Sheet wadding	2 cases
Underwrap	
Gauze pads, 4 × 4 inch	2 cases
Adhesive strips	
Moleskin	
Surgical soap	½ case
Oxygen tanks with regulators and masks	2
ECG monitors with defibrillators	
Ice in small plastic bags	
Small instrument kits	

SUGGESTED READINGS

American College of Sports Medicine: Position Stand. Prevention of Thermal Injuries During Distance Running. American College Sports Medicine, 1984

Mellion MB: Sports Injuries and Athletic Problems. CV Mosby, St. Louis, 1988

Noble HB, Bachman D: Medical aspects of distance race planning. Physician Sports Med 7:78, 1979

APPENDIX V
Preparticipation Health Screening

Many individuals participate in activities simply with the goal of improving health and fitness, not for competition. Usually they exercise in a nonmedical setting. A preparticipation examination may be requested or indicated.

1. *Purpose*
   a. Identify and advise individuals with medical contraindications to exercise.
   b. Identify individuals with risk factors that require further investigation before activity and those who may require a medically supervised program.
   c. Identify persons with special needs for safe exercise such as the elderly or pregnant women.
2. *Criteria:* Screening should be valid, cost-effective, and time-efficient to avoid unnecessary barriers to participation.
3. *Recommendations*
   a. Apparently healthy men over 40 years of age and women over age 50 require a medical examination and diagnostic exercise test before commencing a vigorous exercise protocol.
   b. Preparticipation screening is effectively carried out for the above group by a validated self-administered questionnaire such as the PAR-Q (Physical Activity-Readiness Questionnaire).
   c. Asymptomatic individuals over 40 years beginning mild to moderate programs may not require physical screening but should at least be able to give a negative response to all questions on the PAR-Q.
4. Limitations of PAR-Q
   a. It may fail to alert individuals with premature aging.
   b. It has limited ability to detect contraindications to exercise in individuals not fully informed who give false-positive answers.
   c. There is no provision to identify pregnant women.
   d. There is no provision to identify some indi-

Clinical Point

PHYSICAL ACTIVITY READINESS QUESTIONNAIRE

For most people, physical activity does not pose any problem or hazard. PAR-Q has been designed to identify the small number of adults for whom physical activity might be inappropriate or those who should have medical advice concerning the type of activity most suitable.

1. Has your doctor ever said you have heart trouble?
2. Do you frequently suffer from pains in your chest?
3. Do you often feel faint or have spells of severe dizziness?
4. Has a doctor ever said your blood pressure was too high?
5. Has a doctor ever told you that you have a bone or joint problem such as arthritis that has been aggravated by exercise or might be made worse with exercise?
6. Is there a good physical reason not mentioned here why you should not follow an activity program even if you wanted to?
7. Are you over age 65 and not accustomed to vigorous exercise?

If a person answers yes to any question, vigorous exercise or exercise testing should be postponed. Medical clearance may be necessary.

(From PAR-Q Validation Report. British Columbia Department of Health, June 1975, modified version, with permission.)

viduals who may be on medications that alter the safety of exercise.

e. Nevertheless, it is still a reasonable first screen and is useful prior to the administration of a fitness test by nonmedical but trained personnel.

A second screening instrument, the Physical Activity Readiness Examination (PAR-X) was later developed to facilitate medical examinations resulting from positive responses to the PAR-Q. It includes a checklist of recommended procedures for use during preactivity medical examinations and incorporates a Physical Activity Prescription form (PAR$_x$). The latter form lists absolute and relative contraindications to exercise, includes a summary of guidelines for exercise prescription, and provides special prescriptive advice for use in conjunction with common medical, pharmacologic, and environmental conditions. An important feature of this form is that it aids in the education of physicians who may not be familiar with the principles of preactivity screening and exercise prescription. Copies of the PAR-Q and PAR-X can be obtained by writing to:

> Government of Canada
> Fitness and Amateur Sport
> 365 Laurier Avenue West
> Ottawa, Ontario
> Canada
> K1A 0X6

SUGGESTED READING

American College of Sports Medicine: Guidelines for Exercise Testing and Prescription. 4th Ed. Lea & Febiger, Philadelphia, 1991

APPENDIX VI
Selected Protocols and Standards for Fitness Testing

This section outlines basic tests that may be performed in an office or clinic setting without the need for particularly specialized equipment other than a hand dynamometer and skin calipers. Depending on the level of participation, these tests may be used to assist in predicting risk factors for exercise or incorporated into a preseason screening examination. The data are mostly from publications of the government of Canada, and the standards must be modified for any specific group.

MUSCLE STRENGTH (GRIP STRENGTH) WITH HAND DYNAMOMETER

1. The participant grasps the dynamometer in the appropriate hand. The grip is taken between the fingers and the palm at the base of the thumb. Adjust the grip of the dynamometer so the second joint of the fingers fits snugly under the handle and takes the weight of the instrument. Lock the grip in place. The participant holds the dynamometer in line with the forearm at the level of the thigh. The dynamometer is then squeezed vigorously to exert maximum force (Fig. A-1).
2. The participant exhales while squeezing (to avoid buildup of intrathoracic pressure).
3. During the test neither the hand nor the dynamometer should touch the body or any other object. Measure both hands alternately, allowing two trials per hand. Record the scores for each to the nearest kilogram. Combine the maximum score for each hand and record.
4. Normal values and percentiles given in Table A-2.

Appendix VI is based on material acquired from the references listed at the end of the appendix, with kind permission.

MUSCLE ENDURANCE (PUSH-UPS AND SIT-UPS)

Push-Ups

Caution: Individuals suffering from lumbar spine problems or shoulder joint and periarticular pathology should not perform this test.

1. Test is performed on a gymnasium mat.
2. Correct style and adequate instruction are imperative (Fig. A-2).
3. Push-ups are to be performed consecutively and without a time limit.
4. Have the participants practice one or two repetitions to check for proper technique.
5. Advise the participant that incorrect repetitions, those not meeting the above criteria, are not counted. The test is stopped when the participant is seen to strain forcibly or is unable to maintain the proper push-up technique over two consecutive repetitions. The participant should also be advised to avoid breath-holding by breathing rhythmically and to "exhale on effort," i.e., exhale during upward phase of the push-up.
6. Technique for male athletes.
   a. The participant lies on his stomach, legs together. His hands, pointing forward, are positioned under the shoulders. The participant pushes up from the mat by fully straightening the elbows and using the toes as the pivotal point.
   b. The upper body must be kept in a straight line. The participant returns to the starting position, chin to the mat. Neither stomach nor thighs should touch the mat.
7. Technique for female athletes.
   a. The participant lies on her stomach, legs together. The hands, pointing forward, are posi-

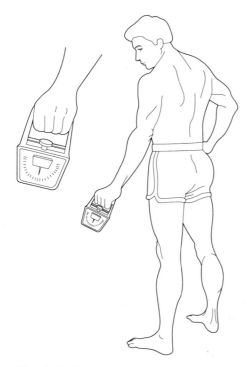

Fig. A-1. Correct use of a dynamometer.

tioned under the shoulders. The participant pushes up from the mat by fully straightening the elbows and using the knees as the pivotal point.

   b. The upper body must be kept in a straight line. The participant returns to the starting position, chin to the mat. The stomach should not touch the mat. The lower legs remain in contact with the mat, ankles plantar-flexed.

8. Normal values and percentiles are shown in Table A-3.

Sit-Ups

Caution: This test should not be performed by individuals suffering from lower back ailments or significant cervical spine pathology.

1. Test is performed on a gymnasium mat.
2. Correct style and adequate instruction are mandatory (Fig. A-3).
3. The participant lies in a supine position, knees bent at a right angle, and feet shoulder-width apart. The hands are placed at the side of the head with the fingers over the ears. The elbows are pointed toward the knees. The hands and elbows must be maintained in these positions for the duration of the test. The ankles of the participant must be held throughout the test by the appraiser to ensure that the heels are in constant contact with the mat.

4. The participant is required to sit up, touch the knees with the elbows, and return to the starting position (shoulders touch floor). *The participant performs as many sit-ups as possible within the minute.* The participant may pause to rest whenever necessary.

5. It is imperative that the participant is well instructed in the correct performance of the sit-up. The participant should be informed to initiate the sit-up by flattening the lower back followed by actively contracting the abdominal muscles and then continuing the movement with a well controlled "curling up" of the trunk to the point where the elbows touch the knees. This action is followed by a "curling down" of the trunk with particular emphasis on the lower back fully contacting the mat before the upper back and shoulder touch the mat.

6. A "rocking" or "bouncing" movement is not permitted. Also, the participant's buttocks must remain in contact with the mat and the fingers in contact with the side of the head at all times. Have the participant practice one or two repetitions to check for proper technique.

7. Advise the participant that incorrect repetitions, those not meeting the above criteria, are not counted. The participant should also be advised to avoid breath-holding by breathing rhythmically and to "exhale on effort," i.e., exhale during "curling-up" phase of the sit-up.

8. When the participant is fully informed of the preceding details and is ready to start the sit-up test, give the command "begin" and start the timer.

9. Normal values and percentiles given in Table A-4.

FLEXIBILITY (SIT AND REACH)

Caution: Individuals with back ailments may not be suitable for this test.

1. Perform forward trunk flexion.
2. When possible a flexometer should be used (modified Wells and Dillon).

TABLE A-2. Norms by Age Groups and Gender for Combined Right and Left Hand Grip Strength

Parameter	15–19 Years		20–29 Years		30–39 Years		40–49 Years		50–59 Years		60–69 Years	
	M	F	M	F	M	F	M	F	M	F	M	F
Norms												
Excellent	≥113	≥71	≥125	≥71	≥123	≥73	≥119	≥73	≥110	≥65	≥102	≥60
Above average	103–112	64–70	113–123	65–70	113–122	66–72	110–118	65–72	102–109	59–64	93–101	54–59
Average	95–102	59–63	106–112	61–64	105–112	61–65	102–109	50–64	96–101	55–58	86–92	51–53
Below average	84–94	54–58	97–105	55–60	97–104	56–60	94–101	55–58	87–95	51–54	79–85	48–50
Poor	≤83	≤53	≤96	≤54	≤96	≤55	≤93	≤54	≤86	≤50	≤78	≤47
Percentiles												
95	125	78	136	78	135	80	128	80	119	72	111	67
90	119	74	127	74	127	76	123	76	114	69	106	62
85	113	71	124	71	123	73	119	73	110	65	102	60
80	110	69	120	70	120	71	117	71	108	63	99	58
75	108	67	118	68	117	69	115	69	105	62	96	56
70	105	65	115	67	115	68	112	67	103	60	94	55
65	103	64	113	65	113	66	110	65	102	59	93	54
60	101	63	111	64	111	65	108	64	100	58	91	53
55	99	61	109	63	109	63	106	62	99	57	89	52
50	97	60	107	62	107	62	104	61	97	56	88	52
45	95	59	106	61	105	61	102	59	96	55	86	51
40	93	58	104	59	104	60	100	58	94	54	84	50
35	90	57	102	58	101	59	98	57	92	53	82	49
30	87	56	100	56	99	58	96	56	90	53	81	49
25	84	54	97	55	97	56	94	55	87	51	79	48
20	81	53	95	53	94	55	91	53	85	50	76	47
15	77	51	91	52	91	53	89	51	83	48	73	45
10	73	49	87	50	87	51	84	49	80	46	69	43
5	67	45	81	47	81	48	76	46	74	42	62	39

Results are given in kilograms.
(Based on data from the Canada Fitness Survey, 1981.)

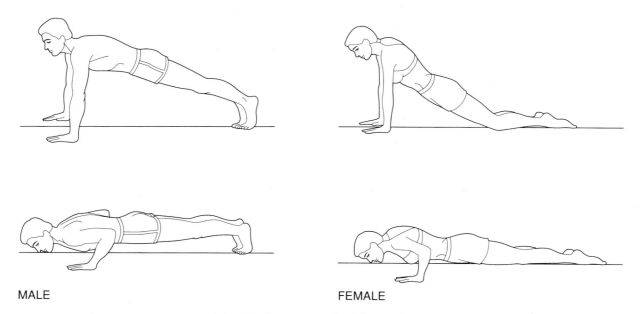

MALE

FEMALE

Fig. A-2. Correct method for push-ups.

3. Have the participant warm up for this test by performing slow stretching movements (modified hurdle stretch held for 20 seconds and repeated twice on each leg) before making the measurements (Fig. A-4).

4. The participant, barefoot, sits with legs fully extended with the soles of the feet placed flat against the two horizontal crossboards of the flexometer. The flexometer should be adjusted to a height at which the balls of the feet rest against the upper crossboard. The inner edge of the soles are placed 2 cm from the edge of the scale. Keeping knees fully extended, arms evenly stretched, and palms down, the participant bends and reaches forward (without jerking), pushing the sliding marker along the scale with the fingertips as far forward as possible. The position of maximum flexion must be held for approximately 2 seconds. Advise the participant that lowering the head maximizes the distance reached (Fig. A-4).

5. If the knees flex, the trial is not counted. Do not attempt to hold the knees down. In addition, do not allow a jerking, bouncing action.

6. The test is repeated twice. Record both readings and use the maximum reading to the nearest 0.5 cm.

7. Normal values and percentiles are given in Table A-5.

ANTHROPOMETRY (STANDING HEIGHT, BODY WEIGHT, GIRTH, BODY COMPOSITION, SKINFOLD)

Standing Height

1. Position and secure a metric tape vertically against a wall. Ensure that it is perfectly straight and even with the floor. If the floor is carpeted, place a 0.5-inch wooden board on the floor against the wall and measure from the top of the board with the participant standing on it.

2. The participant (without footwear) stands erect, arms hanging by the sides, feet together, the heels and back in contact with the wall. The participant is then instructed to look straight ahead, stand as tall as possible, and take a deep breath while the measurement is taken (Fig. A-5).

3. The set square is place on the head, depressing the hair to make firm contact, and a mark is made at the level of the lower boarder of the square on the wall. Ensure that the participant's heels remain in contact with the floor. The distance from the floor to the pencil mark is recorded to the nearest 0.5 cm, e.g., 176.5 cm.

4. Normal values and percentiles are shown in Table A-6.

TABLE A-3. Norms and Percentiles by Age Groups and Gender for Push-Ups

Parameter	15–19 Years		20–29 Years		30–39 Years		40–49 Years		50–59 Years		60–69 Years	
	M	F	M	F	M	F	M	F	M	F	M	F
Norms												
Excellent	≥39	≥33	≥36	≥30	≥30	≥27	≥22	≥24	≥21	≥21	≥18	≥17
Above average	29–38	25–32	29–35	21–29	22–29	20–26	17–21	15–23	13–20	11–20	11–17	12–16
Average	23–28	18–24	22–28	15–20	17–21	13–19	13–16	11–14	10–12	7–10	8–10	5–11
Below average	18–22	12–17	17–21	10–14	12–16	8–12	10–12	5–10	7–9	2–6	5–7	1–4
Poor	≤17	≤11	≤16	≤9	≤11	≤7	≤9	≤4	≤6	≤1	≤4	≤1
Percentiles												
95	50	46	48	37	36	36	30	32	28	30	25	30
90	43	38	41	32	32	31	25	28	24	23	24	25
85	39	33	36	30	30	27	22	24	21	21	18	17
80	35	31	34	26	27	24	21	22	17	17	16	15
75	32	28	32	24	25	22	20	20	15	15	13	13
70	31	26	30	22	24	21	19	18	14	13	11	12
65	29	25	29	21	22	20	17	15	13	11	11	12
60	27	23	27	20	21	17	16	14	11	10	10	10
55	26	21	25	18	20	16	15	13	11	10	10	9
50	24	20	24	16	19	14	13	12	10	9	9	6
45	23	18	22	15	17	13	13	11	10	7	8	5
40	22	16	21	14	16	12	12	10	9	5	7	4
35	21	15	20	13	15	11	11	10	8	4	6	3
30	20	14	18	11	14	10	10	7	7	3	6	2
25	18	12	17	10	12	8	10	5	7	2	5	1
20	16	11	16	9	11	7	8	4	5	1	4	—
15	14	9	14	7	10	6	7	3	5	1	3	—
10	11	6	11	5	8	4	5	2	4	—	2	—
5	8	4	9	2	5	1	4	—	2	—	—	—

Results are given as the number of push-ups.
(Based on data from the Canada Fitness Survey, 1981.)

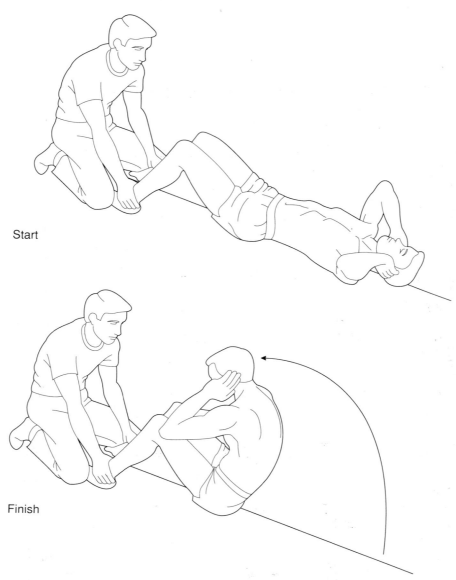

Start

Finish

Fig. A-3. Correct method for sit-ups.

TABLE A-4. Norms and Percentiles by Age Groups and Gender for Sit-Ups

Parameter	15–19 Years		20–29 Years		30–39 Years		40–49 Years		50–59 Years		60–69 Years	
	M	F	M	F	M	F	M	F	M	F	M	F
Norms												
Excellent	≥48	≥42	≥43	≥36	≥36	≥29	≥31	≥25	≥26	≥19	≥23	≥16
Above average	42–47	36–41	37–42	31–35	31–35	24–28	26–30	20–24	22–25	12–18	17–22	12–15
Average	38–41	32–35	33–36	25–30	27–30	20–23	22–25	15–19	18–21	5–11	12–16	4–11
Below average	33–37	27–31	29–32	21–24	22–26	15–19	17–21	7–14	13–17	3–4	7–11	2–3
Poor	≤32	≤26	≤28	≤20	≤21	≤14	≤16	≤6	≤12	≤2	≤6	≤1
Percentiles												
95	53	47	49	43	42	34	36	28	34	26	26	20
90	50	43	45	39	38	31	33	26	28	22	24	18
85	48	42	43	36	36	29	31	25	26	19	23	16
80	46	40	41	34	34	27	30	23	25	17	21	15
75	44	39	40	32	33	26	29	22	24	16	19	14
70	43	37	38	31	32	25	27	21	23	14	18	13
65	42	36	37	31	31	24	26	20	22	12	17	12
60	41	35	36	29	30	23	25	18	21	11	15	10
55	40	34	35	28	29	22	24	17	20	10	15	9
50	39	33	34	27	28	21	23	16	20	7	13	5
45	38	32	33	25	27	20	22	15	18	5	12	4
40	36	31	32	24	26	18	21	13	17	4	11	2
35	35	29	31	23	24	17	20	12	16	3	10	—
30	34	28	30	22	23	16	19	10	15	—	10	—
25	33	27	29	21	22	15	17	7	13	—	7	—
20	32	25	27	19	21	13	16	5	11	—	2	—
15	30	23	26	17	20	11	14	3	10	—	—	—
10	28	21	24	15	17	7	11	—	8	—	—	—
5	23	15	20	11	14	—	6	—	—	—	—	—

Results are given as the number of sit-ups performed in 60 seconds.
(Based on data from the Canada Fitness Survey, 1981.)

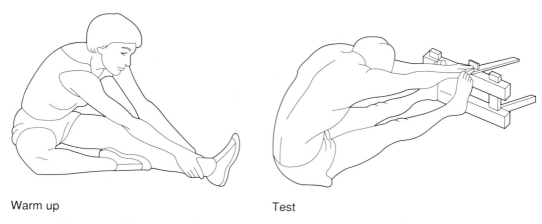

Warm up   Test

Fig. A-4. Warm-up and test positions for testing flexibility (sit and reach).

Body Weight

1. Ensure that the spring or beam scale is on a flat surface. If the floor is carpeted, use a 0.5 inch wooden board under the scale. The participant must be without footwear and in light clothing (shorts and T-shirt or blouse for women).
2. Record the weight in kilograms to the nearest 0.1 kg; e.g., 67.2 kg.

Girth Measurements

1. An adequate-quality tape measure is essential.
2. The participant stands erect in a relaxed manner, arms hanging loosely at the sides. The appraiser holds the tape between the thumb and index finger with the second finger stabilizing and leveling the tape. A cross-handed technique is used to bring the zero line of the tape in line with the measuring aspect of the tape.
3. Ensure that the tape is properly located in the horizontal plane in accordance with the instructions listed below (Fig. A-6).
4. Apply tension to the tape sufficient to maintain its position but not to cause indentation of the skin surface.
5. All measurements are recorded to the nearest 0.1 cm, e.g., 98.7 cm.
   a. Chest girth. Have the participant raise both arms and pass the tape around the chest positioned at the level of the mesosternum (approximately the midlevel of the sternum, midway between the axilla and the horizontal nipple line) (Fig. A-6A). Ensure that the tape is

perfectly horizontal. The participant lowers both arms so they hang relaxed. The reading is taken at the end of a normal expiration.
   b. Waist (abdomen) girth. The participant stands erect. The appraiser uses a cross-handed technique to position the tape horizontally at the level of noticeable waist narrowing (Fig. A-6B). The tape is then placed in the recording position, and the measurement is made at the end of a normal expiration. For some participants, an indeterminate waist can be approximated by taking the girth at the estimated lateral level of the twelfth (or lower floating) rib.
   c. Hip (gluteal) girth. The participant stands erect with feet together. The tape is positioned around the hips at the level of the symphysis pubis and the greatest gluteal protuberance (Fig. A-6C).
   d. Right thigh girth. The participant stands erect, feet slightly apart. The tape is positioned around the right thigh to a level 1 cm below the gluteal line (Fig. A-6D).

Body Composition

Hydrostatic (Underwater) Weight

The criterion measure for assessing body composition is hydrostatic (underwater) weighing. The procedure is described elsewhere. This technique is based on Archimedes' principle, which states that when a body is immersed in water, it is buoyed up by a counterforce equal to the weight of the water displaced. Bone and muscle tissue are more dense than water,

TABLE A-5. Norms and Percentiles by Age Groups and Gender for Trunk Forward Flexion

Parameter	15–19 Years		20–29 Years		30–39 Years		40–49 Years		50–59 Years		60–69 Years	
	M	F	M	F	M	F	M	F	M	F	M	F
Norms												
Excellent	≥39	≥43	≥40	≥41	≥38	≥41	≥35	≥38	≥35	≥39	≥33	≥35
Above average	34–38	38–42	34–39	37–40	33–37	36–40	29–34	34–37	28–34	33–38	25–32	31–34
Average	29–33	34–37	30–33	33–36	28–32	32–35	24–28	30–33	24–27	30–32	20–24	27–30
Below average	24–28	29–33	25–29	28–32	23–27	27–31	18–23	25–29	16–23	25–29	15–19	23–26
Poor	≤23	≤28	≤24	≤27	≤22	≤26	≤17	≤24	≤15	≤24	≤14	≤23
Percentiles												
95	44	47	44	45	43	45	40	43	41	43	44	40
90	42	44	42	43	40	42	37	40	38	40	35	37
85	39	43	40	41	38	41	35	38	35	39	33	35
80	38	42	38	40	37	39	34	37	32	37	30	34
75	36	41	37	39	35	38	32	36	30	36	28	33
70	35	40	36	38	34	37	30	35	29	35	26	31
65	34	38	34	37	33	36	29	34	28	33	25	31
60	33	37	33	36	32	35	28	33	27	32	24	30
55	31	36	32	35	31	34	26	32	26	31	23	28
50	30	35	31	34	29	33	25	31	25	30	22	28
45	29	34	30	33	28	32	24	30	24	30	20	27
40	28	33	29	32	27	31	23	29	22	29	18	26
35	27	32	27	31	26	30	21	28	20	28	17	25
30	26	31	26	29	24	28	20	26	18	26	16	24
25	24	29	25	28	23	27	18	25	16	25	15	23
20	22	27	23	26	21	25	16	24	15	23	14	23
15	19	25	21	25	20	23	14	22	14	22	13	20
10	17	23	18	22	17	21	12	19	12	19	11	18
5	13	18	14	18	13	16	8	14	7	13	8	13

Results are given in centimeters.
(Based on data from the Canada Fitness Survey, 1981.)

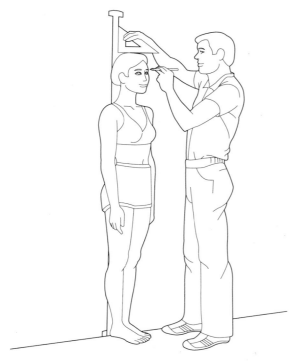

Fig. A-5. Standing height measurement.

whereas fat tissue is less dense than water. Therefore a person with more lean body mass for the same total body weight weighs more in water and has a higher body density and thus a lower percentage of body fat. The residual volume of the lungs is needed to calculate body density and can be measured directly or estimated. Body density can be derived from the following formula.

Body density =

$$\frac{\text{weight in air}}{\text{weight in air} - \text{weight in water}/\text{density of water} - \text{residual volume}}$$

Prediction equations are then used to convert body density to percent body fat (BF). Two formulas are commonly used.

$$BF\% = (457/\text{body density}) - 414.2^9$$

$$BF\% = (495/\text{body density}) - 450^{47}$$

Hydrostatic weighing is the gold standard, but the technique requires special equipment; moreover, the procedure is expensive, complicated, time-consuming, and subject to great error if conducted improp-

erly. Therefore skinfold measurements are used more frequently.

Skinfold Measurements

1. During skinfold measurements it is essential that the participant relax the underlying musculature as much as possible.
2. Use Harpenden or Lange calipers. Skinfold measurements correlate fairly well with hydrostatic weighing. The principle behind this technique is that approximately one-half of stored fat is located as subcutaneous fat, which is closely related to overall fat.
3. When the site of the skinfold has been determined, a fold of skin plus the underlying fat is grasped between the thumb and forefinger with the back of the hand facing the appraiser. Keeping the jaws of the calipers always at right angles to the body surface, the contact faces of the calipers are placed 1 cm below the point where the skinfold is raised. While maintaining the pressure of the fingers on the skinfold, the trigger of the calipers is fully released and the measurement taken.
4. The measurement is noted when the indicator stabilizes, which is approximately 2 seconds after the full pressure of the caliper jaws is applied to the skinfold. The reading is recorded to the nearest 0.2 mm, e.g., 16.8 mm.
5. Complete the first set of skinfold measurements for all sites. Then repeat the procedure to obtain a second set of measurements for each skinfold site.
6. Record the mean of the two measurements unless the difference between the first and second measurements of that particular skinfold site is found to be more than 0.4 mm. If so, take a third measurement of that skinfold site and choose from among the three values the two measurements that most closely match each other in value. Determine the mean of those two measurements. Should the three measurements be equidistant, e.g., 18.6, 19.2, 19.8, determine the mean of all three values.
7. Note that the accuracy of skinfold measurements depends on the following.
   a. Precise identification of the site of the skinfold (Fig. A-7)
   b. Forming the skinfold prior to application of the caliper jaws
   c. Standardization of the alignment of the skinfold crest

TABLE A-6. Percentiles by Age Groups and Gender for Standing Height (cm) and Body Weight (kg)

Percentiles	15–19 Years		20–29 Years		30–39 Years		40–49 Years		50–59 Years		60–69 Years	
	M	F	M	F	M	F	M	F	M	F	M	F
Standing height												
95	191	175	191	175	190	175	190	175	190	174	188	174
90	189	174	189	174	188	174	188	174	187	173	184	172
85	187	173	188	173	186	172	186	172	185	171	180	169
80	185	171	186	171	184	171	183	171	183	170	176	167
75	183	170	184	170	183	169	181	169	180	168	175	165
70	181	169	182	169	181	168	179	168	179	166	174	163
65	179	168	181	167	179	167	177	167	176	165	173	160
60	177	166	179	166	177	165	175	165	175	163	172	159
55	175	165	177	165	175	164	174	164	173	161	171	158
50	174	164	176	163	174	162	172	162	172	160	170	156
45	172	162	174	162	172	161	171	161	171	158	169	155
40	171	161	173	161	171	159	170	159	169	157	168	154
35	169	160	171	159	169	157	169	158	168	155	166	152
30	168	157	169	157	168	156	167	156	167	153	165	151
25	167	155	168	155	167	154	166	154	166	152	164	150
20	165	153	166	153	165	152	165	152	164	150	163	148
15	164	151	165	150	164	150	163	150	163	149	162	147
10	162	148	163	148	162	148	162	148	162	147	161	146
5	161	146	161	146	161	146	161	146	161	145	160	145
Body weight												
95	86	74	96	74	100	82	101	86	97	87	101	85
90	81	70	89	69	94	76	95	78	93	79	94	78
85	78	66	86	66	89	71	92	75	89	75	90	75
80	75	64	83	63	87	69	88	71	87	72	87	72
75	73	62	80	62	85	67	86	70	85	71	85	70
70	71	60	79	61	83	64	85	68	84	69	83	69
65	70	59	77	59	81	63	83	66	82	68	81	67
60	69	58	76	58	79	61	81	65	81	67	79	65
55	67	57	74	57	78	60	79	63	79	65	78	63
50	66	56	73	56	76	59	78	62	78	64	77	62
45	65	55	71	55	75	58	76	60	76	63	76	61
40	64	54	70	54	73	57	75	59	75	62	74	60
35	62	53	69	53	72	56	73	58	73	61	73	59
30	61	52	67	52	70	55	72	57	72	59	72	58
25	60	51	66	51	68	54	70	55	70	58	70	56
20	58	49	65	50	67	53	68	54	68	56	68	55
15	56	48	63	49	65	51	66	53	66	54	66	54
10	54	46	61	47	62	50	64	51	64	53	65	53
05	52	44	57	45	58	47	60	49	60	50	62	50

(Based on data from the Canada Fitness Survey, 1981.)

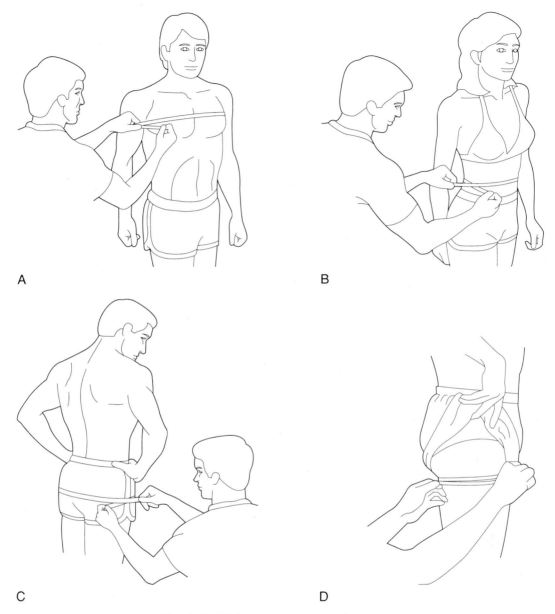

A

B

C

D

Fig. A-6. Girth measurements. See text.

d. Maintenance of the pressure by the fingers on the skinfold when the measurement is taken

e. Complete release of the caliper jaws

Triceps Skinfold. The participant stands with the arms relaxed by the sides. The triceps skinfold is taken on the back of the right arm at the point midway between the tip of the acromion (right shoulder) and the tip of the olecranon (right elbow). The midpoint is determined by placing the fifth finger of the right hand on the tip of the olecranon (right elbow) and the fifth finger of the left hand on the acromion. The thumbs are then placed together to determine the midpoint. The skinfold is then raised at the mid-arm point, so the fold runs vertically along the midline of the back of the arm.

Biceps Skinfold. The biceps skinfold is measured on the right extended upper arm over the biceps at the same level as the mid-arm point for the triceps. The

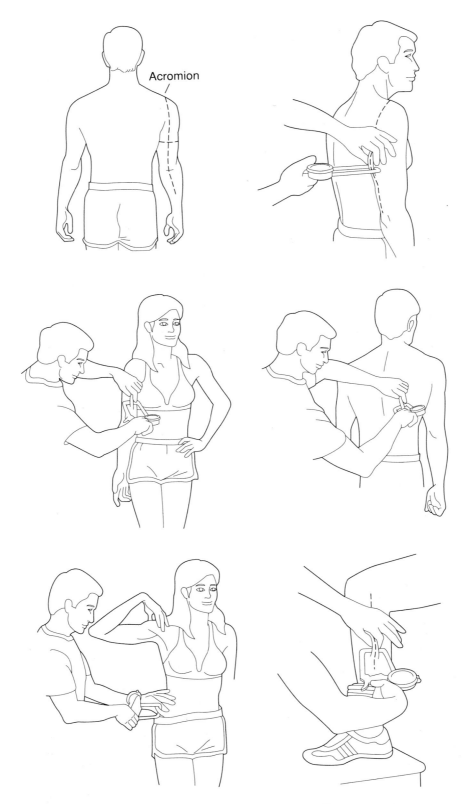

Fig. A-7. Skinfold measurements. See text.

skinfold is then raised at the mid-arm point, so the fold runs vertically along the midline of the front of the arm.

Subscapular Skinfold. The participant stands with the shoulders relaxed and the arms by the sides. The skinfold is raised so it can be measured on a diagonal line coming from the vertebral border of the scapula to a point 1 cm underneath the inferior angle. The skinfold runs downward and outward at an angle of approximately 45 degrees to the spine.

Iliac Crest Skinfold. The participant stands in a normal erect position. The participant then abducts the right arm so it is horizontal and places the right hand on the right shoulder. If the participant is unable to place the hand on the shoulder, keep the horizontal arm extended. The skinfold is then measured 3 cm above the crest of the ilium at the midline of the body so the fold runs forward and slightly downward.

Medial Calf Skinfold. Have the participant place the unweighed (relaxed) right foot flat on a step so the knee is at 90 degrees. The skinfold is raised on the inside of the right calf just above the level of the maximum calf girth so the fold runs vertically along the midline.

Body Weight, Adiposity, and Fat Distribution

It has become increasingly evident that the evaluation of body weight and composition, traditionally based on weight and height tables and percentage of body fat estimates, is subject to a considerable degree of error. For instance, the assumptions underlying the equations used for the prediction of body fat, from simple anthropometric measurements, have not proved universally applicable.

It was suggested by Fitness Canada in 1984 that one should assess body weight by taking into account a number of factors, including primary skinfolds, anthropometric measurements and ratios, and the age and gender of the individual.

The following method requires the consideration of four indicators for a comprehensive assessment of body weight, adiposity, and fat distribution.

1. Body mass index (BMI): The ratio of body weight divided by height squared (kg/m^2)
   Example: Weight = 77.3 kg
   Height = 171.5 cm = 1.72 m
   $$\text{BMI} = \frac{77.3}{(1.72)^2} = \frac{77.3}{2.96} = 26.1$$

2. Sum of (five) skinfolds (millimeters) (SOS): triceps, biceps, subscapular, iliac crest, and medial calf
   Example: Add triceps (12.4) + biceps (10.6) + subscapularis (23.8) + iliac crest (19.2) + medial calf (14.4) = 80 mm

3. Waist/hip ratio (WHR): ratio of waist (abdomen) girth divided by hip (gluteal) girths
   Example: Waist = 85.8
   Hip = 88.9
   WHR = 83.8/88.9 = 0.94

4. Sum of (two) trunk skinfolds (SOTS).

The amount and the distribution of body fat have been identified in several studies as being closely related to morbidity and mortality data. Table A-7 identifies estimated health risk zones (hereafter referred to as risk zones), which are trends in indicators of body fat content and distribution associated with the highest incidence of morbidity and mortality.

First, consider the BMI, an indicator of proportional weight. Should an individual have a high BMI value (i.e., within the risk zones), one must then determine if it is a result of excessive body fat content or elevated muscle mass. The latter can be determined by considering the SOS. If the SOS value is also high, it is a definite indication of too much body fat and corresponding health risk. Conversely, should an individual have a low BMI, within the risk zones, one must determine if that individual has too little fat by considering the SOS. Hence the SOS value facilitates a more accurate interpretation of the BMI value.

Within the past few years, it has been shown that total body fat content is an important factor in assessing body weight, but perhaps even more so is the pattern of fat distribution. An excessive amount of fat in the trunk region has been shown to be associated with increased morbidity, i.e., glucose intolerance, hyperinsulinemia, blood lipid disorders, and mortality. Some investigators have suggested that the WHR provides a valid representation of this pattern of fat distribution and have incorporated this procedure.

The SOTS measurement provides a direct measure of subcutaneous fat in the trunk region. Therefore this value is also considered, adding to the discriminatory capacity of this procedure.

In summary, one must first establish if an individual with a high BMI value has too much fat or if a low BMI value indicates too little fat by considering the SOS value. If an individual has high BMI and SOS values, considering the WHR and SOTS can establish if the pattern of fat distribution is one that carries

TABLE A-7. Percentiles and Associated Health Risk Zones by Age Groups and Gender for Body Weight, Adiposity, and Fat Distribution Measures

15–19 Years

Percentiles	BMI M	BMI F	SOS M	SOS F	WHR M	WHR F	SOTS M	SOTS F
95	18	17	25	36	.73	.65	11	13
90	19	18	27	40	.75	.67	12	14
85	19	19	28	43	.76	.68	13	16
80	20	19	29	46	.77	.69	13	17
75	20	19	31	49	.79	.71	14	18
70	20	20	32	51	.80	.72	15	19
65	21	20	33	54	.81	.73	15	20
60	21	20	35	56	.81	.73	16	21
55	21	21	36	58	.82	.74	17	22
50	22	21	38	61	.83	.75	17	23
45	22	22	40	63	.83	.75	18	24
40	22	22	42	66	.84	.76	19	26
35	22	22	44	69	.85	.77	21	27
30	23	23	47	72	.85	.78	22	29
25	23	23	51	77	.86	.78	24	31
20	24	24	54	83	.87	.79	27	33
15	25	25	61	89	.87	.80	28	37
10	26	26	69	97	.88	.82	32	42
5	28	28	82	116	.92	.86	42	49

20–29 Years

Percentiles	BMI M	BMI F	SOS M	SOS F	WHR M	WHR F	SOTS M	SOTS F
95	19	18	26	37	.76	.65	13	13
90	20	18	29	40	.80	.67	14	14
85	21	19	30	43	.81	.68	16	16
80	21	19	32	46	.81	.69	17	17
75	22	20	34	49	.82	.71	18	18
70	22	20	36	51	.83	.72	19	19
65	22	20	38	53	.83	.73	20	20
60	23	21	40	56	.84	.73	21	21
55	23	21	43	58	.85	.74	23	22
50	23	21	46	60	.85	.75	25	23
45	24	22	49	63	.86	.76	27	24
40	24	22	52	65	.87	.76	28	26
35	25	22	55	69	.87	.77	30	27
30	25	23	58	72	.88	.78	32	29
25	26	23	62	76	.89	.78	35	31
20	27	24	68	81	.91	.79	38	33
15	27	25	74	86	.93	.80	41	36
10	28	26	82	95	.94	.82	46	42
5	30	28	94	111	.96	.85	54	48

BMI (body mass index) = body weight (kg) ÷ height^2 (meters).
SOS [sum of (five) skinfolds (mm)] = triceps + biceps + subscapular + iliac crest + medial calf.
WHR (waist/hip ratio) = waist girth ÷ hip girth.
SOTS [sum of (two) trunk skinfolds (mm)] = subscapular + iliac crest.
Estimated health risk zones according to trends in morbidity and mortality data are in boldface type.
(Based on data from the Canada Fitness Survey, 1981.)

additional health risks. It is also possible that an individual may have acceptable BMI and SOS values and still have excessive trunk fatness, as determined by high WHR and SOTS values. Finally, one must not overlook the importance of a visual appraisal of the individual, which can be a useful adjunct to the assessment of body weight, adiposity, and fat distribution as outlined in this procedure.

CANADIAN AEROBIC FITNESS TEST

The aerobic component of fitness may be assessed by the administration of the Canadian Aerobic Fitness Test (CAFT) and measurements of postexercise heart rate and blood pressure. The CAFT (formerly known as the Canadian Home Fitness Test: Advanced Version) consists in a series of stepping sequences performed on double 20.3 cm steps to a six-count musical rhythm set by a cassette tape with progressive increase in tempo. The CAFT is structured such that a participant begins by performing a 3-minute "warm-up" exercise at a cadence intensity of 65 to 70 percent of the average aerobic power expected of a person 10 years older. Instructions and time signals are given by the cassette tape as to when to start and stop exercising and for counting the 10-second measurement of the postexercise heart rate.

If a predetermined ceiling postexercise heart rate is not attained or exceeded, the participant performs another 3 minutes of exercise at 65 to 70 percent of the average aerobic power expected for his or her age group. Again, if the participant does not attain or exceed the ceiling heart rate, another 3 minutes of stepping is performed at an intensity equivalent to 65 to 70 percent of the average aerobic power for a person 10 years younger.

Equipment needed include a stethoscope, sphygmomanometer, ergometer steps, CAFT cassette tape, cassette recorder, timer or stopwatch, masking tape, and metronome (for calibration of the cassette).

Procedure

1. Verify that the pretest screening items have been completed, i.e., PAR-Q, consent and release form, observations, resting blood pressure and resting heart rate (see Appendix V).
2. Briefly explain the purpose of the CAFT and how it is conducted.

3. Apply the blood pressure cuff to the participant's left arm. The cuff should be wrapped firmly and smoothly around the arm with the lower margin 2 to 3 cm above the antecubital space. It is suggested that the participant wear the cuff throughout the step test. If it tends to slip, tape it to the upper arm or shoulder with masking tape.
4. Determine the starting stage for the participant, based on current calendar age, using the following table.

Age	Starting Stage	
(years)	Males	Females
60–69	1	1
50–59	2	1
40–49	3	2
30–39	4	3
20–29	5	3
15–19	5	4

5. The appraiser should have the participant perform mild calf stretches before and after the stair stepping to prevent muscle cramping.

Stepping Exercise Sequence

1. Demonstrate and have the participant practice the stepping sequence as described below. If handrails are not available on the ergometer steps, the appraiser should step with older participants as a precaution against falls.
2. Have the participant practice the stepping sequence, first without the music and then with the music, but not more than twice each time. Ensure that the participant places both feet completely on the top step, the legs are completely extended, and the back is upright during this phase of the movement.
3. Also, ensure that the participant maintains the proper cadence. Count or step a few steps with any participant who is experiencing difficulty.
4. A participant may start stepping with either foot. The example given begins with the right foot. Reverse right and left in the example if the participant prefers to begin with the left foot.
5. Stepping sequence: Stand in front of the first step with feet together (Fig. A-8).

    STEP — STEP — UP!
    STEP — STEP — DOWN
    UP — 2 – 3! DOWN — 2 – 3!
    UP — 2 – 3! DOWN — 2 – 3!

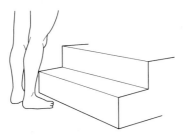

1 Start
Both feet together on ground level.

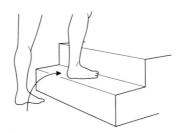

2 Step
Place right foot on first step.

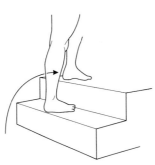

3 Step
Place left foot on the second step.

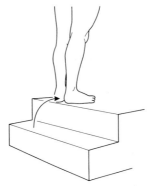

4 Up
Place right foot on the second step alongside left.

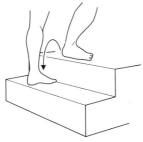

5 Step
Start down with left foot to the first step.

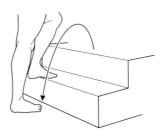

6 Step
Place right foot on ground level.

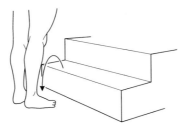

7 Down
Place left foot down on ground level so that both feet are together.

Fig. A-8. Stepping exercise sequence.

6. Inform the participant that the first stepping session lasts 3 minutes. When the music stops, the participant ceases to step and remains motionless. Indicate that you will then inform the participant whether to proceed to the second session of stepping depending on the heart rate response. If the participant is to proceed, explain that this procedure will be repeated at the end of the second session.

7. Indicate that the participant is free to stop stepping anytime discomfort is experienced.

8. Discontinue the test if the participant begins to stagger or complains of dizziness, extreme leg pain, nausea, chest pain, or shows facial pallor. Have the participant lie down in a supine position and check the heart rate and blood pressure.

9. If it becomes obvious that the participant is unable to maintain the proper cadence after the first minute of stepping, step with the participant or maintain the rhythm by clapping.

10. If the difficulty in stepping appears to be related to some physiologic dysfunction, discontinue the test.

11. When the music stops, have the participant remain motionless while standing. Determine the postexercise heart rate with the stethoscope placed either on the sternum or over the second intercostal space on the left side. Start counting the pulse at the termination of the command word "count" and continue until the first sound of the command word "stop." It is a 10-second timing sequence, and the first beat is counted as one.

12. Do not count a heartbeat that occurs during the command word "count." In such cases, the next heartbeat is counted as "one."

13. Determination of an accurate postexercise heart rate is the critical measurement for deciding if the participant should continue to the next session and for predicting aerobic fitness or maximum oxygen consumption (VO_{2max}). Quickly ascertain whether the participant is to continue or stop the test. The participant *does not* continue if the heart rate is *equal to* or *exceeds* the ceiling postexercise heart rate (Table A-8).

14. If there are no contraindications, have the participant complete the second session. Repeat the postexercise heart rate measurement. Determine if the participant is to continue for a third session. The participant may complete a maximum of three stepping sessions.

TABLE A-8.   Ceiling Postexercise Heart Rate

Age (years)	Heart Rate (10 seconds)	
	After First Session	After Second Session
60–69	24	—
50–59	24	23
40–49	26	24
30–39	28	25
29–29	29	26
15–19	30	27

15. After the participant completes the last session of stepping, determined by the postexercise heart rate response, have him or her sit down. Once seated, if the participant appears fatigued or light-headed, elevate the legs to rest on the ergometer steps.

16. Record the postexercise systolic and diastolic (D4) blood pressure reading.
   a. Between 0:30 and 1:00 minute
   b. Between 2:30 and 3:00 minutes

17. Measure and record the postexercise heart rate again between 3:00 and 3:30 (15 second count).

18. The above postexercise measures are taken after the last session is completed to ensure that the heart rate and blood pressure drop below the resting ceiling levels before the participant leaves the site, i.e., heart rate less than 100 beats/minute, systolic blood pressure less than 150 mmHg, diastolic blood pressure less than 100 mmHg.

Prediction of Maximal Aerobic Power (VO_{2max})

1. Predicted VO_{2max} can be calculated from the results of the step test by utilizing the following regression equation.

$$VO_{2max} \ (ml \cdot kg^{-1} \cdot min^{-1}) = 42.5 + [16.6 \ (VO_2)] - [0^2.12 \ (W)] - [0.12 \ (H)] - [0.24 \ (A)]$$

where:

   VO_2 = average oxygen cost of the last completed exercise stage (liters per minute) (Table A-9)
   W = body weight (kilograms)
   H = heart rate after final stage of stepping (beats/minute)
   A = participant's age (years)

TABLE A-9. Energy (Oxygen) Requirements of Various Stages of CAFT

CAFT Stage	Oxygen Requirement (L/min)	
	Males	Females
1	1.1391	0.9390
2	1.3466	1.0484
3	1.6250	1.3213
4	1.8255	1.4925
5	2.0066	1.6267
6	2.3453	1.7867
7	2.7657	—

(From Jette M, Campbell J, Mongeon J et al: The Canadian Fitness Test as a predictor of Aerobic capacity. Can Med Assoc J 114(April 17), 1976, with permission.)

2. The CSTF "aerobic calculator" was devised in the original CSTF package to simplify these calculations. The calculator also provides instructions on how to determine a walk–jog exercise prescription to assist those first beginning an exercise program. However, there are certainly activities other than walking or jogging that may have greater appeal to the participant. In such cases, the heart rate target zone (see CSTF Interpretation and Counselling Manual) would be useful when prescribing aerobic exercise intensity. As a fitness counselor, the appraiser should take special care to adapt the exercise prescription to meet the needs and interests of the participants.

3. The calculator has disadvantages.
   a. It may underestimate the VO_{2max} for fit participants, females in the 20 to 29 years age group, and heavy individuals.
   b. It may overestimate the VO_{2max} for unfit participants. See CAFT limitations (item 5, below) for further explanation and references at the end of this section for suggested further reading.

4. See Table A-10 for norms and percentiles for predicted VO_{2max} norms. Percentiles for heart rate final scores (i.e., heart rate after final session of stepping) are presented in Table A-11. Using this table to interpret aerobic fitness levels may be preferable for participants whose VO_{2max} scores are used as a comparative "check" with VO_{2max} scores and for participants who have difficulty understanding the concept of VO_{2max}.

5. CAFT limitations. The CAFT, as originally de-

vised, was intended to be a motivational tool that could also provide a gross estimate of fitness, i.e., undesirable, minimum, recommended. Later, a regression equation was validated against a maximal treadmill test; however, concerns have been voiced about mode-specific validity, i.e. maximal step test. As a result, the prediction of VO_{2max} was addressed by an ad hoc Advisory Committee convened by Fitness Canada. This committee subsequently made recommendations for necessary research to improve and extend the application of the CAFT. These research results and how they may affect the present form of the CAFT will be reported when they become available and appropriate changes will be incorporated into the fourth edition of the CSTF Operations Manual.

SUBMAXIMAL CYCLE ERGOMETER TESTS

An estimate of VO_{2max} can be derived from the heart rate response to standard submaximal exercise performed on a calibrated cycle ergometer. The procedure is based on the well established linear relation between heart rate and VO_2 and on the fact that the maximal heart rate and VO_{2max} tend to be attained at similar rates of power output. Because cycle ergometer exercise is not a weight-bearing activity, absolute VO_2 ($1 \cdot min^{-1}$) at a particular rate of power output is fairly similar in most persons. However, body weight is a major determinant of the relative VO_2 ($ml \cdot kg^{-1} \cdot min^{-1}$) during cycle exercise, and individuals with greater muscle mass have a performance advantage. Therefore when selecting rates of power output, modifications must be made for the individual's body weight.

Protocol Selection Criteria

Body Weight kg (lb)	Protocol	
	Not Very Active	Very Active
<73 (160)	A	A
74–90 (161–199)	A	B
>91 (200)	B	C

Activity status is subjectively determined by the test administered from reviewing questionnaire data provided by the participant or by verbal query. Individuals who have been regularly participating (the last 3 months) in vigorous activities for at least 15 minutes, three times per week, are classified as very active.

TABLE A-10. Norms and Percentiles by Age Groups and Gender for Predicted VO$_{2max}$

Parameter	15–19 Years		20–29 Years		30–39 Years		40–49 Years		50–59 Years		60–69 Years	
	M	F	M	F	M	F	M	F	M	F	M	F
Norms												
Excellent	≥60	≥43	≥57	≥40	≥48	≥37	≥42	≥35	≥38	≥30	≥30	≥25
Above average	58–59	40–42	52–56	37–39	46–47	34–37	40–42	32–34	36–38	27–29	29–30	24–25
Average	54–57	37–39	43–51	35–37	42–45	31–33	37–39	26–31	34–35	25–27	27–28	22–23
Below average	44–53	35–37	40–42	32–34	38–41	29–31	34–37	24–25	31–33	22–25	26–27	20–22
Poor	≤43	≤34	≤40	≤31	≤37	≤29	≤33	≤23	≤30	≤21	≤26	≤19
Percentiles												
95	62	45	59	43	51	39	44	36	40	31	32	26
90	61	43	58	41	50	38	43	35	39	30	31	26
85	60	43	57	40	48	37	42	35	38	30	30	25
80	59	42	56	39	47	37	42	34	38	29	30	25
75	59	41	55	39	47	36	41	33	37	28	29	24
70	58	40	54	38	46	35	40	33	36	28	29	24
65	58	40	52	37	46	34	40	32	36	27	29	24
60	57	39	48	37	45	33	39	31	35	27	28	23
55	57	38	44	36	44	32	38	30	35	26	28	23
50	56	38	43	35	43	32	38	28	34	26	28	22
45	54	37	43	35	42	31	37	26	34	25	27	22
40	52	37	42	34	41	31	37	25	33	25	27	22
35	47	36	42	34	40	30	36	25	33	24	27	21
30	46	35	41	33	39	30	35	24	32	23	27	21
25	44	35	40	32	38	29	34	24	31	22	26	20
20	43	34	40	31	37	29	32	23	28	21	26	19
15	42	34	39	31	36	28	31	22	26	20	25	19
10	41	33	38	30	34	28	30	22	25	19	24	18
5	40	32	37	29	33	27	29	21	24	18	23	17

Data are given as maximal volume of oxygen consumption (VO$_2$): ml · kg^{-1} · min^{-1}.
(Based on data from the Canada Fitness Survey, 1981.)

TABLE A-11. Norms and Percentiles by Age Groups and Gender for Heart Rate Final Scores (Beats/10 Seconds)

	15–19 Years		20–29 Years		30–39 Years		40–49 Years		50–59 Years		60–69 Years	
	M	F	M	F	M	F	M	F	M	F	M	F
Norms												
Excellent	7 ≤25	6 ≤28	7 ≤26	5 ≤25	6 ≤24	5 ≤26	5 ≤21	4 ≤23	4 ≤20	3 ≤22	2 ≤16	2 ≤19
Above average	7 26–27	6 ≥29 / 5 27	7 27–29	5 26–28	6 25–27	5 27–30	5 22–24	4 24–26	4 21–22	3 23–24	2 17–18	2 20–21
Average	7 28–30	5 28–29	6 26–28	5 29–30 / 4 26	6 28–29	4 25–27	5 25–26	4 27–28 / 3 24–25	4 23–24	3 25–26	2 19	2 22–23
Below average	6 26–29	5 30–31	6 29–30	4 27–29	5 25–27	4 28–29	5 27–28 / 4 24–25	3 26–27	4 25–26 / 3 23	3 27 / 2 23–24	2 20	2 24
Poor	6 ≥30 / 5 ≥30	5 ≥32 / 4 ≥30	6 31–34 / 5 ≥29	4 30–32 / 3 ≥29	5 28–31 / 4 ≥28	4 30–31 / 3 ≥28	4 26–29 / 3 ≥26	3 28–29 / 2 ≥26	3 24–26 / 2 ≥25	2 25–29 / 1 ≥25	2 21–26 / 1 ≥24	2 25–29 / 1 ≥24
Percentiles[b]												
95	23	26	24	23	22	23	18	21	18	21	15	17
90	24	27	25	25	23	25	21	22	19	21	15	18
85	25	28	26	25	24	26	21	23	20	22	16	18
80	25	29	26	26	25	27	22	24	20	23	16	19
75	26	30	26	27	25	27	23	25	21	23	17	20
70t	27	31	28	27	26	29	23	25	21	24	17	20
65	27	27	29	28	27	30	24	26	22	24	18	21
60	28	28	26	29	28	25	24	27	22	25	18	21
55	28	28	27	30	28	26	25	28	23	25	18	21
50	29	29	27	26	28	26	25	24	23	26	19	22
45	30	29	26	26	29	27	26	25	24	26	19	23
40	27	30	28	27	25	27	27	25	24	27	19	23
35	27	30	29	27	25	27	28	26	25	23	20	23
30	28	31	29	28	26	28	24	26	26	24	20	24
25	29	31	30	29	27	29	25	27	23	24	20	24
20	30	32	31	29	27	29	26	27	23	25	21	24
15	30	33	31	30	28	30	26	28	24	25	22	25
10	31	34	32	30	29	30	28	28	25	27	22	26
5	32	■	34	32	31	31	29	29	26	29	26	29
<5	■		■	■	■	■	■	■	■	■	■	■

[a] **Bold** numbers for norms indicate final stepping stage completed. Values in boldface obtained after the second session of stepping. Other values obtained after the third session of stepping.

[b] ■ After first session of stepping.

(Based on data from the Canada Fitness Survey, 1981.)

1201

Test Protocols

Protocol	Workload in Watts (Kilogram Meters Per Minutes)			
	I (1–2)	II (3–4)	III (5–6)	IV (7–8)
A	25 (150)	50 (300)	75 (450)	100 (600)
B	25 (150)	50 (300)	100 (600)	150 (900)
C	50 (300)	100 (600)	150 (900)	200 (1200)

Exercise heart rates are monitored during the test by palpating the pulse or by electronic monitoring. Heart rate is checked during the last 15 seconds of each test stage, and the test is terminated when the heart reaches 65 to 70 percent of the predicted age-adjusted maximal heart rate. These percentages of maximal heart rate are inaccurate in individuals taking drugs that blunt the heart rate response to exercise (e.g., β-blockers).

Target Heart Rate for Cycle Ergometer

Age (years)	Heart Rate (beats/minute)
<20	140
20–29	135
30–39	130
40–49	120
50–59	115
60–65	110

The heart rate is measured for at least two and preferably three test stages. A rough estimate of VO_{2max} can then be extrapolated using the predicted age-adjusted maximal heart rate as illustrated in Figure A-9.

OTHER TESTS

There are several other widely used submaximal cycle ergometer tests of cardiorespiratory endurance, two of which are the distance run and the walking test.

Distance Runs

Various field tests of cardiorespiratory endurance can be employed when equipment is not available or mass testing is required.

1. 1.5-Mile run. This run is best suited for active in-

dividuals because it requires maximal effort. Participants are to run 1.5 miles on a level course as fast as possible after a light warm-up. Proper pacing and high motivation are required for best performance. The VO_{2max} is estimated from the performance time recorded.

2. 12-Minute run. This test is used to estimate VO_{2max}. Participants are told to run as far as possible in 12 minutes. The distance is used to determine VO_{2max}. Norms are available for males and females of various age groups.

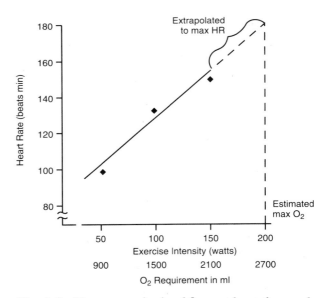

Fig. A-9. Heart rate obtained from at least three submaximal exercise intensities may be extrapolated to the age-predicted maximal heart rate. A vertical line to the intensity scale estimates maximal exercise intensity. (Adapted from Blain SN: p. 438. Metarazzo, et al. (eds): Behavioral Health: A Handbook of Health Enhancement and Disease Prevention. John Wiley & Sons, New York, 1984. With permission.)

Walking Tests

1. 1-Mile walk test. This test has been developed for adults, especially older adults. The test consists in a warm-up and a 1-mile walk as fast as possible. Only walking is allowed. Postexercise heart rate and performance time are used to predict VO_{2max}. Tables of normal values are available.

2. Rockport fitness walking test. This test has been validated as a fitness test. Participants walk 1 mile as fast as possible, record their time, and count their heart rate immediately after finishing. Generalized and gender-specific regression equations have been developed to estimate VO_{2max}.

SUGGESTED READINGS

ACSM Manual. Guidelines for Exercise Testing and Prescription. pp. 40, 44. 4th Ed. Lea & Febiger, Philadelphia, 1991

MacDougal JD, Wenger HA, Green JH (eds): Physiologic Testing of the Elite Athlete. Canadian Association of Sports Sciences in collaboration with The Sports Medicine Council of Canada, 1989

Magee DJ: Sports Physiotherapy. University of Alberta Press, Edmonton, 1988

Mueller FO, Ryan AJ (eds): Prevention of Athletic Injuries: The Role of the Sports Medicine Team. F.A. Davis, Philadelphia 1991

Sutton JR, Brock RM (eds): Sports Medicine for the Mature Athlete. Benchmark Press, Indianapolis 1986

Eponyms

Index

Page numbers followed by *f* indicate figures; those followed by *t* indicate tables.

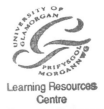